NOTICE

Because of the dynamic nature of medical practice and drug selection and dosage, users are advised that decisions regarding drug therapy must be based on the independent judgment of the clinician, changing information about a drug (e.g., as reflected in the literature and manufacturer's most current product information), and changing medical practices.

While great care has been taken to ensure the accuracy of the information presented, users are advised that the authors, editors, contributors, and publisher make no warranty, express or implied, with respect to, and are not responsible for, the currency, completeness, or accuracy of the information contained in this publication, nor for any errors, omissions, or the application of this information, nor for any consequences arising therefrom. Users are encouraged to confirm the information contained herein with other sources deemed authoritative. Ultimately, it is the responsibility of the treating physician, relying on experience and knowledge of the patient, to determine dosages and the best treatment for the patient. Therefore, the author(s), editors, contributors, and the publisher make no warranty, express or implied, and shall have no liability to any person or entity with regard to claims, loss, or damage caused, or alleged to be caused, directly or indirectly, by the use of information contained in this publication.

Further, the author(s), editors, contributors, and the publisher are not responsible for misuse of any of the information provided in this publication, for negligence by the user, or for any typographical errors.

Internal Medicine

Edited by **Bruce F. Scharschmidt, MD**

ASSOCIATE EDITORS

Robert J. Alpern, MD

Edward J. Benz, Jr., MD

Devron H. Char, MD

Richard A. Jacobs, MD, PhD

Emmet B. Keeffe, MD

Stephen C. Lazarus, MD

Susan Philip, MD, MPH

Michael J. Aminoff, MD, DSc, FRCP

Jeffrey P. Callen, MD, FACP

Andrew R. Hoffman, MD

Joel S. Karliner, MD

Fredric B. Kraemer, MD

Biff F. Palmer, MD

Shaun Ruddy, MD

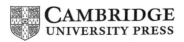

CAMBRIDGE
UNIVERSITY PRESS

CAMBRIDGE UNIVERSITY PRESS
Cambridge, New York, Melbourne, Madrid, Cape Town, Singapore,
São Paulo, Delhi

Cambridge University Press
32 Avenue of the Americas, New York, NY 10013-2473, USA

www.cambridge.org
Information on this title: www.cambridge.org/9780521709408

First published 2007

Printed in the United States of America

A catalog record for this publication is available from the British Library.

Library of Congress Cataloging in Publication Data

Internal medicine / [edited by] Bruce F. Scharschmidt.
    p. ; cm.
ISBN-13: 978-0-521-70940-8 (pbk.)
ISBN-10: 0-521-70940-7 (pbk.)
    1. Internal medicine – Handbooks, manuals, etc.   I. Scharschmidt,
Bruce. II. Title.
    [DNLM: 1. Internal Medicine – Handbooks. WB 39 I5985 2007]
    RC55.I475   2007
    616 – dc   222007016973

ISBN   978-0-521-70940-8 paperback

WB 100

AO7 1962

AFFILIATIONS

EDITOR

Bruce F. Scharschmidt, MD

Vice President, Clinical Development
Chiron Corporation

ASSOCIATE EDITORS

CARDIOLOGY

Joel S. Karliner, MD

Professor of Medicine
School of Medicine
University of California, San Francisco
Associate Chief of Medicine for Research and Staff Cardiologist
VA Medical Center, San Francisco

DERMATOLOGY

Jeffrey P. Callen, MD, FACP

Professor of Medicine (Dermatology)
Chief, Division of Dermatology
University of Louisville School of Medicine
Louisville, Kentucky

ENDOCRINOLOGY, METABOLISM AND BONE DISORDERS

Andrew R. Hoffman, MD

Professor of Medicine
Associate Chair for Academic Affairs
Department of Medicine
Stanford University and VA Palo Alto Health Care System
Stanford, California

Fredric B. Kraemer, MD

Associate Chief of Staff for Research and Development
VA Palo Alto Health Care System
Palo Alto, California
Professor of Medicine
Chief, Division of Endocrinology, Gerontology and Metabolism
Stanford University School of Medicine
Stanford, California

GASTROENTEROLOGY, HEPATOLOGY AND NUTRITION
Emmet B. Keeffe, MD

Professor of Medicine
Chief of Hepatology
Co-Director, Liver Transplant Program
Stanford University Medical Center
Stanford, California

HEAD, EYE, EAR, NOSE AND THROAT
Devron H. Char, MD

President, Tumori Foundation
Clinical Professor, Department of Ophthalmology
Stanford University School of Medicine
Stanford, California

HEMATOLOGY
Edward J. Benz, Jr., MD

Richard and Susan Smith Professor of Medicine
Harvard Medical School
Boston, Massachusetts
President, Dana-Farber Cancer Institute
Boston, Massachusetts

INFECTIOUS DISEASES
Richard A. Jacobs, MD, PhD

Clinical Professor of Medicine and Infectious Diseases
School of Medicine
University of California, San Francisco

Susan Philip, MD, MPH

Medical Director, San Francisco City Clinic
San Francisco Department of Public Health
Assistant Clinical Professor of Medicine
School of Medicine
University of California, San Francisco

KIDNEY AND UROLOGIC DISEASE
Robert J. Alpern, MD

Ensign Professor of Medicine
Dean, Yale School of Medicine
Yale University
New Haven, Connecticut

Biff F. Palmer, MD

Professor of Internal Medicine
Director of Renal Fellowship Program
Department of Medicine
Division of Nephrology
University of Texas Southwestern Medical School
Dallas, Texas

NEUROLOGY

Michael J. Aminoff, MD, DSc, FRCP

Professor of Neurology and Executive Vice Chair
Department of Neurology
School of Medicine, University of California San Francisco
Attending Neurologist
UCSF Medical Center
San Francisco

with contributions by Dr. Aminoff and

Chad Christine, MD

Assistant Clinical Professor of Neurology
Department of Neurology
School of Medicine
University of California, San Francisco

PULMONARY MEDICINE

Stephen C. Lazarus, MD

Professor of Medicine
Director, Fellowship Program in Pulmonary and Critical Care Medicine
Associate Director, Adult Pulmonary Laboratory
Senior Investigator, Cardiovascular Research Institute
School of Medicine
University of California, San Francisco

RHEUMATOLOGY, ALLERGY AND IMMUNOLOGY

Shaun Ruddy, MD

Elam C. Toone Professor Emeritus
Department of Internal Medicine
Medical College of Virginia
VCU Health Systems
Richmond, Virginia

Contents

Preface

Internal Medicine is designed to provide the busy clinician with precisely the information needed where and when it is needed. The Associate Editors and contributors are internationally recognized authorities, and they have organized the content specifically so as to convey the essentials necessary for diagnosis, differential diagnosis, management, treatment and follow-up. Many topics start with a "What To Do First" heading which brings the collective experience and guidance of top experts to bear on the "up front" considerations the clinician must face. We are excited about *Internal Medicine* and hope you share our view that it is an essential resource, particularly in our current era of shortened physician-patient encounters and the need for rapid clinical decision-making.

Bruce F. Scharschmidt

ABDOMINAL AORTIC ANEURYSM (AAA)

RAJABRATA SARKAR, MD

HISTORY & PHYSICAL
- Male:female ratio is 4:1
- 5–10% of males over 65 years of age have AAA
- High incidence in patients with peripheral arterial aneurysm (popliteal, femoral)
- Ruptured AAA – clinical suspicion
  - elderly male with severe back or abdominal pain
  - may radiate to groin.

Signs & Symptoms
- Most are asymptomatic and found on other imaging studies
- pulsatile abdominal mass in less than 30% of patients with significant AAA
- Tender abdominal mass is suggestive of symptomatic aneurysm
- examine for associated peripheral aneurysms (femoral, popliteal)
- Unusual presentations:
  - atheroembolism to lower extremities
  - thrombosis (sudden severe ischemia of legs)
  - high output CHF from aortocaval fistula
  - GI bleeding from primary aorto-enteric fistula
- Ruptured AAA
  - Pulsatile mass + hypotension
  - abdominal/back/groin pain + hypotension

TESTS

Laboratory
- None

Imaging
- Ultrasound for screening
- CT scan is best test for aneurysms being considered for repair
- Defines : associated iliac aneurysms, eligibility for endovascular repair, possible suprarenal extension
- Conventional MRI has no advantage over CT for AAA
- Angiography is not used for diagnosis (can miss AAA due to normal lumen)

- Angiography (contrast or MR) indicated preoperatively in patients with:
  - clinical suspicion of concurrent renal artery stenosis (severe hypertension, elevated creatinine)
  - mesenteric occlusive disease (post-prandial pain)
  - significant lower extremity occlusive disease (claudication + ankle/brachial index<0.7).
- Ruptured AAA: if diagnosis is unclear (no mass):
  - Emergency ultrasound
    - helpful only if aorta is clearly seen and completely normal
    - often not helpful due to bowel gas and patient discomfort
    - cannot rule out a leak from AAA
  - CT scan
    - Best test when diagnosis of AAA is unclear
    - Emergency non-contrast scan of abdomen
    - Intravenous contrast increases post-op renal failure and is not needed to see AAA or leak
    - Oral contrast not required

DIFFERENTIAL DIAGNOSIS

Ruptured AAA

- most common misdiagnosis is kidney stone
- second most common is musculoskeletal back pain; high suspicion of AAA with new onset or change in chronic back pain
- other:
  - appendicitis (associated GI symptoms)
  - diverticulitis (fevers, GI symptoms, focal left sided tenderness)
  - aortic dissection (ripping pain, extends into chest and upper back)
  - incarcerated hernia (physical exam, CT scan if exam inconclusive)

MANAGEMENT

What to Do First

- Emergent (immediate) operation in patients with abdominal pain and hypotension due to ruptured AAA
- Emergent non-contrast CT scan in patients with symptoms suggestive of ruptured AAA

General Measures

- Rule out ruptured AAA first in all patients with suggestive symptoms, as it is the most rapidly lethal diagnosis if missed

■ Risk/benefit ratio of elective repair is contingent upon low operative mortality (less than 5%)

SPECIFIC THERAPY

Indications

■ Most patients
➤ Elective repair if diameter in any orientation is 5 to 5.5 cm
➤ Repair if serial scans (either ultrasound or CT) demonstrate rapid growth (> 1 cm/year) or saccular growth
➤ Urgent repair in patients with symptoms (tenderness)
➤ Repair associated lesions (renal, visceral or peripheral occlusive disease) concurrently if indicated

■ Poor-risk patients
➤ consider endovascular repair
➤ discuss with patient/family outcome if not repaired
➤ (Risk of rupture is 2–3% per year at 5 cm, and may not be significant relative to other co-morbidities)

Treatment Options

■ Operative repair
➤ Most durable treatment
➤ Little difference between transperitoneal and retroperitoneal repairs
➤ Intraoperative pulmonary artery catheters in patients with poor ejection fraction or CHF

Side Effects and Contraindications

■ Operative repair
➤ Perioperative mortality should be less than 5%
➤ Complications
  • Myocardial infarction:
  • Clinical indices (Goldman criteria, Eagle criteria) are predictive of risk, but persantine thallium scanning is not.
  • MI after elective repair is rarely fatal
➤ Ischemic colitis
  • Seen more often after ruptured AAA with hypotension
➤ Renal failure
  • Seen after repair of ruptured and suprarenal AAA. Associated with high mortality (50%)

■ Contraindications
➤ Expected survival less than 50% at 5 years due to associated cardiovascular disease
  • Endovascular Repair

- Lower mortality and morbidity than open repair
- Less durable than standard repair
- Absolute Contraindications
  - ➤ Bilateral common iliac artery aneurysms
  - ➤ Pararenal or suprarenal aneurysm
  - ➤ Angulation, thrombus or dilation of infrarenal neck
  - ➤ Iliac occlusion or stenosis precluding transfemoral access
- Relative contraindications
  - ➤ Long term anticoagulation (higher risk of endoleak [see below])
  - ➤ Associated occlusive disease requiring treatment

Specific Complications
- Endoleak
  - ➤ Persistent arterial flow in aneurysm sac due to: failure of device to seal to arterial wall (Type I), back flow from branch vessel (Type III) or leak through graft material (Type III)
- Post-implant fever
  - ➤ Occurs 12–48 hours after implant; not due to infection

FOLLOW-UP

During Treatment
- Follow AAA less than 5 cm with serial ultrasound or CT scans q6–12 months, or more frequently if there is rapid change in size

Routine
- Patients undergoing endovascular repair require lifelong yearly CT scan to monitor position and seal of device

COMPLICATIONS AND PROGNOSIS

Complications
- Myocardial Infarction
- Renal failure
  - ➤ Poor prognosis (50% mortality). Treatment is supportive. Usually resolves (ATN)
- Ischemic colitis
  - ➤ Diagnose by bedside sigmoidoscopy. Colectomy for full-thickness ischemia; serial endoscopy for mucosal ischemia which often resolves. May cause late ischemic strictures.
- Endoleak (seen only after endovascular repair)
  - ➤ Diagnosed on post-op CT scan or angiogram. Treatment is usually endovascular
- Graft Infection

➤ Can occur after either open or endovascular repair. Symptoms: persistent fever or aorto-enteric fistula (upper GI bleeding). Diagnosis: CT scan. Treatment: graft excision and extra-anatomic bypass. Mortality: 50%.

Prognosis
- Ruptured AAA
  - ➤ Most die en route to hospital or on arrival
  - ➤ 50% of those undergoing surgery survive
  - ➤ Preoperative predictors of poor survival:
    - age > 80
    - preoperative hypotension
    - elevated creatinine preop or postop renal failure
- Elective Repair
  - ➤ Perioperative mortality approximates 5%
- Endovascular Repair
  - ➤ Requires life-long follow-up for late complications
    - Late onset endoleak:
    - Graft migration or disruption
  - ➤ Late complications
    - Graft infection (1%)
    - Secondary aorto-enteric fistula

ABSCESSES AND FISTULAS

EMMET B. KEEFFE, MD

HISTORY & PHYSICAL

Risk Factors
- Recent abdominal surgery
- Penetrating or blunt abdominal trauma
- Perforation of appendix or colonic diverticulum
- Perforation associated w/ intraabdominal malignancy
- Crohn disease
- Chronic diseases, eg, cirrhosis, renal failure
- Drugs, eg, corticosteroids, chemotherapy
- Prior radiotherapy

History
- High spiking fevers w/ chills
- Abdominal pain

- Nausea & vomiting
- Hiccups
- Chest pain
- Dyspnea
- Shoulder pain

Signs & Symptoms
- Tachycardia
- Abdominal tenderness
- Ileus
- Pleural effusion
- Basilar rales

TESTS

Basic Blood Tests
- Leukocytosis w/ left shift
- Anemia
- Nonspecific elevation of bilirubin & liver enzymes

Specific Diagnostic Tests
- Positive blood cultures
- Positive cultures from aspiration of abscess
- Most common aerobes: E coli & Enterococcus
- Most common anaerobes: Bacteroides

Imaging
- Plain abdominal & chest films: air-fluid levels in area of abscess; elevation of right diaphragm in subphrenic abscess
- Gallium scan: useful for smaller abscess not well seen on imaging
- CT: imaging modality of choice for identification of abscess; also allows aspiration for culture
- US: less sensitive for abdominal abscesses
- Charcoal or methylene blue: oral administration with detection in drainage from fistula

DIFFERENTIAL DIAGNOSIS
- Necrotic tumors

MANAGEMENT

What to Do First
- Complete diagnostic studies, particularly imaging, for localization & aspiration

General Measures

- Initiate general supportive care: fluid & electrolyte replacement, establish feeding (TPN if fistula present), oxygenation if needed
- Swan-Ganz catheter, mechanical ventilation &/or vasopressors if unstable

SPECIFIC THERAPY

- Adequate drainage of abscess either percutaneously or by surgery
- Surgery indicated if pt fails to respond to percutaneous drainage in 1–2 d
- Establish adequate drainage of enterocutaneous fistulas, eg, open recent surgical excision, use of percutaneous catheters
- Surgery for complex fistulas or failure to resolve w/ external drainage & TPN
- Antibiotics: broad spectrum initially, & then based on culture results

FOLLOW-UP

- Frequent clinical evaluation early after drainage
- Serial imaging when treated w/ catheter drainage to confirm catheter w/i abscess & abscess closed

COMPLICATIONS AND PROGNOSIS

Complications

- Multiorgan failure leading to death
- Recurrent abscess
- Fistula formation
- Bowel obstruction
- Pneumonia
- Pleural effusion

Prognosis

- Good w/ adequate drainage & response to antibiotic therapy

ACANTHOSIS NIGRICANS

JAMES SEWARD, MD and JEFFREY P. CALLEN, MD
REVISED BY JEFFREY P. CALLEN, MD

HISTORY & PHYSICAL

History

- A cutaneous marker of insulin resistance states
- Other etiologies: hereditary, endocrine disorders, obesity, drugs, and malignancy

- Seen in blacks > Hispanics > whites
- Five types:
  - Type I (Familial)
    - Exceedingly rare
    - Autosomal dominant
    - Present at birth or develops during childhood
    - Worsens at puberty
    - Not associated with an internal cancer
  - Type II (Benign AN)
    - Associated with various endocrine disorders
    - Examples include acromegaly, gigantism, Stein-Leventhal syndrome, Cushing's, diabetes mellitus, hypothyroidism, Addison's disease, hyperandrogenic states, and hypogonadal syndromes
  - Type III (formerly called Pseudo-AN; however, this probably is the result of an endocrinopathy, namely insulin resistance)
    - Most common form
    - Associated with obesity and insulin resistance states
    - Not associated with malignancy
  - Type IV (Drug-induced):
    - Nicotinic acid, niacinamide, diethylstilbestrol, triazineate, oral contraceptives, testosterone, topical fusidic acid, and glucocorticoids
    - Seen in 10% of renal transplant patients
  - Type V (Associated with malignancy):
    - Rare
    - Most often in adults
    - Highly suspected if occurs in non-obese male
    - Tends to be more widespread and involve mucosal surfaces
    - Precedes 18%, accompanies 60%, or follows 22% the internal malignancy
    - Most often associated with adenocarcinoma of gastrointestinal tract (60% stomach)
    - Also associated with lung and breast adenocarcinoma
    - Other cancers also seen

Signs & Symptoms
- Often asymptomatic; skin looks "dirty"
- Velvety brown thickening of skin on intertriginous surfaces, most commonly the axilla, the neck
- Other sites: genitalia, knuckles, lips, submammary area, umbilicus, eyelids, and conjunctiva

TESTS
■ Use history and physical as guide to appropriate workup

Basic Tests:
■ Check blood glucose and possibly an insulin level

Other Tests:
■ Exclude malignancy in non-obese patients with no obvious cause
■ Screen for malignancy as appropriate for patients age, risk factors, and symptoms
■ Screen for endocrinopathy if suspected

DIFFERENTIAL DIAGNOSIS
n/a

MANAGEMENT
■ Depends on cause:
  ➤ Weight loss if obese
  ➤ Treat underlying endocrinopathy
  ➤ Discontinue offending drug
  ➤ Treat underlying malignancy
■ Topical urea, lactic acid, tretinoin, and oral etretinate used with varied success

SPECIFIC THERAPY
Urea-containing products may give symptomatic relief.

FOLLOW-UP
■ Varies dependent upon the association with an underlying disorder or disease

COMPLICATIONS AND PROGNOSIS
■ Depends on underlying cause
■ Obesity related AN improves with weight loss
■ Endocrinopathy associated AN improves with treatment of underlying disease
■ Removal of malignancy may be followed by regression of AN

ACNE

ALFRED L. KNABLE, MD

HISTORY & PHYSICAL
■ May exist transiently during neonatal period
■ Commonly begins during early puberty with increased activity throughout the teens with spontaneous resolution thereafter (strong genetic influence recognized)

- May begin at or persist into later ages
- May result from exposure to various oils, greases, etc. found in cosmetics, pomades, or industry
- May result from or be exacerbated by hormones - Polycystic ovary disease, insulin resistance, hyperandrogenism, Cushing's disease
- Complication of various drugs: corticosteroids, lithium, iodide/bromide, anticonvulsants

Signs & Symptoms

- Primary lesion = microcomedo (clinically unrecognizable = microscopic plugging of pilosebaceous unit)
- First clinically recognizable lesions are open comedones ("blackheads") and/or closed comedones ("whiteheads")
- Earliest stages most common on forehead and across nose and chin
- Later stages of development include inflammatory papules (1–5 mm) and pustules
- Most advanced lesions are cystic and/or nodular (> = 5 mm) with a predilection for lateral cheeks, chin and in more severe cases the chest and upper back (acne conglobata)
- Evaluate for signs of endocrinologic disease – hirsutism, striae, Cushingoid facies

TESTS

- Laboratory – routine: none except when indicated for specific therapies
- Screening. Woman with severe or recalcitrant acne (or the onset or recurrence of acne beyond their late twenties) should have at least a measurement of their free testosterone and dehydroepiandrosterone sulfate levels to consider polycystic ovarian disease or Stein-Leventhal syndrome.

DIFFERENTIAL DIAGNOSIS

- Pityrosporum or bacterial folliculitis more likely to occur on trunk, buttocks, and proximal extremities with follicular-based papules or pustules
- Acne keloidalis nuchae occurs as firm 2- to 5-mm papules on the occiput of African-American men
- Pseudofolliculitis barbae occurs as firm papules and occasionally pustules to beard areas of African-American men
- Hidradenitis suppurativa occurs within the axillae, under the breasts and the inguinal areas with larger cysts and sinus tract formation.
- Rosacea – more central facial and/or perioral, more common in adults, lack of comedones

MANAGEMENT

What to Do First
- Assess type and distribution of acne lesions – comedonal v. inflammatory v. cystic

General Measures
- Keratolytic or antibacterial cleansers: salicylic acid, benzoyl peroxide, sulfur
- Topical vitamin A acid (and similar agents): tretinoin, Adapalene, tazarotene
- Topical antibiotics: erythromycin, Clindamycin, sulfacetamide preparations (both erythromycin and clindamycin may be combined with benzoyl peroxide)
- Oral antibiotics: Tetracycline, Doxycycline, or Minocycline
- Less commonly: sulfones, sulfamethoxazole-trimethoprim, Erythromycin, ampicillin or cephalosporins
- Oral retinoids: Isotretinoin 1 mg/kg/d for 16–20 weeks for severe cases
- Other Therapies
- Azaleic acid (topical), spironolactone, intralesional triamcinolone acetonide for individual inflamed lesions, very rarely oral corticosteroids
- No role for dietary manipulation has been proven

SPECIFIC THERAPY
- Keratolytic agents: Indicated for early acne forms, side effects may include irritation
- Topical vitamin A acid: indicated for early and more advanced acne stages. For pregnant patients discuss use with obstetrician.
- Topical antibiotics: Best for early papulopustular acne. Cream, lotion and gel bases
- should be matched with patient's tolerance and preference, irritation possibly
- Oral antibiotics: Indicated for moderate to severe papulopustular acne and early stages
- of cystic acne.
  - ➤ Minocycline use rarely complicated by pigment deposition, a lupus-like syndrome and reports of depression.
- Oral Retinoids
  - ➤ Indication: Severe, recalcitrant nodulocystic acne +/− scarring

■ Laser/related modalities: limited by availability and cost restraints at present

FOLLOW-UP

■ Allow 6–8 weeks for topical or oral antibiotic therapies to take effect
■ Expect gradual improvement over months with these agents
■ Add to or alter these regimens at 6–8 week intervals
■ Once control is established, may need to see patient only every 6–12 months
■ With oral retinoid use, patients should be seen monthly with appropriate laboratory studies to include: CBC, liver function panel, lipid panel, +/– pregnancy test, +/– BUN and creatinine (Note: registration in the "iPLEDGE" program now mandatory for those prescribing, taking or dispensing Isotretinoin.)
■ Standard course of Isotretinoin is 5 months, but may be repeated in selected individuals

COMPLICATIONS AND PROGNOSIS

Complications

■ Scarring: Occurs in nearly 100% of untreated cystic acne patients
  ➤ Occurs in approximately 25–50% of papulopustular patients (increased risk if lesions are excoriated or otherwise manipulated)
■ Keloid formation: 10–20% of cystic patient, especially prominent on central chest and shoulders
■ Psycho-social considerations
  ➤ Depression or withdrawal occurs in a minority of patients
  ➤ Does not necessarily correlate with severity of acne
  ➤ Should be monitored for at each visit with early intervention, if indicated

Prognosis

■ Excellent with early, appropriate level of intervention

ACROMEGALY

ANDREW R. HOFFMAN, MD

HISTORY & PHYSICAL

History

■ Enlargement of hands and feet
■ Prognathism and loose teeth
■ Increased sweating

- Sleep apnea and snoring
- Diabetes mellitus
- Coarsening change in facial appearance
- Frontal bossing
- Carpal tunnel syndrome
- Infertility
- Amenorrhea or oligoamenorrhea
- Family history of pituitary tumor
- Excessive linear growth (in children)

Signs & Symptoms
- Headache
- Arthralgias
- Impotence
- Skin tags
- Decreased libido
- Visual field cut
- Hypopituitarism
- Galactorrhea in some women

TESTS

Laboratory
- Basic blood studies:
  - ➤ Insulin-like growth factor-I (IGF-I) single best test
  - ➤ growth hormone (GH) 1 h after 75-g glucose load: <5 ng/dL in normals
- Ancillary blood tests:
  - ➤ LH, FSH, prolactin, free T4, TSH
  - ➤ Testosterone
  - ➤ Estradiol
  - ➤ GH-releasing hormone
  - ➤ Fasting serum glucose, HgA1c

Imaging
- MRI of the pituitary to determine if there is pituitary mass

DIFFERENTIAL DIAGNOSIS
- GH-secreting pituitary tumor
- GH- and prolactin-secreting pituitary tumor
- GH- or GHRH-secreting neuroendocrine tumor (e.g., islet cell tumor of the pancreas)
- Acromegaloidism: acromegalic facies in patient with severe insulin resistance

MANAGEMENT

What to Do First
- Assess size and resectability of tumor

SPECIFIC THERAPY
- Surgical resection of tumor (usually transsphenoidal), esp. if there is visual field cut
- Medical therapy:
  - ➤ Somatostatin analog (octreotide or long-acting octreotide) given parenterally; can normalize serum IGF-I and GH; some tumor shrinkage
- Dopamine agonists (bromocriptine or cabergoline): may lower IGF-I and GH in some cases; often require high doses
- GH antagonists (pegvisomant): very effective at lowering serum IGF-I; increases serum GH. Follow LFTs.
- Radiation therapy if surgery and medical therapy fail; may take up to 10 y to normalize serum IGF-I and GH; often causes hypopituitarism
- Observation with repeated pituitary MRI to determine if tumor is growing

Treatment Goals
- Normalize serum IGF-I level
- Normalize GH response to glucose load
- Diminish size of pituitary tumor
- Maintain normal pituitary function
- Fertility
- Cessation of galactorrhea
- Restoration of libido and potency

Side Effects & Contraindications
- Surgery and radiation: hypopituitarism
- Octreotide: gallstones and gastric upset
- Bromocriptine and cabergoline: gastric upset, nasal stuffiness, orthostatic hypotension with initial doses

FOLLOW-UP
- Serum IGF-I postoperatively or 2 wks after changing dose of medicine
- Repeat pituitary MRI after 3–6 mo to assess pituitary growth

COMPLICATIONS AND PROGNOSIS
- Pituitary apoplexy (in patients with macroadenomas):
  - ➤ Presents as very severe headache, altered consciousness, coma
  - ➤ Requires emergent surgical intervention and resection of tumor

- Visual field changes signify tumor growth
- Patients require lifelong observation
- Increased risk of colonic polyps and perhaps colon cancer
- Osteoarthritis
- Increased risk of early mortality (cardiac) if not cured (normal IGF-I levels)

ACTINIC KERATOSIS

MICHAEL DACEY, MD and JEFFREY P. CALLEN, MD
REVISED BY JEFFREY P. CALLEN, MD

HISTORY & PHYSICAL
- also called solar keratosis, senile keratosis
- This disorder is the earliest clinical manifestation of squamous cell carcinoma
- disease of the older adult with chronic sun-damaged skin
- risk factors: fair skin, blue eyes, red or blonde hair, years of ultraviolet radiation exposure through work (e.g., farmers, mail carriers, etc.) or through leisure activities (tanning bed use, tanning)
- Patients who are organ transplant recipients are prone to developing many actinic keratoses, and malignant transformation (progression) is much more common in this setting.
- sun-exposed distribution – most often on the head, neck, forearms or dorsal hands of men, and these areas plus the legs in women
- poorly circumscribed erythematous macules, papules, or plaques, several millimeters to a centimeter in diameter
- adherent, "sandpaper-like" scale
- may form a hypertrophic, verrucous surface and become a horn
- occasionally hyperpigmented
- may be tender

TESTS
- The diagnosis is clinical.
- If the diagnosis is in question, a biopsy may be performed.

DIFFERENTIAL DIAGNOSIS
- Bowen's disease (squamous cell cancer in situ)
- Squamous cell cancer
- Basal cell cancer
- Seborrheic keratosis – sharp demarcation, stuck on appearance, verrucous surface

MANAGEMENT
- Suncreens, sun protective clothing and alteration of behavior lessen the chance of development of new lesions.
- Low-fat diet may also result in a lower rate of appearance of new lesions.
- Smoking cessation

SPECIFIC THERAPY
- Liquid nitrogen application (destructive)
- Curettage with desiccation
- topical application
  - 5-Fluorouracil
  - imiquimod
  - diclofenac
  - tretinoin
- Photodynamic therapy

FOLLOW-UP
- 6–8 weeks after therapy the patient should be re-examined.
- 6 months to 1 year for treatment response and examination for new lesions

COMPLICATIONS AND PROGNOSIS
- patient population is prone to develop new lesions despite avoidance of further ultraviolet exposure
- estimated 10% chance of at least one lesion developing into squamous cell cancer after 10 years (if left untreated)

ACUTE ACALCULOUS CHOLECYSTITIS

SUSAN A. CUMMINGS, MD

HISTORY & PHYSICAL

History
- 5–10% of cholecystectomies
- More fulminant than calculous cholecystitis; may present w/ gangrene, perforation, & empyema
- Risk factors: sepsis, ICU, TPN, immunosuppression, major trauma, burns, diabetes, infections, mechanical ventilation, opiates, CHD & CABG, prolonged fasting, childbirth, nonbiliary surgery, & AIDS; rarely seen in systemic vasculitides due to ischemic injury to gallbladder

- Insidious presentation in already critically ill pts
- Elderly
- Male predominance (80%)

Signs & Symptoms
- Clinical presentation variable, depending on predisposing conditions
- RUQ pain absent in 75% of cases
- Fever or hyperamylasemia may be only clue
- Unexplained sepsis w/ few early localizing signs
- Half of patients already have experienced complication: gangrene, perforation, abscess
- RUQ pain, fever, & positive Murphy sign seen in minority

TESTS

Laboratory
- Leukocytosis w/ left shift in 70–85%
- Hyperamylasemia common
- Abnormal aminotransferases, hyperbilirubinemia, mild increase in serum alkaline phosphatase more common in acalculous than calculous cholecystitis

Imaging
- Plain x-ray: exclusion of a perforated viscus, bowel ischemia, or renal stones
- US: absence of gallstones, thickened gallbladder wall
  - (>5 mm) w/ pericholecystic fluid, failure to visualize
  - gallbladder, perforation w/ abscess, emphysematous cholecystitis; sensitivity of 36–96%; high false-negative rate
- CT: thickened gallbladder wall (>4 mm) in absence of ascites or hypoalbuminemia, pericholecystic fluid, intramural gas, or sloughed mucosa; superior to US w/ sensitivity of 50–100%
- Radionuclide cholescintigraphy (HIDA) scan: failure to opacify gallbladder; sensitivity almost 100%; false-positive rate of up to 40% in which gallbladder not visualized in spite of nonobstructed cystic duct seen in severe liver disease, prolonged fasting, biliary sphincterotomy, hyperbilirubinemia; important not to allow test to delay treatment in very ill pts

DIFFERENTIAL DIAGNOSIS
- Calculous cholecystitis, peptic ulceration, acute pancreatitis, right-sided pyelonephritis, hepatic or subphrenic abscess

MANAGEMENT

What to Do First

- CT: best test to exclude other pathology
- If suspect biliary sepsis, radionuclide study first; otherwise, CT first

General Measures

- Blood cultures, IV broad-spectrum antibiotics
- Early recognition & intervention required due to rapid progression to gangrene & perforation

SPECIFIC THERAPY

- Cholecystectomy; both open & laparoscopic
- If evidence of perforation, then open cholecystectomy urgently; inflammatory mass may preclude successful laparoscopy
- US-guided percutaneous cholecystostomy may be first choice in critically ill pts; success rate 90%; no surgery necessary if postdrainage cholangiogram normal; catheter usually removed 6–8 wk
- Transpapillary endoscopic drainage of gallbladder may be done when pt too sick for surgery & unsuitable for percutaneous drainage (massive ascites or coagulopathy)

FOLLOW-UP

- Routine postop follow-up

COMPLICATIONS AND PROGNOSIS

- <10% mortality in community-acquired cases
- Up to 90% in critically ill pts

ACUTE BACTERIAL MENINGITIS

RICHARD A. JACOBS, MD, PhD

HISTORY & PHYSICAL

History

- Increased risk with exposure to meningococcal meningitis or travel to meningitis belt (sub-Saharan Africa), but most cases sporadic
- Increased incidence with extremes of age, head trauma, immuno-suppression

Signs & Symptoms

- Prodromal upper respiratory tract infection progresses to stiff neck, fever, headache, vomiting, lethargy, photophobia, rigors, weakness, seizures (20–30%)

- Fever, nuchal rigidity, signs of cerebral dysfunction; 50% with Neisseria meningitidis meningitis have an erythematous, macular rash that progresses to petechiae or purpura
- Cranial nerve palsies (III, VI, VII, VIII) in 10–20%
- Elderly may to have lethargy or obtundation without fever, $+/-$ meningismus

TESTS

Laboratory
- Basic Blood Tests:
  - Elevated WBC
- Specific Diagnostic Tests:
  - Blood cultures are often positive
  - Typical cerebrospinal fluid (CSF) in bacterial meningitis (normal): opening pressure >180 mm H_2O (50–150); color turbid (clear); WBC >1000/mm^3 with polymorphonuclear cell predominance (<5); protein >100 mg/dL (15–45); glucose <40 mg/dL (40–80); CSF/blood glucose ratio <0.4 (>0.6); Gram stain of CSF shows organisms in 60–90%
  - Culture of CSF is positive in 70–85%; community-acquired acute bacterial meningitis caused by Streptococcus pneumoniae, Neisseria meningitidis, Listeria monocytogenes, Haemophilus influenzae, Escherichia coli, group B streptococcus
  - Antigen testing for specific pathogens appropriate when a purulent CSF specimen has a negative Gram stain and culture, sensitivity 80%
- Other Tests:
  - Patients with evidence of ICP such as coma or papilledema or focal neurologic findings (seizures, cranial neuropathies) should have a noncontrast CT scan prior to lumbar puncture (LP); begin antibiotics before CT scan

DIFFERENTIAL DIAGNOSIS
- Bacteremia, sepsis, brain abscess, seizure disorder, aseptic meningitis (CSF WBC usually 100–1000/mm^3, eventually with lymphocyte predominance), skull fracture, chronic meningitis, encephalitis, migraine headache, rickettsial infection, drug reaction

MANAGEMENT

What to Do First
- Medical emergency: do not delay appropriate antibiotic therapy
- Quick neurologic exam looking for focality or evidence of increased ICP

- Blood culture × 2
- If increased ICP or focality, start empiric antibiotics based on patient's age and circumstances and send for CT of head without contrast
- If CT nonfocal and safe for LP, proceed to lumbar puncture
- If neurologic exam normal, LP and base therapy on STAT Gram stain of CSF
- If CSF consistent with bacterial meningitis and positive Gram stain, start specific antibiotics. If consistent with bacterial meningitis with a negative CSF Gram stain, start empiric antibiotics

General Measures
- Rigorous supportive care
- Dexamethasone IV before antibiotics and q6h × 2 d for children >1 mo and consider for adults with increased ICP or coma

SPECIFIC THERAPY
Indications
- If strongly suspect meningitis, start IV antibiotics as soon as blood cultures drawn

Treatment options
- Empiric antibiotics (1):
  - ➤ Age 18–50: ceftriaxone or cefotaxime +/− vancomycin (2)
  - ➤ >50 years: ampicillin + ceftriaxone or cefotaxime +/− vancomycin (2)
  - ➤ Immunocompromised: vancomycin + ampicillin + cetazadime
  - ➤ Skull fracture: ceftriaxone or cefotaxime +/− vancomycin (2)
  - ➤ Head trauma, neurosurgery, CSF shunt: vancomycin + ceftazadime
- Positive CSF Gram stain in community-acquired meningitis (1):
  - ➤ Gram-positive cocci: ceftriaxone or cefotaxime + vancomycin (1)
  - ➤ Gram-positive rods: ampicillin or penicillin G +/− gentamicin
  - ➤ Gram-negative rod: ceftriaxone or cefotaxime
    - (1) Modify antibiotics once organism and its susceptibility are known; organism must be fully sensitive to antibiotic used.
    - (2) If prevalence of third-generation cephalosporin-intermediate + resistant S. pneumoniae exceeds 5%, add vancomycin until organism proved susceptible; if intermediate or resistant to cephalosporins, continue vancomycin and ceftriaxone or cefotaxime for possible synergy; if penicillin-susceptible, narrow to penicillin G; if penicillin-non-susceptible

and cephalosporin-susceptible, narrow to third-generation cephalosporin
- If dexamethasone used with vancomycin, consider adding rifampin to increase vancomycin entry into CSF.

FOLLOW-UP

During Treatment
- Look for contiguous foci (sinusitis, mastoiditis, otitis media) or distant infection (endocarditis, pneumonia) with S pneumoniae
- Narrow coverage as culture results and susceptibility data allow
- If patient on adjunctive corticosteroids and not improving as expected, or if pneumococcal isolate, repeat LP 36–48 hours after starting antibiotics to document CSF sterility
- Treat close contacts of patients with N meningitidis to eradicate carriage. If not treated with a third-generation cephalosporin, the patient should receive chemoprophylaxis as well.

COMPLICATIONS AND PROGNOSIS

Complications
- Seizures, coma, sensorineural hearing loss, cranial nerve palsies, obstructive hydrocephalus, subdural effusions, CSF fistula (especially likely with recurrent meningitis), syndrome of inappropriate antidiuretic hormone
- Consider placing ICP monitoring device
- ICP >15–20, elevate head to 30 degrees, hyperventilate adults

Prognosis
- Average case fatality: 5–25%
- N meningitidis: 3–13%
- S pneumoniae: 19–26%
- L monocytogenes: 15–29%

ACUTE FATTY LIVER OF PREGNANCY

CAROLINE A. RIELY, MD

HISTORY & PHYSICAL

History
- Nausea and vomiting, bleeding from gums or elsewhere, signs and symptoms of preeclampsia, coma, either hepatic or hypoglycemic
- Third trimester of pregnancy, or post partem. Often primipara.
- Rare

Signs and Symptoms
- Jaundice, asterixis, may be preeclamptic

TESTS

Laboratory
- True hepatic failure with prolonged PT, low fibrinogen (usually high in pregnancy)
- AST<ALT, usually <1,000
- Elevated bilirubin
- Hyperammonemia, hypoglycemia
- Normal platelet count unless severe and DIC

Liver Biopsy
- Central pallor with microvesicular fat on special stains (plan these with Pathology before doing the biopsy), disarray of hepatocytes, may mimic viral hepatitis; biopsy usually not needed as diagnosis based on clinical grounds.

DIFFERENTIAL DIAGNOSIS
- HELLP syndrome (not true hepatic failure, low platelet count)
- Viral hepatitis (+ serologies, risk factors on history; possible hepatitis E if from endemic area, or herpes simplex hepatitis) or drug induced fulminant hepatic failure (eg acetaminophen ingestion)

MANAGEMENT

What to Do First
- Obstetric consultation, consider delivery

General Measures
- Maximal support, may require ICU, dialysis, etc

SPECIFIC THERAPY
- Delivery/support
- Liver transplantation not indicated except very rarely

FOLLOW-UP
- R/O associated defect in beta oxidation of fatty acids, DNA testing available for the most common defect associated with acute fatty liver of pregnancy, long chain 3-hydroxyl-acyl CoA dehydrogenase. Test patient, her baby and baby's father
- Expect full recovery. May recur in subsequent pregnancies

COMPLICATIONS AND PROGNOSIS

■ Acute hepatic failure, with ascites, renal failure, GI bleeding, prolonged jaundice
■ Nephrogenic diabetes insipidus may occur

ACUTE HEART FAILURE

JOHN R. TEERLINK, MD

HISTORY & PHYSICAL

[see also Gheorghiade M, et al. Acute heart failure syndromes: Current state and framework for future research. *Circulation* 2005;112:3958–68; Niemenen MS, et al. Executive summary of the guidelines on the diagnosis and treatment of acute heart failure. *Eur Heart J* 2005;26:384–416.]

History

■ >1 million hospitalizations for heart failure per year in US alone
■ Acute heart failure (AHF): catastrophic loss of cardiac function (loss of myocyte function: ischemia/ infarction, inflammation, edema, trauma, post-cardiac bypass, alcohol binge or other toxic substance use/ exposure; structural: papillary muscle rupture, VSD)
  ➤ Rapid onset of symptoms
  ➤ Preceding viral illness
  ➤ Angina or anginal equivalent
■ Acute heart failure syndrome (AHFS): gradual or rapid change in heart failure signs and symptoms resulting in a need for urgent therapy. Approximately 30–60% of patients will have normal systolic function.
  ➤ Preceding viral illness
  ➤ Angina or anginal equivalent
  ➤ Prior myocardial infarction or systolic dysfunction
  ➤ Hypertension or other restrictive cardiomyopathy
  ➤ Progressive increase in weight, peripheral edema, bloating, dyspnea
  ➤ Relatively gradual onset of symptoms
■ AHFS clinical presentations
  ➤ Acute decompensated heart failure, de novo or decompensation of chronic heart failure (40–50% of patients)
  ➤ Hypertensive acute heart failure (40–50%)
  ➤ Pulmonary edema (<3%)

➤ Cardiogenic shock (<1%)
➤ High-output failure (<1%)
➤ Right heart failure (?)

Signs & Symptoms

- Dyspnea: exertional, orthopnea, paroxysmal nocturnal, "cardiac asthma"
- Non-productive cough
- Reduced exercise capacity
- Generalized weakness and fatigue
- Nocturia, oliguria
- Confusion, poor memory, insomnia, anxiety, headache, delirium
- Nausea, abdominal discomfort, anorexia
- Consistent with underlying or inciting pathophysiology
- General: distressed, dyspneic, pallor, diaphoresis, cardiac cachexia, jaundice (acute hepatic congestion)
- Vital signs: tachycardia (frequent), hypotension or transient hypertension, narrow pulse pressure, tachypnea, low grade fever.
- Respiratory: rales, pleural effusion, Cheyne-Stokes respiration pattern
- CV: jugular venous distension, hepato/abdominojugular reflux, pulsus alternans (severe), cardiomegaly, LV heave, RV lift, soft S1, loud P2, S3, S4, systolic murmur (functional MR/TR)
- Abd: hepatomegaly, ascites
- Extrem: peripheral, sacral and scrotal edema

TESTS

- Basic Blood Tests
  - ➤ Often normal, except for other comorbidities, especially indicators of CHF or myocardial infarction
  - ➤ Electrolytes: Hyponatremia (dilutional or secondary hyperaldosteronism), hypokalemia (diuretic use), hyperkalemia (K-sparing diuretic, K replacement, renal failure), hypophosphatemia, hypomagnesemia (diuretics use, alcohol)
  - ➤ BUN/ creatinine: Prerenal azotemia
  - ➤ Cardiac enzymes: elevated troponin or CK-MB (myocardial injury)
  - ➤ BNP (B-type natriuretic peptide) or nt-pro-BNP: suggestive of elevated cardiac filling pressures or ventricular wall stress; in patents with dyspnea, high levels supportive of heart failure etiology; may be elevated in right-sided heart failure (i.e., cor pulmonale, pulmonary embolus)

- ➤ D-dimers: occasionally used to assist in dDx of pulmonary embolus
- ➤ Liver function tests: AST, ALT, LDH, direct and indirect bilirubin elevated in congestive hepatopathy
- ➤ TSH: hypo- or hyperthyroidism
- ■ Basic Urine Tests
  - ➤ Proteinuria, high specific gravity, acellular casts
- ■ Specific Diagnostic Tests
  - ➤ Chest X-ray: cardiomegaly (size and shape can assist with dx); pulmonary vascular redistribution, interstitial pulmonary edema (Kerley B lines, perivascular, subpleural effusion), alveolar edema ("butterfly pattern")
  - ➤ Electrocardiogram: ischemia/ infarction; evidence of LVH, prior MI, arrhythmias
  - ➤ Echocardiogram: Cardiac function, structure, wall motion and valvular abnormalities
- ■ Other Tests as Appropriate
  - ➤ Radionuclide Ventriculogram (RVG; MUGA): Cardiac function, wall motion abnormalities
  - ➤ Exercise or pharmacologic stress testing: assess myocardial ischemia risk
  - ➤ Cardiac catheterization: define coronary anatomy, possible interventions

DIFFERENTIAL DIAGNOSIS
- ■ Abnormal ventricular or atrial rhythm
- ■ Acute bronchitis/ asthma
- ■ Pneumonia
- ■ Sepsis
- ■ Cardiogenic Shock
  - ➤ Other non-cardiogenic pulmonary edema (Intravenous narcotics, increased intracerebral pressure, high altitude, transfusion reactions, DIC)

MANAGEMENT
What to Do First
- ■ Check and monitor vital signs, oxygenation and ECG
- ■ Evaluate for underlying etiology (see differential diagnosis), especially sepsis, myocardial ischemia/ infarction, cardiac mechanical abnormalities (valvular, VSD, etc.)
- ■ Treat underlying etiology (i.e. myocardial infarction – primary PCI, thrombolysis)

General Measures

■ Usually more comfortable sitting upright with legs dangling
■ Restore and maintain oxygenation: supplemental oxygen, non-invasive positive pressure ventilation (BiPAP), mechanical ventilation, morphine
■ Reduce volume overload (preload): diuretics, nitrates, morphine, nesiritide, ultrafiltration
■ Reduce afterload: nitroprusside, nitroglycerin, nesiritide
■ Improve cardiac function: positive inotropes (dobutamine, milrinone), intra-aortic balloon counterpulsation, left ventricular assist device
■ Maintain blood pressure, renal perfusion: dopamine (low dose)
■ Consider Swann-Ganz pulmonary artery catheter to measure cardiac output, PCWP and vascular resistances and guide therapy, especially if:
  ➤ Cardiogenic shock/ near shock unresponsive to fluid challenge
  ➤ Unresponsive pulmonary edema, especially with hypotension or shock
  ➤ Assist in diagnosis between cardiogenic and non-cardiogenic etiology

SPECIFIC THERAPY

Indications for Treatment

■ Poor oxygenation
■ Poor peripheral perfusion
■ Poor central perfusion
■ Volume overload
■ Hypotension

Treatment Options

Including Side Effects and Contraindications: General info on drug classes, check for more complete prescribing information

■ Morphine: intravenous, subcutaneous (in mild cases)
  ➤ Indication: Reduce preload, decrease anxiety and hyperadrenergic state
  ➤ Side Effects and Complications: Decreased ventilatory drive with possible CO_2 retention, hypotension, paralytic ileus, toxic megacolon, seizures, somnolence, constipation, urinary retention, dizziness, dry mouth, headache, nausea/ vomiting, rash.
  ➤ Absolute Contraindications: Narcotic-induced pulmonary edema, respiratory depression, paralytic ileus

➤ Relative Contraindications: Neurogenic pulmonary edema, seizure disorder, increased intracerebral pressure,
■ Intravenous loop diuretics (furosemide, torsemide, bumetanide, ethacrynic acid): bolus and/ or infusion. May be combined with thiazide diuretics (oral or IV) for potentiation of effect
  ➤ Indication: Volume overload, reduce preload
  ➤ Side Effects and Complications: renal failure, thrombocytopenia, orthostatic hypotension, dizziness, dry mouth, headache, nausea/ vomiting, dyspepsia, impotence, rash, hypokalemia, arrhythmias, muscle cramps, ototoxicity.
  ➤ Absolute Contraindications: hepatic coma
  ➤ Relative Contraindications: anuria, severe electrolyte depletion
■ Nitroglycerin: sublingual, intravenous, topical (decreased absorption in shock states); requires careful blood pressure monitoring
  ➤ Indication: Reduce preload, treat ischemia, mild afterload reduction
  ➤ Side Effects and Complications: hemolytic anemia, methemoglobinemia, headache, dizziness, hypotension, syncope, angina, reflex tachycardia, nausea/ vomiting, edema rash
  ➤ Absolute Contraindications: Increased intracerebral pressure, cerebral hemorrhage, symptomatic hypotension, angle-closure glaucoma
  ➤ Relative Contraindications: stroke, hypotension, severe anemia
■ Nitroprusside: IV; careful blood pressure monitoring advised (often invasive), follow thiocyanate levels
  ➤ Indication: Reduces preload and afterload
  ➤ Side Effects and Complications: cyanide/thiocyanate toxicity, methemoglobinemia, headache, dizziness, hypotension, syncope, angina, reflex tachycardia, nausea/vomiting, edema rash
  ➤ Absolute Contraindications: increased intracerebral pressure, cerebral hemorrhage, symptomatic hypotension
  ➤ Relative Contraindications: stroke, hypotension, severe anemia
■ Nesiritide: IV, recombinant human B-type natriuretic peptide; requires careful blood pressure monitoring
  ➤ Indication: Reduce preload, afterload reduction; improve symptoms of dyspnea
  ➤ Side Effects and Complications: headache, dizziness, hypotension, syncope, nausea/vomiting, occasional worsening of renal function
  ➤ Absolute Contraindications: cardiogenic shock, symptomatic hypotension, SBP < 90

> Relative Contraindications: stroke, hypotension, severe anemia, significant valvular stenosis, restrictive or obstructive cardiomyopathy, constrictive pericarditis, pericardial tamponade, or other conditions in which cardiac output is dependent upon venous return, or for patients suspected to have low cardiac filling pressures

- Dobutamine: intravenous; requires blood pressure and ECG monitoring
  > Indication: Increases myocardial contractility, mildly reduces preload, mild afterload reduction
  > Side Effects and Complications: arrhythmias, hypotension, asthma exacerbation, nausea/ vomiting, headache, angina, thrombocytopenia, local injection site reaction
  > Absolute Contraindications: IHSS, severe obstructive valvular disease
  > Relative Contraindications: hypertension, recent MI, arrhythmia, volume depletion

- Milrinone: intravenous, many centers no longer use bolus dose to avoid hypotension; requires careful blood pressure and ECG monitoring; may consider if patient on a beta-blocker.
  > Indication: Increases myocardial contractility, mildly reduces preload, afterload reduction
  > Side Effects and Complications: arrhythmias, hypotension, nausea/ vomiting, headache, angina, myocardial infarction, local injection site reaction
  > Absolute Contraindications: IHSS, severe obstructive valvular disease, myocardial infarction
  > Relative Contraindications: hypertension, arrhythmia, volume depletion

- Dopamine: IV, low dose for "renal effects"; requires careful blood pressure and ECG monitoring
  > Indication: Increases myocardial contractility, mildly reduces preload, afterload reduction
  > Side Effects and Complications: arrhythmias, hypotension, nausea/ vomiting, headache, angina, myocardial infarction, local necrosis at injection site reaction
  > Absolute Contraindications: pheochromocytoma, IHSS, severe obstructive valvular disease
  > Relative Contraindications: hypertension, arrhythmia, volume depletion, myocardial infarction, severe peripheral vascular disease

- Ultrafiltration: may require only peripheral IV lines; may preserve renal function, avoid hypokalemia and reduce rehospitalization
  - Indication: usually used for large volume removal
  - Side Effects and Complications: Hypotension, filter and access complications, risks associated with anticoagulation
  - Absolute Contraindications: Uncontrolled symptomatic hypotension
- Intra-aortic balloon counterpulsation pump: usually inserted via femoral artery; requires invasive blood pressure and ECG monitoring.
  - Indication: Augments diastolic coronary flow and forward output, afterload reduction
  - Side Effects and Complications: arrhythmias, headache, nausea/vomiting, peripheral vascular insufficiency, emboli, infarction and gangrene, aortic dissection, rupture, pericardial tamponade
  - Absolute Contraindications: aortic insufficiency, aortic aneurysm or dissection
  - Relative Contraindications: severe peripheral vascular disease

FOLLOW-UP

During Treatment

- Often requires intensive care or telemetry unit monitoring early in course of treatment
- Monitor electrolytes, especially potassium, and renal function

Routine

- Follow-up after treatment of acute episode: diagnose and treat underlying abnormalities (ischemia, hypertension)
- Emphasize lifestyle changes such as reduced sodium intake, compliance with medications

COMPLICATIONS AND PROGNOSIS

- Complications usually related to underlying pathophysiology
- 3–5% in-hospital mortality
- 10–25% 6-month mortality

ACUTE LYMPHOBLASTIC LEUKEMIA

MICHAEL R. GREVER, MD

HISTORY & PHYSICAL

Etiology

- Children with Down syndrome (trisomy 21) or other inherited disorders (e.g., ataxia telangiectasia) have an increased risk; evidence of some environmental exposures to chemical agents (e.g., pesticides) may be important, but most cases not associated with defined causative factor

Signs & Symptoms

■ Most symptoms relate to bone marrow replacement with leukemia (e.g., patients present with excessive fatigue, infection, fever, bruising, bleeding).

■ Patients may also present with symptoms related to bulk disease (e.g., lymph node enlargement, splenic enlargement, pain) and rarely shortness of breath with very high counts (leukostasis) or from bulk disease in the chest (mediastinal mass, pleural effusions).

■ Patients infrequently (∼3–5%) have symptoms from CNS involvement at presentation (headache, confusion, cranial nerve involvement); rare presentation may also include involvement of the orbit.

■ A thorough history must be taken with a complete review of symptoms, exposure to drugs, environmental agents, and familial diseases.

■ Physical signs associated with bone marrow failure (e.g., pallor, tachycardia, fever, petechiae, ecchymoses, infection)

■ Physical signs associated with bulk disease (lymphadenopathy, splenomegaly, hepatomegaly, pleuro/pericardial effusions, mediastinal mass)

■ Complete physical examination critically important, including testicular examination (painless enlargement of a unilateral testis may occur in a small percentage of male children [∼2%] or in patients with T-cell leukemia or hyperleukocytosis), and a careful baseline neurologic examination is important.

TESTS

Basic Blood Tests

■ Review the peripheral blood smear for evidence of circulating immature cells (lymphoblasts), evidence of decreased platelets and lack of mature normal peripheral blood cells. Consensus is that FAB distinction between L1 and L2 is not useful. ALL is currently classified more on immunophenotype complemented by cytogenetic and molecular genetic subclassification. The major subclassifications are:

(1) Precursor B lymphoblastic leukemia characterized by expression of CD19 and/or CD79a and/or CD22; subsets also include pro-B-ALL with no additional differentiation markers; common (c-ALL) additional expression CD10, and pre-B-ALL with cytoplasmic IgM.

(2) Mature B-ALL characterized by expression of surface immuno globulin sIgM, and cytoplasmic kappa or lambda light chains (this is the former L3 variant or Burkitt's leukemia)

(3) T-lineage ALL characterized by expression of cyCD3 or sCD3. Subsets of T-cell ALL include pro-T-ALL (CD7+), pre-T-ALL (CD2+, and/or CD5+, and/or CD8+), cortical T-ALL (CD1a), and mature T-ALL (sCD3+, CD1a−). Immunophenotypic classification of ALL has importance for prognosis & treatment.

■ Morphologic features of lymphoblasts are important: presence of condensed nuclear chromatin, evaluation of nuclear to cytoplasmic ratio, absence of Auer rods and granules in the cytoplasm are consistent with diagnosis of ALL.

■ Morphologically distinct lymphoblasts in the uncommon (~5%) mature B-ALL sub-type ALL- L3 (relatively homogeneous, medium size, more dispersed chromatin, multiple nucleoli, deep blue cytoplasm with sharply defined vacuoles); these cells are also often TdT negative.

■ Characterize the abnormal peripheral blood cells (Wright stain, morphology, complete immunophenotypic analysis); important to also include cytogenetics and molecular genetic studies

Basic Bone Marrow Testing:

■ Bone marrow aspirate and biopsy examinations include cytochemical and special stains to define the type of acute leukemia infiltrating the marrow (morphologic features, Wright stains) and assessment of normal marrow cells remaining (e.g., red cell and megakaryocyte preservation); specialized stains to define the type of blasts include (at minimum): myeloperoxidase negative; usually PAS glycogen positive in block pattern; terminal deoxynucleotidyl transferase (TdT) positive (except L3), but the PAS & TdT can also be observed in small number of AML cases. Therefore, PAS & TdT not exclusively diagnostic of ALL. However, the use of immunophenotypic analysis has become extremely important in defining the final diagnosis.

■ Bone marrow aspirate collected in anticoagulant should also be sent for flow cytometric full immunophenotypic characterization and molecular analyses.

■ Bone marrow aspirate in a sterile vial MUST also be sent for cytogenetics. However, FISH probes are now available for major cytogenetic abnormalities. FISH analysis does not require cells to undergo division.

■ Bone marrow biopsy is important to define fibrosis and cellularity

- Flow Cytometric Analysis of ALL: Precursor B cell (CD19, CD22, CD79a, CD10+/−): These cells are Tdt positive, in contrast to mature B-ALL.
- Mature B cell (correlates with former L3 classification): CD19+; CD20+; CD22+; CD79a+; sIg+; Others: Tdt-; CD34-; CD10+/−
- Precursor T cell: CD7+; cCD3+; CD5+; CD4+/−; CD8+/−; CD34+; TdT+
- Critically important decisions will be based upon subtype characterization, but essential to confirm that this is ALL.

Other Critical Initial Testing
- Send blood for basic assessment of hematologic and metabolic status including CBC with differential, coagulation profile; chemistries including electrolytes; renal and liver function, uric acid, calcium, phosphate, and magnesium; HLA typing for potential stem cell transplantation including patient, siblings, and parent
- Chest x-ray PA & lateral to evaluate for infection and/or a mediastinal mass

Other Laboratory Tests
- Molecular and immunophenotypic characterization of leukemic cells specifically to monitor disease (e.g., search for minimal residual disease following therapy and potentially useful in follow-up for early relapse)
- Immunophenotypic analysis searching for monoclonal population of leukemic cells as well as RT-PCR important for quantitating minimal residual disease at time of remission (and may be helpful with relapse surveillance)
- Imaging studies to assess bulk disease (e.g., CT scan of chest & abdomen)
- Lumbar puncture to assess for CNS disease: Prophylactic treatment essentially required in every case. If the patient has symptoms at presentation, CSF exam is essential. Therapy should also be administered intrathecally along with diagnostic studies. However, in the asymptomatic patient, CNS examination may be accomplished after the patient is stabilized on systemic therapy because of requirement for serial treatment of the CNS compartment. Recent data show that traumatic lumbar puncture may have an adverse impact on survival, necessitating an experienced person to do the initial lumbar punctures, and rationalizes the introduction of prophylactic chemotherapy with initial diagnostic tap.

■ Cardiac evaluation with ECG and determination of cardiac ejection fraction by scan

DIFFERENTIAL DIAGNOSIS
■ Reactive lymphocytosis (e.g., infectious mononucleosis, cytomegaloviral infection, pertussis); acute myelogenous leukemia; acute leukemic transformation from another underlying hematologic disorder (e.g., myelodysplasia, chronic lymphocytic leukemia; mantle cell lymphoma; plasmablastic myeloma)

MANAGEMENT
What to Do First
■ Initial medical management
■ Following careful physical assessment, patient should be treated for complications of bone marrow failure (e.g., transfusion of red cells and/or platelets for anemia or severe thrombocytopenia and treatment of infection with appropriate antibiotics)
■ Metabolic status must be assessed and stabilized (i.e., administration of adequate hydration to avoid complications of tumor lysis); allopurinol should be used to prevent and treat hyperuricemia, but should be stopped following initial reduction of the tumor load; allopurinol should be stopped after day 6–12, depending on the metabolic parameters. Rasburicase (a recombinant urate-oxidase enzyme) has been approved for the initial management of pediatric patients with leukemia, lymphoma, and malignancies anticipated to result in tumor lysis upon treatment. This agent appears to be effective in preventing hyperuricemia and may reduce the need for alkalinization of the urine, thus improving the negative impact of alkalinization on phosphates in impairing renal function.
■ Patient should have central intravenous access for optimal management during induction chemotherapy.
■ Prophylactic antibiotics & antiviral & antifungal agents should be considered for the uninfected patient until neutropenia has resolved; all patients should receive Pneumocystis prophylaxis starting with the second course of chemotherapy; granulocyte colony-stimulating factor (G-CSF) is given to patients after waiting at least 24 h after the last dose of cytotoxic chemotherapy (e.g., day 4 until neutrophils have recovered to >5,000 after the nadir); caution must be exercised in selecting prophylactic agents to avoid drug allergies. Furthermore, caution must be used in understanding the impact of multiple concomitant medications on chemotherapy agents used throughout

treatment (e.g., impact of agents that alter CYPA4 and other p450 enzymes, agents that may alter plasma pharmacokinetics and intracellular concentrations of major antineoplastic agents).

■ Treatment of leukemia should proceed expeditiously, but metabolic stabilization of the patient may be advisable (for a short period) if the disease is not rapidly progressing or if bulk disease is not critically impinging on vital structures. If disease is rapidly progressing, leukopheresis may be helpful for symptoms of hyperleukocytosis, and initiation of systemic chemotherapy should then begin as soon as possible.

Risk-Based Therapeutic Strategies

■ Prognostic Features & Risk Assessment

■ Several clinical features are associated with a poor outcome, including patient age (e.g., <1 year old or >50–60 years old); WBC at presentation (>50,000); time to remission; patients who have residual disease detected by flow or PCR determination of clonal genotypic abnormalities (at level 0.1% or greater)after being in remission have a high cumulative risk for relapse. Specific cytogenetic abnormalities confer a worse prognosis, including the following: pts w/ t:(9;22) or bcr-abl expression by molecular screening have poor long-term outcome; pts w/ t:(4;11) with MLL-AF4A fusion gene have a worse long-term prognosis; patients with hypodiploidy (< 45 chromosomes/leukemic cell) have a worse prognosis than those with hyperdiploidy (>50 chromosomes/leukemic cell). Patients with the t(12;21) with the TEL-AML1 fusion gene have a favorable prognosis. In patients with T-cell ALL, the presence of t(11;19) with MLL-ENL fusion and overexpression of the HOX11 gene confers a good prognosis.

■ Patients with standard-risk ALL are treated with multiagent induction therapy (vincristine, prednisone, cyclophosphamide, L-asparaginase, and an anthracycline); standard-risk patients require consolidation with CNS treatment (may include CNS irradiation and intrathecal chemotherapy) followed by late intensification with chemotherapy and maintenance chemotherapy for a total duration of therapy from 2.5 to 3 years. Additional agents used during intensification therapy following achievement of a complete remission include cyclophosphamide, high-dose methotrexate, mercaptopurine, and cytosine arabinoside. Different intensification and consolidation regimens have been used but often include drugs other than those received during initial induction.

- Patients with poor-risk ALL associated with t(9;22) have benefited from incorporation of imatinib mesylate (Gleevec) into their regimen. Allogeneic stem cell transplantation should be vigorously pursued for patients with this specific diagnosis, and additional second-generation ABL kinase inhibitors are under development.
- Patients with mature B-cell ALL (L3) associated with characteristic chromosomal abnormalities, including t:(8;14)(q24;q32); t(2;8)(p12;q24); or t(8;22)(q24;q11), often rapidly progress unless therapy is started expeditiously; patients with this type of ALL are susceptible to massive tumor lysis, necessitating adequate metabolic preparation and intervention during therapy.
- Patients with mature B-cell ALL (L3) are treated with intensive chemotherapy (including cyclophosphamide, high-dose methotrexate, and cytosine arabinoside in addition to vincristine, ifosfamide, dexamethasone, VM-26 and Adriamycin) combined in an alternating series of courses administered over 6 months. This has markedly improved the outcome in this disease. CNS treatment is also mandatory.
- Treatment of T-cell ALL has markedly improved with the addition of cyclophosphamide and cytosine arabinoside during induction therapy; current CR rates are ranging from 82% to 93%, with LFS at 3 years now 50%, making this a favorable subtype of ALL.
- Stem Cell Transplantation
- In patients with failure to achieve response by weeks 4 to 6 or those with adverse cytogenetics (e.g., t:9;22 and t:4;11), the plan should include a vigorous search for allogeneic stem cell transplantation (either HLA-matched sibling or a matched unrelated donor [MUD]) during first remission; strategies must include participation in ongoing clinical trials.
- In fact, all patients with ALL should be encouraged to participate in ongoing clinical trials based upon their risk assessment for initial response and duration.

Management Summary
- Patients with ALL should be assigned to specific treatment protocols based upon an assessment of their risk for response to therapy and duration of response.
- Therapeutic strategies can be divided into phases of required treatment, including induction, consolidation, intensification, maintenance therapies; essentially all patients need to be treated for CNS disease; some patients can be treated with disease-specific

approaches and others receive therapy based upon their clinical responsiveness.

■ Allogeneic stem cell transplantation should be considered for patients who either do not respond well or have a predictable poor outcome based upon their biologic and clinical parameters (e.g., poor cytogenetic characteristics).

■ Standard-Risk ALL with no adverse parameters:

■ Induction: Multiple drug therapy including prednisone, vincristine, L-asparaginase, cyclophosphamide, daunorubicin, filgastrim

■ Consolidation: Cytarabine, 6-mercaptopurine, L-asparaginase, vincristine, filgastrim

■ CNS Therapy: Methotrexate (IT); number of doses and duration of therapy depend on chosen protocol; need for CNS irradiation also individualized

■ Late intensification: Dexamethasone, vincristine, cyclophosphamide, then cyclophosphamide, cytarabine, and 6-thioguanine

■ Maintenance: 6-Mercaptopurine; methotrexate; vincristine; prednisone

■ This therapeutic approach requires 2.5 to 3 years of therapy

■ Mature B-Cell ALL (formerly called FAB type L3 or Burkitt's Leukemia)
  ➤ Cytoreductive phase: prednisone; cyclophosphamide
    • Course A: vincristine; ifosfamide; mesna; methotrexate; leucovorin; dexamethasone; VM-26; cytosine arabinoside
    • Course B: vincristine; cyclophosphamide; methotrexate; leucovorin; dexamethasone; Adriamycin
  ➤ Intrathecal therapy is needed with the alternating cycles of intensive therapy
  ➤ All therapy for this form of ALL is completed in approximately 6 months

Side Effects & Complications

■ Treatment Toxicities: Multiple chemotherapeutic agents are used in the successful management of this disease; individual side effects are too numerous to outline.

■ Major considerations requiring attention are drug doses and interactions, toxic effects on normal tissue (e.g., mucositis); modification of doses based upon renal and liver function; constant surveillance for infection and bleeding; and then drug-specific toxicities (e.g., L-asparaginase can deplete normal hemostatic factors; can cause pancreatitis).

SPECIFIC THERAPY
n/a

FOLLOW-UP

Routine

- Response Assessment: Initial bone marrow aspiration and biopsy must be obtained on day 29 of initial therapy to determine response. If no remission, need to move quickly in assessing options for allogeneic stem cell transplantation; if positive response, need to continue with therapeutic plan.
- Surveillance Bone Marrows: Required every 6 months or sooner if relapse is suspected based upon peripheral blood counts; opportunity exists for following molecular probes for minimal residual disease for those in complete remission. Monitoring the bone marrow for evidence of minimal residual disease appears to identify those patients at higher risk for relapse. The bone marrow is the most common site for relapse in ALL.

COMPLICATIONS AND PROGNOSIS

- Long-term disease outcome: Current strategies have resulted in the achievement of a complete remission in 70–90% of adults, with long-term survival in the 25–50% range. Risk-based therapeutic strategies have been attempted to reduce the short- and long-term toxicities associated with the treatment of the disease. Highest risk of death during therapy is related to infection. Long-term risks of disease relate to relapse, which can occur for years after completion of treatment. Extramedullary relapse can occur in the CNS, the skin, the testes in males, and anywhere in the body.
- Late complications: Aggressive prophylactic treatment of the CNS with irradiation and intrathecal chemotherapy may result in severe neurologic toxicity, which has necessitated risk-based therapeutic strategies; long-term complications of intensive chemotherapy may produce end-organ damage in the long-term survivors of successful chemotherapy; patients must be watched closely for evidence of secondary malignancies and consequences of immunosuppression.

ACUTE MYELOBLASTIC LEUKEMIA

JAMES D. GRIFFIN, MD

HISTORY & PHYSICAL

History

- Preleukemic syndrome, radiation, prior chemotherapy
- Family history of leukemia uncommon

Signs & Symptoms
- May be asymptomatic
- Fever, fatigue, bruising, gum bleeding, weight loss, rash
- Less common – headache, confusion, frank bleeding
- Pallor, petechiae, leukemia cutis, swollen gums, retinal hemorrhages, signs of infection, lymphadenopathy
- Extramedullary mass (myeloblastoma) – skin, bone, paravertebral, intraspinal
- Less common – jaundice, splenomegaly, CNS signs

TESTS

Laboratory

Basic Studies:
- Blood: CBC, platelets, blood smear,
- Electrolytes (elevated K+ may be spurious if WBC is high)
- Metabolic screen, liver and renal function tests, uric acid
- Coagulation tests: PT, PTT, fibrinogen
- Infection: if febrile, blood, urine, throat, stool cultures (fungal infections uncommon at presentation, non-infectious fever common)
- Urinalysis
- Specific Diagnostic Tests: bone marrow aspirate and biopsy for morphology and cytochemistry, cytogenetics, immunophenotype by flow cytometry
  - ➤ Important to identify Acute Promyelocytic Leukemia (APL;M3)
  - ➤ Cytogenetics is a major predictor of outcome:
    - Good risk: t(15;17), t(8;21), normal
    - Poor risk: 11q23 abnormalities, −7, −5, +8, complex karyotype, mutations in FLT3
- Other Tests as Appropriate: CXR, lumbar puncture, cardiac scan if prior anthracycline use

DIFFERENTIAL DIAGNOSIS
- Acute infection, leukemoid reactions, megaloblastic anemias, myelodysplasia distinguished by bone marrow examination
- Cytopenias can be caused by aplastic anemia, ITP, severe infections, drug reactions, marrow failure syndromes, etc.

MANAGEMENT

What to Do First
- General Measures: While confirming diagnosis, start hydration, correct electrolytes, treat infection, start allopurinol
- Correct anemia with red blood cell transfusions

- Renal failure may be due to hypovolemia, leukemic infiltration, uric acid nephropathy
- Prophylactic platelet transfusions may be given if platelet count <10–20,000/ul, or for bleeding. CNS bleeding is of particular concern
- DIC usually associated with APL
- HLA typing if patient is a candidate for Stem Cell Transplant (SCT)
- Severe neutropenia (<500 neutrophils/ul) with fever requires antibiotic therapy; surveillance cultures of throat, nasopharynx, blood, skin, urine, and stool useful in induction therapy.

SPECIFIC THERAPY
- Chemotherapy and intensive supportive care are required
- Oncologic emergencies
  - Symptomatic leukostasis (CNS symptoms, renal failure, pulmonary insufficiency)
  - Renal or liver failure due to leukemic infiltration may improve rapidly with initiation of chemotherapy
  - Myeloblastomas resulting in organ dysfunction, such as spinal cord compression, can be treated with local irradiation in addition to chemotherapy
  - DIC in association with APL requires urgent treatment.

Induction Therapy
- APL (M3)
  - All-trans-retinoic acid (ATRA) + anthracycline-based chemotherapy
  - At least 2 cycles of consolidation therapy after complete remission
  - Maintenance therapy recommended
- AML (adult)
  - Age <60, standard dose cytarabine + anthracycline (7+3); or high-dose cytarabine + anthracycline or mitoxantrone
  - For age >60, standard-dose cytarabine + anthracycline
  - If history of MDS, clinical trial or SCT
  - If no remission, change therapy

Post Remission Treatment
- For age <60, consolidation therapy with high-dose cytarabine, other consolidation regimen, or SCT
- For age <60 and poor risk cytogenetics or prior MDS, clinical trial or SCT
- For age >60, consolidation therapy with standard-dose cytarabine + anthracycline or clinical trial

Relapse Therapy
- APL (M3)
  - ➤ Arsenic or Anthracycline + ATRA, followed by SCT or clinical trial
- AML
  - ➤ Early (<6 mo), clinical trial or SCT
  - ➤ Late (>6 mo), clinical trial, SCT, or repeat induction regimen

Special Situations
- Children should be treated on pediatric clinical protocols.
- CNS involvement requires intrathecal chemotherapy.

Side Effects & Contraindications
- Cytarabine
  - ➤ Nausea, vomiting, severe neutropenia with risk of life-threatening infections, severe thrombocytopenia with risk of bleeding, alopecia, liver dysfunction, cerebellar ataxia (high dose, age related), rash, renal and neural toxicity less common
- Anthracycline
  - ➤ Nausea, vomiting, severe pancytopenia, cardiac dysfunction (cumulative), alopecia, rash, tissue necrosis with extravasation, mucositis
  - ➤ Dose reductions for severe renal, hepatic dysfunction
- ATRA
  - ➤ "Retinoic Acid Syndrome"
  - ➤ Respiratory distress, fever, weight gain, edema, effusions, hypotension, renal failure
  - ➤ Prevent with chemotherapy, treat with high-dose corticosteroids.
  - ➤ Transient coagulopathy
  - ➤ Increased transaminases, triglycerides, bone pain
  - ➤ Headache
  - ➤ **Contraindications**
    - patient choice, debility from other medical problems

FOLLOW-UP

During Therapy
- Regular assessment of blood counts, renal, liver function
- Bone marrow day 14–21 of induction therapy to assess response and cellularity
- Bone marrow if relapse suspected
- Aggressive evaluation for fever and neutropenia.
- Consolidation and maintenance therapy: weekly to monthly blood tests

COMPLICATIONS AND PROGNOSIS

Complications

- Infection: usually bacterial during induction therapy, bacterial or fungal during relapse
- Bleeding: due to thrombocytopenia or DIC, CNS or GI may be severe
- Drug reactions: cytarabine, antibiotics, allopurinol
- Relapse

Prognosis

- Varies with age, cytogenetics, history of preceding preleukemic disorder
- Long-term survival about 25–35% with chemotherapy alone, somewhat higher with SCT
- Immunotherapy and oncogene-targeted drugs under development

---

ACUTE MYOCARDITIDES

JOHN R. TEERLINK, MD

HISTORY & PHYSICAL

History

- Presentation may be acute, subacute or chronic, but often rapid onset with acute heart failure or cardiogenic shock
- Often previously asymptomatic or symptom onset days to weeks after acute febrile illness or upper respiratory infection.

Signs & Symptoms

- See also acute and chronic heart failure chapters, and chapters pertaining to specific etiology
- Chest pain, often pleuritic or non-specific
- See also acute and chronic heart failure chapters, and chapters pertaining to specific etiology

TESTS

- Basic Tests
  - ➤ See acute and chronic heart failure chapters, and chapters pertaining to specific etiology
- Specific Diagnostic Tests
  - ➤ Chest X-ray: cardiomegaly (size and shape can assist with dx); pulmonary vascular redistribution, interstitial pulmonary

edema (Kerley B lines, perivascular, subpleural effusion), alveolar edema ("butterfly pattern")
- ➤ Electrocardiogram: non-specific ST/T wave changes, conduction abnormalities (especially Chagas')
- ➤ Echocardiogram (2-D with Doppler flow study): single most useful diagnostic test; cardiac function, structure, wall motion and valvular abnormalities, assess wall thickness, exclude other disease
- ■ Other Tests as Appropriate
  - ➤ Radionuclide ventriculogram (RVG; MUGA): Cardiac function, wall motion abnormalities
  - ➤ Exercise or pharmacologic stress testing: assess myocardial ischemia risk
  - ➤ Cardiac catheterization: define coronary anatomy
  - ➤ Endomyocardial biopsy: insensitive and often non-specific; most useful for monitoring anthracycline cardiotoxicity and detection and monitoring of myocarditis, especially Giant cell.
  - ➤ Machado-Guerreiro complement-fixation test or ELISA (Chagas' disease); viral culture from body fluids, viral-neutralizing antibody titers, complement fixation, PCR of viral genes from biopsy samples (viral)

DIFFERENTIAL DIAGNOSIS
- ■ Multiple infectious etiologies: partial listing of most common pathogens
  - ➤ Viral: About 24 viruses associated with myocarditis, including coxsackieviruses (over 50% of cases), HIV, CMV, viral hepatitis, poliomyelitis
  - ➤ Rickettsial: Rocky Mountain spotted fever, scrub typhus, Q fever (endocarditis most common)
  - ➤ Bacterial: diphtheria (about 25% cases and most common cause of death with diphtheria), brucellosis, Legionnaires disease, mycoplasma pneumoniae, streptococcal (see Rheumatic fever)
  - ➤ Spirochetal: Lyme carditis (tickborne; 10% with cardiac involvement, usually degrees of heart block; ventricular dysfunction rare)
  - ➤ Fungal: most frequent in patients with malignancy and/ or immunosuppressive therapy; aspergillosis (not uncommon in generalized infection), mucormycosis (about 20% in patients with disseminated form; invasion of arteries causes infarction), candidiasis (endocarditis most common), cryptococcosis (most common in HIV)

> Protozoal: Trypanosomiasis (Chagas' disease, caused by T. cruzi, reduviid bug vector, Central/ South America, decade(s) latent period; associated with megaesophagus, megacolon, apical and multiple LV aneurysms), toxoplasmosis

> Metazoal: echinococcus (hydatid cyst: intramyocardial), trichinosis

- Toxin exposure: anthracyclines, cytotoxic drugs, emetine, catecholamines (cocaine, pheochromocytoma), heavy metals (lead, cobalt, antimony, arsenic), venoms (snake, scorpion), anaphylaxis, and others
- Giant cell myocarditis: possibly immune or autoimmune etiology, usually rapidly fatal, often young-to-middle aged adults
- Hypersensitivity reactions: sulfonamides, hydrochlorothiazide, penicillins, methyldopa, and others

MANAGEMENT
(See also acute and chronic heart failure chapters, and chapters pertaining to specific etiology)

What to Do First
- Check and monitor vital signs, oxygenation and ECG
- Evaluate for underlying etiology (see differential diagnosis), especially sepsis, myocardial ischemia/ infarction, cardiac mechanical abnormalities (valvular, VSD, etc)
- Treat underlying etiology (i.e. myocardial infarction- thrombolysis, primary PTCA)
- Treat acute heart failure with management as described in acute heart failure chapter
- Attempt to define etiology (if giant cell myocarditis, consider early empiric course of immunosuppressive therapy)

General Measures
- Usually more comfortable sitting upright with legs dangling
- Restore and maintain oxygenation: morphine, supplemental oxygen, non-invasive positive pressure ventilation (BiPAP), mechanical ventilation
- Reduce volume overload (preload): morphine, diuretics, nitrates
- Reduce afterload: nitroglycerin, nitroprusside
- Improve cardiac function: positive inotropes (dobutamine, milrinone), intraaortic balloon counterpulsation, left ventricular assist device
- Maintain blood pressure, renal perfusion: dopamine (low dose)

- Consider Swann-Ganz pulmonary artery catheter to measure cardiac output, PCWP and vascular resistances and guide therapy, especially if:
- Cardiogenic shock/ near shock unresponsive to fluid challenge
- Unresponsive pulmonary edema, especially with hypotension or shock
- Assist in diagnosis between cardiogenic and non-cardiogenic etiology
- Bed rest/ restricted physical activity for 6 months and until normal function

SPECIFIC THERAPY
- Corticosteroids: controversial; in general felt not to be useful
- Immunosuppressive therapy: consider in Giant cell myocarditis
- NSAIDs: contraindicated during acute phase (first 2 weeks), but may be useful in later

Treatment Options
- Amiodarone: May consider for atrial and ventricular arrhythmias and perhaps to prevent death/ sudden death (also consider AICD)
  - Indication: Atrial arrhythmias, symptomatic ventricular arrhythmias
  - Side Effects and Complications: arrhythmias, SA and AV block, hepatic failure, severe pulmonary toxicity, corneal deposits; blue-gray skin discoloration, peripheral neuropathy, ataxia, edema, dizziness, hyper/ hypothyroidism
  - Absolute Contraindications: Severe SA node disease, 2nd/3rd degree AV block, sick sinus syndrome, bradycardia-induced syncope
  - Relative Contraindications: Thyroid disease, pulmonary disease, impaired liver or renal function, elderly

FOLLOW-UP
During Treatment
- Observe for progression of ventricular dysfunction
- Observe for progression of conduction system disease

Routine
- Reassess LV function in 6 months or if marked change in clinical status

COMPLICATIONS AND PROGNOSIS
- Many cases spontaneously resolve; some develop CHF
- Thromboembolic events (50% of Chagas' patients)
- Death due to sudden death and progressive pump dysfunction

ACUTE PANCREATITIS

ANSON W. LOWE, MD

HISTORY & PHYSICAL

Risk Factors
- Obstruction:
  - Gallstone disease (~45%)
  - Pancreatic cancer
- Toxins & drugs:
  - Alcohol abuse (35%)
- Drugs:
  - Immunosuppressives (eg, azathioprine, 6-mercaptopurine); most common drug-induced cause (3–5% incidence)
  - Anti-retrovirals
  - Many others implicated w/ lower frequencies (eg, furosemide, estrogens, etc)
- Genetic causes:
  - Familial history of hereditary pancreatitis or cystic fibrosis
  - Metabolic causes:
  - Hypertriglyceridemia (>1000mg/dL or 11.3 mmol/L)
  - Hypercalcemia
- Vascular:
  - Ischemia
  - Vasculitis (eg, SLE)

Signs & Symptoms
- Abdominal or back pain
- Epigastric tenderness
- Nausea & vomiting
- Jaundice

TESTS

Basic Blood Tests
- Serum amylase and lipase are the most sensitive & widely used; amylase cleared rapidly & may be normal if pt presents >24–48 h after onset of symptoms
- LFTs may suggest presence of biliary tract or gallbladder disease
- Serum triglyceride level
- Other tests useful in managing & clinically staging pt: CBC, electrolytes, BUN/creatinine, glucose, calcium, LDH

Imaging
- Plain chest & abdominal films to exclude perforation or intestinal obstruction
- US:
  - Detection of inflammation useful in validating diagnosis
  - Determination of presence of biliary tract disease such as cholelithiasis & choledocholithiasis
- CT:
  - Useful when diagnosis unclear
  - Useful in determining severity & risk of complications: presence of significant pancreatic necrosis (>50% of gland) predicts increased risk of mortality & subsequent complications
  - Useful in identifying complications: pseudocyst, fluid collections, hemorrhage

DIFFERENTIAL DIAGNOSIS
- Gallbladder disease
- Peptic ulcer disease
- Intestinal ischemia
- Intestinal perforation
- Biliary tract disease must be considered in pts w/ jaundice or increased LFTs; possible diseases:
  - Choledocholithiasis
  - Cholangiocarcinoma
  - Bile duct strictures

MANAGEMENT
What to Do First
- Initial management should emphasize fluid resuscitation & electrolyte management
- Severe cases require ICU hospitalization to manage fluid & respiratory status

General Management
- Analgesics
- Consider treatment w/ antibiotics (eg, imipenem) for severe acute pancreatitis as determined by clinical staging criteria (Ranson criteria) or abdominal CT revealing extensive necrotizing pancreatitis (>50% involvement of gland)
- Antibiotic treatment in severe cases may decrease incidence of subsequent sepsis

SPECIFIC THERAPY

- Consider ERCP for biliary pancreatitis caused by gallstones in common bile duct (choledocholithiasis)
- Diagnosis suggested by elevated bilirubin or AST
- Consider endoscopic therapy for severe biliary pancreatitis; it may reduce incidence of subsequent biliary sepsis
- Surgery rarely necessary early in course of disease, but may be indicated for infected fluid collections or hemorrhage; later complications such as pseudocysts, ascites, & fistulas often surgically managed

FOLLOW-UP

- Dictated by clinical symptoms & extent of complications (eg, pseudocysts, fistulas, ascites)
- Full recovery expected for most pts w/ mild pancreatitis; patients should be monitored until recovery complete; no long term follow-up required for pts who exhibit full recovery & for whom clear cause of pancreatitis has been identified & corrected
- Evaluate all pts should to identify cause of disease:
  - ➤ History of alcohol abuse
  - ➤ Cholelithiasis: assessed by abdominal US
  - ➤ Serum triglyceride assay
- Consider pts w/o identifiable cause to have idiopathic pancreatitis
- ERCP may be indicated to more carefully look for causes of obstruction (eg, strictures, common bile duct stones, cancers of ampulla of Vater)

COMPLICATIONS AND PROGNOSIS

- Initial staging by clinical criteria (eg, Ranson, Glasgow, or APACHE II) or CT useful in determining risk of complications:
- Shock: usually in first days after presentation:
  - ➤ Acute renal failure
  - ➤ Multiorgan failure
- Acute respiratory distress syndrome: usually 4–5 d after presentation
- Infection:
  - ➤ Usually >7 d after presentation
  - ➤ Evaluate fluid collections by abdominal CT followed by needle aspiration w/ gram stain
  - ➤ Infected fluid collections surgically treated w/ drainage & debridement
- Hemorrhage

- Pseudocysts: represent collections of pancreatic enzymes secondary to ruptured pancreatic duct:
  - ➤ Major complications include rupture, hemorrhage, & infection
  - ➤ Initially pseudocysts followed conservatively; size monitored preferably for 4–6 wk w/ abdominal CT
- Drainage indicated for growing or symptomatic pseudocysts, signs of infection, or hemorrhage; depending on expertise of institution, drainage can be performed by endoscopy, interventional radiology, or surgery
- Ascites secondary to ruptured pancreatic duct:
  - ➤ Diagnosis established by presence of high levels of amylase & protein in fluid
  - ➤ W/ adequate nutrition, ascites may resolve spontaneously
  - ➤ Refer pts w/ persistent ascites to gastroenterologist or pancreatic surgeon
- Fistulas:
  - ➤ May resolve spontaneously w/ adequate nutrition &/or somato-statin to decrease secretions
  - ➤ Closure may require repair by pancreatic surgeon

ACUTE PERICARDITIS

ANDREW D. MICHAELS, MD

HISTORY & PHYSICAL

Signs & Symptoms
- prodrome of fever, myalgia, malaise
- chest pain: pleuritic, sharp, retrosternal, improves when sitting up
- dyspnea
- pericardial friction rub
- distant heart sounds may indicate pericardial effusion

TESTS
Laboratory
- routine: electrolytes, renal panel, CBC, PT, PTT, ESR
- cardiac enzymes if myocarditis/MI suspected
- blood cultures if bacterial pericarditis suspected

ECG
- early (hours-days): widespread ST elevation and PR depression
- late (days-weeks): diffuse T wave inversions

Echo
- pericardial effusion in 60% of cases

DIFFERENTIAL DIAGNOSIS

- idiopathic
- infectious (viral, bacterial, fungal, protozoal)
- neoplastic (primary mesothelioma; metastatic breast, lung, melanoma, lymphoma)
- inflammatory (connective tissue disease, Dressler's syndrome, postradiation)
- traumatic (blunt trauma, iatrogenic, e.g., cardiac surgery)
- metabolic (uremia, myxedema)
- medications (hydralazine, procainamide, isoniazide, anticoagulants)
- congenital (pericardial or thymic cysts)
- other (aortic dissection, amyloid, sarcoid, familial Mediterranean fever)

MANAGEMENT

What to Do First
- assess for clinical evidence of tamponade
  - ➤ (elevated neck veins, pulsus paradoxus either palpable or >10–15 mm Hg by blood pressure cuff, hypotension)

General Measures
- symptomatic relief with NSAIDs
- some patients may require steroids
- avoid anticoagulation

SPECIFIC THERAPY

- for bacterial pericarditis: IV antibiotics
- for tuberculous pericarditis: start 4-drug anti-TB therapy
- for neoplastic pericarditis: chemotherapy against underlying malignancy
- for uremic pericarditis: dialysis

FOLLOW-UP

- during treatment, regularly assess for development of new pericardial effusion/tamponade

COMPLICATIONS AND PROGNOSIS

Complications
- 60% develop pericardial effusion
- <10% develop tamponade or constrictive pericarditis

Prognosis
- largely depends on underlying etiology

ACUTE RENAL FAILURE

MICHAEL J. RYAN, MD and RICHARD ZAGER, MD
REVISED BY MICHAEL J. RYAN, MD

HISTORY & PHYSICAL
- Date onset of ARF
- Define clinical setting – Fever, malaise, arthritis, rash, cough, hemoptysis, rash, livedo reticularis, microinfarctions of distal digits
- Difficulty urinating, hesitancy, decreased stream, BPH
- Blood pressure
- Determine volume status
  - History of volume loss
  - Orthostatic changes in pulse and blood pressure
  - Central venous pressure as determined by neck veins
  - S3 gallop
  - Rales
  - Peripheral edema
  - Documented decreased weight or output > input
- Abdominal exam
  - Bladder palpable
  - Rectal/pelvic
    - Enlarged prostate, pelvic masses

TESTS
Laboratory
- Basic blood studies:
  - High BUN/creatinine ratio (>20) suggests prerenal ARF
  - but also seen with obstruction, steroids, GI bleed
- Basic urine tests:
- *1. Urinalysis*
  - Prerenal failure
  - Arterial occlusion
  - Post renal failure
    - Minimal findings (absence of protein, blood, leukocytes on dip; absence of cells, casts in sediment)
  - ATN
    - Coarse granular and darkly pigmented (muddy brown) granular casts, intact tubular epithelial cells
  - Allergic interstitial nephritis
    - Pyuria, WBC casts, urine eosinophils

- ➤ Acute glomerulonephritis
  - Protein, blood on dipstick; RBCs (often dysmorphic), RBC casts, WBCs on sediment
- ➤ Intrarenal obstruction
  - Large number of crystals (oxalate, uric acid, etc)
- ▣ *2. Urine chemistries (urinary indices)*
  - ➤ Most helpful if oliguric
  - ➤ Only use in conjunction with history, physical and urine sediment – not in isolation
  - ➤ FENa = (UNa/PNa divided by UCr/PCr) × 100
    - U is urine concentration
    - P plasma sodium (Na) or creatinine (Cr)
  - ➤ Prerenal: UNa, <20, FENa <1
  - ➤ ATN: UNa >20, FENa >2

FeUN = (UBUN/PBUN divided by UCr/PCr) × 100. FEUN <35% may be more sensitive and specific index than FENa in differentiating between prerenal ARF and ATN, especially if diuretics have been used.

Urine Neutrophil gelatinase-associated lipocalin (NGAL) levels are increased in children with ischemic ATN after cardiac surgery; further studies necessary to clarify role in diagnosis.

Imaging
- ▣ 1. Ultrasound
  - ➤ Useful to evaluate the urinary collecting system, rule out urinary obstruction
- ▣ 2. Doppler scans, nuclear scans
  - ➤ Only useful to rule out vascular occlusion – otherwise, not useful
- ▣ 3. MRI
  - ➤ Gold standard for diagnosis of renal vein thrombosis; may also be useful to diagnose renal artery stenosis or occlusion

Renal Biopsy
- ▣ Should be considered in any patient with ARF in whom etiology is unknown, and whom treatment may be instituted (i.e., possible rapidly progressive glomerulonephritis)

DIFFERENTIAL DIAGNOSIS
- ▣ ARF or CRF?
  - ➤ Sometimes difficult to distinguish
  - ➤ Prior BUN, creatinine, urinalyses invaluable
  - ➤ Prolonged history of fatigue, anorexia, pruritus suggests chronic renal failure.

➤ Small, contracted kidneys on ultrasound indicate renal disease is chronic.
➤ If unsure, assume acute.
■ Etiology of ARF – Divide into prerenal, intrarenal, postrenal

Prerenal
■ Volume depletion
➤ Hemorrhage
➤ GI losses
➤ Renal losses (diuretics)
■ Decreased effective circulating volume with increased extracellular fluid volume (edematous disorders)
➤ Decreased cardiac function
➤ Systemic vasodilation
  • Sepsis
  • Liver failure
  • Anaphylaxis
■ Decreased renal perfusion
➤ NSAID (afferent artery constriction)
➤ Cyclosporine A
➤ ACE-I (efferent artery vasodilation)

Intrarenal
■ ATN
➤ Hypotension
➤ Nephrotoxic drug exposure, poisons
  • Aminoglycosides
  • Amphotericin B
  • Radiocontrast
  • Rhabdomyolysis (myoglobin)
  • Cisplatin
  • Pentamidine
  • Foscarnet
  • IVIG
  • Mannitol
  • Tenofovir
■ Interstitial nephritis
➤ NSAID
➤ Other drug exposure
■ Atheroembolic disease
■ Glomerulonephritis/microvascular disease

- Cast nephropathy
  - ➤ Multiple myeloma
  - ➤ Protease inhibitors
  - ➤ Acyclovir

Post Renal
- See chapter on obstruction
- History, physical, ultrasound, urine chemistries, urine sediment usually pinpoint cause

MANAGEMENT

What to Do First
Stabilize the patient; treat any life-threatening features.
- Thorough history, physical, chart review
  - ➤ 1. Are there reversible causes?
    - Rule out volume depletion
    - Consider central venous monitoring (CVP or Swan-Ganz catheter)
    - Consider trial of IV fluids
  - ➤ 2. Is there obstruction?
    - Renal ultrasound
  - ➤ 3. Urine sediment
  - ➤ 4. Stop all nephrotoxins
  - ➤ 5. Monitor drug levels if possible, and dose medications for reduced GFR

SPECIFIC THERAPY

Prevention
- Correct extracellular fluid volume deficits
- Avoid nephrotoxins (aminoglycosides, radiocontrast, NSAID), esp in high-risk patients
  - ➤ Prehydration with sodium bicarbonate therapy prior to radiocontrast may be better than saline, but more data are needed.
  - ➤ N-acetylcysteine (NAC) 600 mg po BID before and day of procedure is low cost and safe, and may help prevent contrast nephropathy.

Established ATN
Tight control of blood glucose reduces the need for dialysis.
- No specific therapy for established ATN
  - ➤ Renal dose dopamine, fenoldopam, diuretics, mannitol: No conclusive experimental evidence these agents are beneficial in patients with established ATN

Indications for Dialysis
- Life-threatening hyperkalemia
- Hypervolemia
- Metabolic acidosis unresponsive to conservative management
- Prevention of symptoms of uremia (Confusion, nausea/vomiting, pericardial rub), severe azotemia (BUN>120–130)

Type of dialysis
- Hemodialysis often used in hemodynamically stable patients
- Continuous therapies (eg, continuous venovenous hemofiltration) and peritoneal dialysis are used in selected cases.

FOLLOW-UP
- Usually necessary to hospitalize patient
- Assess volume status, need for dialysis daily

COMPLICATIONS AND PROGNOSIS

Complications
- Volume overload
  - ➤ Restrict Na+, water (<1.0 L/d) loop diuretics may be beneficial
  - ➤ Lasix 40 mg IV. If no response, use high dose or constant drip.
  - ➤ Complications of loop diuretics: ototoxicity
  - ➤ Dialysis if respiratory compromise and no response to diuretics
- Hyperkalemia: potentially life-threatening
  - ➤ Mild hyperkalemia (5.5–6.4)
    - Restrict dietary K+. Stop ACE inhibitors and K-sparing diuretics.
    - Kayexalate
  - ➤ Severe (>6.5), or symptomatic with EKG changes
    - Temporizing measures until dialysis initiated:
    - Sodium bicarbonate
      - Side effect: sodium load (volume overload)
    - Calcium gluconate IV
    - D50 and insulin
      - Side effect: hypoglycemia
- Metabolic acidosis
  - ➤ Most advocate maintaining pH >7.2, serum bicarbonate >12, but optimum pH not known.
  - ➤ Limit protein intake
  - ➤ Sodium bicarbonate po or IV
    - Complications: sodium load, volume overload
- Hypocalcemia
  - ➤ No treatment unless symptomatic

- Hyperphosphatemia
  - Phosphate binders (Calcium Carbonate, Calcium Acetate)
  - Dietary phosphate restriction

Prognosis
- Length of stay doubled if ARF present.
- Most who survive ARF recover renal function.
- *Mortality*
  - 7–23% non-ICU patients with ARF
  - 50–80% ICU patients with ARF
  - Major causes of death: infections, cardiovascular disease

---

ACUTE RESPIRATORY ACIDOSIS

F. JOHN GENNARI, MD

HISTORY & PHYSICAL
- Acute respiratory distress
- Nausea and vomiting, headache
- Confusion, restlessness
- Coma, seizures
- Abnormal findings on chest exam

TESTS

Laboratory
- Arterial blood gases are diagnostic – PCO2 >45 mmHg, pH usually <7.30 (see below for rule of thumb for [HCO3−])

Imaging
- Chest X-ray, CT of chest if necessary

DIFFERENTIAL DIAGNOSIS
- Conditions to distinguish from acute respiratory acidosis
  - Metabolic acidosis
  - Mixed disorders
  - Acute on chronic respiratory acidosis
  - Acute respiratory acidosis plus metabolic alkalosis
- Rule of Thumb:
  - Expected [HCO3−] in acute respiratory acidosis:
  - [HCO3−](expected) − 24 mEq/L + 0.1 × (PCO2 − 40, mmHg)

  Observed [HCO2−] should be within 4 mEq/L of the expected value in uncomplicated acute respiratory acidosis, almost always −30 mEq/L

■ Causes of Acute Respiratory Acidosis
➤ Airway obstruction – laryngospasm, bronchospasm (severe asthma), obstructive sleep apnea
➤ Circulatory catastrophes – cardiac arrest, severe pulmonary edema, massive pulmonary embolus
    Note: In severe circulatory failure or cardiac arrest, arterial blood may show a low PCO2 even though venous blood PCO2 is high (termed "pseudorespiratory alkalosis") due to preservation of ventilation in the face of a marked reduction in pulmonary perfusion. Should be treated as respiratory acidosis.
➤ CNS depression – anesthesia, sedatives, cerebral trauma
➤ Neuromuscular impairment – Guillain-Barré, myasthenic crisis, cervical cordotomy, drugs and toxins
➤ Ventilatory restriction – pneumothorax, flail chest, adult respiratory distress syndrome (ARDS)
➤ Iatrogenic mishaps – anesthesia equipment failures

MANAGEMENT
■ Reestablish airway.
■ Relieve bronchospasm.
■ Ensure adequate oxygen delivery.
■ Assisted ventilation as needed
■ Use bicarbonate only when other approaches fail to improve ventilation, as a temporizing measure to increase pH.

SPECIFIC THERAPY
n/a

FOLLOW-UP
■ Correct underlying cause.

COMPLICATIONS AND PROGNOSIS
■ Excellent if cause can be corrected, otherwise poor with limited survival, death, if process not rapidly reversed

ACUTE RESPIRATORY ALKALOSIS

F. JOHN GENNARI, MD

HISTORY & PHYSICAL
■ Air hunger
■ Numbness (circumoral), tingling in extremities

■ Lightheadedness, confusion
■ May be asymptomatic
■ Respiratory rate and/or depth of inspiration increased by definition, but not always detected on exam

TESTS

Laboratory
■ Arterial blood gases are diagnostic – PCO2 <35 mmHg, pH >7.50 (see below for rule of thumb for [HCO3−])

DIFFERENTIAL DIAGNOSIS
■ Conditions to distinguish from Acute Respiratory Alkalosis
  ➤ Metabolic acidosis
  ➤ Mixed disorders
    • Metabolic acidosis and respiratory alkalosis
    • Metabolic alkalosis and chronic respiratory alkalosis
■ Rule of Thumb
  ➤ Expected [HCO3−] in acute respiratory alkalosis:
  ➤ $[HCO3-](expected) = 24 \text{ mEq/L} - 0.2 \times (40 - PCO2, \text{mmHg})$
  Observed $[HCO_3^-]$ should be within 4 mEq/L of the expected value in uncomplicated acute respiratory alkalosis.
■ Causes of Acute Respiratory Alkalosis
  ➤ Hypoxemia
  ➤ Pneumonia
  ➤ Congestive heart failure
  ➤ Pulmonary embolism
  ➤ CNS disorders – infection, trauma
  ➤ Sepsis, particularly with gram negative organisms
  ➤ Anxiety-hyperventilation syndrome
  ➤ Drugs – salicylate intoxication

MANAGEMENT
■ Determine cause of hyperventilation – e.g., hypoxemia, pulmonary injury, metabolic acidosis, before intervening
■ Ensure adequate oxygen delivery

SPECIFIC THERAPY
■ For anxiety-hyperventilation syndrome, recirculating device to increase PCO2 (e.g., paper bag) should produce immediate relief from symptoms
  ➤ Side effects – if diagnosis incorrect can worsen hypoxemia or acidemia

■ Other causes – no specific treatment – use disorder as a sign to help identify underlying illness (e.g., gram-negative sepsis, pulmonary embolism

FOLLOW-UP
■ Counseling for anxiety-hyperventilation, other causes, appropriate follow-up as needed

COMPLICATIONS AND PROGNOSIS
■ Excellent if cause reversible

ACUTE RESPIRATORY FAILURE/MONITORING

THOMAS SHAUGHNESSY, MD

HISTORY & PHYSICAL
Risk Factors
■ Hypercapnea – Ventilation Failure
■ Hypoxia – Oxygenation Failure
■ Impaired consciousness -Airway compromise
■ Hypersecretion – Impaired secretion clearance
■ Cardiac – CHF, pulmonary edema
■ Pulmonary – Infection, Obstructive and/or Restrictive Disease
■ CNS – Stroke, Infection, Acute/Chronic Neuropathy, Encephalopathy
■ Inadequate Secretion Clearance – Malnutrition, CF, bronchitis

Signs and Symptoms
■ Tachypnea, tachycardia, dyspnea, diaphoresis, altered mental status, use of accessory muscles of respiration (SCM, diaphragm, intercostals)

TESTS
■ Acute Respiratory Failure is predominately diagnosed by clinical observations

Laboratory

Basic Studies
■ ABGs:
  ➢ Suggestive of impending resp failure:
    • pH: <7.25
    • PaO_2 <60
    • $PaCO_2$ above baseline with pH <7.30
■ Sustained Minute Ventilation >15 l/min, RR >30

Advanced Studies

- RR/TV >105 ("Tobin Index") – likely requires mechanical ventilation
- PaO_2 / FiO_2 <300 – Acute Lung Injury
- PaO_2 / FiO_2 <200 – ARDS

Other Tests

- ECG – signs of ischemia, MI
- CXR – Infiltrate, increased heart size, pulmonary edema, pneumothorax

DIFFERENTIAL DIAGNOSIS

- Agitation: Sepsis, "sundowning", cerebral vascular accident, drug toxicity, renal or hepatic encephalopathy, acute somatic pain.
- Cardiac: Pulmonary edema, CHF
- Pulmonary: Acute exacerbation of obstructive or restrictive disease, asthma, COPD, pneumonia.

MANAGEMENT

What to Do First

- Secure airway
  - ➤ If upper airway is obstructed – Chin lift/Jaw Thrust maneuver
  - ➤ Oral Nasal Airway, or Laryngeal Mask Airway
- Monitor oxygenation with pulse oximetry
- Treat airflow obstruction with albuterol MDI or nebulizer and IV steroids
- Endotracheal intubation if mental status altered
  - ➤ Institute respiratory support with bag-valve mask ventilation
- Serial ABGs with arterial catheter

General Measures

- Monitor in an intensive care setting
- Consider noninvasive ventilation with CPAP or BiPAP by nasal or facemask
- Consider mechanical ventilation with Assist Control, Intermittent Mandatory Ventilation or Pressure Support Ventilation
- Prompt resuscitation is essential to avoid end organ damage

SPECIFIC THERAPY

Indications for Treatment

- Institute therapy upon diagnosis while etiology is sought
- Treat hypoxic and hypercarbic failure with positive pressure assistance

- Treat airway compromise, impaired secretions, or persistent dyspnea with intubation and ventilation

Treatment Options
- Airway Maneuvers:
  - Relieve upper airway obstruction with chin lift and/or jaw thrust maneuvers
  - Consider oral or nasal airway
- Noninvasive mechanical ventilation:
  - A temporary bridge when resolution is expected in <24 hours
    - CPAP nasal or mask
      - Start at 5 cm H_2O
    - BiPAP Nasal or Mask
      - Start at 10 CM H_2O inspiration/5 cm H_2O expiration
- Endotracheal intubation and Ventilation:
  - Assist Control: Machine delivers preset tidal volume with each spontaneous or ventilator-initiated breath
  - Intermittent Mandatory Ventilation: Provides preset tidal volumes only on ventilator-initiated breaths
  - Pressure Support: Only spontaneous breaths are augmented
  - Initial ventilator settings:
    - FiO2 −1.0
    - Tidal Volume- 6–10 ml/kg
    - RR 10 −12
    - PEEP− 5 cm H_2O
    - Pressure Support − 5 cmH_2O

Side Effects and Complications
- Airway maneuvers: Inadequate relief of obstruction; clinical deterioration; regurgitation and aspiration of gastric contents
- Noninvasive mechanical ventilation:
  - Inadequate delivery of positive pressure support
    - Pressure leak around mask
    - Gastric insufflation with aspiration
  - Pressure necrosis of nose and mouth by continuous mask pressure
  - Inadequate enteral nutrition
  - Agitation requiring sedation
- Endotracheal Intubation:
  - Esophageal intubation
  - Failure to intubate trachea after paralysis
  - Mainstem bronchial intubation with intrapulmonary shunt

➤ Agitation requiring sedation
➤ Hypotension due to decreased venous return
➤ Regurgitation and aspiration of gastric contents
➤ Nosocomial pneumonia

Contraindications

Absolute
■ Airway Maneuvers – None
■ Noninvasive mechanical ventilation – severe agitation and poor cooperation
■ Endotracheal intubation – none

Relative
■ Airway Maneuvers - oral airway in conscious patient may induce emesis
  ➤ Consider cervical traction in the setting of unstable C-spine
■ Noninvasive ventilation – obesity, impaired consciousness, GE reflux, nasogastric nutrition
■ Endotracheal intubation – terminal prognosis with advance directives

FOLLOW-UP

During Treatment
■ Titrate pressure support levels in increments of 2–5 cm H_2O
■ Wean FiO_2 and Pressure support to keep SpO_2 >90% or PaO_2 >60 mmHg
■ Modify RR and TV to keep pH >7.30 and $PaCO_2$ ~40 mmHg

Routine
■ Serial CXRs to assess ETT placement
■ Sedation as needed with narcotics and benzodiazepines
■ Treat dyspnea or tachypnea with a trial of increased ventilation support
■ Resolution indicates fatigue; persistent symptoms suggest agitation
■ Address etiology of failure

COMPLICATIONS AND PROGNOSIS

Complications
■ Aspiration of gastric contents; chemical pneumonitis
■ Nosocomial pneumonia
■ Pneumothorax
■ Hypoxia: Encephalopathy, MI, ARDS, arrhythmia, cardiovascular collapse

■ Hypercarbia: Somnolence, narcosis, respiratory acidosis, myocardial depression

Prognosis
■ Depends on underlying cause
■ 1-year survival after acute respiratory failure 28–72%
■ Mortality from ARDS is 40–50%

ADENOCARCINOMA OF THE AMPULLA OF VATER

SUSAN A. CUMMINGS, MD

HISTORY & PHYSICAL
Risk Factors
■ slowly growing; high cure rate if resected; thus important to distinguish from cholangiocarcinoma and pancreatic cancer
■ adenoma of the ampulla
■ familial polyposis and Gardner's syndrome

Signs & Symptoms
■ same as cholangiocarcinoma with jaundice and pruritus
■ acholic stools
■ silver bullet stool (acholic stool and blood)
■ melena
■ cholangitis

TESTS
Routine Tests
■ high alkaline phosphatase and bilirubin
■ occasional iron deficiency anemia

Special Tests
■ Ultrasound and CT
  ➤ dilated intra and extrahepatic bile ducts
■ ERCP
  ➤ mass at ampulla; biopsy yield may be increased with sphincterotomy

DIFFERENTIAL DIAGNOSIS
■ pancreatic carcionoma
■ distal cholangiocarcinoma
■ duodenal carcinoma

MANAGEMENT

What to Do First
- establish diagnosis by ERCP with biopsy
- assess patient's ability to undergo attempted resection

General Measures
- support nutrition
- provide biliary drainage

SPECIFIC THERAPY
- Whipple resection for 75% of patients will lead to a 5 year survival up to 60% if marginsfree of tumor
- radiation and chemotherapy not very effective

FOLLOW-UP
- serial visits with physical examination, liver chemistries

COMPLICATIONS AND PROGNOSIS
- as high as 40% 5-yr survival, but combined 5-yr survival for all stages is ~10%.
- slowly growing compared to cholangiocarcinoma

ADENOVIRUS

CAROL A. GLASER, MD

HISTORY & PHYSICAL

History
- *DNA viruses; 51 distinct serotypes*
- Humans only host
- Types 31, 40, 41 causes of gastroenteritis (especially younger)
- Spread person-to-person, respiratory, fecal-oral and contaminated fomites
  - ➤ Epidemic keratoconjunctivitis: usual method of spread is by contaminated ophthalmic instruments + eye solutions, hand – to – eye contact, swimming pools
- Incubation period 4–12 days
  - ➤ Account for 2–5% total respiratory illness (higher% children) Epidemics of disease associated with- contaminated swimming pools, day care centers, hospitals, military recruits

Signs & Symptoms

■ *Spectrum of disease very broad—mostly associated with respiratory illness and gastroenteritis but cardiac neurologic, cutaneous, urinary and lymphatic manifestations also occur. Disease more severe in immunodeficient patients*

Respiratory:
■ Common cold – only rarely associated with cold.
■ *Acute febrile pharyngitis (types 1, 2, 3, 5, 6, 7) – mostly infants/young children*
■ with fever, exudative tonsillitis cervical adenopathy and sometimes dry hacking cough
■ Laryngotracheitis – occasionally
■ Acute respiratory disease – syndrome well described in military recruits
■ With fever, pharyngitis, non-productive cough, malaise, chills and headache
■ Pneumonia – most common in young children and military recruits
■ Atypical pneumonia – fever, sore throat, rhinorrhea and chest pain
■ Pertussis-like syndrome – most common in infants <36 months
■ Pharyngoconjunctival fever – fever, pharyngitis, conjunctivitis, malaise and cervical lymphadenopathy
■ Bronchiolitis obliterans

Eye:
■ Acute follicular conjunctivitis
  ➤ usually unilateral
  ➤ follicular lesions on conjunctival surface
  ➤ subconjunctival hemorrhages
■ Epidemic keratoconjunctivitis:
  ➤ highly contagious, more severe than follicular conjunctivitis
  ➤ corneal epithelial inflammation
  ➤ photophobia, lacrimation, discharge, hyperemia
  ➤ often pharyngitis, rhinitis and fever
  ➤ preauricular adenopathy
  ➤ outbreaks often due to types 8, 19, or 37
■ Gastrointestinal
  ➤ Acute gastroenteritis
  ➤ Types 40/41 most frequently involved
  ➤ Children and infants most frequently affected
  ➤ Complications; intussusception, acute mesenteric lymphadenitis, appendicitis

- Genitourinary tract
  - Acute hemorrhagic cystitis; sudden onset of gross hematuria, dysuria, urgency of urination, self limited (Types 11, 21)
  - Herpes-like genital lesions, may be associated with orchitis, cervicitis and/or urethritis
- Cardiovascular
  - Myocarditis/pericarditis

TESTS
- *Viral isolation from affected site – respiratory samples, eye swabs, urine, stool/rectal swab**
- *note that fecal shedding may occur for months after primary infection
  - Enteric adenovirus (40/41) cannot be isolated, antigen detection (EIA) available
  - Immunofluorescence (IF) assays useful for direct detection respiratory secretions or conjunctival swab
  - PCR available on experimental basis for affected site (e.g., spinal fluid from aseptic meningitis, respiratory secretions from pharyngitis, serum used for generalized infection)
  - Serologic studies are of limited utility for acute diagnosis, mostly useful for epidemiologic studies or retrospective diagnosis (EIA, CF used for diagnosis of adenovirus group, HI and neutralization tests are used for type-specific)

DIFFERENTIAL DIAGNOSIS
- *Adenoviruses are often impossible to distinguish clinically from other viral infection and even some bacterial infections, and specific diagnostics must be used when a specific diagnosis is warranted*
  - Respiratory: fever is often higher in adenoviral infections than parainfluenza and RSV, similar to influenza A/B, if high and prolonged fever must also distinguish from bacterial infection
  - Pharyngitis: distinguish from EBV, parainfluenza, influenza, enterovirus and strep
  - Pneumonia: adenovirus more likely bilateral than bacterial
  - Pertussis-like syndrome: clinically indistinguishable from Bordatella pertussis, must distinguish by culture (do viral and specific bacterial)
  - Gastrointestinal: clinically resemble other viral causes of diarrhea, need EIA for adenovirus

MANAGEMENT
- Supportive care
- Nosocomial spread in hospital and clinics (especially eye clinics) can be decreased by isolating infected patients, good handwashing, properly disinfecting instruments, equipment and surfaces.
- Healthcare personnel with adenoviral conjunctivitis should avoid patient contact.

SPECIFIC THERAPY
- No specific antiviral available. Benefit with cidofovir has been reported in a few cases of immunocompromised patients with severe disease.
- Supportive

FOLLOW-UP
n/a

COMPLICATIONS AND PROGNOSIS
Most complications listed above under specific type of illness
- Most self-limiting; occasional deaths, especially due to pneumonia
- Residual lung disease may be seen in some children after recovery from adenoviral pneumonia.
- Special hosts; in immunocompromised hosts adenovirus are often severe – disseminated disease in BMT patients, and involvement of the donor organ in solid organ transplant

Prevention
- Acute respiratory disease has been substantially reduced in the US by live adenovirus type 4 & 7 vaccine in military recruits.
- No vaccine widely available in community settings

ADRENAL INSUFFICIENCY

RICHARD I. DORIN, MD

HISTORY & PHYSICAL

History
- **Acute Adrenal Insufficiency (AI)**
  - Shock (resistant to pressor agents)
  - Tachycardia, high-output circulatory failure
  - Fever, confusion, nausea, vomiting
  - Abdominal, back, flank, or chest pain

- Retroperitoneal hemorrhage
- Anticoagulation, antiphospholipid syndrome, thromboembolic disease
- Sepsis (eg, meningococcus, pseudomonas), severe stress
- Postoperative (esp. cardiac surgery)
- Anemia, hyponatremia, hyperkalemia
- Pituitary apoplexy
- Acute headache, visual field deficit, 3–6 cranial neuropathies
- **Chronic AI:**
  - Weight loss, nausea/vomiting
  - TB, fungal infections, fever
  - Autoimmune disorders, HIV/AIDS, progestational agents
  - Past, recent, or current glucocorticoid administration
  - Cutaneous/buccal pigmentation, vitiligo
  - Salt craving, hypotension, orthostatic hypotension
  - Family history endocrine deficiencies
  - Electrolyte abnormalities
  - Enlarged or calcified adrenals
  - Coagulopathy, anticoagulants
  - Pituitary tumor, visual field abnormalities, galactorrhea
  - Infiltrative disorders (eg, hemochromatosis, amyloidosis, sarcoidosis)
  - Malignancy: cigarette smoking, weight loss, bone or abdominal pain

Signs & Symptoms
- Weight loss, decreased appetite, fatigue
- Salt craving
- Orthostatic dizziness
- Hyperpigmentation: cutaneous hyperpigmentation, buccal hyperpigmentation, calcified ears
- Decreased libido
- Hypotension, orthostatic hypotension
- Decreased axillary and pubic hair

TESTS

Laboratory
- Basic blood studies:
  - Hyponatremia, eosinophilia, lymphocytosis, hypercalcemia (mild)
  - Primary AI only: hyperkalemia, metabolic acidosis, azotemia
  - Low cortisol (<7 mcg/dL) with high ACTH (>50 pg/mL) at 8 AM in Primary AI

➤ Low cortisol (<7 mcg/dL) with low or normal ACTH (0–50 pg/ml) at 8 AM in secondary AI
■ Specific Diagnostic Tests
  ➤ Cosyntropin stimulation test: cortisol before, 30, 60 min after Cosyntropin (250 mcg) IM or IV; post-Cosyntropin cortisol <20 mcg/dL suggestive of AI, always abnormal in primary AI, good specificity but limited sensitivity in secondary AI
■ Other Tests
  ➤ Insulin tolerance test (gold standard for secondary AI): regular insulin 0.1U/kg IV, with plasma cortisol, glucose at 15, 30, 45 min, requires medical supervision, potentially dangerous in setting of seizure history, CV disease, elderly
  ➤ Metyrapone test (gold standard for secondary AI): 3 g metyrapone at midnight with 8 AM serum cortisol, 11-deoxycortisol, and plasma ACTH – rarely done, metyrapone may be difficult to obtain
  ➤ Anti-adrenal antibodies (antibodies directed against 21-hydroxylase in autoimmune primary AI)
  ➤ Anterior pituitary function tests (TSH, free T4, prolactin, IGF-1)

Imaging
■ CT or MRI of adrenals if indicated
■ MRI or CT of sella if indicated

DIFFERENTIAL DIAGNOSIS
■ Primary AI:
  ➤ Autoimmune
  ➤ Infectious: esp TB, fungal (esp. histoplasmosis), opportunistic (CMV adrenalitis, M intracellulare)
  ➤ Genetic (X-linked adrenoleukodystrophy)
  ➤ Congenital adrenal hyperplasia
  ➤ Adrenal hemorrhage
  ➤ Metastastic malignancy, lymphoma
  ➤ Infiltrative (amyloidosis, sarcoid)
  ➤ Drugs: suramin, ketoconazole, etomidate, aminoglutethimide, metyrapone, anticonvulsants (Dilantin, phenobarbital, rifampin)
■ Secondary AI:
  ➤ Pituitary tumor, apoplexy, irradiation, parasellar tumors
  ➤ Metastases to pituitary
  ➤ Autoimmune (lymphocytic hypophysitis)

➤ Infiltrative
➤ Trauma (head injury)
➤ Exogenous/endogenous glucocorticoid excess, progestational agents (eg, medroxyprogesterone), following successful surgical cure of endogenous Cushing's syndrome

MANAGEMENT

What to Do First
■ Acute AI:
  ➤ Give dexamethasone (Decadron) IV, can change to hydrocortisone after Cosyntropin testing is complete; note that DEX does not cross-react in the assay for cortisol
  ➤ Normal saline for volume expansion
  ➤ Do Cosyntropin stimulation test simultaneously with dexamethasone
  ➤ Search for precipitating factors: infection
■ Chronic AI:
  ➤ Establish diagnosis, cause

General Measures
■ Distinguish clinical syndromes of chronic vs. acute AI
■ Assess for a priori evidence of primary vs. secondary AI
■ Assess level of physiologic stress: cortisol requirements increase 10-fold with severe stress (e.g., ICU illness)
■ Medical alert bracelet, patient education

SPECIFIC THERAPY
■ Acute AI: hydrocortisone (= cortisol)
■ Chronic AI: hydrocortisone (= cortisol), higher doses required during stress; fludrocortisone PRN in primary AI

Side Effects & Contraindications
■ Cortisol:
  ➤ Side effects: weight gain, Cushingoid features, metabolic alkalosis, osteoporosis
  ➤ Contraindications: none
■ Fludrocortisone
  ➤ Side effects: hypokalemia, edema, hypertension
  ➤ Contraindications: hypokalemia, hypertension

FOLLOW-UP
■ Assess clinical response, weight, skin pigmentation
■ Follow blood pressure, orthostatic vital signs, serum electrolytes

- Establish etiology of AI, treat associated conditions
- Educate patient to increase hydrocortisone during minor/major illnesses, clinical alert bracelet
- Plasma ACTH may remain elevated despite appropriate replacement therapy

COMPLICATIONS AND PROGNOSIS
- Adrenal crisis: development of acute AI when unable to take oral medications or in setting of superimposed illness
- Cortisol excess: weight gain, Cushingoid features, metabolic syndrome
- Mineralocorticoid excess; edema, hypertension, hypokalemia
- With appropriate adrenocortical hormone replacement, lifespan similar to healthy population

---

ADRENAL TUMORS

RICHARD I. DORIN, MD

HISTORY & PHYSICAL

History
- Abdominal mass
- TB or fungal infection
- Review of prior CT and MRI reports (note: most chest CT studies include imaging of the adrenals)
- Adrenal "incidentaloma"
- History of malignancy, site and cell type of prior tumors
- Multiple endocrine neoplasia syndrome (MEN I and MEN II) and related family history
- Abdominal/flank pain
- Menstrual history, skin and hair changes
- Hypertension, edema
- Weight gain, muscle weakness, polyuria
- Electrolyte abnormalities (esp. hypokalemia)
- Family history of adrenal tumors
- Osteoporosis, loss of height, bone fracture
- Medications: diuretics, glucocorticoids, oral contraceptives, progestational agents
- Cigarette smoking
- Fluid/electrolyte loss: vomiting, diarrhea

Signs & Symptoms

- Glucocorticoid excess: weight gain, central obesity, moon facies, purple striae, proximal muscle weakness, osteoporosis, menstrual irregularities, hypogonadism, hypertension, diabetes mellitus
- Mineralocorticoid excess: hypokalemia (spontaneous or easily provoked), muscle cramps, muscle weakness, nocturia, polyuria, hypertension, edema
- Androgen excess: hirsutism, menstrual irregularities, infertility, acne, male pattern balding, breast atrophy
- Catecholamine excess: hypertension, paroxysms, headache, tachycardia, increased sweating, orthostatic hypotension, constipation, abdominal/chest pain

Routine Laboratory Test Findings

- Glucocorticoid excess: hypokalemia, alkalosis, hyperglycemia
- Mineralocorticoid excess: hypokalemia, alkalosis, mild hypernatremia, anemia, hypomagnesemia
- Catecholamine excess: increased hematocrit; hyperglycemia

TESTS

Laboratory

- Cortisol excess (Cushing syndrome):
  - ➤ Basic:
    - 1.0 mg overnight dexamethasone suppression test
    - 24-h urine free cortisol (UFC)
- Confirmatory: 8 AM plasma ACTH level
- Mineralocorticoid excess:
  - ➤ Basic:
    - Plasma renin activity (PRA)
    - Serum aldosterone
    - Aldosterone/PRA ratio
  - ➤ Confirmatory:
    - 24-h urine aldosterone and cortisol
    - 18-OH corticosterone
    - Saline suppression test (serum aldosterone after 2L IV normal saline)
    - Supine (8 AM) and standing (noon) aldosterone, 18-OH corticosterone, and PRA
- Androgen excess:
  - ➤ Serum testosterone, DHEA-S, androstenedione, prolactin, LH, FSH

- Catecholamine excess:
  - ➤ Basic: 24-h urine for metanephrine, VMA, and free catecholamines
  - ➤ Confirmatory: plasma catecholamines, clonidine suppression test, chromagranin
- Adrenocortical carcinoma: 24-h urine 17-keto-steroids (17-KS), 24-h UFC

Imaging

- CT or MRI of abdomen
- MRI: adrenal adenomas, pheochromocytomas hypointense relative to liver on T2-weighted image; adrenal carcinomas hyperintense on T2 image
- Nuclear Medicine Studies
  - ➤ Fluorodeoxyglucose (FDG) positron emission tomography (PET)
  - ➤ Iodine-131-meta-iodobenzylguanidine (MIBG) for suspected pheochromocytomas
  - ➤ 19-[131I]iodocholesterol (NP59) scan: functional imaging of adrenocortical tissues (labeling compound may be difficult to obtain)

DIFFERENTIAL DIAGNOSIS

- Adrenocortical tumors:
  - ➤ Hypokalemia from GI losses, diuretic use
  - ➤ Cushingoid appearance from exogenous glucocorticoids
  - ➤ Cortisol excess in association with depression, stress, alcoholism (pseudo-Cushing syndrome)
  - ➤ Androgen excess from polycystic ovarian syndrome (PCOS), late-onset congenital adrenal hyperplasia (CAH), androgen ingestion, oral contraceptives, or progestational agents
- Adrenomedullary tumors: catecholamine excess from anxiety, panic attacks, illicit drugs/medication withdrawal, hypoglycemia, thyrotoxicosis
- Metastasis to adrenal
- Bilateral adrenal enlargement:
  - ➤ Endocrine: CAH, ACTH excess, hyperaldosteronism due to bilateral adrenal hyperplasia, Cushing syndrome due to bilateral micronodular or macronodular adrenocortical hyperplasia, Carney's syndrome
  - ➤ Infectious (TB and fungal) and infiltrative disorders (amyloidosis, hemachromatosis); usually associated with hypoadrenalism
  - ➤ Other adrenal tumors: myelolipoma uniformly benign

MANAGEMENT

General Measures
- Search for indication of primary malignancy
- Assess size of adrenal tumor
- Assessment of radiological features; irregular contour, inhomogeneity or necrosis, calcification, unenhanced CT with high attenuation value (>10 HU), local invasion raise suspicion for adrenocortical carcinoma
- Biochemical evaluation of incidentally discovered adrenal tumors: many functioning tumors clinically silent

What to Do First
- Exclude pheochromocytoma
- Cushingoid features: assess for cortisol excess
- Hypertension, hypokalemia, alkalosis: assess for mineralocorticoid/cortisol excess
- Hirsutism, menstrual irregularities: assess for androgen excess
- CT/MRI of abdomen: if <4 cm and 24-h urine 17-KS normal, not primary adrenocortical carcinoma
- Diagnostic biopsy of the adrenal can distinguish primary vs. metastatic lesion, but not benign from malignant adrenocortical neoplasm

SPECIFIC THERAPY
- Cortisol excess: cortisol synthesis inhibitors (ketoconazole, metyrapone, aminoglutethimide)
- Mineralocorticoid excess: mineralocorticoid receptor antagonist (eg, spironolactone) or potassium-sparing diuretic (eg, amiloride, triamterene)
- Androgen excess: enzymatic inhibitors (eg, ketoconazole) or receptor antagonists (eg, spironolactone)
- Pheochromocytoma: alpha-, then beta-adrenergic receptor blockade, catecholamine synthesis inhibitors (eg, alpha-methyl tyrosine)
- Adrenocortical carcinoma: medical management of cortisol excess, surgical resection, radiation, adrenolytic therapy with mitotane
- Surgery indicated:
  - ➤ Pheochromocytoma
  - ➤ Unilateral functional adrenocortical adenoma
  - ➤ Tumor >4 cm
  - ➤ Enlarging tumor, suspicious radiological features
  - ➤ Elevated urinary 17-KS
  - ➤ Not indicated for hyperaldosteronism from bilateral hyperplasia

FOLLOW-UP
- Nonfunctioning adrenal adenoma <4 cm: repeat CT in 3 and 12 mo, then less frequently if radiographically stable
- Functioning adenoma, medical therapy:
  - Electrolytes, PRA, and aldosterone levels for hyperaldosteronism
  - Electrolytes, clinical manifestations, 24-h UFC, and plasma ACTH for Cushing syndrome
- Adrenocortical carcinoma: 17-KS, other hormone levels if functional, and serial CT or MRI scans
- Postoperative:
- Suppression of the hypothalamic-pituitary-adrenal axis requiring glucocorticoid replacement therapy for up to 1 y after resection of cortisol-producing adenoma
- Transient hyponatremia and hyperkalemia may follow cure of aldosteronoma; increased dietary sodium and mineralocorticoid replacement

COMPLICATIONS AND PROGNOSIS
- Benign adrenocortical adenoma: surgery curative
- Adrenocortical carcinoma: poor long-term prognosis; micrometastases common at diagnosis; median survival with surgery, 14–36 mo

---

ADULT OPTIC NEUROPATHIES

BARRETT KATZ, MD, MBA

HISTORY & PHYSICAL
Optic atrophy is a generic term: proxy statement for histologic integrity of neural tissue remaining – AXONS of retinal ganglion cells

Any process that affects blood supply to, supporting glia of, or axons themselves can unfold into

Atrophy
Clinically, must differentiate
- whether the process is bilateral or unilateral
- the nerve head is swollen
- whether atrophy is actually present

Inflammation of the nerve may be demyelinative, immune-related, infective, idiopathic, due to inflammation of contiguous structures (i.e., sinuses, brain, meninges), infiltration (i.e., sarcoid) or shared response with retina (i.e., neuro-retinitis).

Onset of visual symptoms:

- Acute
  - over minutes and hours
  - Ischemic
  - Inflammatory
  - Traumatic
- Sub-acute
  - over a few days
- Chronic
  - over weeks and months
  - Compressive
  - Heredofamilial and Degenerative
  - Indolent inflammation Toxic/nutritional
  - Infiltration of the nerve

Systemic history of import:

- Headache – R/O Temporal Arteritis
- Weight loss- R/O Temporal Arteritis
- Obesity – R/O raised ICP
- Jaw claudication- R/O Temporal Arteritis
- Temporal tenderness- R/O Temporal Arteritis
- Systemic malignancy – metastatic process can cause compression; paraneoplastic syndromes can cause visual loss
- Diabetes – can produce diabetic papillopathy
- Hypertension – associated with AION

Systemic medications that affect optic nerve

- Isoniazid
- Ethambutol
- Hydroxyquinolones
- Chloramphenicol
- D-Penicillamine
- 5-Fluorouracil
- Hexachlorophene
- Cyclosporine

Systemic medications associated with papillederma and raised intracranial pressure:

- Steroids
- Vitamin A
- Heavy metals
- Tetracyclines
- CO_2 retention – chronic lung disease
- Uremia

Nutritional associations to look for
- Tobacco usage
- Alcoholism
- Folate deficiency
- Vitamin B12 deficiency
- Toxins that affect optic nerve
- Methyl alcohol Toluene
- Cisplatin
- BCNU
- Interferon alpha

Signs & Symptoms
- Perception of whiteness of the disc (our best parameter for atrophy) is influenced by disc's cup size – the larger the cup size, the more "white" the disc appears
- Ophthalmoscopic features of disc change
  - Is the disc swollen? – if so must rule out papilledema (disc swelling from raised intracranial pressure) – a medical emergency
  - Are venous pulsations present spontaneously? if so, intracranial pressure < 200 mm H20 and swollen disc is not likely papilled-erna
  - Is there a pressure related optic neuropathy – anything to suggest glaucoma?
    - Glaucoma is the most prevalent optic neuropathy of adults
    - Glaucomatous optic atrophy is characterized by
  - undermining of neuroretinal rim
    - vertical bias to cup configuration
      - asymmetry of disc excavation
- Decreased vision
- Decreased color perception
- Dimness of vision
  - Constriction of peripheral field
    - Trouble with tasks requiring fine steropsis
- Trouble with reading – can be declaration of homonymous hemi-anopia
- Pain on eye movement – characteristic of optic neuritis
  - Transient obscurations of vision – sudden visual loss with valsalva maneuver – characteristic of the swollen disc
- Loss of central vision
- Loss of color vision
- Constriction of visual field

- Asymmetry of pupillary function – a Marcus-Gunn pupil (relative afferent pupillary defect) indicates asymmetry between eyes of functioning axons which subserve afferent limb of pupillary reflex; speaks to unilateral involvement of one optic nerve, or asymmetric involvement of both optic nerves; its presence is NEVER normal

TESTS
- Ophthalmologic consultation for determination of intraocular contribution to process
- Snellen acuity measured with best refraction
- Bedside acuity determination done with pinhole viewing
- Measure color vision
- Measure intraocular pressure
- Formal automated perimetry to characterize visual field change and narrow differential diagnosis

Laboratory
Work-up is driven by working diagnosis
- ESR and C – reactive protein to look for temporal arteritis
- Temporal artery biopsy if clinical suspicion for temporal arteritis
- Measurement of opening pressure on LP for raised ICP (after neuro-imaging to rule out mass)
- CSF analysis to look for more widespread CNS process
- CSF immunoglobulins to look for markers of multiple sclerosis
- FTA-ABS and RPR to screen for syphilis
- B 12 and Folate levels to screen for hematologic etiology
- Toxicology screen to look for endogenous poisons
- Thyroid function tests to screen for dysthyroid contribution to optic neuropathy

Imaging
- MR scan of head and orbits – MR better than CT for fine detail, imaging myelin
- CT scan of head and orbits – CT better for imaging calcifications
- MR angiography – look for vascular cause and associated findings

Ancillary Ophthalmologic Testing
- Visual Evoked Response (VER) - may help in recognizing subtle optic nerve dysfunction, and characterizing defect as demyelinative, if major (P 100) waveform is delayed
- ERG, EOG, Dark adaptation – useful in defining retinal contribution to process

DIFFERENTIAL DIAGNOSIS

- Congenital anomaly of nerve mistaken for atrophy or inflammation – nerve hypoplasia, pits, crescents, colobomas (fusion defects), optic disc drusen
  - ➤ Heredofamilial Optic Atrophies- recessive, dominant, complicated, mitochondrial (Leber's),
    - neurodegenerative

Swollen disc can be caused by:

- Congenital anomaly:
  - ➤ due to ocular disease (hypotony, uveitis)
  - ➤ inflammatory (papillitis, retrobulbar neuritis)
  - ➤ infiltrative (leukemic, sarcoidosis)
  - ➤ from systemic process (anemia, Grave's Dz)
  - ➤ optic nerve tumor (glioma, meningioma)
  - ➤ vascular (non-arteritic AION, arteritic AION, temporal arteritis)
  - ➤ orbital tumor (hemangioma, glioma)
  - ➤ papilledema – due to raised intracranial pressure
- Inflammatory Optic Neuropathies-Multiple Sclerosis, immune-related, infections
- Ischemic Optic Neuropathies-ischemic optic neuropathy, giant cell arteritis, diabetic papillopathy
- Glaucomatous Optic Neuropathies – chronic open angle glaucoma
- Neoplasms and related issues – disc infiltration, optic gliomas, perioptic meningiomas, secondary
- neoplasms to anterior visual pathways
- Nutritional Optic Neuropathies – vitamin deficiencies, tobacco-alcohol amblyopia
- Toxic Optic Neuropathies-drugs, toxins, misc. exposures
- Traumatic Optic Neuropathies – direct, indirect, to orbit, head and from radiation

MANAGEMENT

What to Do First

- decide if disc is swollen – may need ophthalmologic consultation
- decide if raised intracranial pressure is a consideration, and if so deal with emergently
- decide if temporal arteritis is consideration – if so, must address emergently, treat with systemic steroids (to protect the non-involved eye) as you plan temporal artery biopsy
- decide if patient is a vasculopath and treat other systemic risk factors for vascular compromise

General Measures
- if ICP is elevated, must be lowered
- if intraocular pressure is elevated, must be lowered
- if intraocular inflammation is detected, must be addressed directly and with anti-inflammatories let the eye docs decide
- if temporal arteritis is suspected, pt must be begun on steroids, either high dose PO, at least 80–100 mgm Prednisone daily until results of temporal artery bx back
- if Optic Neuritis, results of Optic Neuritis Treatment Trial showed no role for PO steroids, but IV steroids administered in hospital 250 mgm methylprednisolone QID for 3 days, following by 11 days of tapering oral prednisone had no effect on eventual visual outcome of eye, but served to decrease likelihood of another neurological event within the ensuing 2 years, and so decreased risk of patient's meeting clinical criterion for Multiple Sclerosis
- if Optic Neuritis is confirmed, CHAMPS study suggests patient may benefit from long term interferon therapy to further decrease risks of future neurologic events.

SPECIFIC THERAPY
n/a

FOLLOW-UP
n/a

COMPLICATIONS AND PROGNOSIS
- Once optic atrophy ensues, treatment does not bring back dead axons, rather, treatment would only serve to protect damaged and functioning neural tissue
- Often, treatment is directed at protecting the axons that remain, protecting the other (non-involved) eye, or decreasing likelihood of a further neurologic/ophthalmolgic event in the future
- Nonetheless, aggressive treatment is often indicated
- Cannot judge visual rehabilitative potential by amount of optic atrophy present – a totally pale and white disc may be able to generate 20/20 vision
- Even vision of "hand motion" is much preferred to "no light perception" by the patient, so do not give up too early
- Many toxic processes are reversible or partially reversible, once offending agent is discontinued

AGE RELATED MACULOPATHY

SAAD SHAIKH, MD and MARK S. BLUMENKRANZ, MD

HISTORY & PHYSICAL

History

- Elements of history recommended at initial visit:
  - Symptoms
  - Medications
  - Medical and ocular history
  - Family & social history
  - Risk Factors
    - genetic predisposition in AMD appropriate environmental influences
    - Cardiovascular disease, specifically hypertension
    - Smoking history
    - Caucasian ethnicity
    - Older age (6.4% of persons aged between 65 and 74 years, and 19.7% of persons 75 and over had evidence of AMD in one or both eyes)
- Physical Examination
  - Assessment of best corrected visual acuity
  - Vision testing with an Amsler grid
  - Refererral to an ophthalmologist for:
    - biomicroscopic examination of the macula
    - peripheral retinal examination
    - evaluation of treatment options

Signs & Symptoms

- Early ARM
  - The presence of drusen alone may not give rise to symptoms
- Later ARM
  - Distortion, decrease in visual acuity, or scotomas are common symptoms of choroidal neovascularization or secondary hemorrhage, or as scarring or geographic atrophy occur.

TESTS

- Comprehensive eye examinations every one to two years in patients more than 65 years of age who do not have conditions requiring intervention. Daily at home Amsler's grid usage for detecting the progression of age-related macular degeneration

- patient is given a copy of the grid and is instructed to focus one eye on the center dot in the grid from a distance of 35 cm (112 in) with the other eye covered; the procedure is then repeated for evaluation of the other eye.
- patient is instructed to call the physician if line distortions or scotomas are detected.
- Biomicroscopic (Funduscopic) Examination (Classification of ARMD or more specifically ARM (Age Related Maculopathy) as defined by the International ARM Epidemiological Study)
- Early ARM
  - presence of drusen and retinal pigmented epithelium (RPE) pigmentary abnormalities (hypopigmentation and hyperpigmentation).
- Late ARM
  - includes geographic atrophy and exudative disease (detachment of the retinal pigment epithelium or choroidal neovascularization)
- Types of Choroidal Neovascular Membranes (CNVM)
  - Classic (well-defined) or occult (poorly defined)
  - Extrafoveal, Juxtafoveal, or Subfoveal

Fluorescein Angiography
- used to confirm diagnosis and to help determine whether a patient has the atrophic or exudative form of the disease in order to dictate management

DIFFERENTIAL DIAGNOSIS
- Drusen
  - diseases with retinal flecks simulating drusen include Stargardt's disease and fundus albipunctatus
- Geographic Atrophy/Pigmentary Changes
  - can also be caused by Central serous chorioretinopathy, ocular toxoplasmosis, retinal detachment, North Carolina Macular Dystrophy, Central Areolar Dystrophy, & others.
- Choroidal Neovascularization – other causes of CNVMs include ocular histoplamosis, myopic fundus changes, idiopathic choroidal neovascularization, polypoidal choroidopathy, endogenous posterior uveitis syndromes, and others.

MANAGEMENT
- All patients with vision loss should be referred to an ophthalmologist; those with acute loss of vision should be referred urgently.

- Diagnosis of Age Related Maculopathy is established by funduscopic examination and fluorescein angiography
- Treatment dictated by type of disease: early or late, and by subtype of choroidal neovascularization

SPECIFIC THERAPY
- Early AMD
  - Observation
- Later AMD
  - Geographic atrophy (of the RPE)
  - Observation
- Choroidal neovascularization & related complications (i.e. hemorrhage, RPE detachment)
- "classic" juxtafoveal and extrafoveal CNV
  - conventional laser photocoagulation
- subfoveal and/or occult CNV
  - photodynamic therapy
    - whereby a photosensitive dye is injected into a peripheral vein and activated with laser light
    - once it reaches the neovascular complex, reactive free radicals are produced that selectively occluding the leaking new vessels
- Side effects/complications of laser photocoagulation.
  - Loss of visual acuity acutely with the understanding that in the long term more is preserved
  - Epiretinal membrane formation
- Investigational Approaches
  - Subretinal Surgery
  - Macular Translocation
  - Radiation Treatment
  - Pharmacologic Therapies

FOLLOW-UP
- based on extent of AMD and treatment
- The follow-up history should take into account the following:
  - Symptoms
  - Changes in medication
  - Changes in medical and ocular history
  - Changes in family history & social history
- The follow up examination visit should include the following.
  - Assessment of best corrected visual acuity
  - Vision testing with an Amsler's grid
  - Biomicroscopic examination of macula

- Follow-Up Guidelines
  - Early AMD and Geographic Atrophy
    - Complete ophthalmic examination every 6–24 months if no symptoms, varies on other coexistent ocular morbidities
    - Daily monitoring of monocular vision by patient using Amsler's grid.
  - Late AMD with Exudative Findings after Laser or Photodynamic Therapy
    - Visits at 2 to 4, 4 to 6, 6 to 12 weeks, and 3 to 6 months
    - Thereafter, every 6 months for exam (fluorescein angiography optional)
    - Treated patients who report new symptoms may need to be re-examined before their next scheduled follow-up visit.
    - Consider retreatment at each visit for reoccurrence of exudative disease

COMPLICATIONS AND PROGNOSIS

- Complications of progressive exudative disease
  - Exudative RPE and retinal detachment
  - Vitreous hemorrhage
  - RPE tear
  - Disciform scar formation
- Prognosis
  - recurrence rate of approximately 50% after conventional laser treatment of classic lesions
  - reopening by 4–12 months common after photodynamic therapy of subfoveal lesions requiring repeat treatment
  - photocoagulation and photodynamic therapy delay severe visual loss rather than represent a permanent cure in most of cases

AIR EMBOLUS

RAJABRATA SARKAR, MD

HISTORY & PHYSICAL

History

- Most common during operative procedures involving major veins or cardiopulmonary bypass
- Penetrating trauma to chest (air from lung)
- Insertion or removal of large bore venous lines

- Carbon dioxide embolus from laparoscopic insufflation
- Can occur with right to left shunt (VSD, etc.)
- Source of air usually massive

Signs & Symptoms
- Cardiovascular collapse
- Failure to respond to usual resuscitation

TESTS

Specific Tests
- EKG may show ischemic changes with coronary air embolus
- If intraoperative TEE is in use, intracardiac air will be seen

DIFFERENTIAL DIAGNOSIS
- Pulmonary embolism
  - ➤ Usually in ward patient with DVT
  - ➤ Rarely occurs intraoperatively
- Stroke
  - ➤ Intraoperative embolic stroke rarely causes cardiovascular collapse
- Myocardial Infarction
  - ➤ Severe ischemia seen on EKG
- Traumatic cardiac tamponade
  - ➤ Echocardiogram or surgical exploration
- Tension pneumothorax
  - ➤ Hyperresonant breath sounds
  - ➤ Diagnose + treat with needle thoracostomy

MANAGEMENT

What to Do First
- Position patient head down, left side down
  - ➤ Keeps air in apex of right ventricle where slow reabsorption occurs
- Cardiorespiratory support
  - ➤ Intubation + mechanical ventilation
  - ➤ 100% FiO2 to help reabsorption (creates nitrogen gradient)
  - ➤ Volume + pressors as needed
- Find and correct source of air embolism
  - ➤ Close hole in vein
  - ➤ Flush all lines
  - ➤ Check bypass machine and connections

General Measures
- Avoid air embolism
  - Backbleed or aspirate all venous lines during insertion
  - Flush or vent any potential air sources prior to unclamping
  - Check and tap all bypass lines prior to instituting flow

SPECIFIC THERAPY
- If venous lines are in RA or RV, aspirate out the air
- If chest is open, aspirate RV apex with needle after positioning
- If chest is open, cardiac massage to relieve RV outflow obstruction

FOLLOW-UP
- Treat survivors as status-post myocardial infarction

COMPLICATIONS AND PROGNOSIS

Complications
- Myocardial Infarction
  - Secondary to air embolus entering coronary artery
- Anoxic brain injury
  - Secondary to prolonged cerebral hypoperfusion

Prognosis
- If patient presents with cardiovascular collapse, most do not survive
- If air is noticed during embolization (i.e. line placement) and aspirated, prognosis is good
- Air embolism in trauma (penetrating lung injury) is usually lethal

---

ALCOHOL ABUSE, DEPENDENCE, AND WITHDRAWAL

JOSE R. MALDONADO, MD

HISTORY & PHYSICAL

History
- Lifetime prevalence of alcohol abuse or dependence 14%
- Family history increases risk of alcoholism 4–5 fold
- Metabolism:
- 90–98% via hepatic oxidation
- Slow rate (10 mL/h or 1.0 oz liquor/1.5 h)
- CNS depressant effects proportional to blood concentration

Signs & Symptoms
- Alcohol intoxication:
  - ➤ Depends on absolute blood levels, rate & duration of consumption, & tolerance of individual
    - In nonhabituated individuals, blood alcohol levels of & cause:
    - 30 mg/100 mL: mild euphoria
    - 50 mg/100 mL: mild coordination problems
    - 100 mg/100 mL: ataxia
    - 200 mg/100 mL: confusion & decreased consciousness
    - 400 mg/100 mL: anesthesia, coma, & death
- Blackouts:
  - ➤ Transient episodes of amnesia associated to acute intoxication
  - ➤ Dense anterograde amnesia for events & behaviors during intoxication
  - ➤ Occur late in course of alcoholism
  - ➤ Directly correlated w/ severity & duration of alcoholism
- Alcohol withdrawal syndromes:
  - ➤ Syndromes emerges after period of relative or absolute abstinence from alcohol
  - ➤ May occur during period of continuous alcohol consumption
- Early withdrawal:
  - ➤ Onset: first day, peaking 24–48 h after abstinence
  - ➤ Uncomplicated: tremulousness, general irritability, nausea & vomiting
    - Associated w/ eye openers in order to calm nerves
    - Usually subside in 5–7 d
    - Irritability & insomnia may persist >10 d
    - Complicating symptoms may last for 10–14 d:
      - Nausea
      - Vomiting
      - Tension
      - General malaise
      - Autonomic hyperactivity
      - Tachycardia
      - Insomnia
- Alcohol hallucinosis:
  - ➤ Onset: first day, peaking 72 h after abstinence
  - ➤ Usually auditory or visual hallucinations
  - ➤ Sensorium clear & vital signs stable

- Alcohol withdrawal seizures:
  - Generalized motor seizures occurring w/ no underlying seizure disorder
  - Onset: first day, peak 12–48 h after cessation
  - Associated w/ hypomagnesemia, respiratory alkalosis, hypoglycemia, & increased intracellular sodium
  - Its presence has important prognostic value in predicting a complicated withdrawal period: 1/3 of patients go on to develop DTs
- Alcohol withdrawal delirium:
  - Also known as delirium tremens (DTs)
  - Onset 1–3 d after abstinence, peak on 4–5th d
    - Mortality rate:
      - 1% treated
      - 15% untreated
  - Confusion, disorientation, clouded consciousness, perceptual disturbances, agitation, insomnia, fever, autonomic hyperactivity
  - Terror, agitation, & visual hallucinations can occur
  - In 50% of cases, delirious states may alternate w/ lucid intervals
  - Uncomplicated course: symptoms subside after 3 d of full-blown DTs
- Minor symptoms may last as long as 4–5 wk
- When complicated by medical conditions, mortality rate increases to 20%
- Causes of death: infections, cardiac arrhythmias, fluid & electrolyte abnormalities, hyperpyrexia, poor hydration, hypertension, or suicide

TESTS
- CAGE inventory:
  - Have you ever felt the need to CUT DOWN on drinking?
  - Have you ever felt ANNOYED by criticisms of drinking?
  - Have you ever had GUILT about drinking?
  - Have you ever taken a morning EYE OPENER?
  - A score of 2 or higher indicates possible alcohol problem (eg, alcoholism)

DIFFERENTIAL DIAGNOSIS
- Intoxication: abuse of any CNS depressant
- Withdrawal: withdrawal of selected CNS depressants, incl benzodiazepines & barbiturates

MANAGEMENT
Alcohol intoxication

Supportive Measures
- Time-limited phenomenon
- Stop alcohol ingestion
- Provide protective environment
- No methods for accelerating alcohol removal or elimination
- In potentially fatal cases, hemodialysis can be used

Alcohol Withdrawal Syndromes
Supportive Measures
- Abstinence from alcohol
- Rest
- Adequate nutrition
- Restrain combative/agitated pts
- Monitor & correct: fluid balance, electrolytes, & vital signs frequently

SPECIFIC THERAPY
- Adequate hydration: avoid overhydration
- Vitamin supplementation:
  - Thiamine IM/PO daily
  - Folate PO daily
  - Multivitamins
  - B complex vitamin daily
  - Vitamin K for bleeding disorder
- Sedation:
  - Benzodiazepines: gold standard treatment for alcohol withdrawal
  - Benefits:
    - Excellent cross-coverage w/ all CNS depressants
    - Effective in ALL facets & degrees of alcohol withdrawal
      - Low mortality rate, minimal complication rate
  - Long-acting agents (long T1/2), allow for self-taper
  - In severe hepatic damage (& elderly), use lorazepam or oxazepam, primarily metabolized by conjugation
- Alcohol withdrawal – diazepam loading protocol:
  - Mild withdrawal: diazepam 20 mg PO q 1h ×3
  - Moderate/severe withdrawal:
    - Diazepam 5–10 mg IV q 5–10 min
    - Repeat doses until sedation has been achieved

- Average required doses range between 30–160 mg
- For mild re-emergence of withdrawal symptoms or severe insomnia, use small diazepam for 1–2 wk (e.g., Valium 10–20 mg PO q HS)

FOLLOW-UP
■ Long-term involvement in recovery program

COMPLICATIONS AND PROGNOSIS
■ Medical syndromes:
  ➤ Nutritional & vitamin deficiencies (ie, Korsakoff psychosis)
  ➤ Gastritis
  ➤ Respiratory suppression
  ➤ Cardiomyopathy
  ➤ CHF
  ➤ Fatty liver
  ➤ Hepatic cirrhosis
  ➤ Impotence
  ➤ Gynecomastia
■ Neurologic syndromes:
  ➤ Acute alcohol intoxication
  ➤ Alcoholic dementia
  ➤ Wernicke encephalopathy

ALCOHOLIC LIVER DISEASE (ALD)

RAMSEY C. CHEUNG, MD

HISTORY & PHYSICAL

History
■ Alcohol consumption & duration: threshold for ALD = 40 g/d for men, 10–20 g/d for women (10–12 g alcohol: 1.0 oz spirit, 12 oz beer, 4 oz wine)
■ CAGE questionnaire for screening (2 or more suggests alcohol dependence):
  ➤ CUTTING DOWN on drinking
  ➤ ANNOYANCE at others' concern about drinking
  ➤ Feeling GUILTY about drinking
  ➤ Using alcohol as an EYE OPENER

- History of trauma, DUI, withdrawal seizure, pancreatitis
- Family history of alcoholism
- Spectrum of ALD: fatty liver (usually asymptomatic); alcoholic hepatitis (usually symptomatic as described below); alcoholic cirrhosis (compensated or decompensated)

Signs & Symptoms
- Fatigue, malaise, anorexia, fever, RUQ pain & tenderness, encephalopathy, GI bleeding, ascites, jaundice
- Telangiectasia, palmar erythema, Dupuytren contracture, gynecomastia & testicular atrophy (in men), hepatomegaly, splenomegaly, asterixis, fetor hepaticus

TESTS
Basic Blood Studies
- AST>ALT (both usually <300 IU/L; AST/ALT > 2)
- Elevated alkaline phosphatase, elevated GGT, elevated uric acid
- Elevated WBC, increased MCV
- Chemistry panel (elevated glucose, elevated triglyceride, decreased K+, decreased phosphorus, decreased Mg++)

Specific Diagnostic Tests
- Blood alcohol level
- Rule out other liver diseases, eg, anti-HCV antibody, iron studies

Imaging
- Abdominal US or CT: not diagnostic:
  - Rule out other hepatic lesions
  - Cirrhosis & collaterals w/ advanced disease

Liver Biopsy
- Confirm diagnosis if atypical features
- Determine prognosis by staging
- Determine relative contribution of concomitant hepatitis (eg, HCV)
- Differentiate hepatic siderosis from hemochromatosis

DIFFERENTIAL DIAGNOSIS
- Nonalcoholic steatohepatitis (NASH)
- Chronic hepatitis C alone or coexisting w/ ALD (25–65%)

- Hereditary hemochromatosis
- Acetaminophen toxicity w/ alcohol consumption

MANAGEMENT

What to Do First

- Establish diagnosis & assess severity of liver disease, rule out infection
- Determine risk of alcohol withdrawal
- Delirium tremens: temperature, tremor, tachycardia

General Measures

- Adjust or avoid potentially hepatotoxic medications
- Correct electrolyte abnormality & dehydration
- Correct nutritional deficiencies
- Thiamine, folate, pyridoxine, vitamin K (if PT prolonged)
- Benzodiazepines for acute alcohol withdrawal
- Diagnostic paracentesis in pts w/ ascites & abdominal pain

SPECIFIC THERAPY

- Corticosteroids for selected pts w/ severe alcoholic hepatitis:
  - ➤ Prednisolone or methylprednisolone for 4 wk followed by taper & discontinuation over 2–4 wk
  - ➤ Indications: severe alcoholic hepatitis w/ discriminant function [4.6 × (PT in seconds minus control) + bilirubin in mg/dL] >32 &/or hepatic encephalopathy
  - ➤ Contraindications:
    - Absolute: mild alcoholic hepatitis w/ discriminant function <32 & absence of hepatic encephalopathy
    - Relative: corticosteroid use either dangerous or benefit not proven in pts w/ active infection, renal failure, pancreatitis, active GI bleeding
- Liver transplantation:
  - ➤ Indication: cirrhosis w/ Child-Turcotte-Pugh score 7 or more, or evidence of decompensation, & minimum of 6 mo of sobriety
  - ➤ Contraindication: active alcohol use or other contraindication for liver transplant
- Nutritional supplementation:
  - ➤ Enteric feeding before PPN or TPN; multivitamins & minerals
  - ➤ Indication: protein calorie malnutrition &/or to maintain positive nitrogen balance
  - ➤ Side effects & contraindications: severe hepatic encephalopathy

- Abstinence from alcohol:
  - ➤ Counseling, alcohol rehabilitation, &/or naltrexone
  - ➤ Indication: reduce risk of relapse, improve long-term prognosis
- Naltrexone:
  - ➤ Side effects: opiate withdrawal, nausea, vomiting, abdominal cramps, anxiety, headache, insomnia, nervousness, arthralgia
  - ➤ Contraindications: w/ caution in pts w/ hepatic or renal impairment, liver failure, opiate use

FOLLOW-UP

During Treatment

- Monitor for alcohol withdrawal, infection, GI bleed, renal insufficiency, glucose intolerance, side effects of therapy, progression of liver disease
- LFT, CBC, PT, electrolytes regularly

Routine

- Alpha-fetoprotein & abdominal US q 6–12 mo in alcoholic cirrhosis (survival benefit of screening still uncertain)

COMPLICATIONS AND PROGNOSIS

Complications

- Steatosis: 90–100% of all heavy drinkers, reversible w/ abstinence
- Steatohepatitis: 10–35% of heavy drinkers:
- 10–20%/y progress to cirrhosis, 24–68% w/ continued alcohol abuse
- Not completely reversible, can progress despite abstinence
- Cirrhosis: 8–20% of heavy drinkers, more than 8X increased risk w/ chronic HCV infection, = 10–20%/y of alcoholic hepatitis progress to cirrhosis
- HCC: increased risk w/ HCV coinfection

Prognosis

- Average survival of ALD: 80% 1 y, 50% 5 y
- Continued alcohol consumption (single most important risk factor for progression of liver disease)
- Severe alcoholic hepatitis: >50% mortality during hospitalization (corticosteroids reduce mortality risk ~25%)
- 4–5 y survival rate:
- Fatty liver alone: 70–80%
- Alcoholic hepatitis or cirrhosis w/o hepatitis: 50–75%
- Cirrhosis w/ hepatitis: 30–50%
- Cirrhosis: 40–48% if continued alcohol use, 60–77% if stopped

ALLERGIC RHINITIS

PAMELA DAFFERN, MD

HISTORY & PHYSICAL

History

- Personal or family history of atopic dermatitis, allergic rhinitis, or asthma (~15% of population)
- Seasonal symptoms, especially while outdoors during pollen season, usually due to plant pollens or molds
- Perennial symptoms, often worse upon arising, usually due to dust mites or other insect allergens, molds, animal allergens, or occupational exposure

Signs & Symptoms

- Acute: nasocular itching, tearing, rhinorrhea, repetitive sneezing, nasal blockage
- Chronic: postnasal drainage & congestion
- Ocular signs include conjunctival injection, chemosis, "allergic shiners"
- External nasal crease indicative of nasal itching ("allergic salute")
- Nasal exam reveals pale, boggy nasal mucosa w/ clear secretions, enlarged turbinates, narrowed nasal airway
- Chronic mouth breathing may lead to high-arched palate & micrognathia

TESTS

- CBC may reveal peripheral eosinphilia
- Nasal smear reveals metachromatic cells & eosinophils, useful for distinguishing allergic from other forms of rhinitis
- Identify specific IgE antibodies to suspected allergens by skin testing or in vitro (RAST) tests. These are helpful when they corroborate the history of exposure.

DIFFERENTIAL DIAGNOSIS

- Infectious rhinitis: viral or bacterial
- Vasomotor rhinitis: nonspecific triggers (cold air, odors)
- Nasal polyps
- Rhinitis medicamentosa: OTC decongestants or cocaine
- Hormonal rhinitis: thyroid disorders, menopausal
- Wegener's granulomatosis

MANAGEMENT

What to Do First

- Assess exposures & assess for any complicating conditions (asthma or acute sinusitis)

General Measures

- Avoidance of known allergens
  - ➤ Stay indoors when pollen counts are highest (usually early AM & windy conditions)
  - ➤ Encase mattress & pillow for dust mite allergy
  - ➤ Remove or limit contact w/ pet
  - ➤ Identify & remove sources of mold exposure
  - ➤ Occupation? Some jobs are high risk.

SPECIFIC THERAPY

Treatment Options

- Nonsedating antihistamines
  - ➤ Cetirizine
  - ➤ Fexofenadine
  - ➤ Loratidine
- Pseudoephedrine as needed for nasal congestion
- Intranasal corticosteroids
  - ➤ Budesonide
  - ➤ Fluticasone
  - ➤ Mometasone

Topical Nasal Antihistamines

- Azelastine
- Topical antihistamine/vasoconstrictor for ocular symptoms: cromolyn sodium
  - ➤ Nedocromil
  - ➤ Levocobastine
  - ➤ Olopatadine

Immunotherapy

- Should be reserved for pts w/ severe symptoms unresponsive to pharmacotherapy

Side Effects & Contraindications

- Cetirizine may cause sedation & fatigue in a minority of pts
- Epistaxis may result from intranasal corticosteroids
- Pseudoephedrine may cause nervousness, insomnia, blood
- pressure elevations

FOLLOW-UP

During Treatment
- Assess response to therapy & review/reinforce avoidance measures w/in 1 month of initial visit

Routine
- Review symptoms & response to meds during pollen season & at least yearly thereafter

COMPLICATIONS & PROGNOSIS

Complications
- Sinusitis: common. Treatment: mucolytic agents, decongestants, saline lavage; amoxicillin ± clavulanate for 3-wk course for refractory cases
- Asthma: Assess w/ office spirometry & treat w/ inhaled beta-agonist & inhaled or systemic steroids as warranted
- Otitis media: Amoxicillin ± clavulanate for 10-day course
- Snoring/sleep disruption/apnea: during pollen season in 10–30% of pts. Treat underlying inflammation; add decongestants
- Nasal polyps: obstructive symptoms. May require polypectomy if unresponsive to prednisone

Prognosis
- About 80% of pts improve w/ avoidance measures & medical therapy
- Complications generally improve w/ treatment of allergic rhinitis
- Nasal polyps recur in 40% of pts after polypectomy
- Pts not responding to medical management & avoidance measures may benefit from immunotherapy.
- Indications include:
  - Severe & prolonged seasonal or perennial allergic rhinitis
  - Symptoms unresponsive to meds
  - Intolerance of or inability to take meds
  - Unavoidable allergens
    - Contraindications to immunotherapy
  - Severe or poorly controlled asthma
  - Compromised lung function
  - Poorly controlled hypertension
  - Coronary artery disease
  - Use of beta-blockers (topical or systemic)

ALOPECIA

JILL S. WAIBEL, MD and MICHAEL J. WHITE, MD

HISTORY & PHYSICAL

History

■ Onset sudden vs gradual
■ Childhood vs. adult
  ➤ Infantile may be congenital, even with normal-appearing hair at birth.
■ Recent physical or emotional stress (e.g., pregnancy, illness)
■ Exposure history (e.g., medication, chemicals, radiation)
■ History of a systemic disease or high fever (e.g., lupus, STDs)
■ Family history of hair loss

Signs & Symptoms

■ Pattern of hair loss:
  ➤ Generalized vs. Localized
    • Generalized: diffuse or global hair loss affecting hair throughout scalp in a uniform pattern
    • Localized: focal or patchy hair loss, most or all hair missing from involved area
    • If patchy, what is the pattern?
  ➤ Scarring vs. nonscarring – although traditionally used for classification, it is often difficult to assess – late nonscarring may be indistinguishable from scarring
■ Inflammatory vs. non-inflammatory
■ Hair density: normal or decreased
■ Presence of follicular plugging
■ Presence of other dermatologic disease on the scalp or elsewhere

TESTS

Basic Test

■ Hair pluck vs. light hair pull
  ➤ Light hair pull: ~20 hairs grasped between thumb and forefinger and gently pulled
    • Normal result: < 2 telogen (club) hairs per light pull; more hairs = telogen shedding
    • Most useful in early hair loss in central scalp; less useful in hair loss of long duration

> Hair pluck: forceful grasping and extraction of hair, intentionally removing both anagen and telogen hair and then determining ratio; test is uncomfortable and error-prone

Specific Diagnostic Tests
- Hormone studies
  > Female pattern alopecia: consider: DHEA-S, testosterone, testosterone-estradiol-binding globulin (TeBG), prolactin
- Metabolic studies
  > TSH, Hct, Hgb, Fe,%Saturation, total Fe-binding capacity, ferritin
- Fungal tests
  > Potassium hydroxide preparation (Chlorazol Black-E, other special forms available)
  > Fungal culture – often limited by poor collection methods, false negatives common

Other Tests as Appropriate
- Scalp (punch) biopsy for patients with inflammatory lesions

DIFFERENTIAL DIAGNOSIS
Generalized Hair Loss
TELOGEN EFFLUVIUM: sudden stressor causes ~30% of hair follicles to enter resting (telogen) stage (normal = 10%); about 3 months later club hairs are actively shed as new hair growth begins. Full recovery is expected.
- **Systemic**
- Acute illness
- Systemic lupus erythematosus, AIDS trichopathy
- Physical stress: surgery; trauma, acute blood loss
- Hypo/hyperthyroidism – lateral eyebrow hair loss seen in hypothyroidism
- Childbirth
- Significant psychological stress (chronic or acute)
- **Environmental**
- Crash diets with inadequate protein
- Drugs – Coumarins, Heparin, propanolol, Vitamin A, multiple other drugs associated

ANAGEN EFFLUVIUM – abrupt loss of normally growing (anagen) hair; Up to 90% of scalp follicles may be in anagen phase, extensive hair loss may result. Usually occurs 1–4 weeks after the insult.
- Cancer chemotherapeutic agents
- Poisoning – Thallium (rat poison), Arsenic
- Radiation therapy

Generalized Patchy
- Secondary syphilis, "moth-eaten appearance;" usually with a scaly scalp

ALOPECIA TOTALIS (total scalp)/UNIVERSALIS (total body) – more severe forms of alopecia areata. Usually preceded by localized alopecia areata. Spontaneous remissions and recurrences are the hallmark of limited alopecia areata. Recovery in alopecia totalis/universalis is unusual.

Localized Hair Loss
Nonscarring (follicles not destroyed)
- Androgenetic alopecia in men (male-pattern baldness) – genetic, frontotemporal recession. Loss then occurs on vertex, then density decreases over top of the scalp.
- Androgenetic in women (female-pattern baldness) – central scalp regression with retention of frontotemporal hairline
- Alopecia areata – localized hair loss in limited area, usual onset in young adults and children. Often short broken hairs toward the periphery of the lesion; noninflamed skin.
- Seborrheic dermatitis

Scarring
- Lichen planus
- Pustular follicular scarring alopecias
  - ➤ Dissecting cellulitis
  - ➤ Acne keloidalis nuchae
  - ➤ Folliculitis decalvans
- Follicular degeneration syndrome
- Localized Scleroderma (en coup de sabre)
- Discoid lupus erythematosus – discrete bald patches showing follicular plugging, erythema, atrophy, scale
- Sarcoidosis
- Amyloidosis

Infection
- Fungal
- Bacterial

Neoplasm
- Metastatic carcinoma
- Lymphomas
- Non-melanoma skin cancer – Basal cell carcinoma or squamous cell carcinoma

Physical/Environmental
- Injury – burns, chemical hair treatments
  - More common in African-Americans with hair relaxers
- Traction alopecia – chronic tension on hair with various hairstyles (corn rows, ponytails)
- Trichotillomania-repeated manual extraction of hair; often frontoparietal region of the scalp or occipital

MANAGEMENT
- Treat underlying cause of hair loss – medical, infectious, psychosocial.
- Consider referral to dermatologist.
- Scarring is irreversible – the follicle is gone.

SPECIFIC THERAPY
- Androgenic alopecia
  - Topical minoxidil can be applied twice daily.
  - Propecia – effective for men, limited data for use in women
  - Wigs
  - Surgical procedures include hair transplants, scalp reduction and flaps.
- Alopecia areata
  - No curative treatment available; some cases resolve spontaneously
  - Corticosteroids
    - Topical – class 1 or 2 strength – penetration of Rx is the limiting factor
    - Intralesional injection of triamcinolone acetonide
    - Systemic corticosteroids should be avoided
      - pulsed methylprednisolone has been used
  - Refer to a dermatologist for anthralin, PUVA, squaric acid, dyphencyprone, or cyclosporin
  - Hair weaves and wigs
- Tinea capitis/Kerion – see Tinea chapter

FOLLOW-UP
- Dependent on underlying cause or management modality

COMPLICATIONS AND PROGNOSIS
- Dependent upon the disease/condition

ALPHA-1-ANTITRYPSIN

ERIC LEONG, MD, FRCPC

HISTORY & PHYSICAL

Symptoms and Signs
- Neonates: jaundice at 1–2 months of age; hepatomegaly
- Infants: may present with symptoms and signs of chronic liver failure; fewer patients present with acute liver failure; a few present with cholestasis
- Children & adolescents: may present with liver failure
- Adults: may present with symptoms and signs of chronic hepatitis, cirrhosis, portal hypertension, HCC, or emphysema

TESTS

Basic Tests: Blood
- Liver biochemistry: ALT, AST, and GGT elevated in half of infants with homozygous deficiency & in up to 10% of young adults
- Serum alpha-1-AT concentration: often low; can be misleading due to elevation in setting of inflammation

Specific Diagnostic Test
- Serum alpha-1-AT phenotype: PiMM phenotype present in 90–95% of population associated with normal serum alpha-1-AT level; PiZZ phenotype associated with severe alpha-1-AT deficiency and potential development of pulmonary emphysema or liver disease; PiMZ and PiSZ associated with intermediate deficiency

Imaging
- Abdominal sonogram or CT scan: nondiagnostic
- Chest roentgenogram: emphysematous changes

Liver Biopsy
- Accumulation of eosinophilic, periodic acid-Schiff-positive, diastase-resistant globules in endoplasmic reticulum of periportal hepatocytes

DIFFERENTIAL DIAGNOSIS
- Viral hepatitis, biliary atresia in neonates & infants, cystic fibrosis, autoimmune hepatitis, Wilson's disease, Gaucher's disease, glycogen storage diseases

MANAGEMENT

What to Do First
- Evaluate severity of liver and lung disease and complications

General Measures
- Adjust or avoid potentially hepatotoxic drugs
- Discourage smoking to slow progression of lung disease
- Assess status of liver and lung disease
- Check serum alpha-1-AT concentration & phenotype

SPECIFIC THERAPY
- Liver transplantation: treats progressive hepatic dysfunction; should perform before pulmonary disease precludes surgery

FOLLOW-UP

Routine
- Liver biochemistry, INR, CBC every 6–12 months
- Chest roentgenogram & pulmonary function test yearly in patients with evidence of lung disease

COMPLICATIONS AND PROGNOSIS
- Cirrhosis: treat as per liver failure due to other causes
- HCC: can screen with serum AFP and ultrasound every 6 months
- Emphysema: avoidance of smoking most important; can consider alpha-1-antitrypsin replacement therapy and/or lung transplantation for severe lung disease

Prognosis
- 90% 1-year and 80% 5-year survival rates among children after liver transplantation

ALZHEIMER'S DISEASE

CHAD CHRISTINE, MD

HISTORY & PHYSICAL
- Acquired, generalized impairment of cognitive function
- Slowly progressive disorder (typically over years)
- Rare hereditary forms
- Not assoc w/ alteration of level of consciousness
- May be personality changes
- Immediate recall intact, but delayed recall & recent memory impaired

- Parietal lobe dysfunction (pictorial construction, calculations, right left discrimination, performance of complex motor tasks)
- Frontal lobe dysfunction (judgment, social skills, grasp reflexes)

TESTS

Lab Tests
- Diagnosis made clinically
- Serum & CSF studies normal
- Apoliprotein E e4 allele is a risk factor
- Brain imaging may show atrophy

DIFFERENTIAL DIAGNOSIS
- Degenerative disorders: Pick's disease, Creutzfeldt-Jacob disease, normal-pressure hydrocephalus, dementia w/ Lewy bodies, corticobasal ganglionic degeration, progressive supranuclear palsy excluded clinically

Systemic Disorders
- Cancer: primary or metastatic excluded by neuroimaging & CSF cytology
- Infection: serology studies differentiate AIDS dementia & neurosyphilis
- Metabolic disorders: blood studies differentiate hypothyroidism, vitamin B12 deficiency, hepatic & renal failure
- Vascular disorders: brain imaging excludes chronic subdural hematoma & multi-infarct dementia
- Head trauma: severe open or closed head injury
- Behavioral disorders: history & neuropsychological testing exclude pseudodementia

MANAGEMENT
- Reduce or stop meds that may exacerbate cognitive problems
- Follow Mini-Mental Status Examination

SPECIFIC THERAPY
- Indication: cognitive loss
- Cholinesterase inhibitors: mild improvement in cognitive function in early Alzheimer's
  - Donepezil
  - Galantamine
  - Rivastigmine
    - Memantine

FOLLOW-UP
N/A

COMPLICATIONS AND PROGNOSIS
- Early diagnosis allows for planning
- Advanced stage of dementia may require nursing facility
- Prognosis: disease is chronic & progressive

AMAUROSIS FUGAX

MICHAEL J. AMINOFF, MD, DSc

HISTORY & PHYSICAL
- Sudden onset of painless monocular blindness
- Clears within 30 min (usually 1–5 min)
- May be history of TIAs, especially contralateral limb weakness
- Microemboli may be present in retinal vessels
- May be evidence of peripheral vascular disease
- May be carotid bruit or cardiac source of emboli

TESTS
- Basic: CBC, differential count, ESR, PT, PTT, FBS, lipid profile, RPR, electrolytes; consider also SPEP, fibrinogen, proteins C & S, ANA, antiphospholipid antibody, antithrombin III, factor V Leiden
- Chest x-ray
- Cranial MRI; cranial & cervical MRA (may show evidence of diffuse or localized vascular disease); carotid duplex ultrasonography may reveal localized disease
- Cardiac studies: ECG, echo

DIFFERENTIAL DIAGNOSIS
- Other causes of transient monocular visual loss include papilledema, refractive error, episodic hypotension, migraine, vasculitis, poly-cythemia, coagulopathy; exclude them by history, physical exam or tests as above

MANAGEMENT
- Aspirin (optimal dose not established)
- Ticlopidine
- For cardiogenic embolism, initiate anticoagulant treatment w/ hep-arin & introduce warfarin (to INR 2–3)

SPECIFIC THERAPY

- Carotid endarterectomy for ipsilateral localized stenotic lesion (70% or more)
- Treat or control cardiac arrhythmia or continue warfarin
- General measures: stop cigarette smoking, treat underlying medical disorders (polycythemia, hypertension, diabetes, hyperlipidemia)

FOLLOW-UP

- As necessary to control anticoagulants for disturbance of cardiac rhythm
- Every 3 months to ensure no further TIAs or episodes of amaurosis fugax

COMPLICATIONS AND PROGNOSIS

- Stroke may occur w/o treatment; see "Transient Ischemic Attacks"

AMBLYOPIA

CREIG S. HOYT, MD

HISTORY & PHYSICAL

History

- Loss of visual acuity:
  - ➤ More profound when snellen isotypes read in series equaling crowding phenomenon
  - ➤ More profound in recognition acuity than spatial frequency tests
  - ➤ More profound in reducing background luminance or w/ neutral-density filter in front of involved eye

Signs & Symptoms

- Afferent pupil may be positive in 1/4 to 1/3 of cases

TESTS

Color Vision

- Normal w/ usual clinical suspects

Electrophysiologic

- ECG normal
- VEP (pattern) normal or ? amplitude

Screening
- Form deprivation: evaluate red light reflex form in both pupils <6 mo of age
- Strabismic: examine eye alignment by light reflex or cover test in first few years of life
- Anisometropic: visual acuity testing in preschool years

DIFFERENTIAL DIAGNOSIS
- Monocular:
  - Form deprivation: eg, congenital monocular cataract
  - Strabismic: eg, esotrope w/ fixation; preference for 1 eye
  - Anisometropic: eg, high myopia in 1 eye
- Binocular:
  - Form deprivation: eg, congenital binocular cataracts
  - Ametropic: eg, high hyperopia in both eyes
- Sensitive period for each type (when vision can be recovered toward normal):
  - Monocular:
    - Form deprivation: <6 mo
    - Strabismic: <6 y
    - Anisometropic: <8–9 y
  - Binocular:
    - Form deprivation: <6 mo
    - Ametropic: <8–9 y

MANAGEMENT
- Reverse unequal inputs:
  - Form deprivation: remove cataract
  - Strabismic: realign eyes w/ glasses, contacts, eye drops, surgery
  - Anisometropic: correct refractive error w/ glasses or contacts
- Decrease visual input to nonamblyopic eye:
  - Patching: part- or full-time
  - Penalization for cycloplegic eyes: drop in fixing eye (pt must be hyperopic in fixing eye)
  - Black contact lens: must be removed daily

SPECIFIC THERAPY
n/a

FOLLOW-UP
- Monitor visual acuity in amblyopic eye until it returns to normal

COMPLICATIONS AND PROGNOSIS
n/a

AMEBIASIS

J. GORDON FRIERSON, MD

HISTORY & PHYSICAL

History

■ Exposure: ingestion of food or water contaminated by cysts of Entamoeba histolytica, direct fecal-oral contamination (seen in mental institutions and day care centers), oral-anal sexual practices. Insects may contaminate food. Entamoeba dispar is identical to E. histolytica in appearance but does not cause disease.

Signs & Symptoms

■ Intestinal amebiasis: gradual onset of diarrhea which varies from mild to severe, sometimes with blood and pus (dysentery), abdominal pain. Fever, weight loss, dehydration seen in severe cases. Perforation and stricture can occur. Ameboma is a proliferative response to the amebae, resulting in a mass effect in colon wall. Some patients have no symptoms.

■ Systemic amebiasis:
➤ a) hepatic: presents as liver abscess, with fever, weight loss, right upper quadrant pain. Course can be acute or chronic. Rupture can produce empyema, peritonitis, pericarditis.
➤ b) Pericardial amebiasis: usually due to rupture of liver abscess into pericardium. Presents as chest pain, dyspnea, tachycardia, pulsus paradoxicus, hypotension.
➤ c) Amebic brain abscess: acute illness resembling pyogenic abscess with headache, fever, neurologic signs indicating mass
➤ d) Cutaneous amebiasis: usually seen near anus or on genitals. Presents as painful skin ulcerations.

TESTS

■ Basic tests: blood: Intestinal disease: CBC may show anemia, sometimes elevated neutrophils.
➤ Systemic disease: CBC shows anemia, elevated WBC. LFTs altered, usually with elevated alkaline phosphatase and transaminases.

■ Basic tests: urine: not helpful

■ Specific tests: Intestinal disease: Stool examination for O&P demonstrates trophozoites and cysts. May need up to 3, rarely more, stools to show it. Less sensitive than Ag tests, cannot distinguish E. histolytica from E. dispar.

E. histolytica-specific antigen tests (fecal or serum) – ELISA, IF, or radioimmunoassay – very useful in diagnosis.

Serology – Abs to E. histolytica (not formed to E. dispar) usually in 1 week of acute infection and can last years; therefore less useful in patients from endemic areas

■ Systemic disease: Ultrasound or CT scan locates abscess. Serology, done as IHA or CIE, is positive in 95% of cases of liver abscess. For cutaneous disease, use biopsy. Stool O&P exam positive in about 50% of cases.

■ Other tests: Intestinal disease: serology, done as IHA, positive in 85%. PCR not widely available. Barium enema can suggest ulcerative disease, and will locate amebomas (which can resemble carcinoma). Sigmoidoscopy or colonoscopy with biopsy of ulcer (which is typically well demarcated with undermined edges) shows amebae.

➤ Systemic disease: Chest X-ray can show elevated right diaphragm and fluid in right chest.

DIFFERENTIAL DIAGNOSIS

■ Intestinal disease: Entamoeba dispar, which looks identical to E histolytica but is non-pathogen. Ulcerative colitis, Crohn's disease, infectious diarrheas, carcinoma of colon.

■ Systemic disease: Pyogenic liver abscess (main distinguishing feature is positive IHA test), tumors. Skin ulcers resemble pyoderma, tuberculosis, fungal disease.

MANAGEMENT

What to Do First

■ All forms: assess severity, correct fluid and electrolyte problems, transfuse if needed.

General Measures

■ Investigate others who may have shared contaminated items.

SPECIFIC THERAPY

Indications

■ All infected persons, even asymptomatic since they can spread the infection. When E. histolytica and E. dispar cannot be distinguished, probably best to treat as histolytica.

Treatment Options

- Intestinal disease:
  - ➤ asymptomatic (eliminate intraluminal cysts): paromomycin for 7 days or: Iodoquinol for 20 days or: diloxanide furoate for 10 days (obtainable only from the CDC)
  - ➤ mildly to moderately symptomatic disease: metronidazole for 7–10 days or tinadazole 3 days followed by one of the intestinal regimens above
  - ➤ severe dysentery or systemic disease: metronidazole for 10 days or tinadazole 3–5 days followed by one of the intestinal regimens. Large abscesses may require aspiration or surgical drainage, as does pericardial disease.

Side Effects & Complications

- Iodoquinol: occasional mild GI distress. Only about 1% is absorbed. Possible myelo-optic neuropathy in excessive doses. Avoid in those with iodine intolerance.
- Paromomycin: sometimes nausea, cramps, diarrhea. Only about 1% absorbed.
- Diloxanide furoate: flatulence, mild GI distress. Poorly absorbed.
- Metronidazole: dizziness, nausea, malaise, metallic taste in mouth, tingling in extremities, Antabuse-like reaction with alcohol

Tinadazole: GI distress, metallic taste, fatigue. Contraindicated in first trimester of pregnancy (C).

- Contraindications to treatment: absolute: allergy to drug
- Contraindications to treatment: relative: first trimester of pregnancy. In severe disease metronidazole can be used. Paromomycin is intestinal agent of choice, only after ulcerative disease controlled by metronidazole.

FOLLOW-UP

During Treatment

- Intestinal disease: in severe disease monitor fluids, watch for hemorrhage and perforation
- Systemic disease: hospital care until stable

Routine

- Intestinal: check stool O&P 4 weeks after end of chemotherapy. Retreat if needed.
- Systemic disease: follow liver abscess with ultrasound. Retest stools 4 weeks after therapy if positive originally or if not done.

COMPLICATIONS AND PROGNOSIS

- Intestinal disease: perforation, hemorrhage, stricture. Prognosis good with treatment.
- Systemic disease: rupture of liver abscess into peritoneum or pleuropericardial spaces. This requires surgical drainage (possibly needle drainage for pericardial rupture).

AMEBIC LIVER ABSCESS

AIJAZ AHMED, MD

HISTORY & PHYSICAL

History

- Prevalence <1% in industrialized countries; 50–80% in tropical areas
- Fecal-oral spread by poor sanitation, contamination of food by flies, unhygienic food handling, contaminated water, use of human feces as fertilizer
- High-risk groups: lower socioeconomic status, immigrants, travelers, male homosexuals & institutionalized populations
- Host factors predisposing to increased severity: age (children >adults), pregnancy, malignancy, malnutrition/alcoholism, corticosteroid use

Signs & Symptoms

- Fever, rigors, night sweats, nausea, anorexia, malaise, right-sided abdominal discomfort, weight loss, dry cough, pleuritic pain, shoulder pain, hiccups, tender hepatomegaly, dull right lung base (raised hemidiaphragm), pleural rub, right basilar crackles
- Amebic colitis in 10%, past diarrhea/dysentery in 20%, & 50% w/ parasite in stool

TESTS

Laboratory

- Leukocytosis, anemia, – serum alkaline phosphatase, – AST/ALT, – ESR
- Serologic tests:
- Indirect hemagglutination assay (IHA) 90–100% sensitive; combination of immunofluorescent antibody test (IFAT) & cellulose acetate precipitin test (CAP) 100% sensitive; IHA positive for 2 y after therapy

& IFAT for 6 mo; CAP can be negative as early as 1 wk after start of treatment
- Aspiration of abscess: yellow/brown (anchovy), odorless fluid; aspirate only if diagnosis uncertain or rupture imminent

Imaging
- US/CT: round/oval, mostly single (sometimes multiple); hypoechoeic/low density compared to normal liver
- CXR: right hemidiaphragm w/ blunted costophrenic angle, atelectasis

DIFFERENTIAL DIAGNOSIS
- Pyogenic abscess, hydatid cyst

MANAGEMENT
What to Do First
- Obtain history (incl geographic), physical exam, imaging
- Imaging confirms diagnosis of cyst or abscess

General Measures
- Suspected amebic abscess: start therapy while awaiting serologic confirmation
- Aspirate if diagnosis unclear, rupture imminent, or pt critically ill

SPECIFIC THERAPY
Treatment options
- Metronidazole for 5–10 d (alternative options tinidazole or chloroquine), followed by luminal amebicides: diloxanide furoate for 10 d or diiodohydroxyquin for 20 d
- Surgical drainage: ruptured abscess

FOLLOW-UP
- Clinical: resolution of fever & pain
- Imaging: abscess shrinkage

COMPLICATIONS AND PROGNOSIS
Complications
- Rupture of abscess into chest, pericardium, or peritoneum
- Secondary infection (usually after aspiration)
- High risk for complications: age >40, corticosteroid use, multiple abscesses, abscess w/ diameter >10 cm

Prognosis
- Excellent prognosis w/ prompt diagnosis in absence of complications
- Delay in diagnosis can result in rupture & higher mortality: 20% mortality w/ rupture into chest or peritoneum; 30–100% w/ rupture into pericardium

---

AMYLOIDOSIS

KEITH STOCKERL-GOLDSTEIN, MD

HISTORY & PHYSICAL
multiple etiologies-associated with deposition of insoluble protein in organs

    primary amyloidosis (AL) – plasma cell dyscrasia; amyloid: immunoglobulin light chains

    secondary amyloidosis (AA) – chronic infections or inflammation; amyloid A protein

    familial amyloidosis (ATTR) – mutation in transthyretin

    beta2-microglobulin amyloid (B2M) – in renal dialysis

History
- chronic dialysis (B2M)
- family history – family history of amyloidosis or progressive neuropathy suggests ATTR
- chronic inflammatory processes: Crohn's, RA, juvenile RA, ankylosing spondylitis, familial Mediterranean fever (FMF)
- chronic infections including tuberculosis, osteomyelitis, bronchiectasis, IV drug use

Signs & Symptoms
- variable depending on type of amyloid and organ involvement
- renal: proteinuria (AL and AA)
- cardiac: heart failure, conduction abnormalities, low voltage on EKG, orthostatic hypotension; rare in AA
- GI: macroglossia, hepatomegaly, splenomegaly
- neurologic: carpal tunnel syndrome, peripheral neuropathies and autonomic insufficiency
- integument: periorbital purpura, easy bruising, arthropathies
- less commonly: GI bleeding, diarrhea malabsorption, bleeding diathesis, endocrine abnormalities

TESTS

Basic Blood Tests:
- low protein and albumin
- elevated cholesterol/triglyceride
- hyperbilirubinemia

Basic Urine Tests:
- proteinuria

Specific Diagnostic Tests
- Serum/urine electrophoresis/immunoelectrophoresis (AL)
- 24 hour urine protein > 0.5 g/d in >70% patients with AL or AA amyloid
- Imaging:
  - echocardiography: cardiomegaly, diastolic abnormalities, increased wall thickness, restrictive cardiomyopathy
  - "speckled" pattern with increased echo signal
- Radiographs: bone lesions in myeloma
- CT: hepatomegaly, splenomegaly

Other Tests
- Biopsy: tissue required for diagnosis.
- biopsy site based on affected organs and suspected type
- Congo red-green birefringence under polarized light
- abdominal fat pad biopsy in systemic amyloidosis
- bone marrow biopsy
- rectal biopsy
- cardiac, renal, carpal tunnel, peripheral nerve biopsy may be required
- Protein/gene analysis: transthyretin mutations

DIFFERENTIAL DIAGNOSIS
- multiple myeloma should be distinguished from AL
- other plasma cell abnormalities can have similar findings without amyloid

MANAGEMENT

What to Do First
- assess specific organ involvement

General Measures
- manage heart failure

- ➤ calcium channel blockers, beta blockers and digoxin contraindicated in cardiac amyloidosis
- diuretics useful

SPECIFIC THERAPY
Primary Amyloidosis (AL)
- indicated for all patients with AL amyloid
- **Treatment Options**
- high-dose melphalan with autologous stem cell transplant
- melphalan-prednisone
- VAD (vincristine, doxorubicin, dexamethasone)
- thalidomide/dexamethasone
- **Side Effects & Contraindications**
- high-dose melphalan
  - ➤ side effects: mortality rate > 10%, myelosuppression, infectious complications, organ toxicity
  - ➤ contraindications: poor performance status, uncontrolled heart failure, active infections
- melphalan-prednisone
  - ➤ side effects: myelosuppression, myelodysplastic syndrome or acute leukemia
  - ➤ contraindications: poor performance status, active infections
- VAD
  - ➤ side effects: myelosuppression, cardiac toxicity
  - ➤ contraindications: poor performance status, active infections
  - ➤ relative contraindication: based upon cardiac function
- Thalidomide/dexamethasone
  - ➤ side effects: peripheral neuropathy, constipation, fatigue
  - ➤ relative contraindications: peripheral neuropathy

Follow-Up
During Treatment
- chemotherapy should be performed by hematologist/oncologist

Routine
- assessment of cardiac function, renal function, etc based on organ involvement and severity of disease

Complications & Prognosis
Complications
- progression of cardiac disease
- renal failure
- thrombotic events

Prognosis
- survival dependent on organ involvement
- survival less than 6 months from onset of heart failure
- prolongation of survival possible with autologous stem cell transplant

Secondary Amyloidosis (AA)
- **Treatment options**
- treat underlying inflammatory/infectious etiology.
- colchicine: for FMF and inflammatory conditions
- chlorambucil and cyclophosphamide
- **Side Effects & Contraindications**
- colchicine
  - ➤ side effects: GI toxicity, myelosuppression
  - ➤ contraindications: active infections
- cytotoxic drugs
  - ➤ side effects: myelosuppression, infectious complications
  - ➤ contraindications: active infections

Follow-up
During Treatment
- CBC q 2–3 weeks
Routine
- assessment of underlying condition as indicated

Complications & Prognosis
Complications
- progression of infectious or inflammatory condition
- renal failure
Prognosis
- dependent on cause of AA
- prevention of AA with FMF using colchicine

Familial Amyloidosis (ATTR)
- supportive care based on organ involvement and clinical symptoms
- **Treatment options**
- liver transplantation considered definitive therapy

Follow-Up
Routine
- assessment of underlying condition as indicated

Complications & Prognosis
Complications
- progression of disease except following transplantation

Prognosis
- dependent on mutation; survival typically 10–15 years
- improved survival following liver transplant

Beta-2 Microglobulin Amyloid (B2M)
- therapy indicated for all patients with B2M amyloid
- Treatment options
- renal transplantation

Follow-Up
Routine
- assessment of underlying condition as indicated

Complications & Prognosis
Complications
- progression of localized amyloid deposits likely to occur

Prognosis
- deposits regress following renal transplantation
- use of newer dialysis membranes may prevent/reverse this type of amyloidosis

FOLLOW-UP
n/a

COMPLICATIONS AND PROGNOSIS
n/a

AMYOTROPHIC LATERAL SCLEROSIS (ALS)

MICHAEL J. AMINOFF, MD, DSc

HISTORY & PHYSICAL
- Diffuse weakness, wasting, muscle "flickering"
  - ➤ Limb onset in 75%
  - ➤ Bulbar onset in 25%
- May be cramps & vague sensory complaints
- No sphincter disturbance
- Family history somctimes present

- Diffuse weakness, wasting & fasciculations of at least 3 limbs or 2 limbs & bulbar muscles
- Mixed upper & lower motor neuron deficit
- Babinski signs
- Bulbar palsy
- No sensory deficit

TESTS

- EMG: chronic denervation & reinnervation in at least 3 spinal regions (cervical, thoracic, lumbosacral) or 2 spinal regions & bulbar muscles
- NCS: motor conduction normal or slightly slow; no conduction block
- Sensory conduction normal
- CSF normal
- Muscle biopsy: signs of denervation

DIFFERENTIAL DIAGNOSIS

- Compressive lesion excluded by imaging studies
- Familial form excluded by genetic studies
- Multifocal motor neuropathy excluded by NCS
- Infective diseases (poliovirus or West Nile virus infection) distinguished by acute onset & monophasic illness

MANAGEMENT

- Ensure ventilation & nutrition
- Anticholinergics for drooling
- Baclofen or diazepam for spasticity
- Palliative care in terminal stages

SPECIFIC THERAPY

- Riluzole may slow progression (monitor liver enzymes, blood count, electrolytes)

FOLLOW-UP

- Regularly assess ventilatory function & nutritional status
  - ➤ May require semiliquid diet, nasogastric feeding, gastrotomy or cricopharyngomyotomy
  - ➤ May require ventilator support

COMPLICATIONS AND PROGNOSIS

Complications

- Dysphagia is common
- Dysarthia or dysphonia
- Aspiration pneumonia
- Respiratory insufficiency

Prognosis

- Mean survival is 3 years
- Only 25% of pts survive for 5 years

ANALGESIC NEPHROPATHY AND NSAID-INDUCED ARF

CHARLES B. CANGRO, MD, PhD and WILLIAM L. HENRICH, MD

HISTORY & PHYSICAL

Classic Analgesic Nephropathy

- History of long term habitual use of combination analgesic preparations
- minimum total dose required unknown. Some suggest a cumulative dose of 3 kg or a daily ingestion of 1 g per day for more than three years
- female:male 6:1
- consider in any patient with chronic renal failure and a history of multiple somatic complaints, chronic headaches, backache, etc.
- 85% of patients deny heavy analgesic use on initial questioning
- cumulative ingestion of several kilograms of combination analgesics (aspirin and phenacetin or its metabolite acetaminophen) associated with increased risk
- aspirin alone appears to pose little risk
- nonspecific : slowly progressive chronic renal failure
- present with increased creatinine
- anemia
- gastrointestinal symptoms
- may present with end stage renal disease
- flank pain and hematuria if papillary necrosis occurs NSAID – Induced Acute Renal Failure
- most common with propionic acid derivatives (fenoprofen, ibuprofen and naproxen)
- may occur at any time after starting drug use (2 weeks–18 months)
- acute renal failure secondary NSIAD inhibition of renal prostaglandin synthesis and subsequent intra-renal vasoconstriction
- sodium and water retention (presents as edema or hyponatremia)
- hypertension
- nephrotic-range proteinuria (80% of cases)
- hyperkalemia (low renin, Type IV RTA picture)
- papillary necrosis (due to ischemia of inner medulla)

TESTS

Laboratory

- Basic studies
  - ➤ Blood: CBC,
    - Na, K+, Cl−, CO2, BUN, creatinine, Ca++, Mg++, Phos.
  - ➤ Urinalysis
    - Possible findings include:
      - normal
      - sterile pyuria
      - hematuria,
      - low specific gravity
      - mild proteinuria (<2+by dipstick)
      - less 1 gram protein /24 hours
      - proteinuria may be nephrotic with NSAID tubulointerstitial nephritis
      - inability to acidify urine

Imaging

- Renal ultrasound – garland pattern of calcification around the renal pelvis suggestive of prior papillary necrosis
- Non Contrast CT – has been proposed as modality of choice to diagnose or exclude analgesic nephropathy- further research to validate this technique is needed

Renal Biopsy

- infrequently needed. as diagnosis made primarily by history and exposure
- shows interstitial nephritis; with NSAID there may be additional minimal change disease or membranous nephropathy

DIFFERENTIAL DIAGNOSIS

Chronic Analgesic Nephropathy

- urinary tract obstruction
- polycystic kidney disease
- hypertensive nephrosclerosis
- chronic tubulo-interstial renal disease
- hypercalcemia
- sarcoid nephropathy
- medullary cystic kidney disease
- lead nephropathy
- myeloma kidney

NSAID – Induced Acute Renal Failure

- rapidly progressive renal failure
- Membranous nephropathy
- Minimal change disease
- acute renal failure secondary to hypovolemia/hypotension
- vasculitis
- Membranoproliferative glomerulonephritis
- Lupus
- Wegener's granulomatosis
- Goodpasture's syndrome
- acute interstial nephritis secondary to drugs, infection
- any acute glomerulonehritis

MANAGEMENT

What to Do First

- discontinue analgesic use. This may require considerable psychological support and guidance

General Measures

- increase fluid intake
- control blood pressure
- monitor for progressive decline in creatinine clearance
- monitor for transitional cell carcinoma of renal pelvis and ureters
  using checks for hematuria

SPECIFIC THERAPY

- stop or minimize analgesic use.

FOLLOW-UP

- course depends on severity of renal damage at the time of presentation
- decline in renal function will continue if analgesic use is continued
- check periodic serum creatinine values.
- urinalysis (especially for proteinuria and hematuria)
- blood pressure control
- increased atherosclerotic disease

COMPLICATIONS AND PROGNOSIS

- prognosis is good if caught early and analgesic use stopped.
- progression to end stage renal failure can occur

ANAPHYLAXIS

PAMELA DAFFERN, MD

HISTORY & PHYSICAL

History
■ Antigen or substance exposure immediately before the event
> ➤ Antibiotics
> ➤ Medications: insulin, progesterone, protamine, anesthetics
> ➤ Vaccines
> ➤ Latex
> ➤ Blood components or biological products
> ➤ Insect stings
> ➤ Exercise
> ➤ Foods: shellfish, peanuts, fish, nuts

Signs & Symptoms
■ Urticaria
■ Angioedema
■ Flushing
■ Pruritus
■ Sense of impending doom
■ Difficulty swallowing
■ Hoarseness
■ Inspiratory stridor
■ Wheezing
■ Chest tightness
■ Dyspnea
■ Hypotension
■ Arrhythmias
■ Shock
■ Seizures
■ Nausea
■ Abdominal cramping
■ Palpitations
■ Lightheadedness

TESTS

Lab Tests
■ Serum tryptase levels obtained w/in 2 hours of an event are elevated in anaphylaxis but not in other causes of shock or respiratory emergencies

- Skin testing or RAST testing w/ specific allergens
  - Helpful for suspected allergy to foods, some drugs, insects, latex

DIFFERENTIAL DIAGNOSIS
- Vasovagal syncope
- Flushing syndromes (carcinoid)
- Systemic mastocytosis
- Panic attacks
- Angioedema (hereditary, acquired, secondary to ACE inhibitors, idiopathic)
- "Restaurant syndromes" (eg, MSG, sulfites)
- Vocal cord dysfunction syndrome
- Other causes of shock, cardiovascular or respiratory events

MANAGEMENT
What to Do First
- Maintain adequate airway & support blood pressure
  - Administer epinephrine 1:1,000 dilution, IM or SC
  - Repeat every 15 min for 3 doses
  - Add plasma volume expanders if hypotension persists
  - Administer oxygen to maintain O2 saturation
  - Administer diphenhydramine, repeat q4–6h
  - Treat bronchospasm w/ inhaled beta-2 agonist

General Measures
- Consider systemic steroids if initial response is inadequate or reaction is severe
- Monitor for several hours; biphasic reactions may occur after apparent recovery
- Hospitalize pts w/ protracted anaphylaxis unresponsive to therapy

SPECIFIC THERAPY
- Identify & teach avoidance of responsible allergen
- Educate in early symptom recognition
- Prescribe epinephrine for self-administration
- Have pt wear a medical alert bracelet
- Make available an antihistamine preparation for injection

FOLLOW-UP
- Assess risk factors
  - Atopy
  - Asthma
  - Hidden allergens

Special Situations
- Pregnancy
  - Severe uterine cramping may accompany anaphylaxis
  - Miscarriage or premature delivery is uncommon
  - Epinephrine remains treatment of choice
- Operating room
  - Hypotension or difficulty ventilating may be only signs
  - Many sources of exposure
- Pts on beta-blockers
  - May be unresponsive to epinephrine
  - Administer glucagon
- Exercise-induced
  - May be associated w/ specific food allergy or to ingestion of any food w/in 4 hours prior to exercise; caution pt not to exercise alone

COMPLICATIONS & PROGNOSIS
- Further events can be eliminated when precipitating factors are identified & avoided
- Idiopathic reactions may require chronic oral corticosteroids

---

ANEMIAS SECONDARY TO SYSTEMIC DISEASE

LAWRENCE B. GARDNER, MD

HISTORY & PHYSICAL
- Most common anemia seen in hospitalized patients not bleeding or hemolyzing. Common in outpatient rheumatologic conditions.
- Associated primarily with inflammatory states: infection, rheumatologic diseases, vasculitis, cancer, inflammatory bowel disease, renal failure
- Pathophysiology includes increased cytokines, which inhibit hematopoiesis, interfere with iron utilization, decrease red survival, and diminish erythropoietin levels and function.
- Severity of anemia correlates with severity of underlying condition.
- History and physical most significant for underlying condition, not the anemia
- Anemia is usually mild and chronic, so generally compensated. Pallor, fatigue and poor exercise tolerance common.
- Note: Anemia may occur with thyroid disorders, malabsorption (e.g., sprue, achlorhydria), liver disease ± 1 – hypersplenism, and

autoimmune disorders, but the etiologies and treatments are different than those for the classic anemia of chronic disease. The anemia of renal failure is primarily due to erythropoietin deficiency, though hyperparathyroidism aluminum toxicity, and increases in inflammatory cytokines may contribute.

TESTS

- Diagnosis based on correlating an inflammatory condition with the onset of anemia
- Usually a mild normocytic anemia, but microcytosis can be seen. If additional blood lineages are affected, other diagnoses should be considered.
- Anemia of hypoproduction, so reticulocyte count should be inappropriately low
- Iron tests are most helpful: Low serum iron, high ferritin, low transferrin and total iron-binding capacity (differentiates from iron deficiency)
- Erythropoietin often elevated, but not elevated in proportion to the degree of anemia (i.e., lower than the physiological response in simple iron deficiency). Therefore epo levels are usually lower than "standard" levels below.

Hbg (g/dl) in simple iron deficiency	Average epo level (mU/ml)
>13	<10
12	15
11	20
10	40
9	80
8	100
7	200
<6	>1,000

DIFFERENTIAL DIAGNOSIS

n/a

MANAGEMENT

What to Do First

- Treatment is generally not urgent.
- Determine the underlying disease state. Diagnosis is often one of exclusion. Ensure other causes of anemia are not present: evaluate for presence of blood loss and iron deficiency, hemolysis, folate or

B12 deficiency, plasma cell dyscrasia (serum protein electrophoresis), true thyroid abnormalities, myelodysplasia, serum creatine and erythropoietin level. Sedimentation rate or C-reactive protein may be helpful.

- Bone marrow generally useful only lto rule out other conditions
- Age-appropriate cancer screening always indicated

SPECIFIC THERAPY

- Correcting underlying condition is best treatment.
- Other treatment may not be necessary if hematocrit >30% and patient is not symptomatic. However, studies have suggested that quality of life is improved in cancer patients whose anemias are rigorously treated. Beware of risks of anemia in older patients or those with cardiac disease.
- If treatment is needed, pharmacologic doses of erythropoietin should be given: 5–10,000 U 3X week or 40,000 Units once a week subcutaneously. Alternatively, longer-acting forms of erythropoietin (aranesp) may be equally effective (100 units every 1–2 weeks to start).

   Because of poor iron utilization with systemic inflammation, iron administration, intravenous or oral, may increase the response to erythropoietin, even in the presence of high serum ferritin (NB: Both are off-label indications.)
- Patients with low pretreatment erythropoietin levels and without bone marrow or hematologic malignancies respond best. However, there is no pretreatment erythropoietin level that should preclude a pharmacologic trial of erythropoietin, if indicated.

FOLLOW-UP

- A response to erythropoietin should be seen in 4–6 weeks.
- Response rates: 40–80%
- If no response, erythropoietin may be increased to 60,000 Units q week subcutaneously.
- Studies suggest that if after 2 weeks the serum epo is >100 mU/ml and the hemoglobin has not increased by >0.5 gIdl, or after 2 weeks of treatment the serum ferritin is >400 ng/ml, then patient is less likely to respond.

COMPLICATIONS AND PROGNOSIS
n/a

ANISAKIASIS

J. GORDON FRIERSON, MD

HISTORY & PHYSICAL

History

■ Exposure: Ingestion of poorly cooked fish, resulting in ingestion of larval forms of Anisakis simplex or Pseudoterranova decipiens. The larvae invade intestinal wall of stomach or small bowel to level of submucosa, causing inflammatory swelling. Occasionally perforation of small bowel occurs.

Signs & Symptoms

■ Depending on location of worms: Worm may migrate to pharynx in absence of other symptoms. May see epigastric pain, abdominal pain, nausea, vomiting. Abdominal examination may be normal, or may show tenderness over affected bowel, sometimes peritoneal signs (especially in case of perforation). Allergic reactions, including anaphylaxis, can occur.

TESTS

■ Basic tests: blood: normal, or eosinophilia. High WBC in case of perforation.
■ Basic tests: urine: normal
■ Specific tests: If worm appears in pharynx, identify worm.
■ Gastroscopy in case of gastric anisakiasis. Otherwise diagnosis is clinical unless surgery required for peritoneal signs.
■ Other tests: In intestinal form: barium studies may show narrowed inflamed area in ileum. Serology available on research basis, not usually helpful at bedside. Skin testing if allergic reaction present.

DIFFERENTIAL DIAGNOSIS

■ Gastric form: peptic ulcer, cholecystitis, pancreatitis
■ Intestinal form: appendicitis, Crohn's disease, diverticulitis, mesenteric adenitis, Angiostrongylus costaricensis infection

MANAGEMENT

What to Do First

■ Assess severity and need for possible surgery. IV fluids if needed.

General Measures

■ Ascertain source of infection

SPECIFIC THERAPY

Indications
- Gastric form: patients with moderate or severe pain, nausea
- Intestinal form: If surgical indications exist

Treatment Options
- Gastric form: Gastroscopic removal of worms. Pretreatment with H2 blocker may help.

Side Effects & Complications
- Gastric form: same as complications of gastroscopy
- Intestinal form: peritonitis, complications of surgery
- Contraindications to treatment: absolute: asymptomatic patients, and patients with worm migration to mouth and no other symptoms
- Contraindications to treatment: relative: mild symptoms

FOLLOW-UP

During Treatment
- Monitor symptoms, possible surgical problems.

Routine
- Educate patient about mode of acquisition.

COMPLICATIONS AND PROGNOSIS
- Gastric form: Generally there is recovery, worms die off or removed, inflammation subsides.
- Intestinal form: Intestinal perforation, local abscess, peritoneal signs. Surgery is frequent with these presentations. Prognosis good after surgery.

ANORECTAL TUMORS

MARK A. VIERRA, MD

HISTORY & PHYSICAL

History
- Adenocarcinoma of rectum most common anorectal malignancy (~98%)
- Arises in adenomas
- Incidence increases w/ age, uncommon before age 40
- Approximately equal incidence men & women

- More common in developed countries; associated w/ high-fat diet, red meat consumption
- Anal canal tumors most commonly squamous cancer (~70%) & cloacogenic cancer
- Traditional predominance in women; now may be more common in men due increased homosexuality
- Associated w/ HPV & receptive anal intercourse

Signs & Symptoms
- Rectal cancers usually present w/ bleeding, less often obstruction; pain & significant change of bowel habits rare until advanced
- Squamous cancers present as palpable/visible lesions
- May be visible externally (anal canal tumors) or palpable if w/i ~6 cm; sigmoidoscopy or colonoscopy usually used to make diagnosis

TESTS

Laboratory
- Anemia may be present (low MCV)
- ? CEA late, usually sign of advanced disease, not helpful for screening
- LFTs not helpful for detection of occult liver metastases; CT much more sensitive
- Consider HIV testing in pts w/ anal canal tumors

Imaging
- Remainder of colon must be screened w/ colonoscopy
- CT of abdomen & CXR/CT of chest to exclude distant metastases (unless only palliative treatment undertaken)
- Endorectal US of rectal cancer may distinguish tumor stage (T,N), which can be important for deciding treatment: local excision, low anterior resection w/ anastomosis, abdominal-perineal resection

DIFFERENTIAL DIAGNOSIS

Consider Unusual Tumors:
- Rectum:
  - Carcinoid, GI stromal tumor, melanoma
  - Occasionally, ovarian cancer, prostate cancer, endometriosis may mimic rectal cancer
- Anal canal:
  - Condyloma, KS, melanoma, Paget disease of anus
  - Consider HIV

MANAGEMENT

What to Do First

- Confirm diagnosis

SPECIFIC THERAPY

- Rectal cancer:
  - ➤ Small, well-differentiated T1 lesions may be treated w/ local excision +/− XRT
  - ➤ Most lesions treated w/ neoadjuvant chemotherapy & XRT followed by surgery, either low anterior resection w/ anastomosis or abdominal-perineal resection
- Squamous cancer:
  - ➤ Chemotherapy/radiation followed by surgery if response incomplete or in event of recurrence
  - ➤ Earliest lesions may be treated by surgery alone, but this is uncommon

FOLLOW-UP

- Rectal cancer pts at risk for metachronous adenocarcinoma of colon should undergo periodic colonoscopy
- Digital exams, sigmoidoscopy to exclude anastomotic recurrence
- Value of surveillance for metastases not established: consider follow-up evaluation of liver/lung w/ CT, CXR, CEA
- Local recurrence after low anterior resection may be treated w/ abdominal-perineal resection or pelvic exenteration
- Follow anal cancer pts for local recurrence or inguinal node disease

COMPLICATIONS AND PROGNOSIS

- Low anterior resection produces irregular bowel habits, occasionally severe, esp w/ low anastomoses; changes likely greater in pts who also receive XRT
- Minor incontinence occasional; major incontinence very rare; radiation proctitis common but usually self-limited
- Impotence common after low anterior resection or abdominal-perineal resection common; minor bladder disturbance also common, but major difficulties rare
- Surgical complications: bleeding, infection, anastomotic leak or stricture, ureteral injury
- Rectal stricture, troublesome radiation proctitis, fissure may occur after XRT for squamous cancer of anus

ANOREXIA NERVOSA

JOSE R. MALDONADO, MD

HISTORY & PHYSICAL

Demographics

- Lifetime prevalence: 0.5 & 1%
- Females > males (90% occur in females)
- Peak onset usually during adolescence, rarely before puberty
- Mean age of onset: 17 y
- Genetics:
  - ➤ Concordance rate: 70% monozygotic & 20% for dizygotic twins
  - ➤ Anorexia 8-fold more common in relatives of anorexics

History

- Individual's refusal to maintain minimal normal body weight
- Pts usually weigh <85% of ideal body weight for age & height
- Intense fear of gaining weight
- Perception of being fat even at low weight
- Amenorrhea (due to abnormally low estrogen levels)
- In childhood & early adolescence, failure to make expected weight gains instead of weight loss
- Degree of weight loss & fatigue usually denied
- Initial visit usually prompted by family concern
- Few pts present w/ secondary physical complaints (ie, stress fractures, joint problems, or cardiac problems)
- Low body weight achieved through relentless pursuit of thinness through:
  - ➤ Dieting or food restriction
  - ➤ Excessive exercise
  - ➤ Purging
  - ➤ Diuretic misuse
  - ➤ Laxative misuse
  - ➤ Thyroid hormone misuse

Subtypes:

- Restricting type: weight loss accomplished mostly by dieting, fasting, or excessive exercise, w/o binge eating or purging
- Binge-eating/purging type: frequent binge eating or purging, or both

Signs & Symptoms
- Mental status exam:
  - Intense preoccupation w/ food
  - Slow eating
  - Depression
  - Loss of energy
  - Loss of sexual interest
  - Social withdrawal
  - Cognitive impairments: impaired concentration & poor judgment
  - 50% of all anorexics also binge-eat & purge
- Physical exam:
  - Cachexia
  - Slow pulse rate
  - Hypotension
  - Cold & blue extremities
  - Dry skin
  - Fine body hair (lanugo)
  - Scars or abrasions in the knuckles (associated w/ self-induced emesis)
  - Wasting of dental enamel (associated w/ self-induced emesis)
  - Constipation
  - Cold intolerance
  - Lethargy

TESTS

Laboratory
- Usually show alterations in metabolic function:
  - Decreased gonadotropin levels:
    - LH (to prepubertal pattern)
    - FSH
    - Estrogen
  - Elevated growth hormone
  - Elevated resting plasma cortisol
  - Decreased fT3
  - Elevated cholesterol & carotene
- Dehydration
- Elevated BUN
- Elevated LFTs
- Leukopenia
- Anemia

- Decreased potassium levels, particularly associated w/ purging (may lead to cardiac arrhythmias)
- Hypomagnesemia, hypozincemia, hypophosphatemia, hyperamylasemia
- Metabolic alkalosis, hypochloremia, hypokalemia: vomiting
- Metabolic acidosis secondary to laxative abuse
- ECG: sinus bradycardia

DIFFERENTIAL DIAGNOSIS
- GI disorders
- Brain tumors
- Occult malignancies
- HIV/AIDS
- Superior mesenteric artery syndrome
- Major depression
- Schizophrenia
- Body dysmorphic disorder
- Obsessive-compulsive disorder
- Bulimia nervosa
- Delusional disorder, somatic type

MANAGEMENT
What to Do First
- Persuade both pt & family that treatment is necessary

General Measures
- Most pts initially require hospitalization in specialized inpatient unit to correct weight loss & electrolyte abnormalities

SPECIFIC THERAPY
Hospitalized Treatment
- First step: begin weight restoration
- Behavior modification:
  - Systematic reinforcement of weight gain, making access to certain activities contingent on specified daily amount of weight gain (eg, 0.2 kg/d)
  - Reward activities tailored to level of success
  - Behavioral contract specifying amount of weight to be gained
- Family therapy: aims to gain independence, social skills training, & improved communication patterns & more mature defense mechanisms
- Individual psychotherapy

Medical Complications

- Fluid retention may occur during initial stages of refeeding
- First 7–10 d: caloric intake should not exceed 2000 calories/d; monitor fluid intake carefully

Pharmacotherapy

- Medication provides little in treatment of anorexia
- Treat comorbid psychiatric conditions, ie, depression
- Appetite stimulants: cyproheptadine (serotonin antagonist that stimulates appetite) or megestrol (synthetic derivative of progesterone) may help

Tube Feeding

- Indications:
  - Dehydration & electrolyte imbalance
  - Intercurrent medical emergency necessitating weight gain
  - Failure to gain weight after adequate treatment trial
  - Negative reinforcement (ie, weight gain above certain threshold may prevent or discontinue tube-feeding)
- Complications:
  - Aspiration pneumonia
  - Negative transference

FOLLOW-UP

- Long-term outpatient treatment:
- Usually follows discharge from in-patient unit
- Minimal duration 6 mo if weight stable
- Cognitive-behavioral therapy (CBT):
  - Provide suppor
  - Modify distorted patterns of thinking about weight & shape
  - Dealing w/ ongoing problems of living
- Family therapy recommended for children & adolescents

COMPLICATIONS AND PROGNOSIS

Complications

- Amenorrhea: metabolic adaptation to weight loss & hormonal changes
- Orthopedic problems due to excessive exercise
- Cardiovascular problems secondary to starvation & potassium deficiency

Prognosis
- Treatment success rate: <50% of pts fully recover from disorder
- Vocational functioning often preserved
- Mortality: 5–15%:
  - ➤ 50% due to suicide, others to starvation & electrolyte abnormalities

ANTIBIOTIC-ASSOCIATED AND PSEUDOMEMBRANOUS COLITIS

MARTA L. DAVILA, MD

HISTORY & PHYSICAL

History
- Diarrhea a frequent adverse effect of antibiotics; can develop from a few hours up to 2 months after antibiotic intake
- Only 10–20% of all cases of antibiotic-associated diarrhea caused by infection with C. difficile
- Other infectious organisms: C. perfringens, Staphylococcus aureus, Klebsiella oxytoca, Candida species, and Salmonella species

Signs & Symptoms
- Acute watery diarrhea, lower abdominal pain, fever and leukocytosis
- Reactive arthritis a rare complication of C. difficile infection
- Asymptomatic carrier state: 2/3 of infected hospitalized patients asymptomatic; carrier state eliminated by treatment with vancomycin
- Diarrhea without colitis: symptoms usually mild and resolve when the initiating antibiotic discontinued
- Colitis without pseudomembrane formation: more serious illness with systemic manifestations such as fever, malaise, anorexia and leukocytosis; sigmoidoscopic examination – nonspecific erythema without pseudomembranes
- Pseudomembranous colitis: sigmoidoscopy-classic pseudomembranes, which appear as raised yellow or off-white plaques covering the mucosa
- Atypical or rare presentations: fulminant colitis with or without megacolon, pseudomembranous colitis with protein-losing enteropathy, relapsing infection

TESTS

Basic Tests
- blood: CBC
- stool for culture, O&P to rule out other possibilities

Imaging
- plain films of the abdomen to rule out toxic megacolon

Specific Diagnostic Tests
- ELISA assay (stool)
  - ➤ rapid test to detect the presence of C. difficile toxin in stool
  - ➤ most commonly used and widely available
  - ➤ sensitivity: 70–90%; specificity: 99%
- Cytotoxicity assay (stool)
  - ➤ gold standard for the identification of C. difficile cytotoxins
  - ➤ sensitivity: 94–100%; specificity: 100%
  - ➤ expensive with turn-around time of 2–3 days
  - ➤ Sigmoidoscopy or colonoscopy
    - recommended when diagnosis in doubt and has to be established quickly
    - look for pseudomembranes

DIFFERENTIAL DIAGNOSIS
n/a

MANAGEMENT

What to Do First
- discontinue inciting antibiotic if possible

General Measures
- assess severity

SPECIFIC THERAPY

Initial Therapy
- oral metronidazole 500 mg TID or 250 mg QID for 10–14 days is the initial choice for treatment
- alternative first-line agent is oral vancomycin 125 mg QID
- both metronidazole and vancomycin equally effective but metronidazole is much less expensive; vancomycin can lead to selection of vancomycin-resistant enterococci
- oral Bacitracin alternative but not readily available
- for severe infections: oral metronidazole first; if no response in 48 hr, switch to oral vancomycin; if still no improvement, escalate the vancomycin dose at 48-hour intervals up to 500 mg QID

- severely ill patients who cannot tolerate oral medication: metronidazole IV and/or vancomycin enemas
- surgery reserved for those with peritoneal signs, impending perforation, persistent toxic megacolon and refractory septicemia
- surgery of choice subtotal colectomy with ileostomy; can be converted to an ileorectal anastomosis once the patient has recovered

Treatment of Recurrent Infection
- first relapse treated the same way as the initial episode with 10–14 days of oral metronidazole or vancomycin
- treatment for multiple relapses:
  - ➤ tapering and pulsed antibiotic treatment: metronidazole or vancomycin administered every other day or every third day as they are tapered over the course of 4–6 weeks
  - ➤ use of oral anion-binding resins such as colestipol or cholestyramine; given in addition to antibiotics, usually vancomycin, for a period of two weeks
  - ➤ other alternatives: oral lactobacillus strain GG, oral Saccharomyces boulardii with or without antibiotics, intravenous gamma globulin

Side Effects & Complications
- antibiotics used for the treatment of C. difficile are known to also cause C. difficile infection
- anion-binding resins can cause significant abdominal bloating

FOLLOW-UP
- no need to confirm a patient is C. difficile toxin negative after completion of treatment as long as patient is asymptomatic

COMPLICATIONS AND PROGNOSIS
- good, particularly for those who do not experience relapse

ANTIPHOSPHOLIPID ANTIBODIES

MICHELLE A. PETRI, MD MPH

HISTORY & PHYSICAL
- Antiphospholipid antibodies (lupus anticoagulant, anticardiolipin, anti-beta2 glycoprotein I) are a marker for hypercoagulability.
- Fifty percent of patients with antiphospholipid antibodies have systemic lupus erythematosus.

- Three to five percent of the general population has antiphospholipid antibodies.
- Antiphospholipid antibody syndrome (APS) is the presence of: venous or arterial thrombosis or pregnancy morbidity (miscarriages, severe pre-eclampsia; pre-term birth due to placental insufficiency), in the setting of either the lupus anticoagulant or moderate to high titer IgG or IgM anticardiolipin or anti-beta2 glycoprotein I.
- APS should be considered in young people with deep venous thrombosis or stroke.
- Cutaneous manifestations of APS include livedo reticularis, superficial thrombophlebitis, splinter hemorrhages, and leg ulcers.
- Non-thrombotic manifestations of antiphospholipid antibodies include transverse myelitis and chorea.

TESTS

Basic Blood Studies
- Lupus anticoagulant (LA) is a clotting assay performed on plasma.
  - A PTT can miss 50% of lupus anticoagulants.
  - More sensitive screening tests are the modified Russell viper venom time and sensitive PTT.
  - Once a prolonged clotting time is ascertained, two other steps are necessary to confirm a LA: lack of correction with a mixing study and demonstration of phospholipid dependence (such as a platelet neutralization procedure).
- Anticardiolipin and anti-beta2 glycoprotein I are ELISA assays.
  - IgG is the isotype most closely associated with risk of thrombosis and pregnancy loss.
  - 24% of patients with APS are thrombocytopenic.

Specific Diagnostic Tests
- Fifty percent of patients with APS have SLE ("secondary" APS).
- Helpful serologic tests for SLE include ANA, anti-DNA, anti-RNP, anti-Sm, anti-Ro, anti-La, C3, and C4.

Other Tests as Appropriate
- Imaging studies to diagnose thrombosis: brain MRI, brain CT, arteriogram, biopsy, and EKG.
- One-third of patients with APS may have heart valve vegetations or thickened valves on transesophageal echo (TEE).

DIFFERENTIAL DIAGNOSIS
- Genetic causes of hypercoagulability: Factor V Leiden, prothrombin mutation, Protein C deficiency, Protein S deficiency, anti-thrombin III deficiency, homocysteinemia

- Heparin-induced thrombocytopenia
- Thrombotic thrombocytopenic purpura (TTP)
- Disseminated intravascular coagulation (DIC)

MANAGEMENT

What to Do First
- Send lupus anticoagulant tests BEFORE starting heparin/warfarin.
- Treat thrombosis with heparin, thrombolytics, angioplasty, etc.

General Measures
- Rule out other causes of hypercoagulability.
- Eliminate contributing causes of hypercoagulability, such as exogenous estrogen (oral contraceptives), smoking, etc.

SPECIFIC THERAPY

Indications
- Venous or arterial thrombosis secondary to APS is treated with long-term high-intensity (INR 2 to 3) anti-coagulation.
- After ONE late or TWO or more early pregnancy losses, the next pregnancy is treated with low-dose aspirin and heparin.

Treatment Options
- Prophylactic treatment can be considered in patients with LA or moderate-to-high titer anticardiolipin or anti-beta2 glycoprotein I who have not had thrombosis: low-dose aspirin in the general population, low-dose aspirin and hydroxychloroquine in SLE patients.
- Venous thrombosis: treatment of choice is long-term warfarin, with an INR goal of 2 to 3.
  - ➤ Option 1: Regular-intensity warfarin
  - ➤ Option 2: 6 months warfarin; long-term warfarin for recurrent VTE only, OR if antiphospholipid antibodies remain present
- Arterial thrombosis: treatment of choice is long-term high intensity warfarin.
  - ➤ Option 1: Low-dose aspirin AND warfarin (INR 2 to 3)
  - ➤ Option 2: Aspirin only for stroke; long-term warfarin for recurrent stroke only
- Pregnancy loss: regular heparin 5–10,000 units sc bid plus aspirin 81 mg
  - ➤ Option 1: Lovenox 20 mg sc bid plus aspirin 81 mg
  - ➤ Option 2: Aspirin 81 mg alone if there has been only ONE early pregnancy loss

■ Catastrophic APS: multiple organ thrombosis requiring plasma-pheresis or intravenous immunoglobulin in addition to heparin and immunosuppression (corticosteroids)

Side Effects & Complications
■ Bleeding risk increases with warfarin AND with addition of low-dose aspirin.

Contraindications
■ Profound thrombocytopenia (platelets <35,000) greatly increases risk of bleeding; increase platelet count to safer levels with corticosteroids, intravenous immunoglobulin or other therapy, before considering anticoagulation.
■ Warfarin is not used during pregnancy; substitute heparin.

FOLLOW-UP
■ Monitor prothrombin time every 2 weeks to try to keep warfarin in therapeutic window (INR goal is 2 to 3).
■ Antibiotics may lead to marked changes in INR.
■ Elective surgical procedures require switch to heparin before/after.

COMPLICATIONS AND PROGNOSIS
■ 75% of pregnancies treated with heparin and aspirin are successful; 40% of pregnancies treated with aspirin alone are successful.
■ Recurrent thrombosis rate is less with long-term warfarin.

AORTIC COARCTATION

KENDRICK A. SHUNK, MD, PhD

HISTORY & PHYSICAL

History
■ Risk factors
 ➤ Male (2:1)
 ➤ Gonadal dysgenesis
 ➤ Other congenital cardiac disease (commonly bicuspid Aortic valve)

Signs & Symptoms
■ Headache, epistaxis, claudication or cold extremities with exercise
■ Unequal upper extremity blood pressure (R>L)
■ Right arm hypertension

- Murmur mid systolic at anterior chest, back and spinous process, may progress to continuous
- Occasionally poor lower extremity development

TESTS
Specific Diagnostic Tests:
- ECG: LVH
- chest x-ray: rib notching and "3" sign of aortic notch

Other Imaging Tests
- MRI/MRA offers good anatomic definition
- Echocardiography useful to assess gradient
- In adults, angiography remains gold standard to allow assessment of coronaries before coarctation repair

DIFFERENTIAL DIAGNOSIS
- Takayasu's or related aortitis, pseudocoarctation

MANAGEMENT
What to Do First
- surgery

General Measures
- R/O CAD by coronary angiography if any suspicion

SPECIFIC THERAPY
Indication for surgical therapy: detection of significant coartation

Treatment Options
- Surgical repair (usually excision with end-to-end anastomosis)

Side Effects & Contraindications
- Side effects: bleeding, infection, pneumothorax, death
  - Contraindications
    - Absolute: Contraindication to thoracotomy

FOLLOW-UP
- Complications, residua and sequelae are frequent, require indefinite follow-up.

COMPLICATIONS AND PROGNOSIS
- Complications: residual hypertension and increased risk of CAD, MI, CHF, bicuspid aortic valve, re-coarctation
- Prognosis: generally good but CHF, MI are major causes of death at 11–25 years of follow-up

AORTIC DISSECTION

KENDRICK A. SHUNK, MD, PhD

HISTORY & PHYSICAL

History
- Hypertension, Atherosclerosis, Cystic medial necrosis (Marfan's Ehlers-Danlos, others)

Signs & Symptoms
- Severe anterior or posterior chest pain often described as "ripping" or "tearing", often radiating to intrascapular region and migrating with the propagation of the dissection, diaphoresis, syncope, weakness, dyspnea, hoarseness, dysphagia
- Hypertension or hypotension
- Aortic regurgitation (occurs in 50% of type I dissections)
  - Diastolic AR murmur
  - Widened pulse pressure, bounding pulse
- Loss of pulses
- Pulmonary rales
- Neurologic findings
  - Hemiplegia, hemianesthesis (carotid occlusion), paraplegia (spinal artery occlusion), Horner's syndrome

TESTS
- Basic blood tests:
  - Often non-contributory
- Specific diagnostic tests:
  - ECG
    - Usually no ischemia (rarely acute MI from extension into RCA or Left main)
    - Low voltage: suspect hemopericardium
  - CXR
    - May show widened mediastinum and/or left pleural effusion
- Other imaging tests
  - Transthoracic echocardiography successful at identifying 70–90%
  - TEE and CT and MRI all offer excellent sensitivity (~98%)
    - TEE has lesser ability to fully define aortic arch anatomy
    - CT and MRI require movement of critical patient out of ICU
    - Common practice: pursue all three, take first available

➤ Angiography remains gold standard and allows coronary angiography in preparation for surgery

DIFFERENTIAL DIAGNOSIS

■ Occasionally misdiagnosed as acute coronary syndrome, generally with disasterous results

MANAGEMENT

What to Do First

■ Think of it, work to exclude it

General Measures

■ Once diagnosis made, begin immediate medical therapy while further assessing classification
  ➤ Stanford type A
    • Involves ascending aorta
  ➤ Stanford type B
    • Does not involve ascending aorta
  ➤ DeBakey type I
    • Involves ascending through descending aorta
  ➤ DeBakey type II
    • – Involves ascending and arch, not descending aorta
  ➤ DeBakey type III
    • Involves descending aorta only
■ Medical therapy, hemodynamic control is cornerstone for reducing propagation
  ➤ Control BP
  ➤ Control dP/dt

SPECIFIC THERAPY

Indication for surgical therapy: DeBakcy type I and II (Stanford type A) or sometimes propagating type III with end organ effects

Indication for medical therapy: non-surgical candidates and those awaiting surgery

Treatment Options

■ Surgical reconstruction if indicated
■ Medical therapy
  ➤ Labetalol is drug of choice with Beta and Alpha blocking properties dose: Goal HR ~60 and SBP <120
  ➤ Alternatively another IV beta blocker can be used but must be accompanied by sodium nitroprusside, titrate the combination to same therapeutic goal (HR ~60 and SBP <120)

➤ Direct vasodilators (hydralazine, diazoxide) are contraindicated because they increase shear and may propagate dissection

Side Effects & Contraindications
■ Surgery
   ➤ Side effects: major hemorrhage, stroke, MI, spinal cord injury, sepsis, death (15–20% perioperatively)
      • Contraindications
         • relative: emergent need-surgical risk may decrease after several days of medical stabilization (confounded by culling effect)
■ Beta blockers
   ➤ Side effects: dizziness, tiredness, severe bradycardia, hypotension, rales, bronchospasm, heart block.
   ➤ Contraindications
      • Absolute: cardiogenic shock, severe COPD
   ➤ Relative: heart rate <45, AV conduction defects, COPD
■ Sodium Nitroprusside
   ➤ Side effects: precipitous drop of BP with accompanying sequelae, cyanide toxicity-risk increases with dose, duration of therapy-monitor thiocyanate levels
   ➤ Contraindications
      • Absolute: continued infusion beyond 10 minutes at maximum dose
      • Relative: renal or liver impairment, hypothyroidism, hyponatremia, B12 deficiency, increased intracranial pressure, hypovolemia, thiosulfate thiotransferase deficiency (congenital Leber's optic atrophy, tobacco amblyopia)

FOLLOW-UP
■ If nitroprusside is used, thiocyanate levels must be followed closely. Metabolic acidosis is also a (delayed) indication of Cyanide toxicity.
■ Monitor patients for propagation with end organ effects which may be indication for surgery even in type III.

COMPLICATIONS AND PROGNOSIS
■ Complications: tamponade, renal failure, bowel ischemia, stroke, MI, death, sepsis, paraplegia
■ Prognosis: In-hospital mortality of surgically managed type A dissection is 15–20%. In-hospital mortality of medically managed type B dissection is also 15–20%. 10 year survival for non-Marfan's aortic dissection is 60%, worse in Marfan's

AORTIC INSUFFICIENCY (AI)

JUDITH A. WISNESKI, MD

HISTORY & PHYSICAL

Etiology
- Abnormality in AV leaflets
  - Endocarditis
  - Rheumatic heart disease
  - Collagen vascular disease
  - Congenital bicuspid valve
- Dilation of aortic root
  - Marfan syndrome
  - Annuloaortic ectasia
  - Aortic dissection
  - Syphilis
  - Ankylosing spondylitis

History
- Acute
  - Pulmonary congestion/pulmonary edema
- Chronic
  - Pulmonary congestion (most common)
  - Angina (less common with AI than AS)
  - Syncope (rare)
  - Carotid artery pain (rare)

Signs & Symptoms
- Acute
  - Diastolic murmur
  - Soft S1
- Chronic
  - Diastolic blowing murmur at left sternal border (best appreciated with patient sitting, leaning forward)
  - Diastolic murmur at right sternal border (suggests very dilated aortic root)
  - Diastolic murmur at apex (severe AI, Austin-Flint murmur)
  - PMI – hyperdynamic, displaced to left and downward
  - Normal S1 and S2
  - S3 (left ventricular dysfunction)
  - Systolic hypertension

➤ Wide pulse pressure
- Waterhammer pulse (Corrigan's pulse)
- Carotid pulse (prominent sharp upstroke; occasionally bisferiens)
- Head bobbing (DeMusset's sign)
- Capillary pulsations in nail bed (Quincke's sign)

TESTS
ECG
■ Acute AI
➤ Maybe normal
■ Chronic AI
➤ Left atrial abnormality
➤ Left ventricular (LV) hypertrophy

Chest X-Ray
■ Acute AI
➤ Maybe normal
■ Chronic AI
➤ Cardiac enlargement
➤ Aortic dilatation
➤ Calcification of ascending aorta (suggests syphilis as etiology)
➤ Aortic valve usually not calcified with AI

Echo/Doppler *(Extremely Important Test)*
■ Severity of AI
■ LV systolic function
■ LV diastolic and systolic dimensions
■ Aortic root size
■ Premature closure of mitral valve (often seen in acute severe AI)

Cardiac Catheterization
■ Hemodynamics
➤ Width of arterial pressure
➤ LV end-diastolic pressure
➤ Premature closure of mitral valve (LV diastolic pressure higher than pulmonary capillary wedge)
■ Left ventriculography
➤ LV systolic function (LVEF)
➤ LV diastolic and systolic volume index
■ Aortography
➤ Severity of AI

- Coronary angiography (required prior to aortic valve replacement in older patients)

DIFFERENTIAL DIAGNOSIS
- Mitral stenosis (Austin-Flint murmur may be mistaken for mitral stenosis)

MANAGEMENT
n/a

SPECIFIC THERAPY
Medical
- Antibiotic prophylaxis in all patients
- Mild symptoms and preserved LV function and dimensions on echo
  - ➤ Vasodilator therapy (may delay need for aortic valve replacement)
  - ➤ Diuretics

Surgical (usually aortic valve replacement (AVR))
- Moderate to severe symptoms
- Mild symptoms or asymptomatic with deterioration of LV function: LVEF < 55% or LV end-systolic dimension > 50 mm
  - ➤ **Extremely important – asymptomatic patients or patients with mild AI must have serial echo/Doppler studies to assess LV function and size:**
    - End-systolic dimension < 40 mm – echo/Doppler every 2 years
    - End-systolic dimension 40–50 mm–echo/Doppler every 6 months

FOLLOW-UP
n/a

COMPLICATIONS AND PROGNOSIS
Complications
- Medical
  - ➤ See complications under vasodilator therapy (section on Heart Failure)
  - ➤ LV function deteriorates when AVR delayed
- Surgery (AVR)
  - ➤ Acute
    - Complications associated with cardiopulmonary bypass and major surgery
  - ➤ Long-term
    - Thromboembolism
    - Valve failure
    - Bleeding from anticoagulation therapy
    - Endocarditis

Prognosis
- Degree of LV dysfunction prior to AVR major determinant of long-term prognosis (end-systolic dimension > 55 mm, worse prognosis)

AORTITIS

KENDRICK A. SHUNK, MD, PhD

HISTORY & PHYSICAL

History
- Asian, female (Takayasu's arteritis)
- Prior untreated Syphilis
- Rheumatologic disease (ankylosing spondylitis as prototype, others as well)
- Black, female (Giant cell arteritis)

Signs & Symptoms
- Fever, anorexia, malaise, weight loss, night sweats, arthralgias, fatigue, pleuritic pain, localized pain over other affected arteries, polymyalgia rheumatica, headaches, claudication, paresthesias, TIA, tender arteries, unequal pulses

TESTS
- Basic blood tests:
  - ➤ Often elevated: ESR, CRP, WBC, IgG, IgM, C3 and C4 complement, alpha2 globulin (Takayasu's, Giant cell, rheumatolgic)
  - ➤ Anemia of chronic disease often present
  - ➤ Occasionally present: rheumatoid factor, ANA (Takayasu's, rheumatologic)
  - ➤ Luetic: serology negative in 15–30% (e.g. VDRL), fluorescent treponemal (FTA-ABS) almost always positive.
- Specific diagnostic tests: Takayasu's criteria
  - ➤ Age < 40 at diagnosis or onset
  - ➤ *and* either 2 major, 1 major + 2 minor, or 4 minor criteria
    - Major (2): left mid subclavian stenosis, right mid subclavian stenosis
    - Minor (9): high ESR, Carotid tenderness, HTN, aortic regurgitation or aortoannular ectasia, pulmonary artery lesion, left mid common carotid lesion, distal brachiocephalic trunk lesion, descending thoracic aorta lesion, abdominal aorta lesion

- Other tests
  - MRI/MRA useful for defining aneurysm or stenosis
  - Biopsy of an involved artery to confirm Giant cell arteritis

DIFFERENTIAL DIAGNOSIS

- broad, consider:
  - thromboembolic disease
  - other causes of systemic inflammatory response
  - dissection

MANAGEMENT

What to Do First

- Diagnose and treat underlying condition
- Manage acute problems

General Measures

- Establish working diagnosis by history, physical, tests described above
- For Takayasu's,
  - establish type
    - Type I: primarily involves aortic arch and brachiocephalic arteries
    - Type II: primarily involves thoracoabdominal aorta and renal arteries
    - Type III: features of both Type I and Type II
    - Type IV: shows pulmonary artery involvement
  - Treat manifestations

SPECIFIC THERAPY

Takayasu's

- Treatment options (none shown to modify disease progression)
  - Prednisone with gradual taper
  - Methotrexate can be considered if patient's constitutional symptoms not relieved with steroids
  - Cyclophosphamide can also be considered, adjusted for WBC > 3000/mm^3 in refractory cases
  - Aspirin possibly of benefit

Syphilitic Aortitis

- Treatment options
  - Penicillin G for 3 weeks
  - If Penicillin allergic, Doxycycline × 21 days
  - If intolerant of Doxycycline confirm Penicillin allergy, consider erythromycin for 30 days

Giant Cell Aortitis
- Treatment options
  - Prednisone, when ESR and symptoms resolve, taper gradually for 1–2 y
  - Methotrexate can be considered for a steroid sparing effect

Other Rheumatologic Aortitis
- Treatment underlying disease as usual

Side Effects & Contraindications
- Prednisone
  - Side effects: many including glucose intolerance, Cushingoid changes, adrenocortical insufficiency, increased susceptibility to infection, muscle wasting, skin atrophy, peptic ulcer, dependence
  - Contraindications
    - Absolute: abrupt discontinuation in a steroid dependent patient
    - Relative: tntc
- Methotrexate and Cyclophosphamide are both antineoplastic agents and should only be prescribed by physicians specifically trained in their use.
- Aspirin
  - Side effects: GI upset, bleeding
  - Contraindications
    - Absolute: significant aspirin allergy

FOLLOW-UP
- Aggressive respond to vascular crises with arterial bypass or angioplasty is felt to increase longevity in Takayasu's. Aortic valve replacement or aneurysm repair occasionally indicated.

COMPLICATIONS AND PROGNOSIS

Complications
- aortic valve regurgitation, aneurysm formation, sequelae of branch vessel occlusion depend on areas of involvement (stroke, limb ischemia, renovascular hypertension, gut ischemia, coronary ischemia), blindness (Giant Cell),

Prognosis
- Takayasu's: unpredictable course, generally slowly progressive: In older series, 97% 5 year survival if no major complications, 59% after development of major complications. Aggressive management of vascular crises likely improves survival
- Relevant survival data for other etiologies is scarce

APHASIA

MICHAEL J. AMINOFF, MD, DSc

HISTORY & PHYSICAL

Expressive (Broca) aphasia
■ Speech telegrammic or lost; repetition, reading aloud & writing impaired
■ Associated features may include right hemiparesis, hemisensory disturbance

Receptive (Wernicke) Aphasia
■ Impaired comprehension & speech repetition; fluent but meaningless spontaneous speech; word salad; paraphasic errors; dysnomia
■ Associated features may include right hemianopia

Global Aphasia
■ Motor + receptive aphasia

Conduction Aphasia
■ Impaired repetition

TESTS
■ Cranial MRI or CT: lesion in inferior frontal region (expressive aphasia) or posterior part of superior temporal gyrus (receptive aphasia); may be diffuse cerebral atrophy if aphasia is part of global cognitive impairment

DIFFERENTIAL DIAGNOSIS
■ Aphasia is symptom, not diagnosis
■ Most common causes are stroke, tumor, dementing disorder

MANAGEMENT
■ Depends on cause (nature of lesion on imaging study)

TREATMENT
■ Treat underlying cause
■ Speech therapy

SPECIFIC THERAPY
N/A

FOLLOW-UP
N/A

COMPLICATIONS AND PROGNOSIS
■ Depend on cause

APLASTIC ANEMIA

ROBERT A. BRODSKY, MD

HISTORY & PHYSICAL

History
- Drugs (anti-epileptics, chloramphenicol, etc.) account for <10% of cases.
- viruses (EBV, seronegative hepatitis, etc.)
- benzene
- radiation
- idiopathic (> 80% of cases)

Signs & Symptoms
- anemia (fatigue, dyspnea), thrombocytopenia (petechiae, easy bruising, bleeding), neutropenia (fever/infection)
  - ➤ Family history of cytopenias

TESTS
- CBC with differential × 2
- Reticulocyte count
- Bone marrow aspirate and biopsy
- Bone marrow cytogenetics
  - ➤ Bone marrow CD34 count
- Liver enzymes
- HLA typing
- Chromosomal breakage studies (DEB) in patients <40 years old
- Flow cytometry (CD59 or FLAER) for paroxysmal nocturnal hemoglobinuria (PNH)

DIFFERENTIAL DIAGNOSIS
- MDS (cytogenetics, morphology, flow cytometry)
- PNH (flow cytometry for loss of GPI-anchors, aerolysin-based assays)
- Fanconi anemia (chromosomal breakage studies, DEB)
- Hairy cell leukemia
  - ➤ Dyskeratosis congenita

MANAGEMENT

What to Do First
- transfuse only if symptomatic

- transfuse only CMV negative, irradiated blood products, avoid family members as donors
- treat any underlying infections
- consider referral to specialized center

SPECIFIC THERAPY
- indicated for patients with severe aplastic anemia defined as:
  - hypocellular bone marrow (< 25% cellularity) and
  - at least two markedly depressed peripheral blood counts:
    - neutrophils <500
    - platelets <20,000
    - corrected reticulocytes <1% (<60,000/microliter)

Treatment Options
1) allogeneic bone marrow transplantation (Rx of choice in children and young adults who have an HLA-matched sibling)
- Advantages:
  - Restores normal hematopoiesis (curative potential, 80–90%)
  - Little risk of relapse or secondary clonal disease
  - Prompt hematopoietic recovery
- Disadvantages:
  - High morbidity/mortality (GVHD, infections) especially in patients >40
  - cure rate <50% in patients >40
  - Not available to most patients (age restriction, requires HLA-identical sib for best results)
  - alternative donors (unrelated or mismatch grafts) have lower cure rates because of GVHD and generally are not recommended for initial therapy.
2) antithymocyte globulin and cyclosporine (ATG/CSA)
- Advantages:
  - Does not require a stem cell donor
  - No risk of GVHD
  - No age restrictions, available to virtually all patients with SAA
- Disadvantages:
  - Does not usually restore normal hematopoiesis (not curative)
  - majority of patients will relapse, become dependent of cyclosporine or develop secondary clonal disease (PNH, MDS, leukemia)
  - Slow hematopoietic improvement
  - Serum sickness, requirement for high-dose steroids, risk of avascular necrosis (up to 10%)

3) High-dose cyclophosphamide (50 mg/kg/d × 4 days)
- Advantages:
  - ➤ Restores normal hematopoiesis (curative potential): Low risk of relapse. Best results (~70% cure rate) if used as initial therapy; lower response rate in patients previously treated with ATG/CSA
  - ➤ Does not require a stem cell donor
  - ➤ No risk of GVHD
  - ➤ Few age restrictions, available to virtually all patients with SAA
- Disadvantages:
  - ➤ Slow hematopoietic improvement
  - ➤ Intensive supportive care required during first 2 months

FOLLOW-UP
- Regularly assess potential complications of disease and therapy.
- bone marrow transplantation: daily blood counts
  - ➤ monitor for infections/bleeding
  - ➤ monitor for GVHD
- ATG/CSA: daily blood counts
  - ➤ monitor for infections/bleeding
  - ➤ allergic reactions to ATG

Monitor for development of PNH or MDS
- high-dose cyclophosphamide: daily blood counts
  - ➤ monitor for infections/bleeding

Monitor for development of PNH or MDS

Routine
- bone marrow aspirate, biopsy and cytogenetics are discretionary.

COMPLICATIONS AND PROGNOSIS
- ATG/CSA:
  - ➤ serum sickness
    - hyperglycemia
    - PNH (10% to 30%)
    - MDS (10% to 20%)
    - relapse (20% to 40%)
    - aseptic necrosis (5% to 10%)
- bone marrow transplantation GVHD (acute and chronic)
  - ➤ second cancers (rare)

Prognosis
- 1 year mortality > than 70% with supportive care alone
- mortality following therapy is greatest in the first three months

■ complete responders to therapy (normalization of blood counts off all therapy) probably have a normal life expectancy

APPARENT MINERALOCORTICOID EXCESS

MICHEL BAUM, MD

HISTORY & PHYSICAL
■ Hypertension

TESTS
■ Hypokalemic alkalosis with low plasma aldosterone and renin
■ Elevated urinary cortisol metabolites

DIFFERENTIAL DIAGNOSIS
■ Autosomal recessive: Absence of 11-beta hydroxysteroid dehydrogenase (11-beta OH dehydrogenase), which inactivates cortisol – in the absence of 11-beta OH dehydrogenase, cortisol binds to the mineralocorticoid receptor, resulting in mineralocorticoid action in distal nephron
■ Acquired: 11-beta OH steroid dehydrogenase inactivated by glycyrrhizic acid in black licorice and chewing tobacco
■ Distinguish from other causes of hypertension

MANAGEMENT
■ Low-salt diet

SPECIFIC THERAPY
■ Low-salt diet
■ Amiloride or triamterene to block sodium channel in distal nephron

FOLLOW-UP
■ To ensure control of hypertension

COMPLICATIONS AND PROGNOSIS
■ Complications secondary to hypertension

APPENDICITIS

MARK A. VIERRA, MD

HISTORY & PHYSICAL

History
■ Most common in younger age groups

Signs & Symptoms
- Pain most common presenting symptom
- Early pain visceral; often periumbilical or diffuse, may not be recalled by pt
- Later pain may be more localized, typically to RLQ
- Late pain may be atypical if appendiceal location unusual: eg, if retrocecal, in low pelvis, in LLQ, or other locations
- Anorexia very common
- Nausea common but almost never precedes pain
- Vomiting variably present & not usually severe
- Duration of symptoms important: perforation unusual w/ symptoms <24 h; high fever & toxicity unusual w/ short history of symptoms
- Localized tenderness in RLQ most reliable sign
- Fever variably present: less common w/ shorter duration of symptoms, more likely w/ perforation
- CVA tenderness suggests retrocecal appendicitis (or other diagnosis)
- If right adnexal tenderness or anterior rectal tenderness present, consider pelvic appendicitis
- Distal small bowel obstruction in young pt w/o prior abdominal surgery likely to be appendicitis w/ abscess
  - ➤ Difficult hosts to diagnose appendicitis:
    - Pregnancy
    - Diabetes
    - Infants & young children

TESTS

Laboratory
- WBC more likely ? or left shifted w/ greater duration of appendicitis: may be normal in 1/3 or more of pts

Imaging
- Plain abdominal x-ray: highly suggestive of appendicitis if fecalith present; distal small bowel obstruction in young pt w/o prior surgery likely to be appendiceal abscess
- Appendiceal US >90% sensitive in thin pts by experienced ultrasonographer; normal appendixes not usually identified
- Abdominal CT +/− contrast probably >90% sensitive & specific for appendicitis

DIFFERENTIAL DIAGNOSIS
- Mesenteric lymphadenitis
- Diverticulitis

- Crohn disease
- Pelvic inflammatory disease
- Ovarian cyst
- Omental torsion or infarction
- Gastroenteritis
- Cancer of appendix or cecum: be especially wary in older pt or in presence of iron deficiency anemia
- Urinary tract infection or stone
- Abdominal wall pain (Houdini died of a perforated ulcer after mistakenly undergoing operation for appendicitis)
- No clear diagnosis found in many pts thought to have appendicitis

MANAGEMENT

What to Do First

- If diagnosis uncertain, may improve accuracy to observe pt in hospital

General Measures

- Uncomplicated appendicitis:
- Early operation usually recommended
- Most resolve w/ antibiotics, but recurrence common
- Complicated appendicitis:
- Perforation w/ peritonitis: proceed to appendectomy
- Abscess/phlegmon: usually treat w/ percutaneous drainage &/or antibiotics followed by interval appendectomy 6–12 wk later

SPECIFIC THERAPY

- Appendectomy:
- Performed either by laparotomy or laparoscopy
- If diagnosis secure, RLQ incision appropriate; if not, midline incision or laparoscopy provides better exposure of entire abdomen
- Negative appendectomy rates of ~10–15% generally considered acceptable; diagnosis much more difficult in women of childbearing age
- Perioperative antibiotics routinely given: 1 dose or 24 h for uncomplicated appendicitis, longer for abscess or perforation
- Third-generation cephalosporin or extended-spectrum penicillin w/ anaerobic coverage appropriate for most pts
- Percutaneous drainage of appendiceal abscess & antibiotics:
- Treatment of choice for established abscess w/o toxicity
- Antibiotics alone:

- Appropriate for selected cases of appendiceal phlegmon, followed by interval appendectomy

FOLLOW-UP
- No specific follow-up needed

COMPLICATIONS AND PROGNOSIS
- Wound infection most common complication, esp if appendix gangrenous, perforated, or in presence of abscess
- Pelvic abscess more common w/ advanced appendicitis, may require percutaneous drainage
- Small bowel obstruction may occur even years later after any laparotomy
- Cecal fistula relatively uncommon; may be more common in Crohn disease

---

ARTERIAL EMBOLUS

RAJABRATA SARKAR, MD

HISTORY & PHYSICAL
Sources for arterial embolus

Most Common
- Atrial fibrillation
- Myocardial infarction within 6 weeks
- History of prior arterial embolus

Less Common
- Rheumatic heart disease
- Left ventricular aneurysm
- Prosthetic cardiac valve
- Endocarditis
- Dilated cardiomyopathy
- Atrial myxomas
- Aortic aneurysm
- Aortoiliac occlusive disease
- Paradoxical embolus (venous origin)

Signs & Symptoms
- 5 P's
  - ➤ Pain

➤ Pallor
➤ Paresthesia
➤ Pulselessness
➤ Paralysis (ominous + late sign)
▣ Level of clinical ischemia is generally one anatomic level below the arterial occlusion

TESTS
Blood
▣ Creatine kinase (rhabdomyolysis)
▣ Blood gas and electrolytes (lactic acidosis, hyperkalemia)

Urine
▣ Urine myoglobin (from muscle necrosis)

Specific Tests
▣ Doppler determination of pulses
▣ Allows comparison with other limb when those pulses are not palpable

Angiogram
▣ Usually unnecessary when clinical presentation is obvious
▣ Needed in patients with underlying peripheral occlusive disease where question of arterial thrombosis vs. embolus arises

DIFFERENTIAL DIAGNOSIS
Arterial Thrombosis
▣ Chronic ischemic changes in contralateral limb as atherosclerosis is usually symmetrical (but 40% of embolus pts have occlusive changes due to assoc. athero)
▣ History of prior peripheral vascular bypass
▣ Generally has slower onset
▣ May require angiogram to differentiate from embolus

Aortic Dissection
▣ Back, chest and abdominal pain
▣ Both legs are usually involved in dissection
▣ Rarely causes severe peripheral ischemia
▣ Confirm diagnosis with aortic imaging (MR, CT, TEE, etc.)

Neurological Paralysis
▣ Check pulses in all pts alleged to have neuro cause of paralysis or paresthesia

■ Erroneous attribution of weakness and paresthesia to stroke or other neuro cause is most frequent reason for limb loss after arterial embolus

MANAGEMENT

What to Do First

■ Intravenous heparin
  ➤ Give regardless of arterial embolus or thrombosis
  ➤ Prevents propagation of thrombus
■ Hydration
  ➤ Prevent intravascular depletion and prerenal azotemia
  ➤ Alkalinize urine with IV sodium bicarbonate (prevent myoglobin precipitation and acute tubular necrosis)

SPECIFIC THERAPY

Indications for Treatment

■ All patients require specific therapy to avoid limb loss

Surgical Embolectomy

■ Treatment of choice for most extremity emboli
■ Quickest way to restore flow (important if there are sensory or motor changes indicative of advanced ischemia)
■ Requires anesthesia and associated risk
■ Complications
■ Severe hyperkalemia upon reperfusion (cardiac arrest)
■ Compartment syndrome after reperfusion (fasciotomy if preoperative ischemia > 4 hrs)
■ Amputation (15%)
■ Related to duration and level of ischemia
■ Mortality (7–34%)
■ Renal failure (10%)
■ Contraindications (Relative)
■ Systemic illness too severe to tolerate anesthesia (embolectomy can be done under local anesthesia with sedation)

Thrombolytic Therapy

■ Avoids anesthesia, stress and blood loss of surgery
■ Allows lysis of thrombus in small vessels and branches
■ Requires 24–48 hours for restoration of flow
■ Risk of bleeding (puncture site, intracranial)
■ Complications
  ➤ Similar to surgical embolectomy

➤ Bleeding at puncture site
➤ Intracranial bleeding
➤ Systemic fibrinolysis
■ Contraindications (Absolute)
➤ Severe ischemia with neuromuscular changes requiring immediate revascularization
➤ Contraindications (Relative)
➤ Bleeding or risk of bleeding (recent surgery or catheterization)

Expectant Therapy (Amputation)
■ Reserved for clearly nonsalvagable limbs (muscle rigor, extensive gangrene)
■ Usually requires above-knee amputation
■ Little chance of ambulation afterwards

FOLLOW-UP

During Treatment
■ Surgical Embolectomy
■ Postoperative long-term anticoagulation (heparin and then coumadin)
■ Echocardiogram and TEE to evaluate source of embolus
■ Study aorta (Angio, MRA) if cardiac w/u negative for thrombus
■ Thrombolytic therapy
■ Serial angiograms and neurological exams to assess progression of lytic therapy
■ Serial fibrinogen levels to assess systemic fibrinolysis

Routine
■ Long-term anticoagulation reduces recurrent emboli

COMPLICATIONS AND PROGNOSIS

Complications
■ Hyperkelemia from reperfusion
➤ Vent first 500cc of venous blood to prevent Compartment syndrome
➤ Common if ischemia > 4 hrs
➤ Not seen until 12–24 hrs after reperfusion
➤ First sign is pain on passive motion of foot or decreased sensation between 1st/2nd toes
➤ Compartment pressures can be measured if exam is unreliable
➤ Prevent with prophyactic fasciotomy

- Renal failure
  - ➤ Prevent with alkalinization of urine
  - ➤ Injury is acute tubular necrosis, resolves with support (dialysis)
- Amputation
  - ➤ Establishing flow to deep femoral artery may allow below-knee rather than above-knee amputation
  - ➤ Above-knee amputation usually prevents later ambulation
- Bleeding complications (thrombolytic therapy)
  - ➤ Require discontinuation of thrombolytic therapy

Prognosis
- Short-term
  - ➤ Mortality ranges from 7–34%, proportional to underlying disease
  - ➤ Amputation required in 15% despite aggressive therapy
- Long term
  - ➤ Recurrent emboli in 40–45% without anticoagulation and 10% with anticoagulation
  - ➤ Long-term survival is limited (<60% at 5 years)

ASCARIASIS

J. GORDON FRIERSON, MD

HISTORY & PHYSICAL

History
- Life cycle: Eggs of Ascaris lumbricoides passed in the stool must incubate in soil at least 2 weeks to be infectious, are ingested in contaminated food or water, hatch in small intestine. Larvae penetrate gut wall, migrate to lungs in blood stream, penetrate alveolar-capillary barrier, migrate up tracheobronchial tree, are swallowed and mature in small intestine, where they mate and produce eggs. It takes 10–12 weeks from ingestion of eggs to production of eggs.
- Exposure: ingestion of food or water contaminated with infectious eggs (i.e., after soil incubation)

Signs & Symptoms
- During migration, cough, wheeze, fever, and rales may appear. In intestinal phase, usually no symptoms, or non-specific indigestion, epigastric discomfort. Worms may be passed rectally, or may migrate up esophagus and be expectorated.

TESTS
- Basic tests: blood: eosinophilia present in migration phase
- Basic tests: urine: normal
- Specific tests: Stool for O&P will diagnose all but single male infections. Identification of passed worm is diagnostic.
- Other tests: In migration phase, chest X-ray may show patchy infiltrates (Loeffler's syndrome). Worms may be seen on upper GI series, and ultrasound will usually detect worms in biliary tree.

DIFFERENTIAL DIAGNOSIS
- In migratory phase, a similar syndrome is seen with hookworm, strongyloidiasis, and schistosomiasis in their migratory phases. Other causes of Loeffler's syndrome, asthma, industrial exposures, etc., can be confused with pulmonary ascariasis.
- In intestinal phase, mild symptoms mimic almost any mild GI disorder.

MANAGEMENT

What to Do First
- Assess severity of infection, look for worms in ectopic positions.

General Measures
- Find source of infection. Instruct on hygiene.

SPECIFIC THERAPY

Indications
- Probably all patients should be treated, as the worms may migrate, leading to complications.

Treatment Options
- Mebendazole for 3 days
- Pyrantel pamoate
- Albendazole

Side Effects & Complications
- Mild nonspecific intestinal complaints may occur, and pyrantel pamoate may rarely cause headache, dizziness, rash. Occasionally a worm will migrate during treatment.
- Contraindications: First-trimester pregnant women. Treat them later in pregnancy, preferably with pyrantel pamoate.

FOLLOW-UP

Routine

- Stool O&P 2 or more weeks after treatment

COMPLICATIONS AND PROGNOSIS

- Worms in biliary tree may cause symptoms of cholecystitis; more rarely, pancreatitis occurs from worms in pancreatic duct. Intestinal obstruction may occur in small children.
- Worms in biliary or pancreatic systems may necessitate surgery. Intestinal obstruction requires surgery.

ASCITES

ANDY S. YU, MD and EMMET B. KEEFFE, MD

HISTORY & PHYSICAL

History

- Risk factors for liver disease: excessive alcohol consumption, injection drug use, blood transfusion, multiple sexual partners, occupational exposure, Asian country of origin, family history
- Risk factors for nonhepatic causes of ascites: TB, cancer

Signs & Symptoms

- Lower extremity edema; anasarca
- Physical findings of chronic liver disease: firm liver, splenomegaly, jaundice, gynecomastia, vascular spiders, palmar erythema, asterixis
- Physical findings of heart disease: abnormal jugular venous distention
- Physical findings indicative of malignancy: nodule in umbilicus or supraclavicular region

TESTS

Basic Tests

- Ascitic fluid cell count:
  - ➤ Neutrophil count >250/mm3 presumed to be infection
  - ➤ Tuberculous peritonitis & peritoneal carcinomatosis predominantly lymphocytic WBC count
- Ascitic fluid albumin to calculate serum-ascites albumin gradient (SAAG) (serum albumin minus ascitic fluid albumin)

➤ SAAG ≥1.1 gm/dL (high gradient) = portal hypertension
➤ SAAG ≤1.1 gm/dL (low gradient) = absence of portal hypertension

■ Ascitic fluid total protein (AFTP):
  ➤ AFTP >2.5 gm/dL in 20% of uncomplicated ascites
  ➤ DDx of high AFTP: peritoneal carcinomatosis, tuberculous peritonitis, cardiac ascites, Budd-Chiari syndrome, myxedema, biliary ascites, & pancreatic ascites

■ Culture:
  ➤ Results optimized by bedside inoculation of 10 mL of ascitic fluid into each of two culture bottles

Optional Tests
■ Glucose: may drop to 0.0 mg/dL in gut perforation
■ LDH:
  ➤ Pts w/ neutrocytic ascites & 2 of following 3 ascitic fluid findings may have surgical peritonitis:
  ➤ Total protein >1.0 gm/dL
  ➤ Glucose <50 mg/dL
  ➤ LDH >upper limit of normal for serum

■ Amylase:
  ➤ Amylase in uncomplicated ascites less than half of serum
  ➤ Ascitic fluid amylase level averages 2000 IU/L in pancreatic ascites

■ Triglyceride: = 200 mg/dL & usually >1000 mg/dL in chylous ascites
■ Cytology:
  ➤ Positive only in peritoneal carcinomatosis
  ➤ Negative in hepatocellular carcinoma, massive liver metastases, or lymphoma w/o peritoneal metastases

DIFFERENTIAL DIAGNOSIS
■ High SAAG ascites: cirrhosis, alcoholic hepatitis, hepatocellular carcinoma, massive liver metastases, fulminant hepatic failure, cardiac ascites, myxedema, Budd-Chiari syndrome, portal vein thrombosis, veno-occlusive disease of liver, acute fatty liver of pregnancy, mixed ascites

■ Low SAAG ascites: peritoneal carcinomatosis, tuberculous peritonitis, pancreatic ascites, biliary ascites, peritonitis from connective tissue disease, bowel infarction or perforation

MANAGEMENT

What to Do First
- Establish cause
- Determine SAAG

General Measures
- Low SAAG: management disease-specific & pts do not respond to dietary salt restriction & diuretics
- High SAAG: dietary salt restriction & diuretics

SPECIFIC THERAPY

Treatment Options: Routine
- Dietary sodium restriction to 2 g daily
- Oral diuretics, including spironolactone & furosemide
- Single 5 L paracentesis for tense ascites

Treatment Options: Refractory Ascites
- Liver transplantation
- Large-volume paracentesis: albumin infusion of 6–10 g/L of ascitic fluid removed optional for paracentesis of >5 L
- Transjugular intrahepatic portosystemic shunt (TIPS)
- Peritoneovenous shunt

Side Effects & Contraindications
- Oral diuretics:
  - Side effects: renal failure, electrolyte disturbances, hepatic encephalopathy and, with spironolactone, gynecomastia
  - Contraindications:
    - Absolute: serum creatinine >2.0 mg/dL, serum sodium <120 mmol/L
    - Relative: serum creatinine 1.5–2.0 mg/dL
- Liver transplantation:
  - Side effects: allograft rejection/dysfunction, surgical complications, infections
  - Contraindications: absolute: advanced cardiopulmonary diseases, HIV seropositivity, extrahepatic malignancy, active substance abuse, medical noncompliance, anatomic anomalies precluding transplant surgery
- Large-volume paracentesis:
  - Side effects: asymptomatic changes in electrolytes & creatinine, procedure-related complications

➤ Contraindications: absolute: clinically evident disseminated intravascular coagulopathy or fibrinolysis
- TIPS:
  ➤ Side effects: hepatic encephalopathy (23%), liver failure, post-procedural bleed, stent occlusion, heart failure, hemolysis
  ➤ Contraindications: absolute: advanced liver disease, heart failure, pulmonary hypertension, advanced renal dysfunction
- Peritoneovenous shunt:
  ➤ Side effects: shunt thrombosis, consumptive coagulopathy, heart failure, bowel obstruction
  ➤ Contraindications: absolute: active or prior spontaneous bacterial peritonitis, heart failure, renal failure

FOLLOW-UP

During Treatment
- Regularly monitor serum electrolytes & creatinine
- Daily body weight:
  ➤ No limit to weight loss in presence of pedal edema
  ➤ Diuresis limited to 750 mL/d once edema resolved

Routine
- Clinical follow-up & renal chemistry q 1–3 mo
- Medical compliance reinforced

COMPLICATIONS AND PROGNOSIS

Complications
- Spontaneous ascitic fluid infection:
  ➤ 27% of pts w/ cirrhotic ascites on admission
  ➤ Long-term outpt prophylactic antibiotic after 1 episode of infection
- Hepatic hydrothorax:
  ➤ 5% of all pts w/ cirrhotic ascites
  ➤ Principles of management same as those for cirrhotic ascites; TIPS & liver transplant if conservative measures fail
- Abdominal wall hernia:
  ➤ 20% among all pts w/ ascites
  ➤ Surgical repair considered electively, postponed until transplant surgery for transplant candidates, but performed emergently for incarceration or rupture of hernia

Prognosis
- 50% 2-y survival once ascites occurs

■ 25% 1-y survival once ascites becomes refractory
■ 20% 1-y survival after first episode of spontaneous ascitic fluid infection

ASPERGILLOSIS

RICHARD A. JACOBS, MD, PhD

HISTORY & PHYSICAL

History
■ Aspergillus species ubiquitous molds found in every country
■ Found in soil and decomposing vegetable matter
■ Aspergillus fumigatus cause about 90% of invasive disease
■ Nosocomial infection via airborne transmission has been suggested after case clusters in transplantation wards have been reported
■ Airborne conidia or spores can enter the alveoli, nose, paranasal sinuses, ear or skin if traumatized (IV sites, occlusive dressings, etc)

Signs & Symptoms
■ Continuum of colonization to invasive disease
■ Three main spectra of disease: allergic bronchopulmonary aspergillosis (ABPA), pulmonary aspergilloma and invasive aspergillois (lungs, sinuses, central nervous system, ears, eyes, skin, other sites)
■ Allergic bronchopulmonary aspergillosis (ABPA):
  ➤ Hypersensitivity pulmonary disease
  ➤ Usually caused by A fumigatus
  ➤ Suspect in corticosteroid-dependent asthmatic with wheezing, pulmonary infiltrates, fevers, eosinophilia in sputum and blood and sputum with brown flecks or plugs
■ Pulmonary aspergilloma:
  ➤ Comprised of matted tangle of Aspergillus hyphae, mucus, fibrin and cellular debris in a pulmonary cavity (eg, as in bullous emphysema or cavitary tuberculosis)
  ➤ Hemoptysis is common; cause of mortality in 25% patients with aspergilloma
■ Invasive aspergillosis:
  ➤ Think of risk factors for invasive disease: neutropenia, long-term corticosteroid therapy, bone marrow or solid transplantation patients

- ➤ Extremely high mortality (up to 100%) despite prompt surgical and medical therapy
- ➤ High mortality may reflect rapid growth and angio-invasiveness of organism
- ■ Manifestations depend on site of infection:
  - ➤ Lung:
    - • Most common site of primary invasive disease
    - • Neutropenic patients may have a fulminant course with high fevers and dense infiltrates on chest x-ray
    - • Cavitation can occur during bone marrow recovery as seen on CT
    - • Hemoptysis, pneumothorax and dissemination may occur
  - ➤ Sinus:
    - • Indolent or fulminant based on host factors
    - • Can present as headaches, sinus tenderness, proptosis or monocular blindness
    - • Neutropenic patients may progress rapidly with spread to contiguous structures, vascular invasion and necrosis
  - ➤ Central nervous system:
    - • May be seen as brain or epidural abscesses, meningitis (more unusual) or subarachnoid hemorrhage
    - • Strokes may occur with cerebral vessel invasion and infarction
  - ➤ Skin:
    - • Usually via hematogenous spread; primary infection is less common
    - • Present as erythematous papules that progress to pustules; eventually an ulcer covered by a black eschar forms
    - • Primary skin infections associated with burn wounds and contaminated adhesive dressings

TESTS

Laboratory
- ■ Blood cultures and CSF rarely positive
  - ➤ Isolation in urine, sputum, stool or wound interpreted in context of the host (eg, sputum culture in a neutropenic patient with an infiltrate may suggest invasive disease)
  - ➤ Basic studies: histopathology
    - • Acute angle, septated, branching and non-pigmented hyphae
    - • Best seen with Gomori methenamine silver and Periodic acid-Schiff stains

➤ Basic studies: culture
  • Important for definitive diagnosis of invasive disease together with histopathology
➤ Other studies: serology
  • Antibodies to Aspergillus traditionally not helpful in diagnosis of invasive disease
  • However, precipitating antibodies to Aspergillus antigen a criterion in diagnosis of ABPA EIA, ELISA and immunoblot methods may show promise in the future
    Galactomannan – carbohydrate component of Aspergillus cell wall. FDA-approved antigen assay in serum. Sensitivity 81–94%, specificity 84–99% depending on cutoff values used. Useful as adjunct to clinical, radiologic, and microbiologic findings but does not replace these.

Imaging
■ CXR:
  ➤ Late findings include cavities or wedge-shaped pleural-based densities for invasive pulmonary disease.
■ CT:
  ➤ May precede CXR findings
  ➤ A "halo sign" is an early sign, seen as a pulmonary nodule surrounded by an area of low attenuation; may be caused by bleeding or edema surrounding an area of ischemia.
  ➤ The "crescent sign" is a later sign referring to lung tissue that has infarcted and contracted around a nodule, leaving an air crescent.

DIFFERENTIAL DIAGNOSIS
■ Histopathologically, Aspergillus hyphae are very difficult to distinguish from Pseudallescheria boydii, Fusarium and some other molds.
■ Culture is key to confirm the histopathologic appearance in tissue because treatment may be different depending on the mold isolated.

MANAGEMENT
What to Do First
■ First assess risk factors for invasive disease: neutropenia, prolonged use of corticosteroid and other immunosuppressive therapy, bone marrow or solid organ transplant patient.

- If present, have a low threshold for instituting high-dose amphotericin, even in absence of conclusive data.
- Think of involving surgical services early if surgical excision for biopsy or therapy (brain abscess, sinus disease) may be needed.

General Measures
- General supportive care, reverse neutropenia, dose reduction of corticosteroids and other immunosuppressives if possible; await bone marrow recovery

SPECIFIC THERAPY

Indications
- Everyone for whom invasive disease is suspected; this is a rapidly progressive disease with a high mortality even if therapy is initiated promptly.

Treatment Options
- Medical Therapy:
  - Voriconazole: Has replaced amphotericin as the initial agent of choice. Start IV, can switch to PO after 7 days if improvement seen.
  - Amphotericin:
    - Use at maximally tolerated doses.
    - Lipid-based formulations of amphotericin may be substituted if the patient develops nephrotoxicity on therapy, or has baseline impaired renal function.
  - Itraconazole:
    - Itraconazole oral therapy may be an option to initiate therapy if the patient is not ill, for pulmonary disease, or as follow-up therapy to amphotericin once the progression of disease is halted.
    - Itraconazole cyclodextran solution may have increased bioavailability.
  - Caspofungin:
    - In the echinocandin class, approved for invasive aspergillosis. No PO form available. Commonly has been used in salvage therapy.
  - Other agents:
    - New triazoles such as posaconazole and ravuconazole may be effective alternatives for invasive disease.

- Combination therapy – observational studies have suggested some benefit in salvage regimens (ampho + itra, liposomal ampho + caspofungin, vori + caspofungin) but there have been no randomized controlled trials to show efficacy.
- Corticosteroids are used for exacerbations of ABPA.

■ Surgery:
➤ Excision may be helpful for some cases of localized pulmonary disease.
➤ Surgical debridement can be curative in invasive sinus disease but may increase mortality in neutropenic patients.
➤ In brain abscesses, surgical drainage has an important diagnostic and therapeutic role.

Side Effects & Contraindications

Voriconazole:
  Side effects: vision changes, nausea, fever, rash, elevated LFTs
Contraindications: many drug-drug interactions

■ Amphotericin B:
➤ Side effects: fevers, chills, nausea, vomiting and headaches; rigors may be prevented by the addition of hydrocortisone to bag, meperidine may treat rigors; nephrotoxicity; electrolyte disturbance (renal tubular acidosis, hypokalemia, hypomagnesemia)
➤ Contraindications: if Cr 2.5–3.0, may consider giving lipid-based amphotericin product

■ Itraconazole:
➤ Side effects: nausea, vomiting, anorexia, abdominal pain, rash; rarely hypokalemia and hepatitis
➤ Contraindications: end-stage renal disease for cyclodextran solution; lower cyclosporin dose when concomitantly given; may dangerously increase serum levels of digoxin and loratadine, causing fatal arrhythmias

FOLLOW-UP

■ Duration of therapy is unknown, but for severe invasive disease, most treat with voriconazole IV then PO or amphotericin IV +/− follow-up itraconazole therapy depending on clinical response.
■ Follow patients for clinical improvement, resolution of underlying risk factors (this may be the most important factor) and radiographic resolution of lesions.

COMPLICATIONS AND PROGNOSIS

Prognosis
- Invasive disease:
  - ➤ Extremely high mortality in the immunocompromised host, even with prompt therapy
  - ➤ Sinus: 50% mortality
  - ➤ CNS: up to 100% mortality

Prevention
- Use of rooms with high-efficiency particulate air filters (HEPA) in severely neutropenic patients (such as bone marrow transplant) may have efficacy.

ASTHMA

STEPHEN C. LAZARUS, MD

HISTORY & PHYSICAL

History
- Recurrent chest tightness, dyspnea, wheezing, cough (may be only symptom)
- Onset in childhoold or as adult
- Frequent or severe "chest colds"
- Associated with family/personal history of atopy, allergic rhinitis
- More prevalent in male children, female adults
- Samter syndrome ("triad asthma"): nasal polyps, ASA sensitivity; asthma (3–10%)
- Early childhood infections may protect against asthma by favoring TH1 (vs TH2) phenotype (hygiene hypothesis)

Signs & Symptoms
- Exam may be normal
- Prolonged expiratory phase, wheezes, sternocleidomastoid retractions
- With severe obstruction, chest may be quiet
- Neither symptoms nor exam are predictors of severity of airflow obstruction

TESTS

Laboratory
- Basic blood tests: CBC (eosinophilia common)

Specific Tests
- Pulmonary function:
  - Every patient should have complete PFTs once to confirm diagnosis
  - Follow with spirometry and/or peak flow
  - May be normal between attacks
  - Variable airflow obstruction (decreased FEV_1, FVC, peak flow)
  - Reversible ($\geq$12% and $\geq$200 mL) with inhaled beta-agonist
- IgE elevated in most patients
- Allergy skin tests useful to identify triggers to avoid, or for hyposensitization in severe cases

Other Tests
- Bronchoprovocation (histamine or methacholine):
  - Asthmatics unusually sensitive ($PC_{20} = 8$ mg/mL)
  - Useful to confirm diagnosis if PFTs normal

DIFFERENTIAL DIAGNOSIS
- Children: bronchiolitis, cystic fibrosis
- Adults: COPD, vocal cord dysfunction, allergic bronchopulmonary aspergillosis, Churg-Strauss syndrome, polyarteritis nosodum, cardiac asthma

MANAGEMENT
- See NHLBI National Asthma Education and Prevention Program, Expert Panel Report 2: Guidelines for the Diagnosis and Management of Asthma (http://www.nhlbi.nih.gov/guidelines/asthma/asthgdln.htm)

Chronic Asthma

What to Do First
- Assess severity:
  - Mild intermittent: symptoms $\leq$2 d/wk; $\leq$2 nights/mo;
    - $FEV_1 \geq$80%; PEF variability <20%
  - Mild persistent: symptoms >2 d/wk; >2 nights/mo;
    - $FEV_1 \geq$80%; PEF variability 20–30%
  - Moderate persistent: symptoms daily; >1 night/wk;
    - FEV_1 60–80%; PEF variability >30%

➤ Severe persistent:symptoms continuously; frequently at night; FEV_1 ≤60%; PEF variability >30%

General Measures

■ Therapy aimed at reducing chronic inflammation ubiquitous in asthma
■ Goals: reduce symptoms, prevent exacerbations, normalize pulmonary function
■ Classes of pharmacotherapy:
➤ Relievers (albuterol, bitolterol, ipratropium, pirbuterol, metaproterenol, terbutaline)
➤ Controllers (inhaled corticosteroids, LTRAs, long-acting beta-agonists)

Acute Exacerbation of Asthma

What to Do First

■ Quick history and physical
■ Chest x-ray (only if suspect pneumonia, pneumothorax)
■ Assess SaO_2, PEF, or FEV_1
■ Administer oxygen if SaO_2 <93%
■ Albuterol MDI or nebulizer q 20–30 min × 4
■ Levalbuterol by nebulizer may be useful if $beta_2$ side effects a problem
■ Ipratropium may add to $beta_2$ effect
■ All patients should receive systemic steroids (oral = IV unless GI problem)
■ Continue inhaled corticosteroid
■ PEF or FEV_1 to assess response
■ Arrange follow-up within 48 h
■ Fatigue, altered mental status, $PaCO_2$ ≥42 suggest respiratory failure
■ Intubation, ventilation can be difficult

SPECIFIC THERAPY

■ Mild intermittent:
➤ rescue beta-agonist PRN
■ Mild persistent:
➤ low-dose inhaled steroid + rescue beta-agonist PRN, or
➤ LTRA + rescue beta-agonist PRN
■ Moderate persistent:
➤ Moderate dose inhaled steroid + rescue beta-agonist PRN, or

➤ Low-dose inhaled steroid + long-acting beta-agonist + rescue beta-agonist PRN, or

➤ Low-dose inhaled steroid + LTRA + rescue beta-agonist PRN

■ Severe persistent:

➤ High-dose inhaled steroid + long-acting beta-agonist + rescue beta-agonist PRN, or

➤ High-dose inhaled steroid + LTRA + rescue beta-agonist PRN, or

➤ High-dose inhaled steroid + long-acting beta-agonist +LTRA + rescue beta-agonist PRN, or

➤ Oral steroids + high-dose inhaled steroid + long-acting beta-agonist + LTRA + rescue beta-agonist PRN

■ Nonresponsive patients rare; some respond better to one agent than another

■ Most failures due to undertreatment, or failure to appreciate severity

■ Theophylline or nedocromil: alternative but less-effective controllers

■ Salmeterol should not be used as monotherapy: more exacerbations than with inhaled steroids

■ If symptoms resolve with treatment, continue × 1–3 mo before stepping down slowly

■ If symptoms persist, step-up; consider other diagnosis

Other Measures

■ Environmental controls (mattress covers; no pets, smoke, carpets, draperies) reduce bronchial hyperresponsiveness, frequency and severity of asthma

■ Annual influenza vaccine

■ Peak flow monitoring detects asymptomatic deterioration; reinforces improvement with therapy; increases adherence to prescribed medication regimen

■ Smoking cessation

■ Patient education (inhaler skills, rationale for meds, self-management) improves asthma control, reduces morbidity and mortality and costs

■ Action plan = specific written instructions:

➤ Daily medication regimen

➤ How to recognize exacerbation

➤ How to adjust medications

➤ When to seek help

■ Consider ASA, sulfite sensitivity, beta-blockers

■ Treat comorbid conditions (allergic rhinitis, sinusitis, GERD)

- Immunotherapy (shots) more useful for allergic rhinitis than asthma, but consider in severe disease
- For refractory disease consider macrolides (putative role of mycoplasma, chlamydia)
- Monoclonal antibody against IgE promising
- Refer to asthma specialist for life-threatening exacerbation, refractory symptoms, frequent or continuous steroids

FOLLOW-UP
- Q 6–12 mo if stable; more frequent if not
- Assess control by:
  - Spirometry or PEF at each visit
  - Rescue medication use
  - Frequency of nocturnal symptoms (ask!)
  - Exercise limitation
  - BID or periodic PEF monitoring in selected patients

COMPLICATIONS AND PROGNOSIS

Complications
- Inhaled steroids:
  - Local (thrush, dysphonia): dose- and technique-dependent; usually prevented by use of spacer and rinsing mouth
  - Systemic (adrenal suppression, osteoporosis, cataracts, growth retardation): rare at doses $\leq$400–800 mcg/d; titrate dose downward to minimize risk
- Beta2-agonists:
  - Tremor, tachycardia, hypokalemia (levalbuterol useful if these are problems)
  - Little evidence for deleterious effects from regular use
- Leukotriene receptor antagonists:
  - Transaminitis uncommon; assess for symptoms at each visit
  - Rare Churg-Strauss syndrome probably reflects unmasking of preexisting disease
- Respiratory failure:
  - 20–30% of near deaths occur in patients thought previously to be mild
  - Barotrauma major complication of mechanical ventilation; dramatically less with permissive hypercapnea

Prognosis
- Normal life expectancy

- Most patients can achieve good control with no limitation of function
- Asthmatics appear to lose lung function throughout life at a rate slightly faster than normals
- Chronic undertreatment may lead to nonreversible (fixed) airflow obstruction (remodelling)

ATELECTASIS

THOMAS SHAUGHNESSY, MD

HISTORY & PHYSICAL

Risk Factors
- Hypoventilation: impaired consciousness, obesity, supine position, general anesthesia, postop splinting after thoracic and upper abdominal surgery
- Hypersecretion: impaired secretion clearance, cystic fibrosis, bronchitis
- Cardiac: pulmonary edema
- Pulmonary: pneumonia, restrictive lung disease

Signs & Symptoms
- Tachypnea, shallow tidal volumes, hypoxia unresponsive to supplemental oxygen, consolidation on CXR, impaired cough and secretion clearance

TESTS
- Atelectasis often diagnosis of exclusion based on history, exam, and radiography

Basic Studies
- Auscultation and percussion: decreased breath sounds and tones over affected area
- SpO2 <90% on supplemental oxygen
- CXR:
  - ➤ Blunting of costophrenic angle, heart borders
  - ➤ Consolidation with circumscribed edges esp at fissures
  - ➤ Shifting of cardiac silhouette toward affected side

Advanced Studies
- CT: well-circumscribed consolidation

DIFFERENTIAL DIAGNOSIS
- Cardiac: unilateral or bilateral pulmonary edema
- Pulmonary: pneumonia, pleural effusion, interstitial lung disease, carcinoma, unilateral diaphragm paralysis

MANAGEMENT

What to Do First
- Supplemental oxygen
- Ensure adequate analgesia: consider regional anesthesia (epidural, intercostal blocks)
- Incentive spirometry and/or PEP therapy
- Institute respiratory support with bag-valve mask ventilation if mental status impaired

General Measures
- Tidal volume and FRC recruited through:
  - Enhanced spontaneous ventilation
  - Expectoration of secretions
  - Positive pressure ventilation
- Monitoring in ICU and serial ABG analysis with arterial catheter may be required if SpO2 remains <90%

SPECIFIC THERAPY

Indications
- Therapy should be instituted once diagnosis considered and work-up initiated

Treatment Options
- Incentive spirometry: q 2–4 h
- Aerosol therapy (saline, N-acetylcysteine) q 2–4 h
- PEP maneuvers by mask q 2–4 h
- Percussion therapy q 4 h (most effective for CF)
- Noninvasive ventilation support with CPAP: start by mask at 5 cm H_2O; 15 min q 3–4 h
- BiPAP by nasal or facemask: start at 10 cm H_2O inspiration/5 cm H_2O expiration
- Nasotracheal suctioning q 1–4 h, preferably via nasal airway
- Endotracheal intubation and mechanical ventilation and sighs if mental status/gag reflex impaired:
  - Initial ventilator settings:
    - FiO_2: 1.0
    - Tidal volume: 10–12 mL/kg

- RR: 10–12
- PEEP: 5–10 cm H_2O
- Pressure support: 5–10 cm H_2O
- Bronchoscopy:
  - Relatively ineffective if plug distal to mainstem bronchus
  - Reserve for life-threatening hypoxia with complete lung collapse (suggestive of treatable plug at mainstem bronchus)

Side Effects & Complications
- PEP/CPAP/BiPAP:
  - Inadequate delivery of positive pressure support
  - Pressure leak around mask
  - Gastric insufflation with aspiration
  - Pressure necrosis of nose and mouth by continuous mask pressure
  - Agitation requiring sedation
- Aerosol therapy: bronchospasm
- Percussion therapy: rib fracture
- Nasotracheal suction: epistaxis, bronchospasm, emesis, aspiration
- Endotracheal intubation:
  - Esophageal intubation
  - Failure to intubate trachea after suspending respiration with neuromuscular blocking agents
  - Mainstem bronchial intubation with intrapulmonary shunt
  - Agitation requiring sedation
  - Hypotension due to decreased venous return
  - Regurgitation and aspiration of gastric contents
  - Nosocomial pneumonia
  - Bronchoscopy: pneumothorax, bronchospasm
- Contraindications
  - Absolute:
    - Nasotracheal suctioning: coagulopathy, recent pharyngeal surgery
    - PEP/CPAP/BiPAP: severe GE reflux, recent pharyngeal surgery, severe agitation and poor cooperation
    - Percussion therapy: rib fracture
    - Endotracheal intubation: none
  - Relative:
    - PEP/CPAP/BiPAP: obesity, depressed consciousness, GE reflux, nasogastric nutrition

- Endotracheal intubation: terminal prognosis with advance directives

FOLLOW-UP

During Treatment
- ▓ Titrate pressure support levels in increments of 5 cm H_2O to achieve visible chest wall expansion
- ▓ Wean FiO2 and pressure support to keep SpO_2 >90% or PaO >60 mm Hg
- ▓ Treat bronchospasm with albuterol aerosol

Routine
- ▓ Serial CXRs
- ▓ Sedation as needed with narcotics and benzodiazepines for agitation
- ▓ Track progress with serial tidal volume and vital capacity measurements

COMPLICATIONS AND PROGNOSIS
- ▓ Respiratory failure

ATHEROSCLEROTIC OCCLUSIVE DISEASE

RAJABRATA SARKAR, MD

HISTORY & PHYSICAL

History
- ▓ Risk factors for atherosclerosis
  - ➤ Smoking (present in >90% of patients)
  - ➤ Hypertension
  - ➤ Hyperlipidemia
  - ➤ Hypercoaguable state (suspect in patients <50 years of age)
  - ➤ Diabetes
- ▓ Most have symptoms of atherosclerosis in another vascular bed (coronary, cerebrovascular, etc.)

Signs & Symptoms
- ▓ Cerebrovascular
  - ➤ Acute stroke
  - ➤ transient ischemic attacks (TIA)
    - transient monocular blindness
    - amourosis fugax – "curtain coming down partway across one eye"

- weakness or numbness of arm or leg
- dysarthria, aphasia
■ Visceral (mesenteric)
  ➤ Intestinal angina: Post-prandial abdominal pain, occurs 20 minutes after ingestion and resolves after several hours
  ➤ Weight loss + fear of food
■ Renal
  ➤ Ischemic nephropathy (elevated creatinine)
  ➤ Hypertension (poorly controlled by medication)
■ Extremity
  ➤ Claudication
    - Aching pain usually in upper calf reproducibly induced by exercise; never present at rest
    - Relieved by rest while standing (does not require sitting for relief)
    - Can radiate to buttocks and thighs with proximal (iliac) disease
    - Can occur in arm with subclavian stenosis
  ➤ Impotence
    - Suggests aorto-iliac occlusive disease
  ➤ Limb threat
    - Rest pain
      - Burning pain across ball of foot
      - awakens patient at night
      - relieved by dangling leg from bed or walking
      - does NOT radiate into calf or leg
      - NEVER starts in knee or upper leg
    - Gangrene
    - Non-healing arterial ulcers
      - Usually on distal aspects of foot
      - very tender
■ Embolism
  ➤ "Blue toe" syndrome
■ Carotid Bruit
  ➤ Associated (40%) with carotid stenosis
  ➤ Often not present with critical carotid stenosis
■ Abdominal bruit
  ➤ Suggestive of mesenteric or renal stenosis
■ Peripheral pulses
  ➤ Usually decreased in most patients with symptomatic occlusive leg disease
  ➤ Palpable pedal pulses may be present

- ■ Elevation on pallor
  - ➤ Cadaveric pallor on elevating foot 3 feet with patient supine
- ■ Ischemic changes in limb
  - ➤ Muscle atrophy, shiny skin
  - ➤ Loss of secondary skin structures (hair follicles)
- ■ Ankle/brachial index:
  - ➤ Ratio of blood pressure at ankle to that in arm. Put cuff on upper arm, Doppler (not palpate) the radial pulse and inflate cuff until Doppler signal is gone. Repeat at each ankle with cuff immediately above ankle.
  - ➤ Normal >0.9
  - ➤ Claudication 0.3–0.9
  - ➤ Limb Threat < 0.3
  - ➤ Falsely elevated (and not helpful) in diabetics with severely calcified non-compressible vessels

TESTS

Laboratory
- ■ Blood
  - ➤ Hypercoaguable evaluation for patients less than 50 years of age
  - ➤ Lipid profile

Non-Invasive Vascular Studies
- ■ Carotid Duplex (ultrasound imaging + Doppler velocity analysis)
  - ➤ Determines extent and severity of extracranial carotid stenosis
- ■ Captopril-renal scan
  - ➤ Useful as screening test for functional significance of renal artery stenosis
  - ➤ Can be false-negative in bilateral disease
- ■ Lower extremity segmental pressure and waveforms
  - ➤ Multiple cuffs on lower extremity
  - ➤ Defines extent and level of occlusive disease
  - ➤ Pressures and ratios not useful in diabetics with severely calcified vessels
    - • Pulse waveforms and toe pressures useful in diabetics
  - ➤ Magnetic resonance angiography (MRA)
  - ➤ Replaces angiography for diagnosis in many vascular beds (mesenteric, carotid)

Invasive Studies
- ■ Cerebral angiography

> Used if discrepancy between duplex and MRA findings
> Risk of stroke (1%)
- Angiography: Aortogram + runoff (lower extremities)
  > Often required to confirm diagnosis of mesenteric or renal stenosis
  > Lateral aortogram needed to visualize mesenteric orifices
  > Used only as a preoperative study (not for diagnosis) in lower extremity occlusive disease
  > Can be done with gadolinium (MRA constrast) to minimize renal risk in patients with renal insufficiency

DIFFERENTIAL DIAGNOSIS
Carotid Artery Occlusive Disease (TIA or Stroke)
- Intracranial tumors (often causes global neuro Sx (headache) r/o with CT or MRI)
- Intracranial vascular lesion (i.e. aneurysm, AVM) (may need intracranial views on angio to exclude)
- Arrhythmia causing neuro symptoms (rarely causes unilateral ocular symptoms or focal neuro changes)
- Other source of embolic stroke (usually cardiac) (difficult to prove origin of cerebral embolus if patient has multiple possible sources i.e. aortic and carotid lesions)

Visceral Occlusive Disease (Intestinal Angina)
- Gastroesophageal reflux
- Gallbladder disease
- Variant angina
- Intra-abdominal malignancy
- Chronic pancreatitis

Renal Artery Occlusive Disease (Hypertension, Renal Insufficiency)
- Parenchymal renal disease (appropriate serum and urine tests)
- Diabetic nephrosclerosis (difficult to differentiate from ischemic nephropathy)
- Hypertensive nephrosclerosis (difficult to differentiate from ischemic nephropathy)
- Essential hypertension (usually well-controlled by medications)

Lower Extremity Occlusive Disease
- Neurogenic claudication (requires sitting for relief, brought on by prolonged standing)

- Musculoskeletal causes of limb pain (require longer rest to resolve, rarely originate in calf)
- Diabetic neuropathy (shooting pain or cramps that radiate up and down the leg, occur at night, rarely localized just to foot)
- Venous ulcers (located at malleolus, painless, other stigmata and history of venous disease)

MANAGEMENT

What to Do First

- Determine if urgent revascularization is needed:
- Symptomatic carotid stenosis –
  - ➤ recent TIA
  - ➤ resolving stroke with high grade lesion
- Acute mesenteric infarction –
  - ➤ severe abdominal pain (out of proportion to tenderness) peritoneal signs
    - acidosis
    - leukocytosis
- Renal artery
  - ➤ Severe bilateral disease with volume overload/pulmonary edema
- Critical limb ischemia – as defined above as Limb Threat

General Measures

- Smoking cessation
- Risk factor control: aggressive management of hyperlipidemia, hypertension
- Evaluation for hypercoagulable state – most require lifelong anticoagulation

SPECIFIC THERAPY

Carotid Stenosis

- Symptomatic Patients
  - ➤ Carotid endarterectomy: all patients with stenosis > 70%, and any good-risk patient with stenosis > 50%
  - ➤ Perioperative combined stroke + death rate must be less than 7% to achieve benefit
- Asymptomatic Patients
  - ➤ Perioperative combined stroke + death rate must be less than 5% to achieve benefit
  - ➤ Carotid endarterectomy: for any patient with > 80% stenosis and expected survival greater than 2 years

➤ Anti-platelet therapy for patients with expected survival < 2 years due to co-morbid conditions

➤ Angioplasty + stenting in patients with surgically inaccessible lesions or hazardous comorbidity (irradiated neck, etc.)

■ Visceral occlusive disease

➤ Surgical revascularization (bypass or endarterectomy) in all symptomatic patients or patients with 2 or more involved mesenteric vessels

➤ Percutaneous angioplasty in very high risk patients, recurrent disease or as a bridge to surgery in patients with severe weight loss

■ Renal artery occlusive disease

➤ Angioplasty + stenting for focal stenosis of main renal artery

➤ Renal artery bypass (better long-term results than angioplasty)
  • Younger patients (age <65)
  • Failed stenting or in-stent restenosis
  • Diffuse disease
  • Disease of branch vessels
  • In conjuction with other vascular procedure (aneurysm repair, etc.)

■ Lower Extremity Occlusive Disease

➤ Smoking cessation and graduated walking program for claudication

➤ Revascularization for disabling claudication unresponsive to above measures or limb threat
  • Angioplasty + stenting or aortofemoral bypass for iliac disease
  • Bypass for femoral, popliteal and tibial artery disease

Side Effects & Contraindications

■ Carotid Endarterectomy

➤ Contraindications

➤ Absolute

➤ Occlusion of internal carotid artery
  • must be confirmed by either MRA or angiogram
  • Duplex has 8% false-positive rate for occlusion

➤ Relative

➤ Irradiated or surgically reconstructed neck (muscle flap)

➤ Symptomatic coronary artery disease requiring revascularization first

■ Mesenteric and Visceral Revascularization

➤ Contraindications

➤ Absolute
➤ No distal reconstitution of target vessel
- Lower extremity revascularization
   ➤ Contraindications
   ➤ Absolute
   ➤ No distal reconstitution of target vessel
   ➤ Relative
   ➤ Gangrene too extensive to allow limb salvage
   ➤ Heel gangrene extending to bone
   ➤ Gangrene of thigh or upper calf
   ➤ Inability to ambulate for other reasons
   ➤ Prior stroke or other neurological disease
   ➤ Musculoskeletal disease preventing ambulation
   ➤ Contracture of knee joint greater than 15 degrees

FOLLOW-UP

Carotid Stenosis
- Lesions (both primary and post-endarterectomy): follow by duplex scan every 6 months and then yearly if 2 serial scans demonstrate no change.
- All patients: anti-platelet therapy

Renal and Mesenteric Lesions
- Renal artery lesions (primary and after revascularization): scan with either duplex (technically difficult) or MRA every year for restenosis
- Mesenteric revascularization: post-revascularization MRA or angio; follow clinically for recurrent symptoms

Lower Extremity Occlusive Disease
- Claudication: yearly ABI.
- Post stenting: ABI every 6 months.
- Lower extremity bypass graft: duplex studies yearly to detect focal stenosis before graft thrombosis occurs.

COMPLICATIONS AND PROGNOSIS

Carotid Endarterectomy
- Stroke (<3% in asymptomatic patients, <5% in symptomatic)
- Myocardial infarction (1–4%)
- Perioperative death (1–2%)
- Cranial nerve injury (5–15% transient, <5% permanent)

Renal Artery Stenting/Angioplasty
- Renal artery occlusion or dissection (<5%)
- In-stent restenosis (>30% at 2 years)

Visceral/Renal/Lower Extremity Revascularization
- Perioperative complications (per carotid endarterectomy)
- Embolization (<5%)
- Restenosis of iliac stents (30%)
- Late graft occlusion with recurrent symptoms (variable incidence)
- Graft infection (2% lifetime risk)
- Carotid Stenosis
- Long Term Stroke rates (per year)
- After endarterectomy 1–2%
- After carotid occlusion (not amenable to endarterectomy) – 4%
- High-grade stenosis managed medically – 4–6%

Mesenteric Occlusive disease
- Without revascularization, prognosis is grim – 80% dead at 2 years
- After revasc, 15% will have recurrent disease and symptoms long term

Renal Artery Occlusive Disease
- 80–95% have relief of HTN, stabilization of creatinine with surgery
- Stenting has 30–40% long-term failure rate; trials show no benefit to stenting versus medical management
- Surgical bypass has better long-term patency

Lower Extremity Occlusive Disease
- Claudication is not predictive of future limb loss (7% limb loss at 5 years)
- Patients with limb threat (see above) have high rates of limb loss without revascularization and high long-term mortality
- Renal artery stenting/angioplasty
  - Renal artery occlusion or dissection (<5%)
  - In-stent restenosis (<30% at 2 years)
- Visceral/renal/lower extremity revascularization
  - Perioperative complications (per carotid endarterectomy)
  - Embolization (<5%)
  - Restenosis of iliac stents (30%)
  - Late graft occlusion with recurrent symptoms (variable incidence)
  - Prosthetic graft infection (2% lifetime risk)

ATOPIC DERMATITIS

J. MARK JACKSON, MD

HISTORY & PHYSICAL

History
- Dry, scaly, itchy, red patches and plaques
- Sensitive skin asthma, hay fever, family history of atopy

Signs & Symptoms
- Erythematous, scaly, thickened (lichenified) patches and plaques
- Flexural areas, creases of extremities, and neck
- Face and diaper areas in infants

TESTS
- Tests-elevated IgE levels and eosinophils
- No tests necessary

DIFFERENTIAL DIAGNOSIS
- seborrheic dermatitis
- contact dermatitis
- irritant dermatitis
- pityriasis rosea
- drug eruption cutaneous T-cell lymphoma psoriasis

MANAGEMENT

What to Do First
- Determine patient discomfort to determine therapy.
- Discontinue skin irritants (fragrances, chemicals, etc.).

General Measures
- Moisturizers (creams/emollients), particularly after bathing
- Relieve itching

SPECIFIC THERAPY
- First line – topical emollients, topical corticosteroids, topical tacrolimus or pimecrolimus, soporific antihistamines (non-sedating antihistamines have limited benefit)
- Second line – oral/IM corticosteroids, ultraviolet light (either Psoralen + UVA [PUVS], UVB, or narrow-band UVB phototherapy)
- Third line – Methotrexate, cyclosporin, mycophenolate mofetil, or other immunosuppressives

- Side Effects & Complications
- Emollients – irritation, contact allergy
- Topical corticosteroids – atrophy, contact allergy
- Ultraviolet light – sunburn, irritation, skin cancer (long-term use), and nausea and vomiting with psoralens typical side effects of immunosuppressive agents

FOLLOW-UP
- During Rx, monitor for irritation from topicals or side effects from systemic medications
- Topical corticosteroids – monitor progress, evaluate for atrophy/ irritation
- Systemic corticosteroids
- Long-term use – complete physical exam, ppd, chest X-ray, blood sugars periodically, blood pressure, and eye exam

COMPLICATIONS AND PROGNOSIS
This tends to be a life-long condition with exacerbations and remissions that tend toward slow resolution with age.

ATRIAL FIBRILLATION (AF)

EDMUND C. KEUNG, MD

HISTORY & PHYSICAL

History
- Chronic or paroxysmal
- Remodeled atria from rheumatic, coronary, hypertensive, congenital heart disease; mitral valve prolapse
- Occurs in 5–40% post-coronary artery bypass operations; 70% on day 2 and 3 postop
- Acute alcohol intake ("holiday heart")
- Heart disease absent (lone atrial fibrillation)
- Increases with age (from 1.5% at age 60 to 10% at age 80)
- Irregularly irregular pulse. Variable first heart sound intensity inversely related to the preceding cycle length.

Signs & Symptoms
- No symptoms or palpitation; irregularly irregular tachycardia and pulse

■ If rapid: dizziness and hypotension, shortness of breath, chest pain

TESTS

■ Basic Test: 12-lead ECG: no recognizable discrete P waves. Irregularly irregular QRS complexes, may be wide from aberrant conduction. Ventricular response <40 to >180 bpm.

■ Specific Diagnostic Test: Echocardiogram: identify structural heart disease, left atrial thrombus (with transesophageal echo) and measure atrial and LV size and function

DIFFERENTIAL DIAGNOSIS

■ Frequent atrial premature complexes may mimic AF but P waves easily recognized on 12-lead ECG.

■ Multifocal atrial tachycardia: irregularly irregular rate and pulse but multiple (>2) P wave morphologies.

MANAGEMENT

What to Do First

■ Vital signs to assess hemodynamic response to rapid AF; 12 lead ECG to measure ventricular rate and to assess acute myocardial ischemia, infarction or pericarditis.

General Measures

■ Avoid caffeine and alcohol if correlated with AF occurrence

SPECIFIC THERAPY

Indicated for rapid ventricular response and restoration of normal sinus rhythm (NSR)

Acute

■ Emergency DC cardioversion (synchronized to R wave) to restore NSR when a rapid ventricular response results in hypotension, pulmonary edema, or ischemia.

■ In stable patients: beta blockers or calcium channel blockers (verapamil, diltiazem), either IV or PO, to slow ventricular response. Digoxin less effective.

■ Cardioversion to NSR without anticoagulation if AF <48 hours duration or atrial clot is excluded by transesophageal echo (92% sensitivity and 98% specificity).

■ Cardioversion: DC shock, IV ibutilide (30% success rate), IV or PO procainamide, sotalol, propafanone or PO amiodarone. (IV amiodarone not established).

Chronic

■ Warfarin for all patients with high-risk factors (TIA, embolism, CVA, hypertension, heart failure or poor LV systolic function, age ≥75, age ≥60 with diabetes mellitus or coronary artery disease, thyrotoxicosis, rheumatic valve disease, prosthetic valves, persistent atrial thrombus). Aspirin for age <60 with lone AF, or with heart disease but no risk factors (no heart failure, hypertension, or LVEF <0.35) and age ≥60 without above risk factors

■ Restore NSR: DC cardioversion or antiarrhythmic Rx. Before cardioversion rule out atrial clot by transesophageal echo; otherwise warfarin Rx; goal: INR of 2–3 for 4 weeks before cardioversion.

■ 12 months after successful cardioversion: without antiarrhythmic Rx: 20–40% in NSR; with antiarrhythmic Rx: 40–50% in NSR. If NSR, discontinue warfarin after 2–3 mos.

■ Maintain NSR:

■ Propafenone, sotalol (in patients without reduced LV function or prior infarction), or amiodarone. In AF <6 mos, amiodarone more effective than propafenone or sotalol (69% vs 39% in NSR after 1 year).

■ Control of ventricular response in chronic AF:

■ Beta-blockers and calcium channel blockers. Digoxin much less effective in ambulatory patients. Try amiodarone + beta blocker when rate control difficult.

■ Radiofrequency (RF) ablation of AV node (AVN) with implantation of a permanent cardiac pacemaker. Selected patients with paroxysmal AF: ablation of ectopic atrial focus from pulmonary veins, or isolation of pulmonary veins around the ostia with RF ablation, with a success rate of 70–90% (6–24 month follow-up). The long-term success rate of RF ablation in patients with persistent or chronic AF has not been established.

Side Effects & Contraindications

■ Potentially life-threatening pro-arrhythmic event due to antiarrhythmic therapy, especially with reduced LV function

■ Clinically significant AV nodal block with combination of beta blocker and amiodarone

■ Drug toxicity

FOLLOW-UP

■ Beta-blockers and calcium channel blockers during acute treatment: monitor BP and HR

- Chronic antiarrhythmic therapy: Routine ECG at regular intervals to monitor AV conduction, QRS and QT duration and ventricular arrhythmias. Holter to identify asymptomatic atrial fibrillation or heart block.
- Ibutilide, sotalol and propafenone require ECG telemetry monitoring at start of Rx.
- Amiodarone: Biannual thyroid function tests and chest x-ray

COMPLICATIONS AND PROGNOSIS
- Thromboembolism from left atrial clots 5–8%/yr in high-risk patients
- Cardiomyopathy in AF with chronic rapid ventricular response

---

ATRIAL FLUTTER

EDMUND C. KEUNG, MD

HISTORY & PHYSICAL

History
- Chronic or paroxysmal
- Underlying heart disease: rheumatic, coronary, hypertensive heart disease, mitral valve prolapse, after surgery for congenital heart disease (incisional reentry)
- COPD, acute alcohol ingestion, digoxin toxicity

Signs & Symptoms
- Palpitation, regular rapid pulse
- No symptoms; or dizziness and hypotension, shortness of breath, chest pain
- Atrial rate 250 to 300/min. Typical ventricular response: 150 bpm (2:1 AV conduction)

TESTS
- Basic Tests:
  - ➣ 12-lead ECG:
  - ➣ Cavotricuspid isthmus (CTI) dependent counterclockwise atrial flutter: predominantly negative flutter waves in leads II, III and F; (+) flutter waves in V1 and (−) in V6
  - ➣ Cavotricuspid isthmus (CTI) dependent clockwise atrial flutter: predominantly positive flutter waves in II, III and F, (−) in V1 and (+) in V6

➤ Atypical atrial flutter: includes a wide variety of non-CTI-dependent flutter. Not easily diagnosed by surface ECG: may mimic CTI-dependent flutter or no identifiable discrete flutter waves due to extensive atrial disease. Flutter wave rate >300/min. Unstable and may deteriorate to AF.

■ Specific Diagnostic Tests:

➤ Echocardiogram to identify structural heart disease

➤ Electrophysiology study to confirm type of atrial flutter (usually performed in conjunction with RF ablation)

DIFFERENTIAL DIAGNOSIS

■ Sinus tachycardia, supraventricular tachycardia (SVT), and atrial tachycardia

■ Carotid sinus message or adenosine IV: increased AV block enables better identification of flutter waves. May terminate reentrant SVTs such as AV nodal reentrant tachycardia, AV reentrant tachycardia and atrial tachycardia, but not atrial flutter.

■ Distinguish from atrial tachycardia by characteristic form and rates of the flutter waves on surface ECG.

■ Diagnostic electrophysiology study possibly required

MANAGEMENT

What to Do First

■ Vital signs to assess hemodynamic response to rapid atrial flutter; 12-lead ECG to assess for acute myocardial ischemia, infarction or pericarditis

General Measures

■ Avoid caffeine and alcohol, if correlated with atrial flutter occurrence.

SPECIFIC THERAPY

Indicated for rapid ventricular response and restoration of sinus rhythm

Acute

■ Emergency DC cardioversion (synchronized to R wave) to restore NSR when rapid ventricular response results in hypotension, pulmonary edema, or ischemia

- In stable patients: beta blockers or calcium channel blockers (verapamil, diltiazem), either IV or PO, to slow ventricular response. Digoxin usually ineffective.
- Cardioversion to NSR: use DC shock, IV ibutilide (1–2 h), IV or PO procainamide, sotalol, flecainide, propafenone or amiodarone

Chronic

- Exclude atrial clot by transesophageal echo; or warfarin Rx with INR of 2–3 for 4 weeks before cardioversion (see AF)
- Chronic anticoagulation with warfarin (see guidelines for AF)
- Radiofrequency ablation: best Rx for chronic atrial flutter. In CTI-dependent atrial flutter, 90–100% cure with RF ablation in the tricuspid annulus-inferior vena cava isthmus.
- Maintenance of NSR:
- Propafenone (absence of structural heart disease), sotalol (LVEF > 30%) or amiodarone.
- Control of ventricular response: beta blockers > calcium channel blockers

Side Effects & Contraindications

- Potentially life-threatening proarrhythmia possible with antiarrhythmic therapy. Rapid ventricular response from 1:1 AV conduction with propafenone or flecainide.

FOLLOW-UP

During Treatment

- Beta blockers or calcium channel blockers during acute Rx: monitor BP and HR
- Chronic antiarrhythmic Rx: ECG at regular intervals to monitor AV conduction, QRS and QT duration and ventricular arrhythmias. Holter to identify asymptomatic atrial flutter or heart block.
- Ibutilide, sotalol and propafenone require ECG telemetry monitoring at start of Rx.
- Amiodarone: Biannual thyroid function tests and chest x-ray

COMPLICATIONS AND PROGNOSIS

- Risk of thromboembolism uncertain. No consensus on use of warfarin or aspirin. Same anticoagulation protocol as patients with atrial fibrillation recommended.
- Cardiomyopathy in atrial flutter with chronic rapid ventricular response

ATRIAL PREMATURE COMPLEXES

EDMUND C. KEUNG, MD

HISTORY & PHYSICAL

History
■ Most common cause of an irregular pulse. Often induced by stress, tobacco, excessive caffeine or alcohol intake. Common in structural heart diseases.

Signs & Symptoms
■ Often asymptomatic. Palpitation and irregular pulse. Rarely, fatigue and exacerbation of heart failure.

TESTS
■ Basic Tests
  ➤ 12-lead ECG:
  ➤ Premature P wave with or without conduction to ventricle (blocked APC). Premature P wave morphology and P-R interval differ from sinus P wave and conduction. Premature P wave often masked by preceding T wave. Post-premature pauses usually non-compensatory
■ Specific Diagnostic Test
  ➤ none

DIFFERENTIAL DIAGNOSIS
■ Ventricular premature complex, junctional premature complex.

MANAGEMENT

What to Do First
■ 12-lead ECG

General Measures
■ Abstin from alcohol and caffeine

SPECIFIC THERAPY
■ Generally requires no treatment. In symptomatic patients, reassurance, digoxin, beta and calcium channel blocker.

Side Effects & Contraindications
■ Excessive suppression of AVN or sinus node activity with beta blockers or calcium channel blockers.

FOLLOW-UP
- Holter to ascertain effectiveness of treatment.

COMPLICATIONS AND PROGNOSIS
- Can be precursor of atrial fibrillation or flutter.

ATRIAL SEPTAL DEFECT (ASD)

MARIA ANSARI, MD

HISTORY & PHYSICAL

History
- Sinus Venosus (defect in superior portion of atrial septum)
  - ➤ Associated with partial anomalous pulmonary venous return
- Ostium secundum (defect in central portion of atrial septum)
  - ➤ Most common adult congenital heart disease after bicuspid aortic valve
  - ➤ Females: Males 2:1
  - ➤ Mitral valve prolapse present in up to 1/3
- Ostium primum (defect in lower portion of atrial septum)
  - ➤ Associated with clefts of AV valves, particularly MV cleft or regurgitation

Signs & Symptoms
- May not be symptomatic until age 40–50
- Symptoms of heart failure with exertional dyspnea may develop
- Atrial arrhythmias, especially atrial fibrillation are common
- Rarely cyanosis develops when there is shunt reversal (right-to-left)
- RV lift, palpable PA, fixed split S2 with mid systolic murmur
- Ejection click is common

TESTS

Screening
- Physical exam

Imaging
- EKG
  - ➤ Ostium primum: RSR' on EKG with LAD and 1st degree AVB in 75% of cases
  - ➤ Ostium secundum: rsR' or RSR' in V1 common with RAD
- Transthoracic echocardiogram

➤ Left-to-right shunt by color and Doppler flow or using saline contrast; level of shunt readily identified in most cases
- Transesophageal echocardiography
  ➤ Helps identify shunt level if not well visualized by surface echo
  ➤ Sinus venosus: diagnosis often made by TEE (better visualization of pulmonary veins)
- Cardiac catheterization
  ➤ Required if magnitude of left-to-right shunt is uncertain or associated coronary anomalies or disease are suspected

DIFFERENTIAL DIAGNOSIS
- Patent foramen ovale (present in 15–20% of normal adults)

MANAGEMENT
- Endocarditis prophylaxis necessary in sinus venosus and ostium primum defects
- Risk of endocarditis is low in isolated ostium secundum defects and routine prophylaxis is not recommended

SPECIFIC THERAPY
- Operative repair (suture or patch closure) indicated in all patients with significant left to right shunt (generally pulmonary to systemic shunt ration greater than 1.7: 1) or if there is evidence of right ventricular dilation

FOLLOW-UP
- Leak of ASD patch may occur-detected by echocardiography
- Endocarditis prophylaxis for first 6 months after surgery

COMPLICATIONS AND PROGNOSIS
Complications
- Heart failure-due to chronic left-to-right shunting
- Atrial arrhythmias
- Cerebral vascular accidents from paradoxical emboli
- Pulmonary artery hypertension (occurs in 15% of patients)
- Eisenmenger's syndrome: development of pulmonary hypertension and subsequent reversal of shunt right-to-left (occurs in 5% of patients)

Prognosis
- Repair in early adulthood (<24 years of age) have normal long-term survival
- Later repair associated with an 85% 10-year survival

ATRIAL TACHYCARDIA (AT)

EDMUND C. KEUNG, MD

HISTORY & PHYSICAL

History

- Underlying structural heart disease: coronary, hypertensive heart disease, mitral valve prolapse, after surgery for congenital heart disease (incisional reentry).
- COPD, acute alcohol ingestion and digoxin toxicity.

Signs & Symptoms

- Palpitation, regular or irregular rapid pulse.
- Dizziness, hypotension, syncope, shortness of breath, chest pain.

TESTS

- Basic Tests
  - 12-lead ECG:
  - Narrow QRS tachycardia unless pre-existing conduction defect or rate-related aberrant ventricular conduction. Atrial rate 150–200 bpm. Ectopic P wave precedes each QRS complex (long RP tachycardia). AV nodal block frequent.
  - Positive P wave in lead V1 predicts a left atrial focus (93% sensitivity and 88% specificity).
  - Positive or biphasic P wave in lead AVL predicts a right atrial focus (88% sensitivity and 79% specificity).
- Specific Diagnostic Test
  - Electrophysiology study to confirm AT (usually performed in conjunction of RF ablation)

DIFFERENTIAL DIAGNOSIS

- Sinus tachycardia, atrial flutter, AV re-entry tachycardia, and atrial tachycardia. Diagnostic electrophysiology study often required to differentiate three types of AT: automatic, triggered and reentrant.

MANAGEMENT

What to Do First

- Vital signs to assess hemodynamic response; 12 lead ECG to assess acute myocardial ischemia, infarction

General Measures
- Identify and initiate treatment of underlying conditions responsible for AT. Avoidance of caffeine and alcohol, if correlated with SVT occurrence

SPECIFIC THERAPY
Restore sinus rhythm

Acute
- Slow rapid ventricular response with IV beta blockers (metoprolol, esmolol) or calcium channel blockers (verapamil, diltiazem), or digoxin. 56% termination with adenosine. If AT occurs in the presence of digoxin, discontinue digoxin and administer KCl to maintain normal serum K+ level.

Chronic
- Class IA, IC and III antiarrhythmic agents to restore and maintain NSR.
- Radio frequency ablation of atrial ectopic focus (a different focus may occur after initial success)

Side Effects & Contraindications
- Excessive suppression of AVN or sinus node activity with beta blockers or calcium channel blockers. Pro-arrhythmic effects from antiarrhythmic agents.

FOLLOW-UP
- During beta blocker and calcium channel blocker Rx monitor BP and HR and AV conduction. Periodic ECG to monitor AV conduction, QRS and QT duration during Class I and III treatment. Holter to ascertain effectiveness of treatment.

COMPLICATIONS AND PROGNOSIS
- Cardiomyopathy with incessant AT

ATRIOVENTRICULAR BLOCK

EDMUND C. KEUNG, MD

HISTORY & PHYSICAL

History
- Ischemic heart disease and myocardial infarction

- Degenerative: Lenegre disease, Lev disease
- Infection: rheumatic fever, myocarditis, Lyme borreliosis, Chagas disease and endocarditis
- Immune/inflammatory processes: ankylosing spondylitis, rheumatoid arthritis, scleroderma and Reiter disease
- Infiltrative processes: amyloidosis, sarcoidosis
- Iatrogenic: medications: digoxin, beta and calcium channel blockers, Class I and III antiarrhythmic drugs. Post-heart surgery (CABG and aortic valve replacement).
- AV Wenckebach second-degree block
  - Progressive increase in the A-C venous pulse interval before the non-conducted P wave
  - Progressive decrease in the intensity of the first heart sound
- AV dissociation
  - Intermittent cannon A wave in the venous pulse and variable intensity of the first heart sound

Signs & Symptoms
- Rarely symptomatic in first-degree AV block or Type I second-degree (Wenckebach) AV block
- High-degree AV block:
  - Transient dizziness, lightheadedness, near-syncope or syncope, fatigue, worsening of congestive heart failure

TESTS
- Basic Tests
  - 12-lead ECG:
  - First-degree AV block: PR interval > 0.21 sec
  - Second degree AV block:
  - Type I AV block (Mobitz I or Wenckebach AV block):
    - Regular sinus P-P intervals
    - Progressive prolongation of PR intervals (but with decreasing increment) before non-conduction of P wave occurs
    - Progressive decrease in R-R intervals; the longest R-R interval (pause) is shorter than 2 times the shortest R-R interval. QRS occurs in groups.
  - Atypical AV Wenckebach: several unchanged PR intervals or irregular change in PR intervals
  - Type II AV block (Mobitz II AV block): Constant regular sinus P-P intervals and R-R intervals before the AV block

- P-P interval encompassing the block is twice the regular P-P interval.
- A bundle branch block or intraventricular conduction delay almost always present
- Third-degree (complete) AV block: All P waves fail to conduct to ventricle.
- No relationship between P wave and QRS complexes
- Both P-P and R-R intervals are constant.

■ Specific Diagnostic Test
➤ Holter monitoring
➤ Electrophysiology study to diagnose infra or intra-Hisian block usually not required

DIFFERENTIAL DIAGNOSIS
■ Second-degree AV block: from blocked APC
■ Third-degree (complete) AV block is a form of AV dissociation. P-P intervals > R-R intervals in third-degree AV block.
■ In 2:1 AV block (either constant or isolated), surface ECG cannot distinguish Mobitz I from II.
■ Evidence for Mobitz II: presence of IVCD or BBB

MANAGEMENT
What to Do First
■ Vital signs to ascertain hemodynamic effect of AV block

General Measures
■ Identify and initiate treatment of underlying conditions responsible for AV block. Establish relationship between symptoms and presence of AV block. Review and readjust drug treatment accordingly.

SPECIFIC THERAPY
Pacemaker implantation:

First-degree AV block: No pacemaker implantation except when markedly prolonged PR interval (>0.3 s)
■ results in dizziness, lightheadedness and fatigue (Class IIa indication)
■ occurs in patients with LV dysfunction and CHF (Class IIb)
Second-degree AV block:
■ Symptomatic bradycardia with second-degree AV block (Class I)
■ Asymptomatic Type II second-degree AV block with wide QRS (Class I)

- Asymptomatic Type II second-degree AV block with narrow QRS (Class IIa)
- Asymptomatic Type I AV block with EP documented intra- or infra-Hisian block (Class IIa)

Third-degree AV block:

- Symptomatic bradycardia (Class I)
- Asymptomatic patients: asystole >3 sec or escape rate <40 bpm while awake, especially if LV dysfunction is present (Class I)
- AV block from neuromuscular diseases (Class I)
- Asymptomatic patients with rate >40 bpm while awake (Class IIa)

Side Effects & Contraindications
- None

FOLLOW-UP
- ECG and Holter monitoring if symptoms appear. Pacemaker follow-up after implantation.

COMPLICATIONS AND PROGNOSIS
- Pacemaker: cardiac perforation; lead dislodgement; infected pacemaker pocket; lead fracture; failure to sense; failure to pace; pulse generator depletion. Requires specialized pacemaker follow-up.

AUTOIMMUNE HEPATITIS (AIH)

ANDY S. YU, MD and JOANNE C. IMPERIAL, MD

HISTORY & PHYSICAL

History
- Disease of young (age 15–35) & perimenopausal women
- Classified into types 1, 2, 3
- Strong relationship w/ HLA A1-B8-DR3, DR4
- Often associated w/ extrahepatic immunologic diseases: thyroiditis, vasculitis, Coombs-positive hemolytic anemia, uveitis, connective tissue disorders
- Must exclude other liver diseases in order to confirm diagnosis (hepatitis B & C, excessive alcohol use, hepatotoxic medications, biliary tract disease)

Signs & Symptoms
- Fatigue (85%) & jaundice (50%) common

- Vague upper abdominal pain, pruritus, anorexia, polymyalgia, epistaxis, bleeding gums, easy bruisability are also frequent complaints
- Triad of acne, amenorrhea, & arthralgia may be seen in adolescent females
- Acute hepatitis: uncommon & often predated by chronic symptoms
- Chronic hepatitis: associated w/ variable physical signs & symptoms; may be detected when patient is asymptomatic
- Advanced liver disease: liver failure (jaundice, hepatomegaly, pruritus, ascites, encephalopathy) may be first presentation in many patients

TESTS

Basic Blood Studies
- Early disease:
  - Moderately increased AST and ALT (range, 200–1000U), bilirubin, & alkaline phosphatase
  - Serology (important for classification of AIH):
    - Positive ANA (50%) & SMA (70%) in classic type 1 AIH
    - Positive anti-LKM1 seen in type 2 AIH; rare in U.S. patients; subgroup of patients w/ anti-LKM1 may have antibodies to HCV & GOR (usually Mediterranean men)
    - Positive antibodies to soluble liver antigen (anti-SLA ab) & liver/pancreas (anti-LP): type 3 AIH
    - Gamma-globulin $= 1.5 \times$ upper limit of normal & as high as 50–70 g/L
  - Advanced disease:
    - Increased serum bilirubin and INR; decreased serum albumin

Liver Biopsy
- Performed prior to treatment to assess severity of liver disease & differentiate between alternative liver diseases
- Early disease: periportal/lobular hepatitis; plasma cell infiltration
- Moderate or advanced disease: fibrosis, cirrhosis

Imaging
- Abdominal US or CT: nonspecific/nondiagnostic:
  - Early disease: often normal
  - Advanced disease: small shrunken liver, venous collaterals suggestive of portal hypertension

DIFFERENTIAL DIAGNOSIS
- PBC

- PSC
- Chronic HBV & HCV infection
- Autoimmune cholangitis
- Cryptogenic chronic active hepatitis
- Wilson disease
- Drug-induced hepatotoxity

MANAGEMENT

What to Do First
- Establish firm diagnosis before treatment
- Classify AIH according to type based on serologic tests

General Measures
- Use history, physical exam, liver chemistry, liver biopsy to confirm AIH & to assess degree of histologic injury
- Decision to treat based on clinical, biochemical, & histologic severity of illness
- Close monitoring of biochemistry (esp CBC & liver enzymes), side effects while on medications

SPECIFIC THERAPY

Indications
- All patients w/ evidence of hepatic inflammation; may be deferred for pts w/ mildly increased AST and ALT (<2.5 × normal), intolerance to steroids & azathioprine, inactive &/or decompensated cirrhosis, severe cytopenias; early treatment prolongs survival (87% at 5 y)

Treatment Options
- Treatment delays, but does not prevent, development of cirrhosis & end-stage liver disease
- Combination therapy w/ prednisone/azathioprine:
  - Azathioprine daily for 18–24 mo
  - Prednisone daily (80% of patients successfully maintained on azathioprine as single agent after initial response induced by steroid therapy)
- Prednisone monotherapy (more steroid-related side effects; indicated in pts w/ azathioprine intolerance or severe cytopenias: high dose or low dose at onset of therapy dependent upon disease severity & patient profile
- Overall response ~80%
- Cyclosporine, 6-mercaptopurine, mycophenylate mofetil, tacrolimus unproven therapies for unresponsive AIH

■ Liver transplantation (OLT) for treatment failures or end-stage disease

FOLLOW-UP

During Therapy

■ Regular monitoring of CBC, liver chemistry; gamma-globulin at end of treatment
■ Repeat liver biopsy to assess histologic response prior to cessation of therapy; goal of therapy: normal biopsy or mild CAH; AST/ALT <2.5X normal
■ Relapse rate of 60–85% w/in 3 y, esp if histology still active at time of treatment; rebound AST & gamma-globulin after cessation of therapy predict histologic recurrence 75–90%; relapse requires retreatment

COMPLICATIONS AND PROGNOSIS

■ Cirrhosis:
  ➤ 40% progress to cirrhosis w/in 10 y despite therapy
  ➤ Consider OLT for patients w/ liver failure (CTP score = 7) or those unresponsive to medical therapy
■ Important risk factors for progression & need for OLT:
  ➤ Male gender
  ➤ Younger patients w/ type 2 AIH
  ➤ Failure to achieve remission w/ 4 y of immunosuppression
  ➤ Fulminant hepatic failure
■ 96% 5-y survival post-OLT
■ AIH recurrence post-OLT (5–33%): HLA-DR3 (+) recipients of HLA-DR3 (−) allografts; during or after prednisone taper or withdrawal
■ Higher frequency of acute rejection post-OLT
■ HCC: 7% w/ cirrhosis for = 5 y

AUTONOMIC DYSFUNCTION

MICHAEL J. AMINOFF, MD, DSc

HISTORY & PHYSICAL

■ Postural dizziness
■ Syncope (especially postural & postprandial)
■ Hypo- or hyperhidrosis
■ Urinary incontinence, urgency, frequency, hesitancy or retention

- Impotence
- Vomiting, dysphagia, constipation, diarrhea, gastric fullness
- Postural hypotension or paroxysmal hypertension
- Fixed heart rate or paroxysmal, postural or persistent tachycardia
- Impaired thermoregulatory sweating
- Hyperthermia
- Pupillary abnormalities
- Somatic neurologic abnormalities sometimes present, indicating involvement of CNS or PNS

TESTS
- Blood studies: normal
- CT or MRI: may reveal structural cause for symptoms in brain stem or cervical cord; usually normal in Shy-Drager syndrome or primary autonomic failure
- Autonomic function studies: abnormal BP and heart rate response to standing, Valsalva maneuver; abnormal heart rate or cutaneous vasomotor response to deep inspiration; abnormal thermoregulatory sweating; impaired sympathetic skin response
- NCS: may reveal dysfunction of PNS

DIFFERENTIAL DIAGNOSIS
- Postural hypotension may occur in cardiac, metabolic, toxic or endocrine disorders; w/ hypovolemia; w/ certain meds (eg, dopaminergics, antidepressants, hypnotics, antihypertensives, etc); after prolonged bed rest
- Dysautonomia resulting from peripheral neuropathy (eg, diabetic or amyloid neuropathy, Guillain-Barre syndrome) is suggested by the clinical & electrodiagnostic findings
- Associated signs of parkinsonism or cerebellar deficit suggest Shy-Drager syndrome or multisystem atrophy

MANAGEMENT
- Asymptomatic
  - ➤ No treatment needed
  - ➤ Avoid alcohol & likely precipitants
- Symptomatic postural hypotension
  - ➤ Treat underlying cause; use following measures as needed
  - ➤ Make postural changes gradually
  - ➤ Copious fluids: salt supplements
  - ➤ Waist-high elastic hosiery
  - ➤ Sleep w/ head of bed propped up

> Florinef; increase daily dose every 2 weeks; may need 1 mg/day; watch for recumbent hypertension, ankle edema, worsened diabetes
> Prostaglandin synthase inhibitors
> Midodrine
Ephedrine
■ Other symptoms
> Air-conditioning to avoid hyperthermia

SPECIFIC THERAPY
■ Treat underlying cause

FOLLOW-UP
■ As needed

COMPLICATIONS AND PROGNOSIS
■ Treatment may be required indefinitely unless underlying disorder recovers

---

AUTOSOMAL DOMINANT POLYCYSTIC RENAL DISEASE

WILLIAM M. BENNETT, MD

HISTORY & PHYSICAL
■ family history of PKD in a parent or sibling
■ if parent not tested, query early death from stroke, history of hypertension or renal failure
■ associated findings: hypertension, mitral valve prolapse, hepatomegaly (liver cysts), inguinal or umbilical hernias, colonic diverticula
■ ask specifically about hematuria, proteinuria, symptoms of urinary tract infection, passage of stones or previous blood pressure elevation
■ kidneys may be palpable, enlarged and tender but this is unusual in early disease

TESTS
■ urinalysis
■ serum electrolytes
■ uric acid
■ BUN
■ creatinine

- creatinine clearance as a baseline to measure progression
- diagnosis is made by renal imaging: ultrasound, CT, MRI
- false positives rare
- false negative common through third decade (15–20%) with ultrasound
- CT and MRI more sensitive

DIFFERENTIAL DIAGNOSIS
- simple cysts (tend to be single and unilateral)
- von Hippel Lindau syndrome – diagnosis by extrarenal manifestations; cerebellar tumors, pheochromocytoma
- tuberous sclerosis – diagnosis by extrarenal manifestations; adenoma sebaceum

MANAGEMENT
- establish baseline renal function and imaging (MRI or CT best) for longitudinal follow-up
- introduce patient and family to Polycystic Kidney Research Foundation (1.800.PKD.CURE)
- genetic counseling imperative for autosomal dominant disorder
- screen patients with family history of cerebral aneurysms or neurological symptoms with MRA or CT

SPECIFIC THERAPY
- none available
- blood pressure management: goal is normal pressure for age. Some theoretical considerations favor ACE inhibitors, angiotensin receptor blockers. Few comparative studies available.
- nephrolithiasis: usually uric acid or calcium oxalate – manage as usual
- lower urinary tract infection: treat as usual patient
- upper urinary tract infection – treat with antibiotics that are known to penetrate cysts: trimethoprim-sulfamethoxazole, fluoroquinolones, chloramphenicol; avoid instrumentation of the urinary tract
- pain & discomfort – non-narcotic analgesics preferably acetaminophen, avoid aspirin and NSAIDs (except for short courses with good hydration), opiates as needed, rule-out obstruction and infection; if pain becomes chronic consider multidisciplinary pain clinic, antidepressants, cyst aspiration/sclerosis, laparoscopic cyst decompression or open cyst reduction. Absolute contraindications for surgical approaches are advanced renal insufficiency and inability to tolerate general anesthesia.

■ hepatic involvement – pain management issues are the same as with renal pain. Aspiration/sclerosis if there are a few dominant cysts.

FOLLOW-UP

Routine
■ annual assessment of renal function, blood pressure control and imaging
■ as needed to manage complications

COMPLICATIONS AND PROGNOSIS
■ 50% of patients progress to end-stage renal disease.
■ risk factors for progression – male sex, gross hematuria, hypertension before age 35, total renal volume >500 mL on imaging, women with >3 pregnancies and 24-h urine protein >500 mg

---

AUTOSOMAL RECESSIVE POLYCYSTIC RENAL DISEASE

WILLIAM M. BENNETT, MD

HISTORY & PHYSICAL
■ Parents are unaffected; there may be disease in a sibling, usually presents in childhood with hypertension, renal dysfunction, failure to thrive
■ associated liver fibrosis, more prominent in older children
■ no specific physical findings

TESTS
■ urinalysis
■ serum electrolytes
■ uric acid
■ BUN
■ creatinine
■ creatinine clearance as baseline to measure progression
■ diagnosis is made by renal imaging: ultrasound, CT, MRI
■ best imaging modality unsettled, probably ultrasound especially in young children

DIFFERENTIAL DIAGNOSIS
■ renal dysplasias
■ obstructive uropathy
■ ADPKD early onset

MANAGEMENT
- referral to pediatric nephrologist
- introduce patient and family to Polycystic Kidney Research Foundation (1.800.PKD.CURE)
- genetic counseling for recessive disease

SPECIFIC THERAPY
- none available
- management of renal dysfunction
- aggressive blood pressure control

FOLLOW-UP
- every 6–12 months by pediatric nephrologist

COMPLICATIONS AND PROGNOSIS
- progressive renal failure in most
- with modern management by dialysis, transplantation and liver replacement if necessary, survival into adulthood is more common

---

AV REENTRANT TACHYCARDIA (AVRT)

EDMUND C. KEUNG, MD

HISTORY & PHYSICAL

History
- Re-entrant circuit producing supraventricular tachycardia. Involves one or more atrioventricular accessory (bypass) tracts or pathways.
- Wolff-Parkinson-White (WPW) or pre-excitation syndrome: antegrade conduction over accessory pathway.
- Can have concealed pathways that conduct only from ventricle to atrium.
- No structural heart disease in most adult patients.
- Long history of intermittent palpitation and tachycardia with abrupt onset and termination.

Signs & Symptoms
- Abrupt onset and termination of tachycardia. Shortness of breath, chest discomfort and near- or frank syncope. Rarely, cardiac arrest.

TESTS
- Basic Tests

- ➤ 12-lead ECG:
- ➤ Delta waves with short PR interval (<100 ms, depends on degree of pre-excitation) from antegrade ventricular pre-excitation.
- ➤ ECG with full pre-excitation, Rs in lead V1: left-sided accessory pathways.
- ➤ rS to Rs transition > lead V2: reight-sided accessory pathways.
- ➤ Positive delta wave and QRS in lead V1: LV accessory pathway.
- ➤ Negative delta wave and QRS in V1: RV accessory pathway.
- ➤ No delta wave: concealed accessory pathway; ventriculo-atrial conduction.
- ➤ Antidromic AVRT: Wide QRS complex SVT using the accessory pathway as the antegrade limb and the AVN as the retrograde limb of the reentrant circuit.
- ➤ Orthodromic AVRT: Narrow QRS tachycardia with antegrade conduction over the AVN and retrograde conduction over the accessory pathway.
- ➤ Retrograde P waves during AVRT follow QRS (short RP tachycardia).
- ■ Specific Diagnostic Test:
  - ➤ Electrophysiology study to characterize and map the location of the pathway (usually performed in conjunction with RF ablation).

Differential Diagnosis
- ■ Sinus tachycardia, atrial flutter, and atrial tachycardia. Diagnostic electrophysiology study often required.

MANAGEMENT
What to Do First
- ■ Vital signs to assess hemodynamic response.
- ■ 12 lead ECG to rule out atrial fibrillation and flutter with pre-excitation during AVRT.

General Measures
- ■ In adult, no treatment or diagnostic electrophysiology study if delta wave only but no history of tachyarrhythmias.
- ■ Avoid caffeine and alcohol, if correlated with SVT occurrence

SPECIFIC THERAPY
Restore NSR
Acute

- Emergency DC cardioversion (synchronized to R wave) to restore NSR if rapid ventricular response causes hemodynamic instability, especially atrial fibrillation with very rapid response or atrial flutter with 1:1 AV conduction.
- Vagal maneuvers (carotid sinus massage, Valsalva) followed by IV adenosine. IV beta blockers (metoprolol, esmolol) or calcium channel blockers (verapamil, diltiazem), or IV procainamide.

Chronic

- RF ablation of pathway is Rx of choice.
- Otherwise: beta blockers or calcium channel blockers (verapamil, diltiazem), or Class IA, IC and III antiarrhythmic drugs.

Side Effects & Contraindications

- Betab blockers and calcium channel blockers contraindicated in atrial fibrillation and flutter in WPW syndrome (VF from increased ventricular rate). AF possible after adenosine Rx.

FOLLOW-UP

- Holter to monitor presence of AVRT, atrial fibrillation or flutter

COMPLICATIONS AND PROGNOSIS

- None if no tachycardias and delta wave only. Rapid ventricular response leading to ventricular fibrillation and sudden death in WPW syndrome.

AV-NODAL REENTRANT TACHYCARDIA (AVNRT)

EDMUND C. KEUNG, MD

HISTORY & PHYSICAL

History

- Most common form of SVT. More frequent in women (66%). Heart disease often absent. Rare atypical form often incessant.

Signs & Symptoms

- Palpitation, usually regular rapid pulse. Depending on co-existing cardiac conditions and rate of ventricular response:, dizziness, hypotension, syncope, shortness of breath (with reduced left ventricular function), chest pain (with significant coronary heart disease).

TESTS
- Basic Tests
  - ➤ 12-lead ECG:
  - ➤ Narrow QRS tachycardia unless pre-existing conduction defect or rate-related aberrant ventricular conduction. Commonly at 180–200 bpm (range 150–250 bpm).
  - ➤ Typical AVNRT (Slow-Fast): retrograde P wave buried in the QRS or in the S wave (short RP tachycardia). Begins with an APC with a long PR interval (antegrade conduction down slow pathway). Generally not initiated with a VPC. Usually terminates with a retrograde P wave (86%).
  - ➤ Atypical AVNRT (Fast-Slow): retrograde P wave before the next QRS complex (thus, long RP tachycardia).
- Specific Diagnostic Test
  - ➤ Electrophysiology study to confirm AVNRT (usually performed in conjunction with RF ablation).

DIFFERENTIAL DIAGNOSIS
- Sinus tachycardia, atrial flutter, AV re-entry tachycardia, and atrial tachycardia. Carotid sinus massage or adenosine IV: terminates AVNRT, AVRT (bypass tracts) and AT (56%) but increases AV block in atrial flutter and in AT, thus enabling better identification of p waves. Diagnostic electrophysiology study often required.

MANAGEMENT
What to Do First
- Vital signs to assess hemodynamic response; 12 lead ECG to assess acute myocardial ischemia, infarction.

General Measures
- Avoid caffeine and alcohol if correlated with SVT occurrence

SPECIFIC THERAPY
Restore NSR
Acute
- Restoration of NSR when a rapid ventricular response results in hypotension, pulmonary edema, or ischemia. Vagal maneuvers (carotid sinus massage, Valsalva) followed by IV adenosine.
Chronic
- For frequent occurrence, beta blockers or calcium channel blockers (verapamil, diltiazem), or digoxin PO for chronic suppression. Class I and III antiarrhythmic agents often not required.

- Radio frequency ablation of the slow or fast (rare) AVN pathway often best Rx.

Side Effects & Contraindications
- Excessive suppression of AVN or sinus node activity with beta blockers or calcium channel blockers. Inadvertent ablation of the AVN during RF ablation requiring permanent pacemaker.

FOLLOW-UP
- During chronic Rx with beta blockers and calcium channel blockers monitor BP and HR and AV conduction. Holter to identify asymptomatic AVNRT or heart block from drug Rx.

COMPLICATIONS AND PROGNOSIS
- Cardiomyopathy with incessant AVNRT

BACK OR NECK PAIN

MICHAEL J. AMINOFF, MD, DSc

HISTORY & PHYSICAL
- Pain in back or neck, sometimes w/ radiation to limbs
- May be segmental weakness, numbness or paresthesias in limbs
- May be sphincter or sexual dysfunction
- May be history of trauma or unaccustomed activity
- May be past history of malignancy, structural spinal disorder, osteoporosis, inflammatory disease, predisposition to infection
- Spasm of paraspinal muscles commonly present
- Spinal movement may be limited
- Spinal tenderness common
- Focal neurologic deficit may indicate root or cord involvement
- Rectal or pelvic exam may reveal local cause of back pain
- May be evidence of underlying psychiatric disorder

TESTS
- MRI will reveal bone or joint disease, disc herniation, local infection
- CBC may suggest infection or coagulopathy
- ESR may be increased in infective, inflammatory or neoplastic disorders

DIFFERENTIAL DIAGNOSIS
- Mode of onset & duration of pain may suggest underlying disorder
  - ➤ Acute disorder: disc prolapse or local infection
  - ➤ Chronic disorder: musculoskeletal or neoplastic cause
- Cutaneous pain over back or neck may be due to shingles; development of skin rash indicates diagnosis
- Primary infection of other sites (eg, lungs, bladder, skin) suggests spinal osteomyelitis
- Osteoporosis common in the elderly or inactive, or in those w/ family history or taking steroids
- Secondary tumors of spine more common than primary tumors

MANAGEMENT
- Analgesics or NSAIDs for pain
- If fracture suspected, immobilize spine/neck for imaging studies

SPECIFIC THERAPY
- Treat underlying disorder
- Surgical drainage for acute hematoma or abscess
- Spinal injury w/ cord compression may require decompression & spinal fusion; high-dose steroids helpful in first 24 hrs
- Irradiation & steroids for tumors
- Soft collar for cervical spondylosis; surgery sometimes needed

FOLLOW-UP
- Depends on causal disorder

COMPLICATIONS AND PROGNOSIS
- Depend on causal disorder

BACTERIAL ARTHRITIS

STEVEN R. YTTERBERG, MD

HISTORY & PHYSICAL

History
- Bacteremia
- Extra-articular infections: skin infections, SBE, abscess

Risk Factors
- Pre-existing joint damage by inflammatory arthritis, joint prostheses, joint surgery
- Very young or elderly

- Immunosuppressed conditions: immunosuppressive medications, HIV, diabetes mellitus
- IV drug abuse

Sign & Symptoms

- Abrupt onset of inflammatory arthritis, monoarticular 80–90%
- Any joint possible; knee most often in adults & hip frequent in children
- Joint pain, moderate to severe; worse w/ motion
- Marked limitation of active & passive range of motion
- Distinguish septic bursitis (eg, prepatellar or olecranon) from true joint sepsis
- Systemic signs & symptoms of infection: fever (~60%), chills (~10%)
- Presentation varies w/ age/risk factors & organism involved
  - Children: younger–systemic symptoms w/ high fever, often associated osteomyelitis; hip often involved, held in flexion; H. influenzae common in younger children (incidence declining due to vaccination)
  - Adults: lower extremity joints especially
  - Elderly: gram-negative bacteria a concern
  - Prosthetic joint infections: early after surgery–acute signs & symptoms (Staphylococcus sp & Streptococcus sp), late infections more indolent
  - N. gonorrhoeae: most common form of infectious arthritis (~1% of patients w/ GC); vesicopustular or hemorrhagic skin lesions often present; monoarthritis, oligoarthritis, migratory arthritis, tenosynovitis possible

TESTS

Lab Tests

- CBC: leukocytosis w/ shift to left
- Elevated ESR & CRP

Specific Diagnostic Tests

- Arthrocentesis required: examine for cell count, crystals, Gram stain & cultures for routine & anaerobic bacteria, consider mycobacterial & fungal smears & cultures
- Joint fluid inflammatory: WBC typically >50,000 cells/cc, >80% neutrophils; glucose less than half serum level
- Synovial fluid Gram stain often positive (50–70%), but not sensitive (<60%) for presence of bacteria; culture diagnostic (positive in 70–90% of cases but only 10–50% w/ N. gonorrhoeae)

- Blood cultures positive in about 50%
- Cultures of other sites of infection
- PCR for bacterial DNA in fluid or tissue, especially for N. gonorrhoeae, mycobacterial or partially treated infections

Imaging
- Joint radiographs should be done early
  - Usually show only soft tissue swelling initially
  - Helpful to exclude associated osteomyelitis
  - Provide baseline to assess treatment response
- Destructive arthritis w/in days to weeks if untreated
- Bone scans can show joint inflammation in joint before radiographic change but are nonspecific & not usually necessary
- CT & MRI can aid in diagnosis, showing local extension of infection or presence of osteomyelitis

DIFFERENTIAL DIAGNOSIS
- Trauma: history helpful; radiograph to exclude local bone pathology
- Crystalline arthritis: gout, pseudogout; may have history of previous episodes of acute inflammatory arthritis; diagnosis depends on seeing crystals in synovial fluid
- Initial onset of a chronic arthropathy such as RA or a seronegative spondyloarthropathy, although onset is usually not as abrupt

MANAGEMENT

What to Do First
- Arthrocentesis to obtain specimen to establish specific diagnosis & determine antibiotic sensitivities, & to remove pus
- Empiric IV antibiotics based on clinical picture; consider age, risk factors, exposure, extra-articular infections; Gram stain important:
  - Neonates: S. aureus, Enterobacteriaceae, group B streptococci
  - Children <5 yrs: H. influenzae, S. aureus, streptococci
  - Children >5 yrs: S. aureus, streptococci
  - Adolescents/adults: N. gonorrhoeae, S. aureus, streptococci, Enterobacteriaceae
  - Prosthetic joints, recent joint procedure or surgery: S. epidermidis, S. aureus, streptococci, gram-negative bacilli

General Measures
- Drainage of reaccumulating pus by:
  - Arthrocentesis
  - Arthroscopic lavage & debridement

> Arthrotomy: consider especially for hips or shoulders, infection in pts w/ RA, or joints responding poorly to other means
- Stop any immunosuppressive meds
- Establish a specific diagnosis based on cultures
- Obtain cultures from other potential sites of infection, esp. if N. gonorrhoeae suspected
- Avoid weight bearing in lower extremity joints, but physical therapy helpful to avoid contractures

SPECIFIC THERAPY

Indications
- All pts w/ septic arthritis require antibiotic therapy

Treatment Options
- Antibiotic therapy, initially vancomycin for gram-positive & ceftriaxone for gram-negative, later guided by microbial sensitivity studies
- IV antibiotics initially; intra-articular antibiotic therapy not necessary
- Optimal duration of parenteral therapy not clear; suggest 1 week for N. gonorrhoeae, 3 weeks for S. aureus, 2 weeks for other infections; subsequent oral antibiotics for a total of 4–6 weeks therapy suggested by some for more virulent organisms & 2–4 weeks for less virulent

Side Effects & Complications
- Typical antibiotic complications need to be considered

FOLLOW-UP

During Treatment
- Assessment daily or more often during initial stage of infection
- Repeat arthrocenteses indicate success of treatment w/ diminishing synovial fluid volumes, diminished WBC counts, diminished neutrophil percentages, sterility of cultures

Routine
- Assessment for recurrent infection
- Physical therapy for possible contractures

COMPLICATIONS & PROGNOSIS

Complications
- Infection-related
  > Osteomyelitis
  > Disseminated infection

- Joint-related
  - Contractures
  - Joint erosions & destruction

Prognosis
- Poor prognosis w/ increased mortality & poor joint outcomes in elderly, RA, those w/ prosthetic joints
- Poor prognosis w/ delayed institution of therapy

BACTERIAL PNEUMONIA

RICHARD A. JACOBS, MD, PhD

HISTORY & PHYSICAL

History
- Predisposing factors-smoking, altered mental status (aspiration), excessive alcohol, older age, immunosuppression, viral upper respiratory tract infections, endotracheal and nasogastric tubes (nosocomial pneumonia)
- Etiology depends on clinical setting:
  - Outpatient: S pneumoniae, H influenzae, C pneumoniae, M pneumoniae, Legionella
  - Nosocomial: S aureus, Pseudomonas, other Gram-negative bacilli
  - Aspiration: aerobic and anaerobic "mouth flora"
  - Immunocompromised: any of above plus Pneumocystis carinii (PCP), fungi (aspergillus, Cryptococcus, coccidioidomycosis), nocardia

Signs & Symptoms
- Fever, cough, pleuritic chest pain, tachycardia, tachypnea, dyspnea, rales, evidence of consolidation (dullness, decreased breath sounds, bronchial breath sounds)

TESTS
- CXR to confirm infiltrate
- Determine etiology with 2 pretreatment blood cultures and sputum for Gram stain and culture; thoracentesis for culture if pleural effusion
- Urine antigen for Pneumococcus. Also, Legionella if diagnosis is suspected.

- Serologic studies not helpful in acute management
- CBC, electrolytes, glucose, creatinine and oxygen saturation to determine need for hospitalization

DIFFERENTIAL DIAGNOSIS
- Other noninfectious causes of pulmonary infiltrates (tumor, collagen vascular diseases, atalectasis, congestive heart failure, etc)

MANAGEMENT
What to Do First
- Determine need for hospitalization:
- Elderly with comorbid diseases (neoplastic, liver, CHF, renal) have high mortality and should be admitted; altered mental status, tachypnea (RR>30), hypotension (BP<90), tachycardia (P>125), temperature <35 or >40, acidosis (pH<7.35), hyponatremia (Na<130), hyperglycemia (glucose >250), elevated BUN (>30) and hypoxia (oxygen saturation <90%) associated with poor prognosis-presence of several of these, even in otherwise healthy young adult, should prompt admission
- Supplemental oxygen, as needed
- Obtain specimens for culture

SPECIFIC THERAPY
- Empirical:
  - Outpatient: doxycycline, a macrolide, ketolide or a fluoroquinolone with activity against S pneumoniae (levofloxacin, moxifloxacin, gatifloxacin). Fluoroquinoles and ketolides generally not necessary in young, otherwise healthy adults unless macrolide-resistant S. pneumo is prevalent in the community.
  - Hospitalized (ward): extended-spectrum cephalosporin (ceftriaxone, cefotaxime) plus a macrolide or a fluoroquinolone alone
  - Hospitalized (ICU): extended-spectrum cephalosporin or beta-lactam + beta-lactamase inhibitor (ampicillin-sulbactam, piperacillin-tazobactam) in combination with a macrolide or a fluoroquinolone
  - Aspiration: amoxicillin or clindamycin
  - Nosocomial: piperacillin-tazobactam or ceftriaxone or vancomycin plus fluoroquinolone (choice depends upon local microbiology and resistance patterns)
- Organism-specific therapy:
  - S pneumoniae: susceptibilities should be determined because of increasing prevalence of resistance; penicillins, doxycycline,

macrolides, fluoroquinolones active against sensitive strains (MIC <0.1); penicillins, fluoroquinolones, cephalosporins active against intermediate strains (MIC 0.1–1.0); vancomycin, fluoroquinolones active against resistant strains (MIC >1.0)

- ➤ H influenzae: second- or third-generation cephalosporin, fluoroquinolones, amoxicillin-clavulanic acid, azithromycin, clarithromycin, trimethoprim-sulfamethoxazole
- ➤ C pneumoniae: macrolide, doxycycline, or fluoroquinolone
- ➤ Legionella: azithromycin or a fluoroquinolone (+rifampin in severe disease)
- ➤ M pneumoniae: doxycycline or a macrolide

FOLLOW-UP

- ■ Clinical improvement in 3–5 d
  If using telithromycin (ketolide), monitor for signs of liver toxicity; three severe cases have recently been reported.
- ■ Follow-up CXR if symptoms persist (exclude empyema, cavitation) and in elderly in 8–12 wks (to exclude malignancy)

COMPLICATIONS AND PROGNOSIS

- ■ Empyema and abscess occur infrequently.
- ■ Mortality 10–15%: mainly in elderly with comorbid illnesses and immunocompromised
- ■ Prevention with pneumococcal vaccination in those >50 y or with underlying diseases; yearly influenza vaccination

BALANITIS

KEY H. STAGE, MD, FACS

HISTORY & PHYSICAL

Signs & Symptoms

- ■ Balanitis is inflammation of the glans penis; balanoposthitis refers to inflammation of both the glans penis and prepuce.
- ■ Physical signs of balanitis and balanoposthitis include erythema, scaling, aculopapular exanthem, moist discharge, fissuring, and ulceration with or without induration.
  - ➤ Benign lesions: Pearly penile papules (may look like genital warts), Fordyce spots (yellow submucosal sebaceous glands),

sclerosing lymphangiitis (perhaps related to trauma of intercourse, transitory)

TESTS
- HLA-B27 for possible Reiter's syndrome
- KOH and wet prep for possible Candidal infection
- dark field examination with antibody testing for syphilis
- viral culture and Tzanck prep for Herpes simplex
- culture for possible chancroid (Haemophilus ducreyi)
- biopsy makes diagnosis if conservative management fails or diagnosis uncertain

DIFFERENTIAL DIAGNOSIS
- Balanitis mostly seen in uncircumcised males; may be secondary to poor hygiene, accumulated smegma beneath the foreskin. Other causes include diabetes mellitus, infection (candida, gardnerella, trichomonas, group B streptococcus, anaerobic microbials)), systemic disease, or neoplasia. Erythematous areas adjacent to the glans penis – candidal infection, Bowen's disease, erythroplasia of Queyrat, plasma cell balanitis (Zoon's balanitis), balanitis xerotica obliterans, squamous cell carcinoma in situ (Bowen's disease).
- Dry maculopapular exanthem suggests psoriasis, contact dermatitis, possible Reiter's syndrome.
- If ulcerated area adjacent to the glans penis, consider syphilis chancroid, granuloma inguinale, lymphogranuloma venereum.
- Punctate clusters of small vesicles suggest herpes simplex.
- Single large (usually >2 cm), bright-red, moist patch on the glans penis or inner aspect of the foreskin suggests plasma cell balanitis (Zoon's balanitis).
- Definitive dx made with biopsy, serology, and/or culture

MANAGEMENT
- Incorporates attention to proper diagnosis, as well as initial general measures for treatment
- If infection suspected, appropriate topical antifungal or antibacterial ointment or cream applied (bacitracin, imidizole)
- Warm soaks also helpful
- Appropriate cultures taken, follow-up appointment made to assess initial success of general treatment measures

SPECIFIC THERAPY

- Specific therapy is possible only after appropriate diagnosis made
  - ➤ Candidal balanitis: Patient should be screened for possible diabetes. Careful cleansing and use of topical imidizole cream, or BID application of nystatin-triamcinolone cream for 2 weeks often successful.
  - ➤ Genital herpes: Acyclovir drug of choice. Oral acyclovir more effective than topical therapy. Oral prophylaxis can be used long-term. Alternative medication – famciclovir, valacyclovir.
  - ➤ Zoon's balanitis (plasma cell balanitis): Circumcision or Mohs micrographic surgery for excision is usual treatment.
  - ➤ Balanitis xerotica obliterans: Initial conservative management with topical steroids and antibacterials. Consider biopsy, circumcision, partial resection, or Mohs micrographic surgery if topical medication unsuccessful.
  - ➤ Bowen's disease and erythroplasia of Queyrat: May be precursor to squamous cell carcinoma. Diagnosis should be made based on biopsy and histology. Treatment includes circumcision, partial resection, or Mohs micrographic surgery.
  - ➤ Contact dermatitis: Attempt to remove causative irritant from exposure. Common causes: iatrogenic application of various topicals, latex condoms, spermicides, nickel allergy, various cleansing agents and disinfectants. Topical corticosteroids may provide relief, combine with oral antihistamines for pruritus. Occasional use of oral steroids required.
  - ➤ Reiter's syndrome: Treatment involves appropriate use of antibiotic therapy – multidisciplinary approach to disease.
  - ➤ Psoriasis: Improvement of genital lesions seen with application of topical steroids and emollients, dermatologic evaluation necessary.
  - ➤ Condyloma: Treated most often topically using a variety of agents. 5% imiquimod cream used primarily. Alternatively, 20% podophyllin/benzoin or trichloroacetic acid. Goal of therapy to remove lesion; total eradication of human papilloma virus most often impossible. Electrocautery or laser therapy necessary for large lesions not responding to topical agents; liquid nitrogen also used as cryotherapy.

FOLLOW-UP

- If initial conservative measures fail, biopsy is mandatory.

- With infectious lesions such as chancroid, syphilis, or gonorrhea, complete resolution of the lesion should be documented after treatment.
- Follow-up for condyloma – patient instructed to present to the office whenever recurrence is noted. This enables early topical treatment before lesion progresses in size.
- Follow-up for premalignant lesions of the penis mandatory
- If diagnosis of Bowen's disease, erythroplasia of Queyrat, or balanitis xerotica obliterans made, periodic self-inspection as well as regular examination in the office required after excision

COMPLICATIONS AND PROGNOSIS
- Complications due to lack of appropriate diagnosis
- Unrecognized squamous cell carcinoma of the penis may progress and metastasize.

BARTTER'S SYNDROME

MICHEL BAUM, MD

HISTORY & PHYSICAL
- may have a history of polyhydramnios and prematurity
- polydipsia, polyuria, failure to thrive, constipation, muscle cramps, salt craving

TESTS
- Hypokalemia, metabolic alkalosis, with or without hypomagnesemia
- Fractional excretion of Na and Cl >1%, usually UCa/UCr >0.20
- Elevated plasma renin, aldosterone and urinary prostaglandins
- Nephrocalcinosis common

DIFFERENTIAL DIAGNOSIS
- Autosomal recessive defect in thick ascending limb transport due to mutation in thick ascending limb Na/K/2Cl cotransporter, Cl channel, K channel, Barttin (Cl^- channel beta-subunit necessary for renal Cl^- reabsorption – associated with deafness due to defect in inner ear K^+ secretion)
  Very rarely, autosomal dominant hypocalcemia, caused by gain-of-function mutations in calcium sensing receptor, is associated with Bartter's.

- Distinguish from other causes of salt wasting, including diuretic abuse, cystic fibrosis and Gitelman's syndrome

MANAGEMENT
n/a

SPECIFIC THERAPY
- KCl supplements, indomethacin – may need Mg supplements
  - NaCl supplements (in neonates)
  - May need growth hormone

FOLLOW-UP
To ensure growth and response to therapy

COMPLICATIONS AND PROGNOSIS
Short stature, failure to thrive, constipation and volume depletion
Nephrocalcinosis and renal insufficiency

BELL'S PALSY

CHAD CHRISTINE, MD

HISTORY & PHYSICAL
- Acute or subacute onset of unilateral facial weakness
- May progress over several hours or even a day
- Often preceded or accompanied by periaural pain
- Impairment of taste, lacrimation or hyperacusis common
- Weakness interferes w/ eyelid closure
- Difficulty eating & drinking
- Variable lower motor neuron weakness
- Other cranial nerves spared
- Examine ear & acoustic foramen to evaluate for herpes zoster infection (Ramsay Hunt syndrome)

TESTS
- Diagnosis made clinically
- Brain imaging performed if atypical presentation

DIFFERENTIAL DIAGNOSIS
- Tumors, trauma, stroke, bacterial infection, Ramsay Hunt syndrome, sarcoidosis excluded clinically
- Lyme disease & AIDS differentiated serologically

MANAGEMENT
- General measures: tape eyelid closed at night & use Lacrilube to avoid corneal drying

SPECIFIC THERAPY
- Indications: symptom onset within 72 hrs
  - Prednisone
  - Treatment w/ both prednisone & acyclovir may improve the degree of recovery

FOLLOW-UP
- Not always necessary; depends on severity of symptoms

COMPLICATIONS AND PROGNOSIS
- Most pts show recovery within 1–3 months
  - Some are left w/ mild to severe facial weakness
  - Aberrant reinnervation: jaw-winking, hemifacial spasm, crocodile tears
- 85% of pts recover completely; 95% recover satisfactorily within weeks to months

---

BENIGN DISORDERS OF THE RECTUM AND ANUS

MARK A. VIERRA, MD

HISTORY & PHYSICAL

History
- Hemorrhoids:
  - More common w/ age, during pregnancy, associated w/ constipation
  - Grade 1: internal hemorrhoids, physiologic & universally present to some degree
  - Grade 2: spontaneously prolapse w/ defecation but self-reduce
  - Grade 3: spontaneously prolapse w/ defection, must be manually reduced
  - Grade 4: prolapsed, unable to be reduced
- Fissure: associated w/ constipation; all ages
- Prolapse: occasionally present in children; more common in elderly (women > men) & institutionalized pts

- Incontinence: most common in women w/ sphincter injury after vaginal delivery; less commonly associated w/ other injury, XRT, prior anorectal surgery, neurologic disease
- Condyloma (HPV): associated w/ anorectal intercourse

Signs & Symptoms
- Hemorrhoids do not hurt unless acutely thrombosed; most commonly present w/ bleeding (blood on toilet paper, in toilet bowl); rarely may cause anemia
- Fissure causes severe pain w/ or immediately after defecation; usually few symptoms apart from defecation; small amount of blood on toilet paper or stool may occur; linear mucosal tear usually present in posterior midline; if located at other parts of rectum, consider Crohn disease, venereal disease
- Rectal prolapse: should be demonstrable during straining; pt may not always be able to distinguish hemorrhoid prolapse from true rectal prolapse
- Incontinence: associated w/ poor or absent sphincter pressure &/or sensation; incontinence w/o sensation differs from rectal urgency w/ loss of control

TESTS
Laboratory
- Unimportant except rarely anemia from bleeding hemorrhoids
- Incontinence may require cinedefecography, nerve conduction studies
- Pathology on condyloma important to exclude malignancy

Imaging
- Cinedefecography may be helpful for incontinence
- If fissure unusual in appearance or location, consider imaging remainder of GI tract to look for Crohn disease

DIFFERENTIAL DIAGNOSIS
- All pts w/ bleeding per rectum or guiaic positive (can occur w/ hemorrhoids, fissure, prolapse) should undergo colonoscopy
- Most fissures benign, but consider Crohn disease, venereal disease, trauma if appearance or location of fissure unusual
- Cause of incontinence usually apparent from history & physical exam
- Consider associated squamous cell carcinoma in pts w/ condyloma

MANAGEMENT

What to Do First
- Establish diagnosis

General Measures
- Pain relief w/ sitz baths & local therapy

SPECIFIC THERAPY
- Hemorrhoids:
  - Most pts require no treatment except counseling for high-fiber diet
  - Grade 2 & 3 hemorrhoids often may be treated w/ hemorrhoid banding; sclerotherapy less commonly used
  - Surgery may be used for grade 2–4 hemorrhoids but not necessary unless pt dissatisfied w condition
  - Thrombosed hemorrhoids may be treated expectantly if small, or may require opening & evacuation of clot or urgent hemorrhoidectomy
- Fissure:
  - Initial trial of fiber & stool softeners; trial nitroglycerine ointment to anus TID if persists
  - Surgical options include botulinum toxin injection or division of internal sphincter or rectal dilatation under anesthesia
- Condyloma:
  - Topical podophylin, laser therapy, coagulation, or surgical excision (rare)
- Rectal prolapse:
  - Transabdominal rectopexy; sigmoid resection & rectopexy; Altmeier procedure (transanal resection of prolapse) +/– levatoroplasty
- Incontinence:
  - Mild incontinence may be manageable w/ diet & bulk agents to produce firmer stools
  - If caused by sphincter injury, pt may benefit from sphincter reconstruction Limited experience to date w/ artificial sphincters; arely, colostomy may be appropriate

FOLLOW-UP
- Hemorrhoids, prolapse, & incontinence do not require follow-up except for symptomatic recurrence
- Typical fissures that resolve w/ management do not require follow-up

- Condyloma may require repeated treatment; if perianal disease cannot be eradicated, consider intrarectal involvement that may require treatment

COMPLICATIONS AND PROGNOSIS

- Hemorrhoidectomy:
  - ➤ Bleeding uncommon but not rare complication of hemorrhoidectomy or hemorrhoid banding; may occur up to 2 wk after procedure
  - ➤ Infection may occur & present only w/ urinary retention; fever, pain may be relatively late &/or subtle
  - ➤ Lateral internal sphincterotomy may produce incontinence, esp in women
- Prolapse:
  - ➤ W/ surgery, bleeding, infection may occur
  - ➤ Recurrence of prolapse may be common
  - ➤ Transabdominal surgery may rarely result in impotence in men
  - ➤ Prolapse may produce incontinence
- Condyloma: at risk for late squamous cancer
- Incontinence:
  - ➤ Inadequate resolution of symptoms w/ surgery may occur
  - ➤ Bleeding & infection uncommon acute complications

BENIGN PROSTATIC HYPERPLASIA

CLAUS G. ROEHRBORN, MD

HISTORY & PHYSICAL

History

- Disease affects usually men >40 years
- Increasing incidence with advancing age (60% men in their 60s, 80% men in their 80s)
- Ask about lower urinary tract symptoms (LUTS): frequency, urgency, nocturia, weak stream, straining, incomplete emptying, intermittency
- Duration of symptoms and onset
- Medications affecting bladder and sphincter function: anticholinergics, alpha sympathomimetics, cold medicines containing sympathomimetics, antihistamines, steroid hormones

- Unrelated surgeries or anesthetic interventions worsening symptoms
- Prior surgery or other treatment for BPH

Signs & Symptoms
- On digital rectal examination (DRE), soft, non-tender, non-nodular gland; estimate in increments of 10 ml (range 20–>100 ml)
- Check anal sphincter tone during DRE to rule out gross neurologic deficits.
- Check suprapubic area for distension suggestive of retention.

TESTS
Basic Blood Tests
- Serum prostate specific antigen (PSA): evaluate if elevated. Recent evidence suggests that any value >2.5 ng/ml should be further assessed by urologist.
- Serum creatinine to assess baseline kidney function; continue evaluation if elevated by imaging (ultrasound), etc.

Basic Urine Tests
- Urinalysis to check for infection or hematuria; continue appropriate evaluation if indicated
- Specific Tests: Urine
- Urinary flow rate recording: maximum flow rate
  - ➤ <10 ml/sec: clear indication for obstruction
  - ➤ 10–15 ml/sec: suspicious for obstruction
  - ➤ >15 ml/sec: unlikely to be obstructed
- Residual urine measurement after voiding: prefer to use noninvasive methods such as ultrasound
- Calculate voiding efficiency: voided volume/(residual + voided volume) × 100.
  - ➤ Voiding efficiency <50%: suspect significant obstruction
  - ➤ Residual urine >300 ml total: suspect near-complete urinary retention and consider urgent treatment

DIFFERENTIAL DIAGNOSIS
- All causes of LUTS and/or obstructed voiding
  - ➤ Other prostate conditions (prostatitis and prostate cancer)
  - ➤ Urethral stricture disease
  - ➤ Neurogenic bladder (MS, parkinsonism, diabetes, etc)

- ➤ Prior surgery of the lower urinary tract
- ➤ Screen for concomitant medications (see above)

MANAGEMENT
What to Do First
- ■ Rule out common indications for surgery
  - ➤ Gross hematuria (may be treated first with a trial of a 5-alpha reductase inhibitor such as finasteride or dutasteride)
  - ➤ Bladder stones (may not require treatment of prostate by surgery after successful removal; often medical therapy is sufficient for LUTS)
  - ➤ Refractory urinary tract infection
  - ➤ Refractory retention after one attempt at catheter removal
  - ➤ Upper urinary tract compromise (elevated creatinine, hydro by ultrasound)

General Measures
- ■ Rule out all differential diagnoses, specifically prostate cancer by serum PSA and DRE.

SPECIFIC THERAPY
Indications
- ■ Indications for surgical intervention (see above)
- ■ If no absolute indications exist, decision for or against treatment depends on the patient's degree of bother.

Treatment Options
- ■ Watchful Waiting
- ■ Yearly follow-up with standard evaluation

Medical Therapies: Alpha Blocker
- ■ First-line medical therapy: tamsulosin (Flomax); doxazosin (Cardura); terazosin (Hytrin), alfuzosin (Uroxatral)
- ■ Improve all symptoms by about 30%, improve flow rate and emptying
- ■ Adverse events: dizziness, asthenia (more common w/ doxazosin and terazosin), fatigue, ejaculatory abnormalities (particularly tamsulosin)
- ■ Medical Therapies: 5-alpha reductase inhibitor
- ■ Finasteride (Proscar), dutasteride (Avodart)
- ■ Reduces prostate volume by 20%, serum PSA by average of 50% by blocking key enzyme in testosterone metabolism

■ Improves symptoms and flow rate less than alpha blocker
■ Adverse events: impotence, reduced libido, reduced ejaculate volume (all sexual related adverse events, about 15% in first year)

Minimally Invasive Therapies
■ Most available therapies are heat-based; only mechanical device currently available is Urolume Endoprosthesis permanent stent
■ TUMT (Transurethral microwave thermotherapy)
  ➤ administer microwave-generated heat via an antenna placed in prostatic urethra
■ TUNA (Transurethral Needle Ablation)
  ➤ administer radiofrequency-generated heat via a needle placed into the prostate
■ ILTT (Interstitial laser thermal therapy)
  ➤ administer laser energy via needles into the prostate

Surgical Therapies
■ TUIP (Transurethral Incision of the Prostate): indicated for glands <30 ml
  ➤ Single or double incision into bladder neck by electrocautery or laser energy
■ KTP or "Green Light Laser" Prostatectomy > KTP laser used to ablate prostate tissue by transurethral approach, no tissue available for histology, nearly bloodless procedure
■ TURP (Transurethral Resection of the Prostate): indicated for glands >30 but <60 ml (transition zone)
  ➤ Resection of the periurethral part of the prostate by electrocautery or laser (holmium) energy for either resection or enucleation
■ Open surgery: indicated for glands with a transition zone >60 mL or total volume >100 mL

FOLLOW-UP
■ Yearly follow-up with symptom and bother assessment, DRE and serum PSA (as long as >10 years life expectancy)
■ After initiation of treatment, 3 months
■ Standard for each follow-up visit: quantitative symptom assessment and assessment of adverse events; serum PSA if >10 years life expectancy; flow rate and residual urine optional

COMPLICATIONS AND PROGNOSIS
■ Acute and total urinary retention

- Gross hematuria: recurrent urinary tract infection
- Bladder stones
- Upper tract obstruction and azotemia: rare

BENIGN TUMORS OF THE LIVER

EMMET B. KEEFFE, MD

HISTORY & PHYSICAL

History

- Cavernous hemangioma most common benign tumor of liver
- Other two common benign tumors of liver: focal nodular hyperplasia & hepatic adenoma
- Most benign tumors asymptomatic & detected on abdominal imaging
- Cavernous hemagiomas occur in all ages, mostly in third to fifth decade of life; male/female ratio 4:1 to 6:1
- FNH much less common than cavernous hemangioma, but more common than hepatocellular adenoma
- FNH usually asymptomatic, but up to 1/3 may be associated w/ abdominal pain
- FNH 2:1 female predominance
- Hepatocellular adenoma primarily in users of oral contraceptives, w/ estimated prevalence of 1–3/100,000
- Hepatocellular adenoma has significant risk of rupture & malignant degeneration

Signs & Symptoms

- All 3 lesions most commonly detected asymptomatically
- Widespread use of abdominal imaging often leads to detection
- Occasionally, tumors identified on routine laparotomy for other indications

TESTS

Basic Blood Tests

- Routine LFTs typically normal

Imaging

- Cavernous hemangioma: well-defined hyperechoic mass on US; hypodense lesion w/ peripheral contrast enhancement followed by complete filling in on CT; & low signal density on T1-weighted images & very high signal density (light bulb) on T2-weighted images; cotton wool pooling of isotope on technetium-labeled RBC scan

- FNH hypoechoic; hyperechoic or mixed on US; central scar in some but not all cases by CT; central scar more often detected by MR than CT; 50% of lesions take up isotope or fill in on routine technetium sulfur colloid liver scan
- Hepatocellular adenoma diagnosed on basis of clinical awareness in association w/ use of oral contraceptives & imaging studies not characteristic of other benign or malignant lesions; can also be diagnosed by hepatic arteriography, although not often used

Biopsy
- Liver biopsy not performed for cavernous hemangioma because of ease of diagnosis by imaging & risk of bleeding
- Percutaenous liver biopsy often not diagnostic for FNH or hepatocellular adenoma, but can exclude malignant lesion

DIFFERENTIAL DIAGNOSIS
- Hepatocellular carcinoma: usually associated w/ chronic underlying chronic liver disease, (incr.) LFTs, (incr.) AFP
- Hepatic metastasis: usually associated w/ multiple rather than 1 lesion, (incr.) LFTs & known primary
- Other epithelial tumors: bile duct adenoma, hepatobiliary cystadenoma
- Other mesenchymal tumors: infantile hemangioendothelioma, liomyoma
- Other misc tumors: carcinoid, teratoma

MANAGEMENT
What to Do First
- Assess likelihood that tumor benign based on presence of single lesion, normal LFTs, & no underlying liver disease

General Measures
- Use history, physical exam, LFTs, & imaging to exclude underlying chronic liver disease, & CEA & AFP to exclude malignant tumor
- Assess size, presence of symptoms and potential need for resection based on symptoms or clarification of diagnosis

SPECIFIC THERAPY

Treatment Options

- Cavernous hemangiomas: small, asymptomatic lesions generally observed; large, symptomatic lesions resected if anatomically feasible & operative risk reasonable
- FNH: if confirmed or strongly suspected by clinical, radiologic or biopsy features, generally observed
- Hepatocellular adenoma: surgical resection generally recommended whenever possible, particularly if tumor >4–6 cm in diameter, which is associated w/ risk of intraperitoneal hemorrhage; whether or not resected, oral contraceptives should be discontinued, which may be associated w/ spontaneous tumor regression

FOLLOW-UP

- Tumors suspected to be cavernous hemangioma or FNH: repeat imaging, typically US, in 6 mo & then annually for 1 or 2 y to confirm stability & lack of progression
- LFTs q 6–12 m

COMPLICATIONS AND PROGNOSIS

Complications

- Cavernous hemangioma may be associated w/ episodes of severe, acute abdominal pain from bleeding or thrombosis of tumor; rupture w/ hemoperitoneum rare
- FNH only rarely associated w/ intralesional bleeding, necrosis or hemoperitoneum, typically w/ use of oral contraceptives
- Hepatocellular adenoma may be associated w/ tumor rupture in hemoperitoneum in 25–40% of cases

Prognosis

- Cavernous hemangioma: good, w/ no complications resulting from smaller lesions; lesions >4–6 cm have some risk of thrombosis or bleeding, but only few spontaneous ruptures reported; no reports of malignant transformation
- FNH: good, w/ only rare complications of rupture & no reports of malignant degeneration
- Hepatocellular adenoma: depends on size, w/ lesions >4–6 cm having substantial risk of rupture w/ intraperitoneal bleeding; few reports of malignant transformation

BILIARY TRACT MOTILITY DISORDERS

GEORGE TRIADAFILOPOULOS, MD

HISTORY & PHYSICAL

- clinical syndromes of biliary or pancreatic obstruction related to mechanical or functional abnormalities of the sphincter of Oddi (SO)
- terms papillary stenosis, sclerosing papillitis, biliary spasm, biliary dyskinesia, post-cholecystectomy syndrome and sphincter of Oddi stenosis or dysfunction (SOD) used interexchangeably
- sphincter of Oddi stenosis an anatomic abnormality associated with narrowing of the SO; sphincter of Oddi dyskinesia a spastic disturbance of the SO, leading to intermittent biliary obstruction
- female gender and generalized intestinal dysmotility most frequent risk factors
- SOD may affect patients who have undergone cholecystectomy (post-cholecystectomy syndrome)

Signs & Symptoms

- sphincter of Oddi dysfunction may cause biliary pain and pancreatitis
- RUQ pain most common symptom: steady, not colicky and subsides within a few hours
- radiation of pain to back, epigastrium and the right shoulder may occur
- nausea and vomiting may be present
- pain may be in the epigastrium radiating to the back and relieved with fetal position
- complaints of gas, bloating or dyspepsia nonspecific and should not be attributed to a biliary motor disorder
- localized tenderness in the RUQ or epigastrium with or without a positive Murphy's sign
- jaundice unusual

TESTS

Basic Tests

- increased bilirubin, amylase, lipase, aminotransferases and alkaline phosphatase

Specific Diagnostic Tests

■ SO manometry = gold standard; performed during ERCP; basal pressure and phasic wave contractions recorded from the common bile duct and pancreatic duct segments of the sphincter of Oddi

➤ patients with SO stenosis have abnormally elevated basal SO pressure (>40 mmHg) that does not relax following administration of smooth muscle relaxants

➤ patients with SO dyskinesia also have elevated basal SO pressure but the pressure decreases following amyl nitrite or glucagon and increases paradoxically following CCK

➤ Milwaukee classification system for SOD recognizes three types of patients:

➤ Type I patients have: a) pain associated with abnormal serum aminotransferases; b) a dilated common bile duct >10 mm on ultrasound or >12 mm on ERCP; and c) delayed drainage of contrast from the common bile duct after more than 45 minutes in the supine position

➤ Type II patients have one or two of the above 3 criteria

➤ Type III patients have none of the above criteria

Other Tests

■ Ultrasound accurate for gallstones and bile duct dilation; unexplained dilation of the common bile duct associated with SOD predicts a favorable response to sphincterotomy

■ Hepatobiliary scintigraphy using technetium-99m labeled dyes may reveal delayed biliary drainage; clearance rates in patients with SOD overlap with those in a normal controls; scintigraphy may be falsely positive in patients who have extrahepatic biliary obstruction, or falsely negative in patients with intermittent bile flow obstruction.

DIFFERENTIAL DIAGNOSIS

■ Cholelithiasis, pancreatitis, chronic intestinal pseudoobstruction, biliary or pancreatic malignancies, irritable bowel syndrome, peptic ulcer disease and non-ulcer dyspepsia should be considered.

MANAGEMENT

What to Do First

■ Exclude acute cholecystitis, pancreatitis and cholangitis

General Measures

■ For severe attacks, admit the patient for hydration, NPO, analgesia;

NG tube suction may be needed for abdominal distention, nausea and vomiting.

SPECIFIC THERAPY

Indications

■ All symptomatic patients should be offered medical, endoscopic or surgical therapy aimed at reducing the impaired flow of biliary and pancreatic secretions into the duodenum

Treatment Options

■ Patients who are classified as Milwaukee type I usually respond to sphincterotomy. For type II patients in whom sphincterotomy is being considered, biliary manometry is recommended. Type III patients may not have SOD and need careful evaluation.

■ Smooth muscle relaxants may reduce basal SO pressure and improve patients with SOD. Nifedipine improves pain, and decreases the frequency of pain episodes, use of oral analgesics, and emergency room visits. Nitrates decrease both basal and phasic SO activity and may improve pain.

■ Endoscopic injection of botulinum toxin for SO dysfunction has also been successfully used. Improvement in biliary pain and recurrent pancreatitis can be achieved in 50 to 60 percent of patients treated by surgical sphincterotomy.

Side Effects & Complications

■ SO manometry associated with a high rate of pancreatitis

Contraindications

■ Because endoscopic sphincterotomy carries risks (bleeding, perforation and pancreatitis), it should be used only in patients who have been thoroughly investigated

FOLLOW-UP

During Treatment

■ After sphincterotomy patients observed for possible complications

Routine

■ Limited use of narcotic analgesics may prevent addiction

COMPLICATIONS AND PROGNOSIS

Complications

■ Pancreatitis, cholangitis, narcotic addiction from chronic analgesic use

Prognosis
- Most reliable finding predicting a favorable response to sphinctero-tomy is elevated SO basal pressure
- In general, biliary tract motility disorders are chronic and relapsing, impair quality of life and lead to frequent use of health care resources, emergency room visits and potential for narcotic addiction

BIOTIN DEFICIENCY

ELISABETH RYZEN, MD

HISTORY & PHYSICAL

History
- prolonged raw egg white consumption, prolonged TPN

Signs & Symptoms
- dermatitis, glossitis, in children retarded physical, mental development, alopecia, defects in cell-mediated immunity, keratoconjunctivitis

TESTS

Laboratory
- Basic studies: none

DIFFERENTIAL DIAGNOSIS
n/a

MANAGEMENT
n/a

SPECIFIC THERAPY
- Biotin

Side Effects & Contraindications
- None

FOLLOW-UP
n/a

COMPLICATIONS AND PROGNOSIS
- Reversible with replacement

BLADDER TUMORS

MARKLYN J. JONES, MD and KENNETH S. KOENEMAN, MD

HISTORY & PHYSICAL

History

- Tobacco most common cause (>30–50% of cases)
- Fourth leading cause of cancer death
- M > F (2.5X), White > African American
- Incidence increases with age
- Chronic cystitis, especially squamous cell Ca (indwelling catheter, stones, Schistosoma haematobium)
- Cyclophosphamide, radiation exposure to bladder, or chemical exposure (aromatic amines; aniline dyes most common)

Signs & Symptoms

- Hematuria, microscopic or gross, often painless in up to 80%
- Irritative voiding symptoms (frequency, urgency, dysuria), with sterile urine
- Flank pain secondary to hydronephrosis/ureteral obstruction
- Bone pain (mets) or pelvic pain (mass)
- Sites of metastasis from transitional cell Ca (most to least): pelvic lymph nodes, liver, lung, bone, and adrenal gland

TESTS

- History and Physical – include bimanual examination
- Urine: hematuria (always refer patient to urologist for work-up of gross hematuria or 2 of 3 UAs with microscopic hematuria [>3 RBCs/hpf]); can have pyuria, but rule out cystitis
  - ➤ Cytology, especially positive in high-grade TC Ca or CIS
  - ➤ Special tests: BardTM BTA-STAT, NMP-22 (nuclear matrix protein), hyaluronidase ELISA, FISH, tumors with p53 overexpression more likely to progress and less likely to respond to chemotherapy
- Blood: CBC (anemia), and LFTs to rule out bone or liver mets, and alkaline phosphatase to rule out bone mets; if gross hematuria, check PT/PTT, platelets
- Screening – Only for high-risk populations (tobacco), can perform UA, urine cytology or special urine tests (BTA-STAT, NMP-22, hyaluronidase ELISA, or FISH)
- Imaging

- IVP (intravenous urogram) with tomogram, or retrograde urogram is gold standard to evaluate upper tract for filling defects (tumors), but CT urogram also useful and popular
- Bladder ultrasound, IVP, abdominal/pelvic CT often not diagnostic, but can reveal large masses or large polypoid filling defects
- CT scan is useful in metastatic work-up to check for lymph nodes and liver mets; PET CT useful with indeterminate CT; pelvic MRI can be used for determination of local invasion
- CXR or CT chest to rule out lung mets
- Bone scan is indicated if alkaline phosphatase is abnormal or osseous pain is present

Diagnostic Procedures
- Cystoscopy (fluorescent cystoscopy increases sensitivity), transurethral resection of the bladder tumor (TURBT), and site-directed bladder biopsy to rule out carcinoma in situ

DIFFERENTIAL DIAGNOSIS
- For hematuria or irritative voiding symptoms
  - Intravesical calculi
  - Cystitis (bacterial or fungal, etc.)
  - Interstitial cystitis (noninfectious)
  - BPH or prostatitis
  - Radiation, chemical or exogenous injury
- For Bladder Masses
  - Transitional cell carcinoma, TC Ca >90%
  - Squamous cell, SC Ca, 5% US cases: poorer prognosis except bilharzial (secondary to schistosomiasis), which are well differentiated
  - Adenocarcinoma, <2%
    - Most common in exstrophic bladders
    - Common in urachal tumor, often cystic, poorly differentiated, poor prognosis
    - Must be evaluated for other sites of origin – bladder metastasis (most to least common): melanoma, colon, prostate, lung, and breast
  - Lymphoma, pheochromocytoma, and small cell carcinoma are all rare.
  - Leiomyosarcoma in adults, or rhabdomyosarcoma in children
  - Benign Lesion

- Nephrogenic adenoma: metaplastic response to trauma, resembles primitive collecting tubules, often have irritative symptoms
- Inverted papilloma: benign lesion associated with TC Ca

➣ Carcinoma in situ (CIS) – Flat, high-grade, noninvasive lesion; usually velvety patch of erythematous urothelium; often irritative symptoms; urine cytology positive in 95%; often recurrent and progressive; BCG intravesical immunotherapy after TURBT is standard first-line local therapy

MANAGEMENT

What to Do First

■ Perform accurate tissue diagnosis and staging.

General Measures

■ Assess general health and comorbidities of patient (i.e., performance status concerning cardiac, pulmonary, liver, GI, renal function, etc.).

SPECIFIC THERAPY

Refer to urologist to manage

■ CIS: TURBT + bacillus Calmette-Guerin (BCG) intravesical immunotherapy (BCG or other) +/− interferon; for diffuse recurrence, consider radical cystectomy
■ Noninvasive: TURBT, 50% recur, 5% progress to muscle invasion
■ Invasion into lamina propria: >70% recur after TURBT, >40% may progress to muscle invasion, TURBT +/− intravesical BCG or chemotherapy
■ Invasion into muscle and local pelvic structures: TURBT for diagnosis, then radical cystectomy + pelvic lymphadenectomy
■ Invasion into pelvic or abdominal wall, lymph nodes, or metastasis: chemotherapy (Cisplatinum combination – gemcitabine + cisplatin best tolerated vs. MVAC), possible adjuvant surgery or XRT

FOLLOW-UP

■ Cystoscopy protocol at lengthening intervals q 3–4 to q 6–12 months for localized, low-grade and -stage disease, often followed 5–15 years for recurrence
■ 1- to 2-yearly intervals for upper tract imaging (U/S, IVP, CT) for local disease
■ Higher-stage cancer, S/P cystectomy: Needs lifelong surveillance for progression, recurrent UTI, upper tract cancer, urethral recurrence

or obstruction/pyelonephritis, and possible B12 or absorption (GI) problems secondary to bowel used for "neobladder/ileal conduit"

COMPLICATIONS AND PROGNOSIS
- Natural History of Bladder TC Ca
  - ➤ >70% are low-grade noninvasive or invasion into lamina propria
  - ➤ Recurrences and progression are common, especially with grade III or >T1 stage
  - ➤ Life expectancy for metastatic disease - no greater than 12–16 months
  - ➤ 1–5% of pts with bladder TC Ca can develop upper tract TC Ca; 15–20% for CIS

BLASTOCYSTIS HOMINIS INFECTION

J. GORDON FRIERSON, MD

HISTORY & PHYSICAL

History
- Exposure: Ingestion of contaminated food and water is presumed mode of infection (full cycle not worked out yet). It is controversial whether Blastocystis hominis is a pathogen, and it is found frequently in absence of symptoms. With careful search, another cause of symptoms frequently found.

Signs & Symptoms
- Unclear whether it causes any symptoms. If so, mild chronic diarrhea most often reported. Abdominal examination usually normal.

TESTS
- Basic tests: blood: normal
- Basic tests: urine: normal
- Specific tests: Stool exam for O&P shows organism.
- Other tests: none

DIFFERENTIAL DIAGNOSIS
- Any cause of mild chronic diarrhea

MANAGEMENT

What to Do First
- Determine presence of symptoms. Look for other causes of symptoms, as another cause is frequently found.

General Measures
- None

SPECIFIC THERAPY

Indications
- A symptomatic patient in whom no other cause of diarrhea can be found (after proper search) can be treated empirically (no treatment trials yet published).

Treatment Options
- Metronidazole for 10 days
- Iodoquinol for 20 days

Side Effects & Complications
- As for amebiasis, giardiasis
- Contraindications to treatment: absolute: allergy to medications
- Contraindications to treatment: relative: asymptomatic patient, and some feel no one should be treated

FOLLOW-UP

Routine
- If treated, stools can be re-examined.

COMPLICATIONS AND PROGNOSIS
- Prognosis is good for symptoms, though organism may persist or re-appear after an interval (? reinfection).

BLASTOMYCES DERMATITIDIS

RICHARD A. JACOBS, MD, PhD

HISTORY & PHYSICAL

History
- In North America: southeastern, south-central states, especially bordering Mississippi and Ohio River basins; Great Lakes region; St. Lawrence River area of New York and Canada
- Middle-aged men with outdoor occupations that expose them to soil may be at highest risk.

Signs & Symptoms
- Blastomycosis is a systemic disease with a wide variety of pulmonary and extrapulmonary manifestations.

- Acute infection:
  - ➤ Acute pulmonary infection often unrecognized
  - ➤ 1/2 develop symptomatic disease, incubation 30–45 d
  - ➤ Nonspecific symptoms, mimic influenza
- Chronic/recurrent infection – most common course:
  - ➤ Pulmonary: chronic pneumonia, productive cough, hemoptysis, weight loss, pleuritic chest pain
  - ➤ Skin: most common extrapulmonary manifestation (40–80% cases), verrucous lesions (similar to squamous cell ca) or ulcerative-type; occur mucosa of nose/mouth/larynx
  - ➤ Subcutaneous nodules: cold abscesses in conjunction with pulm and other extrapulm disease, often with acutely ill patient
  - ➤ Bone/Joint: long bones, vertebrae, ribs most common with well-circumscribed osteolytic lesion
  - ➤ Genitourinary tract: 10–30% of cases in men, prostate and epididymis
  - ➤ CNS: Uncommon in normal host (<5% cases)
  - ➤ AIDS: more common complications, usually as abscess or meningitis

TESTS

Laboratory
- Microbiology – culture
  - ➤ Standard fungal media
- Serology
  - ➤ Serum comp fix neither specific nor sensitive, as are the other antibody-dependent modalities
- Skin testing
  - ➤ No reagent currently available
- Histopathology
  - ➤ Direct examination of sputum/pus/secretions with or without KOH, bronchoscopy only for patients not producing sputum
  - ➤ Pyogranuloma on tissue section (GMS stain)

Imaging
- CXR
  - ➤ Acute pulmonary: nonspecific, lobar or segmented consolidation
  - ➤ Chronic pulmonary: lobar or segmental infiltrates, with or without cavitation; intermediate-sized nodules, solitary cavities, fibronodular infiltrates

DIFFERENTIAL DIAGNOSIS

- Distinguish from other fungal infections of the lung (Histo, Cryptococcus, Cocci)
- Distinguish from mycobacterial diseases of the lung, other chronic pneumonias, pyogenic pneumonia, malignancy
- Skin disease similar to pyoderma gangrenosum, leishmaniasis, M marinum infection, squamous cell carcinoma

MANAGEMENT

What to Do First

- Establish diagnosis, differentiate from malignancy and other fungal infections

General Measures

- Withholding therapy for acute pulmonary disease in normal host is controversial

SPECIFIC THERAPY

Treatment Options

- Itraconazole or ketoconazole or fluconazole for mild to moderate pulmonary disease and mild to moderate non-CNS disseminated disease, usually for at least 6 mo
- Amphotericin B for serious pulmonary, CNS disease, or serious non-CNS disseminated disease, change to itraconazole after patient's condition has stabilized

Side Effects & Complications

- Amphotericin B (conventional): infusion-related toxicities (often ameliorated with hydrocortisone in IV bag), nephrotoxicity, hypokalemia, hypomagnesemia, nephrotoxicity (can be dose-limiting)
- Azoles: transaminitis, many drug interactions

FOLLOW-UP

During Treatment

- Close clinical follow-up

Routine

- Relapses can be common, close follow-up especially in first two years after stopping azole therapy
- Consider long-term suppressive therapy in AIDS patients, other severely immunosuppressed patients

COMPLICATIONS AND PROGNOSIS

Complications
- Relapse in immunosuppressed
- Disseminated disease, especially to bone/joint, rarely to CNS

Prognosis
- Good for normal hosts with acute disease
- Much poorer for end-stage AIDS (mortality upward of 20%)

BLEPHARITIS

AYMAN NASERI, MD

HISTORY & PHYSICAL

History
- Symptoms of bilateral, chronic ocular burning, itching, and/or irritation
- More common in older adults
- Frequently no associated illnesses or exposures
- Seen in younger patients with rosacea or atopy
- Commonly, no Hx of other ocular disease

Signs & Symptoms
- Screening ophthalmic exam often normal (ie, vision, pupils, eye movements, visual fields, etc.)
- Classic eyelid margin findings: debris on lashes, thickened eyelid margin with telangiectasias
- Unilateral symptoms or conjunctivitis very uncommon

TESTS
- Clinical diagnosis
- No diagnostic lab test
- Need baseline ophthalmic exam
- Slit-lamp examination very helpful
- Eyelid margin cultures useful in some patients

DIFFERENTIAL DIAGNOSIS
- Unlikely blepharitis if unilateral or markedly asymmetric disease
- Malignancy

➤ Sebaceous cell carcinoma
➤ Squamous cell carcinoma
■ Dry eyes/keratitis sicca
■ Atopic disease
■ Roscaea
■ Allergic conjunctivitis
■ Medication toxicity
■ Herpes simplex infection (usually unilateral)

MANAGEMENT

What to Do First

■ Document baseline ophthalmic exam (ie, vision, pupils, eye movements, visual fields, etc.)
■ Assess for signs and symptoms of rosacea, atopy, medication toxicity
■ If symptoms are unilateral or acute, refer to ophthalmologist

General Measures

■ Warm compresses to both eyes BID
■ Gentle cleansing of eyelid margin with mild soap (e.g. baby shampoo)

SPECIFIC THERAPY

■ After failure of general measures, consider referral to ophthalmologist
■ Ophthalmologist may consider empiric topical antibiotic therapy
■ Eyelid cultures with organism susceptibility and directed therapy sometimes necessary
■ Management of concomitant atopy or rosacea
■ Topical antibiotic/steroid combination may be used by ophthalmologist but patients must be followed for complications including glaucoma and cataract

FOLLOW-UP

■ Four to six weeks after initial therapy (see general measures)
■ Refer to ophthalmologist if no improvement in 2–3 months after therapy

COMPLICATIONS AND PROGNOSIS

■ Misdiagnosis may delay appropriate therapy
■ Toxicity may result from topical medications
■ Cataract and glaucoma from antibiotic/steroid preparations

BRAIN ABSCESS

MICHAEL J. AMINOFF, MD, DSc

HISTORY & PHYSICAL

- Primary infection often present either adjacent to cranial infection (eg, ears, teeth, nasal sinuses) or at distant site (eg, lungs); may relate to cyanotic congenital heart disease
- Symptoms of expanding intracranial mass–eg, headache, somnolence, lethargy, obtundation, focal deficits, seizures
- Fever may be absent (40% of cases)
- Signs depend on location of abscess & on ICP
- Common signs include fever, confusion, somnolence, obtundation, papilledema, extraocular palsies, neck stiffness, weakness, visual disturbances, dysphasia, dysarthria
- May be signs of primary infection or of congenital heart disease

TESTS

- Blood studies: leukocytosis (absent in 25% cases)
- Cranial CT or MRI: one or more rim-enhancing lesions, w/ perilesional edema; shift of midline structures
- CSF is at increased pressure; may show pleocytosis, increased protein concentration; cultures usually negative
- Blood cultures & culture of specimens from likely sites of primary infection to identify causal organism

DIFFERENTIAL DIAGNOSIS

- Other expanding focal lesions usually excluded by imaging appearance, but metastatic disease may be simulated
- If abscess suspected clinically, perform imaging studies first; do not perform LP as herniation & clinical deterioration may result

MANAGEMENT

- Control cerebral edema w/ steroids (eg, dexamethasone); mannitol is also effective in short term
- Control infection w/ antibiotics
- Needle aspiration to identify organism if poor response to antibiotics
- Consider surgical drainage (excision or aspiration) if significant mass effect; periventricular location; poor response to antibiotics

SPECIFIC THERAPY

- Antibiotics

FOLLOW-UP
- Imaging studies every 2 wks for 6 months or until contrast enhancement disappears

COMPLICATIONS AND PROGNOSIS
- Mortality depends on condition when effective antibiotics initiated: 5–10% if pt alert, 50% if pt comatose
- Intraventricular rupture has 90% associated mortality
- Persisting contrast enhancement has 20% recurrence rate
- 30% of survivors have residual neurologic deficit

BRAIN DEATH

MICHAEL J. AMINOFF, MD, DSc

HISTORY & PHYSICAL
- Coma
- Unresponsive to external stimulation (but spinal reflex responses may occur)
- No brain stem reflex responses: absent pupillary, oculocephalic, corneal, gag reflexes; no response on cold-caloric testing; no spontaneous respiration on apnea test
- No reversible causes of clinical state (eg, temperature exceeds 32C, no exposure to CNS depressant drugs)
- Clinically stable for at least 6 hr

TESTS
- Ancillary tests sometimes required to confirm brain death
  - EEG: isoelectric
  - Radionuclide brain scan or cerebral angiography: no cerebral blood flow

DIFFERENTIAL DIAGNOSIS
- Exclude hypothermia, coma w/ preserved brain stem reflexes or drug overdose

MANAGEMENT
- Discuss w/ family
- Discontinue life support

TREATMENT
- None

SPECIFIC THERAPY
N/A

FOLLOW-UP
N/A

COMPLICATIONS AND PROGNOSIS
■ Recovery will not occur

BRONCHIECTASIS

PRESCOTT G. WOODRUFF, MD, MPH

HISTORY & PHYSICAL

History
■ Typical symptoms: chronic cough, purulent sputum, fever, weakness, weight loss, hemoptysis
■ Clues to associated diagnoses: history of TB or severe necrotizing pneumonia, recurrent sinopulmonary infections, infertility

Signs & Symptoms
■ Crackles, rhonchi, wheezes
■ Fetid breath
■ Digital clubbing (inconstant)
■ Clues to associated diagnoses: nasal polyps or chronic sinusitis

TESTS
■ Imaging (critical to making diagnosis of bronchiectasis)
  ➢ Chest xray: may show tram tracks (thin parallel markings that radiate from the hili), bronchial dilatation, cystic spaces, peribronchial haziness, atelectasis, or consolidation.
  ➢ HRCT: preferred; may show bronchial dilatation, bronchial wall thickening, lack of normal bronchial tapering, air-fluid levels
  ➢ Sputum analysis: Pseudomonas, other gram-neg organisms, S aureus, or atypical mycobacterial disease may influence prognosis and guide treatment
  ➢ Serum protein electrophoresis (for alpha-1-antitrypsin deficiency)
  ➢ Immunoglobulin levels, including IgG subclasses, for hypogammaglobulinemia
  ➢ Sweat test or genotyping for cystic fibrosis

➤ *Aspergillus* precipitins or specific immunoglobulins for ABPA
➤ Light or electron microscopic exam of respiratory epithelium or sperm for primary ciliary dyskinesia

Other Specific Tests
■ PFTs:
  ➤ Spirometry to evaluate severity of airway obstruction
  ➤ Bronchoscopy: not routine, but may be indicated if aspirated foreign bodies or obstructing lesions suspected

DIFFERENTIAL DIAGNOSIS

Underlying Conditions
■ Bronchial obstruction/ bronchopulmonary sequestration
■ Necrotizing infections/tuberculosis
■ Atypical mycobacterial infection (as primary cause or associated condition)
■ Cystic fibrosis
■ Immunodeficiency (immunoglobulin deficiency or phagocyte dysfunction)
■ HIV infection
■ Allergic bronchopulmonary aspergillosis (ABPA)
■ Alpha-1-antitrypsin deficiency
■ Primary ciliary dyskinesia
■ Aspiration
■ Rheumatoid arthritis
■ Congenital cartilage deficiency
■ Tracheobronchomegaly
■ Unilateral hyperlucent lung
■ Yellow nail syndrome

MANAGEMENT

What to Do First
■ Establish underlying condition, if possible
■ Evaluate degree of airway obstruction with spirometry and response to bronchodilator

General Measures
■ Smoking cessation
■ Influenza and pneumococcal vaccines
■ Inhaled beta-agonists or anticholinergics

SPECIFIC THERAPY

Indications
- Treatment based on symptoms and underlying conditions

Treatment Options
- General therapies:
  - Inhaled beta-agonists or anticholinergics
  - Antibiotics for recurrent or persistent lower respiratory infections or hemoptysis using prolonged course (eg, oral broad-spectrum antibiotic for 3 mo) or rotating course (eg, one of three oral antibiotics for first wk of every mo)
  - IV antibiotics (2–3 wks) may be required for *Pseudomonas*
  - Chest physical therapy with postural drainage
  - Inhaled tobramycin (28 d on/28 d off) may be helpful with chronic *Pseudomonas*
  - Consider resection for single bronchiectatic area with recurrrent infection
  - Bronchial artery embolization or, less commonly, resection for massive or recurrent hemoptysis (see complications)
  - Therapies for specific underlying conditions (specialist referral recommended):
  - Aerosolized recombinant DNase and tobramycin for cystic fibrosis
  - IV immunoglobulin for immunoglobulin deficiency
  - Replacement enzyme therapy for alpha-1-antitrypsin deficiency

Side Effects & Complications
- Chronic antibiotic therapy can lead to resistant organisms; thus extended-spectrum antibiotics generally discouraged for rotating regimens unless indicated by sputum microbiology
- Bronchial artery embolization may be complicated by ischemia of spinal or thoracic nerves, pulmonary infarct, or mediastinal hematoma
- Surgical complications associated with general anesthesia and thoracic surgery

Contraindications
- Relative: resectional therapy requires adequate pulmonary function (specialist referral recommended)

FOLLOW-UP

During Treatment

■ Regular office visits if on rotating antibiotics

Routine

■ Depending on severity of symptoms and airway obstruction

COMPLICATIONS AND PROGNOSIS

Complications

■ Hemoptysis:
  ➤ If nonmassive (>500 mL/d), antibiotics and bronchoscopic evaluation should be considered
  ➤ If massive, patient should be positioned bleeding side down with attention to airway management, and bronchial artery embolization or, rarely, lobectomy considered

Prognosis

■ Overall, good; minority has severe physical and social problems as result of bronchiectasis
■ Decreased pulmonary function and cor pulmonale associated with increased mortality
■ After bronchial artery embolization for hemoptysis, rebleeding may occur in 50% as long as 3 y after procedure

BRONCHIOLITIS

STEPHEN C. LAZARUS, MD

HISTORY & PHYSICAL

Difficult to identify early because involvement of peripheral airways produces few symptoms

History

■ Bronchiolitis:
  ➤ Common in infants and small children: usually due to virus (especially RSV); begins as acute viral illness; cough, dyspnea, fever later
  ➤ Uncommon in adults: industrial, environmental exposures to poorly soluble irritants (nitrogen dioxide, phosgene) from silo gas, jet and missile fuel, fires; may occur with *Mycoplasma, Legionella*, viruses

- Bronchiolitis obliterans:
  - After inhalation of toxic fumes
  - After respiratory infections
  - Associated with connective tissue disorders (rheumatoid arthritis, SLE, polymyositis, dermatomyositis)
  - After bone marrow transplantation: occurs in 10% of patients with chronic graft-vs-host disease; preceded 2–3 mo after transplantation by mucositis, esophagitis, skin rash
  - After lung or heart-lung transplantation: occurs in 30–50% of lung transplant recipients; probably reflects chronic rejection
- Bronchiolitis obliterans with organizing pneumonia (BOOP):
  - Usually follows flu-like illness
  - Often thought to be slowly resolving pneumonia
- Respiratory bronchiolitis: smokers and patients with mineral dust exposure
- Panbronchiolitis:
- Most cases in Japan; also non-Japanese Asians and caucasians
- Predominantly males, nonsmokers
- Associated with chronic sinusitis

Signs & Symptoms
- Despite widespread involvement of small bronchi and bronchioles, symptoms may occur late
- Gradual onset of dyspnea and nonproductive cough
- Fever may be present with acute bronchiolitis
- Physical exam typically normal
- Wheezing uncommon; may be diffuse or localized
- Crackles or "Velcro" rales in 68% of patients with BOOP
- Rales common with respiratory bronchiolitis

TESTS

Laboratory
- Routine blood tests: usually normal

Imaging
- CXR, CT:
  - Variable pattern
  - Miliary or diffuse nodular; reticulonodular; normal
  - Hyperinflation or air trapping may be present

- ➤ BOOP: bilateral ground glass densities in 81%; also miliary nodules and symmetric lower lobe interstitial infiltrates
- ➤ Respiratory bronchiolitis: diffuse interstitial infiltrates or reticulonodular opacities
- ➤ Panbronchiolitis: diffuse small centrilobular nodular opacities and hyperinflation
- PFTs
  - ➤ ABG often normal; hypoxemia and hypercapnia late
  - ➤ Because total cross-sectional area of bronchioles large and changes in bronchiolar caliber contribute little to airway resistance (silent zone of lung), PFTs may be normal until late
  - ➤ Bronchiolitis obliterans: progressive obstruction, often with reduced diffusing capacity
  - ➤ BOOP: restrictive pattern, with reduced diffusing capacity in 72%
  - ➤ Respiratory bronchiolitis: restrictive pattern, with reduced diffusing capacity
  - ➤ Panbronchiolitis: progressive obstruction or restriction, with reduced diffusing capacity
- Lung Biopsy
  - ➤ Often required for specific diagnosis, esp to distinguish BOOP from ILD
  - ➤ Consider in any patient with progressive disease

DIFFERENTIAL DIAGNOSIS

- Asthma: reversible airflow obstruction
- Bronchiolitis: clinical history most helpful
- Bronchiolitis obliterans
- BOOP: usually requires lung biopsy for diagnosis; steroid responsive, important to confirm diagnosis
- Respiratory bronchiolitis: HRCT (diffuse or patchy ground glass opacities or fine nodules) useful to distinguish from ILD (peripheral reticulation, honeycombing)
- Panbronchiolitis: characteristic HRCT: diffuse small centrilobular nodular opacities and hyperinflation
- Interstitial lung diseases
- Pneumonia

MANAGEMENT

What to Do First

- Symptomatic treatment (oxygen, cough suppressants, hydration for acute bronchiolitis)

General Measures

- Early recognition is important; once fibrosis occurs, it is not reversible
- Look for etiology, comorbid conditions
- No proven role for bronchodilators, though empiric trial may provide relief
- Corticosteroid trial for progressive disease

SPECIFIC THERAPY

- For bronchiolitis after lung transplantation: treat for rejection
- BOOP:
  - Very steroid responsive (often improves within days)
  - Continue high dose for 2–3 mo
  - Taper slowly, as relapses may occur
  - Chronic steroids sometimes required

FOLLOW-UP

- PFTs and HRCT frequently, as symptoms not helpful for monitoring response

COMPLICATIONS AND PROGNOSIS

Complications

- Bronchiolitis can lead to bronchiolitis obliterans, bronchiolectasis, localized emphysema
- Early diagnosis and treatment key to preventing irreversible loss of lung function
- Can lead to oxygen dependence and respiratory failure and death

Prognosis

- Without complications, bronchiolitis usually self-limited; recovery in days-weeks
- Bronchiolitis obliterans after bone marrow transplantation usually does not improve with therapy
- Bronchiolitis obliterans after lung transplant may respond if treated early; may stabilize if treated later; major cause of death in long-term survivors
- BOOP has best prognosis: 60–70% respond to steroids, with nearly 60% demonstrating complete response

BRONCHITIS, ACUTE

IVAN W. CHENG, MD

HISTORY & PHYSICAL

History

- Reversible inflammation and edema of the trachea and bronchial tree
- Most commonly due to infection, but can also result from allergic or environmental exposures, smoke or chemical fumes
- Most commonly (up to 95%) viral: influenza, adenovirus, respiratory syncytial virus, rhinovirus, coronavirus, measles, and HSV
- Most viral cases develop between the early fall and spring
- Viral incubation period brief: 1–5 d
- Bacterial etiologies include Mycoplasma and Chlamydia pneumoniae and *Bordetella pertussis*
- Bacterial infections generally have longer incubation periods, up to 3–4 wks

Signs & Symptoms

- Cough, sputum production, rhinitis, pharyngitis, laryngitis common
- Hemoptysis, fever less common
- Lungs usually clear to auscultation, but may reveal wheezing, rhonchi and prolonged expiratory phase

TESTS

- Gram stain and culture of sputum generally not helpful
- WBC count usually normal
- No definitive tests for diagnosis
- Chest x-ray may be appropriate in some cases (abnormal exam, elderly, immunocompromised) to rule out pneumonia
- Chest CT generally not indicated
- Pulmonary function tests may demonstrate obstructive physiology, but this finding probably not useful diagnostically

DIFFERENTIAL DIAGNOSIS

- Sinusitis
- Allergic rhinitis
- Asthma
- Pneumonia
- Allergic aspergillosis
- Occupational exposure

- Chronic bronchitis
- Upper respiratory infection, "common cold"
- Congestive heart failure
- Reflux esophagitis
- Bronchogenic tumor
- Aspiration

MANAGEMENT

- Treatment generally supportive, based on symptoms: antipyretics, analgesics, cough suppressants, decongestants, fluids

SPECIFIC THERAPY

- Scant evidence that antibiotics have any advantage over placebo
- Placebo-controlled studies using doxycycline, erythromycin, and trimethoprim-sulfamethoxazole have not shown consistent, significant benefit
- Liberal use of antibiotics may contribute to development of bacterial resistance
- Specific antiviral treatment of bronchitis due to influenza may shorten duration of illness if therapy is begun within first 48 h of illness
- Reserve antibiotics for those with underlying disease (COPD, IPF) and those with significant fever and purulent sputum
- Inhaled bronchodilators may speed improvement of symptoms and return to work

FOLLOW-UP

Assess for:
- Secondary bacterial infection
- Exacerbation of asthma, COPD

COMPLICATIONS AND PROGNOSIS

- Acute bronchitis may trigger exacerbations of asthma, COPD
- Bronchial hyperresponsiveness may develop and last for weeks; may cause persistent cough
- Generally no long-term sequelae; link has been postulated between acute bronchitis caused by Chlamydia and adult-onset asthma

BUDD-CHIARI SYNDROME

MINDIE H. NGUYEN, MD

HISTORY & PHYSICAL

History
- membranous occlusion of the hepatic vein:
  - ➤ congenital or acquired as a post-thrombotic event
  - ➤ most common cause worldwide
- underlying thrombotic diathesis:
  - ➤ myeloproliferative disorder: most common cause in U.S.
  - ➤ other hematological disorder: antiphospholipid syndrome, lupus anticoagulant, paroxysmal nocturnal hemoglobinuria, protein C or S or antithrombin III deficiency
  - ➤ miscellaneous: pregnancy or high-dose estrogen use, chronic infections (eg, aspergillosis, amebic abcess), tumors (eg, HCC, renal cell carcinoma), chronic inflammatory disease (eg, IBD, Behcet's disease), trauma
- idiopathic: 30% of cases

Signs & Symptoms
- classic triad: hepatomegaly, ascites, abdominal pain
- presentation: acute, subacute, or chronic

TESTS

Basic Studies
- blood (CBC, INR, LFT's): abnormal but nonspecific
- ascitic fluid: high protein concentration (>2.0 g/dL); low white blood cell (< 500); serum-ascites albumin gradient usually >1.1

Imaging
- ultrasound: sensitivity and specificity: 85–90%
- CT: less sensitive and specific than color Doppler ultrasound
- MRI: sensitivity and specificity: 90%
- hepatic venography (gold standard):
  - ➤ thrombus within hepatic veins, "spider-web" pattern of collaterals, or inability to cannulate the hepatic veins

Liver Biopsy
- valuable in evaluating the extent of fibrosis and guiding therapy
- pathologic findings:
  - ➤ necrotic and pale centrilobular areas

> high-grade venous congestion
> heterogenous involvement of liver is occasionally problematic; caudate lobe usually spared

DIFFERENTIAL DIAGNOSIS
- right-sided congestive heart failure
- constrictive pericarditis
- metastatic and infiltrative disease involving the liver
- granulomatous liver disease

MANAGEMENT
What to Do First
- assess severity of portal hypertension and liver disease
- identify and evaluate for potential predisposing conditions

General Measures
- provides only short-term, symptomatic benefit
- diuretics: effective for ascites
- anticoagulation: to prevent recurrent thrombosis

SPECIFIC THERAPY
- TIPS:
  > successful as a bridge to transplantation for acute/fulminant BCS
  > successful for long-term treatment for portal hypertension
  > many patients required repeated stent revisions
- angioplasty, stent placement in hepatic veins and/or inferior vena cava
- transcardiac membranotomy for membranous obstruction
- surgical shunts: patency rate: 65–95%
- liver transplantation: for fulminant course or end-stage cirrhosis

FOLLOW-UP
- monitor for signs of portal hypertension: ascites, varices, encephalopathy
- monitor liver synthetic dysfunction and signs of progressive liver disease
- monitor shunt patency
- removal or control of predisposing risk factors

COMPLICATIONS AND PROGNOSIS
Complications
- TIPS: shunt stenosis or occlusion; hepatic encephalopathy

- surgical shunt: liver failure; hepatic encephalopathy
- OLT: usual complications

Prognosis
- 2-year mortality with supportive medical therapy alone: 85–90%
- 5-year survival with surgical shunt: 38–87% depending on continued patency of graft, degree of fibrosis, type of shunt
- 5-year survival with liver transplantation: 70%

BUERGER'S DISEASE

RAJABRATA SARKAR, MD

HISTORY & PHYSICAL

History
- Young male smokers with finger or toe gangrene
- More common in Middle Eastern, Mediterranean and Far Eastern populations
- Foot or calf claudication
- Ulceration or gangrene of toes or fingers
- Superficial venous thrombophlebitis
- Raynaud's syndrome

Criteria for Clinical Diagnosis
- Smoking history
- Age less than 50
- Occlusive lesions below popliteal or brachial artery
- No trauma or proximal embolic source
- Normal proximal arteries
- Absence of risk factors for atherosclerosis (besides smoking)
  - ➤ Negative collagen vascular disease workup
  - ➤ No diabetes
  - ➤ No hyperlipidemia
- Negative hypercoagulable workup

Signs & Symptoms
- 50% have gangrene of distal toes or fingers
- Pulses at wrist or ankle may be present
- Cold and tender fingers or toes
- Phlebitis in extremities
- Normal proximal pulses (femoral, axillary)

TESTS

Blood

- Serological studies to rule out:
  - Diabetes
  - Collagen vascular disease
  - Hyperlipidemia
  - Hypercoagulable state

Specific Diagnostic Studies

- Noninvasive vascular studies
- Decreased finger or toe pressures
- Normal proximal pressure (elbow or knee)
- Contrast arteriography
  - Rules out proximal lesions and defines:
  - Multiple distal obstructions
  - "corkscrew" collaterals

DIFFERENTIAL DIAGNOSIS

- Thromboembolic disease
- Popliteal artery entrapment
- Adventitial cystic disease
- Arteritis
  - All ruled out by angiography
- Accelerated atherosclerosis due to hypercoagulable state or diabetes
  - Ruled out by serum studies

MANAGEMENT

What to Do First

- Smoking cessation is primary therapy
- Cessation of smoking is necessary and often sufficient for Buerger's disease to abate

General Measures

- Patient education regarding risk of limb loss and role of smoking
- Nicotine replacement therapy
- Formal smoking cessation program
- Skin care, careful fitting of shoes, cold avoidance
- Pain control
- Local wound care
  - Debridement of wet gangrene
  - Antibiotics for associated cellulitis
  - Dressing changes

SPECIFIC THERAPY
- Vasodilators, anticoagulants, prostaglandins are not beneficial
- Surgical bypass and sympathectomy are not useful

FOLLOW-UP
- Close followup of any gangrene is needed to determine later need for subsequent amputation

COMPLICATIONS AND PROGNOSIS
- Limb Loss
  - 50% of those who keep smoking
- Other vascular beds
  - Buerger's disease rarely affects coronary arteries or other areas

BULIMIA NERVOSA

JOSE R. MALDONADO, MD

HISTORY & PHYSICAL

History
- Lifetime prevalence: 1%–3% in females, 0.1%–0.3% in men
- Females >> males (90% occurs in females)
- **Repeated episodes of binge eating, followed by compensatory inappropriate methods to prevent weight gain (purging & dietary restrictions)**
- At least twice a week for 3 months
- Dissatisfaction about body weight and shape
- Fear of weight gain
- A sense of lack of control over eating patterns
- Binges: usually high-calorie foods, usually until person feels uncomfortable or develops abdominal pain
- Secrecy: patients are usually ashamed of their eating patterns and attempt to hide their symptoms
- Binges are often preceded by dysphoria and/or anxiety induced by daily stress, interpersonal stressors, intense hunger caused by dietary restrictions
- Binges are usually followed by feelings of guilt and depressed mood
- Purging:
  - Seen in 80–90% of bulimia cases
  - Provides relief from physical discomfort and reduces the fear of gaining weight following a binge episode

➤ Methods: fingers, instruments, syrup of ipecac, laxatives (1/3 of bulimics), enemas, diuretics

Subtypes
- Purging type: regular self-induction of emesis or the misuse of laxatives, diuretics or enemas after a binge
- Non-purging type: use of non-purging compensatory methods (i.e., fasting or excessive exercise after a binge

Signs & Symptoms
- Loss of dental enamel: lingual surface, front teeth
- Increased frequency of dental cavities
- Enlarged salivary (parotid) glands
- Calluses or scars on dorsal surface of hands from repeated trauma from the teeth during emesis induction and gagging
- Cardiac and skeletal myopathies secondary to repeated ipecac misuse

TESTS
- Fluid and electrolyte abnormalities:
  ➤ Hypokalemia
  ➤ Hyponatremia
  ➤ Hypochloremia
- Metabolic alkalosis (following repeated emesis):
- Metabolic acidosis (following laxative abuse)

DIFFERENTIAL DIAGNOSIS
- Anorexia nervosa, binge-eating/purging type
- Kleine-Levin syndrome
- Major depressive disorder
- Borderline personality disorder
- Body dysmorphic disorder
- Delusional disorder, somatic type

MANAGEMENT

What to Do First
- Persuade patient that treatment is necessary

General Measures
- Referral to psychiatrist with experience in pharmacologic and behavioral therapy of eating disorders

SPECIFIC THERAPY

Pharmacological Treatment

- Antidepressants:
  - ➤ Bulimics without depression respond as well to antidepressant treatment as do depressed bulimics
  - ➤ All antidepressant agents have proven effective to some extent
  - ➤ On average:
    - Binge eating and purging decline about 80%
    - 35–50% of patients become symptom-free for some period of time
  - ➤ Relapse to binging often occurs when medication is withdrawn, and occasionally even when medication is maintained
  - ➤ Long-term efficacy with current medications has not been established

Cognitive-Behavioral Therapy (CBT)

- Goals:
  - ➤ Enhance food intake
  - ➤ Decrease avoidance of specific foods
  - ➤ Deal with distorted thinking about foods, body image, and weight
- Binge eating and purging usually decline once dietary restriction is eased
- Initial stages of treatment include a detailed self-monitoring of food intake and the precipitants and consequences of binge eating
- In the later stages of treatment, relapse-prevention techniques are used (e.g., learning how to cope with high-risk situations)
- Average treatment course: weekly for about 20 sessions over a 6-month period
- CBT vs. medication:
  - ➤ CBT is the preferred initial approach to the treatment of bulimia nervosa
  - ➤ Medication is considered only when the patient does not respond to an adequate course of CBT
  - ➤ 50% of the patients will become symptom-free following treatment
  - ➤ 25% will demonstrate significant improvement

FOLLOW-UP

Long-term treatment for 6 months:

- Cognitive-behavioral therapy (CBT), aims:
  - ➤ Provide support

➤ Modify distorted patterns of thinking about weight and shape
➤ Dealing with ongoing problems of living
■ Family therapy recommended for children and adolescents

COMPLICATIONS AND PROGNOSIS

Complications
■ Menstrual irregularities (25%)
■ Hypokalemia
■ GI problems related to self-induced emesis: chronic hoarseness, esophageal tears and gastric rupture, GERD
■ GI problems associated with chronic laxative use: physiologic adaptation of colon leading to slowed GI motility, an enlarged colon, and constipation

Prognosis
■ Usually begins in late adolescence with dieting and binge eating preceding the onset of purging by several months
■ Usually a chronic, sometimes episodic, course

BULLOUS PEMPHIGOID

DANIEL J SHEEHAN, MD; ROBERT SWERLICK, MD; and
JEFFREY P. CALLEN, MD

HISTORY & PHYSICAL
■ Highest incidence in elderly
■ Severe pruritus
■ Urticarial papules and plaques with tense vesicles
■ Mucosal lesions in < 1/3 of patients

TESTS

Basic Blood Tests:
■ Eosinophilia

Specific Diagnostic Tests
■ Skin biopsy: subepidermal bullae
■ Direct immunofluorescence (DIF): IgG and C3 deposits at the basement membrane zone (BMZ)
■ Indirect immunofluorescence (IIF): anti-basement membrane IgG antibodies

DIFFERENTIAL DIAGNOSIS

- Bullous impetigo – impetigo bullae are flaccid
- Other Immunologically mediated blistering diseases: See below

MANAGEMENT

What to Do First

- Skin biopsy of intact blister and adjacent normal skin

General Measures

- Antibiotics for secondary infections, wet dressings, anti-pruritics

SPECIFIC THERAPY

- Localized disease: potent topical corticosteroids
- Widespread disease: systemic corticosteroids (e.g., prednisone)
- Consider corticosteroid-sparing agents such as tetracycline, dapsone, azathioprine, mycophenolate mofetil, cyclophosphamide, methotrexate, intravenous immune globulin, rituximab

Side Effects & Contraindications

- Topical corticosteroids
  - Side Effects
    - Atrophy, striae, purpura, telangiectasia, hypopigmentation, delayed wound healing
  - Contraindications
    - Absolute: none
- Prednisone
  - Side Effects
    - Hypertension, myopathy, osteoporosis, peptic ulcers, impaired wound healing, growth suppression, diabetes mellitus, suppression of the hypothalamic-pituitary-adrenal axis, cataracts, mood alterations
  - Contraindications
    - Absolute: none
    - Relative: Systemic infection, Pregnancy, nursing mother
- Tetracycline
  - Side Effects
    - Tooth discoloration, photosensitivity, pseudotumor cerebri, decreased effectiveness of OCP's, anorexia, nausea, vomiting, and diarrhea
  - Contraindications
    - Absolute: hypersensitivity to any tetracycline, last $1/2$ of pregnancy, infancy to 8 years of age

- Relative: impaired renal function
- Dapsone
  - Side Effects
    - Idiosyncratic: Hepatitis, mononucleosis-like illness, psychosis, agranulocytosis/leukopenia
    - Dose-related: Hemolytic anemia, peripheral neuropathy
  - Contraindications
    - Absolute: History of dapsone allergy, G6PD deficiency
    - Relative: History of sulfa allergy, severe anemia or hemoglobin abnormality, ischemic heart disease, peripheral vascular disease, severe COPD
- Azathioprine
  - Side Effects
    - Leukopenia, thrombocytopenia, bone marrow suppression, macrocytic anemia, serious infections, nausea, vomiting, diarrhea, increased liver enzymes, fertility impairment
  - Contraindications
    - Absolute: hypersensitivity to azathioprine, pregnancy, nursing mother, thiopurine methyltransferase deficiency
    - Relative: systemic infection
- Mycophenolate mofetil
  - Side Effects
    - Nausea, vomiting, diarrhea, dysuria, sterile pyuria, bone marrow suppression is uncommon, hyperlipidemia
  - Contraindications
    - Absolute: hypersensitivity to mycophenolate mofetil
    - Relative: systemic infection, pregnancy
- Cyclophosphamide
  - Side Effects
    - Bladder malignancy, myeloproliferative or lymphoproliferative malignancies, sterility, hemorrhagic cystitis, infection, anaphylaxis, nausea, vomiting, alopecia, leukopenia
  - Contraindications
    - Absolute: bone marrow depression, hypersensitivity to cyclophosphamide, pregnancy, nursing mother
    - Relative: leukopenia, thrombocytopenia, decreased liver function, decreased kidney function
- Methotrexate
  - Side Effects
    - Transient liver enzyme abnormalities, vomiting, diarrhea, stomatitis, malaise, fatigue, fever, chills, anemia, leukopenia,

thrombocytopenia, liver fibrosis, liver cirrhosis, opportunistic infection, leukoencephalopathy, pulmonary disease

➤ Contraindications
  • Absolute: pregnancy, nursing mother, alcoholism, alcoholic liver disease, chronic liver disease, immunodeficiency, blood dyscrasia, hypersensitivity to methotrexate
  • Relative: decreased renal function, ascites, pleural

■ Rituximab (375 mg/m2 weekly for 4–8 weeks)
  ➤ Side Effects
    • Infusion reaction
  ➤ Contraindications
    • Absolute: hypersensitivity to rituximab, hepatitis B carrier, concomitant cisplatin use
    • Relative: systemic infection

FOLLOW-UP

During Treatment

■ Chest x-ray and/or skin testing for tuberculosis is recommended at the onset of systemic therapies.

■ Corticosteroids: monitor blood pressure, blood sugar and electrolytes. Baseline bone densitometry and follow-up evaluation should be performed and calcium and vitamin D along with a bisphosphonate is advised for patients on 5 mg/d or higher doses for >3 months.

■ Azathioprine and mycophenolate mofetil: CBC and differential biweekly × 2 months, monthly for third and fourth months. Liver function studies q month × 4 months. CBC and differential and LFTs q 2–3 months thereafter.

■ Cyclophosphamide: CBC with differential, UA for RBCs

■ Methotrexate: CBC with differential monthly, BUN/Cr q 1–2 months, liver enzymes q 1–2 months

Routine

■ Monitor for presence of new active blistering

COMPLICATIONS AND PROGNOSIS

■ Tends to be chronic, but complete remissions do occur

■ Low mortality even without aggressive treatment, except in very elderly patients

CANDIDIASIS

RICHARD A. JACOBS, MD, PhD

HISTORY & PHYSICAL

History

- Candida are yeast that reproduce by budding, appear as large oval Gram positive organisms on Gram stain and grow on routine culture media
- Found in nature and as part of the normal skin, vaginal, and gastrointestinal flora of humans
- Diabetes, neutropenia, broad-spectrum antibiotics, HIV, intravascular devices and Foley catheters predispose to infection
- Important human pathogens include C albicans, C tropicalis, C parapsilosis, C glabrata, C krusei and C lusitaniae

Signs & Symptoms

- Oral mucosa: thrush refers to white, raised patches on the tongue and mucous membranes; other lesions include plaques, atrophy of the tongue and angular cheilitis (cracks at the corners of the mouth)
- Esophageal: presents as dysphagia, nausea or chest pain; can occur without thrush
- Other gastrointestinal sites of infection: stomach, small and large bowel (ulcerations or plaques)
- Cutaneous: lesions include balanitis (white patches on the penis usually resulting from intercourse with partner with candida vaginitis), paronychia (inflammation around nail bed common in those with prolonged water exposure), onychomycosis (involvement of nail), intertriginous (inflammation with erythema, fissures and maceration in warm moist areas of skin opposition, such as groin or under breasts) and subcutaneous nodules that are firm, sometimes painful nodules that are multiple and widespread and represent hematogenous dissemination
- Candidemia: usually associated with intravascular device and presents as acute onset of fever without localizing findings; also seen in neutropenic patients
- Genitourinary: asymptomatic candiduria most common and seen in those with long term, indwelling Foley catheters, on broad spectrum antibiotics; cystitis and pyelonephritis less common; vaginitis discussed elsewhere

- Hepatosplenic: multiple abscesses in the liver and/or spleen seen in immunocompromised patients, especially those with prolonged neutropenia; presents with fever, nausea and vomiting
- Less common manifestations: endocarditis, pneumonia, meningitis, arthritis, osteomyelitis, peritonitis and endophthalmitis

TESTS
- Diagnosis made by seeing organism on KOH preparation (skin, mucous membranes, vaginal secretions) or by culture; endoscopy, biopsy of liver or aspiration of subcutaneous nodule may be needed to obtain appropriate material
- Abdominal CT in neutropenic patients with elevated alkaline phosphatase and fever usually shows multiple abscesses or "bull's-eye" lesions in liver and/or spleen
- Echocardiogram in patients with persistent candidemia without focus (especially IV drug users)

DIFFERENTIAL DIAGNOSIS
- Other bacterial and fungal infections can produce similar clinical manifestations and are differentiated by culture

MANAGEMENT
- Assess risk factors for infection
- Obtain material for microscopic examination and/or culture
- If immunocompromised or seriously ill, empirical therapy should be started before results of studies known

SPECIFIC THERAPY
- Different species of Candida have different sensitivities: amphotericin B and lipid formulations of amphotericin B are active against most species except C lusitaniae; azoles (miconazole and ketoconazole) and triazoles (fluconazole and itraconazole) active against C albicans, C tropicalis and C parapsilosis, but have unreliable activity against C glabrata and are inactive against C krusei
- Superficial infections of skin and mucous membranes treated with topical agents such as nystatin, clotrimazole or miconazole; refractory cases treated with fluconazole
- Esophageal candidiasis treated with fluconazole, or for refractory cases amphotericin B
- Line-related candidemia can be treated with fluconazole for at least 2 weeks after last positive culture; C glabrata and C krusei should be treated with amphotericin B; line removal critical for successful outcome

- Candiduria rarely associated with candidemia; candiduria with a Foley catheter does not require therapy
- Other invasive disease, especially in the immunocompromised patient, treated with amphotericin B; once clinical improvement occurs, fluconazole orally can be used if the organism is sensitive

FOLLOW-UP
- Symptoms usually resolve in several days with appropriate therapy.
- With candidemia, blood cultures should be obtained every other day until negative.

With candidemia, once blood cultures are clear, obtain ophthalmologic evaluation to rule out candida chorioretinitis or endophthalmitis.

COMPLICATIONS AND PROGNOSIS
- Complications uncommon in competent host; esophageal or bowel perforation, secondary seeding in candidemia (joints, CNS, heart, eye, liver and spleen) occur infrequently even in compromised host
- Prognosis superb for superficial infections; invasive disease associated with significant mortality, especially if immunosuppression cannot be reversed

CANDIDIASIS: ORAL

SOL SILVERMAN JR, DDS

HISTORY & PHYSICAL
- recent onset associated with discomfort, pain, halitosis, dysgeusia
- can appear as white (pseudomembranous), red (erythematous), or white-red combination
- can be isolated or wide-spread on any mucosal surface
- risk increased in immunosuppression, diabetes, anemia, xerostomia, antibiotics, dentures

TESTS
- clinical appearance and response to antifungal medications
- smear for hyphae or culture

DIFFERENTIAL DIAGNOSIS
- leukoplakia, dysplasia, carcinoma, hypersensitivity, immunosuppression

MANAGEMENT
- rule out xerostomia, hyperglycemia, anemia, immunosuppression, antibiotic use

SPECIFIC THERAPY
- stabilize patients and frequent mouth rinses (water and/or antiseptic)
- systemic antifungals
- topical antifungals
- sialogogues if necessary

FOLLOW-UP
- watch for recurrence; search for causative factor(s)

COMPLICATIONS AND PROGNOSIS
- prognosis depends upon eliminating or controlling causative factors
- complications include discomfort, halitosis, dysgeusia, transmission to partners,
- genital/anal/skin spread

CARCINOID

MAY CHEN, MD and GEORGE A. FISHER, MD, PhD

HISTORY & PHYSICAL

History
- Carcinoid ("cancer-like") neoplasms least aggressive of neuroendocrine tumors
- Incidence 0.5–1.5 per 100,000
- Median age at presentation ~60 years of age
- Female predominance in younger age groups
- Familial association with MEN type I

Signs & Symptoms
- Local symptoms: depend on site of disease
- Gastric carcinoids: dyspepsia, nausea or anemia
- Midgut carcinoids: 40–60% asymptomatic (e.g. found in 1 of 200 appendectomy specimens)
- Most frequent symptoms those of carcinoid syndrome
- Carcinoid syndrome most common with liver metastases; occasionally crampy abdominal pain due to obstruction

■ Rectal carcinoids: abdominal cramping and changes in bowel habits
*Note: rectal carcinoids do not cause carcinoid syndrome

Carcinoid Syndrome
■ Flushing sensation lasting 2–5 minutes with warmth and erythema
of upper body, head and neck; often spontaneous; sometimes precipitated by stress, alcohol, cheeses
■ Diarrhea up to 30 watery stools/day, often with crampy abdominal
pain
■ Wheezing or asthma
■ Cardiac manifestations: endocardial fibrosis predominantly of right
ventricle, causing tricuspid regurgitation, and less commonly pulmonic stenosis.

TESTS

Basic Laboratory Tests
■ elevated 24 h urine for 5-HIAA (75% sensitive and 100% specific for
carcinoid syndrome)
■ elevated platelet 5-HIAA (more sensitive in combination with urinary
5-HIAA)

Other Tests
■ plasma chromagranin A and B (not specific, can occur in patients
with pancreatic endocrine tumors)
■ plasma HCG (elevated in 28% pts with carcinoid)

Radiographic Tests
■ Octreotide scan (somatostatin receptor scintigraphy)
■ I-MIBG
■ Biphasic CT scan: for determining stage of disease, particularly to
determine if liver metastases present

Pathology
■ although elevated urinary 5-HIAA pathognomonic, biopsy should
always be obtained for confirmation (and exclude other poorly differentiated neuroendocrine tumors)

DIFFERENTIAL DIAGNOSIS
■ Any tumor located in stomach, small bowel or rectum – the usual
sites of carcinoid tumors

MANAGEMENT

What to Do First
- obtain 5-HIAA and CT scan of abdomen if carcinoid tumor suspected based on symptoms

General Measures
- stage disease with CT scan of abdomen and obtain biopsy for confirmation

SPECIFIC THERAPY

Localized Disease
- resection in all medically operable patients
- hepatic resection in patients with limited liver disease
- liver transplantation in younger patients with extensive liver metastases and no extrahepatic disease (one study of 15 pts with 5 year survival 69% after liver transplant for carcinoid)

Metastatic or unresectable disease without carcinoid syndrome
- follow with serial CT scans, as many will have indolent courses; treat only for symptoms or more rapid growth

Carcinoid Syndrome
- octreotide: alleviates carcinoid syndrome in 85% of patients
- progression of tumor, symptomatic disease, or carcinoid syndrome refractory to octreotide
- liver-dominant disease
  - limited liver lesions: resection or thermal ablation (percutaneous radiofrequency ablation), or hepatic arterial embolization (with or without chemotherapy)
- interferon with or without octreotide:
- chemotherapy
  - progressive disease refractory to other treatment
  - active agents: doxorubicin, 5-FU, DTIC, actinomycin D, cisplatin VP-16, streptozotocin.
  - combination chemotherapy no advantage over single agent (responses in <30% of patients, duration of response usually <1 year)

FOLLOW-UP
- Serial visits with symptom survey for pain, weight loss or symptoms carcinoid syndrome
- Serial urinalyses for 5-HIAA and abdominal CT scans to determine stability vs progression

COMPLICATIONS AND PROGNOSIS

- Overall median survival of years to decades
- Early stage carcinoid tumors (any site): highly curable (>90%) with surgery alone
- Midgut carcinoid: preferential metastases to liver
- Foregut and hindgut carcinoid: may metastasize to bone
- Metastatic or unresectable carcinoid tmors typically slow-growing with indolent course
  - regional metastasis: overall 5-yr survival rate of 64% (23% for stomach, 100% for appendix).
  - distant metastases: overall 5-yr survival ~20% (0% for stomach, ~10% for rectum and bronchus, 20% for small intestine, 27% for appendix)
- 70% of patients with midgut carcinoids develop carcinoid syndrome, most often in association with liver metastases
- Carcinoid crisis: immediate and life-threatening complication of carcinoid
  - spontaneously or with stress, anesthesia, certain foods (e.g. cheese, alcohol)
  - intense flushing, diarrhea, abdominal pain, mental status changes from headache to coma, tachycardia, hypertension, or profound hypotension
- Complications due to carcinoid-induced fibrosis:
  - cardiac fibrosis associated with right heart abnormalities: tricuspid regurgitation and pulmonic stenosis with CHF (up to 50% with carcinoid syndrome).
  - retroperitoneal fibrosis causing ureteral obstruction
  - Peyronies disease
- Causes of death:
- liver failure (extensive metastases), CHF, carcinoid crisis, malnutrition
- Rare complications:
  - pellegra with hyperkeratosis and pigmentation
  - intrabdominal fibrosis and occlusion of mesenteric arteries or veins
  - sexual dysfunction in men
  - endocrine abnormalities: Cushings syndrome from ectopic ACTH (most common in foregut carcinoids); acromegaly secondary to GH release
  - others: rheumatoid arthritis arthralgias, mental status changes, ophthalmic changes secondary to vessel occlusion

CARDIAC ARREST

MICHEL ACCAD, MD

HISTORY & PHYSICAL

History
- Determine time of arrest (if witnessed)
- Antecedent complaints: chest pain, breathlessness, palpitations, choking, abdominal pain. severe headache. Underlying condition: sepsis, renal failure, known heart/lung disease, toxic exposure.
- Was death anticipated (known terminal illness)?

Signs & Symptoms
- Unresponsiveness ("are you alright?")
- Absent breathing (look, listen, feel), or agonal breathing (not effective breathing)
- Absent circulation: absent carotid pulse, no breathing, coughing or movement.
- Signs of irreversible death: rigor mortis, dependent lividity

TESTS
n/a

DIFFERENTIAL DIAGNOSIS
n/a

MANAGEMENT

What to Do First
- Call CODE, check for valid DNR order
- Primary ABCD survey:
- Airway: position patient supine on firm surface. Head tilt-chin lift or jaw-thrust maneuver. If foreign body aspiration suspected, tongue-jaw lift and finger sweep, followed by Heimlich maneuver.
- Breathing: bag-mask device, produce visible chest rise. Additional rescuer to provide bag-mask seal, cricoid pressure as needed. If cannot ventilate, consider foreign body aspiration.
- Circulation: chest compressions. Elbows locked, $1\frac{1}{2}''$ to $2''$ excursions, ~100 compression/min
- Defibrillation: attach monitor/defibrillator. If rhythm VT/VF, deliver shock (200J, 200–300J, 360J)

General Measures
- Secondary ABCD survey:
- Airway: intubate as soon as possible
- Breathing: confirm tube placement by auscultation, pulse oximetry, or end-tidal CO_2
- Circulation: establish IV access (peripheral is ok). Assess for adequacy of compressions. Administer drugs according to specific algorithm (see below).
- Differential diagnosis. Consider reversible causes of cardiac arrest (see below).

SPECIFIC THERAPY
- Pulseless VT/VF
  - Single shock (360 J for monophasic defibrillator, 150–200 J for biphasic truncated exponential waveform, or 120 J for biphasic rectilinear waveform), then resume CPR for one cycle before checking for pulse and rhythm.
  - Organize therapies around 5 cycles (or 2 minutes) of CPR. Administer shock between therapies. Give drug therapies during CPR.
  - Epinephrine IV push q 3–5 min and/or vasopressin IV push (one time only)
  - Consider antiarrhythmics:
    - Amiodarone: bolus IV over 10 min, then drip
    - Lidocaine: bolus
  - Consider buffers: Na-bicarbonate IV push
- Pulseless electrical activity (PEA)
  - Organize therapies around 5 cycles (or 2 minutes) of CPR.
  - Epinephrine IV push q3–5 min
  - If PEA rhythm slow, atropine IV push q3–5 min
  - Na-bicarbonate for tricyclic overdose, hyperkalemia, metabolic acidosis, or prolonged arrest
  - Review most frequent reversible causes – "5Hs and 5Ts"
    - Hypovolemia (include hemorrhage, sepsis, anaphylaxis)
    - Hypoxia
    - Hydrogen ion (acidosis)
    - Hyper-/hypokalemia
    - Hypothermia
    - "Tablets" (i.e., drug overdose)
    - Tamponade
    - Tension pneumothorax

- Thrombosis (coronary)
- Thrombosis (pulmonary)

■ Asystole
  ➤ Confirm asystole: check lead placement, power, gain
  ➤ Dismal prognosis; consider DNR order
  ➤ Epinephrine 1 mg IV push q3–5 min
  ➤ Consider transcutaneous pacing.

Consider allowing family member presence during resuscitative efforts (shown to ease the grieving process). Assign staff person to accompany family member and answer questions.

FOLLOW-UP

Termination of Resuscitative Efforts

■ In the absence of mitigating factors, resuscitation unlikely to be successful and can be discontinued if there is no return of spontaneous circulation during 30 minutes of Advanced Cardiac Life Support (15 min for newborn infants).

■ Debriefing of code team. Review and analyze sequence of interventions. Allow free discussion and constructive criticism from all members. Allow expression of feelings.

■ Notify family/friends. Do not announce death over the phone. Allow time for shock, grieving. Answer questions about circumstances of death, disposition of body. Allow family to see body.

■ Consider autopsy or organ/tissue donation.

■ Training practice of lifesaving procedures on newly dead patients only under defined educational programs

Successful Resuscitation

■ Survival to discharge after an in-hospital cardiac arrest usually <15%

■ Prognostic factors: most important factor is *time of resuscitative efforts*. Time to CPR, time to defibrillation, comorbid disease, prearrest state, and initial arrest rhythm *are not clearly predictive of outcome*.

■ Prognosis for neurologic outcome in comatose patients best assessed 2–3 days after arrest. 3 factors associated with poor outcome:
  ➤ absence of pupillary response to light on the 3rd day
  ➤ absence of motor response to pain by the 3rd day
  ➤ bilateral absence of cortical response to somatosensory evoked potentials within the first week

- Post-resuscitation syndrome:
  - ➤ Cardiovascular dysfunction (12–24 h post arrest)
  - ➤ Reperfusion failure
  - ➤ Reperfusion injury with release of toxic metabolites
  - ➤ Coagulopathy
  - ➤ Infection
  - ➤ Systemic Inflammatory Response Syndrome (SIRS)
- Routine measures:
  - ➤ intensive cardiac care monitoring
  - ➤ change IV lines placed without sterile technique during code
  - ➤ administer IV fluids (NS)
  - ➤ correct hypoglycemia, acidosis, and electrolyte abnormalities
  - ➤ stress ulcer and DVT prophylaxis
  - ➤ continue anti-arrhythmic therapy (VF/VT arrest) and monitor drug toxicity (eg QT interval, procainamide/NAPA level, etc.)
  - ➤ treat fever aggressively (decrease cerebral oxygen demand)
  - ➤ address underlying condition based on differential diagnosis
  - ➤ periodic assessment of neurologic status

COMPLICATIONS AND PROGNOSIS
n/a

CARDIAC TRAUMA

JUDITH A. WISNESKI, MD

HISTORY & PHYSICAL
- Recent blunt or sharp, penetrating trauma to chest or back
- Trauma resulting in an increase in intravascular pressure
- Sudden rapid decelerative force

Cardiac Trauma Can Result in Injury to Following Structures:

Pericardium
- Acute pericarditis (see Pericardial diseases)
- Pericardial effusion or tamponade (see Pericardial diseases)

Myocardium
- Contusion
  - ➤ Symptoms & Signs
    - Chest pain, arrhythmias (ventricular tachycardia, ventricular fibrillation, atrial fibrillation)

TESTS
- ECG – ST changes (*very common*), new Q waves
- Blood – Elevation of Troponin I and other cardiac enzymes similar to acute MI
- Echo/Doppler – May show decreased left ventricular function, pending severity of contusion
- Coronary angiography – may be indicated to define coronary anatomy
- MRI – define region of injury (severe, large contusions)

DIFFERENTIAL DIAGNOSIS
n/a

MANAGEMENT
- Avoid anticoagulation and GPllb/llla inhibitors
- Avoid non-steroidal agents
- Treatment for chest pain (does not respond to nitroglycerin)
- Bed rest (similar to acute MI)
- Monitor and treat for arrhythmias

SPECIFIC THERAPY
n/a

FOLLOW-UP
n/a

COMPLICATIONS AND PROGNOSIS
- Ventricular aneurysm
- Late rupture

CARDIAC TUMORS

PRISCILLA HSUE, MD

HISTORY & PHYSICAL
Primary Cardiac Tumors – 75% benign, remainder are malignant
- Benign:
  - ➤ Atrial myxoma
    - most common primary cardiac neoplasm – benign or malignant
    - peak incidence age 40–60
    - familial myxoma syndrome – Carney complex
    - 75% in left atrium
    - treat with prompt surgical removal

- recurrences rare, occurring within 4 years of surgery
- followup echo recommended

➤ Rhabdomyoma
  - most common benign cardiac tumor of childhood – most younger than 1 year of age
  - associated with tuberous sclerosis
  - usually located in multiple areas of ventricular myocardium; can cause hypoxic episodes, syncope, heart failure, or arrythmias
  - surgical removal usually successful

➤ Papillary fibroelastoma
  - resembles sea anemone
  - most frequently located on aortic or cardiac valves
  - up to 30% have systemic embolization
  - treat with anticoagulation
  - surgery reserved for patients with recurrent embolization

➤ Fibromas (located near septal myocardium) and lipomas (occur in both myocardium and pericardium)
  - size up to several centimeters
  - symptoms related to local tissue encroachment rather than obstruction

■ Malignant:
  ➤ Angiosarcoma
    - most common malignant primary cardiac neoplasm
    - 2–3 × more frequent in men
    - ages 20–50
    - most from right atrium or pericardium with resultant signs/symptoms of right–sided heart failure
    - hemorrhagic pericardial effusion or obliteration of pericardial space by tumor cells and thrombus occurs
    - intracavitary mass effects and local metastases are common
    - precordial chest pain similar to pericarditis
    - poor prognosis – mean survival under 1 year after diagnosis
    - surgical therapy usually not possible secondary to extensive disease at time of diagnosis
    - combined treatment with radiation and chemotherapy

  ➤ Rhabdomyosarcoma
    - more common in men ages 20–50
    - can arise in any cardiac chamber; often multiple
    - poor prognosis – most die within 1 year of diagnosis

- limited success with resection of localized tumors and adjuvant therapy
> Mesothelioma
  - primary; usually diffuse, pericardial tumors
  - involve both parietal and visceral pericardial layers
  - extend only superficially into myocardium and rarely involve cardiac chambers
  - symptoms are typically pericarditis or tamponade with characteristic hemorrhagic effusion
  - poor prognosis with surgical excision usually not possible
  - radiation and chemotherapy result in only temporary improvement

Secondary Cardiac Tumors

- 20–40× more common than primary cardiac neoplasms
- most common to metastasize to heart are from lung, breast, lymphoma, leukemia, renal cell carcinoma, and melanoma (latter has highest frequency of secondary involvement of the heart)
- mechanisms: direct extension, through lymphatic systems, or by bloodstream
- signs/symptoms not common – appreciable cardiac dysfunction occurs in only 10% of patients, the majority from pericardial involvement resulting in constriction and inflammation
- pericardial involvement – pericarditis, pericardial effusion, pericardial constriction
- EKG: nonspecific ST-T abnormalities, low voltage, and atrial arrhythmias
- if effusion, pericardiocentesis to obtain fluid for cytology

Signs & Symptoms

- systemic findings including fever, cachexia, malaise, rash, clubbing, Raynaud's phenomenon, arthalgias – similar to presentation of endocarditis, malignancy or collagen vascular disease
- systemic signs/symptoms resolve when tumor is removed
- peripheral emboli with stroke, myocardial infarction, abdominal pain, or pulseless extremity
- symptoms caused by anatomic location of tumor if it is located near valve such as symptoms of valvular stenosis, regurgitation or new onset heart failure
- infiltrative tumors may cause arrythmias, conduction defects, and hemodynamic compromise

■ physical exam depends on location of tumor and may be positional
  ➤ tumor plop – low pitched sound occurring after S2, occurring later than an opening snap
  ➤ if tumor located near tricuspid valve – symptoms of right-sided failure such as hepatomegaly, ascites
  ➤ tumor located in left atrium (usually myxoma) – symptoms of mitral stenosis such as opening snap, loud first heart sound, rales, and diastolic rumble

TESTS
■ Basic blood tests
  ➤ hypergammaglobulinemia
  ➤ elevated erythrocyte sedimentation rate
  ➤ thrombocytosis or thrombocytopenia
  ➤ polycythemia
  ➤ leukocytosis
  ➤ anemia

Imaging
■ CXR
  ➤ alterations in cardiac contour, chambers, mediastinal widening, calcifications
■ Transthoracic echo (TTE)
  ➤ provides information regarding tumor size, attachment, and mobility to allow operative resection
  ➤ sensitive for detection of small tumors, especially in left ventricle or non-prolapsing tumors
  ➤ can differentiate between left atrial thrombus and myxoma
■ Transesophageal echo (TEE)
  ➤ obtain if TTE study is suboptimal or confusing
  ➤ improved resolution of tumor and attachment
  ➤ can detect some masses not visualized by TTE
  ➤ improved visualization of right atrial tumors
  ➤ superior for anatomic details such as tumor contour, cysts, calcification, and stalk
■ Radionuclide imaging
  ➤ Lower rate of resolution than echo or angiography
■ CT
  ➤ use to determine the degree of myocardial invasion and the involvement of pericardial and extracardiac structures
  ➤ high degree of tissue discrimination and evaluation of extracardiac structures

- MRI
  - ➤ provides larger field of view
  - ➤ can be useful to define tumor prolapse, secondary valve obstruction, and cardiac chamber size
  - ➤ may depict size, shape, and surface characteristics of tumor more clearly than TTE
- Cardiac Catheterization
  - ➤ obtain if noninvasive evaluation is inadequate
  - ➤ suggested if malignant cardiac tumor considered likely
  - ➤ findings include compression of cardiac chambers or large vessels, intracavitary filling defects, variations in myocardial thickness, pericardial effusion, and wall motion abnormalities
  - ➤ risk of peripheral embolization due to dislodgement
- Pericardiocentesis with fluid cytology if large pericardial effusion is present
- Endomyocardial biopsy to diagnose metastatic tumors

DIFFERENTIAL DIAGNOSIS
- Rheumatic heart disease
- Pulmonary hypertension
- Cerebrovascular disease
- Endocarditis
- Vasculitis
- Pericarditis
- Pulmonary embolus
- Mural thrombus
- Carcinoid heart disease
- Valvular heart disease (i.e. MS, MR, etc.)
- Cardiomyopathy

MANAGEMENT
What to Do First
- visualization usually with echocardiography

General Measures
- refer for prompt surgical removal if appropriate
- followup echocardiography to exclude recurrence

SPECIFIC THERAPY
- Benign Tumors
  - ➤ operative excision (Rx of choice)
  - ➤ in many cases, results in complete cure

➤ should carry out operation promptly after diagnosis
➤ complications – dislodgement of tumor fragments resulting in peripheral emboli or dispersion of micrometastasis is major risk
■ Malignant Tumors
➤ surgery is Rx of choice if feasible
➤ partial resection
➤ chemotherapy
➤ radiation therapy
■ Metastatic tumors
➤ no definitive Rx of choice
➤ chemotherapy
➤ radiation therapy
➤ surgery
➤ if recurrent pericardial effusion occurs, pericardial window or percardiectomy

FOLLOW-UP
■ Repeat TTE to exclude recurrence

COMPLICATIONS AND PROGNOSIS

Prognosis
■ Benign tumors – surgery generally curative with perioperative mortality of about 5%
■ Malignant tumors – most pts die within 1 year of diagnosis
■ Metastatic tumors – ranges from 6 months for pts with solid tumors to greater than 15 months for pts with lymphoma

CAT SCRATCH DISEASE

RICHARD A. JACOBS, MD, PhD

HISTORY & PHYSICAL

History
■ caused by Bartonella henselae, a slow-growing, fastidious, aerobic gram-negative rod
■ up to 55% of cats have serologic evidence of infection with B. henselae and 40% of randomly sampled healthy cats are bacteremic with the organism (prevalence of seropositivity and bacteremia higher in kittens and feral cats)
■ exposure to cats almost universal

- disease usually follows bite or scratch of kitten or feral cat, most commonly seen in children and young adults
- fleas important in transmission between cats; role of fleas in transmission to humans unclear

Signs & Symptoms

- A cutaneous papule or pustule develops at the site of animal contact within 10 days of exposure
- The hallmark of CSD, regional lymphadenopathy without lymphangitis, develops several weeks after the primary cutaneous lesion
- Single node involvement most common, but multiple nodes at single or multiple sites can occur
- Suppuration occurs in a minority of cases
- Nonspecific systemic symptoms (low-grade fever, fatigue, malaise, headache) may accompany adenopathy
- Less common manifestations include Parinaud's oculoglandular syndrome (granulomatous conjunctivitis with ipsilateral preauricular lymphadenopathy), neuroretinitis (acute unilateral decrease in visual acuity with papilledema and stellate macular infiltrates), granulomatous hepatitis and/or splenitis osteitis and encephalopathy

TESTS

- For classic CSD and Parinaud's oculoglandular syndrome, diagnosis made clinically and by exposure history
- For less common manifestations, diagnosis often made pathologically or serologically:
  - ➤ Neuroretinitis: single elevated antibody titer or four-fold rise in titer to B. henselae confirms diagnosis
  - ➤ Granulomatous hepatitis/splenitis: abnormal liver function tests prompt ultrasound or CT scan that demonstrates multiple hypoechoic or hypodense lesions. Biopsy shows granulomas with or without necrosis and stellate abscesses; silver stain may reveal bacilli; serum serology positive
  - ➤ Osteitis: biopsy with granulomas as above, and serology positive
  - ➤ Encephalopathy: CSF nondiagnostic – may be normal or have elevated protein and/or mild pleocytosis. Serum serologies positive.

DIFFERENTIAL DIAGNOSIS

- Other causes of lymphadenopathy – infectious mononucleosis, CMV, toxoplasmosis, typical and atypical tuberculosis, syphilis, brucella, fungal infections, malignancies, etc.

MANAGEMENT
- Symptomatic treatment for pain, fever

SPECIFIC THERAPY
- Classic CSD – a benign, self-limited disease that resolves spontaneously in several months
- Azithromycin may hasten resolution of adenopathy, but is not routinely recommended. Consider for severe systemic symptoms or suppuration.
- Unclear if therapy affects resolution of retinitis, hepatosplenic granulomatous disease, osteitis or encephalopathy, but many would treat with doxycyline or erythromycin with or without rifampin

FOLLOW-UP
- Spontaneous resolution may be slow and intermittent clinical assessment is indicated, particularly when the diagnosis is clinical.

COMPLICATIONS AND PROGNOSIS
- Full recovery is the rule.
- Suppuration of lymph nodes in 15%
- Rare permanent loss of vision, but most recover full visual acuity even without therapy

---

CECAL VOLVULUS

BASSEM SAFADI, MD and ROY SOETIKNO, MD, MS

HISTORY & PHYSICAL

Risk Factors
- incomplete fixation of the right colon mesentery to the lateral abdominal wall
- two types: ileocolic (90%), cecal bascule (10%)
- cecal volvulus causes small bowel obstruction

Symptoms & Signs
- crampy abdominal pain, nausea, vomiting and abdominal distention.
- acute, but can sometimes be insidious
- abdominal distention and tympany
- peritoneal signs, fever, and leukocytosis suggest ischemia and perforation

TESTS
- abdominal X-ray: dilated loops of small bowel with air/fluid levels (small bowel obstruction)
- dilated air filled cecum projecting from the right lower quadrant to the left upper quadrant
- Gastrograffin enema: abrupt blockage at the torsion point
- abdominal CT scan can be diagnostic

DIFFERENTIAL DIAGNOSIS
- Small bowel obstruction
- Ileus

MANAGEMENT

What to Do First
- Confirm diagnosis with abdominal X-ray, barium enema or CT scan

General Management
- Assess patient for comorbidities and suitability for surgery

SPECIFIC THERAPY
- urgent laparotomy to reduce volvulus and fix the cecum
- right hemicolectomy if gangrene or perforation is present
- reduction and placement of cecostomy tube has high complications rates from the cecostomy tube and a higher recurrence rate (20%)

FOLLOW-UP
- Usual postoperative visits to ensure wound healing

COMPLICATIONS AND PROGNOSIS
- Mortality 15% with viable and 40% with non-viable bowel

CELIAC SPRUE AND MALABSORPTION

GARY M. GRAY, MD

HISTORY & PHYSICAL

History
- Fatigue; abdominal bloating, distention and borborygmi; large volume, loose and malodorous stools; anorexia; weight loss
- Family history of growth failure, celiac sprue or malabsorption

Physical

- mooth, red tongue; cracking at mouth corners; blistering skin rash (dermatitis herpetiformis); protrusion of abdomen ("pot belly" in children); pallor; bruising; edema

TESTS

Basic Blood:

- anemia (iron deficiency; folate/vitamin B12 deficiency); hypoalbuminemia; elevated alkaline phosphatase; reduced serum calcium, magnesium, zinc

Basic Urine:

- none usually helpful; see xylose test under specific diagnostic tests

Specific Diagnostic:

- Blood: Total serum IgA; IgA antibodies: transglutaminase (more sensitive than endomysial; alpha-gliadin and reticulin have lower specificity)
- Functional tests of malabsorption: elevated quantitative fecal fat (72-hour); reduced xylose absorption (25 g ingested; 5-hour urine excretion)
- Small intestinal biopsy (via upper GI endoscopy to distal duodenum): flat villi with change of elongated columnar cells to cuboidal shape; lymphocyte infiltration of enterocyte surface layer; lymphocyte and plasma cell infiltration of subepithelium (lamina propria)

DIFFERENTIAL DIAGNOSIS

- maldigestion due to pancreatic insufficiency (chronic pancreatitis) or pancreatic duct obstruction (pancreatic carcinoma); fecal fat elevated but xylose absorption normal
- other intestinal enteropathies (extensive small intestinal Crohn's disease, hypogammaglobulinemia, tropical sprue, Whipple's disease; carcinomatosis; these diseases rarely produce the completely flat intestinal biopsy seen in celiac sprue)
- drugs that cause malabsorption: colchicine, neomycin, cholestyramine, laxatives
- post-gastric surgery malabsorption
- systemic diseases associated with malabsorption: thyrotoxicosis, hypothyroidism, Addison's disease, diabetes with autonomic neuropathy, systemic sclerosis

■ irritable bowel syndrome (multiple stools but scanty quantity and no malabsorption)

MANAGEMENT

What to Do First

■ Consider differential diagnosis of sprue vs. other causes of malabsorption

■ Eliminate gluten-containing foods from the diet (wheat, barley, rye, some oat preparations–if contaminated with wheat, barley or rye during manufacturing or for the occasional patient with a toxic reaction to this grain); consultation with a nutritionist/dietitian is essential at the onset

General Measures

■ Add vitamin supplements (multivitamins, folic acid, fat-soluble vitamins [A,D,E]) and calcium (usually as the carbonate); vitamin B12 supplementation is usually not necessary

SPECIFIC THERAPY

■ All patients with sprue are treated with dietary gluten exclusion, even if symptom-free, because of risk of osteoporosis, intestinal lymphoma and cancer.

■ If gluten exclusion fails to achieve remission within a few weeks, corticosteroids (prednisone 10–20 mg/day) given for 1–4 months

■ No nutritional risk of gluten exclusion; meats, fish, vegetables and rice allow adequate oral nutrition

■ For refractory disease not responding to corticosteroids, immunosuppressants such as 6-mercaptopurine, azathioprine, methotrexate, or cyclosporine may be indicated

■ Specific treatment of other causes of malabsorption dependent on condition

FOLLOW-UP

■ Response to gluten elimination usually prompt, days to a few weeks

■ Monitoring of improvement in functional absorptive parameters (xylose, fecal fat) usually sufficient; serial intestinal biopsies not indicated routinely

■ Long-term monitoring: brief yearly visits for global assessment

■ Prompt thorough evaluation for any anorexia, fatigue, weight loss

COMPLICATIONS AND PROGNOSIS

■ Most common complications: osteoporosis due to calcium malabsorption and iron deficiency anemia

- Refractory celiac sprue: intestinal ulcerations; risk of intestinal lymphoma or carcinoma increased but not common; physician must be alert for these developments
- Long-term prognosis is usually excellent if gluten-free diet is maintained.

CELLULITIS

RICHARD A. JACOBS, MD, PhD

HISTORY & PHYSICAL

History

- Predisposing factors include trauma, IV drug use, underlying skin disease (psoriasis, eczema), peripheral edema (CHF, venectomy for CABG, lymph node dissection), diabetes, peripheral vascular disease and bites (human, dogs, cats)
- Epidemiology determines bacteriology:
  - ➤ Community-acquired – 90% group A streptococcus (S. pyogenes), 10% Staphylococcus aureus. Increasing reports of community-acquired methicillin-resistant S. aureus skin and soft tissue infections, especially in athletes, gay men, drug users, prisoners.
  - ➤ Nosocomial (surgical wounds, IV sites, decubitus ulcers) – S. aureus, enterococcus, enteric Gram-negative rods, group A streptococcus
  - ➤ IV drug use – S. aureus, streptococci, Eikenella corrodens, other mouth flora
  - ➤ Diabetes/peripheral vascular disease – localized cellulitis surrounding ulcer in patient without systemic symptoms due to group A strep and/or S. aureus; extensive cellulitis with systemic symptoms polymicrobial including S. aureus, group A strep, anaerobes, enteric Gram-negative rods
  - ➤ Dog and cat bites – S. aureus, streptococci, anaerobes, Pasteurella multocida and other Pasteurella species, Capnocytophagia species
  - ➤ Human bites – viridans streptococci, mouth anaerobes, Eikenella corrodens, S. aureus

Signs & Symptoms

- Pain, tenderness and erythema (pain absent in diabetics with neuropathy); may spread rapidly with systemic symptoms, local adenopathy and bullous formation in severe cases

TESTS

- Blood cultures low yield and rarely alter therapy or outcome; indicated in drug users, immunocompromised and those with clinical sepsis
- Aspiration of leading edge (using non-bacteriostatic saline) useful in immunocompromised, those suspected of having an unusual organism, those failing to respond to therapy
- Culture bite wound aerobically and anaerobically, if infected
- X-rays (plain films/MRI) if suspect osteomyelitis or foreign body; in diabetes and peripheral vascular disease, probing ulcer to bone has 89% positive predictive value for osteomyelitis

DIFFERENTIAL DIAGNOSIS

- Uncomplicated cellulitis versus cellulitis associated with osteomyelitis or deep tissue infection (necrotizing fasciitis, myositis)
- Tissue necrosis, cloudy drainage, crepitance, anesthesia of involved skin (from dermal nerve infarction) suggest deep tissue infection
- Osteomyelitis excluded by probing wound and x-rays

MANAGEMENT

- Assess severity of illness and hospitalize, if indicated
- Elevate involved area and treat predisposing condition (edema, tinea pedis)
- Diabetic and vascular ulcers with localized cellulitis may need minor debridement; if systemic symptoms present, surgical consultation for more aggressive debridement
- Human bites usually hospitalized
- All bites should be irrigated and debrided of devitalized tissue
- Tetanus and rabies immunization, if indicated, in animal bites

SPECIFIC THERAPY

- Community-acquired – dicloxacillin, cephalexin or clindamycin (severe penicillin allergy); if hospitalized – nafcillin, cefazolin or vancomycin (severe penicillin allergy)

  If suspect community-acquired MRSA (see epi above) – TMP-SMX, doxycycline, clindamycin
- Nosocomial – second- (cefuroxime) or third- (ceftriaxone) generation cephalosporin
- IV drug use – dicloxacillin, cephalexin (or Augmentin if Eikenella suspected); in penicillin-allergic patient, clindamycin (plus doxycycline if Eikenella suspected); hospitalized – third-generation cephalosporin

- Diabetic/vascular insufficiency – dicloxacillin, cephalexin or clindamycin; if hospitalized, Unasyn or Zosyn alone or with a fluoroquinolone
- Human bites – Augmentin or, in the penicillin-allergic patient, clindamycin plus a fluoroquinolone; hospitalized – Unasyn or Zosyn; clindamycin plus a fluoroquinolone if penicillin-allergic
- Dog/cat bites – same as human bites

FOLLOW-UP
- Improvement in 48–72 h expected in uncomplicated cellulitis; if not improved, consider osteomyelitis, abscess (especially IV drug user), deep tissue infection or unusual organism
- Bites – assess every 24–48 hours until improvement; Pasteurella infections slow to resolve (over weeks)
- Diabetes/vascular insufficiency – assess every 48–72 hours; cellulitis improves in days; ulcer takes weeks to resolve

COMPLICATIONS AND PROGNOSIS
- Chronic recurrent cellulitis a rare complication associated with predisposing conditions (tinea pedis, edema); treat underlying condition and consider prophylaxis with monthly benzathine penicillin or daily oral penicillin or macrolide
- Bites – septic arthritis, osteomyelitis, sepsis (seen in asplenia, severe liver disease) and endocarditis; prophylaxis indicated in high-risk bites (cat and human bites, bites of the hand) and high-risk patients (immunosuppressed, asplenic, cirrhosis); Augmentin for 5 days drug of choice
- Diabetes/vascular insufficiency – localized disease successfully treated in >90%; invasive disease results in amputation in up to 50%

CEREBROVASCULAR DISEASE & STROKE

MICHAEL J. AMINOFF, MD, DSc

HISTORY & PHYSICAL
- Sudden onset of focal motor or sensory deficit
- Altered consciousness common; coma may occur
- May be headache or seizures
- May be past history of TIA, amaurosis fugax, hypertension, diabetes or other predisposing disorder

- Focal signs depend on site of cerebral ischemia
  - Anterior circulation: hemiparesis, hemisensory loss, aphasia, homonymous hemianopia
  - Posterior circulation: dysarthria, dysphagia, ataxia, homonymous hemianopia, vertigo, nystagmus, cranial neuropathies, monoparesis, hemiparesis or quadriparesis
  - Lacunar: pure motor or sensory deficit, ataxic hemiparesis, clumsy hand
- May be retinal emboli, cardiac arrhythmias or murmurs, carotid bruit, tender temporal arteries or evidence of hypertension
- Neck stiffness may signify intracranial hemorrhage or increased ICP

TESTS
- Blood studies: CBC & differential count, ESR, PT/PTT, FBS, LFT, RPR, cardiac enzymes, cholesterol & lipids, antiphospholipid antibodies
- Chest x-ray
- ECG
- Cranial CT scan in first 24 hr to detect hemorrhage & mass lesion (tumor, abscess) simulating stroke
- Cranial MRI & MRA (including neck vessels) after 24 hr to define extent of lesion & status of affected vasculature
- Doppler ultrasonography of neck vessels

DIFFERENTIAL DIAGNOSIS
- Acute myocardial infarct may present as stroke: requires immediate ECG & cardiac enzyme studies
- Cardiogenic embolism suspected: echo & Holter monitoring as needed
- Hypercoagulable state: assess for sickle cell disease, polycythemia, protein C or S deficiency, afibrinogenemia, antithrombin III deficiency, homocystinemia, TTP, etc, depending on age, ethnicity, family history
- Vasculopathy (eg, necrotizing vasculitis, collagen vascular disease, syphilis, giant cell arteritis): check ESR, CSF (for pleocytosis, VDRL)
- In hemorrhagic stroke, exclude vascular anomalies (eg, AVM, aneurysm, cavernoma) or underlying tumor by MRI; recreational drug use (amphetamines, cocaine, ephedrine, others) by toxicology screen & history
- Other structural lesions: detected by brain imaging studies

MANAGEMENT
- Supportive care

- Anticonvulsant drugs if seizures occur
- Assess type of stroke (ischemic or hemorrhagic) & candidacy for therapy
- Reduce ICP w/ mannitol (1 g/kg IV over 30 min) if necessary after intracerebral hemorrhage; consider surgical decompression of cerebellar hematomas or superficial cerebral hematoma exerting mass effect

SPECIFIC THERAPY
- IV thrombolytic therapy indicated for ischemic stroke within 3 hours of onset; contraindications include:
  - CT evidence of hemorrhage
  - Recent hemorrhage
  - Treatment w/ anticoagulants
  - Hypertension (systolic pressure >185 mm Hg or diastolic pressure >110 mm Hg)
- Anticoagulants for cardiogenic embolism: heparin + warfarin (aim for INR 2–3); contraindications include:
  - CT evidence of hemorrhage
  - Blood-stained CSF
- Treatment of underlying hyperviscosity states, bleeding disorders, vasculopathy or structural lesions as required; antihypertensive medication if needed after 3 wk (do not give in acute phase after stroke, as cerebral ischemia may be exacerbated)

FOLLOW-UP
- Aim is to reduce risk of recurrence
  - Control hypertension, hyperlipidemia, cigarette smoking, diabetes
  - Consider antithrombotic agents (aspirin [optimal dose not determined], ticlopidine or clopidogrel) to prevent ischemic stroke
  - Warfarin for persisting cardiac source of embolism
  - Consider carotid endarterectomy for stenosis >70% in pts w/ TIA, amaurosis fugax or nondisabling completed stroke (not for asymptomatic stenosis)

COMPLICATIONS AND PROGNOSIS
- Prognosis depends on age, cause of stroke, general medical condition, severity of deficit
- Among survivors, 15% require institutional care

CERVICAL SPINE DISORDERS

MICHAEL J. AMINOFF, MD, DSc

HISTORY & PHYSICAL
- Neck pain, sometimes radiating to arm or head
- Weakness, numbness or paresthesias occur in arms w/ radicular involvement
- Leg weakness, gait disorder or sphincter dysfunction occurs w/ cord compression
- May be history of trauma or other precipitating cause (eg, coagulopathy, osteoporosis, malignant disease, predisposition to infection)
- Spasm of cervical paraspinal muscles
- Restriction of neck movements, esp. lateral flexion
- Focal tenderness over spinous process (esp. w/ tumor or infection)
- May be segmental motor, sensory or reflex deficit in arms
- Spurling's sign may be positive
- With cord compression, may be spastic paraparesis & sensory disturbances in legs, w/ brisk reflexes & extensor plantar responses

TESTS
- If fracture suspected, neck must be immobilized immediately & then imaged
- MRI detects structural abnormalities of spine & suggests their nature & severity
- EMG may indicate whether MRI abnormalities are of clinical relevance

DIFFERENTIAL DIAGNOSIS
- MRI distinguishes btwn different spinal disorders–eg, disc protrusion, cervical spondylosis, metastatic deposits, osteoporosis, epidural infection

MANAGEMENT
- Analgesics or NSAIDs for pain
- Use of soft collar sometimes helpful

SPECIFIC THERAPY
- Treat underlying cause
- Spinal stenosis, cervical spondylosis or prolapsed disc may require surgery
- Metastatic disease may require irradiation

FOLLOW-UP
- Depends on underlying cause
- Close follow-up important if sphincters or neurologic function at risk

COMPLICATIONS AND PROGNOSIS
- Depend on underlying disorder

CHEDIAK HIGASHI SYNDROME

NANCY BERLINER, MD

HISTORY & PHYSICAL
- Manifests in childhood or infancy with infections of the skin, lungs, and mucous membranes
- Family history: inherited as autosomal recessive
- Non-hematologic manifestations: partial oculocutaneous albinism, progressive peripheral and cranial neuropathies, and mental retardation

TESTS
- Peripheral smear: neutrophils and monocytes contain giant primary granules
- Functional studies: impaired degranulation and fusion with phagosomes. Defective chemotaxis.

DIFFERENTIAL DIAGNOSIS
- Evaluate for other immunodeficiency syndromes and neutrophil functional defects

MANAGEMENT
- Early or stable phase: prophylactic antibiotics and aggressive parenteral antibiotics for infections
- Ascorbic acid may also be of benefit

SPECIFIC THERAPY
- Allogeneic hematopoietic cell transplantation only potentially curative therapy for CHS.

FOLLOW-UP
n/a

COMPLICATIONS AND PROGNOSIS
- Majority of patients develop accelerated phase with lymphohistiocytic proliferation in the liver, spleen, bone marrow, and lymphatics.

■ Accelerated phase: treated with vinca alkaloids and glucocorticoids, but often responds poorly

---

CHEILITIS

SOL SILVERMAN JR, DDS

HISTORY & PHYSICAL
■ chronic cracking, scaling of vermilion border
■ often asymptomatic when mild

TESTS
■ none

DIFFERENTIAL DIAGNOSIS
■ allergic response (erythema multiforme)
■ actinic cheilitis with dysplasia, carcinoma
■ candidiasis (scraping, antifungal trial)

MANAGEMENT
■ keep lips lubricated, e.g. vaseline
■ sun screen

SPECIFIC THERAPY
■ topical, systemic corticosteroids

FOLLOW-UP
■ for control

COMPLICATIONS AND PROGNOSIS
■ chronic, recurrent nature; lubrication
■ monitor for dysplasia, malignant transformation

CHOLANGIOCARCINOMA

SUSAN A. CUMMINGS, MD

HISTORY & PHYSICAL

History
■ average age 60 yr; males >females
■ more than 20% associated with PSC, usually after 10 yr of disease; 85% with pancolitis; can occur after
  ➤ colectomy

➤ choledochal cysts
➤ Caroli's disease
➤ Oriental cholangiohepatitis due to Clonorchis sinensis, also Opisthorchis
➤ chronic choledocholithiasis
➤ exposure to thorium dioxide

Signs & Symptoms

- abdominal pain
- pruritus
- jaundice
- anorexia and weight loss
- weakness and fatigue
- cholangitis
- Courvoisier's sign: palpable, nontender gallbladder accompanied by
- jaundice if the tumor is below the cystic duct takeoff
- jaundice
- abdominal mass.
- hepatomegaly
- 1% involve only intrahepatic ducts and present as liver mass

TESTS

Basic Tests

- elevation of alkaline phosphatase
- elevated bilirubin, often >20 mg/dl
- CA 19–9 >100 U/ml in ~60%
- aminotransferases variably normal or mildly elevated
- increased prothrombin time with prolonged obstruction
- rarely hypercalcemia

Special Tests

- Ultrasound
  ➤ dilatation of the biliary system to the level of the obstruction, extensive intrahepatic dilatation except in PSC; may or may not show a mass
- CT scan
  ➤ similar to ultrasound
- ERCP
  ➤ able to locate the area of obstruction and get brush cytology (positive in 50~75%).

> false negative cytology due to scirrhous nature of tumor; confirmation of tissue diagnosis can be difficult.
> allows stenting of the area
- Percutaneous cholangiography
  > may be needed in more proximal tumors
- MRCP, PET, endoscopic ultrasound, or intraductal ultrasound techniques undergoing development

DIFFERENTIAL DIAGNOSIS
- choledocholithiasis
- bile duct stricture after surgery
- primary sclerosing cholangitis
- metastases that obstruct the bile ducts
- chronic pancreatitis
- pancreatic carcinoma

MANAGEMENT

What to Do First
- establish diagnosis by imaging studies, cholangiography, and/or CA 19–9
- assess patient's ability to undergo attempted resection

General Measures
- support nutrition
- provide biliary drainage

SPECIFIC THERAPY
- chemotherapy ineffective
- radiation results variable, may double the length of survival
- internal radiation or brachytherapy undergoing study
- surgery: only chance for cure
  > 25% resectable
  > 20% distal common bile duct, 25% mid-bile duct, 50% upper bile duct
  > tumor at the bifurcation of the common hepatic duct = Klatskin's tumor
  > 1% entirely intrahepatic.
  > distal tumors: Whipple resection, small tumor best chance of long-term survival and highest rate of resectability; up to a 50% 5-year survival.
  > middle third tumors. slightly lower resectability.

➤ proximal tumors: hardest to resect as the adjacent structures, i.e., portal vein, liver are involved; procedure = resection and Roux-en-Y hepaticojejunostomy

FOLLOW-UP
- serial visits with physical examination, liver chemistries, CA 19–9

COMPLICATIONS AND PROGNOSIS
- median survival after surgery: 2 years
- median survival without surgery: 6–12 mo
- stenting of the biliary tree for palliation; metal stents patent for 8 months; operative biliary-enteric bypass can also be offered but no difference in survival
- liver transplantation: 5-yr survival 17%; high recurrence; usually not done

---

CHOLEDOCHAL CYSTS

AIJAZ AHMED, MD

HISTORY & PHYSICAL

History
- biliary cysts: choledochal cysts, gallbladder cysts, and cystic duct cysts
- choledochal cysts may involve any segment of the bile duct
- classification (Todani et al.)
  ➤ type I A choledochal cyst
  ➤ type I B segmented choledochal dilatation
  ➤ type I C diffuse or cylindrical duct dilatation
  ➤ type II extra hepatic duct diverticula
  ➤ type III choledochocele
  ➤ type IVA multiple intra- and extrahepatic duct cysts
  ➤ type IVB multiple extrahepatic duct cysts
  ➤ type V intrahepatic duct cysts (Caroli's disease)
- type I cysts are the most common, accounting for 40% to 60% of all cases, followed by type IV; type II, III and V are rare
- Type V divided into two subtypes:
  ➤ simple type (Caroli's disease) cyst, limited to the larger intrahepatic bile ducts without cirrhosis/portal hypertension
  ➤ periportal fibrosis type (Caroli's syndrome) with cirrhosis/portal hypertension (more common than Caroli's disease)

- incidence:1/15,000 in the Western countries and as high as 1/1000 in Japan
- not familial; female to male ratio 3:1
- two thirds of the patients present before the age of 10

Signs & Symptoms

- classic clinical presentation of choledochal cyst disease Type I, II, and IV: triad of abdominal pain (>50%), mass (50%) and jaundice (one third)
- adults with persistent and unexplained symptoms, including jaundice, recurrent abdominal pain, fever, nausea, vomiting, cholangitis and pancreatitis
- typical presentation often includes only one or two findings of the triad
- type III: recurrent biliary pain or pancreatitis
- type V: recurrent cholangitis and liver abscesses, pain, and fever

TESTS

Laboratory

- elevated total bilirubin, liver enzymes, amylase and lipase
- tumor markers: CA19–9, alpha-fetoprotein

Imaging

- ultrasound: best way to establish diagnosis of choledochal cyst
- ERCP: confirm diagnosis, help classify cyst, and may be therapeutic (type III)
- abnormal pancreatobiliary duct junction suggestive of choledochal cysts

DIFFERENTIAL DIAGNOSIS

- cholangitis, Caroli's disease, CBD obstruction secondary to stone or stricture

MANAGEMENT

What to Do First

- rule out biliary obstruction
- classify and confirm diagnosis (ultrasound and/or ERCP)
- rule out cholangiocarcinoma: ERCP, CT scan, tumor markers
- identification of pancreatic duct insertion by ERCP critical to plan surgical management

General Measures

- history, physical, LFTs and imaging studies to determine liver damage and assess surgical candidacy

SPECIFIC THERAPY

Indications

- initial management depends on the age, presentation and type of the cyst
- ERCP plays a major role in the diagnosis and classification of biliary cystic disease and, in fewer instances, in its therapy (type III)
- cholecystectomy must be performed with cyst resection in all patients to reduce the risk of cancer, with type III cysts as the only possible exception
- acute suppurative cholangitis: broad-spectrum, intravenous antibiotics and endoscopic/percutaneous biliary decompression
- severe biliary pancreatitis: ERCP followed by resection of the cyst
- type III cysts varies with the presentation:
  - ➤ endoscopic sphincterotomy for biliary and pancreatic symptoms
  - ➤ resection for duodenal obstruction (malignancy rare with type III cysts)

Therapeutic Options

- Type/Procedure of choice
- gallbladder cysts/cholecystectomy
- cystic duct cysts/cholecystectomy
- choledochal cyst type I/Roux-en-Y hepaticojejunostomy
- choledochal cyst type II/excision of diverticulum
- choledochal cyst type III/endoscopic sphincterotomy
- choledochal cyst type IV/Roux-en-Y hepaticojejunostomy
- choledochal cyst type V/hepatic resection/ liver transplantation

FOLLOW-UP

- postoperative surveillance: incomplete resection

COMPLICATIONS AND PROGNOSIS

- complications of choledochal cyst disease:
  - ➤ gallstones
  - ➤ acute cholecystitis
  - ➤ pancreatitis
  - ➤ recurrent cholangitis
  - ➤ liver abscesses

➤ cholangiocarcinoma (15% overall; 2.5% with type III cysts)
➤ cancer of the gallbladder
➤ rare complications: portal hypertension, portal vein thrombosis, spontaneous cyst rupture, cirrhosis, pancreatic cancer

Prognosis
■ incidence of carcinoma does not fall to zero even with excision
■ type V: recurrent episodes of bacterial cholangitis (2 to 20 per year)
■ prognosis poor with frequent episodes of cholangitis

CHOLESTASIS

AIJAZ AHMED, MD

HISTORY & PHYSICAL

History
■ gender and comorbid conditions: a 50-year-old woman with thyroiditis and cholestasis is likely to have primary biliary cirrhosis (PBC); a 35-year-old man with ulcerative colitis and cholestasis is suspicious for primary sclerosing cholangitis (PSC)
■ familial causes of cholestasis/jaundice
■ cholestasis of pregnancy
■ recent hepatitis or infectious mononucleosis virus; foreign travel
■ history of alcohol use
■ hepatotoxic drug exposure
■ herbal remedies: mistletoe and bush tea
■ recent surgery (multiple transfusions, resorption of hematoma, hepatic ischemia, decompensation of subclinical liver disease), Gilbert's syndrome, total parenteral nutrition, sepsis
■ occupation: leptospirosis in farm/sewer workers; chemicals in refuse handlers; carbon tetrachloride in dry cleaning; vinyl chloride in plastic industry

Signs & Symptoms
■ fatigue most common early symptom
■ pruritus, dark urine and pale/clay colored stools
■ skin pigmentation, excoriations, xanthelasma and xanthomas

- palmar erythema, spider nevi, bruising, gynecomastia, parotid enlargement, Dupuytren's contracture, firm/hard/irregular liver edge suggests cirrhosis
- splenomegaly suggests portal hypertension
- abdominal pain (viral hepatitis); abdominal pain with arthralgia (autoimmune hepatitis); abdominal with backache (pancreatic cancer); abdominal pain with fever rigors (cholangitis or hepatic abscess)
- marked weight loss with jaundice a concern for malignancy

TESTS

Laboratory
- alkaline phosphatase out of proportion to aminotransferases
- when aminotransferases normal, confirm hepatic source of alkaline phosphatase with GGT or 5'-nucleotidase level
- AMA are present in 95% of patients with PBC
- serum bilirubin level typically normal in early cholestatic disorders
- when hyperbilirubinemia present, determine if unconjugated (hemolysis, Gilbert's syndrome, and heart failure) or conjugated (hepatocellular diseases and extrahepatic biliary obstruction)
- hemolysis: associated with increased reticulocyte count, decreased serum haptoglobulin, and peripheral blood smear showing spherocytes and fragmented cells
- hyperlipidemia

Imaging
- ultrasonography: to exclude extrahepatic biliary obstruction or gallstones
- CT scan: when malignancy is suspected
- ERCP: diagnostic for PSC; to obtain brushings from strictures; for decompression of biliary tract in cholangitis
- magnetic resonance cholangiopancreatography (MRCP): less invasive than ERCP, but lacks therapeutic options
- liver biopsy: usually diagnostic in PBC and alcoholic hepatitis, and often helpful in the diagnosis of PSC, viral and drug-induced hepatitis; severity (grade and stage) of liver diseases can be determined

DIFFERENTIAL DIAGNOSIS
- primary differential: obstructive from nonobstructive biliary tract disease

MANAGEMENT

What to Do First
- determine demographics, history and clinical manifestations provide important clues to a cost-effective diagnostic approach
- obtain tests: CBC, LFTs (including direct/conjugated and indirect/unconjugated bilirubin) and ultrasound; this information leads to more specific/sensitive diagnostic tests

General Measures
- avoid or discontinue hepatotoxic drugs
- appropriate treatment depends on the underlying cause
- liver transplant evaluation: decompensated chronic cholestatic disorders (PBC and PSC)

SPECIFIC THERAPY
- pruritus: oral cholestyramine, antihistamines, opiate antagonists (naloxone and naltrexone), ursodeoxycholic acid, rifampin and phenobarbitol
- malabsorption: oral supplementation of fat-soluble vitamins; in severe cases, parenteral injections may be required; medium chain triglycerides to improve caloric intake
- osteopenia: vitamin D and calcium supplementation, estrogen replacement, calcitonin and biphosphonates; avoid tobacco use and corticosteroids

FOLLOW-UP
n/a

COMPLICATIONS AND PROGNOSIS

Complications
- cirrhosis and liver failure (PBC, PSC); secondary biliary cirrhosis (extrahepatic biliary obstruction); cholangiocarcinoma (PSC); biliary strictures (PSC); cholangitis (PSC, extrahepatic cholestasis)

Prognosis
- prognosis are excellent with acute cholestatic disorders: postoperative jaundice, cholestasis of pregnancy, benign recurrent intrahepatic cholestasis, drug/TPN induced cholestasis
- PBC and PBC can recur in small number (<10%) of patients after liver transplantation

CHOLESTASIS OF PREGNANCY

CAROLINE A. RIELY, MD

HISTORY & PHYSICAL

History
- Itching, typically worse at night, on palms and soles, beginning in the third, or late second, trimester
- May have + family history, or itching with previous pregnancies

Signs and Symptoms
- Excoriations. Pruritus may vary, but doesn't resolve until delivery
- Jaundice very rarely

TESTS

Laboratory
- Elevated AST, ALT, may be > 1,000
- Elevated bile acids
- Normal GGTP, alk phosphatase only modestly abnormal
- Hyperbilirubinemia rarely

Liver Biopsy
- Bland cholestasis. Biopsy usually not indicated, diagnosis based on clinical grounds

DIFFERENTIAL DIAGNOSIS
- Viral hepatitis (+ serologies, risk factors)
- Cholestasis due to drugs, other liver diseases (PBC, PSC)

MANAGEMENT

What to Do First
- Reassure

General Measures
- Associated with an increased risk of prematurity/still birth
- Consider early delivery, by 38 weeks, or in very severe cases, at 36 weeks if fetal lung mature

SPECIFIC THERAPY
- Consider treatment with ursodeoxycholic acid, 15 mg/kg/day in divided dose. Sedative antipuritics may help (eg hydroxyzine)

FOLLOW-UP
- Cholestasis resolves with delivery
- No sequellae other than a slight increase in risk for gall stones

COMPLICATIONS AND PROGNOSIS
- Increased risk of prematurity/stillbirth

CHORDAE TENDINEAE RUPTURE

JUDITH A. WISBESKI, MD

HISTORY & PHYSICAL

History
- Idiopathic
- Endocarditis
- Trauma
- Connective tissue disorders
- Rheumatic heart disease
- Congenital
- Sudden onset of pulmonary congestion or acute pulmonary edema
- Chest pain may be present

Signs & Symptoms
- Crescendo early or mid systolic murmur, radiates to base of heart (rupture of chordae to posterior leaflet) or radiates to spine (rupture of chordae to anterior leaflet)
- Signs of pulmonary congestion
- Hypotension may be present

TESTS
- ECG
  - May be normal
- Blood
  - Cardiac enzymes usually normal
- Chest X-Ray
  - Heart size may be normal
  - Normal left atrial size
  - Pulmonary congestion present
- Echo/Doppler
  - Detects and quantitates mitral regurgitation
  - Flail mitral valve leaflet may be visualized

➤ Normal left ventricular (LV) systolic function and dimensions
➤ Normal left atrial dimensions
■ Cardiac Catheterization
➤ Prominent V wave in pulmonary capillary wedge pressure
➤ LV and left atrial (or pulmonary capillary wedge) pressures equal in late systole
➤ Low cardiac output and index
➤ Detect and quantitate mitral regurgitation during left ventriculography
➤ Normal LV function and no segemental wall motion abnormalities

DIFFERENTIAL DIAGNOSIS
■ Aortic stenosis

MANAGEMENT
■ see section under Papillary Muscle Dysfunction and Rupture
■ Medical and surgical treatment for acute MR due to chordae tendinae
■ rupture similar to papillary muscle rupture

SPECIFIC THERAPY
n/a

FOLLOW-UP
n/a

COMPLICATIONS AND PROGNOSIS
n/a

CHROMIUM DEFICIENCY

ELISABETH RYZEN, MD

H&P
Abnormal glucose tolerance in chromium-deplete animals, but no clear relevance of animals studies to humans, no evidence chromium needed for insulin action. Glucose intolerance and peripheral neuropathy rarely occur in patients receiving long-term TPN.

Tests/DDx/Mgt/Specific Therapy/FU/Complications & Prognosis:
N/A

CHRONIC ACALCULOUS CHOLECYSTITIS

SUSAN A. CUMMINGS, MD

HISTORY & PHYSICAL

- Loose clinical syndrome; also known as dyspepsia, biliary dyskinesia, & acalculous biliary pain
- RUQ pain associated w/ nausea in absence of peptic disease or gallstones
- 90% of gallbladders removed w/ this syndrome show chronic ➤ cholecystitis
- 75–90% of gallbladders removed incidentally at autopsy or surgery show similar changes
- 30–50% of carefully chosen pts somewhat better w/ cholecystectomy

TESTS

Basic Blood Tests
- Usually normal

Specific Diagnostic Tests
- Hepatobiliary scintigraphy to visualize gallbladder & IV CCK to evaluate gallbladder ejection fraction; abnormal is <35 EF; some studies advocate this test, others have found it of no use in predicting who will improve w/ surgery

DIFFERENTIAL DIAGNOSIS
- Peptic ulcer disease, GERD, IBS, biliary motility abnormality

MANAGEMENT

What to Do First
- Exclude alternative differential diagnoses
- Hepatobiliary scintigraphy

SPECIFIC THERAPY
- Cholecystectomy

FOLLOW-UP
- Clinical to determine resolution of pain

COMPLICATIONS AND PROGNOSIS
- Usual complications of surgery
- Prognosis good if pain resolves

CHRONIC BUNDLE BRANCH BLOCK AND HEMI-BLOCKS

EDMUND C. KEUNG, MD

HISTORY & PHYSICAL

History

■ Associated with high incidence of cardiac disease and sudden death (from complete heart block and ventricular tachycardia or fibrillation), especially LBBB.

■ RBBB: widely split second heart sound (delayed P2)

■ LBBB: reversed splitting of second heart sound (P2 before A2)

Signs & Symptoms

■ Rarely symptomatic but may develop syncope or near syncope with progression to complete heart block or with ventricular tachyarrhythmias.

TESTS

■ Basic Tests

➤ 12-lead ECG:

➤ RBBB:

• QRS ≥120 ms. rsR' (90%) or notched R (10%) in V1.

• Deep and broad S wave in leads I and V6 (may be masked by LAFB

• Incomplete RBBB: waveforms similar to RBBB but QRS <120 ms

➤ LBBB:

• QRS ≥120 ms.

• Absence of q in I and V6.

• Monophasic and usually notched R wave in lead I and a dominant S wave (rS, 67%; QS, 33%) in V1–2.

• Incomplete LBBB: waveforms similar to LBBB but QRS <120 ms. Often seen in LVH.

➤ Intraventricular conduction delay (IVCD):

• QRS ≥120 ms but characteristic waveforms for LBBB or RBBB not present (often seen in severe dilated cardiomyopathy).

➤ Left anterior fascicular block (LAFB):

• left QRS axis deviation ($-30°$ to $-90°$) with rS or QS in leads II, III and F, qR in lead aVL with onset of Q to peak of R ≥45 ms

- ➤ Left ventricular posterior fascicular block (LPFB):
  - right QRS axis deviation (90° to 180°), qR in III and F, rS in I and aVL, q wave ≤ 40 ms in the inferior leads.
  - Exclude RVH by echo.
- ➤ Bifascicular block: RBBB + LAFB or LPFB.
- ■ Specific Diagnostic Test
  - ➤ Electrophysiology study to measure HQ intervals (not indicated for this measurement alone) or to assess inducibility of VT with syncope and bifascicular block.

DIFFERENTIAL DIAGNOSIS

- ■ Secondary degree AV block: from blocked APC.
- ■ Third degree (complete) AV block is a form of AV dissociation. P-P intervals > R-R intervals in third degree AV block.
- ■ In 2:1 AV block (either constant or isolated), surface ECG cannot distinguish Mobitz I from II.
- ■ Evidence for Mobitz II: presence of IVCD or BBB.

MANAGEMENT

What to Do First
- ■ No acute intervention required unless syncope occurs.

General Measures
- ■ Identify and initiate treatment of underlying conditions responsible for BBB block.

SPECIFIC THERAPY

Pacemaker Implantation
- ■ Intermittent third degree or second degree AV block in chronic bi- or trifascicular block (Class I)
- ■ Syncope when VT is excluded with EP study (Class IIa).
- ■ Incidental finding at EP study of non-physiologic paced induced infra-Hisian block (Class IIa)
- ■ Incidental finding at EP study of HV interval ≥ 100 ms (Class IIa)

Side Effects & Contraindications
- ■ none

FOLLOW-UP

- ■ ECG and Holter monitoring if symptoms appear to search for heart block and ventricular tachyarrhythmias. Pacemaker follow-up after implantation

COMPLICATIONS AND PROGNOSIS
- Progression of bifascicular block to complete heart block: slow.
- Syncope in the presence of bifascicular block: increased incidence of sudden cardiac death.

CHRONIC CORONARY ARTERY DISEASE (CAD)

JOEL S. KARLINER, MD

HISTORY & PHYSICAL

History
- Risk factors: hypertension, abnormal lipids, smoking, diabetes, prior MI, revascularization, obesity, family history
- Associations: peripheral vascular and cerebral vascular disease, chronic renal disease, especially dialysis
- Complaint: chest discomfort with exertion, and/or at rest (mixed angina)
- Squeezing, burning, substernal. Can radiate to throat, jaws, shoulder, arm (usually left), back
- Emotion (anger) also a cause
- Anginal equivalent: exertional dyspnea due to LV ischemia

Signs & Symptoms
- May be normal. Hypertension common.
- Signs of valvular heart disease (e.g., aortic stenosis)
- Mitral insufficiency usually secondary
- Signs of CHF (see CHF chapter)

TESTS
- *Basic blood tests*
    - Hct, Hgb, smear (R/O anemia)
    - Lipid and renal panels
    - Glucose, Hgb A1C
- *Basic test*
    - resting ECG
- *Specific Diagnostic Tests*
    - Treadmill exercise test: alone or with imaging
    - If pt unable to walk, do pharmacologic imaging test (e.g., dobutamine echocardiography, persantine-thallium study).
    - Gold standard: coronary angiography

DIFFERENTIAL DIAGNOSIS

- Non-cardiac:
  - ➤ Gastroesophageal reflux: do EGD
  - ➤ Chest wall pain: may be apparent on physical exam.
  - ➤ Cervical spondylitis: do x-ray or MRI
- Cardiac:
  - ➤ Pericarditis (especially after CABG): do ECG and echo.
  - ➤ Tachyarrhythmias: 24-h Holter monitor; event monitor
  - ➤ Substance abuse, especially cocaine: toxicology screen

MANAGEMENT

What to Do First

- Resting ECG
- Exercise test with or without scintigraphy; pharmacologic stress echo or scintigram
- If younger with convincing history, coronary angiography may be indicated without stress test

General Measures

- Dietary counseling: reduce fat intake, weight loss
- Discontinue tobacco; may need group Rx
- Exercise prescription
- Optimal diabetes control

SPECIFIC THERAPY

- Indication for following is diagnosis of chronic CAD:
  - ➤ ASA
  - ➤ Statin, fibrate, and/or niacin depending on lipid profile
  - ➤ Prophylactic and therapeutic sublingual nitroglycerin
  - ➤ Beta-blocker Rx
  - ➤ Optimal BP control with additional medications as necessary (long-acting dihydropyridine calcium channel antagonist, ACE inhibitor, hydrochlorothiazide, angiotensin II antagonist, clonidine [oral or patch])
  - ➤ If ACE inhibitor not necessary for BP control, add low-dose ACE inhibitor for cardiac and renal protection, especially in patients with left ventricular dysfunction. Patients with normal left ventricular function may not benefit.
  - ➤ Long-acting nitrates
  - ➤ Hormone replacement therapy: controversial. May have adverse cardiovascular effects. Use only for serious menopausal symptoms, not for prevention of heart attack or stroke.

> Revascularization if symptoms not controlled or patient has progressive symptoms despite optimal Rx and is not febrile, anemic, or thyrotoxic, and is compliant with mediations (see ACS chapter).
- Drug eluting stent, bare metal stent, or balloon angioplasty (see ACS chapter)
- Coronary bypass surgery

Side Effects & Complications
- ASA: bleeding, allergy
- Statin, fibrate: abnormal LFTs; rhabdomyolysis
- Niacin: abnormal LFTs; glucose intolerance
- NTG and long-acting nitrates: headaches; nitrate tolerance; hypotension
- Beta-blockade: bradycardia, hypotension, fatigue, decreased libido and cognition; exacerbation of asthma; decreased LV function and diabetes are not contraindications
- Calcium antagonists: bradycardia (except dihydropyridines); orthostatic hypotension; amlodipine OK in CHF; short-acting preparations contraindicated
- ACE inhibitors: renal dysfunction; hyperkalemia; cough
- Hydrochlorothiazide: worsening diabetes, gout, renal insufficiency, hypokalemia
- Angiotensin II receptor antagonists: renal dysfunction; hyperkalemia
- Clonidine: bradycardia, fatigue, decreased congnition
- Hormone replacement therapy: higher morbidity and mortality vs. control in pts when started long after menopause. Long-term benefit not proved if started at time of menopause(see above).
- Angioplasty/stent: Acute MI. Restenosis with recurrent angina (usually in first 6 months, more likely in diabetics; incidence less with drug eluting stents and clopidogrel Rx)
- Coronary bypass surgery: Acute: arrhythmias, bleeding, pericarditis, MI, stroke. Chronic: graft occlusion (usually venous graft); diminished cognition.
- Avoid COX-2 inhibitors unless arthritic symptoms are otherwise not controllable; if used, employ lowest possible dose for shortest possible time.

FOLLOW-UP
- History at each visit regarding stability of symptoms,
  > compliance with medications and lifestyle changes

- Vital signs to assure optimal heart rate and BP control
- Yearly renal panel in diabetes
- Yearly lipid panel in all patients
- Exercise test every 1–3 years depending on symptoms.

COMPLICATIONS AND PROGNOSIS
- Chronic stable angina by itself: good prognosis
- Prognosis worse with increasing age, diabetes, prior MI with decreased LV function, multivessel disease, poorly controlled BP, continued smoking, female gender, renal failure, noncompliance with medications, and progressive symptoms despite optimal medical management

CHRONIC GRANULOMATOUS DISEASE

NANCY BERLINER, MD

HISTORY & PHYSICAL
- Severe bacterial and fungal infections from early childhood
- Family history of the disorder: usually X-linked, but autosomal recessive inheritance also occurs
- Examine for evidence of infection. Most common infections: pneumonia, lymphadenitis, cutaneous infections, hepatic abscesses, osteomyelitis, aphthous ulcers, perirectal abscesses

TESTS
- Diagnosis confirmed by tests of neutrophil oxidative metabolism: nitroblue tetrazolium (NBT) slide test or measurements of superoxide or peroxide production.

DIFFERENTIAL DIAGNOSIS
- Heterogeneous group of rare disorders
- Defective production of superoxide (O_2^-) by neutrophils, monocytes, and eosinophils
- Caused by mutations in any of four genes encoding the respiratory burst oxidase.
- Also evaluate for other immunodeficiency syndromes and neutrophil functional defects

MANAGEMENT
- Aggressive prophylaxis with prophylactic trimethoprim-sulfamethoxazole or dicloxacillin

- Prompt treatment of infection with parenteral antibiotics
- Surgical interventions including drainage of abscesses and resection of infected tissue

SPECIFIC THERAPY
- Prophylaxis with interferon-gamma helps decreases infections in some patients
- Stem cell transplantation
  - A potential target for gene therapy

FOLLOW-UP
n/a

COMPLICATIONS AND PROGNOSIS
- Life-threatening infections shorten life expectancy

CHRONIC HEART FAILURE

JOHN R. TEERLINK, MD

HISTORY & PHYSICAL

History
- Prior/current evidence of coronary artery disease (and related risk factors, such as smoking, dyslipidemias, etc.), valvular disease, congenital heart disease, hypertension, myocarditis, thyroid disease, alcohol or other cardiotoxic (cocaine, anthracyclines) ingestion or exposure, infiltrative disease (amyloid, hemochromatosis, etc.)
- Family h/o cardiomyopathy, myocardial infarction
- Progressive increase in weight, peripheral edema, bloating, dyspnea
- Relatively gradual onset of symptoms
- Episodic symptoms suggestive of underlying ischemia
- Exacerbations often preceded by:
  - Excessive salt and/or fluid intake
  - Changes in therapy (or non-compliance)
  - Excessive activity
  - Progression of disease
  - Other precipitating causes (arrhythmias, infection, pulmonary emboli)

Signs & Symptoms
- Dyspnea: exertional, orthopnea, paroxysmal nocturnal, "cardiac asthma"

- Chronic non-productive cough
- Reduced exercise capacity
- Generalized weakness and fatigue
- Nocturia, oliguria
- Confusion, poor memory, insomnia, anxiety, headache, delirium
- Nausea, abdominal discomfort, anorexia, right upper quadrant pain
- Consistent with underlying or inciting pathophysiology
- General: distressed, dyspnea, pallor, diaphoresis, cachexia, jaundice (acute hepatic congestion)
- Vital signs: tachycardia (usually), hypotension or hypertension, narrow pulse pressure, tachypnea, diaphoresis, low grade fever.
- Respiratory: rales, pleural effusion, Cheyne-Stokes respiration pattern
- CV: jugular venous distension, hepatojugular reflux, pulsus alternans (indicates severe LV dysfunction), cardiomegaly, LV heave, RV lift, loud P2, S3, S4, systolic murmur (functional MR/TR)
- Abd: hepatomegaly, ascites
- Extrem: peripheral edema, cool/ poorly perfused

TESTS
- Basic Blood Tests
  - Usually normal, except for other comorbidities
  - Electrolytes: Hyponatremia (dilutional), secondary hyperaldosteronism, Hypokalemia (diuretic use), hypophosphatemia, hypomagnesemia (diuretics, alcohol)
  - BUN/creatinine: Prerenal azotemia
  - BNP (B-type natriuretic peptide) or nt-pro-BNP: suggestive of elevated cardiac filling pressures or ventricular wall stress; usually only used for acute exacerbations; may be elevated in right-sided heart failure (i.e., cor pulmonale, pulmonary embolus)
  - Cardiac enzymes: elevated troponins or CK-MB (myocardial injury)
  - Liver function tests: AST, ALT, LDH, direct and indirect bilirubin elevated in congestive hepatopathy
  - TSH: hypo- or hyperthyroidism
- Basic Urine Tests
  - Proteinuria, high specific gravity, acellular casts
- Specific Diagnostic Tests
  - Chest X-ray: cardiomegaly (size and shape can assist with dx); pulmonary vascular redistribution, interstitial pulmonary

edema (Kerley B lines, perivascular, subpleural effusion), alveolar edema ("butterfly pattern")
➤ Electrocardiogram: ischemia/infarction; evidence of LVH, prior MI
➤ Echocardiogram(2-D with Doppler flow study): single most useful diagnostic test; cardiac function, structure, wall motion and valvular abnormalities
■ Other Tests as Appropriate
➤ Radionuclide ventriculogram (RVG; MUGA): cardiac function, wall motion abnormalities
➤ Exercise or pharmacologic stress testing: assess myocardial ischemia risk
➤ Cardiac catheterization: define coronary anatomy, possible interventions;
➤ Good distal targets, absent scintigraphic perfusion + radioactive glucose uptake in "dead" region = hibernating myocardium; good response to revascularization likely.

DIFFERENTIAL DIAGNOSIS
■ Abnormal ventricular or atrial rhythm
■ Chronic pulmonary emboli
■ Chronic obstructive pulmonary disease
■ Pneumonia
■ Sepsis
■ Cardiogenic shock

MANAGEMENT
[also see Heart Failure Society Of America. Executive summary: HFSA 2006 Comprehensive Heart Failure Practice Guideline. J Card Fail. 2006 Feb;12(1):10–38; Hunt SA, et al. ACC/AHA 2005 guideline update for the diagnosis and management of chronic heart failure in the adult: a report of the American College of Cardiology/American Heart Association Task Force on Practice Guidelines (Writing Committee to Update the 2001 Guidelines for the Evaluation and Management of Heart Failure). J Am Coll Cardiol. 2005 Sep 20;46(6):e1–82; and Swedberg K, et al. Guidelines for the diagnosis and treatment of chronic heart failure: executive summary (update 2005): The Task Force for the Diagnosis and Treatment of Chronic Heart Failure of the European Society of Cardiology. Eur Heart J. 2005 Jun;26(11):1115–40.]

What to Do First
■ Identify nature and severity of cardiac abnormality: combine history and physical examination with echocardiographic and other diagnostic studies, as necessary

- Assess nature and degree of patient's functional limitation, NYHA Class (a dynamic scale)
  - I: no limitation of physical activity, no symptoms with ordinary physical activity
  - II: slight limitation of physical activity, comfortable at rest, symptomatic with ordinary activity
  - III: marked limitation of physical activity, comfortable at rest, symptomatic with less than ordinary activity
  - IV: inability to perform physical activity without discomfort, symptoms may be present at rest
- Assess ACC/AHA clinical stage of heart failure (a one-way scale)
  - A: High risk for developing heart failure without current structural heart disease or symptoms of heart failure (i.e., patients with hypertension, atherosclerosis, diabetes, obesity, metabolic syndrome, etc.)
  - B: Structural heart disease without signs or symptoms of heart failure (prior myocardial infarction, left ventricular hypertrophy or enlargement, reduced ejection fraction, valvular disease)
  - C: Structural heart disease with prior or current signs or symptoms of heart failure (known structural heart disease and dyspnea, exercise intolerance, etc.)
  - D: Refractory heart failure requiring specialized interventions (marked symptoms at rest despite maximal therapy)
- Assess presence and severity of fluid retention: body weight (may decrease long-term solely due to cardiac cachexia), physical examination, especially jugular venous distention, hepatojugular reflux, rales, hepatomegaly, edema

General Measures

- Prevent development of heart failure:
  - Control coronary risk factors (smoking, hyperlipidemia, hypertension, weight reduction in obese patients, diabetes)
  - Discontinue alcohol use
  - In acute MI patients, limit MI size with reperfusion (thrombolytics, PTCA) and adverse ventricular remodeling/neurohormonal activation (ACE inhibitors, beta blockers, aldosterone antagonists, ARB)
  - In patients with asymptomatic LV dysfunction, limit adverse ventricular remodeling/neurohormonal activation (ACE inhibitors [ARB if intolerant to ACE inhibitor], beta blockers)
- Correct reversible causes: valvular, ischemia, arrhythmia, alcohol or drug use, high output states, cardiac shunts, drugs that cause/

exacerbate heart failure (NSAIDs, calcium channel blockers, anti-arrhythmics), treat hemochromatosis, sarcoidosis, amyloidosis, pericardial disease hypertension
- Maintain fluid balance:
  - ➤ Restrict salt intake (≤3 g salt/d)
  - ➤ Daily weights (same time of day, post-voiding, nude)
- Improve physical conditioning: encourage moderate degrees of exercise to prevent/reverse deconditioning
- Specific measures
  - ➤ Control ventricular response in atrial fibrillation or other SVT
  - ➤ Anti-coagulation in atrial fibrillation or previous embolic event
  - ➤ Coronary revascularization in patients with angina or if survival benefit anticipated
- Avoid certain medications
  - ➤ Anti-arrhythmic agents to suppress asymptomatic ventricular arrhythmias
  - ➤ Most calcium channel blockers
  - ➤ Nonsteroidal anti-inflammatory drugs
- Other general measures include influenza and pneumococcal vaccination, close outpatient surveillance

SPECIFIC THERAPY

Treatment Options, including Side Effects and Contraindications: General information on drug classes, check for more complete prescribing information, see also Chapter on Hypertension and Acute Heart Failure
- Approved Therapies:
- Diuretics: thiazides (hydrochlorothiazide), loop diuretics (furosemide, torsemide, bumetanide), metolazone, potassium-sparing. If patient–properly instructed and motivated, may use a prn dose for transient increases in body weight.
  - ➤ Indication: Volume overload, reduce preload. Thiazides or metolazone alone in mild fluid retention, loop diuretics in most patients (mild-severe); metolazone and loop diuretic in severe cases. Rapidly improve symptoms.
  - ➤ Side Effects and Complications: renal failure, thrombocytopenia, orthostatic hypotension, dizziness, dry mouth, headache, nausea/vomiting, dyspepsia, impotence, rash, hypokalemia, muscle cramps, ototoxicity.
  - ➤ Absolute Contraindications: hepatic coma
  - ➤ Relative Contraindications: anuria, severe electrolyte depletion

- ACE inhibitors: Improve morbidity and mortality. Captopril, enalapril, lisinopril, quinapril, fosinopril (ramipril for heart failure after acute MI) FDA approved; full symptomatic improvement may take weeks to months
  - Indication: Left ventricular dysfunction (asymptomatic or symptomatic), heart failure
  - Side effects: Hyperkalemia (especially with Type IV RTA), hypotension, chronic dry cough (causes ~5% to discontinue in blinded trials; should rechallenge later to establish diagnosis), angioedema, dizziness, skin rash, dysgusia (captopril; often resolves spontaneously)
  - Absolute Contraindications: Any prior angioedema, pregnancy, hyperkalemia, renovascular disease
  - Relative Contraindications: Renal failure (although ACE inhibitors may improve renal dysfunction), volume depletion
- Beta-blockers: improve morbidity and mortality, may improve disease progression independent of symptoms; agents with beneficial results in large clinical trials include carvedilol, metoprolol succinate, bisoprolol. "Start low, go slow" titration. Advise patients of possible early side effects which do not generally prevent long-time use. Symptomatic improvement may take months.
  - Indication: Heart failure due to systolic dysfunction (stable NYHA class II–IV)
  - Side effects: hypotension, fluid retention and worsening of heart failure, bradycardia and heart block, worsens bronchospasm, CNS symptoms (depression, nightmares, excitement, confusion), fatigue, lethargy, impotence, increase triglycerides (depression of HDL).
  - Absolute Contraindications: Severe peripheral vascular disease, severe bronchospastic disease, sick sinus syndrome or advanced heart block (unless treated with pacemaker), unstable NYHA IV CHF.
  - Relative Contraindications: Types I and II diabetes, depression, dyslipidemia, peripheral vascular disease.
- Digoxin: improves symptoms, minimal effect on survival; use in conjunction with diuretics, ACE inhibitor, and beta blockers; dose-adjustment required for many medications; serum levels not useful in guiding therapy. Side effects may occur at any level, though more frequent >2 ng/mL and in elderly.
  - Indication: Heart failure due to systolic dysfunction (NYHA class II–IV) for symptom improvement

➤ Side effects: cardiac arrhythmias (ectopic and reentrant tachycardias), bradycardia and heart block, anorexia, nausea, vomiting, visual disturbances ("yellow halo"), disorientation, confusion, hypotension, fluid retention and worsening of heart failure, worsens bronchospasm, CNS symptoms (depression, nightmares, excitement, confusion), fatigue, lethargy, impotence, increase triglycerides (depression of HDL).

➤ Absolute Contraindications: Ventricular fibrillation, ventricular tachycardia, significant AV block, anuria.

➤ Relative Contraindications: Renal failure

■ Angiotensin II receptor blockers: Candesartan and valsartan FDA approved for heart failure treatment. Use in addition to optimal standard therapy (ACE inhibitor, beta blocker) or substitute for ACE inhibitor in patients who are ACE inhibitor intolerant due to cough or angioedema (ARB may also cause angioedema). Improves morbidity; in patients unable to take ACE inhibitor, improves mortality.

➤ Indications: Heart failure due to systolic dysfunction (NYHA class II–IV) for symptom improvement, as add-on to standard care or replace ACE inhibitor (IF ACE intolerant)

➤ Side Effects and Complications: Hyperkalemia (especially with Type IV RTA), hypotension, angioedema (less frequent than ACE inhibitor), dizziness, skin rash (less frequent than ACE inhibitor), hepatotoxicity

➤ Absolute Contraindications: Any prior angioedema, pregnancy, hyperkalemia, renovascular disease

➤ Relative Contraindications: Renal failure, volume depletion

■ Aldosterone antagonists: spironolactone, eplerenone (FDA approved for post-myocardial heart failure), neurohormonal antagonist, weak potassium-sparing diuretic. Improves morbidity and mortality in advanced heart failure patients (spironolactone) and in post-myocardial infarction heart failure patients (eplerenone). Carefully monitor potassium.

➤ Indications: Heart failure due to systolic dysfunction (NYHA class IIIB–IV) or post-myocardial infarction; consider in patients with less severe heart failure symptoms who require potassium supplementation

➤ Side Effects and Complications: Hyperkalemia (especially with Type IV RTA), agranulocytosis, anaphylaxis, gynecomastia, hypotension, headache, dizziness, confusion, skin rash, impotence, irregular menstrual bleeding

- ➤ Absolute Contraindications: Anuria, hyperkalemia, acute renal insufficiency
- ➤ Relative Contraindications: Hepatic insufficiency
- ■ Isosorbide dinitrate and hydralazine: combination of vasodilators, though biochemical effects may be more important. FDA approved for treatment of symptomatic heart failure in addition to standard therapy (ACE inhibitors, beta blockers, etc.).
  - ➤ Indication: Consider if truly intolerant to ACE inhibitors and angiotensin II receptor blockers; addition to ACE inhibitor, diuretic, beta blocker, ARB, digoxin, if still symptomatic
  - ➤ Side Effects and Complications: hemolytic anemia, methemoglobinemia, headache, dizziness, hypotension, syncope, angina, reflex tachycardia, nausea/vomiting, edema, rash, GI distress, rash; agranulocytosis, SLE-like syndrome (hydralazine)
  - ➤ Absolute Contraindications: Increased intracerebral pressure, cerebral hemorrhage, symptomatic hypotension, angle-closure glaucoma, stenotic valvular disease
  - ➤ Relative Contraindications: stroke, hypotension, severe anemia, impaired renal function, acute MI (hydralazine)
- ■ Unapproved drugs used in treatment of patients with heart failure
- ■ Calcium channel blockers: Generally contraindicated in heart failure. May consider Amlodipine, which has demonstrated no adverse effect on survival (also perhaps felodipine).
  - ➤ Indication: Angina, hypertension
  - ➤ Side Effects and Complications: Hypotension, headache, flushing, congestive heart failure, peripheral edema, bradycardia with sinus/AV node depression (especially verapamil and diltiazem), palpitations/reflex tachycardia, constipation (especially verapamil in elderly), GI distress, exacerbate heart failure in patients with systolic dysfunction, possible increase in myocardial infarction in diabetics with renal disease (nisoldipine, amlodipine)
  - ➤ Absolute Contraindications: 2nd/3rd-degree AV block, sick sinus syndrome, systolic dysfunction (perhaps except amlodipine), post-myocardial infarction, hypotension, pulmonary congestion
  - ➤ Relative Contraindications: Impaired liver or renal function
- ■ Anti-arrhythmic therapy: Drugs generally contraindicated in heart failure. Treatment for asymptomatic or nonsustained ventricular arrhythmias not indicated. Beta-blockers reduce sudden death in CHF. Class I agents (quinidine, procainamide, flecainide, encainide) increase risk of death. May consider amiodarone for atrial arrhythmias, but not for general use to prevent death/sudden death.

➤ Indication: Atrial arrhythmias, symptomatic ventricular arrhythmias (consider AICD)
➤ Side Effects and Complications: arrhythmias, SA and AV block, hepatic failure, severe pulmonary toxicity, corneal deposits; blue-gray skin discoloration, peripheral neuropathy, ataxia, edema, dizziness, hyper/hypothyroidism
➤ Absolute Contraindications: Severe SA node disease, 2nd/3rd-degree AV block, sick sinus syndrome, bradycardia-induced syncope
➤ Relative Contraindications: Thyroid disease, pulmonary disease, impaired liver or renal function, elderly

■ Device Therapy
■ Implantable Cardioverter Defibrillators (ICD): Improve survival in selected patients; multiple guidelines and indications; decision must be individualized
➤ Indications: Secondary prevention of sudden death with no known reversible causes; primary prevention in patients with:
  • Class II or III heart failure + LVEF $\leq$35% OR
  • Prior MI LVEF $\leq$30% OR
  • Prior MI LVEF $\leq$35% + inducible sustained VT or VF
➤ Contraindications:
  • Cardiogenic shock or symptomatic hypotension
  • NIDCM with symptoms <3 months
  • CABG or PTCA within the past 3 months
  • Acute MI within the past 40 days
  • Candidate for coronary revascularization
  • Irreversible brain damage from preexisting cerebral disease
  • Noncardiac disease with a likely survival <1 year
➤ Side Effects and Complications: Acute: infection and local wound complications, myocardial perforation with pericardial tamponade, VT/VF induced during testing. Chronic: Infection, inappropriate shocks, system failure (leads, generator).

■ Biventricular pacemakers (BiV)/Cardiac Resynchronization Therapy (CRT): Reduce CHF hospitalizations and improve survival in selected patients; multiple guidelines and indications; decision must be individualized
➤ Indications: Patients with symptomatic Class III–IV heart failure despite stable, optimal heart failure drug therapy AND LV ejection fraction $\leq$0.35 AND QRS $\geq$120 milliseconds
➤ Contraindications: As above for ICD; must be individualized
➤ Side Effects and Complications: Acute: infection and local wound

complications, myocardial perforation with pericardial tamponade, VT/VF induced during placement. Chronic: Infection, inappropriate pacing, pacemaker syndrome, system failure (leads, generator).

FOLLOW-UP

During Treatment

- Often require weekly or bi-weekly visits during titration of medications, especially beta blockers
- Monitor electrolytes, especially potassium, and renal function
- Emphasize lifestyle changes such as reduced sodium intake, aerobic exercise, compliance with medications, daily weights.
- Educate patient about pathophysiology of heart failure and reason for medications (improves outcomes and compliance).

Routine

- Follow-up at least every 6 months
- Improved outcomes noted when followed by cardiologist, heart failure specialist.
- Repeat evaluation of LV function generally not indicated, unless major intercurrent event or deterioration, although rechecking 6 months after beta blocker therapy may demonstrate significant improvement.
- If ICD or CRT device in place, requires follow-up with qualified cardiologist to interrogate and check settings

COMPLICATIONS AND PROGNOSIS

- Complications usually related to underlying pathophysiology, also sudden death (about 50% of overall mortality) and death due to progressive heart failure
- 50% 5-year mortality in some series

CHRONIC KIDNEY DISEASE

ROBERT D. TOTO, MD

HISTORY & PHYSICAL

History

- Infections, toxins, environment: hepatitis B and C, lead, mercury, silicon; Drugs: acetaminophen/paracetamol/caffeine combinations,

NSAIDS, lithium, cancer chemotherapeutic agents, pamidronate, lithium, herbal (e.g., some Chinese herbs) remedies

Risk Factors for Progressive Renal Disease
■ Age, male gender, diabetes mellitus, hypertension, family history (pattern of inheritance); African-American, Hispanic, cigarette smoking, persistent albuminuria, nephrotoxin exposure (e.g., analgesics).

Signs & Symptoms
■ May be asymptomatic; symptoms usual when estimated glomerular filtration rate ≤ 25 mL/min/1.73 m^2
■ General: fatigue, malaise, weakness, fever (systemic diseases and retroperitoneal fibrosis)
■ HEENT: headache, visual disturbances, periorbital edema, retinal changes of hypertensive/diabetic retinopathy, cholesterol emboli, uremic fetor
■ CV and PULM: dyspnea, edema, chest pain, hypertension, hemoptysis, hyperpnea (metabolic acidosis) pulmonary edema
■ GI: dysgeusia, anorexia, nausea, vomiting, diarrhea, occult GI hemorrhage
■ GU: Nocturia, foamy urine, dysuria, hematuria, stranguria, painful urination, flank or back pain, hypospadias, urethral stricture, prostate enlargement
■ MS: lower extremity edema, bone and articular pain, generalized muscle wasting and weakness
■ NS: encephalopathy: difficulty concentrating, insomnia, daytime drowsiness, seizures, coma; peripheral neuropathy
■ SKIN: pruritus, easy bruising, petechiae, cutaneous infarcts, palpable purpura, calcinosis

TESTS

Laboratory
■ Basic blood tests:
  ➤ Early disease: estimated GFR <60 ml/min/1.73 m^2, elevated serum creatinine, elevated BUN
  ➤ Advanced disease: early disease + hyperkalemia, hypobicarbonatemia, hyperphosphatemia, hypocalcemia, hypercalcemia, hypermagnesemia, elevated serum PTH, decreased serum 1,25 (OH)2 vitamin D3, elevated alkaline phosphatase, normochromic normocytic anemia

- Basic urine tests:
  - Early disease: microalbuminuria/proteinuria, microhematuria, pyuria; casts including red blood cells (RBCs), white blood cells (WBCs), granular; crystalluria
  - Advanced disease: same as early and hyaline casts
  - Urinalysis Patterns:
  - Glomerulonephritis: hematuria, dysmorphic RBC, heavy proteinuria (urine protein/creatinine ratio ≥3.0), RBC casts
  - Tubulointerstitial nephritis: microhematuria, pyuria, + WBC casts, mild proteinuria (urine protein/creatinine ratio ≤2.0) and waxy casts
  - Renal ischemia (vasculitis, atheroembolism, renal artery stenosis) or urinary obstruction: minimal cellular elements + proteinuria
  - Urine [Na] and fractional Na excretion (FENa) not helpful in chronic kidney disease

Specific Diagnostic Tests:
- Estimated glomerular filtration rate (eGFR), creatinine clearance (Ccr)
- Spot urine albumin mg/creatinine g ratio (>30 and <300 = microalbuminuria; >300 = macroalbuminuria); spot urine total protein mg/creatinine g ratio, >200 abnormal
- Anti-nuclear antibodies (SLE), anti-glomerular basement membrane antibody, anti-neutrophil cytoplasmic antibody (ANCA), hepatitis B surface antigen, anti-hepatitis C antibody; HIV, complement components 3 and 4, anti-topoisomerase antibody, cryoglobulins, serum and urine protein electrophoresis, urine immunofixation (light chain deposition disease)

Imaging:
- CXR to evaluate heart and lungs (see management)
- Renal ultrasound
  - Early disease: Normal or enlarged kidneys; cystic-autosomal dominant polycystic kidney disease (ADPKD); hydronephrosis, increased echogenicity
  - Advanced disease: small shrunken kidneys, increased echogenicity; normal or enlarged kidneys in ADPKD, diabetes HIV nephropathy: hydronephrosis
- CT/MRI/MRA: angiomyolipomas, ADPKD; papillary necrosis, renal artery stenosis (MRA)

- Voiding cystourethrogram
- Renal Biopsy:
  - ➣ Useful when kidneys normal size to make specific diagnosis – e.g., SLE, glomerulonephritis. When kidneys small (e.g., ≤9 cm) usual finding is end-stage kidney – i.e. global glomerulosclerosis + tubulointerstitial nephritis

DIFFERENTIAL DIAGNOSIS

- *Chronic kidney disease* (CKD) symptoms mimicked by systemic diseases, cancer, wasting illnesses, depression, hypothyroidism, chronic heart failure, chronic liver disease. Elevated BUN and creatinine point to kidney, adrenocortical insufficiency.

Causes of Chronic Kidney Disease

- *Systemic disease*: Diagnosis usually established by history, exam, sonogram and specific laboratory tests: diabetes mellitus, hypertension, systemic lupus erythematosus, Sjogren's syndrome, systemic necrotizing vasculitides, atheroembolic renal disease, myeloma, light chain deposition disease, amyloidosis, genetic disease – e.g., polycystic disease, tuberous sclerosis, cystinosis, Fabry's disease, sickle cell disease, heart failure, cirrhosis
- *Primary renal and urinary tract disease*: Specific glomerular disease usually requires renal biopsy; obstructive uropathy by sonogram or CT scan (e.g., retroperitoneal fibrosis), vesicoureteral reflux (detected by voiding cystourethrogram), prostate disease, recurrent UTI or voiding dysfunction (Hx, exam, voiding study)

MANAGEMENT

What to Do First

- Assess cardiovascular and volume status by physical exam and CXR, and determine if dialysis is indicated because of:
- a) hypertension and/or pulmonary edema; b) hyperkalemia; c) pericarditis; d) metabolic acidosis; e) altered MS

General Measures

- Dialysis not indicated:
  - ➣ Restore volume status with conservative measures (e.g., diuretics in patient with volume overload).
  - ➣ Treat hypertension (present in >90% of cases).
    - Target blood pressure <130/80 mmHg with (in order): ACE inhibitor/angiotensin II receptor blocker + thiazide (serum creatinine ≤1.8 mg/dl) or loop diuretic (serum

creatinine >1.8 mg/dl), calcium channel blocker, central-acting alpha-agonist/peripheral alpha-blocker/beta-blocker, then vasodilator (e.g., minoxidil) and dietary Na restriction (2 g/day).

➤ Treat hyperkalemia and acidosis (see below).

SPECIFIC THERAPY

■ eGFR or Ccr 25–75 ml/min/1.73 m2, see "Preserve renal function"

■ eGFR or Ccr <25 ml/min/1.73 m2, consult access surgeon, dietician and social worker to assist in preparing for dialysis

■ eGFR or Ccr <20 ml/min/1.73 m2, place vascular access (hemodialysis) or plan peritoneal catheter in 6–12 months

■ eGFR or Ccr in range of 8–12 ml/min/1.73 m2, initiate maintenance renal replacement therapy unless: a) patient's weight is stable; b) serum albumin is at least at lower limit of normal range for laboratory; c) patient is symptom-free

Preserve (Remaining) Renal Function for All Levels of CKD

■ Treat underlying disease process – e.g. treat SLE, relieve obstruction, identify and discontinue nephrotoxin (e.g., lithium) whenever possible

■ Normalize BP using ACE inhibitor unless: a) patient has known allergy; b) cough intolerable; c) hyperkalemic with K ≥6.0 on K-restricted diet; d) known or suspected critical renal artery stenosis

■ Optimize glycemic control in diabetic (HgbA1c ≤6.5%)

■ Cease cigarette smoking (hard evidence)

■ Improve dyslipidemia with low-saturated-fat diet and statin drug for LDL-cholesterol (≤70 for highest risk [e.g., diabetic] and ≤100 mg/dl for non-diabetic) and triglyceride <150 mg/dl

■ Dietary protein intake: 0.8 g/kg/day prior to dialysis. After initiation of dialysis 1.0–1.4 g/kg/d for hemodialysis and 1.4–1.6 g/kg/d for peritoneal dialysis.

Preserve Cardiac Function

■ 50% of deaths in patients with ESRD are cardiac in origin.

■ Normalize BP, manage dyslipidemia with statins (see above); fibric acid derivative for uncontrolled hypertriglyceridemia, stop smoking, folic acid 5 mg/day to reduce risk of hyperhomocysteinemia

Manage Acid-Base and Electrolyte Disturbances

■ Hyperkalemia: +EKG changes: IV Calcium gluconate, insulin, inhaled beta-2 agonist, oral or rectal Kayexalate and dietary potassium restriction (0.8 mEq/kg/day). - EKG change: diet/Kayexalate.

■ Acidosis: Check ABG, treat with oral sodium bicarbonate: 1 mEq/kg/day as Shohl's solution (1 mEq/ml); baking soda (60 mEq/tsp) or NaHCO3 tabs (8 mEq/650 mg tab). For pH <7.15. consider intravenous NaHCO3 therapy. Renal osteodystrophy: Goal to normalize calcium and phosphorus, lower PTH and increase vitamin D: Dietary phosphate restriction to 12 mg/kg/day. Add Ca- based binder (Ca Acetate of Ca Carbonate) or non-Ca-based binder such as sevalemer HCl (Renalgel) 1–4 tablets with meals. Measure PTH and 25(OH)2 vitamin D3. If PTH elevated and 25 (OH)2 vitamin D3 low, administer ergocalciferol 50,000 units monthly for 6 months and repeat PTH. If still elevated, administer active vitamin D such as calcitriol or paricalcitriol.

■ Avoid malnutrition: 0.8 g/kg/day protein, 35 kcal/kg/day prior to dialysis (see above). Monitor body weight, muscle mass, serum albumin, BUN (protein intake) and Scr (muscle mass).

Anemia
■ Measure serum Fe, TIBC and ferritin.
■ Treat hemoglobin <11 g/dl with subcutaneous erythropoietin or darbepoietin subcutaneously along with oral or intravenous iron therapy.
■ No contraindications; BP may increase in 20–25% of patients.

FOLLOW-UP
■ Every 3 months for patients with eGFR or Ccr $\leq$25 ml/min/1.73 m^2
■ Increase frequency as needed as patient approaches ESRD
■ Labs at visit: chemistries, iron stores, hemoglobin, spot urine albumin or protein/creatinine ratio. Goals: urine albumin/creatinine ratio <300 mg/g, urine protein/creatinine <200 mg/g.

COMPLICATIONS AND PROGNOSIS
Adverse drug events:
■ ACE inhibitors: cough, hyperkalemia, rarely angioedema (more common in African-Americans)
■ HMG-CoA reductase inhibitors: rhabdomyolysis, muscle pain or asymptomatic CK elevation
■ Active vitamin D3 (e.g., calcitriol) may cause hypercalemia.
■ Loop diuretics: hypokalemia, hypomagnesemia, hypochloremic metabolic alkalosis
■ ESRD: nearly all patients with Ccr <25 ml/min/1.73 m^2 reach ESRD within 2 years. Mortality rate on dialysis at 5 years is about 50%.

CHRONIC LYMPHOCYTIC LEUKEMIA

KANTI R. RAI, MD

HISTORY & PHYSICAL

History
- Characteristically, a disease of elderly
- Predominant in males

Signs & Symptoms
- Often diagnosed in an asymptomatic patient on routine CBC
- Usually has an indolent course
- Patients may present with "B" symptoms and abdominal fullness (secondary to splenomegaly)
- Physical exam may be normal at initial diagnosis
  - ➤ Some patients may have some or all of the following: pallor, lymphadenopathy, splenomegaly, skin involvement

TESTS

Essential Criteria for Diagnosis
- Absolute lymphocytosis ($\geq$5,000/microliter) persistent for >4 weeks
- More than 30% involvement of the bone marrow by CLL
- Characteristic phenotypic profile of the lymphocytes on flow cytometry: CD5(+), CD19(+), CD20(+), CD23(+), dim expression of monoclonal surface immunoglobulin

Other Lab Findings
- Absolute lymphocytosis with mature appearing lymphocytes in peripheral blood
- Anemia, thrombocytopenia may be seen
- Hypogammaglobulinemia may be seen

Bone Marrow
- Hypercellular or normocellular
- Marked lymphoid infiltration
- Flow cytometry: as above

DIFFERENTIAL DIAGNOSIS
- Other lymphoproliferative disorders (see table)

CLL
- sIg: W
- CD5: +
- CD23: +
- CD20: +
- CD10: −
- CD103: −

HCL
- sIg: B
- CD5: −
- CD23: −
- CD20: +++
- CD10: −
- CD103: +

PLL
- sIg: B
- CD5: +/−
- CD23: −
- CD20: +++
- CD10: −
- CD103: −

SLVL
- sIg: B
- CD5: +/−
- CD23: −
- CD20: +++
- CD10: −
- CD103: −

MCL-L
- sIg: B
- CD5: +++
- CD23: −
- CD20: ++
- CD10: −
- CD103: −

FCL-L
- sIg: B
- CD5: −
- CD23: −
- CD20: ++++
- CD10: −
- CD103: −

- SIg – surface immunoglobulin, W – weak, B – bright, HCL – Hairy cell leukemia, PLL – Prolymphocytic leukemia, SLVL – Splenic lymphoma with villous lymphocytes, MCL – Mantle cell lymphoma-leukemic phase, FCC – Follicular center lymphoma-leukemic phase

Staging
- Rai stage Clinical features
  - Stage 0 lymphocytosis only
  - Stage I lymphocytosis + enlarged lymph nodes
  - Stage II lymphocytosis + enlarged spleen or liver with or without enlarged nodes
  - Stage III lymphocytosis + anemia with or without enlarged nodes, liver, spleen
  - Stage IV lymphocytosis + thrombocytopenia with or without enlarged nodes, spleen, liver and anemia
- Modified Rai criteria
  - Stage 0 = low risk; Stage I/II = intermediate risk; Stage III/IV = high risk

MANAGEMENT

What to Do First
- To decide if the patient needs treatment

Indications
- Disease related symptoms (weight loss, fever, fatigue)
- Progressive increase in lymphocytosis with a rapid LDT
- Worsening of anemia and or thrombocytopenia
- Auto-immune anemia or thrombocytopenia
- Symptomatic bulky lymphadenopathy or splenomegaly
- Recurrent infections

Treatment Strategy Based on Stage
- Low risk and Intermediate risk - Observation, unless any of the above indication is present
- High risk – Initiate cytotoxic therapy

SPECIFIC THERAPY
- Chlorambucil PO Q 3–4 weeks or
- Cyclophosphamide PO/iv Q3–4 weeks or
- Fludarabine iv QD × 5 days q month for 4–6 months
- Glucocorticoids: Prednisone alone or combination with alkylating agents (not with Fludarabine)
- Monoclonal antibodies:
  - ➤ Campath-1H (anti-CD52) – for Fludarabine failures given iv or sc at 30 mg each dose 3 times a week (usually Mondays, Wednesdays and Fridays) for up to 8 weeks
  - ➤ Rituximab (anti-CD20) (in clinical trials) – In combination with fludarabine (given at standard dosage as described above, on monthly basis), and rituximab given on day 1 of each month's fludarabine, at 375 mg/M2 iv, for 4–6 months

FOLLOW-UP

During Treatment
- CBC and physical exam at 2–3 weeks
- Coombs, quantitative immunoglobulins periodically
- Bone marrow biopsy at complete remission (CR) by all other criteria

Routine
- Once in CR: CBC, physical exam q 2–3 months

COMPLICATIONS AND PROGNOSIS

Complications
- Pancytopenia
- Opportunistic infections
- Auto-immune hemolytic anemia

Prognosis
- Stage: median survival for stage
  - Stage 0: 12+ yrs
  - Stage I: 8.5 yrs
  - Stage III: 1.5 yrs
  - Stage IV: 1.5 yrs
- Bone marrow histology: diffuse pattern of lymphoid infiltration has worse prognosis
- Lymphocyte doubling time (LDT): a rapid LDT of <12 months has poor outcome
- CD-38 expression on the CLL B lymphocytes is associated with worse prognosis

---

CHRONIC MYELOGENOUS LEUKEMIA

ALAN M. GEWIRTZ, MD

HISTORY & PHYSICAL

Epidemiology
- 15% of all leukemias; incidence 1–2 cases per l00,000 population
- A disease predominantly affecting middle-aged individuals (median age 45–55 yrs old) but all age groups, including children, represented
- Increased incidence in survivors of atomic bomb explosions but otherwise, no definitive link to environmental or infectious causation

Signs & Symptoms
- Fatigue, anorexia, night sweats, weight loss, abdominal fullness, easy bruising and bleeding; infections unusual
- 40–50% of cases asymptomatic, and picked up by routine CBC
- splenomegaly, of variable degree, most common finding – 75% of patients

- hepatomegaly, usually mild, in approx. 50%
- pallor, petechiae, ecchymosis, lymphadenopathy less common

TESTS

Peripheral Blood

- WBC elevated, typically >25,OOO; rarely, WBC is normal
- Differential - blasts (<10% of total WBC) through mature neutrophils
- Absolute basophilia $\pm$ esosinophilia; monocytes decreased
- Thrombocytosis in 30–50%
- Normochromic, normocytic anemia common
- Low, or absent, leukocyte alkaline phosphatase (LAP)

Bone Marrow

- Markedly hypercellular with diminished fat; M:E ratio increased, often dramatically
- Megakaryocytes typically increased, clustered, small, with dysplastic nuclei; dysplasia in other lineages not usual Blasts and promyelocytes <10% of total nucleated cells

Specific Diagnostic Tests

- Cytogenetics: gt;95% + for Philadelphia (Ph) chromosome created by reciprocal translocation between chromosomes 9 and 22. Adds a 3' segment of the ABL gene (chromosome 9q34) to 5' portion of BCR gene (chromosome 22q11) creating BCR-ABL oncogene with intrinsic tyrosine kinase activity lit (9;22)-(q34;q11).
- Molecular Diagnosis: RT-PCR (reverse transcription-polymerase chain reaction) for BCR-ABL mRNA

DIFFERENTIAL DIAGNOSIS

- Leukemoid reactions secondary to sepsis, metastatic carcinoma, chronic inflammatory disorders may occasionally be confused with CML. In these instances, LAP score is high, not low; cytogenetics are normal, molecular tests for bcr-abl are negative
- Other myeloproliferative disorders or myelofibrosis may occasionally present with CML like picture. Cytogenetics and RT-PCR can rule in or rule out CML.

MANAGEMENT

General Measures

- Lower WBC to alleviate symptoms – Hydroxyurea – 0.5 to 6.0 grams/day

- Patient Education – Natural history of disease progression (chronic, to accelerated, to blast phase) must be discussed, along with treatment options (see below)
- HLA type patient and siblings
- Determine if patient is candidate for allogeneic hematopoietic cell transplant; transplant only documented curative modality, but only 20% of patients are allotransplant candidates.

SPECIFIC THERAPY

- Virtually all chronic-phase patients are now treated initially with abl kinase inhibitor, imatinib mesylate (Gleevec). >80% of patients will achieve a complete cytogenetic remission on standard dose of 400 mg/day. Most patients remain PCR+ for bcr/abl. Higher imatinib doses may prove beneficial, but this remains unproven. Approx. 50–70% of patients report nausea, fluid retention, GI upset, including nausea, vomiting, and diarrhea. Hepatotoxicity reported in 1–3%, neutropenia and thrombocytopenia in up to approx 1/3 of patients. More potent second-generation abl kinase inhibitors are actively being investigated in the clinic now.
- Allogeneic hematopoietic cell transplant- Only treatment known to cure disease. Timing of transplant, especially for young patients with matched related donors, remains controversial. Most experts suggest initial trial of imatinib, but move to transplant for patients with suboptimal response to imatinib (failure to achieve a complete hematologic response after 3 months, or failure to achieve any significant cytogenetic response after 6 months, or failure to achieve a major cytogenetic response after 1 year), or development of imatinib resistance.
- **Other useful drugs**
- Hydroxyurea – For patients with inadequate response to imatinib. 0.5–2.0 gm/d as tolerated. WBC and platelet counts need to be monitored frequently.
- Interferon-alpha – up to 9 million units/day as tolerated; may take >3 months to control disease; 20% of patients will become entirely Ph(−) for variable and in some cases prolonged periods of time. Cytarabine – used in conjunction with interferon; benefit suggested but not proven; 2O mg/m2/d × 10 days each month.
- Cytosine arabinoside – dose depends on disease activity. 20 mg/m2 daily × 2 weeks to full dose for blast transformation.

Busulfan – 2–6 mg PO qd until WBC <30–40,000; then half dose until count <20,000, when drug stopped. Observe until counts stabilize.

1–2 mg PO qd as maintenance until count l0,000, then stop. Can compromise the ability of a patient to be transplanted and therefore not used for primary therapy.

Side Effects & Contraindications
- Interferon-alpha: flu-like symptoms (fatigue, myalgia, fever, bone pain), rash, depression
- Contraindication – known hypersensitivity to interferon or vehicle
- Cytarabine: myelosuppression, mucositis, diarrhea, alopecia; Contraindication – known hypersensitivity to cytarabine or vehicle
- Hydroxyurea: myelosuppression, mucositis, diarrhea, rash, nausea
- Contraindication – known hypersensitivity to cytarabine or vehicle
- Busulfan: myelosuppression, marrow aplasia, mucositis, diarrhea, hyperpigmentation

FOLLOW-UP
- For responding patients on imatinib, especially potential transplant candidates, frequent surveillance (~q 3 months) of symptoms, blood counts, and Q-PCR for changes in bcr/abl level are recommended. Evidence for imatinib resistance or disease acceleration should prompt rapid intervention with increased dose of imatinib, second-generation abl kinase inhibitor, or transplantation for those who are candidates.

COMPLICATIONS AND PROGNOSIS
- Patients who respond to imatinib with complete cytogenetic response and 3- to 5-fold reduction of bcr/abl transcripts have excellent prognosis. It is unknown if such patients are "clinically cured," as follow-up times are still relatively short.
  - ➤ ~4% of patients on imatinib will develop resistance per year. Such patients may be salvaged with higher doses of imatinib, second-generation abl kinase inhibitors, use of the above-mentioned cytostatic or cytotoxic agents alone or in combination, or preferably stem cell transplant if the patient is still in chronic phase of disease.
  - ➤ Prognosis is poor for patients who cannot be transplanted and who develop abl kinase inhibitor resistance. GVHD remains the major complication of allogeneic stem cell transplantation.
  - ➤ Patients who relapse after allogeneic stem cell transplantation can be salvaged by donor lymphocyte infusions. Vaccines and other forms of immunotherapy are under investigation and may prove useful.

CHRONIC OBSTRUCTIVE PULMONARY DISEASE

STEPHEN C. LAZARUS, MD

HISTORY & PHYSICAL

History
- Cigarettes account for 80–90% of COPD
- Only 10–20% of smokers develop COPD
- Synergy between smoking and certain inhaled dusts
- More common in men (corrected for smoking)

Signs & Symptoms
- Cough, expectoration (usually scant), dyspnea
- May start as dyspnea with exertion
- Chronic bronchitis most common cause of hemoptysis
- Physical exam often normal
- Rhonchi, wheezes, crackles variably present
- Prolonged expiration common; >4 sec = significant obstruction
- Late: barrel chest, pursed lips, weight loss, tripod posture (leaning forward supported on arms/elbows)
- Loud P2 suggests pulmonary hypertension

TESTS
- PFTs
  - All patients should have spirometry
  - Quantitate severity of obstruction
  - Assess reversibility
  - Follow/document progress/prognosis
  - Decreased FEV1, FEV1/FVC
  - TLC, RV may be increased
  - Decreased DLCO in emphysema

Imaging
- CXR:
  - Not specific for COPD; most useful for complications
  - Bronchial wall thickening, "tram-tracks" suggest chronic bronchitis
  - Hyperinflation, oligemia, bullae suggest emphysema
- CT can demonstrate emphysema, bronchiectasis

Arterial Blood Gases
- Early: mild-moderate hypoxemia
- Late: increased hypoxemia; hypercapnia

Sputum
- Commonly colonized with S pneumoniae, H influenza, M catarrhalis

DIFFERENTIAL DIAGNOSIS
- Asthma (distinguished by reversibility)
- Chronic bronchitis (sputum × 3 mo × $\geq$2 successive y)
- Emphysema (CT or pathologic diagnosis)
- Cystic fibrosis
- Bronchiectasis (CT diagnosis)
- Alpha1-proteinase inhibitor deficiency (<1% of all COPD)

MANAGEMENT
- See Global Initiative For Chronic Obstructive Lung Disease, produced by NIH National Heart, Lung & Blood Institute and World Health Organization: http://www.goldcopd.com

What to Do First
- Assess severity:
  - Spirometry should be routine
  - Hypoxemia influences survival

General Measures
- Eliminate causative factors (smoking, allergens, occupational exposures)
- Improve airway function (bronchodilators, steroids)
- Prevent or treat infectious exacerbations (vaccines, antibiotics)
- Support end-stage COPD
- Look for comorbid conditions (pneumothorax, CHF, PE, hypophosphatemia, hypokalemia)

SPECIFIC THERAPY
- Smoking cessation slows loss of lung function
- Oxygen (only treatment proven to prolong life):
  - Indications:
    - PaO_2 <55; SaO_2 <88%
    - PaO_2 56–59 or SaO_2 89% + right heart failure or Hct >56%
  - Continuous (20–24 h/d) better than 12 h

- ➤ Titrate flow to PaO_2 60–80
- ➤ Most patients require increased flow for exercise, sleep
- ■ Bronchodilators:
  - ➤ Ipratropium or short-acting beta$_2$ or long-acting beta$_2$ or combination
  - ➤ Nebulization usually not necessary with proper inhaler technique and dose
  - ➤ Theophylline may be useful as additional therapy
  - ➤ Long-acting anticholinergics and PDE4 inhibitors look promising for the near future
- ■ Inhaled corticosteroids (ICS):
  - ➤ 4 recent, large, multinational studies:
  - ➤ ICS do not slow progression of disease
  - ➤ May reduce exacerbations and visits
  - ➤ Increased risk of osteoporosis, skin thinning
- ■ Oral steroids effective in exacerbations
- ■ Treat infectious exacerbations:
  - ➤ Unclear when antibiotics needed; meta-analysis suggests pos effect
  - ➤ Treat empirically for *S pneumonia*, *H influenza*, *M catarrhalis*, *Legionella*, *Mycoplasma*; consider *Pseudomonas*, AFB
- ■ Vaccination:
  - ➤ Pneumococcal q 5–10 y
  - ➤ Influenza q 1 y
- ■ Pulmonary rehabilitation improves quality of life, not survival
- ■ Lung volume reduction surgery controversial; benefits may be short-lived; multicenter NIH trial underway
- ■ Lung transplant: COPD most common indication; 1-y survival, ~90%; 5-y, ~50%
- ■ Opiates help relieve dyspnea in some patients

FOLLOW-UP
- ■ Routine, periodic spirometry best objective measure to assess status
- ■ Evaluate frequently for comorbid conditions (CHF, poor nutrition)

COMPLICATIONS AND PROGNOSIS

Complications
- ■ Exacerbation (S pneumoniae, H influenzae up to 80%)
- ■ Pneumonia
- ■ Hemoptysis

- Pneumothorax: suspect with sudden increase in dyspnea
- Respiratory failure
- Cor pulmonale: vasoconstriction due to hypoxemia; LVH may contribute; thromboemboli also
- Depression, anxiety, inactivity
- Sleep abnormalities (less REM, hypercarbia)
- Malnutrition (50%): may affect respiratory muscles
- Giant bullae: usually in smokers, upper lung zones, may become infected, esp with *Aspergillus*
- Lung cancer

Prognosis
- Mild obstruction (FEV_1 >50%): good
- Severe obstruction (FEV_1 ≤0.75 L): 1-y mortality, 30%
- 4th leading cause of death in U.S.
- Natural history: increased rate of decline in FEV_1
- Normal: 20–40 mL/y
- COPD, still smoking: 62 mL/y
- COPD, stopped smoking: 32 mL/y

CHRONIC PANCREATITIS

ANSON W. LOWE, MD

HISTORY & PHYSICAL

History
- Alcohol abuse
- Familial history of hereditary pancreatitis
- Obstruction of the pancreatic duct
- Tropical pancreatitis

Signs & Symptoms
- Abdominal or back pain
- Nausea and vomiting
- Weight Loss
- Diarrhea
- Jaundice

TESTS
In general, highly sensitive and specific tests for chronic pancreatitis in its early stages do not exist
- Blood tests

> serum amylase and lipase are often only slightly elevated or normal.
> glucose levels may be abnormal secondary to diabetes
- Radiology
  > plain abdominal films – calcifications
  > ultrasound
  > CT scan: 75–90% sensitive
- Endoscopy
  > ERCP currently the gold standard
- Pancreatic function tests
  > secretin stimulation test – it requires the collection of duodenal juice secreted after secretin administration followed by the measurement of bicarbonate and protein secreted. Rarely available to most practioners.
  > "tubeless" test is useful for severe disease
    - bentiromide test (BT-PABA)
    - serum trypsin-like immunoreactivity

DIFFERENTIAL DIAGNOSIS
- other common causes of abdominal pain such as biliary tract disease, peptic ulcer disease, and intestinal ischemia.
- pancreatic cancer
- cholangiocarcinoma

MANAGEMENT

What to Do First
- Pain – represents the most common management problem
  > first exclude correctable causes of pain
    - pseudocyst
    - biliary stricture
    - duodenal stenosis
    - peptic ulcer disease
    - pancreatic cancer

SPECIFIC THERAPY
- trial of high-dose pancreatic enzymes along with acid supression (e.g. H_2-antagonist)
- analgesics
- consider therapeutic endoscopy (e.g. sphincterotomy, lithotripsy, pancreatic duct stenting
  > controversial and should be performed in an investigational setting

- thoracoscopic nerve ablation (investigational)
  - ➤ considered in patients who do not have a dilated pancreatic duct that can be surgically drained.
- surgery – reserved for patients with intolerable severe pain. Should be performed in an institution experienced in pancreatic surgery.
  - ➤ surgical decompression of the pancreatic duct. Best candidates are those who exhibit ductal dilation > 6mm in diameter.
  - ➤ pancreatic resection, usually of the pancreatic head, can be considered in patients with non-dilated ducts. Outcomes are not well established.

FOLLOW-UP
- dictated by clinical symptoms and extent of complications (e.g. pseudocysts, fistulas, ascites)
- 50% mortality after diagnosis within 20–25 years. 15–20% die of complications related to pancreatitis
- periodic follow-up for progression of disease. Chronic pancreatitis is usually progressive and thus patients must be monitored for the development of malabsorption or diabetes.

COMPLICATIONS AND PROGNOSIS
- pseudocyst – represent collections of pancreatic enzymes secondary to a ruptured pancreatic duct. Develop in 10% of patients. Major complications include rupture, hemorrhage, and infection.
  - ➤ most pseudocyst resolve spontaneously. Treatment is reserved for growing or symptomatic pseudocysts. Depending on the expertise of the institution, treatment may incorporate surgical resection, external drainage, or internal drainage. Depending on the available expertise, treatment of pseudocyst can be performed by endoscopy, interventional radiology, or surgery.
- malabsorption – treated with pancreatic enzyme replacement.
  - ➤ enzymes are normally given before meals. If non-enteric coated forms are used, they should be administered with bicarbonate or acid secretion should be inhibited.
- pancreatic ascites or pleural effusions: secondary to a ruptured pancreatic duct
  - ➤ diagnosis established by the presence of high levels of amylase and protein in the fluid
  - ➤ medical management may include diuretics, carbonic anhydrase inhibitors, total parenteral nutrition, or octreotide.

> ➤ surgery management: drainage of the pancreatic duct into the intestine.
- ■ duodenal and bile-duct obstruction (5–10% of patients)
  - ➤ usually surgically treated with gastrojejunostomy or choledo-choenterostomy.

CHRONIC RENAL FAILURE

ROBERT D. TOTO, MD

HISTORY & PHYSICAL

History
- ■ Infections, toxins, environment: hepatitis B and C, lead, mercury, silicon, acetaminophen/paracetamol/caffeine combinations, NSAIDS, lithium, pamidronate, herbal (e.g. Chinese herbs) remedies, Balkan nephropathy

Risk Factors for Progressive Renal Disease
- ■ Age, diabetes mellitus, hypertension, Family history (pattern of inheritance); black race, cigarette smoking, persistent albuminuria.

Signs & Symptoms
- ■ May be asymptomatic. Symptoms usual when Ccr $\leq$25 mL/min/1.73 m^2.
- ■ General: fatigue, malaise, weakness, fever (systemic diseases and retroperitoneal fibrosis)
- ■ HEENT: headache, visual disturbances, retinal changes of hypertensive/diabetic retinopathy, cholesterol emboli, uremic fetor
- ■ CV and PULM: dyspnea, edema, chest pain, hypertension, hyperpnea (metabolic acidosis) pulmonary edema
- ■ GI: dysguesia, loss of appetite, nausea, vomiting, diarrhea occult GI emorrhage
- ■ GU: Nocturia, foamy urine, dysuria, hematuria, painful urination, flank or back pain, hypospadias, urethral stricture, prostate enlargement
- ■ MS: lower extremity edema, bone and articular pain, generalized muscle wasting and weakness
- ■ NS: encephalopathy: difficulty concentrating, insomnia, daytime drowsiness; peripheral neuropathy

- SKIN: pruritis, easy bruising, petechiae, cutaneous infarcts, palpable purpura, calcinosis.

TESTS

Laboratory
- Basic blood tests:
  - Early disease: elevated serum creatinine, BUN
  - Advanced disease: early disease + hyperkalemia, hypobicarbonatemia, hyperphosphatemia, hypocalcemia, hypercalcemia, hypermagnesemia, elevated serum PTH, decreased serum 1,25 (OH)2 vitamin D3, elevated alkaline phosphatase, anemia
- Basic urine tests:
  - Early disease: microalbuminuria/proteinuria, microhematuria, pyuria, casts including: RBC, WBC, granular; crystalluria
  - Advanced disease: same as early and hyaline casts
  - Urinalysis Patterns:
  - Glomerulonephritis: hematuria, dysmorphic RBCs, heavy proteinuria (urine protein/creatinine ratio >3.0) and RBC casts
  - Tubulointerstitial nephritis: microhematuria, pyuria, + WBC casts, mild proteinuria (urine protein/creatinine ratio ≤ 2.0) and waxy casts
  - Renal Ischemia (Vasculitis, atheroembolism, renal artery stenosis) or Urinary obstruction: Minimal cellular elements + proteinuria
  - Urine [Na] and fractional Na excretion (FENa) not helpful

Specific Diagnostic Tests:
- Creatinine clearance (Ccr)
- Spot urine albumin mg/gram creatinine mg ratio (> 30 and < 300 = microalbuminuria; > 300 = macroalbuminuria); spot urine total protein mg/creatinine mg ratio (>0.15 abnormal)
- Anti-nuclear antibodies (SLE), Anti-neutrophil cytoplasmic antibody, hepatitis B surface antigen, Anti-hepatitis C antibody; HIV, complement components 3 and 4, anti-topoisomerase antibody, cryoglobulins, serum and urine protein electrophoresis, urine immunofixation (light chain deposition disease)

Imaging:
- Chest X-Ray to evaluate heart and lungs (see management)
- Renal ultrasound
  - Early disease: Normal or enlarged kidneys; cystic-autosomal dominant polycystic kidney disease (ADPKD); hydronephrosis

> Advanced disease: small shrunken kidneys, increased echo-
  genicicty; normal or enlarged kidneys in ADPKD, diabetes HIV
  nephropathy: hydronephrosis
- CT/MRI: angiomyolipomas, ADPKD; papillary necrosis
- Voiding cystourethrogram
- Renal Biopsy:
  > Useful when kidneys normal size to make specific diagnosis, e.g.
    SLE, glomerulonephritis. When kidneys small (e.g. less ($\leq$ 9 cm)
    usual finding is end-stage kidney i.e. global glomerulosclerosis +
    tubulointerstitial nephritis

DIFFERENTIAL DIAGNOSIS
- *Chronic renal failure* (CRF) symptoms mimicked by systemic
  diseases, cancer, wasting illnesses, depression, hypothyroidism,
  chronic heart failure, chronic liver disease. Elevated BUN and creatinine point to kidney.

Causes of Chronic Renal Failure
- *Systemic disease*: Diagnosis usually established by history, exam,
  sonogram and specific laboratory tests diabetes mellitus, hypertension, systemic lupus erythematosus, Sjogren's syndrome, systemic
  necrotizing vasculitis, atheromembolic renal disease, myeloma, light
  chain deposition disease, amyloidosis, genetic disease e.g. polycystic disease, tuberous sclerosis, cystinosis, Fabry's disease, sickle cell
  disease, CHF, cirrhosis.
- *Primary renal and urinary tract disease*: Specific glomerular disease
  usually requires renal biopsy; obstructive uropathy by sonogram or
  CT scan (e.g. retroperitoneal fibrosis), prostate disease, recurrent
  UTI or voiding dysfunction (Hx, exam, voiding study).

MANAGEMENT
What to Do First
- Assess cardiovascular and volume status by physical exam and CXR,
  and determine if dialysis is indicated because of:
- a) hypertension and/or pulmonary edema; b) hyperkalemia; c)
  pericarditis; d) metabolic acidosis; e) altered MS

General Measures
- Dialysis not indicated:
  > Restore volume status

➤ Treat hypertension (present in >80% of cases)
- Target blood pressure 120–130/70–80 mmHg with (in order): ACE inhibitor/angiotensin II receptor blocker + thiazide (serum creatinine ≤1.8 mg/dl) or loop diuretic (serum creatinine >1.8 mg/dl), calcium channel blocker, central-acting alpha-agonist/peripheral alpha-blocker/beta-blocker, then vasodilator (e.g. minoxidil) and dietary Na restriction (2 grams/day).

➤ Treat hyperkalemia and acidosis (see below)

SPECIFIC THERAPY
- Ccr 25–75 ml/min/1.73 m2, see "Preserve renal function"
- Ccr is <25 ml/min/1.73 m2, consult access surgeon, dietician and social worker to assist in preparing for dialysis.
- Ccr <20 ml/min/1.73 m2 place vascular access (hemodialysis) or plan peritoneal catheter in 6–12 months
- Ccr in range of 8–12 ml/min/1.73 m2 initiate maintenance renal replacement therapy unless: a) patient's weight is stable; serum albumin is at least at lower limit of normal range for laboratory; c) patient is symptom-free

Preserve (Remaining) Renal Function for all Levels of CRF
- Treat underlying disease process, e.g. treat SLE, relieve obstruction, discontinue nephrotoxin whenever possible
- Normalize BP using ACE inhibitor unless: a) patient has known allergy; b) cough intolerable; c) hyperkalemic with K ≥6.0 on K restricted diet; d) known or suspected critical renal artery stenosis
- Optimize glycemic control in diabetic (HgbA1c ≤ 5.5%)
- Cease cigarette smoking (hard evidence)
- Improve dyslipidemia, i.e. LDL-cholesterol (≤100 mg/dl for diabetic and ≤130 mg/dl for non-diabetic) and triglyceride <250 mg/dl
- Dietary protein intake: 0.8 g/kg/day represents minimal restriction, no malnutrition in clinical trials

Preserve Cardiac Function
- 50% of deaths in patients with ESRD are cardiac in origin.
- Normalize BP, manage dyslipidemia with HMG coA reductase inhibitor or fibric acid derivative, stop smoking, folic acid 5 mg/day to reduce risk of hyperhomocysteinemia

Manage Acid-Base and Electrolyte Disturbances

- Hyperkalemia: + EKG changes: IV Calcium gluconate, insulin, inhaled beta-2 agonist, oral or rectal kayexalate and dietary potassium restriction (1 mEq/kg/day). – EKG change: diet/kayexalate
- Acidosis: Check ABG, treat with oral sodium bicarbonate: 1 mEq/kg/day as Shohl's solution (1 mEq/ml); baking soda (60 mEq per tsp) or NaHCO3 tabs (8 mEq/650 mg tab). Renal osteodystrophy: Goal to normalize calcium and phosphorus, lower PTH and increase vitamin D: Dietary phosphate restriction to 12 mg/kg/day. Add Ca-based binder (Ca Acetate of Ca Carbonate) or sevalemer HCl (Renalgel) 1–2 tablets with meals. Measure PTH and 1,25(OH)2 vitamin D3 and if elevated and reduced respectively, initiate 1,25(OH) vitamin D3 0.5–1.0 mg/day.
- Avoid malnutrition: 0.8 g/kg/day protein, 35 kcal/kg/day. Monitor body weight, muscle mass, serum albumin, BUN (protein intake) and Scr (muscle mass)

Anemia

- Measure serum Fe, TIBC and ferritin and
- Treat Hct <33% with erythropoietin (EPO) and oral or intravenous iron therapy. EPO SC once or twice weekly.
- No contraindications; BP may increase in 20–25% of patients.

FOLLOW-UP

- Every 3 months for patients with Ccr $\leq$25 ml/min/1.73 m^2
- Increase frequency to as needed as patient approaches ESRD
- Labs at visit: chemistries, iron stores Hgb, spot urine protein/creatinine ratio, goal is ratio of <1.0.

COMPLICATIONS AND PROGNOSIS

Adverse drug events:

- ACE inhibition: cough, hyperkalemia, rarely angioedema (more common in African-Americans)
- HMG-CoA reductase inhibitors: rhabdomyolysis, muscle pain or asymptomatic CK elevation
- Vitamin D3 may cause hypercalemia.
- Loop diuretics: hypokalemia, hypomagnesemia, hypochloremic metabolic alkalosis.
- End-Stage Renal Disease: nearly all patients with Ccr <25 ml/min/1.73 m2 reach end-stage renal disease within 2 years. Mortality rate on dialysis at 5 years is about 50%.

CHRONIC RESPIRATORY ACIDOSIS

F. JOHN GENNARI, MD

HISTORY & PHYSICAL

- CO_2 retention for >3–4 days
- May be asymptomatic
- Exertional dyspnea
- Right-sided heart failure (cor pulmonale)
- Cardiac arrhythmias
- Confusion, fine tremor
- Abnormal chest examination, peripheral edema, papilledema when severe

TESTS

Laboratory

- Arterial blood gases are diagnostic – PCO2 >45 mmHg, pH <7.40 (see below for rule of thumb for [HCO3–])

Imaging

- Chest X-ray, CT of chest if necessary

DIFFERENTIAL DIAGNOSIS

- Conditions to Distinguish from Chronic Respiratory Acidosis
  - ➤ Metabolic alkalosis
  - ➤ Mixed disorders
    - Acute on chronic respiratory acidosis
    - Acute respiratory acidosis plus metabolic alkalosis
- Rule of Thumb:
  - ➤ Expected [HCO3–] in chronic respiratory acidosis:
  - ➤ [HCO3–](expected) = 24 mEq/L + 0.4 (PCO2 − 40, mmHg) Observed [HCO3–] should be within 4 mEq/L of the expected value in uncomplicated chronic respiratory acidosis.
- Causes of Chronic Respiratory Acidosis
  - ➤ Chronic obstructive pulmonary disease (most common cause)
  - ➤ CNS depression
  - ➤ Sleep apnea
  - ➤ Obesity-hypoventilation syndrome
  - ➤ Neuromuscular impairment (see under acute respiratory acidosis)
  - ➤ Restrictive lung diseases

MANAGEMENT
- Treat pulmonary infections aggressively.
- Treat bronchospasm if present.
- Avoid ventilator therapy unless process is rapidly reversible.

SPECIFIC THERAPY
- Minimize fluid accumulation with judicious use of diuretics
  - Side effects – hypokalemia, metabolic alkalosis
- Acetazolamide can reduce edema, serum [HCO3−], stimulating ventilation
  - Side effects – hypokalemia, metabolic acidosis
- Oxygen therapy, used judiciously, prolongs survival.
  - Side effects – decreased ventilatory drive, worsening hypercapnia

FOLLOW-UP
- Stabilize or improve PCO2

COMPLICATIONS AND PROGNOSIS
- Extremely variable, but generally poor

CHRONIC RESPIRATORY ALKALOSIS

F. JOHN GENNARI, MD

HISTORY & PHYSICAL
- Increase in ventilation for >2–3 days
- Usually asymptomatic
- With CNS disease, Cheyne-Stokes respiration or, with mid-brain tumors or injury, metronomic hyperventilation (very regular pattern)
- If symptomatic, symptoms due to underlying illness
- Respiratory rate and/or depth of inspiration increased by definition, but not usually detected on exam, unless abnormal ventilatory pattern present

TESTS

Laboratory
- Arterial blood gases are diagnostic – PCO2 <35 mmHg, pH >7.45 (see below for rule of thumb for [HCO3−])

DIFFERENTIAL DIAGNOSIS
- Conditions to distinguish from Chronic Respiratory Alkalosis

- ➤ Metabolic acidosis
- ➤ Mixed disorders
  - Metabolic acidosis and respiratory alkalosis
  - Acute on chronic respiratory alkalosis
- ■ Rule of Thumb:
  - ➤ Expected [HCO3−] in chronic respiratory alkalosis:
  - ➤ [HCO3−](expected) = 24 mEq/L − 0.4 × (40 − PCO2, mmHg)

  Observed [HCO3−] should be within 4 mEq/L of the expected value in uncomplicated chronic respiratory alkalosis.
- ■ Causes of Chronic Respiratory Alkalosis
  - ➤ Sustained hypoxemia
  - ➤ High altitude exposure
  - ➤ Pregnancy
  - ➤ Hepatic failure
  - ➤ Interstitial pulmonary disease
  - ➤ CNS disease – cerebrovascular disease, tumors
  - ➤ Drugs – progesterone, salicylates

MANAGEMENT
- ■ No treatment necessary for alkalosis per se – disorder is sign helping to diagnose underlying diagnosis (e.g., CNS disease, hepatic failure)

SPECIFIC THERAPY
n/a

FOLLOW-UP
- ■ Dependent on underlying condition

COMPLICATIONS AND PROGNOSIS
- ■ Dependent on underlying condition
- ■ Very poor if secondary to hepatic failure or CNS disease

CHRONIC RESPIRATORY FAILURE

THOMAS SHAUGHNESSY, MD

HISTORY & PHYSICAL

Risk Factors
- ■ Malnutrition
- ■ Catabolic nutritional state: Sepsis, burn, ARDS, multiple organ failure syndrome (MOFS), systemic inflammatory response syndrome (SIRS)

- Hypoventilation: Neurologic injury with impaired consciousness, quadriplegia with C3 or above lesion, chronic progressive myopathy or neuropathy
- Hypersecretion: Impaired secretion clearance, cystic fibrosis
- Pulmonary: Pneumonia, end-stage restrictive lung disease, COPD, ARDS
- Obesity: Pickwickian Syndrome

Signs and Symptoms
- Tachypnea, shallow tidal volumes
- Poor cough, impaired secretion clearance
- Recurrent episodes of acute respiratory failure, or
- Failure to wean from mechanical ventilation

TESTS
- Diagnosis of chronic respiratory failure is based on history

Basic Studies
- ABG: hypercarbia, hypoxia, respiratory acidosis
- CXR: assess reversible causes (pneumonia, CHF, exacerbation of COPD, CF)

Advanced Studies
- RR/TV index (Tobin) >105 – predicts unsuccessful extubation
- Dead space ventilation (%) = $(PaCO_2 - PetCO_2)/PaCO_2 \times 100$
  - ➤ >70% suggests persistent ventilator dependence.

DIFFERENTIAL DIAGNOSIS
- Cardiac: Unilateral or bilateral pulmonary edema
- Pulmonary: pneumonia, pleural effusion, COPD, interstitial lung disease, carcinoma, diaphragm dysfunction, splinting and hypoventilation after thoracic or upper abdominal surgery
- Neuromuscular disorders

MANAGEMENT
What to Do First
- Treat reversible causes of respiratory failure
- Optimize nutrition: enteral route preferred to augment anabolism
- Consider anabolic steroids oxandralone, nandralone
- Initiate physical therapy

General Measures
- Monitoring in an ICU and serial ABGs with arterial catheter is usually appropriate

- If not intubated:
  - Consider non-invasive ventilation (BiPAP) as a bridge while treating underlying etiology
  - Some patients may benefit from intermittent BiPAP (e.g., overnight) at home
- If intubated:
  - Continue serial weaning trials
    - No one method of weaning has been established as superior:
      - T-piece trials
      - Pressure support wean
      - IMV wean
  - Recent literature favors T-piece wean, with daily estimates of suitability for extubation
  - Assure adequate analgesia; Consider regional anesthesia (epidural, intercostal blocks)
  - Assure adequate sleep/wake cycles; Consider increased ventilatory support at night
  - Consider tracheostomy after 14–21 days of weaning attempts
  - Chronic intermittent ventilation if weaning requires > 6 months and patient has been clinically optimized

SPECIFIC THERAPY

Indications for Treatment
- Therapy should be instituted once a diagnosis is considered and work up initiated

Treatment Options

Non-Invasive Ventilation
- BiPAP – nasal or mask
- Start at 10 cm H_2O inspiration/5 cm H_2O expiration

Weaning Protocols
- T-piece:
  - Start with 15–30 mins BID or TID
  - Increase in 15–30 min increments if RR <25
- Pressure Support:
  - Start at PS level that provides an adequate TV
  - Decrease by 2 cm H_2O every 1–2 days
- IMV: Decrease RR by 2 breaths TID to qD if RR <25

Tracheostomy:
- Decreased work of breathing may facilitate weaning

- Enhanced suctioning facilitates nursing care
- Greater patient comfort, less sedation
- Allows aggressive physical therapy

Side Effects and Complications
- Intubation >3 wks: Impaired secretion clearance
  - Nosocomial pneumonia
  - Laryngeal stricture
  - Tracheomalacia
- Tracheostomy:
  - Perioperative hemorrhage
  - Swallowing dysfunction
  - Tracheal stricture
  - Tracheoinominate fistula

Contraindications to Weaning
- Absolut: Sepsis, pulmonary edema, myocardial ischemia, pneumonia, bronchospasm
- Relative:
  - Severe musculoskeletal deconditioning
  - Malnutrition
  - Avoid anabolic steroids in the presence of hepatic dysfunction or active infection.
  - Encephalopathy
  - Bronchitis and Hypersecretion

FOLLOW-UP

During Treatment
- Assess nutrition with serial albumin, nitrogen balance, or respiratory quotient.
- Titrate pressure support levels in increments of 2–5 cm H_2O to achieve RR <25, RR/TV ratio <100
- Wean FiO_2 and pressure support to keep SpO_2 >90% or PaO_2 > 60 mmHg
- Treat bronchospasm with albuterol aerosol.

Routine
- Serial CXRs
- Sedation as needed with narcotics and benzodiazepines for agitation
- Track progress with serial tidal volume and vital capacity measurements q week
- Serial dead space measurement q 2–4 weeks.

COMPLICATIONS AND PROGNOSIS
- Nosocomial pneumonia
- Permanent ventilator dependence

CHURG STRAUSS DISEASE

ERIC L. MATTESON, MD

HISTORY & PHYSICAL
- Similar to Wegener's, with asthma;
- GI complaints more common, renal disease less so

TESTS
Laboratory
- CBC for anemia, thrombocytosis, (eosinophilia in CS)
- ESR and/or C-reactive protein elevated
- Urinalysis
- Anti-neutrophil anti-cytoplasmic antibody (c-ANCA) positive in >90% of patients with WG and many with CS

Other Tests
- Biopsy
  - GCA: Temporal artery shows mononuclear cell infiltration and multinucleated giant cells, intimal proliferation. Histology in TA is similar.
  - WG, CS: Non-caseating granuloma, vasculitis in mucosal, dermal, retroocular, pulmonary lesions; rapidly progressive or focal segmental glomerulonephritis in kidney
- Imaging
  - Chest radiography and CT: Pulmonary nodules, pleural effusions in WG; fleeting infiltrates more common in CS
  - Arteriogram required for diagnosis and follow-up of TA, may be needed in GCA for symptomatic stenosis
  - Echocardiography in TA or GCA may reveal aortic aneurysm

DIFFERENTIAL DIAGNOSIS
- GCA, TA
  - Migraine, especially ophthalmoplegic migraine
  - Cluster headache
  - Viral syndromes
  - Polymyalgia rheumatica in patients >50 years of age

- ➤ Occult infection or malignancy
- ➤ Myocardial ischemia
- ➤ Wegener's granulomatosis and polyarteritis nodosa
- ➤ Central retinal artery occlusion, retinal detachment, glaucoma
- ➤ Thyroid disease
- ➤ Polymyositis, SLE, rheumatoid arthritis
- ➤ Arterial fibrodysplasia
- ■ WG, CS
  - ➤ Chronic sinusitis
  - ➤ Polyarteritis nodosa; microscopic polyangiitis
  - ➤ Fungal, bacterial diseases; syphilis
  - ➤ SLE

MANAGEMENT

What to Do First

- ■ Assess extent and severity of vascular disease by history and physical exam; angiography especially in suspected TA
- ■ Control blood pressure
- ■ With impending organ damage, e.g. visual loss, evolving stroke, begin immediate "pulse" (methylprednisolone, 1 gm/d qd × 3).
- ■ Ophthalmologic consultation in GCA, (eye disease often unilateral initially, but may soon involve the other eye)
- ■ ENT consultation in WG.

SPECIFIC THERAPY

- ■ GCA
  - ➤ prednisone is usually dramatically effective within 2–3 days. Taper slowly
- ■ TA, WG, CS
  - ➤ prednisone, tapering slowly over months.
  - ➤ cyclophosphamide orally
  - ➤ methotrexate may suffice in milder or controlled disease.
  - ➤ trimethoprim-sulfamethoxazole may suffice in patients with WS confined to the upper airways; should be considered even in systemic disease
  - ➤ other options include tumor necrosis factor-alpha antagonists, mycophenolate mofetil, and azathioprine

Side Effects & Contraindications

- ■ As in Nongranulomatous Vasculitis

FOLLOW-UP

During Treatment

■ Regularly assess disease activity by history and physical examination including bilateral blood pressures and heart exam

➤ GCA
- After one month, taper corticosteroid dose by about 5 mg every two weeks to 10–15 mg/day, and more slowly thereafter. Most relapses occur in the first 18 months of treatment. Average duration of therapy is about 2–3 years.

➤ TA
- Therapy may be protracted; $\frac{1}{4}$ of patients will require years of immunosuppression
- Subclavian involvement is common (90%), and blood pressure readings may not reflect aortic root pressure. Angiography and echocardiography may help
- Follow-up vascular imaging required.
- Surgical intervention for critical stenosis or aneurysms.

➤ WG,CS
- Monitor urinalysis, chest radiograph, clinical status
- Long-term immunosuppression is usually required
- c-ANCA roughly correlates with disease activity

COMPLICATIONS AND PROGNOSIS

■ GCA
➤ Thoracic aortic aneurysms 17 times, abdominal aneurysms 2.5 times, more likely than in age-matched controls
➤ Visual loss (6–10%)
➤ Stroke
➤ Patients with GCA have a normal life expectancy

■ TA
➤ Aortic root involvement with valvular insufficiency and congestive heart failure in 20%
➤ Stroke
➤ Progressive arterial and aorta lesions may require surgery
➤ 5 year survival 83%; 10 year survival 58% in patients with severe disease

■ WS, CS
➤ Renal failure, stroke, mononeuritis, vision loss; tracheal stenosis, nasal deformity, infection
➤ 5 year survival >80%

CLOSTRIDIUM INFECTIONS

RICHARD A. JACOBS, MD, PhD

HISTORY & PHYSICAL

History

- Clostridium spp. are anaerobic, spore-forming, Gram-positive bacilli that are ubiquitous in nature and found in soil, dust, air and as part of the normal flora of the intestinal tract and female reproductive tract.
- Common human pathogens include C perfringens, C septicum, C tertium, C novyi, C difficile, C tetani and C botulinum.
- Frequently recovered from infected sites, but usually as part of a polymicrobial infection, making it difficult to determine role in causing disease
- Certain well-defined syndromes have been described (see below).
- Disease follows trauma (open fractures, crush injuries, gunshot wounds), surgery (especially GI procedures), ingestion of contaminated food or occurs spontaneously from endogenous flora.

Signs & Symptoms

- Manifestations depend upon site involved
- Bacteremia: systemic symptoms and sepsis; C perfringens and C septicum most common isolates; C septicum associated with colon cancer and neutropenia and causes particularly severe disease with metastatic infections in up to 25% of patients; up to 50% of blood isolates considered contaminants not associated with infection requiring therapy
- Intra-abdominal infections: usually part of polymicrobial infection and role unclear
- Gallbladder: significance unclear except in emphysematous cholecystitis, a severe form of gallbladder disease seen most commonly in diabetics; presents with severe RUQ pain and sepsis
- Genital tract: part of polymicrobial infection of tubo-ovarian abscesses; cause of uterine gas gangrene, a rare complication of abortion/uterine surgery
- Soft tissue infections: crepitant cellulitis presents with edema and crepitance of the involved area, a foul-smelling discharge and systemic toxicity; myonecrosis (gas gangrene) presents with systemic toxicity, severe pain at the involved site, and as the disease progresses

(usually rapidly within hours) bullous formation of the overlying skin and a foul-smelling discharge

■ Enteric infections: enterocolitis in neutropenic patients with abdominal pain, fever, diarrhea and a distended abdomen; due to invasion of bowel wall (usually the cecum) with clostridia, other enteric Gram-negative bacilli and anaerobes; food poisoning due to eating foods (usually meat) contaminated with C. perfringens; incubation period is short (6–12 h) and the watery diarrhea and cramps are self-limited, lasting <24 h

TESTS

■ Presence of gas on x-rays is best clue to diagnosis, BUT presence of gas is not diagnostic of clostridial infection (many other enteric Gram-negative bacilli can produce gas).

■ Drainage from skin lesions (crepitant cellulitis/myonecrosis) should be sent for Gram's stain and culture; Gram's stain shows characteristic large Gram-positive rods, some with terminal spores, and rare WBCs.

DIFFERENTIAL DIAGNOSIS

■ Crepitant cellulitis and clostridial myonecrosis must be distinguished form other deep tissue infections such as necrotizing fasciitis, staphylococcal pyomyositis, anaerobic cellulitis and synergistic necrotizing cellulitis; distinction made at time of surgery based on structures involved and culture results

■ Other causes of food poisoning producing a similar syndrome include staphylococcal and Bacillus cereus food poisoning; cultures of stool and/or food positive for organism

MANAGEMENT

■ Supportive care with fluids and pressors for those with septic shock

SPECIFIC THERAPY

■ For those with tissue involvement (skin, muscle, gallbladder, uterus) a combination of surgery and antibiotic therapy required

■ Surgical removal of the gallbladder or uterus and wide surgical excision of involved muscle is critical; frequent (sometimes daily or twice-daily) surgical debridement often required; amputation may be required

■ Role of hyperbaric oxygen not well studied, but some feel it is an important modality of therapy that should be employed if available

■ Antitoxin no longer recommended

- Antibiotic of choice is penicillin; metronidazole, imipenem, chloramphenicol also with good activity, but less clinical experience; cefoxitin has variable activity against clostridia and should not be used; clindamycin is active against C perfringens, but other species are less susceptible
- Food poisoning is self-limited and requires no therapy.

FOLLOW-UP
- Patients with clostridial myonecrosis require at least twice-daily follow-up to assess the need for additional debridement or amputation.

COMPLICATIONS AND PROGNOSIS
- Loss of limb and disfigurement from surgery
- Mortality in antibiotic era about 25%
- Early diagnosis and prompt surgical intervention improve outcome.

CLUSTER HEADACHE

CHAD CHRISTINE, MD

HISTORY & PHYSICAL
- Brief, severe unilateral, nonthrobbing pain in & about eye
- Typically 10 minutes to 2 hrs in duration
- More common in men than women (5:1)
- Commonly occurs at night & may awaken pt
- May occur at the same time daily for days to weeks
- Headache-free periods may last months to years
- May be precipitated by alcohol or vasodilators
- Ipsilateral conjunctival injection & facial flushing, ipsilateral lacrimation, nasal congestion, possibly Horner's syndrome (ptosis, miosis, anhidrosis)

TESTS
- Diagnosis made clinically
- Lab tests normal
- Brain imaging normal

DIFFERENTIAL DIAGNOSIS
- Migraine headache disorder & trigeminal neuralgia excluded by history
- Temporal arteritis excluded by history & sed rate
- Carotid aneurysm excluded by history & brain imaging

MANAGEMENT
- General measures: avoid alcohol, vasodilators, smoking

SPECIFIC THERAPY
- Agents to abort an individual headache
  - Oxygen by face mask 7–10 L/min for 15 minutes
  - 5-HT agonists: sumatriptan, rizatriptan, zolmitriptan, naratriptan, almotriptan, eletriptan, frovatriptan
  - DHE, intranasal lidocaine (2% gel) occasionally effective
- Prophylactic agents
  - DHE IM or SC in divided doses
  - Prednisone (episodic cluster) for 3–5 d followed by taper over 1 wk
  - Verapamil SR (episodic cluster)
  - Methysergide (episodic cluster) (may be used qhs for nocturnal attacks)
  - Valproic acid (chronic cluster)
  - Lithium (chronic cluster); must monitor serum level, keep <1.2 mEq/L

FOLLOW-UP
- Indicated if attacks are frequent or ongoing prophylactic therapy

COMPLICATIONS AND PROGNOSIS
- Prognosis good

COCCIDIOIDES IMMITIS

RICHARD A. JACOBS, MD, PhD

HISTORY & PHYSICAL

History
- Endemic to soils of certain regions of Western Hemisphere
- In United States, endemic in desert Southwest (portions of California, esp San Joaquin Valley, southern Nevada, Arizona, New Mexico, western Texas, southwest Utah)
- Other areas: Mexico, Central America, South America
- Most easily recovered at end of winter rains, but new infections peak during summer months with dry soil
- Rate of infection in endemic area: 3%/year

- Epidemics associated with disruption of infected soil, by archaeologic excavation or in severe dust storms or earthquakes
- All infections result from inhaling arthroconidia
- Exposure history is key to diagnosis – incubation usually 1–3 weeks, but even brief/trivial exposures (driving through region, changing planes at airport) have been implicated

Signs & Symptoms
- 50–70% of infections inapparent or mild enough that medical attention not sought
- Many others experience nonspecific, self-limited respiratory illness
- Early respiratory infection:
  - Symptoms first appear 7–21 d after exposure
  - Cough, chest pain, dyspnea, fever, fatigue, weight loss, headache
  - Skin manifestations: nonpruritic fine papular rash (early/transient), also E nodosum and E multiforme (in females)
  - Triad of fever, e. nodosum, arthralgias = "desert rheumatism"
  - Uncommonly, fulminant respiratory failure/sepsis (1/3 of HIV patients present this way)
- Pulmonary Nodules/Cavities:
  - 4% pulmonary infections result in nodule (usually without symptoms), occ. forming a cavity
  - Most cavities do not cause symptoms – occ. pleuritic pain, cough, hemoptysis
  - Can rupture into pleural space – often without immunodeficiency, causes pyopneumothorax (prompt surgery indicated)
- Extrapulmonary Dissemination:
  - 0.5% of all infections in general population
  - Increased risk with immunodeficiency (HIV, post-transplant, high-dose steroids, Hodgkin disease)
  - Men>women, but high risk during third trimester of pregnancy or immediate postpartum period
  - Increased risk among African or Filipino ancestry
  - Increased risk with waning T-cell immunity
  - Extrapulmonary dissemination often exists with no pulmonary disease
  - Most common: skin – superficial maculopapular lesion, often nasolabial fold; joints and bones
  - Most serious: Coccidioidal meningitis – headache, vomiting, altered mental status

TESTS

Laboratory

- Early respiratory: normal, except for increased ESR or eosinophilia
- *CSF examination (meningitis)*:
  - ➤ Elevated CSF pressure
  - ➤ Elevated WBC count, protein
  - ➤ Depressed glucose
  - ➤ Eosinophils may be prominent
- *Microbiology – culture*
  - ➤ Cultures highly infectious to lab personnel – treat with great care, always warn lab if cocci is suspected
  - ➤ Usually grows well after 5–7 d of incubation
- *Serology*
  - ➤ Mainstay for outpatient diagnosis – most highly specific for active infection, one negative test does not exclude diagnosis
  - ➤ Complement-fixing antibodies – blood or other body fluids (esp CSF). 1:16 or greater usually treated as positive, but significant inter-lab variability. Serial determinations by same lab most useful; any + titer in CSF significant
  - ➤ Tube preciptin antibodies – 90% have TP antibodies at some time in first 3 weeks of symptoms, <5% at 7 mo after self-limited illness
  - ➤ Immunodiffusion – IDTP or IDCF detects above antibodies using alternative technique – at least as sensitive
  - ➤ ELISA – IgM or IgG Ab – highly sensitive, but occ. false positives, especially with IgM ELISA. Usually confirm a positive ELISA with IDTP, IDCF or CF before considering truly positive.
- *Skin testing*
  - ➤ DTH quite specific, but remains positive for life (thus, most useful in epidemiology)
- *Histopathology*
  - ➤ Direct examination of sputum secretions or tissue

Imaging (CXR)

- Early respiratory: unilateral infiltrates, hilar adenopathy, effusions
- Fulminant: diffuse infiltrate (ARDS-like)
- Pulmonary nodules and cavities appear on CXR if they are present

DIFFERENTIAL DIAGNOSIS

- Distinguish from other fungal infections of the lung (Histo, Cryptococcus, Aspergillus).
- Distinguish from mycobacterial diseases of the lung, other chronic pneumonias.

MANAGEMENT

What to Do First

- Determine if therapy is warranted, attempt to confirm diagnosis with tissue or good serology data. Obtain excellent travel/exposure history.

General Measures

- Establish extent of disease and risk of future complications.
- Prescribe antifungal agents where indicated, consider surgery for debridement or reconstruction.
- In general population, complications uncommon
- Any risk factors (racial, immunosuppression, third trimester or recent postpartum) should prompt antifungals.

SPECIFIC THERAPY

Treatment Options

- Azole antifungals for mild/chronic disease – probably no efficacy difference between fluconazole, itraconazole, ketoconazole – durations of 3–6 m
- Amphotericin B for severe disease
- Meningitis: fluconazole now used initially, shunting for hydrocephalus

Side Effects & Complications

- Amphotericin B (conventional): infusion-related toxicities (often ameliorated with hydrocortisone in IV bag), nephrotoxicity, hypokalemia, hypomagnesemia, nephrotoxicity (can be dose-limiting)
- Azoles: transaminitis, many drug interactions

FOLLOW-UP

During Treatment

- Close clinical follow-up, serial CXR, can follow serology titers

Routine

- Close clinical follow-up

COMPLICATIONS AND PROGNOSIS

Complications

- Pulmonary complications rare, can rupture a cavity causing pyopneumothorax
- Extrapulmonary disseminated disease, especially meningitis, bones/joints

Prognosis
- Good for normal hosts
- With acute presentation/septic picture, very poor prognosis

---

COLON POLYPS AND TUMORS

DAVID A. LIEBERMAN, MD

HISTORY & PHYSICAL

History
- patients with (+) history should be considered for complete colon exam
- family history of colorectal cancer (CRC) in first-degree relative
- family history of CRC under age 50
- personal history of colon polyps or cancer
- personal history of ulcerative colitis – duration >8 years

Signs & Symptoms
- findings prompting a colon examination:
  - recurrent/persistent rectal bleeding in patient over age 40
  - significant change in bowel habits
  - weight loss
  - iron deficiency anemia
  - rectal exam reveals mass

TESTS

Screening of Asymptomatic, Average Risk
- colon screening is recommended to begin at age 50; screening options include:
  - fecal occult blood test (FOBT) annually
    - home testing performed on 3 stool samples has higher positive predictive value than office test on digital exam; digital exam in office is not an adequate screening test
  - there is controversy regarding rehydration of FOBT slides
  - flexible sigmoidoscopy every 5 years
  - colonoscopy every 10 years
- NOTE: overall health and comorbidities should be considered when assessing risk and benefit of continuing screening beyond age 75

Surveillance
- Positive family history of CRC
  - risk of CRC in family member increased by 2–4 fold

- colonoscopy is recommended
- first exam should occur at an age at least 10 years younger than index family member, and then every 5 years
- if there are two first-degree relatives or a first-degree relative with CRC under age 50, hereditary cancer syndrome should be suspected; if confirmed, colonoscopy every 2 years is recommended
- Prior history of CRC
  - surveillance colonoscopy is recommended
  - cancer in colon: if patient had complete exam prior to resection, follow-up should be within 1 year; if complete exam of the colon was not possible prior to resection, then an exam should be completed within 3–6 months after surgery to rule out synchronous lesions
- Prior history of adenoma: surveillance colonoscopy is recommended as follows:
  - 1 or 2 tubular adenomas <1 cm at baseline: surveillance at 5 years or more; if negative, routine screening for average risk recommended
  - if baseline exam revealed 3 or more adenomas, adenoma >1 cm, villous adenoma or adenoma with high-grade dysplasia: surveillance at 3 years, and if negative every 5 years
  - if baseline exam revealed 10 or more adenomas, surveillance prior to 3 years should be considered
  - History of ulcerative colitis
  - risk of colorectal cancer increased after 8 years of disease
  - surveillance colonoscopy is recommended every 2 years with biopsies from each portion of the colon

DIFFERENTIAL DIAGNOSIS
- signs or symptoms of colonic disease: colon polyp vs. colorectal cancer

MANAGEMENT
- Positive FOBT
  - if any of 3 cards are positive, the test should be considered positive
  - colonoscopy is appropriate follow-up test
- Positive sigmoidoscopy
  - if an adenoma of any size is found in the sigmoid colon, the risk of advanced proximal neoplasia is 2- to 3-fold higher than patients who do not have sigmoid adenomas; small polyps should be biopsied to determine if it is an adenoma

➤ all patients with adenomas found at sigmoidoscopy should undergo colonoscopy

➤ patients with only hyperplastic polyps have similar risk of proximal advanced neoplasia as patients with no polyps and do not need complete colon exam

■ Positive Barium Enema or Virtual CT Colography

➤ colonoscopy should be performed if polyps are found on imaging studies

SPECIFIC THERAPY

■ most polyps can be removed at time of colonoscopy

■ large polyps greater than 2 or 3 cm may require surgical resection

■ pedunculated polyps with cancer localized to mucosa can be resected with polypectomy if the margin is clear of tumor

■ most flat or sessile polyps with cancer must be surgically removed to confirm complete removal

FOLLOW-UP

■ all removed polyps should be examined; follow-up is based on histology:

➤ hyperplastic polyps: no specific follow-up needed

➤ 1 or 2 tubular adenomas <1 cm: low-risk lesion; surveillance colonoscopy recommended at 5 years or more; emerging data from the National Polyp Study may lead to extension of this interval

➤ advanced neoplasia defined as 3 or more adenomas, tubular adenoma >1 cm, villous adenoma, adenoma with high-grade dysplasia: follow-up at 3 years with colonoscopy; if the baseline exam was incomplete, the exam should be repeated at 1 year; if there was any doubt about complete removal of polyps, the exam should be repeated in 6–12 months

COMPLICATIONS AND PROGNOSIS

Risks of Colonoscopy

■ serious bleeding: 1–2/1,000 procedures, most associated with polypectomy

■ perforation: 1/1,000 procedures, most associated with polypectomy

■ death: 1/10,000 associated with either perforation or bleeding

■ cardiopulmonary complications: serious complications rare, but transient hypoxia, hypotension, vagal reactions can occur during colonoscopy

Prognosis
- removal of adenomas is associated with reduced incidence of CRC (National Polyp Study)
- screening asymptomatic individuals over age 50 can reduce CRC mortality (RCTs with FOBT and case-control studies with sigmoidoscopy)

COMA

MICHAEL J. AMINOFF, MD, DSc

HISTORY & PHYSICAL
- Unresponsive & unarousable
- Cause may be suggested by mode of onset (acute or insidious)
- May relate to past medical or psychiatric history, medication or drug use, history of trauma
- Response to pain or other stimuli depends on depth of coma
- Signs of bihemispheric or brain stem dysfunction may be present
- Structural lesions may cause unequal pupils, dysconjugate eye movements, papilledema, focal deficits
- Metabolic or toxic cause, subarachnoid hemorrhage or meningitis produces preserved pupillary & eye movement reflexes, no focal deficits in limbs

TESTS
- See "Confusion"

DIFFERENTIAL DIAGNOSIS
- Sudden onset of coma suggests vascular cause (eg, SAH)
- Rapid progression from focal hemispheric deficit to coma suggests ICH
- Absence of focal or lateralizing signs suggests SAH, meningitis or metabolic/toxic encephalopathy
- Persistent vegetative state is distinguished by occurrence of sleep/wake cycles
- In de-efferented state, pt is awake, alert, mute, quadriplegic; midbrain movements (eg, voluntary eye opening) are preserved & EEG is normal

MANAGEMENT
- Supportive care

SPECIFIC THERAPY
■ Treat underlying disorder

FOLLOW-UP
N/A

COMPLICATIONS AND PROGNOSIS
■ Depends on cause
  ➤ Good for drug-induced coma, w/ supportive care
  ➤ Poor when structural lesions responsible
  ➤ Poor outcome from anoxic encephalopathy if pupillary responses absent after 24 hrs
  ➤ Will not recover if findings indicate brain death

COMPLICATIONS OF HUMAN IMMUNODEFICIENCY VIRUS TYPE 1 (HIV-1) INFECTION

MALCOLM D.V. JOHN, MD, MPH

HISTORY & PHYSICAL

History
Fungi
■ *Pneumocystis carinii*: ubiquitous; pneumonia (PCP) occurs in 20–40% of patients with AIDS today (rarely in those with CD4 >200–250/mm^3); rare cases of person-to-person transmission among immunosuppressed reported (some authorities recommend that HIV+ persons at risk for PCP not share a hospital room with a patient who has PCP)
■ *Candida species*: common on mucosal surfaces and skin; recovered from soil, hospital environments, inanimate objects, and food; no special measures to reduce exposure to these fungi
■ *Cryptococcus neoformans*: cannot completely avoid exposure; no evidence exists that exposure to pigeon droppings is associated with an increased risk for acquisition
■ *Histoplasma capsulatum*: endemic to the Mississippi-Ohio River Valley area and parts of Latin America; activities associated with increased risk (e.g., creating dust when working with surface soil; cleaning chicken coops that are heavily contaminated with droppings; disturbing soil beneath bird-roosting sites; cleaning, remodeling, or demolishing old buildings; and exploring caves)

- *Coccidiodes immitus*: endemic to Southwestern U.S. and Latin America; HIV+ persons living in or visiting endemic areas should avoid activities associated with increased risk (e.g., extensive exposure to disturbed native soil, for example, at building excavation sites or during dust storms)
- *Penicillium marneffei*: primarily seen in S.E. Asia; associated with the bamboo rat; probably acquired via inhalation of aerosolized conidia
- *Aspergillus*: ubiquitous fungus found mainly on decomposing vegetable matter esp. around human habitations esp. in cellars, potted plants, and pepper and spices

Parasites

- *Toxoplasma gondii*: worldwide distribution; found in raw or undercooked meat, particularly undercooked pork, lamb, or venison; also from in soil contaminated with animal feces; and cat feces; can be congenitally acquired if mother infected during pregnancy
- *Cryptosporidium parvum*: probable ubiquitous animal pathogen with human as incidental hosts. Modes of transmission include direct contact with infected adults, diaper-aged children, and infected animals; drinking contaminated water; coming into contact with contaminated water during recreational activities; and eating contaminated food.
- *Isospora belli*: more common in southeastern United States and the Caribbean; occurs in <0.2% AIDS cases in the U.S.
- *Microsporidia*: general attention to hand washing and other personal hygiene measures are recommended to decrease risk of infection; Enterocytozoon bieniusi and Septata intestinalis are main pathogens
- *Giardia lamblia*: transmission by oral ingestion of cysts – e.g., foodborne, contaminated water (esp. cold surface water), person-to-person (esp. children in daycare centers, male homosexuals and institutionalized individuals)
- *Other Parasites*: Leishmania – widespread; spread by sandflies; Strongyloides stercoralis – widely distributed in tropical and southern USA; found in soil and institutionalized individuals

Bacteria

- *Mycobacterium tuberculosis*: almost all transmission due to inhalation of infectious droplets from infected individuals produce by coughing, sneezing or talking; close contact and a highly infectious (smear positive) source increases likelihood of transmission; higher exposure risk include volunteer work or employment in health-care facilities, correctional institutions, and shelters for the homeless, as well as in other settings identified as high risk by local health authorities; skin inoculation and venereal transmission have been reported

- *Mycobacterium Avian Complex (MAC)*: fairly ubiquitous in environmental sources such as food, water, and soil
- *Other atypical mycobacteria*: M. kansasii occurs in the south and midwest with outbreaks among HIV+ patients primarily in the south and midwest esp. among urban IDUs and among those with underlying chronic pulmonary disease; other atypical mycobacteria occur sporadically
- *Bartonella hanselae/quintara*: can be transmitted from cats; esp. <1 yr old by bite, scratch.
- *Syphilis*: transmission can be sexual, congenital, or by kissing/close content w/ active lesions, transfusions, accidental direct inoculation
- *Other bacterial infections*: streptococcus pneumonia (common at al stages of HIV), Haemophilus influenzae (100-fold higher than healthy controls); uncommon agents include Staphylococcus aureus, Legionella species, Rhodococcus equii and Nocardia asteroides

Viruses

- *Cytomegalovirus (CMV)*: ubiquitous; risk groups with relatively low rates of seropositivity include persons who have not had male homosexual contact or used injection drugs; CMV is shed in semen, cervical secretions, and saliva; child-care providers or parents of children in child-care facilities are at increased risk; risk of CMV infection can be diminished by good hygienic practices and safe sex practices
- *Herpes Simplex Virus (HSV)*: use latex condoms during every act of sexual intercourse to reduce the risk for exposure to herpes simplex virus (HSV) and to other sexually transmitted pathogens; specifically avoid sexual contact when herpetic lesions (genital or orolabial) are evident
- *Varicella-Zoster Virus (VZV)*: HIV+ children and adults who are susceptible to VZV (i.e., those who have no history of chickenpox or shingles or are seronegative for VZV) should avoid exposure to persons with chickenpox or shingles; household contacts (especially children) of susceptible HIV+ persons should be vaccinated against VZV if they have no history of chickenpox and are seronegative for HIV, so that they will not transmit VZV to their susceptible HIV-infected contacts
- *JC Virus*: cause of progressive multifocal leukoencephalopathy (PML)
- *Hepatitis C Virus (HCV)*: main route of transmission in the United States is injection drug use (also snorting of drugs has been

associated with transmission); some sexual and blood transfusion related transmission; other modes include blood-borne transmission from tattooing, piercing, sharing razors, dental supplies and other personal items; accelerated progression to cirrhosis esp. if concomitant alcohol use

- *Human Papilloma Virus (HPV)*: worldwide; transmitted by close contact ± minor trauma; anogenital warts transmitted sexually, little evidence exists to suggest that condoms reduce the risk for infection with HPV; HIV+ women are 2-3 times more likely to have detectable HPV DNA in cervicovaginal specimens and 5 times more likely to have squamous intraepithelial lesions (SILs), vulvovaginal condylomata acuminata, or anal intraepithelial neoplasia

- *Epstein-Barr Virus (EBV)*: widespread; acquired early in life; found in oropharyngeal secretions

- *Molluscum contagiosum*: worldwide; spread by direct contact; disease rare in the immunocompetent

Tumors

- *Kaposi Sarcoma (KS)*: The mechanism of transmitting human herpesvirus 8 (HHV-8), the herpesvirus associated with Kaposi's sarcoma (KS), is not known; sexual transmission is likely among men who have sex with men and can occur among heterosexuals as well; however, the virus has been detected more frequently in saliva than in semen

- *Lymphoma*: Hodgkin's lymphoma, Non-Hodgkin's lymphoma (NHL) with most being B-cell lymphomas, and Burkitt's lymphoma found more frequently among HIV+ persons; primary central nervous system lymphoma (PCNSL) 1000-fold more common; evidence that Epstein-Barr virus (EBV) is associated with these lymphomas (not clear for Hodgkin's)

- *PBCL (HHV8)*:

- *Cervical cancer*: associated with HPV infection esp. with types 16 and 18; an AIDS-defining diagnosis; incidence remains low although prevalence of SIL and cervical intraepithelial neoplasia (CIN) is high; more likely to present with advanced disease, have persistent or recurrent disease, short survival after diagnosis, and to die from cervical cancer

- *Anal Cancer*: associated with HPV infection esp. types 16 and 18; HIV+ women and men who have sex with men at increased risk

- *Other Cancers*: increased incidence of leiomyosarcomas and leiomyomas in HIV+ persons esp. HIV+ children, also associated with EBV

Signs & Symptoms

Fungi

- *PCP*: fever, dry cough, dysphagia, high LDH, severe hypoxia
- *Candida*: pseudomembranous thrush – white, creamy plaques on inflamed base, buccal mucosa, tongue, gums, palate; scrapes off easily; erythematous thrush – spotty or confluent red patches; hyperplastic thrush – white lesions that do not wipes off and respond to azole therapy. Oral pain, taste perversion, odynophagia with esophagitis in late-stage disease – dysphagia, odynophagia, thrush, diffuse esophageal pain; also recurrent vulvovaginitis esp. when CD4 <100/mm^3
- *Cryptococcus*: meningitis – fever, headache, alert, nausea and vomiting, malaise, less common are visual changes, stiff neck, cranial nerve deficits, seizures, no focal neurologic deficits; other – nodules or ulcerative skin lesions, may resemble molluscum, is rare complication of disseminated C. neoformans
- *Histoplasma capsulatum*: fever, wasting, adenopathy, skin or mucosal lesion, pancytopenia, diarrhea, meningitis, sepsis-like symptoms, pulmonary infiltrations or cavitations, abnormal LFTs
- *Cocciodes immitus*: diffuse pulmonary infiltrations or cavitations, hilar adenopathy; extrapulmonary disease include skin lesions (maculopapular, keratotic and verrucous ulcers, and subcutaneous abscesses), joint and bone involvement, and meningitis
- *Penicillium marneffei*: fever, pneumonitis, skin and mucosal lesions (nodules, pustules, and papules)
- *Aspergillus*: invasive pulmonary disease with lung consolidation and cavitation, hypoxemia; tracheobronchitis with cough, fever, dyspnea; acute or chronic invasive sinusitis; invasive fungal dermatitis; also, cerebral aspergillosis, post-traumatic keratitis, aspergilloma (fungus ball), allergic sinusitis, allergic bronchopulmonary aspergillosis (ABPA), and dissemination to other sites

Parasites

- *Toxoplasma gondii*: encephalitis (fever, reduced alertness, headache, focal neurologic deficits, seizures), retinitis and adenitis
- *Cryptosporidia*: enteritis, watery diarrhea, no fecal leukocytes, fever uncommon, malabsorption, wasting, large stool volume with abdominal pain
- *Isospora*: enteritis, watery diarrhea, no fecal leukocytes, no fever, wasting, malabsorption

- *Microsporidia*: enteritis, watery diarrhea, no fecal leukocytes, fever uncommon, malabsorption, wasting
- *Entamoeba histolytica*: colitis, bloody stools, cramps, no fecal leukocytes (bloody stools), most are asymptomatic carriers.
- *Giardia*: enteritis, watery diarrhea with/without malabsorption, wasting, bloating, flatulence
- *Cyclospora*: enteritis, watery diarrhea
- *Leishmaniasis*: visceral form – generalized involvement of reticuloendothelial system e.g. spleen, liver, bone marrow, lymph nodes; cutaneous form – skin and mucosal lesions and ulcerations

Bacteria

- *Tuberculosis (TB)*: diverse pulmonary symptoms, freq. extrapulm. disease esp. meningitis and adenitis, usually fever, weight loss, fatigue, reduced alertness, headache, meningismus, focal deficits.
- *MAC*: fever, night sweats, anorexia, weight loss, enteritis, watery diarrhea, no fecal leukocytes, fever and wasting common, diffuse abdominal pain in late stage, hepatomegaly, diarrhea, splenomegaly, abdominal pain, lymphadenopathy,
- *Other atypical mycobacteria*: M. kansasii associated with pulmonary complaints and infiltrates
- *Syphilis*: erythematous macules and papules involving trunk, extremities, palms, and soles, chancre; neurosyphilis – asymptomatic; meningeal: headache, fever, photophobia, meningismus ± seizures, focal findings, cranial nerve palsies; labes dorsalis: sharp pains, paresthesias, decreased DTRs, loss of pupil response; meningovascular syphilis: strokes, myelitis; ocular syphilis – iritis, uveitis, optic neuritis
- *Bartonella hanselae/quintara*: bacillary angiomatosis (flesh colored or red-purple papules and nodules any place on skin, may resemble Kaposi's sarcoma); visceral disease common involving liver (hepatic peliosis), lymph nodes, osteolytic bone lesions, and bacteremia
- *Other bacteria*: Staphylococcus aureus (including community-acquired MRSA): folliculitis ± pruritus in trunk, groin, face; less common: bullous impetigo, ecthyma, cellulitis, and abscesses; less commonly, pulmonary complaints from pneumonia; Rhodococcus equii: cough, dyspnea, cavitary pulmonary lesions; Salmonella: watery diarrhea, fever, fecal leukocytes ; Shigella: watery diarrhea or bloody flux, fever, fecal leukocytes; Campylobacter jejuni: watery diarrhea or bloody flux, fever, fever leukocytes; Clostridium difficile: watery diarrhea, fecal leukocytes, fever and leukocytosis common; E. coli: watery diarrhea

Viruses

- *CMV*: dysphagia, odynophagia, focal chest pain, colitis and/or enteritis, fecal leukocytes and/or blood, cramps, fever, watery diarrhea with/without blood, hemorrhage, toxic megacolon, fever ±, delirium, lethargy, disorientation, malaise, and headache most common, stiff neck, photophobia, cranial nerve deficits less common, no focal neurologic deficits

- *HSV*: small painful ulcers or vesicles on an erythematous base, usually on gingiva and palate; local pain; dysphagia, odynophagia, focal chest pain, vesicles on erythematous base

- *VZV*: vesicles on erythematous base in unilateral dermatomal distribution, sever pain, trgeminal nerve involvement with possible blindness, disseminated disease, VZV pneumonia

- *JC (PML)*: afebrile, alert, no headache, progressively impaired speech, vision, motor fxn, cranial nerve deficit, cortical blindness, cognition affected relatively late.

- *HCV*: acute – malaise, nausea, RUQ pain, jaundice, dark urine; chronic (85%) – fatigue, malaise, cirrhosis (esophageal varices, ascites, coagulopathy, encephalopathy), hepatocellular carcinoma, extrahepatic manifestations (cryoglobulins, glomerulonephritis, vasculitis, porphyria, connective tissue disorders)

- *HPV*: cutaneous warts including deep plantar, common warts (exophytic, hyperkeratotic papules with rough surface), plane or flat warts, anogenital warts (flesh- to gray-colored, hyperkeratotic, exophytic papules that are either sessile or pedunculated); rarer manifestations include epidermodysplasia verruciformis and recurrent respiratory papillomatosis

- *Molluscum contagiosum*: pearly white or flesh-colored papules with central umbilication, may occur any place except palms or soles, but most common on face ± genital region

- *Enteric viruses*: water diarrhea, acute, 1/3 may become chronic

- *HIV-associated*: dementia: afebrile, triad of cognitive, motor, and behavioral dysfunction, early concentration and memory deficits, inattention, lack of motor coordination, ataxia, late global dementia, paraplegic, mutism; myopathy: pain and aching in muscles, usually in thighs and shoulders.

Tumors

- *Kaposi's Sarcoma*: dyspnea, cough; red or purple nodules, usually on palate or gingiva; most have cutaneous lesions also; usually asymptomatic; may be cosmetic concern or disruption of teeth; firm, subcutaneous brown-black or purple macules, papules, plaques, and nodules; any cutaneous site esp. face, chest, genitals with or without oral mucosa, visceral involvement, lymphatic obstruction

- *Non-Hodgkin's Lymphoma (NHL)*: usually widespread disease involving extranodal sites most commonly the GI tract (diarrhea, biliary colic, obstruction, abdominal pain and swelling), CNS, bone marrow, liver, and lungs
- *PCNSL*: afebrile, headache, focal neurologic, mental status change, personality or behavioral changes, seizures
- PBCL (HHV8):
- Cervical cancer: cervical lesions of various types (e.g., hyperemic, hypertrophic, ulcerative)
- Anal cancer: anal lesions of various types (e.g., hyperemic, hypertrophic, ulcerative)

Other Acute Diarrhea

- Idiopathic: variable, noninfectious causes-rule out medications, dietary, irritable bowel syndrome

Other Chronic Diarrhea

- Small bowel overgrowth: watery diarrhea, malabsorption, wasting, hypochlorhydria
- Idiopathic: watery diarrhea, malabsorption, no fecal leukocytes

Other Dermatologic

- Drug reactions: erythematous papular rash with/without pruritus is most common, most frequent onset is 7-10 days after initiating treatment
- Eosinophilic folliculitis: pruritic papules and pustules on face, trunk, and extremities; spontaneous exacerbations and remissions
- Ichthyosis: fish-like scales
- Seborrhea: erythematous, scaling plaques with indistinct margins and yellowish scale on scalp (dandruff), central (butterfly), ears, hairline, chest, upper back, axilla, groin, behind ears

Other Lower extremity symptoms

- Sensory neuropathy: pain and numbness in toes and feet; ankles, calves, and fingers involved in more advanced cases
- Toxic neuropathy: pain and numbness in toes and feet; ankles, calves, and fingers involved in more advanced cases
- Tarsal tunnel syndrome: pain and numbness predominantly in anterior portion of soles and feet
- Vacuolar myelopathy: stiffness and weakness in legs with leg numbness; bowel/bladder incontinence in advanced cases
- Inflammatory demyelinating polyneuropathies: predominantly weakness in arms and legs, with minor sensory symptoms.

■ AZT myopathy: pain and aching in muscles, usually in thighs and shoulders. Weakness with difficulty arising from a chair or reacting above shoulders

TESTS

Laboratory
■ Specific diagnostic tests:
■ See summaries on individual pathogens listed elsewhere for details.

Other Tests
Dermatologic
■ *Bacillary angiomatosis*: Biopsy (vascular proliferation with edema and polymorphonuclear infiltrate); Warthin-Starry stain shows organism B. henselae or quintara.
■ *Cryptococcosis*: Serum cryptococcal antigen assay usually positive; Biopsy (Gomori methanamine-silver stain typically shows budding yeast + positive culture LP to exclude meningitis.
■ *HSV*: Tzanck Prep (multinucleate giant cells and intranuclear inclusions specific for HSV or VZV). Swab or biopsy for viral culture and/or FA stain. Biopsy site: edge of ulcer.
■ *Kaposi's sarcoma*: biospy
■ *Molluscum contagiosum*: Lesions restricted to epidermis; histologic or electron microscopic exam of scraping or vesicle fluid
■ *Syphilis*: Primary: dark field or DFA stain of exudate + VDRL. Secondary: VDRL or RPR with confirmation by antitreponemal antibody (MHATP, FTA-Abs, TPHA)
■ *Staphylococcus aureus*: Swab or aspirate should show gram-positive cocci in clusters and culture S. Aureus in 4+ concentrations
■ *Other*: Eosinophilic folliculitis: Biopsy (intercellular edema of follicular epithelium w/infiltrate of eosinophils, monocytes, and polymorphonuclear neutrophils progressing to eosinophilic abscess; Psoriasis: Histopathologic features may be similar to seborrhea or drug reactions; distinguish by history and clinical features; Drug reaction: rash usually responds at 3-5 days after drug discontinued; Ichthyosis: Clinical features; Seborrhea: Clinical features

Central Nervous System
■ *Toxoplasmosis:* CT/MRI (Location in basal ganglia. Gray-white jct. Sites usually multiple. Enhancement: prominent-usually solid, irregular. Usually edema mass effect)
■ *Lymphoma*: CT/MRI (Location periventricular or anywhere, 2–6 cm. One or many sites. Enhancement: prominent, usually solid,

irregular. Prominent edema mass effect.) CSF (Normal: 20–30%; Protein: 10–150 mg/dL; Leukocytes: 0–100 mononuclear cells; Experimental: EBV PCR or in-situ hybridization; cytology positive in <5%). Suspect with failure to respond to empiric toxoplasmosis treatment.

■ *Cryptococcal meningitis*: CT/MRI (usually normal or increased intracranial pressure; enhancing basal ganglia in cryptococcomanon-hypodense areas. Enhancement: neg. Edema mass effect: ventricular enlargement/obstructive hydrocephalus). CSF (Normal: 20%; Protein: 30–150 mg/dL; Leukocyte: 0–100 mononuclear cells; Glucose: 50–70 mg/dL; India ink positive: 60–80%; cryptococcal antigen nearly 100% sensitive and specific). Cryptococcal antigen in nearly 100%; in serum, 95%. Definitive diagnosis: CSF antigen and/or positive cultures.

■ *CMV*: CT/MRI (Location: periventricular, brain stem. Site: confluent. Enhancement: variable, no prominence). CSF (Protein: 100-1000 mg/dL. Leukocyte: 10-1000 mononuclear cell/uL. Glucose usually decreased. CMV PCR positive. CSF cultures usually neg. for CMV). Definitive diagnosis: brain biopsy with histopathology and/or positive culture. Hyponatremia (reflects CMV adrenalitis). Retinal examination for CMV retinitis.

■ *PML*: CT/MRI (location: white matter, subcortical, multifocal. Variable sites. Enhancement: neg. No mass effect). CSF (Normal or changes associated with HIV infection. Experimental: JC virus PCR). Definitive diagnosis: stereotactic biopsy, antibody stain to SV40 (JC virus). Characteristic inclusions in oligodendrocytes; bizarre astrocytes.

■ *HIV-associated dementia*: CT/MRI (Location: diffuse, deep, white matter hyperintensities. Site: diffuse, ill-defined. Enhancement: negative. Atrophy: prominent. No mass effect.) CSF (Normal: 30–50%. Protein: increased in 60%. Leukocyte: increased in 5–10% (mononuclear cells) beta2-microglobin elevated (>3 mg/L)). Neuropsychological tests show subcortical dementia and typical scan. Mini-mental examination is insensitive; use timed tests.

■ *Neurosyphilis*: CT/MRI (Aseptic meningitis: may show meningeal enhancement). CSF (Protein: 45–200 mg/dL. Leukocyte: 5–100 mononuclear cells. VDRL positive: sensitivity, 65%; specificity, 100% positive. Experimental: PCR). Serum VDRL and FTA-ABS are lue in >90%; false negative serum VDRL in 5–10% with tabes dorsalis or general paresis. Definitive: positive CSF VDRL (found in 60–70%).

■ *TB*: CT/MRI (Intracerebral lesions in 50-70%). CSF (Normal: 5-10%. Protein: normal [40%], up to 500 mg/dL. Leukocytes 5–2000 [avg is 60-70% mononuclear cells]. Glucose: 4–40 mg/dL. AFB Smear positive: 20%). Chest radiographs: active TB in 50%. Tuberculin skin test positive: 20–30%. Definitive diagnosis: positive culture CSF.

Acute Diarrhea

■ *Salmonella*: stool culture, blood culture
■ *Shigella*: Stool culture
■ *Campylobacter jejuni*: stool culture
■ *Clostridium difficile*: endoscopy: polymorphonuclear cells, colitis, or normal. Stool toxin assay: tissue culture of EIA preferred. CT scan: colitis with thickened mucosa.
■ *E. Coli*: Adherence to Hep-2 cells.
■ *Enteric viruses*: Major agents; adenovirus, astrovirus, picornavirus, calicivirus

Chronic diarrhea

■ *Microsporidia*: Special trichrome stain described, biopsy-EM or Giemsa stain
■ *Cryptosporidia*: AFB smear of stool to show oocyst of 4–6 um
■ *CMV*: Biopsy (intranuclear inclusion bodies, pref w/inflammation, vasculitis), CT scan-segmental or pancolitis
■ *MAC*: positive blood cultures; biopsy (may show changes like Whipple's, but w/AFB); CT scan may be supportive; hepatosplenomegaly, adenopathy, antd thickened small bowel
■ *Isospora*: AFB smear of stool; oocytes of 20–30 um
■ *Entamoeba histolytica*: Stool ova and parasite examination
■ *Giardia*: Stool ova and parasite exam ×2 and giardia antigen; rarely need string test
■ *Cyclospora*: Stool AFB smear resembles cryptosporidia
■ *Small bowel overgrowth*: hydrogen breath test; quantitative culture of small bowel aspirate
■ *Strongyloides*: larvae in feces or duodenal contents
■ *Idiopathic*: biopsy shows villus atrophy, crypt hyperplasia plus no identifiable cause despite endoscopy with biopsy and EM for microsporidia

DIFFERENTIAL DIAGNOSIS

■ *Generalized Lymphadenopathy*: syphilis, lymphoma, KS, TB; also MAC and CMV if CD4<100/mm^3

- *Eye*: HIV retinopathy; if CD4<50-100/mm^3, CMV and much less frequently toxoplasma gondii, HSV, VZV, pneumocystis; other agents include syphilis, candida and drugs (rifabutin, cidofivir, clofazamine)
- *Dermatologic Disease*: Bartonella hensela or quintana (bacillary angiomatosis), HSV, VZV (herpes zoster), Kaposi sarcoma (HHV-8), molluscum contagiosum, Staphylococcus aureus, syphilis, eosinophilic folliculitis, psoriasis, drug reaction, also Cryptococcus neoformans and Histoplama capsulatum if CD4 <100–200/mm^3
- *Oral Lesions*: candida (thrush), EBV (oral hairy leukoplakia, OHL), HSV, KS (HHV-8), aphthous ulcers
- *Esophagitis/Esophageal Ulcers*: candida (50–70%), CMV (10–20%), aphthous ulcers (10–20%), HSV (2.5%)
- *Diarrhea* – acute: salmonella (5–15%), shigella (1–3%), Campylobacter jejuni (4–8%), Clostridium difficile (10–15%), E. coli (10–20%), enteric viruses (15–30%), idiopathic (25–40%), drug reaction
- *Diarrhea – chronic*: microsporidia; E. bieneusi, S. intestinalis, cryptosporidium, CMV, MAC, Isospora, Entamoeba histolytica, Giardia lamblia, Cyclospora cayetanensis, idiopathic, small bowel overgrowth, lymphoma, drug reaction
- *Pulmonary Infection* – acute: streptococcus pneumonia, Haemophilus influenzae; uncommonly Staphylococcus aureus, Legionella, and Aspergillus
- *Pulmonary infection – chronic or subacute*: Pneumocytis carinii; M. tuberculosis, rarely M. kansasii or nocardia; cryptococcus, Histoplasma capsulatum, Coccidiodes immitis, Aspergillus, Rhoddococcus; Candida and CMV are common isolates but rare cause of pulmonary disease; MAC may colonize respiratory tract but rarely a cause of pulmonary disease; also lymphocytic interstitial pneumonia (LIP)
- *Central Nervous System Disease*: HIV-associated dementia (20%), cryptococcus meningitis (8-20%), toxoplasmosis (3–10%), JC virus (PMLE, 2–4%), lymphoma (1–2%), neurosyphilis (0.5%), CMV (0.5%), tuberculosis (0.5–1.0%)
- *Constitutional Symptoms*: lymphoma, TB; if CD4 <200/mm^3, think PCP, lymphoma, HIV and if <100/mm^3, MAC, CMV, HIV, and Histoplasma capsulatum
- *Fever of Unknown Origin (FUO) in AIDS*: MAC (31%), PCP (13%), CMV (11%), bacterial pneumonia (9%), lymphoma (7%), sinusitis (6%), bartonella (8.5%), catheter infection (1–10%), drug allergy (2–5%); also disseminated histoplasmosis (7%), leishmaniasis, TB

MANAGEMENT

What to Do First

■ Thorough history & physical (including pap smear, if not done in past year) with attention to history of CD4 counts, AIDS-defining illnesses, TB exposure or risk, prior chicken pox/shingles, sexually transmitted diseases, hepatitis A/B/C, and review of symptoms (weight loss, fever, night sweats, fatigue, anorexia, dysphagia, nausea, vomiting, diarrhea, abdominal pain, chest pain, dyspnea, cough, headaches, weakness, painful extremities, mental status changes, paresthesias or dysesthesias, rashes, insomnia, adenopathy, visual changes)

■ Screening laboratory evaluations should include CBC, CD4 count, toxoplasma IgG, PPD (unless history of positive PPD or TB treatment), hepatitis serologies (HBsAb, HBcAb, HBsAg, HCV IgG, and some advocate HAV IgG), RPR/VDRL; some suggest VZV Ab (if no history of chicken pox or shingles) and CMV serology (if low risk)

General Measures

■ Vaccinate as needed with Pneumovax, influenza vaccine, HBV vaccine, HAV vaccine, & tetanus booster.

■ Review role of pets (sources of diarrhea such as cryptosporidium, salmonella, and campylobacter; also, cats are a source of bartonella and toxoplasma; healthy birds may be a source of cryptococcus or histoplasma; reptiles may carry salmonella), food and water (sources of diarrhea esp. salmonella in eggs and poultry; toxoplasma in uncooked meats, and cryptosporidia in lakes and rivers), travel (contaminated food and water esp. in developing countries; penicillium marneffii in endemic ares), and occupational exposures (esp. TB in healthcare settings, homeless shelters, correctional facilities; cryptosporidia, CMV, HAV, Giardia in child care settings; cryptosporidia, toxoplasma, bartonella, salmonella, and campylobacter in settings requiring animal contact) in risks of acquiring opportunistic infections. In particular:

➤ HIV+ persons should avoid contact with human and animal feces and wash hands after contact with human feces (e.g., diaper changing), after handling pets, and after gardening or other contact with soil. Avoid sexual practices that might result in oral exposure to feces (e.g., oral-anal contact), and use latex condoms during sexual intercourse to reduce risk of sexually transmitted diseases as well (HSV, syphilis, etc.) as CMV and HHV8. Avoid bringing any animal that has diarrhea into households, avoid purchasing a dog or cat aged <6 months (otherwise have veterinarian examine stools for cryptosporidium, etc.; >1 year old better in avoiding Bartonella), and avoid adopting stray pets. Cat litter box should be changed daily, preferably by an HIV-negative, nonpregnant person or should wash hands thoroughly after changing litter box; should try to keep cats inside and should not adopt or handle stray cats (cats should be fed only canned or dried commercial food or well-cooked table food, not raw or undercooked meats). Also, avoid raw or undercooked meat, particularly undercooked pork, lamb, or venison; wash hands after contact with raw meat and after gardening or other contact with soil. In addition, wash fruits and vegetables well before eating them raw; avoid exposure to calves and lambs and to premises where these animals are raised. HIV+ persons should be aware of occupational risks and take appropriate precautions and hygeine measures, but no recommendations to avoid certain forms of employment. Appropriate precautions including any necessary vaccinations or chemoprophylaxis (e.g., for malaria) should be taken when traveling. Intravenous drug users should be encouraged to enter rehabilitation programs; if they continue to use drugs, education regarding cleaning equipment used and not sharing needles should be reviewed. CMV negatives should receive CMV-negative leukopore-filtered blood.

SPECIFIC THERAPY

Indicated for any evidence of active disease (as indicated in "Tests" section); see also primary and secondary prophylaxis

Fungal

- *PCP*: Trimethoprim + sulfamethoxazole; alternative are Trimethoprim, Pentamidine, Clindamycin, Atovaquone, Trimetrexate
- *Candida*: Fluconazole, Clotrimazole oral troches, Nystatin; Amphotericin B, Itraconazole
- *Cryptococcus (meningitis)*: Amphotericin B + flucytosine then fluconazole; alternatives include Fluconazole, Itraconazole, Fluconazole plus flucytosine
- *Aspergillosis*: Amphotericin B; Itraconazole, Amphotec, Abelcet, AmBisome
- *Histoplasmosis*: Amphotericin B, Itraconazole; Fluconazole
- *Cocciodioidomycosis*: Amphotericin B; Fluconazole, Itraconazole
- *Penicillium marneffei*: Amphotericin B; Itraconazole

Parasitic

■ *Toxoplasma gondii (encephalitis)*: Pyrimethamine + folinic acid + sulfadiazine or trisulfapyrimidine; Pyrimethamine + folinic acid + clindamycin, Pyrimethamine + folinic acid and one of Azithromycin, clathromycin or atovaquone, azithromycin

■ *Cryptosporidia*: Paromomycin, Paromomycin + azithromycin then paromomycin alone, anti-diarrheal agents, Nitazoxanide; Octreotide, Azithromycin, Atovaquone

■ *Isospora*: Trimethprim + sulfamethoxazole; Pyrimethamine + folinic acid

■ *Microsporidia*:nutritional supplements and anti-diarrheal agents, Albendazole shown to work for S. intestinalis, the cause of 10–20% of microsporidial diarrhea; alternatives include metronidazole, ato-quavone, thalidomide

Bacteria

■ *TB*: Rifampin-based therapy, Rifabutin-based therapy, Streptomycin-based therapy; usual is to start with rifampin (RIF)/isoniazid (INH)/pyrazinamide (PZA)/ethambutol (EMB) qd × 2 months, then INH/RIF for 18 wks, provided sensitive to both drugs

■ *MAC*: Clarithromycin + ethambutol + rifabutin; Azithromycin, amikacin or ciprofolxacin

■ *Bartonella hanselae/quintara (bacillary angiomatoses)*: Erythromycin; other macrolides

■ *Rhodococcus equii*: Vancomycin, rifampin, ciprofloxacin or imipenem; Erythromycin

■ *Strongyloides*: Thiabendazole, albendozole

■ *Other bacterial infections*: see individual pathogens elsewhere

Virus

■ *CMV*: Foscarnet, Ganciclovir, Vitrasert (q 6 mo) + oral ganciclovir, cidofovir + probenecid, foscarnet and ganciclovir, fomivirsen

■ *HSV*: mild primary/recurrent disease use oral acyclovir or famicyclovir or valacyclovir; severe/visceral/refractory disease use IV acyclovir or foscarnet

■ *VZV*: Acyclovir or famicyclovir or valacyclovir; severe/refractory/visceral disease use IV acyclovir or foscarnet

■ *JC virus (PML)*: highly active antiretroviral therapy (HAART), cidofovir (unclear benefit esp. if already on HAART)

■ *HCV*: alpha interferon + ribavarin; consider PEG-IFN + ribavirin (more effective, but unclear toxicities)

■ *HPV*: intravaginal 5-fluorouracil

Tumors

- *Kaposi Sarcoma (HHV8)*: Topical liquid nitrogen, intralesional vinblastine, Radiation (low dose)
- *NHL*: regiments containing methotrexate, bleomycin, doxorubicin, cyclophosphamide, Adriamycin, vincristine and corticosteroids
- *PCNSL*: cranial radiation, intrathecal cytosine arabinoside, chemotherapy
- *PBCL (HHV8)*:
- *Cervical Cancer (HPV)*: low-grade intraepithelial lesion (LGSIL or LSIL) (CIN 1) evaluated by colposcopy and biopsy or follow-up Pap smears every 4-6 months; high-grade squamous intraepithelial lesions (HGIL or HSIL) (CIN 2 or 3) treated with colposcopy and biopsy and treated with loop excision or conization; invasive carcinoma treated with surgery or radiation therapy
- *Anal CA (HPV)*: chemoradiation with 5-FU + cisplatin; surgery for resistant disease

Side Effects & Contraindications

- See under individual pathogens elsewhere

FOLLOW-UP

Maintenance/suppressive therapy is indicated after treatment for:

- *CMV*: Valganciclovir, Foscarnet, Ganciclovir, Cidofovir, intraocular ganciclovir release device q 6 mo + oral ganciclovir
- *Cryptococcal meningitis*: Fluconazole; alternatives are Amphotericin, Fluconazole and Itraconazole
- *Toxoplasmosis*: Pyrimethamine + folinic acid + sulfadiazine; alternatives are pyrimethamine + folinic acid + clindamycin, pyrimethamine + folinic acid + either atoquavone, dapsone or azithromycin
- *Isospora*: Trimethoprim + sulfamethoxazole; alternatives are Pyrimethamine + sulfadoxine and Pyrimethamine + folinic acid
- *HSV*: Acyclovir 400 mg bid, famciclovir 250 mg bid or valacyclovir 500–1,000 mg qd
- *VZV*: Acyclovir, famciclovir, or valacyclovir With immune reconstitution after therapy for HIV, primary prophylaxis may be stopped in the following settings:
- *Pneumocystis carinii*: CD4 >200/mm^3 for 3–6 months regardless of prior h/o PCP if no thrush or fever
- *Toxoplasma gondii*: CD4 >100/mm^3 for 3–6 months
- *MAC*: CD4 >100/mm^3 for 3–6 months and no symptoms of MAC infection Reinstitute prophylaxis if patient meets criteria again. With

immune reconstitution after therapy for HIV, secondary may be stopped in the following settings:

- *CMV*: consider in patients with CD4 >100/mm^3 after ≥6 months of HAART with quiescent retinitis; if anti-CMV therapy stopped. Should have dilated funduscopic exams on a regular basis and therapy restarted if recrudescence of retinitis or CD4 <50/mm^3.
- *Cryptococcal meningitis*: recent data suggest that may be able to stop maintenance therapy if asymptomatic for >1-2 years and no evidence of cryptococcal infection during that period (though role of ongoing cryptococcemia unclear)
- *MAC*: may be considered if no MAC symptoms
- *Toxoplasmosis*: no data at this time

COMPLICATIONS AND PROGNOSIS

Complications

See under individual pathogens for details.

Be aware of OI "Reversal Syndromes" after beginning HAART:

- *MAC*: Lymphadenitis, high fever, lung infiltrates; onset 1–12 weeks
- *CMV*: Retinitis and vitritis; onset 1-2 months. Uveitis and macular edema, epiretinal membrane formation, cataracts, papillitis; Onset 2 months–2 yrs.
- *TB*: Fever, worsening lung infiltrates/effusion, mediastinal and peripheral lymphadenopathy; Onset 1–6 weeks
- *Crptococcal meningitis*: new meningeal signs and symptoms, increased WBC in CSF, adenopathy; Onset 1 week-8 months.

"Reversal" syndromes can be prevented and managed by obtaining mycobacterial blood culture and ophthalmologic exam and initiating MAC prophylaxis (for at least 1 month, if possible) before initiating HAART inn patients with CD4 <50/mm^3; giving brief course of corticosteroids in severe cases of mycobacerial "reversal" syndrome. Most cases resolve in several weeks by continuing HAART and anti-OI medications. Invasive diagnostic procedures can be avoided if clinical setting and presentation is typical.

Prognosis

- Most important means of improving prognosis from opportunistic infections is improvement of host immune function – i.e. immune reconstitution with HAART. HAART improves T-cell counts but unclear if improves T-cell diversity, which may be the key to complete immune restoration; if HAART does not fully restore T-cell diversity, then HIV+ persons may be at some long-term risk for opportunistic infections and malignancies.

CONDYLOMA ACUMINATA

DAVID OUTLAND, MD and JEFFREY P. CALLEN, MD
REVISED BY JEFFREY P. CALLEN, MD

HISTORY & PHYSICAL

- Usually asymptomatic but can be pruritic or painful
- Sexually transmitted in adults, but may not always be sexually transmitted in children
- The most common STD in the United States
- Caused by human papillomavirus infection
- Most common HPV types are 6 and 11
- Can also be caused by types 16, 18, 31, and 33
- Types 16, 18, 31, and 33 can cause intraepithelial neoplasia that may eventuate into squamous cell carcinoma
- Flesh colored verrucous papules most commonly on the shaft, glans, or corona of the penis in men, or on the vulva or adjacent skin in women
- May also occur on the scrotum, perineum, pubis, groin and anus

TESTS

- 5% acetic acid application may highlight subclinical or small lesions
- Biopsy is diagnostic, but is rarely necessary

DIFFERENTIAL DIAGNOSIS

- Condyloma lata
- Bowenoid papulosis
- Molluscum contagiosum
- Lichen planus
- Pearly penile papules
- Nevi
- Skin tags
- Squamous cell carcinoma

MANAGEMENT

- Discuss with patient viral and infective nature.
- Discuss need for condom usage.
- Tell patient need for partner to be evaluated.
- Counsel and test patients for other sexually transmitted diseases.
- Most therapies are destructive.

SPECIFIC THERAPY

- Destructive therapies
  - ➤ Liquid nitrogen cryotherapy

➤ Liquid nitrogen cryotherapy followed by application of podophyllin
➤ Podophyllin 10–25% in tincture of benzoin (Should be washed off in 3–6 hours)
➤ Trichloroacetic acid
➤ Podofillox 0.5% applied at home per patient
➤ Electrodessication or carbon dioxide laser
■ All destructive therapies carry risk of blistering, ulceration, scarring and infection
■ Immune modulating therapies
  ➤ Topical imiquimod applied per patient 3× weekly
    • Major side effect is local irritation
  ➤ Intralesional interferon-alpha
  ➤ Major side effect is irritation, pain and systemic complaints such as fever, malaise, lethargy

FOLLOW-UP
■ Frequent visits every 3 to 6 weeks to assess response and re-treat as appropriate

COMPLICATIONS AND PROGNOSIS
■ Most common complications are treatment-related – i.e., blistering, ulceration and pain.
■ Many lesions require multiple treatments.
■ Treatment may last months.
■ Recurrence is fairly common.
■ Eventual remission from clinically evident lesions is common; however, recurrence may occur after remission.
■ Follow patients with Pap smears and examinations.

CONFUSION & DELIRIUM

MICHAEL J. AMINOFF, MD, DSc

HISTORY & PHYSICAL
■ Acute change in mental status; disorientation commonly disproportionate to other deficits; reduced attention span; may be drowsiness; agitation or excitement common in delirium; hallucinations typically visual or auditory
■ Other cognitive & behavioral deficits may occur
■ Speech often tangential

- Easy distractibility
- History of predisposing medical cause–eg, infection (esp. respiratory or urinary), recent surgery, malnutrition, drug abuse, seizures, trauma, endocrine disturbance, sensory deprivation; commonly occurs in elderly hospitalized pts

TESTS
- Investigations needed to identify cause
- Laboratory studies: CBC, FBS, electrolytes, BUN, liver & thyroid function tests, urine toxicology screen, ABGs
- CXR to detect pulmonary infection
- ECG to detect recent MI or cardiac arrhythmia
- Cranial CT scan or MRI to detect structural cause
- Spinal tap to exclude infective cause (meningitis, encephalitis)
- EEG if seizure disorder is suspected

DIFFERENTIAL DIAGNOSIS
N/A

MANAGEMENT
- Control symptoms of acute confusional state

SPECIFIC THERAPY
- Treat underlying cause

FOLLOW-UP
N/A

COMPLICATIONS AND PROGNOSIS
- Depends on underlying cause & on occurrence of any injuries while pt is confused

---

CONGENITAL QUALITATIVE PLATELET DISORDERS

MORTIMER PONCZ

HISTORY & PHYSICAL
- Easy bruising, esp palpable bruises & scattered bruises of varying age
- Menorrhagia or recurrent nosebleeds requiring red cell transfusions
- Hemorrhage after injury or surgery, esp late-onset hemorrhage (1 wk later)
- Family history of a bleeding diathesis
- Consanguinity or originating from an in-bred population

TESTS

Laboratory

- CBC; PT; PTT
- Bleeding time
- Review platelet & white cell size/morphology on peripheral smear & mean platelet volume
- Platelet aggregation studies: standard & low-dose ADP, epinephrine, collagen, arachidonic acid, thrombin; ristocetin agglutination; ADP: ATP ratio; ATP &/or serotonin release

Other Tests

- Platelet electron micrographs
- Flow cytometry using antibodies to potentially missing surface proteins

DIFFERENTIAL DIAGNOSIS

- Rule out vWd & acquired defects (aspirin ingestion), which are more frequent
- Glanzmann thrombasthenia: autosomal recessive; normal platelet count; abnormal platelet aggregation studies w/ all agonists, except ristocetin; absence/defect of platelet alpha IIb/beta 3 receptors
- Bernard-Soulier syndrome: autosomal recessive; mild thrombocytopenia w/ large platelets; normal aggregation studies except ristocetin; absence of platelet GPIb/IX/V receptor
- Wiskott-Aldrich syndrome: X-linked recessive, occasionally autosomal recessive; thrombocytopenia w/ small platelets, eczema, immunodeficiency; absence of isohemagglutinins, poor lymphocyte mitogenic response, decreased IgM, increased IgE, WAS protein defect
- Gray platelet syndrome: autosomal recessive; variable platelet aggregation defect; no vWf, fibrinogen, alpha-thromboglobulin or platelet factor 4 release; gray platelets on Wright stains due to lack of alpha granules, abnormal platelet electron micrographs; pulmonary fibrosis in some; some families w/ risk of acute myelogenous leukemia
- Hermansky-Pudlak syndrome: autosomal recessive, common in Puerto Ricans; platelet dense granule deficiency w/ abnormal ATP:ADP ratio; albinism, ceroid deposits in macrophages
- Chediak-Higashi syndrome: autosomal recessive; platelet dense granule deficiency w/ abnormal ATP:ADP ratio; albinism; giant granules in neutrophils

- Scott syndrome: autosomal recessive; prolonged bleeding time; normal platelet aggregation; platelets fail to express negatively charged phospholipids on surface of activated platelets (procoagulant defect)
- Giant platelet disorders w/ thrombocytopenia:
  - ➤ May-Hegglin anomaly: autosomal dominant; pale blue inclusions (Dohle bodies) in leukocytes; variable clinical bleeding
  - ➤ Epstein syndrome: nerve deafness and nephritis
  - ➤ Fechtner syndrome: same as Epstein + cataracts
  - ➤ Sebastian platelet syndrome: same as Fechtner + neutrophil inclusions

MANAGEMENT

General Measures
- No aspirin
- Head injury precautions; avoid contact sports
- Assess efficacy of DDAVP infusion in correcting bleeding time
- Education in prevention/management of nosebleeds
- Hormonal management of menorrhagia

SPECIFIC THERAPY

Treatment Options
- Local measures for nose/mouth bleeds (pressure, topical thrombin, e-aminocaproic acid)
- Platelet transfusions for severe hemorrhage; try to avoid sensitization to platelets; use white cell-poor platelets for transfusions
- DDAVP for bleeding if efficacious
- Recombinant activated factor VII for bleeding, esp in Glanzmann thrombasthenia

FOLLOW-UP
n/a

COMPLICATIONS AND PROGNOSIS

Complications
- Iron deficiency anemia
- Intracranial hemorrhage
- Menorrhagia
- Pregnancy concerns, esp if resistant to platelet transfusions
- Rare joint bleeds
- Development of antibodies to proteins on normal platelets after transfusions ((decr.) transfused platelet half-life)

Prognosis
- Most pts live near-normal life in spite of platelet defect

CONJUNCTIVAL TUMORS

DEVRON H. CHAR, MD

HISTORY & PHYSICAL

- Conjunctival tumors are rare; most common in elderly, sun-exposed patients.
- Older patients with a unilateral, chronic inflammation of conjunctiva and/or eyelid
- Malignancy should be ruled out histologically.

TESTS

- All suspicious lesions should be biopsied.

DIFFERENTIAL DIAGNOSIS

- Most common conjunctival tumors: squamous cell carcinoma, melanoma, benign and malignant lymphoid lesions and KS.

MANAGEMENT

- Management of both squamous cell carcinoma and melanoma usually is surgical.
- Flat, in situ lesions may be treated with topical anti-metabolites.
- Resection with clear margins: <2% recurrences; >60% if partially removed
- In American patients only two reports of metastases in conjunctival squamous cell carcinoma
- Lymphoid lesions; conventional histologic lymphoma work-up
- Flow cytometry & molecular studies to differentiate benign/malignant lymphoid lesions
- Symptomatic isolated conjunctival lymphoid lesion usually irradiated; preliminary results with doxycycline for *Chlamydia psittaci*
- Conjunctival lymphoma with systemic disease: chemotherapy

SPECIFIC THERAPY

n/a

FOLLOW-UP

- Conjunctival melanomas spread (risk factors: thicker tumors, more diffuse lesions, involvement of the caruncle or eyelid) to lymph nodes, lung and liver.
- Lymphoid conjunctiva lesions rarely develop extraocular disease; those that also involve the orbit can have or develop widespread lymphoma.

COMPLICATIONS AND PROGNOSIS
n/a

CONSTIPATION AND FECAL IMPACTION

GEORGE TRIADAFILOPOULOS, MD

HISTORY & PHYSICAL

History
- Constipation: lack of urge for defecation; infrequent and hard stools; difficult and painful defecation with straining; <3 bowel movements per week
- Common predisposing factors: low fiber diet, sedentary lifestyle, old age, previous gynecologic or pelvic surgery, diabetes mellitus, hypothyroidism, depression, chronic pharmacologic therapy with psychotropics, calcium channel blockers, aluminum or calcium antacids, opiates, or anticholinergics, irritable bowel syndrome, diverticulosis, chronic neurological disease, and anorectal dysmotility
- Severe idiopathic chronic constipation: predominantly a disease of women

Signs & Symptoms
- Acute constipation (with or without fecal impaction): nausea, vomiting, abdominal distension and lack of stool evacuation; passage of flatus may or may not be present
- Physical exam not generally helpful, except for rectal examination: fissures or hemorrhoids, abnormal contraction of the puborectalis and external anal sphincter muscles

TESTS

Basic Tests
- CBC, routine chemistries, stool for occult blood, thyroid function tests are important to evaluate metabolic or endocrine causes; plain abdominal film of the abdomen can detect significant stool retention and megacolon

Specific Diagnostic Tests
- Colonic transit study: passage of swallowed radiopaque markers through the colon monitored by abdominal radiograph on day 5 after ingestion distinguishes several subtypes of chronic constipation:

- Normal colonic transit (usually IBS): all markers absent
- Colonic inertia: slow passage of radiopaque markers through the proximal colon; several markers present throughout the colon; dysfunction in the myenteric nerve plexus
- Outlet delay, in which markers move normally through the colon but stagnate in the rectum; markers present in the pelvis; Hirschsprung's disease, fecal impaction, and in abnormal responses of the pelvic floor muscles during defecation (pelvic floor dyssynergia)

■ Flexible sigmoidoscopy or colonoscopy: imperative to exclude colonic obstruction

■ Barium enema: less costly than colonoscopy but useful in detecting structural causes of constipation, and for the diagnosis of megacolon, megarectum and diverticulosis

Other Tests

■ Anorectal motility study for evaluation of rectal sensation and compliance, reflexive relaxation of the internal anal sphincter, and balloon expulsion (pseudodefecation). EMG studies of the external sphincter and puborectalis muscles using needle or surface-electrodes may also be useful

■ Defecography with fluoroscopic monitoring of evacuation of thickened barium; particularly useful in cases of pelvic floor dyssynergia

DIFFERENTIAL DIAGNOSIS

■ Colonic obstruction by anal, rectal or colonic tumor

MANAGEMENT

What to Do First

■ Exclude malignancy, usually colonic, as a cause of constipation Discontinue offending drug(s)

General Measures

■ Treat hypothyroidism, diabetes and metabolic or electrolyte abnormalities if present

SPECIFIC THERAPY

Indications

■ Chronic constipation that compromises quality of life and predisposes to hemorrhoidal bleeding, fecal impaction, or acute colonic pseudoobstruction requires aggressive, chronic therapy. Patients should initially be disimpacted and the colon evacuated effectively by drinking a balanced electrolyte solution containing polyethylene glycol.

Treatment Options
■ Constipation is treated medically with any of the following, used alone or in combination: 1) Stimulant laxatives; 2) Saline cathartics, and hyperosmolar cathartics or osmolar cathartics; 3) Mineral oil; 4) Bulk forming agents; 5) Polyethylene glycol; or 6) Stool softeners.
■ Some patients with severe constipation have been treated successfully with misoprostol, which enhances colonic contractility
■ Enemas or glycerine suppositories may be administered if there is no success with oral therapy, to prevent fecal impaction
■ Behavioral therapy may be effective in patients with neurogenic constipation, dementia, or those with physical impairments
■ Subtotal colectomy with ileorectal anastomosis can dramatically ameliorate incapacitating constipation in patients with colonic inertia
■ Surgical repair of a rectocele and/or rectal intussusception may not alleviate constipation unless improved rectal evacuation when pressure is placed on the posterior wall of the vagina during defecation is evident
■ Surgery is the treatment of choice for Hirschsprung's disease

FOLLOW-UP

During Treatment
■ Increasing fiber may cause gaseousness and bloating over the period of the first 4–6 weeks; increase fluid intake (6–8 glasses per day)

Routine
■ Bowel retraining is useful as it enhances the efficiency of the gastrocolic reflex leading to postprandial defecation

COMPLICATIONS AND PROGNOSIS

Complications
■ Abuse of laxatives: melanosis coli.
■ In elderly and sedentary adults with severe constipation: fecal impaction with acute or subacute intestinal obstruction may occur
■ Acute colonic pseudo-obstruction (Ogilvie's syndrome): urgent medical or endoscopic decompression

Prognosis
- Generally good; if a specific cause is found and removed, constipation resolves; if not, long-term therapy is needed
- Most patients are satisfied with the results of medical therapy or surgery and reported a good or improved quality of life

CONSTRICTIVE PERICARDITIS

ANDREW D. MICHAELS, MD

HISTORY & PHYSICAL

Signs & Symptoms
- dyspnea, fatigue
- enlarging abdominal girth, lower extremity edema
- elevated neck veins with prominent x and y descents
- Kussmaul's sign

TESTS

Chest X-Ray
- pericardial calcification

Echo
- pericardial thickening
- respiratory variation in tricuspid and mitral inflow velocities

MRI
- pericardial thickening

Cardiac Catheterization
- elevated and equalized diastolic pressures in right and left ventricles, right atrium, wedge
- "dip and plateau" pressure pattern in ventricles

DIFFERENTIAL DIAGNOSIS
- restrictive cardiomyopathy may mimic presentation and hemodynamics

MANAGEMENT
- medical therapy is palliative (salt restriction, diuretics)

SPECIFIC THERAPY
- surgical pericardiotomy (pericardial stripping) for highly symptomatic patients
- perioperative mortality 5–15%

FOLLOW-UP
- serial clinical evaluation of neck veins
- serial echos to follow hemodynamics

COMPLICATIONS AND PROGNOSIS

Prognosis
- untreated, generally carries a high mortality rate of 5–25%/year

CONTACT DERMATITIS

J. MARK JACKSON, MD

HISTORY & PHYSICAL
- History – pruritic eruption, patient may consider contact as a possibility
- Physical usually dermatitis in site of exposure, occasionally beyond
  - Linear lesions are common in acute contact dermatitis – e.g., Rhus dermatitis
  - Follows pattern of contactant – e.g., nickel allergy under jewelry
  For eyelid dermatitis, consider agents touched by hands that may the affect the eyes (even if hands are clear).

TESTS
- Patch tests by experienced physician
- ROAT (repeat open application test) on normal uninvolved site – e.g., antecubital fossa

DIFFERENTIAL DIAGNOSIS
- Same as above plus irritant dermatitis, r/o with patch testing

MANAGEMENT

What to Do First?
- Identify causative agent and eliminate
- Treat involved skin same as atopic dermatitis

SPECIFIC THERAPY
- Specific Therapy, Follow-up, and Treatment
- Acute contact dermatitis – 10 to 16-day course of oral prednisone
- Chronic contact dermatitis eliminate cause, topical corticosteroids or other agents, oral antihistamines, systemic therapy similar to atopic dermatitis

FOLLOW-UP
n/a

COMPLICATIONS AND PROGNOSIS
n/a

CONTRACEPTION FOR THE INTERNIST

MAXINE H. DORIN, MD
REVISED BY FREDRIC B. KRAEMER, MD;
ANDREW R. HOFFMAN, MD; and THOMAS F. McELARTH, MD, PhD

HISTORY & PHYSICAL
- Age, last menstrual period, menstrual pattern, birth control method (past/present), number of pregnancies and outcome
- History of STDs, PID, infertility
- Diabetes, hypertension, thromboembolic events, liver and renal disease, migraines, seizure disorder
- Surgical history, esp. abdominal pelvic surgery
- Smoking history
- Total number of sexual partners, current sexual partner(s)
  - ➤ History of depression
  - ➤ History of poor tolerance of progestational agents

TESTS
- Pap smear
- Consider Gonococcus and Chlamydia cultures, syphilis and HIV tests
- Consider fasting lipid profile and LFT

DIFFERENTIAL DIAGNOSIS
n/a

MANAGEMENT

What to Do First
- Review yearly health maintenance program
- Discussion of various contraception options, including risk, benefits, failure/success rates of each method

General Measures
- Assess risk factors

SPECIFIC THERAPY
- Oral contraceptives (OC):

- ➤ Progestin-only pills
- ➤ Combination estrogen/progestin: monophasics, multiphasics
- ➤ Progestins used: norethindrone, norethindrone acetate, desogestrel, norgestrel, levonegestrel, norgestimate
- ➤ Estrogens used: ethinyl estradiol, mestranol
- ■ Benefits:
  - ➤ Protective effect against endometrial cancers
  - ➤ Protection against benign breast disease, salpingitis, ectopic pregnancy, dysmenorrhea and iron deficiency anemia
  - ➤ Fewer menstrual disorders
  - ➤ No overall increased risk of breast cancer for OC users up to age 55 y
  - ➤ OCs containing norgestimate, levonorgestrel, gestodene, and desogestrel may improve acne
- ■ Side Effects
  - ➤ Nausea, vomiting, abdominal cramps, bloating, breakthrough bleeding, altered menstrual flow, breast tenderness, edema, headaches, weight changes, rash, acne, depressive symptoms in some women (reaction to progestin component)
- ■ Contraindications
  - ➤ Pregnancy, migraines with aura, vaginal bleeding of unknown cause, breast, endometrial or hepatic cancer, thromboembolic disorders, smokers >35 y, CAD, CVD, documented history of sensitivity to progestins, history of depression
- ■ Complications
  - ➤ Thromboembolism, MI, hypertension, hepatic adenoma, stroke, depression
- ■ Special Situations
  - ➤ Smokers at increased risk of MI and CVD, esp >35 y
  - ➤ Drugs that decrease efficacy of OCs: rifampin griseofulvin, and anticonvulsants (phenobarbital, phenytoin, carbamazepine, primidone, ethosuximide)
  - ➤ OCs may potentiate corticosteroids, theophylline, aminophylline, metoprolol, cyclosporin action, whereas they decrease efficacy of cyclopenthazide, guanethidine
- ■ Prognosis
  - ➤ With perfect use: progestin-only OCs: failure rate 0.5%; combination OCs: failure rate 0.1%
- ■ Injectable contraception:
  - ➤ Medroxyprogesterone acetate IM q 12 wks
  - ➤ Side Effects

- ➤ Irregular bleeding, amenorrhea, weight gain, headaches, breast tenderness, loss of libido, depression, nervousness, fatigue, delayed return of fertility
- ➤ Contraindications
- ➤ Similar to OCs
- ➤ Complications
- ➤ Thromboembolism, angioedema, anaphylaxis, seizures
- ➤ Prognosis
- ➤ 0.3% failure rate in first y; delay fertility up to 9 mo

■ Subdermal implant:
- ➤ Levonorgestrel placed subdermal for 5 y
- ➤ Side Effects
- ➤ Menstrual irregularities, headaches, acne, weight gain, nausea, depression
- ➤ Contraindications
- ➤ Active thrombophlebitis, undiagnosed vaginal bleeding, acute liver disease, breast cancer, known pregnancy, depression
- ➤ Prognosis
- ➤ 0.2% failure rate in first y

■ Patch
- ➤ Estrogen/progestin patch weekly for 3 weeks and off for 1 week
- ➤ Side Effects
- ➤ Similar to OCs
- ➤ Contraindications
- ➤ Similar to OCs

■ Vaginal Ring
- ➤ Estrogen/progestin ring worn 3 weeks out of 4
- ➤ Side Effects
- ➤ Similar to OCs
- ➤ Contraindications
- ➤ Similar to OCs

■ Intrauterine device (IUD):
- ➤ Copper IUD replaced q 10 y
- ➤ Progestin IUD replaced q 5 y
- ➤ Side Effects
  - • Dysmenorrhea, heavier menses esp with copper IUD
- ➤ Contraindications
  - • Absolute: cervical or uterine cancer, undiagnosed vaginal bleeding, pregnancy, active PID
  - • Relative: high risk of STD
- ➤ Special Situations

- Overall protective effect on risk of ectopic pregnancies
➤ Complications
  - Perforation, infection, and expulsion
  - Increased rates of 2nd trimester abortion, premature delivery, low birth weight and stillbirth when IUD not removed in 1st trimester
➤ Prognosis
  - First year failure rate:
  - Copper, 0.5%
  - Progestin, 0.1%
- Barrier methods:
  ➤ Diaphragm: circular metal ring covered with latex; fitted by provider; used with spermicides; left in 6 h after intercourse
  ➤ Cervical caps: latex rubber, covers only cervix, harder to fit
  ➤ Condoms: latex sheath to cover penis (latex-free condoms available)
  ➤ Female condom: also requires spermicide
  ➤ Sponge: in place up to 24 h
  ➤ Side Effects
    - Allergy to latex or to spermicides
    - Increased incidence of UTIs with diaphragm
    - Increased risk of toxic shock syndrome with diaphragm and sponge
  ➤ Special Situations
    - Condom breakage uncommon
    - Petroleum-based products markedly reduce strength of condoms
    - Both male and female condoms decrease risk of STDs
  ➤ Prognosis
    - First-year failure rate:
      - Diaphragm, 18%
      - Cervical cap, 18%
      - Condoms without spermicides, 12%
      - Female condoms with spermicides, 15%
- Female sterilization:
  ➤ Postpartum sterilization: partial salpingectomy
  ➤ Uni/bipolar coagulation
  ➤ Silicone band application (Falope ring)
  ➤ Hulka or Filshie clips
- Side Effects
  ➤ Concern regarding menstrual irregularities not supported

- Contraindications
  - ➤ Risk of surgery outweighs benefit of sterilization
- Complications
  - ➤ Pregnancies occurring after sterilization usually are ectopic
  - ➤ Poststerilization regret
- Prognosis
  - ➤ 10-year cumulative failure rate:
    - Postpartum, 0.8%
    - Unipolar coagulation, 0.8%
    - Bipolar coagulation, 2.5%
    - Spring clip, 3.7%
    - Falope ring, 2%
    - Filshie clip, 0.7% 2-y cumulative failure rate
    - Vasectomy, 0.15% 1-y failure rate

FOLLOW-UP
n/a

COMPLICATIONS AND PROGNOSIS
n/a

CORNEAL ULCER

DOUGLAS S. HOLSCLAW, MD

HISTORY & PHYSICAL

History
- Contact lens wear, trauma, ocular foreign body, dry eyes, trichiasis, lagophthalmous, neurotropic cornea, topical steroid use, history of atopy or ocular herpes simplex

Signs & Symptoms
- Redness, mild to severe ocular pain, photophobia, blurry vision, ocular discharge
- Critical signs: focal white opacity (infiltrate) cornea stroma, overlying epithelial defect w/ fluorescein staining
- Other signs: eyelid edema, conjunctival injection, ciliary flush, corneal stroma edema, Descemet folds, anterior chamber cells & flare, hypopion
- Severity of symptoms depends on causative organism

TESTS

Laboratory
- Corneal scraping for cytology & culture/sensitivities

DIFFERENTIAL DIAGNOSIS

Infectious:
- Bacterial: most common; corneal infections assumed bacterial unless clinical characteristics or lab studies direct otherwise
- Fungal: consider after trauma, infiltrates feathery edges, satellite lesions
- Acanthamoeba: extremely painful, history of swimming w/contact lenses
- Viral: herpes simplex or zoster, may have eyelid vesicles, dendritic pattern of epithelial staining

Other:
- Corneal abrasion: epithelial defect w/ edema, no stromal opacity
- Corneal scar: stromal opacity w/out epithelial defect, redness, or pain
- Sterile ulcer: not infectious, culture negative, seen in collagen vascular diseases, neurotropic keratopathy, vernal or atopy, vitamin A deficiency
- Subepithelial infiltrates: follow viral conjunctivitis, epithelium intact
- Staphylococcal hypersensitivity: peripheral infiltrates, often multiple
- Residual corneal foreign body or rust ring

MANAGEMENT

What to Do First
- Corneal scraping for culture & sensitivities: blood & chocolate agar (bacteria), thioglycolate broth (aerobic & anaerobic bacteria), Sabouraud medium w/out cyclohexamide (fungi)
- Corneal scraping for cytology: gram & giemsa stains, KOH prep if fungus suspected
- Swab cultures of palpebral conjunctiva & eyelids if significant discharge

General Measures
- Prompt treatment required if suspicion of bacterial corneal ulcer
- Institute local therapy immediately after cultures
- No systemic antibiotics for bacterial corneal ulcers

- No eye patch for corneal ulcers
- Eye shield may be used if significant corneal thinning
- Topical cycloplegics (scopolamine $\frac{1}{4}$%) for comfort

SPECIFIC THERAPY

Indications

- Suspicion of bacterial corneal ulcer requires prompt treatment pending culture results

Treatment Options

- Corneal ulcers treated as bacterial unless high suspicion of other cause
- Initial treatment depends on size, location, severity of ulceration:
  - Small, peripheral, & nonvision-threatening infiltrates: topical quinolones – ofloxacin 0.3%, ciprofloxacin 0.3%, or levofloxacin 0.5% 2 drops q 15 min for 2 hours, then q 1 hour around the clock
  - Large, central, & vision-threatening infiltrates: fortified topical antibiotics (must be compounded by pharmacy) – cefazolin & tobramycin; consider subconjunctival injection of antibiotics in addition to topicals in most severe infections, when fortified topical antibiotics not available in short time, or pt compliance concerns
- Subsequent treatment adjusted by culture & sensitivity results
- Corneal ulcers dues to nonbacterial causes (fungal, herpes simplex virus, or acanthamoeba) as indicted by stains or cultures require specific treatment directed at organism

Side Effects & Contraindications

- Side effects: pain/stinging on drop instillation, toxicity to corneal epithelium, conjunctival sloughing may occur after subconjunctival injection
- Contraindications:
  - Allergy to above antibiotics:
    - Cefazolin allergy: vancomycin
    - Tobramycin allergy: ceftazidime

FOLLOW-UP

During Treatment

- Initially, daily; assess improvement in infiltrate size & density, size of epithelial defect, follow for corneal thinning

Routine

■ Later treatment concerns visual rehabilitation, if necessary

COMPLICATIONS AND PROGNOSIS

Complications

■ Corneal scarring: ? vision, depending on density & location of scar
■ Corneal thinning: ? vision secondary to irregular astigmatism
■ Corneal vascularization: later reduction in vision due to corneal lipid deposits
■ Corneal perforation: may require tissue adhesive, corneal patch graft, or cornea TX
■ Endophthalmitis: may occur due to intraocular extension of infection after perforation

Prognosis

■ Impact on visual acuity depends on location & severity of any corneal scarring, thinning, & vascularization
■ Visual rehabilitation may require glasses, rigid contact lenses, laser phototherapeutic keratectomy, or cornea TX

CORONARY ARTERY INJURY

JUDITH A. WISNESKI, MD

HISTORY & PHYSICAL

■ Myocardial ischemia

TESTS

■ ECG – ST changes and new Q waves
■ Blood – Elevation of Troponin I and other cardiac enzymes
■ Coronary angiography (most important) detect the injury and presence of CAD

DIFFERENTIAL DIAGNOSIS

n/a

MANAGEMENT

■ Surgical intervention essential for laceration
■ Thrombolytics and anticoagulation for acute thrombosis, pending other injuries

SPECIFIC THERAPY
n/a

FOLLOW-UP
n/a

COMPLICATIONS AND PROGNOSIS
■ Similar to acute MI (*see Coronary syndromes*)

CORONARY SYNDROMES, ACUTE

KENDRICK A. SHUNK, MD, PhD

HISTORY & PHYSICAL

History
■ Angina or suspected angina persistent for >20 minutes requires immediate rule-out of STEMI by ECG (within 10 minutes)
■ When STEMI ruled out, perform early stratification of risk of death
  ➤ Clinical assessment of likelihood (high, intermediate, or low) of acute ischemia caused by CAD
  ➤ 5 most important factors for likelihood: Nature of symptoms, H/O CAD, age, sex, # of risk factors
  ➤ Traditional risk factors: diabetes, hypertension, male, age, smoking, high LDL, low HDL, family history
  ➤ Other risk factors: h/o elevated CRP, homocysteine, Lp(a)
■ High risk historical features (1 or more = high risk)
  ➤ Accelerated tempo of ischemic symptoms in preceding 48H
  ➤ Prolonged ongoing (>20 min) rest pain
■ Intermediate risk historical features (1 or more but without high risk features)
  ➤ Prior MI, Peripheral or cerebrovascular disease, CABG, prior Aspirin use
  ➤ Prolonged but resolved (>20 min) rest angina with mod or high likelihood of CAD
  ➤ Rest angina (<20 min or relieved by rest or sublingual nitro)
■ Not a high or intermediate risk historical feature:
  ➤ New-onset in the past two weeks of Canadian Class III or IV angina (angina walking 2 blocks or less)

Signs & Symptoms
(one or more makes pt high risk)

- Pulmonary edema, most likely related to ischemia
- New or worsening MR murmur
- S3 or new/worsening rales
- Hypotension
- Tachycardia
- Bradycardia
- Age >75 (age >70 but not >75 is intermediate risk)
- Physical exam should also aim to exclude other precipitants of angina, e.g. uncontrolled HTN, thyrotoxicosis, aortic stenosis, hypertrophic cardiomyopathy

TESTS
- Basic blood tests:
  - Differentiate UA from NSTEMI by presence of cardiac enzymes
    - Troponins (TnT or TnI)
      - More sensitive and specific that CK-MB
      - Low sensitivity in first 6 hours after symptom onset
      - Useful for selection of therapy / risk stratification
      - Detects recent MI up to 2 weeks after onset
    - CK-MB
      - Prior standard and still acceptable
      - Less sensitive than troponins
      - Less specific in setting of skeletal muscle disease
      - Better ability to detect early re-infarction
    - Myoglobin
      - Highly sensitive
      - Rapid release kinetics-detects MI early
      - Very low specificity in setting of skeletal muscle disease limits value for ruling out MI
  - High risk: TnT or TnI >0.1 ng/ml
  - Intermediate risk: Tn >0.01 but <0.1 ng/ml
  - Low risk: normal troponin
- Specific diagnostic tests
  - 12-lead electrocardiogram (ECG)
  - Important for risk assessment of UA and NSTEMI and exclusion of STEMI
    - High-risk features:
      - Transient ST changes of ≥0.05 mV with angina at rest
      - LBBB or RBBB, new or presumed new
      - Sustained VT

- Intermediate risk features:
  - T wave inversions of >0.2 mV
  - Pathologic Q waves
- Low risk feature:
  - Normal ECG or no change with episode of chest pain

DIFFERENTIAL DIAGNOSIS

- Consider non "plaque rupture" mechanisms of angina
  - ➤ Anemia, sepsis, thyrotoxicosis, etc. (increased O_2 demand or decreased O_2 delivery with stenosis due to stable coronary plaque)
- Consider non-coronary but cardiac chest pain
  - ➤ Uncontrolled hypertension, hypertrophic cardiomyopathy, pericarditis, Mitral prolapse
- Consider noncardiac chest pain
  - ➤ GERD, PUD, esophageal spasm, biliary disease
  - ➤ Musculoskeletal
  - ➤ Cervical disc disease
  - ➤ Pulmonary process
  - ➤ Aortic Dissection

MANAGEMENT

What to Do First

- Assess likelihood of ACS and stratify risk of death by history, physical, ECG, and cardiac enzymes.
- Initiate therapy

General Measures

- Control ischemia
- Control platelets and coagulation
- Consider revascularization

SPECIFIC THERAPY

Indication for therapy: ACS

Treatment Options

- Anti-ischemic therapy
  - ➤ Bed rest (wih continuous ECG monitoring for ischemia, arrhythmia)
  - ➤ Nitroglycerin SL PRN followed by IV, titrate upward to relieve ischemia
  - ➤ Supplemental O_2 if pulse oximetry <90% or respiratory distress or cyanosis present

➤ Morphine IV if symptoms not relieved with nitroglycerin or if pulmonary edema or severe agitation present
➤ Beta blockade IV (metoprolol, atenolol)
➤ Calcium blockade (non-dihydropyridine agents – Diltiazem or Verapamil) if beta blocker contraindicated or ischemia persists despite adequate beta blockade and V dysfunction or other contraindication not present
➤ Consider ACE inhibitor therapy if pt remains hypertensive despite beta blockade and adequate nitrate therapy
➤ Consider intra-aortic balloon counterpulsation if patient refractory to medical therapy

■ Anti-platelet, anticoagulation therapy
➤ Aspirin po chewed STAT, then po qd (Clopidogrel if aspirin allergic)
➤ Clopidogrel, 300 or 600 mg po then 75 mg po qd after coronary anatomy is shown to be "non-surgical" or if patient is not a CABG candidate for other reasons; otherwise benefit of early use is controversial (Clopidogrel use within 5–7 days of CABG increases bleeding risk and may delay CABG)
➤ Heparin, unfractionated to target PTT of 1.5–2.5X control (or LMWH)
➤ GPIIb/IIIa inhibitor added to Aspirin and Heparin if ischemia persists or high risk features present. Eptifibatide or tirofiban appropriate for ACS without definite plan for PCI, Reopro may be used if PCI planned within 24 hours.

Side Effects & Contraindications
■ Nitrates
➤ Side effects: head ache, hypotension, reflex tachycardia, tachyphylaxis
➤ Contraindications
  • Absolute: recent (<24 h) Sildenafil citrate (Viagra) use
  • Relative: hypotension
■ Beta blockers
➤ Side effects: dizziness, tiredness, severe bradycardia, hypotension, rales, bronchospasm, heart block
➤ Contraindications
  • Absolute: cardiogenic shock, severe COPD
  • Relative: heart rate <45, AV conduction defects, COPD
■ Dihydropyridine Calcium channel blockers
➤ Side effects: constipation, hypotension, heart block

➤ Contraindications
- Absolute: cardiogenic shock, heart block without pacemaker, pulmonary edema on CXR
- Relative: combination therapy with beta blocker
- Note: Immediate release dihydropyridine calcium antagonists (e.g., nifedipine) are contraindicated in the absence of adequate beta blockade

▪ Aspirin
➤ Side effects: GI upset, bleeding
➤ Contraindications
- Absolute: significant aspirin allergy

▪ Clopidogrel
➤ Side effects: bleeding, rash, rare neutropenia
➤ Contraindications
- Absolute: active pathological bleeding (ICH, PUD)

▪ Heparin
➤ Side effects: bleeding, thrombocytopenia
➤ Contraindications
- Absolute: severe thrombocytopenia

▪ GPIIb/IIIa agents
➤ Side effects: bleeding, thrombocytopenia
➤ Contraindications
- Absolute: severe hypertension, major surgery in past 6 weeks, stroke within past month or any severe hemorrhagic stroke, active significant bleeding
- Relative: thrombocytopenia, renal impairment (adjust dose), anticipated urgent major surgery

▪ Revascularization therapy for STEMI, immediate PCI preferred if available immediately, otherwise consider thrombolytic therapy.

▪ (Thrombolytic therapy is contraindicated in the absence of STEMI, a true posterior MI, or a presumed new LBBB)
➤ For NSTEMI and UA, consider early conservative versus invasive management
- Any ACS pt without contraindication to coronary angiography may optionally be managed invasively (within 12–24H) unless not a candidate for revascularization
- Any high risk feature should prompt strong consideration of immediate or early invasive management
- Early invasive approach is favored (TIMI-18), especially in NSTEMI (Troponin +) or TIMI risk score >4 (www.timi.org/files/riskscore/ua_calculator.htm).

- Conservative strategy should be mainly reserved for low-risk UA patients (no recurrent ischemia, EF > 40, negative stress test, no prior coronary revascularization).
- Add imaging (nuclear or echo) to stress in presence of:
  - Baseline ST abnormality, LVH, digoxin
  - IVCD (LBBB, RBBB or NSIVCD)
  - Paced rhythm
  - Pre-excitation
- Exercise is preferred, but use pharmacological stress with imaging if pt cannot exercise adequately (adenosine or persantine nuclear; dobutamine echo)
- Prompt coronary angiography for any ACS patient who fails to stabilize
- Prompt coronary angiography for ACS patients with any prior CABG or PCI within past 6 months
- ➤ Revascularization, CABG or PCI
  - CABG favored: Significant left main or multivessel disease with proximal LAD involvement, particularly in diabetics
  - PCI or CABG not recommended if stenosis <50% or if disease not affecting proximal LAD and pt has not been treated with medical therapy or has no evidence of ischemia on non-invasive testing
  - BARI trial – 1829 pts with 2 or 3 vessel disease, 64% with UA, 7 year follow up. Only significant benefit for CABG over PCI was in subgroup of diabetics who received IMA graft. Numerous trials are ongoing to assess CABG vs multivessel PCI with DES.

FOLLOW-UP
- ■ Acute phase of disease (highest risk) usually over by 2 months
- ■ At D/C, all patients should receive nitroglycerin tabs (or spray) with instructions
- ■ Aspirin
- ■ Clopidogrel
- ■ Thorough instructions for any new or adjusted medications
- ■ Multidisciplinary approach with (dietician, rehabilitation) can improve compliance
- ■ Instruct patient to call physician for change in anginal threshold, frequency or severity
- ■ Follow up appointment needed in 1–2 weeks, up to 6 if low risk
- ■ Aggressive attention to modifiable traditional risk factors
  - ➤ D/C tobacco

- ➤ BP < 135/80
- ➤ LDL < 100 (<70 preferred), use statin, escalate dose if necessary, monitor for LFT elevation or rhabdomyolysis, consider adjuncts (e.g., ezetimibe)
- ➤ Tight glucose control in diabetic patients
- ➤ Consider fibrate or niacin if HDL < 40 or TG >200
- ➤ Prescribe appropriate exercise

COMPLICATIONS AND PROGNOSIS

Complications
- Recurrent admissions
- Ischemic cardiomyopathy, leading cause of clinical heart failure, can progress to death or need for transplant.
- Dressler's syndrome, uncommon without transmural infarct, pericariditis usually ~6 weeks post infarction which is treated with steroids or NSAIDS
- Depression: high-risk post-MI and worsens prognosis
- Arrhythmia:
  - ➤ Ventricular tachycardia, re-entry at scar or ischemic
  - ➤ Bundle branch block
  - ➤ Ventricular aneurysm
- Stroke
- Death: risk after NSTEMI > after STEMI

Prognosis
- Determined by risk stratification. Exercise time on treadmill and LVEF are strong predictors.

CORONAVIRUS/COMMON COLD

CAROL A. GLASER, MD

HISTORY & PHYSICAL

History
- Large RNA virus
- At least 2 antigenic groups of respiratory coronavirus
- Human only host
- Spread via resiratory secretions
- Young children have the highest attack rates.
- Incubation period 2–5 days
- Common cause of URI in adults/children

Signs & Symptoms
- Upper respiratory infection
- Sneezing
- Coryza
- Sometimes low-grade fever
- Occasionally lower tract symptoms

TESTS

Specific
- Most strains cannot be isolated in diagnostic virology laboratory.
- Antibody assays not commercially available
- Electron Microscopy (EM) – viral particles can sometimes be visualized by EM, but not routinely available

DIFFERENTIAL DIAGNOSIS
- Other respiratory viruses, particularly rhinovirus
- Allergies

MANAGEMENT
- Good handwashing
- No vaccines available

SPECIFIC THERAPY
- No specific therapy yet available
- Supportive

FOLLOW-UP
n/a

COMPLICATIONS AND PROGNOSIS
n/a

COUGH

DARYA SOTO, MD

HISTORY & PHYSICAL

History
- Time of onset, frequency, timing of cough:
  - ➤ Paroxysmal (pertussis)
  - ➤ Nocturnal (asthma, gastric reflux, chronic aspiration, pulmonary edema)

➤ With meals (aspiration secondary to neurologic dysfunction)
- Character of cough:
  ➤ Dry (pulmonary fibrosis)
  ➤ Productive (chronic bronchitis)
  ➤ Purulent (bronchiectasis)
  ➤ Hemoptysis scant: infectious bronchitis, chronic bronchitis or cancer; massive: bronchiectasis
- Recent respiratory infection (cough may last >2 mo due to transient bronchial hyperreactivity)
- Aggravating factors:
  ➤ Post-nasal drip, rhinitis, sinus tenderness and drainage
  ➤ Dyspepsia
  ➤ Medications (ACE inhibitors)
  ➤ Tobacco (chronic cough in 75% of smokers)
  ➤ Exercise (asthma)
  ➤ Environmental exposures (cold air, fumes, dust, asbestos, mold, animal dander); at home, work or secondary to hobby; does time away alleviate symptoms?
- Alleviating factors: what medications have alleviated symptoms?
- Personal or family history of asthma, eczema or allergies

Signs & Symptoms
- Fluid behind tympanic membranes (TM) suggests otitis media; hair touching TM may cause cough
- Pale, edematous nasal mucosa suggests allergies
- Hoarseness or stridor suggests laryngotracheal disease
- Oropharyngeal secretions and cobblestone mucosa suggests post-nasal drip
- Neck mass or enlarged thyroid may impinge on trachea and cause cough
- Wheezing: asthma, chronic bronchitis and emphysema; when unilateral, it suggests a partially obstructing mass
- Wet rales: pneumonia; "Velcro" rales (usually best heard on slow inspiration): interstitial lung disease
- Evaluate cranial nerves IX and X (gag reflex) to assess risk for aspiration

TESTS

Laboratory
- WBC count with differential (eosinophilia in asthma and allergies)

DIFFERENTIAL DIAGNOSIS

Acute Cough

- Infectious:
    - ➤ Otitis media, acute bronchitis, acute sinusitis, laryngopharyngitis
    - ➤ Pneumonia (CXR)
    - ➤ TB (PPD, CXR, sputum for AFB)
- Pulmonary embolus (50% present with acute cough; arterial blood gas, ventilation/perfusion scan and/or spiral chest CT first tests done)
- Foreign body in large airways (bronchoscopy)
- Pulmonary edema (cardiac evaluation)

Chronic Cough (>3 Wks Duration)

- Most commonly due to postnasal drip/chronic sinusitis, asthma, GERD, chronic bronchitis and bronchiectasis
- Chronic sinusitis (sinus CT)
- Cough variant asthma (spirometry; methacholine bronchoprovocation if spirometry normal)
- GERD (esophageal pH monitoring)
- Chronic bronchitis (cough with daily sputum x 3 mo in 2 consecutive y)
- Bronchiectasis (HRCT)
- Pulmonary fibrosis (pulmonary function tests, HRCT, bronchoscopy, lung biopsy)
- Bronchogenic carcinoma (chest CT, transbronchial or Wang needle biopsy, CT-guided FNA)
- Tracheal narrowing: carcinoma, thyroid enlargement (CT)
- Chronic aspiration (barium swallow)
- Medications (ACE inhibitor)

MANAGEMENT

What to Do First

- Treat potentially rapidly progressive process (infection, asthma, PE, CHF)

General Measures

- Avoid toxins, irritants and allergens (change home or work environment)
- Smoking cessation
- Treat underlying cause

SPECIFIC THERAPY

- Nasal steroids for allergic rhinitis
- Antihistamines for allergies
- Treat bronchoconstriction with beta-2 agonist and steroid inhalers; prednisone for severe bronchoconstriction, to break cough cycle, or as diagnostic test; ipratropium bromide for chronic bronchitis; leukotriene receptor antagonist for exercise-induced asthma
- Trial of H2 blocker or proton pump inhibitor if GERD present or suspected
- Prednisone and other immunosuppressive agents for pulmonary fibrosis
- Antibiotics for URI or pneumonia; intermittent oral and inhaled antibiotics (to cover Pseudomonas) in bronchiectasis
- Antitussives (dextromethorphan, codeine, hydrocodone) should be used with caution in patients with impaired mucociliary clearance

FOLLOW-UP

- Dictated by specific underlying cause

COMPLICATIONS AND PROGNOSIS

- Chronic cough can lead to:
  - ➤ Chest wall pain, rib fractures
  - ➤ Emesis, esophageal perforation
  - ➤ Dizziness, syncope
  - ➤ Cardiac arrythmias
  - ➤ Pneumothorax, pneumomediastinum, pneumoperitoneum
  - ➤ SC, interstitial emphysema
  - ➤ Stress incontinence
  - ➤ Psychosocial stress

CRIGLER-NAJJER SYNDROME TYPE 1

WILLIAM E. BERQUIST, MD

HISTORY & PHYSICAL

- incidence: rare
- inheritance: autosomal recessive
- newborn jaundice beginning by day 3 of life and persisting
- normal physical exam initially
- possible mental status and general neurologic deterioration to coma and death (kernicterus)

TESTS

Basic Tests
- plasma bilirubin from 17–50 mg/dL, all unconjugated and usually >20mg/dL
- normal liver enzymes and hemolytic screen

Special Diagnostic Tests
- phenobarbital therapy fails to decrease bilirubin
- gene probes abnormal: mutations in the gene that encodes UGT1A1 resulting in absent enzyme activity
- liver biopsy: tissue enzyme assay of UGT1A1 shows no activity
- Other Diagnostic
- oral cholecystogram: normal
- liver biopsy: histology normal

DIFFERENTIAL DIAGNOSIS
- sepsis
- hemolysis
- Crigler-Najjer syndrome type 2 and Gilbert's respond to phenobarbital therapy

MANAGEMENT
- monitor bilirubin, hydration, and neurologic exam
- avoid bilirubin-displacing drugs
- phenobarbital trial: 5 mg/kg/day orally

SPECIFIC THERAPY
- phototherapy: basic treatment for >10 hr/d keeping total bilirubin <20 mg/dL (normal birth weight infants) and <35–45 mg/dL (older patients) for kernicterus prevention

Other Specific Therapies
- double-volume exchange transfusion (infants)
- plasmapheresis (older patients)
- liver transplantation
- tin mesoporphyrin inhibits heme oxygenase and decreases bilirubin production (experimental); complications of cutaneous photosensitivity and iron deficiency anemia
- oral agents to decrease enterohepatic circulation of bilirubin: cholestyramine, agar, calcium carbonate and phosphate

FOLLOW-UP
- monitoring and maintaining appropriate bilirubin levels and hydration

COMPLICATIONS AND PROGNOSIS
- high kernicterus risk and infant death without ongoing treatment (phototherapy) or definitive therapy with liver transplantation

CRIGLER-NAJJER TYPE 2

WILLIAM E. BERQUIST, MD

HISTORY & PHYSICAL
- incidence: rare
- inheritance: autosomal dominant, variable penetrance
- jaundice at birth
- normal physical exam and rare incidence kernicterus

TESTS

Basic Tests
- plasma bilirubin: 6–45 mg/dl, all unconjugated ususally >20 mg/dl
- normal liver enzymes and hemolytic screen

Special Diagnostic
- phenobarbital therapy decreases bilirubin
- DNA mutations in encoding gene UGT1A1
- liver biopsy tissue: decreased activity of UGT1A1 enzyme

Other Diagnostic
- oral cholecystogram: normal
- liver biopsy: histology normal

DIFFERENTIAL DIAGNOSIS
- sepsis, hemolysis, breast-milk jaundice
- Crigler-Najjer syndrome type 1: unresponsive bilirubin to phenobarbital therapy
- Gilbert's Syndrome: lower bilirubin and different gene probe analysis

MANAGEMENT
- evaluate and treat any sepsis, hemolysis, or dehydration

General Measures
- trial on phenobarbital orally usually improves bilirubin to 2–5 mg/dl in 7–10 days
- phototherapy and/or double-volume exchange transfusion for kernicterus prevention in infants

SPECIFIC THERAPY
n/a

FOLLOW-UP
- discretional phenobarbital use after neonatal period or if unconjugated bilirubin >35 mg/dL

COMPLICATIONS AND PROGNOSIS
- rare kernicterus cases otherwise excellent prognosis

CROHN'S DISEASE

CHRISTINE A. CARTWRIGHT, MD

HISTORY & PHYSICAL
- History: diarrhea, abdominal pain, fever, nausea, vomiting, weight loss, anemia
- Trigger factors: infection, smoking, NSAIDs, stress
- Physical signs: fever, abdominal tenderness and fullness (usually right lower quadrant)

TESTS

Basic Tests: Blood
- CBC, ESR, albumin, LFTs

Other Tests:
- stool studies: culture, O+P × 3, C. difficile, Giardia EIA antigen
- amebic ELISA serology
- colonoscopy and biopsy
- UGI and SBFT
- abdominal and pelvic CT scan (in some circumstances)

DIFFERENTIAL DIAGNOSIS
- Ulcerative colitis or other causes:
- Infectious diseases (giardiasis, amebiasis, pseudomembranous, CMV)

- Ischemic colitis
- Radiation
- Drugs

Differences between Crohn's disease and ulcerative colitis:

- ulcerative colitis: mucosal, diffuse, continuous, involves the rectum, limited to colon
- Crohn's: transmural, patchy, skip lesions, discrete ulcers, anywhere in the GI tract but usually involves the distal ileum and right colon and spares the rectum; perianal disease, fistulae, abscesses, strictures, obstruction, granulomas

MANAGEMENT

What to Do First

- Assess disease location, type, severity and presence of complications
- location: distal ileum and right colon (50%), small bowel alone (30%), colon alone (20%), perianal (25–30%), or gastro-duodenal (less common)
- type: inflammatory, stenotic and/or fistulizing
- severity:
  - ➤ mild: diarrhea, pain
  - ➤ moderate-severe: fever, weight loss, pain, tenderness, nausea, vomiting, anemia
  - ➤ severe-fulminant: despite steroids, fever, persisting nausea and vomiting, cachexia, signs of obstruction and peritoneal inflammation
- complications: fistulae, abscesses, obstruction, perforation

General Measures

- Complete baseline evaluation: laboratory tests, barium studies, endoscopy, and in some cases abdominal and pelvic CT scan

SPECIFIC THERAPY

Maintenance therapy:

Mild-Moderate Disease

- oral aminosalicylates
- sulfasalazine 2–4 g/d or balsalazide 6.75 g/d (for colonic disease) or
- mesalamine 4–4.8 g/d for small bowel disease
- side effects of sulfasalazine: intolerance to sulfapyridine moiety of sulfasalazine is common (headache, nausea), as are mild allergic reactions (skin rash); severe allergic reactions (e.g., fibrosing alveolitis, pericarditis, pancreatitis, agranulocytosis) are rare

- abnormal sperm count, motility and morphology occur commonly with sulfasalazine (and not mesalamine) but are reversible with discontinuation of medication
- low-grade hemolysis on sulfasalazine is not unusual, but is rarely severe
- sulfasalazine may interfere with folic acid absorption
- side effects of mesalamine: hair loss, rarely interstitial nephritis (may be irreversible)
- antibiotics: metronidazole or ciprofloxacin
- side effects of metronidazole: nausea, diarrhea, metallic taste, peripheral neuropathies (may be irreversible), monilial infections, teratogenic, ?cancer risk
- side effects of ciprofloxacin: diarrhea, teratogenic

Moderate to Severe Disease
- Add azathioprine (Aza) or 6-mercaptopurine (6MP) – start at a low dose (50 mg/d) and slowly increase the dose by adding not more than 25 mg each month until 2.5 mg/kg/day for Aza or 1.5 mg/kg/day for 6MP or until leukopenia or elevated LFTs, whichever occurs first. Check CBC and LFTs every 2 weeks when starting or increasing the dose and every 3 months when on a stable dose. If TPMT enzyme activity is checked initially and is normal, then one can start at a higher dose and increase the dose at a faster rate to achieve earlier effect.
  - ➤ side effects of Aza or 6MP: fatigue, nausea, bone marrow depression, opportunistic infections, pancreatitis, hepatitis, fever, rarely lymphoma
- Methotrexate if intolerant to Aza or 6MP. Induction dose: 25 mg i.m. weekly for 16 weeks. Maintenance dose: 15 mg i.m. weekly
  - ➤ side effects of methotrexate: fatigue, nausea, diarrhea, leukopenia, opportunistic infections, liver disease
- consider adding a TNF blocker if Aza, 6MP or methotrexate fails to hold the disease in remission. TNF blockers will be more effective if pt is on concomitant Aza, 6MP or methotrexate. Caution: Therapy with double or triple immunomodulators increases the risk for life-threatening infections.
  - ➤ side effects of TNF blockers: infusion reactions, infections, immune response, lymphoma

Active disease:
- oral corticosteroids (occasionally)

- oral prednisone with gradual tapering – usually faster at higher doses and slower at lower doses
- short-term side effects include acne, night sweats, sleep and mood disturbances, appetite stimulation
- long-term side include hypertension, diabetes, acne, osteoporosis, osteonecrosis, glaucoma, cataracts, depression and obesity
- Budesonide (9 mg/d); Caution: may not be as effective as prednisone and has long-term steroid toxicities
- There is no place for frequent or long-term systemic steroids (including budesonide) in the management of IBD because the adverse effects outweigh the potential benefits.

Severe-Fulminant Disease
- hospitalization for IV steroids, antibiotics and bowel rest
- surgical consultation if evidence for obstruction
- abscess drainage (open or percutaneous)
- if chronically obstructed: elective surgery
- ?cyclosporine for fistulizing disease
- side effects of cyclosporine include nephrotoxicity, seizures, hypertension, opportunistic infections, hirsutism, tremor and gingival hyperplasia

FOLLOW-UP
- Frequent visits to assess symptoms and laboratory tests, particularly CBC and LFTs

COMPLICATIONS AND PROGNOSIS
- Intestinal complications:
  - obstruction
  - perforation
  - abscess
  - fistulae
    - entero-enteric
    - entero-vesical
    - entero-cutaneous
    - mesenteric
    - retroperitoneal
    - perianal
- Related to small bowel pathophysiology:
  - gallstones
  - malabsorption

➤ renal:
- stones
- fistulae
- hydronephrosis
- amyloidosis

■ Extra-intestinal manifestations:
➤ colitis-related: correlates with inflammatory activity of the bowel
- arthritis:
  - peripheral
  - central – follows an independent course
    - associated with HLA haplotype B27
    - sacro-iliitis
    - ankylosing spondylitis
- skin:
  - erythema nodosum
  - pyoderma gangrenosum
- eye:
  - episcleritis or scleritis
  - uveitis – may follow an independent course
    - often clusters with AS and SI
    - often associated with HLA-B27

CROUP

CAROL A. GLASER, MD

HISTORY & PHYSICAL

History

■ Spasmodic croup and acute laryngotracheitis sometimes both termed laryngotracheitis b/c overlap of syndromes
■ Sometimes referred to as spasmodic croup
■ 3 months to 3 years of age, peak 2nd year of life
■ more common in boys than girls
■ epidemiology patterns of croup reflect seasonal patterns of agents
■ Croup is a distinctive clinical syndrome resulting from involvement of the larynx with resultant edema and stridor (aka laryngotracheobronchitis).
■ Etiologies
➤ Usually viral, in order of frequency;
- Parainfluenza most common cause (1,2,3)

- Influenza A/B
- RSV
- Adenovirus
- Rhinovirus
- Mycoplasma
- Enterovirus
- HSV
- Reovirus

Signs & Symptoms

- Child initially has mild cold symptoms
- Then ACUTE onset of
  - Dyspnea
  - Croupy cough
  - Inspiratory stridor
- Fever-more likely with some agents than others (e.g., influenza)
- Often fluctuating course
- Auscultation of chest: inspiratory stridor, rales, rhonchi, and/or wheezing
- Course of croupy cough generally lasts 3–4 days

TESTS

- WBC is often unremarkable
- Respiratory culture may identify etiology. Multiplex tests, and rapid PCR tests when widely available, will further help.

Clinical presentation usually sufficient for diagnosis. Presence of "steeple sign" on PA chest film reflects subglottic narrowing.

DIFFERENTIAL DIAGNOSIS

- Acute epiglottitis; must be distinguished from epiglottitis: generally lacks croupy cough, in epiglottitis there is a cherry-red epiglottis, child has characteristic sitting posture in epiglottitis. Also laryngeal diphtheria, foreign body aspiration, angioneurotic edema.

MANAGEMENT

- Mild cases: mostly symptomatic, with close observation
- Pt often responds to moist air.
- Mild sedation at bedtime sometimes used
- Symptomatic

SPECIFIC THERAPY

-Mild cases: symptomatic care as above
More severe cases:

Corticosteroids
Dexamethasone
Nebulized budesonide
Nebulized epinephrine requires caution and close cardiac monitoring.

FOLLOW-UP
With primary care within 24 hours for moderate to severe cases

COMPLICATIONS AND PROGNOSIS
- Hypoxemia
- Cardiorespiratory failure rarely requires mechanical ventilation.
- Reactive airway disease later in life

CRYPTOCOCCUS NEOFORMANS

RICHARD A. JACOBS, MD, PhD

HISTORY & PHYSICAL

History
- Worldwide distribution
- High concentration in pigeon feces; soil or decayed wood chips also implicated
- Disease thought to occur after organism aerosolized and inhaled
- Exposure is common: many healthy subjects have positive skin tests
- New cases were rare before emergence of AIDS
- Immunologic defects in T-cell-mediated host defense are at increased risk for progressive disease
- AIDS predisposing factor in 80–90% of cryptococcal infections, usually with CD4 count <100/mm^3
- Transplantation next most common risk factor, peak period 4–6 wks or more post-tx
- Incidence increased in lymphoreticular malignancies (Hodgkin's disease) and sarcoidosis (even without steroids)
- 2 varieties: var. neoformans true opportunistic pathogen; var. gatti also causes disease in non-immunocompromised hosts, more refractory to treatment

Signs & Symptoms
- Central Nervous System:
  - ➤ 85% of cryptococcal infections involve brain or meninges
  - ➤ Acute or insidious (acute more common in AIDS/immunosuppressed)

- Mild/nonspecific symptoms or CNS-referable
- Headache, nausea, dizziness, irritability, somnolence, clumsiness, confusion, or obtundation all possible
- Some HIV-positive pts may be asymptomatic
- Seizures late finding
- Physical findings non-specific: afebrile or mild temp to 39C, minimal to no nuchal rigidity
- Papilledema 1/3, CN palsies 1/5
- Mortality lower with var. gatti, but long-term neurologic sequelae more common
- Pulmonary:
  - Asymptomatic or scant, blood-streaked sputum
  - HIV-positive pts: 5–25% with cryptococcus have cough and dyspnea
  - Rales or pleural friction rub uncommon, empyema extremely rare
  - Nonimmunosuppressed: pulmonary cryptococcosis may progress/regress or remain stable for long periods
  - AIDS: cryptococcal pneumonia can be severe, rapidly progressive (42% acute-phase mortality)
- Other sites:
  - Skin lesions 5–10% of patients, painless on face or scalp – often ignored but frequently first signs of infection
  - In AIDS patients, skin lesions may resemble molloscum contagiosum

TESTS

Laboratory
- No abnormalities in CBC, ESR
- CSF examination
- Always measure opening pressure
- Glucose usually low to very low
- Protein increased
- Leukocyte counts usually $20/mm^3$ or higher with lymphocyte predominance
- In end-stage AIDS, low to absent CSF pleiocytosis possible, carries grave prognosis
- *Microbiology – culture*
  - India ink examination of fluid NOT reliable, many HIV patients have organisms that have hard to see or non-existent capsules
  - CSF, negative cultures do not rule out disease

> Urine – consider
> Sputum – consider
> Blood – most often positive in AIDS, indicative of extensive infection
- *Serology*
  > Cryptococcal antigen (CrAg) – detection of cryptococcal polysaccharide capsular antigen is clinically very useful
  > False-positive results possible, but usually with titer <1:8
  > CSF and serum testing provides >90% sensitivity for CNS cryptococcosis; CSF CrAg has better specificity; serum CrAg specificity for non-CNS infections is lower
  > In HIV patients, a positive serum CrAg always prompts CSF evaluation
- *Histopathology*
  > Organisms easily detected in tissue specimens, especially with special stains

Imaging
- CT or MRI helpful for defining ventricular system and evaluating presence of hydrocephalus
- CNS imaging may reveal "cryptococcomas"
- CXR: without AIDS, resembles tumor; AIDS – lymphadenopathy, pleural effusions, diffuse mixed interstitial and intra-alveolar infiltrates

DIFFERENTIAL DIAGNOSIS
- Early CNS cryptococcosis may resemble other fungal infections, tuberculosis, viral meningoencephalitis, or meningeal metastases
- Distinguish cryptococcal masses from other causes of intracranial lesions: pyogenic, nocardial, aspergillomas, TB, toxo, lymphoma, neoplasm
- Pulmonary disease hard to distinguish from PCP, tuberculosis, Histoplasma capsulatum, others – bronchoscopy helps to clarify

MANAGEMENT
What to Do First
- Examine CSF, manage high intracranial pressure by serial taps or consult neurology/neurosurgery for possible shunting, begin empiric therapy

General Measures
- Begin therapy with Amphotericin B

- Follow patients closely, switch to oral azole for completion of therapy
- Lifelong suppression for HIV-positive patients
- Data on treating HIV-negative patients is sparse – care must be individualized

SPECIFIC THERAPY
- All patients with CNS disease merit treatment
- HIV-positive patients and immunosuppressed treated with any site of infection
- Pulmonary cryptococcosis without immunosuppression or predisposing factors often resolves without treatment

Treatment Options
- Amphotericin B for 2 weeks, then 8 weeks of fluconazole or itraconazole, then lifelong maintenance with flu/itra. This is the regimen for HIV-positive patients; flucytosine was not shown to improve efficacy, so its use is controversial.
- Amphotericin B +/– flucytosine for 6 weeks. This is the non-HIV-infected patient regimen; with continued immunosuppression, the therapy is often extended beyond 6 wks. 4-wk course only with negative cultures at <2 wks of therapy. Unclear if lifelong suppression with azole is needed.
- Fluconazole: unclear if initial therapy with oral azole is appropriate– logically this should work, but it is not yet standard of care
- Liposomal amphotericin B approved for cryptococcosis based on open-label, noncomparative studies; may be substituted if nephrotoxicity precludes standard amphotericin therapy

Side Effects & Complications
- Amphotericin B (conventional): infusion-related toxicities (often ameliorated with hydrocortisone in IV bag), nephrotoxicity, hypokalemia, hypomagnesemia, nephrotoxicity (can be dose-limiting)
- Flucytosine: Leukopenia, thrombocytopenia, GI disturbance/ diarrhea – adjust dose for renal function, especially when used with amphotericin
- Fluconazole: transaminitis, many drug interactions
- Liposomal amphotericin: nephrotoxicity (but rarer than with conventional ampho), mild infusion-related

FOLLOW-UP

During Treatment
- Serial LP if elevated CSF opening pressure

- Document negative CSF cultures, reassess every 1–2 wks until negative
- Value of following serial CSF or serum CrAg debatable: most helpful to run both samples side-by-side as test has some variability during different runs. Different labs often use different kits, which cannot be compared.

Routine
- Close clinical follow-up
- At end of therapy, CSF values should be normalized

COMPLICATIONS AND PROGNOSIS

Complications
- High ICP – more common in end-stage AIDS patients. Treatment somewhat controversial – options: serial LPs, acetazolamide, CSF shunts
- Neurologic deficits – in up to 40% of AIDS patients
- Death – 25–30% of meningitis cases
- Relapse – prostate can be sequestered focus

Prognosis
- Infections rarely cured in AIDS patients, chronically immunosuppressed patients
- 20–25% relapse after initial response with Amphotericin B

CRYPTOSPORIDIOSIS

J. GORDON FRIERSON, MD

HISTORY & PHYSICAL

History
- Life cycle: Oocysts excreted in stool, ingested, develop to sporozoites and gameteocytes in intestinal epithelial cells. New zygotes produced, maturing to oocysts, which complete the cycle.
- Exposure: ingestion of oocysts by fecal-oral route. Water-born outbreaks occur. Auto-inoculation occurs.

Signs & Symptoms
- In immunocompetent host: Incubation period of 2–12 days (median 7), rapid onset of watery diarrhea, cramps, bloating, often mild fever, weight loss, sometimes nausea and vomiting. Duration averages

9 days, can be up to 8 weeks. Cysts shed up to 7–8 weeks. Recovery occurs. In immunosuppressed, symptoms can be prolonged or permanent, and of varying severity.

TESTS
- Basic tests: blood: no specific findings
- Basic tests: urine: normal
- Specific tests:
  - ➤ a) Stool examination, concentrated, stained with acid-fast technique shows oocysts. May need several stools to find parasite. ELISA for cryptosporidium antigen in stool available, which is approximately as accurate.
  - ➤ b) Biopsy of small or large bowel.
- Other tests: Serology (IFA, ELISA) available, but rises slowly, not useful in acute case. PCR not yet widely available.

DIFFERENTIAL DIAGNOSIS
- Most causes of acute diarrhea without blood. Stool exam can resemble cyclospora (also acid-fast).

MANAGEMENT
What to Do First
- Assess need for fluid and electrolyte replacement. Assess overall immunocompetence.

General Measures
- Determine source of infection if possible (could be water supply). Instruction in hygiene to prevent spread.

SPECIFIC THERAPY
Indications
- Severe diarrhea, immunocompromised patients.

Treatment Options
- No specific chemotherapy is reliable. In immunocompetent patients use antimotility agents and rehydration, as infection is self-limited. In immunocompromised patients paromomycin, clarithromycin may be helpful.

Side Effects & Complications
- None beyond dehydration, electrolyte imbalance. For immunocompromised patients, see HIV section.
- Contraindications to treatment: absolute: none.

■ Contraindications to treatment: relative: none.

FOLLOW-UP

During Treatment
■ General status.

Routine
■ Infection is self-limiting in immunocompetent patients, no follow needed after symptoms subside. See HIV section for immunocompromised patients.

COMPLICATIONS AND PROGNOSIS
■ Prognosis is good.

CRYSTAL-INDUCED ARTHRITIS

SHAUN RUDDY, MD

HISTORY & PHYSICAL

History
■ Inflammation caused by crystals of monosodium urate (MSU) (gout) or calcium pyrophosphate dihydrate (pseudogout or CPPD disease)
■ Usually middle-aged men; very rare in premenopausal women
■ Acute arthritis: abrupt onset of intense pain in a single joint, typically the first MTP (podagra) in gout; in knee, ankle or wrist for pseudogout
■ Subacute or chronic gout or CPPD disease: polyarthritis involving fingers, toes, wrists, ankles, elbows, knees, shoulders
■ Tophaceous gout: due to deposition of MSU deposits in distal extremities, ears, erosion of adjacent structures
■ Gout in family, obesity, hyperlipidemia, ethanol excess, hypertension, "syndrome X," trauma, surgery, ketosis
■ Uric acid kidney stones
■ Conditions leading to overproduction of uric acid
■ Congenital disorders of purine salvage pathway (rare)
  ➤ Proliferative disorders
  ➤ Hematologic–eg, myeloma, lymphoma, polycythemia, hemoglobinopathies, treatment of other neoplasms
  ➤ Cutaneous – eg, psoriasis
  ➤ Bone: Paget's disease

- Conditions leading to underexcretion of uric acid
  - Renal failure
  - Drugs: diuretics, cyclosporine
- Metabolic diseases for CPPD: hyperparathyroidism, hypothyroidism, hemochromatosis, gout, amyloidosis

Signs & Symptoms
- Acute: hot, red, swollen, exquisitely tender joint (85% monoarticular); joint effusion
- Chronic: indolent polyarthritis may lead to deformities
- Tophi are irregular hard nodular deposits of MSU in subcutaneous tissue of fingers, toes, ulnar surface

TESTS

Lab Tests
- Serum uric acid
  - Usually elevated in acute gouty arthritis (~85%), less often in alcoholics
  - Invariably elevated in chronic tophaceous gout
  - Asymptomatic hyperuricemia is common, esp. w/ diuretics; requires no treatment
- For CPPD: serum Ca, P, Mg, alkaline phosphatase, transferrin saturation, TSH
- Aspirate synovial fluid
  - WBC usually >10,000/mm3; if >100,000/mm3, suspect infection
  - Polarized light microscopy
    - Strongly negatively birefringent needle-shaped crystals of MSU are diagnostic of gout
    - Weakly positive birefringent rhomboid crystals are diagnostic of CPPD disease
    - Crystals may be found in asymptomatic joints
- Needle & aspirate nodular subcutaneous tophus, examine for MSU crystals

Radiographs
- Soft tissue swelling, effusion in acute arthritis
- Juxta-articular "punched-out" erosive lesions in digits w/ tophaceous gout
- In CPPD disease: chondrocalcinosis, punctate calcifications of hyaline or fibrocartilage of knees, wrists, hips

DIFFERENTIAL DIAGNOSIS
- Septic arthritis: aspirate & culture the joint, treat w/ antibiotics until results are known
- Calcium pyrophosphate deposition disease often co-exists w/ osteoarthritis, disordered calcium metabolism
- Polyarthritis of subacute or chronic crystal-induced disease may be confused w/ rheumatoid arthritis, spondyloarthropathies

MANAGEMENT
What to Do First
- Aspirate the joint for synovial fluid culture & crystal identification
  General Measures
- Put joint at rest
- Pt education: encourage weight loss, decreased alcohol intake

SPECIFIC THERAPY
Acute Attack
- High-dose NSAID
  OR
- Oral colchicine, no more than 3 doses 1 hr apart
  OR
- IV colchicine (single injection)
  OR
- Intra-articular injection of triamcinolone hexacetonide
  OR
- Oral corticosteroid tapering from 40 mg prednisone quickly: the best choice when preceding ones are relatively contraindicated

Preventing Intercurrent Attacks
- Oral colchicine twice daily
  OR
- Moderate-dose NSAID

Chronic Treatment for Elevated Uric Acid and/or Tophi
- Allopurinol, titrated to dose producing serum uric acid of <6.0 mg/dL
- If allopurinol is not tolerated: probenicid; increase monthly until uric acid is normal
  For CPPD disease, correct underlying metabolic abnormality

Side Effects
- NSAIDs: generics (ibuprofen, naproxen, sulindac) are as effective as selective COX-2 inhibitor celecoxib but cause serious GI bleeding

more often. Other side effects, including diminished platelet function, headache, psychosis, impaired renal function, & sodium retention, probably occur w/ the same frequency.

- Colchicine: diarrhea (undesirable in a pt w/ exquisitely painful toe!), nausea, bone marrow suppression; do not use in renal disease
- Corticosteroids: glucose intolerance is the main problem w/ short-term tapering dose. Joint infection is rare after intra-articular injection.
- Beginning treatment of hyperuricemia often precipitates acute attacks of arthritis
- Allopurinol: rashes are frequent, more common in renal disease, include possibly fatal toxic epidermal necrolysis; hepatitis; bone marrow suppression (adjust dose of concomitant azathioprine, 6-mercaptopurine)
- Probenecid: not effective w/ decreased renal function; uric acid stones (advise increased water consumption)

FOLLOW-UP
- Re-evaluate daily for response to treatment during acute attacks
- Monthly, while controlling recurrent acute attacks or adjusting dose of anti-hyperuricemic agent

COMPLICATIONS & PROGNOSIS
- Untreated tophaceous deposits may erode & destroy joints
- Renal calculi occur in 5–10% of pts
- Acute attacks are almost always controlled w/ anti-inflammatory agents
- W/ adequate control of serum uric acid, tophi reabsorb & recurrent attacks become infrequent

CUSHING'S SYNDROME

RICHARD I. DORIN, MD

HISTORY & PHYSICAL

History
- Weight gain, central obesity, increased appetite
- Osteoporosis, fracture, loss of height, renal stones
- Hypertension, diabetes mellitus, metabolic syndrome
- Hypokalemia, alkalosis, polyuria, muscle weakness, cramps

- Muscle weakness, atrophy
- History of exogenous glucocorticoid administration
- Alcoholism
- Family history of Cushing syndrome (CS)
- Cigarette smoking, weight loss, bone/abdominal pain, flushing
- Visual field abnormalities, other pituitary disease, galactorrhea

Signs & Symptoms
- Neuropsychiatric: Depression, insomnia, mania, psychosis
- Muscle weakness, easy bruising, stretch marks (striae)
- Women: hirsutism, virilism, thinning of scalp hair, acne, amenorrhea/menstrual irregularity
- Men: decreased libido, gynecomastia, impotence
- Hyperpigmentation (with ACTH excess)
- Edema, polyuria, nocturia
- Hypertension, acne, hirsutism, easy bruising, hyperpigmentation
- Central obesity, striae (1.0 cm, violaceous), fragile skin, nonhealing ulcerations
- Supraclavicular fat pads, dorsal fat pad, moon facies
- Muscle atrophy, proximal muscle weakness
- Hypokalemia, alkalosis

TESTS
- Screening:
  - ➤ 1.0 mg overnight dexamethasone suppression test (1.0 mg dexamethasone at midnight, check 8 AM cortisol): normal <2 mcg/dL; limited specificity; false-positive with stress, anticonvulsant therapy, oral contraceptives, obesity; concomitant DEX level may be useful
  - ➤ 24-h urine free cortisol (and creatinine to assure adequate 24-hr urine collection)
- Confirmatory:
  - ➤ Evening (10–12 PM) to morning (6–8 AM) serum/salivary cortisol ratios
  - ➤ Serial evaluation of (midnight) salivary cortisol for cyclical/periodic CS
  - ➤ 2-d medium dose (2 mg) dexamethasone suppression test
- Tests to establish the cause of CS:
  - ➤ 8 AM plasma ACTH level:
    - Low in ACTH-independent

- May be normal or elevated in pituitary corticotrophic adenoma
- Normal to marked elevation in ectopic ACTH

■ High-dose (8 mg) dexamethasone suppression test: useful to distinguish between pituitary vs. ectopic source of ACTH in established case of ACTH-dependent CS; suppression of ACTH, serum and 24-hr urine cortisol in pituitary adenoma; may be given as a 2-day test or as an overnight test

■ Inferior petrosal sinus (IPS) sampling:
  ➤ In ACTH-dependent CS, pituitary vs. ectopic source of ACTH
  ➤ Not useful in distinguishing CS from normal or pseudo-Cushing or normal from pituitary corticotrophic adenoma
  ➤ Primary utility is to distinguish between pituitary (Cushing's disease) or ectopic source of ACTH in established case of ACTH-dependent CS, especially when MRI of sella is negative
  ➤ May be useful in lateralizing corticotroph adenoma in pituitary (Cushing's disease)

Imaging
■ ACTH-independent CS: abdominal CT/MRI
■ ACTH-dependent, pituitary adenoma: MRI of sella; often due to microadenoma (often not visualized)
■ Ectopic (nonpituitary) Cushing: CXR, chest CT, 111-Indium-ocreotide (Octrescan), FDG-PET scan

DIFFERENTIAL DIAGNOSIS
■ Pseudo-Cushing's: may be associated with depression, alcoholism, intercurrent stress
■ *ACTH-independent:* adrenal adenoma or carcinoma, nodular hyperplasia, exogenous glucocorticoid administration
■ *ACTH-dependent:*
  ➤ Pituitary corticotroph adenoma (Cushing's disease, CD)
  ➤ Plasma ACTH levels may be normal or elevated
■ **Ectopic ACTH:**
  ➤ Often in setting of known malignancy
  ➤ Small cell carcinoma of the lung
  ➤ Carcinoid tumors (bronchial, thymic, islet, gut)
  ➤ Other neuroendocrine tumors (e.g. pheochromocytoma, medullary CA of thyroid)
  ➤ Plasma ACTH and UFC levels may be dramatically elevated
  ➤ Syndrome of mineralocorticoid excess (hypokalemia, alkalosis, edema) may dominate

MANAGEMENT

General Measures
- Control diabetes, hypertension, hypokalemia, increased cardiovascular risk
- Patients immunosuppressed; vigilance for opportunistic, unusual infections

What to Do First
- Confirm the diagnosis of CS
- Distinguish between ACTH-dependent and independent
- Localize source of ACTH or cortisol excess biochemically, then by imaging

SPECIFIC THERAPY

Surgical Treatment
- Pituitary: transsphenoidal adenomectomy or hemihypophysectomy
- Adrenal adenoma/carcinoma: abdominal, flank, or laparoscopic surgery
- Ectopic: surgical or chemotherapy as indicated by primary disease
- Bilateral adrenalectomy always curative; reserved for ACTH-dependent CS that failed primary surgical and medical therapies; lifelong glucocorticoid and mineralocorticoid replacement
- Radiotherapy
  - Pituitary irradiation for nonresectable adenoma or after bilateral adrenalectomy in CD
- Medical Therapy
  - Enzymatic inhibitors of cortisol synthesis (ketoconazole, metyrapone, aminoglutethimide)
  - Hydrocortisone replacement if steroidogenic blockade complete
  - Mineralocorticoid excess: mineralocorticoid receptor blockers (spironolactone)
  - Adrenal carcinoma: adrenolytic therapy (mitotane)

FOLLOW-UP
- Patients feel worse after cure of CS due to adrenal insufficiency or corticosteroid withdrawal
- Early Postoperative:
  - Early drop in serum cortisol predictive of successful cure; useful if exogenous hydrocortisone is withheld in hemodynamically stable patient post-operative
  - If patient is hemodynamically unstable, give high-dose hydrocortisone immediately postoperative, then taper

➤ May require higher than physiologic doses temporarily

➤ Education and medical alert bracelet for expected course of post-cure adrenal insufficiency

■ Intermediate:

➤ Most patients require maintenance hydrocortisone replacement, plus stress doses for stress, illness, in the year following successful surgical management of CS

■ During medical treatment: follow clinically for symptoms and signs of cortisol excess or deficiency, 24-hr UFC of uncertain value

■ Long-term:

➤ Late recurrences not unusual; assess annually for hypercortisolism, screen for osteoporosis (DXA scan)

➤ Hypopituitarism after pituitary surgery or XRT

➤ Nelson syndrome (invasive corticotrophic adenoma, high ACTH levels) after bilateral adrenalectomy for CS

COMPLICATIONS AND PROGNOSIS

Complications

■ Hypercortisolism: immunosuppression, cardiovascular risk, psychiatric disturbance, severe insulin resistance $+/-$ glucose intolerance

■ Post-cure: $2°/3°$ adrenal insufficiency universal; corticosteroid withdrawal syndrome; stress doses of corticosteroid during medical/surgical illness

■ Chronic: osteoporosis, increased cardiovascular risk, limited adrenal reserve, medical alert bracelet for steroid coverage for stress

Prognosis

■ Untreated CS: 50% mortality at 5 y

■ Cured patients: longstanding adrenal insufficiency for up to 1 y; gradual resolution of weakness, osteoporosis

■ Obesity, hypertension, and glucose intolerance may persist

■ Recurrence rate of 10–30% for transsphenoidal hypophysectomy

CUTANEOUS LARVA MIGRANS

J. GORDON FRIERSON, MD

HISTORY & PHYSICAL

History

■ Exposure: skin exposure to larvae of dog and cat hookworms (Ancylostoma braziliense, Ankylostoma caninum), usually on beaches contaminated with dog or cat feces

Signs & Symptoms
- Serpiginous, red, often pruritic, slightly raised tracks, usually on feet, which advance up to 1–2 cm per day

TESTS
- Basic tests: blood: none helpful
- Basic tests: urine: not helpful
- Specific tests: none
- Other tests: none

DIFFERENTIAL DIAGNOSIS
- Similar tracks can be seen in strongyloidiasis (usually perianal or on buttocks). Human hookworm can migrate short distance, not in distinct track.

MANAGEMENT
What to Do First
- Reassure patient. Larva does not invade.

General Measures
- Keep foot clean, give tetanus booster. Antibiotics if secondarily infected.

SPECIFIC THERAPY
Indications
- Persistent infestation. Larva eventually dies without treatment, but can take months.

Treatment Options
- Ivermectin single dose
- Albendazole for 3 days
- Thiabendazole 15% in water-soluble base, applied tid for 5 days (needs to be compounded, variable results reported)

Side Effects & Complications
- Ivermectin and albendazole: minor intestinal symptoms
- Contraindications to treatment: absolute: pregnancy, except for topical thiabendazole
- Contraindications to treatment: relative: apparently resolving case

FOLLOW-UP
Routine
- Retreatment needed in around 5–10% of cases

COMPLICATIONS AND PROGNOSIS
- Secondary bacterial infection, tetanus. Prognosis otherwise excellent.

CUTANEOUS LUPUS ERYTHEMATOSUS (LE)

RICHARD D. SONTHEIMER, MD and JEFFREY P. CALLEN, MD

HISTORY & PHYSICAL
- Acute Cutaneous LE (ACLE) – rash on cheeks and nose of face. Most often appears after sun exposure. Less common features: scaly, bumpy, edema. Rarely blisters. Can come and go quite quickly. Sometime extends to outer arms, dorsal hands (sparing the knuckles), and other parts of the upper body. Leg involvement rare.
- Subacute Cutaneous LE (SCLE) – psoriasis-like scaly rash or ringworm-shaped scaly rash on the sun-exposed areas of the outer arms, backs of hands, neck, shoulders, upper trunk. Relative sparing of central face. Can be precipitated by treatment with some systemic drugs (e.g., more commonly – hydrochlorothiazide, diltiazem, terbinafine, cinnarizine; less commonly – griseofulvin, naproxen, aldactone, captopril, cilazapril, verapamil, nifedipine, interferon beta, ranitidine, piroxicam, D-penicillamine, sulfonylureas, procainamide, oxyprenolol, gold salts).
- Discoid LE (DLE) – scaly, coin-shaped skin changes that usually develop on the scalp and face. Commonly produces circumscribed hair loss.
  - ➤ All – red skin lesions, photosensitivity, absence of pruritus, pain or tenderness in lesions

Signs & Symptoms
- ACLE – symmetrical, butterfly-shaped erythematous skin on malar eminences and bridge of nose (with or without associated papules and mild scale). Sometimes presents as a predominately papular eruption.
- SCLE – discrete or confluent, non-indurated, scaly psoriasis-like plaques (psoriasiform) or ring-shaped (annular) lesions on the sun-exposed areas of upper trunk, neck and arms with relative sparing of the central face. Central face involvement suggests concurrent presence of ACLE.
- DLE – localized (above the neck only) or generalized (above and below the neck) scaly, coin-shaped plaques or nodules of

variable-size that usually develop one or more of the following features over time: keratotic follicular plugging; hyperpigmentation at the outer borders of lesions; hypopigmentation, telangiectasia and atrophic scarring at the center of lesions. Focal, scarring alopecia with scalp involvement.

➤ All – red skin lesions, sun-exposed distribution

TESTS

Basic Blood Tests

■ ACLE – positive ANA, elevated ESR, anemia, leukopenia, thrombocytopenia, hypocomplementemia, abnormal renal function, increased serum globulins, anti-phospholipid autoantibodies.

■ SCLE – positive ANA, Ro/SS-A (can be present in absence of ANA)

■ DLE – ANA is usually negative, but with human substrates low titers are possible

Basic Urine Tests

■ ACLE – proteinuria, hematuria, cellular casts

■ SCLE – usually normal

■ DLE – normal

Specific Diagnostic Tests

■ ACLE – double-stranded DNA and Sm autoantibodies

■ SCLE – Ro/SS-A and La/SS-B autoantibodies

■ DLE – none

Other Tests as Appropriate

■ All – lesional skin biopsy (routine H&E examination) of skin reveals LE-specific skin disease pattern known as an interface dermatitis

■ All – lesional skin biopsy (direct immunofluorescence examination) for selected patients in whom diagnosis is in question

DIFFERENTIAL DIAGNOSIS

■ ACLE – dermatomyositis, acne rosacea, seborrheic dermatitis, photoallergic or phototoxic drug eruptions

■ SCLE – polymorphous light eruption, photosensitive psoriasis, erythema annulare centrifugum and other annular reactive skin disorders

■ DLE – granuloma faciale, sarcoidosis

MANAGEMENT

What to Do First

1. All – evaluate carefully for evidence of underlying systemic LE (SLE) activity. If found, treat appropriately with systemic immunomodulatory therapy (corticosteroids, antimalarials).
2. SCLE – assess for the possibility of drug induction (as discussed above) as a cause and discontinue in applicable situations.

General Measures

■ All – counsel patient about the relationships between cutaneous and systemic manifestations of LE to allay fears and encourage compliance (ACLE – greatest risk, localized DLE – lowest risk, SCLE – low to intermediate risk). Encourage use of sunscreens. Educate about ultraviolet light avoidance techniques.

SPECIFIC THERAPY

Indications

■ Presence of symptomatic skin disease

Treatment Options

■ All – topical corticosteroid creams, ointments, gels, foams, and solutions with careful attention to location, strength and duration of treatment to prevent atrophogenic side effects in skin. Intralesional injections of triamcinolone acetonide may be useful as an adjunctive therapy.
■ Hydroxychloroquine without or with or other antimalarial agent (quinacrine) for non- or partial responders
■ Alternative systemic therapy: dapsone, retinoids, thalidomide, immunosuppressives, particularly methotrexate, azathioprine or mycophenolate mofetil

FOLLOW-UP

During Treatment

■ All – watch for treatment side effects and development or exacerbation of intercurrent SLE activity. Ophthalmologic examination at baseline and bi-annual while on hydroxychloroquine or chloroquine. Cigarette smoking in some individuals blunts the clinical response of cutaneous LE to antimalarial.

Routine

■ All – actively treat skin disease activity when flaring. Cautious withdrawal of therapy when skin disease activity remits (some patients can have prolonged treatment-free remissions). Watch for development of intercurrent SLE.

COMPLICATIONS AND PROGNOSIS
- ACLE – associated with high risk of SLE. Ultimate prognosis is dependent on severity of SLE.
- SCLE – Post-inflammatory hyperpigmentation and hypopigmentation. Course marked by intermittent periods of skin disease activity. Risk for developing Sjogren's syndrome is approximately 20%; for clinically significant SLE, approximately 10%.
- DLE – severe dystrophic scarring of skin and permanent hair loss that can be psychosocially and occupationally disabling. <5% risk of developing clinically significant SLE when isolated DLE lesions are the presenting manifestation of the disease.

CUTANEOUS VASCULITIS

VICTORIA P. WERTH, MD

HISTORY & PHYSICAL

Risk Factors
- **Infection:** Hepatitis B or C, rarely A, acute respiratory infections (viral or bacterial), streptococcal, bacterial endocarditis, intestinal bypass syndrome, mycobacterial
- **Drugs:** most common – aspirin, sulfonamides, penicillins, barbiturates, amphetamines, propylthiouracil, TNF inhibitors
- **Rheumatic diseases:** Systemic lupus erythematosus, rheumatoid arthritis, dermatomyositis, Sjogren's syndrome
- **Abnormal globulins:** cryoglobulinemia, myeloma
- **Genetic:** complement deficiency
- **Other:** ulcerative colitis, malignancy

Signs & Symptoms
- Small vessel vasculitis:
  - ➤ palpable purpura (often in dependent areas like legs) or urticaria-like, less commonly vesiculobullous, pustules, cutaneous necrosis, ulceration
  - ➤ Can have symptomatic involvement of other organs. Gastrointestinal tract symptoms include colicky pain, hemorrhage, ulceration, and perforation.
  - ➤ Kidney involvement is usually asymptomatic.

> Lung involvement includes pleuritis, effusions, nodules, infiltrates, or cavitation.
> Neurologic involvement has symptoms of neuropathy, cephalalgia, intracranial hemorrhage.
> Henoch-Schonlein purpura (HSP) – palpable purpura, abdominal pain, arthritis, nephritis
■ Medium and large vessel vasculitis:
> livedo reticularis, purpura, nodules, necrosis, ulceration
> Systemic disease is similar to that seen with small vessel vasculitis, but is more frequent and often more serious.

TESTS

Laboratory
■ Basic blood studies:
> Complete blood count, sedimentation rate, cryoglobulin, serum protein electrophoresis, hepatitis profile, anti-nuclear antibody, serum complement levels, tests of renal and liver function
■ Basic urine studies:
> Look for hematuria or proteinuria, which can indicate possible renal involvement.

Screening
■ Confirmatory Tests
> Anti-neutrophil cytoplasmic antibody (ANCA) test to evaluate type of vasculitis
> p-ANCA non-specific, various vasculitides
> c-ANCA is more specific for Wegener's granulomatosis.

Imaging
■ Chest x-ray if there are pulmonary symptoms
■ CT or MRI of head if there are central neurologic findings
■ Mesenteric arteriography if skin findings of medium vessel vasculitis and abdominal symptoms suggesting of polyarteritis nodosa

Biopsy
■ Skin biopsy to confirm vasculitis and type of vessel involved (small or medium)
■ Skin biopsy for direct immunofluorescence to evaluate type of immunoglobulin in vessel wall. IgA is commonly seen in early HSP lesions.
■ Renal biopsy to evaluate possible renal vasculitis if type of renal lesion unclear

DIFFERENTIAL DIAGNOSIS

- Macular purpura can be seen in thrombocytopenia, Rocky Mountain spotted fever, or hemorrhagic disorders
- Pustules may be seen in infections like disseminated gonorrhea and bacterial or fungal endocarditis.
- Palpable purpura can be seen in embolic disorders, such as endocarditis, cholesterol emboli, and left atrial myxoma.

MANAGEMENT

What to Do First

- assess presence of systemic disease, particularly gastrointestinal, renal, or neurologic
- determine type of vasculitis, based on type of skin lesions, other clinical findings, laboratory tests

General Measures

- Determine possible precipitating causes, such as drugs or infection, underlying diseases.

SPECIFIC THERAPY

Indications

- Type of therapy is determined by the extent of skin disease, the type of vasculitis, and involvement of other organs

Treatment Options

- Skin Disease only
  - Mild Disease
    - **Colchicine:** Periodically check CBC.
    - **Dapsone:** Check G6PD at baseline. Recheck CBC, hepatic function panel every week as dapsone dose is increased.
    - Consider combination of Colchicine and dapsone
  - Moderate to severe (extensive skin lesions ± systemic involvement)
    - **Prednisone:** Short course
    - **Methotrexate**: This is especially helpful for cutaneous polyarteritis nodosa.
    - **Azathioprine:** Used as glucocorticoid-sparing agent in patients requiring long-term steroids
    - **Cyclophosphamide:** Used as glucocorticoid-sparing agent in severe disease, certain types of vasculitis (e.g., Wegener's), and severe disease refractory to other therapies
    - **Intravenous immunoglobulin:** severe disease

• **Apheresis:** severe vasculitis. This usually requires an immuno-suppressive agent in addition to prevent rebound

FOLLOW-UP

During Treatment

■ Look for development of systemic symptoms. Follow skin exam and other relevant organs. Monitor blood for toxicity related to drugs and evidence of systemic vasculitis, urinalysis, Hemoccult stool.

Routine

■ After skin lesions resolve, follow patient monthly or bimonthly until off treatment. After that, follow yearly unless there is evidence of active systemic disease or new symptoms develop

COMPLICATIONS AND PROGNOSIS

Complications

■ Can develop systemic disease at any point. Delayed onset of renal involvement after resolution of skin disease can occur in some forms of vasculitis (Henoch-Schonlein purpura). Those with a generalized distribution of lesions, with lesions not just on the lower extremities, are at higher risk of systemic disease.

Prognosis

■ An acute episode of vasculitis will often resolve and not recur. There are certainly patients who have prolonged courses of skin-only leukocytoclastic vasculitis and never progress to systemic disease. Other patients can progress or initially have systemic disease, and occasionally this can be chronic. Therapy must be targeted based on the organs involved, and usually disease can be controlled, if not eradicated.

CYCLOSPORIASIS

J. GORDON FRIERSON, MD

HISTORY & PHYSICAL

History

■ Exposure: ingestion of cysts of Cyclospora cayetanensis via contaminated food and water (presumed mechanism, full life cycle not yet demonstrated). Waterborne outbreaks described.

Signs & Symptoms
- Watery diarrhea, nausea, vomiting, abdominal cramps, belching, sometimes fever. Abdominal exam may show mild tenderness, distention. Symptoms last 6–7 weeks.

TESTS
- Basic tests: blood: usually normal
- Basic tests: urine: normal
- Specific tests: Stool O&P examination, using acid-fast staining. May need several stools.
- Other tests: not easily detected by small bowel biopsy

DIFFERENTIAL DIAGNOSIS
- Other causes of watery diarrhea, especially giardiasis, isosporiasis, cryptosporidial infection, travelers' diarrhea

MANAGEMENT
What to Do First
- Assess need for fluid and/or electrolyte therapy.

General Measures
- Assess source of infection.

SPECIFIC THERAPY
Indications
- All symptomatic patients

Treatment Options
- Trimethoprim-sulfamethoxazole for 7 days. Treat for 10 days in immunosuppressed patients.

Side Effects & Complications
- Allergy to sulfa component may occur. Sometimes GI upset from medications.
- Contraindications to treatment: absolute: allergy to medications
- Contraindications to treatment: relative: asymptomatic patients

FOLLOW-UP
During Treatment
- Observe for tolerance of meds.

Routine
- Stool examination 2–3 weeks after completing therapy

COMPLICATIONS AND PROGNOSIS
- Prognosis good in normal and immunosuppressed patients

CYST OF TUNICA ALBUGINEA OF TESTIS

ARTHUR I. SAGALOWSKY, MD

HISTORY & PHYSICAL
- 1–2 mm, asymptomatic, round mass on surface of testis

TESTS
- ultrasound confirmatory

DIFFERENTIAL DIAGNOSIS
n/a

MANAGEMENT
n/a

SPECIFIC THERAPY
- observation

FOLLOW-UP
n/a

COMPLICATIONS AND PROGNOSIS
n/a

CYSTIC FIBROSIS

ERIC LEONG, MD, FRCPC

HISTORY & PHYSICAL

Symptoms and Signs
- Usually asymptomatic; vague RUQ pain; neonatal cholestasis seen in few patients; cholecystitis or cholangitis with gallstone disease; cirrhosis with liver failure if advanced
- Symptomatic stage: hepatosplenomegaly, variceal bleeding
- Pulmonary disease and pancreatic insufficiency often predominate

TESTS

Basic Tests: Blood
- Early disease: liver biochemistry intermittently abnormal, with 41% prevalence at 12 years of age
- Advanced disease: low albumin, elevated bilirubin and INR

Specific Diagnostic Tests
- Sweat chloride test: low chloride concentration
- Genetic test: no specific gene mutation occurs more frequently in patients with liver disease

Imaging
- Ultrasound: nodular, coarse liver in biliary cirrhosis, or increased echogenicity in hepatic steatosis; gallstones in up to 25%; micro-gallbladder in up to 20%
- Cholangiogram: focal biliary stricturing and dilatation

Liver Biopsy
- Significant sampling error can occur due to patchy fibrosis; focal biliary cirrhosis often seen, leading to multilobular biliary cirrhosis in 10%; may see giant cells, bile plugs, or bile duct proliferation among the 30% with neonatal cholestasis

DIFFERENTIAL DIAGNOSIS
- Neonates & infants: neonatal (giant cell) hepatitis, TORCH (toxoplasma, rubella, cytomegalovirus, herpes virus), syndromic/non-syndromic bile duct paucity, extrahepatic biliary atresia, choledochal cyst, neonatal sclerosing cholangitis, alpha-1-antitrypsin deficiency, tyrosinemia, Gaucher's disease, Niemann-Pick disease, galactosemia, fructosemia, hypothyroidism, Crigler-Najjar syndromes
- Adults: primary biliary cirrhosis, primary sclerosing cholangitis, choledochal cyst, cholangiocarcinoma, ampullary neoplasm, pancreatic neoplasm

MANAGEMENT

What to Do First
- Assess severity of liver disease and complications: history of meconium ileus and pancreatic insufficiency may be predictive of development of liver disease, which predominantly occurs in first decade of life
- Determine candidacy for therapy

General Measures
- Adjust or avoid potentially hepatotoxic drugs
- Optimize pulmonary function; optimize nutritional status in those with pancreatic insufficiency
- Evaluate stage of liver disease
- Sweat chloride test if diagnosis is not established

SPECIFIC THERAPY

Indications for Treatment
- Medical therapy to improve nutritional status
- Liver transplantation for decompensated cirrhosis

Treatment Options
- Pancreatic enzyme replacement: lipase PO with each meal or snack if pancreatic-insufficient
- Ursodeoxycholic acid: improves liver biochemistry and may improve liver histology in early disease
- Liver transplantation: patients with end-stage liver disease and mild pulmonary involvement

FOLLOW-UP

During Treatment and Routine
- Monitor patient's nutritional status, LFTs every 3 to 6 months
- Closely monitor whole blood cyclosporine levels after liver transplantation; intestinal malabsorption and altered drug metabolism may necessitate higher dosages

COMPLICATIONS AND PROGNOSIS
- Gallstones: in up to 25%; consider cholecystectomy if symptomatic
- Hepatic steatosis: frequently seen; improved nutrition appears to reduce incidence
- Cirrhosis: develops in up to 8–10% of all cystic fibrosis patients at a median age of 10 years; accounts for almost all non-pulmonary causes of mortality
- Pulmonary: see Pulmonary section
- Pancreatic insufficiency: frequent

Prognosis
- Median life expectancy almost 30 years

CYSTIC FIBROSIS

MICHAEL S. STULBARG, MD
REVISED BY ANDREA GLASSBERG, MD

HISTORY & PHYSICAL

- Most common inherited disorder in Caucasians; may occur with any ethnicity
- Autosomal recessive inheritance (chromosome 7); more than 800 genetic defects described, but delta F 508 most common.
- Recurrent episodes of cough and purulent sputum, often from childhood; associated with minor hemoptysis, fatigue, weight loss; diagnosis may not be suspected into adulthood
- *S aureus* predominates early, *P aeruginosa*, usually mucoid, later; other gram-negative rods (eg, *Stenotrophomonas maltophilia*, *Burkholderia cepacia*) may become major pathogen
- Colonization with *Aspergillus* and nontuberculous mycobacteria common but usually not significant
- Associated conditions:
  - Pancreatic insufficiency with steatorrhea, weight loss
  - Diabetes mellitus, in about 20%
  - Sinusitis almost universal, may be dominant problem
  - Chronic diarrhea or constipation, sometimes with abdominal pain, nausea, vomiting (if severe = DIOS, distal intestinal obstruction syndrome)
  - Abdominal pain common with increased incidence of gallstones and pancreatitis, DIOS
  - Liver dysfunction common (ie, increased alkaline phosphatase); liver failure rare (< 1%)
  - Azospermia almost uniform in men; women with decreased rates of pregnancy

Signs & Symptoms

- Recurrent cough, purulent sputum, with or without precipitating event; with progression, daily productive cough
- Chronic: symptoms like chronic bronchitis: chronic cough, dyspnea, wheezing; yellow to green sputum, often with blood streaks
- Cachexia, respiratory distress, clubbing; abdomen may have fecal masses, esp in right lower quadrant
- Mild: lungs may be clear
- Advanced: early crackles, esp in upper chest

- Exacerbations:
  - Insidious presentation most common, with increasing cough, dyspnea, fatigue, anorexia and often weight loss
  - Acute presentations after viral infections
  - Fever usually low grade or absent
  - Musculoskeletal or pleural pain

Complications:
- Hemoptysis: may be life-threatening
- Pneumothorax
- Respiratory failure
- Hyperglycemia, hypoglycemia, almost never ketoacidosis
- Bowel obstruction

TESTS

Laboratory
- Basic tests:
  - Sweat chloride: <40 mEq/L = normal; 40–60 mEq/L suggestive, >60 diagnostic
  - Hematology: leukocytosis, mild anemia common
  - ABG: for suspected ventilatory failure
  - Abdominal pain: amylase, liver functions
  - Diabetes: fasting blood glucose, hemoglobin A1C
  - Pancreatic insufficiency: protime, vitamin A and E
- Cultures:
  - Gram stain/culture for bacteria: *S aureus, P aeruginosa, H influenza*, other gram-neg rods
  - Culture for mycobacteria, fungus
  - Blood cultures rarely helpful
- Spirometry:
  - Key to decision making (eg, when worse by 10–20%)

Imaging
- CXR: hyperinflation, bronchial wall thickening, scattered nodular densities, cystic changes; upper lobe predominance; look for pneumothorax, consolidation
- CT rarely helpful

DIFFERENTIAL DIAGNOSIS
- Sinusitis
- Bronchiectasis of other cause
- Pneumothorax

MANAGEMENT

What to Do First
- Assess oxygenation, adequacy of ventilation, need for admission (as for COPD)

General Measures
- Initiate antibiotics (usually 2–3 wks), nutritional assessment and respiratory therapy
- Hospitalization may be more for nutrition, respiratory therapy than antibiotics

SPECIFIC THERAPY

Indications
- Combination of increased symptoms, weight loss, hemoptysis, worsening spirometry
- Patients usually know when inpatient care necessary

Treatment Options
- Bronchodilators: as for COPD
- Inhaled steroids: often tried; high doses may be more effective; titrate down for safety
- Antibiotics: base on recent organism and sensitivities; higher than standard doses are required; use central line (ie, percutaneous or indwelling port):
  - ➤ *S aureus*: usually penicillin resistant
  - ➤ *Pseudomonas*: double drug therapy required (2 of 3 classes)
    - Beta lactam: eg, ceftazadime, piperacillin, meropenem
    - Quinolone: ciprofloxacin
    - Aminoglycoside: gentamicin or tobramycin
- Inhaled tobramycin: useful for chronic Pseudomonas colonization
- Inhaled DNAse: prevents exacerbations; no benefit for acute exacerbation
- Respiratory therapy: patient preference important:
  - ➤ Traditional: chest physiotherapy with postural drainage
  - ➤ Mechanical devices: flutter valve, PEP mask, mechanical percussor, chest vest, positive pressure oscillation (IPV)
- Ventilatory support:
  - ➤ Partial: nasal mask ventilation useful as temporizing maneuver or bridge to lung transplantation
  - ➤ Mechanical ventilation: used for acute respiratory failure when reasonable hope of extubation

■ Nutritional support: diabetes and pancreatic insufficiency
  ➤ Adequate caloric intake (may need calorie count)
  ➤ Avoid fat restriction, ie, give adequate pancreatic enzymes
  ➤ Diabetes: frequent blood glucose and sliding scale

Side Effects and Complications
■ Antibiotics:
  ➤ Side effects: rash, diarrhea, renal dysfunction (check levels of aminoglycoside for safety)

FOLLOW-UP
■ Continue antibiotic therapy until back to baseline (usually 2–3 wk)
■ Repeat spirometry at end of treatment

COMPLICATIONS AND PROGNOSIS
Complications
■ Hemoptysis: if life-threatening or no response to antibiotics, consider bronchial artery embolization
■ Failure to respond to antibiotics: consider drug resistance, unusual organisms (eg, fungus, mycobacteria)
■ Ventilatory failure: consider nasal mask ventilation; full mechanical ventilation used with reluctance because of difficulty weaning

Prognosis
■ Median survival 31 y
■ Consider lung transplantation for advanced disease

CYSTICERCOSIS

J. GORDON FRIERSON, MD

HISTORY & PHYSICAL
History
■ Exposure: ingesting *Taenia solium* eggs in contaminated food or water or from dirty hands. Life cycle: *Taenia solium* (pork tapeworm) acquired by man from eating undercooked pork containing encysted larvae (cysticercoids). After maturing, segments of the tapeworm are passed in stool, the eggs of which are infectious for man and pig. Upon ingestion, larvae from the eggs are absorbed and pass to brain, muscle, and SQ tissue, where they encyst.

Signs & Symptoms
- Neurocysticercosis: often no symptoms. May present with seizures (most common presentation), focal neurologic signs, or chronic headache (from increased intracranial pressure).
- Cysticercosis elsewhere: SQ nodules, about 1–2 cm in size. Occasionally retro-orbital or subretinal.

TESTS
- Basic tests: blood: CBC, chemistries are normal
- Basic tests: urine: normal
- Specific tests: neurocysticercosis: MRI or CT scans are suggestive, and in endemic areas probably diagnostic. MRI preferred as CT will not show cysts in ventricles. MRI and CT also help determine viability and stage of degeneration of cysts, and assess if hydrocephalus present. Serology, using immunoblot technique (done at CDC), about 98% sensitive if multiple cysts, about 70% if one cyst, and highly specific. Immunoblot serology on CSF has same accuracy.
  - ➤ Cysticercosis elsewhere: Biopsy of SQ nodule is diagnostic. Soft tissue X-rays of muscles (or cranium) can show calcified cysts if old enough (>5 years).
- Other tests: CSF exam can be normal or show increased cells, mainly lymphocytes. Eosinophils often present but require staining to see.

DIFFERENTIAL DIAGNOSIS
- Neurocysticercosis: tuberculoma, neoplasm, other types of cysts, abscess or focal area of infection by bacteria, fungus, or toxoplasmosis
- Cysticercosis elsewhere: fibromas, lipomas, sebaceous cysts

MANAGEMENT
What to Do First
- Assess patient for presence of both intracranial and extracranial disease. If intracranial, assess for hydrocephalus, and stage of cysts (ring enhancement implies leakage of antigen and early degeneration, calcium implies later stage or dead cyst). Assess for presence of *Taenia solium* in bowel by stool exam and asking about passing segments (eggs not always seen on stool exam). Treat *T. solium* if present.

General Measures
- Control seizures with anticonvulsants, and hydrocephalus with steroids and possible shunting.

SPECIFIC THERAPY

Indications
- Treat patients with viable cysts (those without ring enhancement) and signs of mass effect. Treatment of patients with cysts in stages of degeneration, with or without focal symptoms or seizures, is controversial.

Treatment Options
- Albendazole for 8–20 days. Repeat if needed.
- Praziquantel for 15 days. Repeat if needed.

Side Effects & Complications
- Death of cysts can cause inflammation, headache, seizures. Control this with dexamethasone, and taper, or administer steroids prophylactically (especially with large number of cysts). Steroids enhance absorption of albendazole, reduce absorption of praziquantel. Albendazole can cause mild GI distress, in longer courses can cause neutropenia, alopecia, liver function abnormalities. Prazquantel can cause mild GI distress, malaise, dizziness, urticaria, all usually mild.
- Contraindications to treatment: absolute: dead, calcified cysts
- Contraindications to treatment: relative: asymptomatic patients with viable or degenerating cysts (this is a controversial area)

FOLLOW-UP

During Treatment
- Observe for headache, seizures, altered consciousness, due to sudden death of parasites.

Routine
- Serial MRI or CT scans. If viable cysts remain, re-treat. If seizure-free in 2 years and EEG normal, can stop anticonvulsants. Educate patient about epidemiology to prevent reinfection.

COMPLICATIONS AND PROGNOSIS
- Prognosis generally good in absence of hydrocephalus, though seizures may be permanent. Shunts frequently clog up due to cyst debris, and outlook poor. Periodic steroids may prevent shunt obstruction.

CYSTINURIA

MICHEL BAUM, MD

HISTORY & PHYSICAL
- History of severe flank pain, may have history of gross hematuria
- Recurrent renal stones – usually start in second and third decade

TESTS
- Urinalysis with hexagonal cystine crystals, hematuria
- Urinary cystine >250 mg/g creatinine

DIFFERENTIAL DIAGNOSIS
- Autosomal recessive disorder due to defect in dibasic amino acid transporter resulting in increased urinary excretion of lysine, arginine, ornithine, and cystine
- Distinguish from other causes of nephrolithiasis.

MANAGEMENT
n/a

SPECIFIC THERAPY
- Fluid intake
- Alkalinize urine to pH 6.5–7.0
- Chelation with Thiola or penicillamine

FOLLOW-UP
- To assess response to cystine excretion and complications of therapy
- To assess renal function
- Sonograms looking for new stones

COMPLICATIONS AND PROGNOSIS
Renal insufficiency results from recurrent stone formation and repeated interventions.

CYSTITIS AND PYELONEPHRITIS

GARY SINCLAIR, MD

HISTORY & PHYSICAL
- It is essential to distinguish between lower urinary tract infections (cystitis) and upper urinary tract infections (pyelonephritis).

- Lower urinary tract infections present with dysuria, urgency, and frequency.
- Upper urinary tract infections present with fever, nausea, rigors, and back pain.
- In males, prostate exam should be considered to rule out prostatitis (gently if acute prostatitis expected).
- In women, pelvic exam should be considered to rule out cervicitis, pelvic inflammatory disease.
- Bladder palpation and percussion should be used to assess for urinary retention.

TESTS
- Dipstick urinalysis – assess for leukocyte esterase and nitrites (leuckocyte esterase is more sensitive, nitrites are more specific)
- Microscopic urinalysis – assess for white blood cells (pyuria ≥ 10 wbc/hpf in a centrifuged urine sample), red blood cells, and casts (WBC can be present in pyelonephritis)
- Urine Gram stain to guide empiric therapy
- Midstream urine and blood (if febrile) cultures – suspect Escherichia coli, Enterococcus sp., Klebsiella sp., Enterobacater sp., Serratia sp., Proteus sp., Morganella sp. and Providencia sp. in outpatient setting, Pseudomonas sp., Candida sp. in hospitalized patient
- Peripheral WBC count (normal in cystitis, elevated in pyelonephritis)
- Post void residual if urinary obstruction is suspected
- Assess for renal calculi by non-contrast CT scan if severe pain or failure to respond to treatment (no dramatic improvement within 24 h of appropriate antibiotics, recurrence after completion of treatment, or persistent bacteriuria, fever, or pain despite appropriate antibiotic selection)
- Assess for perinephric abscess by either ultrasound or CT (same criteria as for renal calculi, see above)

DIFFERENTIAL DIAGNOSIS
- Urethritis, cervicitis, pelvic inflammatory disease, prostatitis, prostatic abscess, renal calculi, urinary obstruction, appendicitis, diverticulitis, ectopic pregnancy

MANAGEMENT
- Hydration
- Relief of urinary obstruction (catheter)
- Removal of foreign object (replace or preferably remove indwelling bladder catheters whenever possible)

SPECIFIC THERAPY

■ Simple cystitis in woman can be treated with a 3-day oral course of an appropriate antibiotic.

■ Generally, do not treat asymptomatic bacteriuria (pregnancy, kidney transplant, immunocompromise, anatomic abnormalities, impending surgery are exceptions to this rule; bladder catheter is not an exception).

■ Complicated urinary tract infections (anatomic abnormality, obstruction, hospital-acquired organism, indwelling bladder catheter) require at least 10 days of therapy.

■ Urinary tract infections in men are always considered complicated (and require evaluation of genitourinary anatomy; stongly consider Urology consultation).

■ Pyelonephritis requires 14 days of IV or IV equivalent (oral quinolone) therapy.

■ Whenever possible, Gram stain should be used to guide empiric choice of antibiotics.

■ Community acquired Gram-negative infections generally respond to third-generation cephalosporins, quinolones, and trimethoprimsulfamethoxazole.

■ Ampicillin (or vancomycin for hospital-acquired organisms) is the agent of choice for Enterococccus sp., though simple cystitis may respond to trimethoprim-sulfamethoxazole, quinolones, Macrodantin, or doxycycline. Linezolid is effective for Vancomycinresistant enterococci but should be reserved for severe or lifethreatening infections.

■ Hospital-acquired urinary tract infections may require antipseudomonal penicillin with or without a beta-lactamase inhibitor, ceftazidime, imipenem, aztreonam, or quinolone therapy.

■ Candidal urinary tract infections can be treated with fluconazole. For resistant Candida sp, a single dose of amphotericin B has been found effective in some patients. Liposomal formulations of amphotericin do not penetrate the renal parenchyma or bladder and should not be used. Newer azoles and echinocandins may play a role in highly resistant infections. Consider ID consultation.

FOLLOW-UP

■ Expect rapid (within 24 h) improvement for treatment of acute urinary tract infections.

■ If improvement not rapid, consider complications (see below).

■ Test of cure not necessary if patient becomes asymptomatic

COMPLICATIONS AND PROGNOSIS
■ Prostatic abscess (requires drainage – can be source of fever of unknown origin), perinephric abscess, bacteremia, urinary obstruction, emphysematous pyelonephritis

---

CYTOMEGALOVIRUS

CAROL A. GLASER, MD

HISTORY & PHYSICAL
■ DNA virus/member of herpesvirus group (herpesvirus 5)
■ Human only reservoir
■ Transmission via:
  ➢ direct personal contact with bodily secretions, saliva, tears, urine, stool, semen
  ➢ Vertical: mother to infant before, during and after birth (including breast milk)
  ➢ Blood transfusion
■ Incubation period; 3–12 weeks following blood transfusion, 1–4 months after tissue transplantation, incubation period unknown in household transmission
■ No seasonal predilection
■ Persists in latent form after primary infection
■ Most common cause of congenital infection
■ Most common cause of posttransplant infection (source can be reactivation, donor organ, or blood products)
■ Infection higher in lower socioeconomic groups
■ Large variation, seroprevalence varies 30–90%

Signs & Symptoms
■ Most asymptomatic in normal hosts or
■ Mononucleosis-like syndrome
  ➢ Prolonged fever; malaise, myalgia, pharyngitis, hepatosplenomegly, mild hepatitis. Can also cause organ-specific disease: colitis, encephalitis, Guillain-Barré, myocarditis.
  In immunocompromised hosts:
More severe organ-specific disease. Pneumonitis can mimic rejection in lung transplant. Chorioretinitis primarily seen in AIDS

TESTS

Nonspecific
- Moderate elevation of transaminases
- Lymphocytosis with atypical monocytes
- Negative heterophils

Specific
- Non-congenital: difficult due to increase number of asymptomatic infection and relapsing infection. May need multiple methods for accurate diagnosis:
  - ➤ 4-fold rise IgG antibody in paired sera
  - ➤ IgM antibody may be helpful (but invariably present)
  - ➤ Recovery of virus from target organ is optimal
  - ➤ Peripheral blood antigenemia in immunocompromised
  - ➤ Nucleic acid amplification techniques commercially available
- Congenital; viral isolation best method – urine is excellent sample

DIFFERENTIAL DIAGNOSIS
Other causes of mononucleosis syndrome in immunocompetent pt; acute rejection post lung transplant; overall differential broad in immunocompromised host

MANAGEMENT
If severe, immunosuppressive agents may need to be changed or dose reduced.

SPECIFIC THERAPY
- DHPG or Ganciclovir phosphonoformate has been used for immunocompromised patients.
  Valganciclovir (oral) – treatment of AIDS retinitis, prevention post-transplant
- Foscarnet another option
  Cidofovir in AIDS (cannot be given with CSA or tacrolimus in post-transplant)
  AIDS retinitis – ganciclovir intraocular implant
- CMV-IgG is available and may be beneficial in some settings.

FOLLOW-UP
Full supportive care in severe disease in immunocompromised pt

COMPLICATIONS AND PROGNOSIS
- Symptomatic congenital; IUGR, jaundice, HSM, thrombocytopenia, microcephaly, mild hepatitis

- In immunocompromised (usually profoundly immunosuppressed), wide spectrum:
  - Asymptomatic
  - Hepatitis
  - Retinitis
  - Pneumonitis

DEEP VENOUS THROMBOSIS

RAJABRATA SARKAR, MD

HISTORY & PHYSICAL

History
- Slow onset of leg or arm swelling, pain and edema
- Predisposing conditions
  - Leg or pelvic trauma
  - Pregnancy
  - Malignancy
  - Obesity
  - Nephrotic syndrome
  - Intravenous drug abuse
  - Oral contraceptive use
  - Indwelling venous catheters
  - History of prior deep venous thrombus (DVT)
  - Prior episode of post-operative "leg swelling" (undiagnosed prior DVT)
  - Known hypercoagulable states
    - Factor V Leyden mutation
    - Protein C or S deficiency
    - Lupus anticoagulant
    - Antithrombin III deficiency
    - Hyperhomocysteinemia

Signs & Symptoms
- Swollen edematous limb with diffuse tenderness on deep palpation
- Severe edema with purple changes of skin
  - Suggestive of arterial obstruction secondary to venous obstruction
  - Can have sensory and eventually motor changes

TESTS

Blood

- Hypercoagulable workup only in pts without predisposing condition; so-called "idiopathic DVT"; blood for w/u must be drawn BEFORE heparin is started
  - D-dimer levels
  - Very sensitive; not very specific
  - Can be used to rule out DVT but not diagnose it

Specific Diagnostic Studies

- Duplex study
  - Highly sensitive and specific
  - Study of choice for DVT
- Contrast venography
  - Currently used only if duplex is nondiagnostic or to separate prior chronic DVT from acute DVT

DIFFERENTIAL DIAGNOSIS

- Cellulitis
  - Warm, red skin
  - Normal duplex study
- Trauma
  - Distinguish by history
  - Duplex to r/o DVT (common in trauma)
- Arterial occlusion
  - Distinguish by history, pulses
  - Duplex may be needed (DVT can occur after arterial thrombosis)

MANAGEMENT

What to Do First

- Immediate anticoagulation
  - Low molecular weight heparin
  - Unfractionated (standard) heparin

General Measures

- Prevent DVT in surgical and bedridden patients with low-dose heparin
- Initial elevation
- Ambulation with elastic stockings

SPECIFIC THERAPY

Indications

▇ Any DVT in the popliteal vein or above
▇ Calf DVT
  ➤ treat with anticoagulation if symptomatic
  ➤ If asymptomatic, anticoagulate, or
  ➤ Observe and document no progression to popliteal v. with serial duplex
  ➤ Only 20% will propagate to higher level
▇ Unfractionated or low-molecule weight (LMW) heparin
  ➤ If using unfractionated heparin, must achieve therapeutic levels within 24 hours
  ➤ Convert to coumadin within 2–3 days
  ➤ LMW heparin allows outpatient treatment, no need to check PTT
  ➤ Contraindications
    • Prior heparin allergy
    • Documented prior heparin-induced thrombocyotpenia
    • Ongoing bleeding from another site
    • Recent neurological surgery
  ➤ Side effects
    • Heparin-induced thrombocytopenia (HIT)
      • Develops in 1–3% of patients
      • Can occur with both unfractionated and
      • Has mild (type I) and severe (type II) forms
      • Mild is asymptomatic drop in platelet count
      • Severe is pro-thrombotic with arterial and venous thromboses
      • Discontinue heparin; check anti-platelet Ab titer
      • Switch to either heparinoid or thrombin inhibitor and then coumadin
  ➤ Bleeding
    • Much lower incidence with LMW heparin
    • Treat with: blood replacement if needed and reversal of heparin (fresh frozen plasma)
▇ Coumadin (warfarin sodium)
  ➤ Dose to keep INR between 2 and 3
  ➤ Continue for 6 months
  ➤ If recurrent, may need lifelong treatment
▇ Contraindications
  ➤ Pregnancy – use LMW heparin (can breastfeed also on heparin)
  ➤ Coumadin allergy

- Side Effects
  - Warfarin-induced skin necrosis
  - Due to depletion of Protein C
  - More common in pts with Protein C or S deficiency
  - Caused by initial large coumadin loading dose
  - Avoid large loading dose
- Bleeding
  - Proportional to degree of anticoagulation
  - Treat with: blood replacement if needed and reversal of coumadin (fresh frozen plasma and/or vitamin K)
- Thrombolytic therapy
  - No decrease in post-thrombotic syndrome, pulmonary embolism compared to heparin therapy
  - Increased risk of bleeding (puncture site and intracranial)
- Surgical Thrombectomy
  - Reserved for ileofemoral DVT with impending venous gangrene
  - High incidence of rethrombosis and venous complications

FOLLOW-UP

During Treatment
- Check coagulation studies as needed for heparin (not for LMW) and coumadin
- Counsel patients regarding other meds that alter coumadin activity

Routine
- Check for later development of post-thrombotic syndrome
- Lifelong anticoagulation for patients with documented hypercoaguable syndrome

COMPLICATIONS AND PROGNOSIS

Complications
- Pulmonary Embolism (PE)
  - Most common cause of preventable in-hospital death
  - 200,000 death/year in US
  - Most pts die within 2 hours of PE
  - Treat with heparin (LMW or unfractionated)
  - Consider placement of IVC filter if PE occurs on adequate anticoagulation
- Post-thrombotic syndrome (Chronic venous insufficiency)
  - Occurs in 25% of patients with DVT despite current therapy
    - Major cause of disability in young patients

➤ Ulceration occurs in 10% of these patients
➤ Treat with graduated pressure stockings, elevation

Prognosis
■ Most patients will avoid PE with anticoagulation treatment; some get chronic venous insufficiency despite adequate treatment

DEMENTIA

CHAD CHRISTINE, MD

HISTORY & PHYSICAL
■ Acquired, generalized impairment of cognitive function
■ Slowly progressive disorder (typically over years)
■ Rare hereditary forms
■ Not assoc w/ alteration of level of consciousness
■ May be personality changes
■ Immediate recall intact, but delayed recall & recent memory impaired
■ Parietal lobe dysfunction (pictorial construction, calculations, right left discrimination, performance of complex motor tasks)
■ Frontal lobe dysfunction (judgment, social skills, grasp reflexes)

TESTS

Lab Tests
■ Diagnosis made clinically
■ Serum & CSF studies normal
■ Apoliprotein E e4 allele is a risk factor for Alzheimer's disease
■ Brain imaging may show atrophy

DIFFERENTIAL DIAGNOSIS
■ Degenerative disorders: Pick's disease, Creutzfeldt-Jacob disease, normal-pressure hydrocephalus, dementia w/ Lewy bodies, corticobasal ganglionic degeration, progressive supranuclear palsy excluded clinically
■ Systemic disorders
   ➤ Cancer: primary or metastatic excluded by neuroimaging & CSF cytology
   ➤ Infection: serology studies differentiate AIDS dementia & neurosyphilis

- Metabolic disorders: blood studies differentiate hypothyroidism, vitamin B12 deficiency, hepatic & renal failure
- Vascular disorders: brain imaging excludes chronic subdural hematoma & multi-infarct dementia
- Head trauma: severe open or closed head injury
- Behavioral disorders: history & neuropsychological testing exclude pseudodementia

MANAGEMENT
- Reduce or stop meds that may exacerbate cognitive problems
- Follow Mini-Mental Status Examination

SPECIFIC THERAPY
- Depends on cause

FOLLOW-UP
N/A

COMPLICATIONS AND PROGNOSIS
- Depend on cause

DENT'S DISEASE

MICHEL BAUM, MD

HISTORY & PHYSICAL
- Recurrent renal stones, may have failure to thrive and rickets
- Progressive renal insufficiency

TESTS
- Low-molecular-weight proteinuria, nephrocalcinosis, may have rickets
- May have glucosuria, amino aciduria and phosphaturia (acidosis is rare)
- Most have hypercalciuria

DIFFERENTIAL DIAGNOSIS
- X-linked recessive defect in proximal tubule chloride channel (CLCN5)
- Distinguish from other causes of proteinuria and nephrolithiasis

MANAGEMENT
- Fluid intake, low-salt diet

SPECIFIC THERAPY
- Thiazide diuretics to prevent stone formation may be of benefit.

FOLLOW-UP
- To ensure growth and follow renal function and nephrocalcinosis

COMPLICATIONS AND PROGNOSIS
- Often results in progressive renal insufficiency secondary to nephro-calcinosis and recurrent renal stones

---

DERMATOFIBROMA

JEFFREY P. CALLEN, MD

HISTORY & PHYSICAL

History
- Asymptomatic or symptoms related to surface trauma such as shaving
- More common in women
- May represent the end stage of an insect bite or folliculitis
- Possibly more common in patients with lupus erythematosus

Signs & Symptoms
- Leg lesions are most common, but the arms and trunk might also be affected.
- Flesh-colored, erythematous or hyperpigmented papule or nodule with little surface change
- When the lesion is pinched, it will dimple centrally.

TESTS
- Skin biopsy is diagnostic

DIFFERENTIAL DIAGNOSIS
- Includes keloid, hypertrophic scar, melanoma, basal cell carcinoma, Kaposi sarcoma, dermatofibrosarcoma protuberans

MANAGEMENT
- Surgical removal for symptomatic lesions

SPECIFIC THERAPY
- None

FOLLOW-UP
- After removal, no follow-up is usually needed.

COMPLICATIONS AND PROGNOSIS
- Dermatofibroma persists if not removed.

DIABETES INSIPIDUS

ANDREW R. HOFFMAN, MD

HISTORY & PHYSICAL

History
- Abrupt onset of severe thirst, esp for cold liquids
- Polyuria, polydipsia (may be >1.0 L/h)
- Nocturia
- History of pituitary tumor, surgery, apoplexy, or irradiation
- Head trauma
- Craniopharyngioma
- Dysgerminoma
- Metastatic cancer, esp. breast and lung
- Histiocytosis X, sarcoidosis, TB
- 3rd trimester of pregnancy

Signs & Symptoms
- Dehydration
- Hypernatremia, hyperosmolality
- Altered mental status, coma
- Orthostatic hypotension

TESTS

Laboratory
- Basic studies:
  - Serum sodium, serum osmolality, calcium, glucose
  - Urine osmolality, urine analysis with specific gravity (<1.005 in DI)
- Ancillary tests:
  - Serum ADH (aka AVP)
  - Lithium level
- Dehydration testing: withhold fluids until serum osmolality rises; treat with parenteral DDAVP to distinguish central (pituitary) DI from nephrogenic DI and primary polydipsia

Imaging

- MRI of the pituitary and brain: normal posterior pituitary bright spot on T1 imaging absent in DI

DIFFERENTIAL DIAGNOSIS

- Idiopathic DI
- Primary polydipsia (psychogenic water drinking)
- Nephrogenic diabetes insipidus: congenital, hypercalcemia, lithium use, hypokalemia
- Diabetes mellitus
- In pregnancy, excess vasopressinase from placenta
- Pituitary tumor
- Hypothalamic mass: craniopharyngioma, dysgerminoma, metastases
- Granulomatous disease and histiocytosis
- Pituitary apoplexy

MANAGEMENT

What to Do First

- Treat with DDAVP (parenteral, nasal spray, or tablet)
- Volume and free water replacement
- Rule out nephrogenic DI, hypercalcemia, and diabetes mellitus
- Evaluate pituitary and hypothalamus by MRI

General Measures

- Normalize serum sodium
- Treat hormone deficiencies and excesses
- Normalize serum calcium, glucose

SPECIFIC THERAPY

- Hormone replacement therapy with DDAVP, which has only ADH activity, not pressor (AVP) or oxytocin-like activity
- Replace other hormones as needed: cortisol, thyroid hormone, testosterone, estrogen/progestin, GH
- Surgery for craniopharyngioma
- Radiation therapy for dysgerminoma

Side Effects & Contraindications

- Surgery and radiation side effects: panhypopituitarism, CNS injury

FOLLOW-UP

- Measurements of serum sodium
- Repeat pituitary MRI after 3–6 mo to assess tumor growth

COMPLICATIONS AND PROGNOSIS

- Overtreatment causes hyponatremia and altered mental status
- Undertreatment leads to persistent DI: oral DDAVP may not be adequate, nasal spray has variable absorption
- Patients require lifelong observation
- If idiopathic, other pituitary deficiencies unlikely
- May occur transiently after pituitary surgery, then may be followed by SIADH within 1 wk; SIADH may resolve or revert to permanent DI ("triple response")
- DI during pregnancy from increased vasopressinase resolves postpartum
- Initiation of glucocorticoid and thyroid hormone replacement in hypopituitarism may unmask or markedly worsen DI
- Lithium-induced nephrogenic DI may persist long after drug stopped

---

DIABETES MELLITUS, TYPE 1

FREDRIC B. KRAEMER, MD

HISTORY & PHYSICAL

History
- Known type 1 diabetes
- Family history of type 1 diabetes
- Recent history of mumps or viral infection
- Pancreatectomy

Signs & Symptoms
- Presentation: polyuria, polydipsia, nocturia, polyphagia, weight loss, fatigue, blurred vision, candidiasis, recurrent furunculosis
- Diabetic ketoacidosis (DKA):
- Symptoms: polyuria, polydipsia, nocturia, polyphagia, weight loss, fatigue, abdominal pain, nausea/vomiting, weakness, drowsiness, stupor, coma
- Signs: tachycardia, hypothermia, dehydration, Kussmaul respiration, altered mental status

Established disease:
- Visual changes: blurred vision, floating specks, loss of vision
- Paresthesias, numbness, lancinating, burning/aching pain, coldness, usually affecting lower extremities, usually worse at night

- Dysphagia, early satiety, bloating, nausea/vomiting, diarrhea, constipation
- Impotence, incontinence
- Claudication
- Foot ulcers
- Microaneurysms, hemorrhages, exudates, cotton wool spots, new vessels
- Loss of sensation, proprioception, temperature discrimination, absent ankle jerks
- Hammerhead deformity of toes, calluses, ulcers
- Miosis, diminished pupillary dilation
- Resting tachycardia, postural hypotension
- Necrobiosis lipoidicum diabeticorum
- Diminished/absent pulses in lower extremities

TESTS

Laboratory
- Basic blood studies:
  - Established disease: elevated glucose, HgbA1c, creatinine, dyslipidemia
  - Ketoacidosis: elevated glucose, electrolyte abnormalities, acidemia, reduced bicarbonate, positive ketones
- Basic urine studies:
  - Established disease: albuminuria
  - Ketoacidosis: glycosuria, ketonuria
- Specific diagnostic tests
  - Anti GAD (glutamic acid decarboxylase), anti-insulin, anti-islet cell antibodies, C-peptide

DIFFERENTIAL DIAGNOSIS
- Type 2 diabetes mellitus
- Diabetic ketoacidosis; alcoholic ketoacidosis; anion gap acidosis; methanol, ethylene glycol, salicylate overdose, uremia, lactic acidosis

MANAGEMENT

What to Do First
- Diabetic ketoacidosis:
  - Start hydration and insulin
  - Search for precipitating factor: omission of insulin most common, infection, MI, stroke

■ Established disease: assess degree of control, presence of complications/associated conditions

General Measures
■ Self-monitoring of glucose
■ Attention to meal planning (diet)
■ Regular exercise
■ Continuing education

Treatment Goals
■ Glucose:
  ➢ Preprandial: 80–120 mg/dL
  ➢ Bedtime: 100–140 mg/dL
  ➢ HgbA1c: <7%
  ➢ Individualized based on ability to understand/carry out treatment regimen, risk of hypoglycemia, advanced age, renal disease, CVD
  ➢ BP: <130/80
  ➢ Lipids: LDL cholesterol <100 mg/dL

SPECIFIC THERAPY
■ Diabetic ketoacidosis:
  ➢ Hydration with normal saline or half-normal saline (3–5 L deficit in adults)
  ➢ IV regular insulin
  ➢ Start replacement if serum potassium normal or low; if serum potassium high, delay replacement until serum potassium normal
  ➢ Consider 1–2 amps bicarbonate in half normal saline if pH <7.0–7.1
■ Established disease:
  ➢ Insulin, 3 or more injections/day or insulin pump
■ Side Effects & Contraindications
■ Insulin:
  ➢ Side effects: hypoglycemia, lipohypertrophy, lipoatrophy, insulin allergy, insulin antibodies
  ➢ Contraindications: none

FOLLOW-UP
■ See well-controlled, stable patients q 3 mo
■ See poorly controlled patients more frequently, PRN
■ Review records of home glucose monitoring (HGM), adherence, symptoms of hyper/hypoglycemia, chronic complications, other illnesses, medications, lifestyle changes, psychosocial issues

- Weight, BP, foot exam at each visit
- HgbA$_{1c}$ quarterly
- Serum lipid profile yearly or more frequently if abnormal
- Dilated eye exam, serum creatinine, urine microalbumin yearly

COMPLICATIONS AND PROGNOSIS

- Diabetic ketoacidosis: 5–9% mortality
- Hypoxia
- Cerebral edema: usually only occurs in children; treat with mannitol, dexamethasone, and mechanical ventilation; 50% mortality
- Venous and arterial thrombosis
- Retinopathy: develops in 50–90%; best treated by near-normal glucose control, BP management, and photocoagulation therapy by ophthalmologist; may lead to blindness in up to 10%
- Neuropathy: develops in 50–90%, best treated by near-normal glucose control; predisposes to foot ulcers and amputations
- Nephropathy: develops in 30–50%, best treated by near-normal glucose control, BP management, ACE inhibitor; end-stage renal disease in 50–75% with nephropathy
- Atherosclerosis: CAD 11-fold higher; peripheral vascular disease 4- to 6-fold higher; CVD 2- to 4-fold higher; best prevented by aggressive BP and lipid management; use aspirin/ACE inhibitor
- 35% mortality by age 55 y

DIABETES MELLITUS, TYPE 2

FREDRIC B. KRAEMER, MD

HISTORY & PHYSICAL

History

- Known type 2 diabetes
- Family history of type 2 diabetes
- Obesity
- Metabolic syndrome (hypertension, obesity, elevated triglycerides, low HDL)
- History of gestational diabetes or delivered baby with birth weight >9.0 lbs
- Increased risk if Native American, Hispanic, African American, Indian (Asia)

Signs & Symptoms

- May be asymptomatic

- Presentation: polyuria, polydipsia, nocturia, polyphagia, weight loss or weight gain, fatigue, blurred vision, candidiasis, recurrent furunculosis
- Established disease:
  - Visual changes: blurred vision, floating specks, loss of vision
  - Paresthesias, numbness, lancinating, burning/aching pain, coldness, usually affecting lower extremities, usually worse at night
  - Dysphagia, early satiety, bloating, nausea/vomiting, diarrhea, constipation
  - Impotence, incontinence
  - Claudication
  - Foot ulcers
  - Microaneurysms, hemorrhages, exudates, cotton wool spots, new vessels
  - Loss of sensation, proprioception, temperature discrimination, absent ankle jerks
  - Hammerhead deformity of toes, calluses, ulcers
  - Miosis, diminished pupillary dilation
  - Resting tachycardia, postural hypotension
  - Necrobiosis lipoidicum diabeticorum
  - Diminished or absent pulses in lower extremities

TESTS

Laboratory
- Basic blood studies: elevated glucose, HgbA1c, creatinine, dyslipidemia; thyroid function tests
- Basic urine studies: glycosuria, albuminuria
- Specific Diagnostic Tests
  - Oral glucose tolerance test (glucose $\geq$200 mg/dL at 2 h)
  - C-peptide, insulin
  - ECG

DIFFERENTIAL DIAGNOSIS
- Fasting glucose $\geq$126 mg/dL on 2 occasions establishes diagnosis

MANAGEMENT

What to Do First
- Assess whether symptomatic or glucose >300 mg/dL
- If asymptomatic, start with diet and exercise alone
- If symptomatic, start medication along with diet and exercise

■ Assess degree of control, presence of complications, or associated conditions

General Measures
■ Self-monitoring of glucose
■ Attention to meal planning (diet), weight loss if indicated
■ Regular exercise
■ Continuing education

Treatment Goals
■ Glucose:
> Preprandial: 80–120 mg/dL
> Bedtime: 100–140 mg/dL
> HgbA1c: <7%
> Must be individualized based on ability to understand and carry out treatment regimen, risk of hypoglycemia, advanced age, renal disease, CVD
> BP: <130/80 mmHg
> Lipids: LDL cholesterol <100 mg/dL

SPECIFIC THERAPY
■ Metformin: currently first-line agent; can be used in combination with other oral agents or with insulin
■ Sulfonylureas:
> Several available: tolazamide, chlorpropamide, glyburide, glipizide, glimepiride, rapaglinide, nateglinide
> Chlorpropamide, glyburide, and glimepiride have long half-lives, glipizide and tolazamide intermediate, and rapaglinide and nateglinide very short
> Add to metformin or use as first-line agent
■ Glitazones (thiazolidinediones):
> Rosiglitazone, pioglitazone
> Add to metformin or sulfonylurea
> Not generally first-line agent, but can be used as monotherapy
■ Alpha-glucosidase inhibitors:
> Acarbose, miglitol
> Add to first-line agents
■ Insulin:
> Use exclusively in pregnant and nursing mothers, in patients with significant liver disease, and in anyone not adequately controlled on oral agents
> Use in combination with oral agents or alone

■ Side Effects & Contraindications
■ Metformin:
  ➤ Side effects: abdominal pain, diarrhea, lactic acidosis
  ➤ Contraindications: pregnancy, breast feeding, renal insufficiency (Cr = 1.5 mg/dL), uncompensated CHF, severe hepatic dysfunction, marked alcoholism
■ Sulfonylureas:
  ➤ Side effects: hypoglycemia, GI, allergy
  ➤ Contraindications: pregnancy, breast feeding
■ Glitazones (thiazolidinediones):
  ➤ Side effects: hepatitis, edema
  ➤ Contraindications: pregnancy, breast feeding, liver disease, severe CHF
■ Alpha-glucosidase inhibitors:
  ➤ Side effects: abdominal pain, diarrhea, flatulence
  ➤ Contraindications: pregnancy, breast feeding, cirrhosis, IBD, intestinal obstruction
■ Insulin:
  ➤ Side effects: hypoglycemia, lipohypertrophy, lipoatrophy, insulin allergy, insulin antibodies
  ➤ Contraindications: none

FOLLOW-UP

■ See well-controlled, stable patients q 6 mo
■ See poorly controlled patients or those well-controlled on insulin q 3 mo or more frequently, PRN
■ Review records of home glucose monitoring (HGM), adherence, symptoms of hyper- or hypoglycemia, chronic complications, other illnesses, medications, lifestyle changes, psychosocial issues
■ Weight, BP, and foot exam at each visit
■ HgbA$_{1c}$ quarterly or q 6 mo
■ Serum lipid profile yearly or more frequently if abnormal
■ Dilated eye exam, serum creatinine, urine microalbumin yearly

COMPLICATIONS AND PROGNOSIS

■ Retinopathy: develops in 50–90%, best treated by near-normal glucose control, BP management, and photocoagulation therapy by ophthalmologist; may lead to blindness in up to 10%
■ Neuropathy: develops in 50–90%, best treated by near-normal glucose control; predisposes to foot ulcers and amputations

- Nephropathy: develops in 10–40%, best treated by near-normal glucose control, BP management, and use of ACE inhibitor; ESRD in 50–75% with nephropathy
- Atherosclerosis:
  - CAD, CVD, 2–4 fold higher
  - Peripheral vascular disease 4–6 fold higher
  - Best prevented by aggressive BP and lipid management, aspirin, ACE inhibitor

DIABETIC RETINOPATHY

LAWRENCE J. SINGERMAN, MD, FACS, FICS and
JOAN H. HORNIK, AB

HISTORY & PHYSICAL

History

- Leading cause of new cases of blindness in working-age people; ~6000/y but possibly higher
- Risk of blindness due to diabetes related to age at diagnosis of diabetes & duration of disease:
  - 12% of pts w/ insulin-dependent diabetes for ≥30 y are blind
  - 97% of pts w/ insulin-dependent diabetes for ≥15 y have retinopathy
  - Increasing incidence of diabetes increases risk of retinal blindness
- Two main categories:
  - Background diabetic retinopathy (BDR) or nonproliferative diabetic retinopathy (NPDR):
    - Characterized by damage to small retinal blood vessels w/ subsequent leakage of blood or fluid into retina
    - Most visual loss at this stage due to macular edema
    - Poor perfusion in macula can cause visual loss
  - Proliferative diabetic retinopathy:
    - Characterized by neovascularization (growth of new blood vessels on optic head or in periphery)
    - Any of manifestations of BDR may be present
    - If untreated, vessels may continue to proliferate & enlarge, leading to visual loss or blindness from
      - Rupture w/ subsequent preretinal or vitreous hemorrhage

- Fibrous tissue formation w/ traction retinal detachment &/or hole

Signs & Symptoms
- Microaneurysms
- Intraretinal hemorrhages
- Lipid exudates (sometimes called hard exudates)
- Intraretinal microvascular abnormalities
- Venous beading & loops
- Cotton wool spots (formerly called soft exudates)
- Capillary nonperfusion (occlusion of fine retinal capillaries)
- Neovascularization:
  - Disc (NVD)
  - Elsewhere (NVE)
- Retinal detachment:
  - Caused by retinal hole or tear (rhegmatogenous)
  - Caused by traction on retina

TESTS

Common
- Ophthalmoscopy
- Fundus photography
- Fluorescein angiography

Less Common
- Ocular coherence tomography
- Retinal thickness analyzer
- Visual fields
- Indocyanine green angiography

DIFFERENTIAL DIAGNOSIS
- Branch &/or central retinal vein occlusion
- Hypertensive retinopathy

MANAGEMENT

General Measures
- Panretinal photocoagulation (PRP) in eyes with high-risk PDR: 1) new vessels with preretinal or vitreous hemorrhage, 20 NVD $\geq$ 1/4 to 1/3 disc area, even without hemorrhage
- Individualize PRP in eyes w/ non-high-risk PDR:
  - Rubeosis requires prompt PRP to prevent neovascular glaucoma
  - Early PDR or severe NPDR may be treated, particularly in

- Pt w/ history of noncompliance or poor follow-up
- PDR that develops during pregnancy
- Moderate to severe NPDR in 1 eye & severe PDR w/ visual loss in other eye
- Juvenile-onset diabetes
- Rapid progression of retinopathy

➤ Most eyes w/ early PDR & severe NPDR require treatment w/in 3–5 y; early treatment, even if light, often prevents disease progression

SPECIFIC THERAPY

Treatment Options

■ Laser techniques: various laser wavelengths – green, red, yellow — all can be effective

■ Vitrectomy:
  ➤ Clears media of opacities & vitreous hemorrhage
  ➤ Allows repair of traction and rhegmatogenous retinal detachment
  ➤ Removes fibrous proliferation
  ➤ Removes scaffold for growth of fibrovascular proliferation; after successful vitrectomy, neovascularization usually does not recur

FOLLOW-UP

■ Monitor eyes w/ high-risk PDR & treated by PRP closely at 6–8 wk intervals until NV has regressed

COMPLICATIONS AND PROGNOSIS

■ Burns of excessive intensity can result in pt discomfort & increase risk of adverse effects (rupturing Bruch's membrane, choroidal hemorrhage, choroidal effusions, visual field loss)

■ Decreased central visual acuity & visual field loss most common & significant complications after PRP; decreased visual acuity after PRP may be due to development or exacerbation of macular edema

■ Inadvertent foveal burns may occur

Clinical Trials – Potential New Treatments

■ Macugen (pegaptanib sodium; OIS/Eyetech) – anti-VEGF (vascular endothelial growth factor) aptamer, injected intravitreally
  ➤ 0.3 mg -> stable or improved vision (73% vs. 51%, $p = .023$), decreased mean retinal thickness ≥ 100 microns (42% vs. 16%, $p < .05$), reduced need for additional laser therapy (25% vs. 48%, $p < .05$)

- Arxxant (ruboxistaurin; Eli Lilly) – promising new protein kinase C beta (PKC-ß) inhibitor, taken orally
  - ➤ May reduce vision loss; ongoing analysis and studies
- DRCR.net studies (NEI/NIH); ongoing studies
  - ➤ Mild grid vs. focal laser
  - ➤ Laser vs. triamcinolone
  - ➤ Peribulbar triamcinolone vs. laser
- Cand5 (Acuity) – small interfering RNA, injected intravitreally, that selectively silences the mRNA encoding for VEGF; ongoing analysis and studies
- Intraocular implants (Posurdex, Retisert) – slow release of steroids; ongoing analysis and studies

---

DIARRHEA

JAYSHREE MATADIAL, MD and SUZANNE M. MATSUI, MD

HISTORY & PHYSICAL

History
- Duration of diarrhea:
  - ➤ acute – acquired within 2–3 weeks of evaluation
  - ➤ chronic – >4 weeks of symptoms
- Character of fecal output: too loose, too frequent, increased volume
- History of exposure to enterotoxins or recent antibiotic use
- History of exposure to poorly absorbed osmotically active agents or new medications
- History of systemic disease: diabetes, pancreatic insufficiency, small bowel disease, endocrinopathy, surgical resection, neoplasms, IBD, AIDS
- History of travel, epidemiological setting in which illness was acquired, family and social history all important

Signs & Symptoms
- Abdominal pain, cramping, bloating, distention, tenesmus
- Fever, rashes
- Dehydration
- Signs of malnutrition, malabsorption, weight loss
- Hematochezia, anemia, watery diarrhea, passage of mucous
- Manifestations of systemic disease

TESTS

Laboratory

Basic Studies: Blood

■ CBC, LFTs, BUN, creatinine, TSH/FT4, chem 7, albumin, calcium, ESR

Basic Studies: Stool

■ Fecal leukocytes, O&P, C&S, stool hemocult, C. difficile toxin, qualitative fecal fat

Specific Diagnostic Tests (Mostly for Chronic Diarrhea)

■ 1. 72 hr quantitative stool collection: evaluate weight, fat, osmolality,
■ electrolytes, Mg, pH, occult blood, laxative screen, and/or fecal
■ chymotrypsin
  ➤ Quantitative fecal fat 7–14 gm/d: low specificity for accurate diagnosis between defective fat digestion and absorption, >14 g/d: more specific for exocrine pancreatic disease, small intestinal mucosal defects, abnormal enterohepatic bile salt circulation
  ➤ Stool electrolytes to calculate osmotic gap: 290−2([Na]+[K])
    • if >125, pure osmotic diarrhea; if <50, pure secretory diarrhea
  ➤ Fecal pH <5.3 carbohydrate malabsorption, >5.6 factors other than carbohydrate malabsorption present
  ➤ Phenolphthalein test: red discolorization after alkylinization in laxative use
■ Urine for 5-HIAA, VMA and metanephrine, serum for gastrin, VIP, PP, calcitonin: detection of hormone producing tumors
■ Endoscopy
  ➤ Small/large intestinal biopsy: colitis, tumor, malabsorption, pseudomembranes, melanosis coli
  ➤ Small intestinal aspirate: bacterial overgrowth ≥10 colonies/ml
  ➤ Barium radiographs (UGI/SBFT) may complement endoscopy
■ Lactose-free diet trial/lactose and other carbohydrate H2 breath tests
■ Therapeutic trial of cholestyramine or pancreatic enzymes, specific bile acid absorption tests or exocrine pancreatic function tests

DIFFERENTIAL DIAGNOSIS

Exudative/Inflammatory Diarrhea

■ IBD, microscopic colitis, infectious diarrheas with invasive organisms, radiation enteritis, ischemic colitis, food allergy, food toxins

Osmotic Diarrhea

- Disaccharidase deficiency, small intestinal mucosal disease, laxative abuse, medication/ETOH induced, malabsorption syndromes, lymphatic obstruction, intestinal resection, bacterial overgrowth

Secretory Diarrhea

- Celiac sprue, enterotoxins, endocrine tumors, medication, neoplasms, colitis, fatty acid/bile acid malabsorption, hyperthyroidism, collagen vascular disease

Diarrhea Due to Dysmotility

- IBS, diabetic diarrhea, blind loop syndrome, malignant carcinoid, post vagotomy, cholecystectomy, gastrectomy, ileocecal valve
- resection

MANAGEMENT

What to Do First

- Assess acuteness, severity of diarrhea, complications and candidacy for therapy
- Determine organic vs functional disorder

General Measures

- Correction of electrolyte disorders and anemia
- Rehydration
- Avoidance of offending agent if possible
- Nutritional support

SPECIFIC THERAPY

- Antibiotics for infectious etiologies: (see section on infectious diarrhea) especially in immunosuppressed patients or those with valvular heart disease, orthopedic prosthesis, or malignancies
- Antimotility agents if not detrimental (see below)
- Octreotide for endocrine tumors
- Cholestyramine for bile acid diarrhea
- Anti-inflammatory agents for IBD/microscopic colitis: glucocorticoids, 5ASA compounds, azathioprine, 6MPClonidine for diabetic diarrhea
- Enzyme replacement therapy for disaccharidase deficiency and pancreatic insufficiency

Side Effects & Contraindications

- Antibiotics: may cause prolongation of microorganism excretion time, allergic reactions, worsening diarrhea
  - ➤ Contraindication: history of allergy to medication

- Antimotility agents: may cause toxic megacolon, sequelae of disease process may occur in the presence of infection
  - ➤ Contraindication: some infectious etiologies
- Octreotide: delays gallbladder emptying predisposing to gallstones, hyperglycemia
- Anti-inflammatory agents/Immunosuppressive agents: Cushing's syndrome, immunosuppression, infectious complications, bone marrow suppression, kidney and liver disease, hyperglycemia, psych disorders, electrolyte disorders, HPA axis suppression, osteoporosis
- Clonidine: rebound hypertension if stopped abruptly, postural hypotension, depression, anticholinergic side effects, impotence, arrhythmias, sedation, myalgias
  - ➤ Contraindication: severe CAD, pregnancy
- Cholestyramine: steatorrhea with high doses, constipation, osteo porosis, rash, vitamin deficiencies, fecal impaction
  - ➤ Contraindication: complete biliary obstruction

FOLLOW-UP
- Ensure maintenance of nutritional status, blood counts, hydration

COMPLICATIONS AND PROGNOSIS
- Dehydration/electrolyte imbalances
- Malnutrition/malabsorption
- Anemia
- Weight loss
- Renal failure/specific complications of certain infections
- Shock/death

DIENTAMOEBA FRAGILIS INFECTION

J. GORDON FRIERSON, MD

HISTORY & PHYSICAL

History
- Exposure: It is presumed that a cyst form of Dientamoeba fragilis is ingested in contaminated food and/or water (cyst form has never been seen).

Signs & Symptoms
- Many patients have no symptoms. Some have low-grade diarrhea, flatulence, abdominal discomfort. Abdominal examination normal, or slight tenderness in lower abdomen.

TESTS
- Basic tests: blood: Usually normal. Eosinophilia occasionally reported.
- Basic tests: urine: normal
- Specific tests: Stool exam for O&P shows trophozoites.
- Other tests: None

DIFFERENTIAL DIAGNOSIS
- All causes of mild diarrhea

MANAGEMENT
What to Do First
- Nothing

General Measures
- None

SPECIFIC THERAPY
Indications
- Symptomatic patients

Treatment Options
- Iodoquinal for 3 weeks.
- or: Paromomycin for 7 days
- or: Tetracycline for 10 days

Side Effects & Complications
- All the medications can cause mild GI distress.
- Contraindications to treatment: absolute: allergy to medications
- Contraindications to treatment: relative: asymptomatic patient

FOLLOW-UP
Routine
- Repeat stool examination if symptoms persist. Repeat stool exams optional if symptoms disappear.

COMPLICATIONS AND PROGNOSIS
- Prognosis is good. Two or three courses of treatment sometimes needed.

DIPHTHERIA

RICHARD A. JACOBS, MD, PhD

HISTORY & PHYSICAL

History

- Etiologic agent Corynebacterium diphtheriae, an aerobic, pleomorphic, Gram-positive bacillus
- Organism not very tissue-invasive; produces disease by local infiltration of mucous membranes of the respiratory tract and by production of toxin that primarily affects the heart and peripheral nerves
- Humans only known reservoir; disease spread by respiratory secretions from those who have active disease or those who are asymptomatic respiratory carriers, and from direct contact with cutaneous lesions

Signs & Symptoms

- Locally invasive disease:
  - Nasal – serosanguinous or purulent nasal discharge; membrane, if present, is minimal; toxin production from this limited form of disease is rare
  - Pharyngeal – fever, sore throat, dysphagia and cervical adenopathy with membrane formation on the tonsils, soft palate and uvula; membrane initially white but becomes gray within days and is associated with bleeding of underlying mucosa when removed
  - Laryngeal – hoarseness, stridor, dyspnea and airway occlusion can result as infection and membrane spread to larynx and tracheobronchial tree; toxin production in pharyngeal and laryngeal disease is common
  - Cutaneous – classic description is chronic ulcer with membrane formation; however, most skin lesions from which C. diphtheriae is isolated look like other chronic, nonhealing ulcers; toxin production rare in cutaneous disease, but skin lesions serve as major reservoir for spread of infection
- Toxin-mediated disease:
  - Local – paralysis of soft palate followed by cranial neuropathies
  - Peripheral neuropathy – usually proximal motor neuropathy of lower extremities; other areas (upper extremities, trunk) less commonly involved; peripheral sensory neuropathy also

uncommon; neuropathy develops weeks to months after onset of respiratory disease

➤ Cardiac – wide spectrum of disease from ST abnormalities to conduction defects, including complete heart block, to arrhythmias; usually occurs within several days to several weeks of onset of respiratory disease

TESTS

- Diagnosis should be considered whenever a membrane is present in association with upper respiratory signs and symptoms, but diagnosis confirmed by culturing C. diphtheriae from appropriate specimens.
- Special medium (Loffler or Tindale) required for culture; if diagnosis considered, notify laboratory so specimen can be plated on appropriate medium
- Confirm toxin production – Elek test (in vitro) or PCR in conjunction with culture

DIFFERENTIAL DIAGNOSIS

- Group A streptococcal pharyngitis (also groups C and G), Arcanobacterium haemolyticum infection, viral pharyngitis, infectious mononucleosis, epiglottitis
- Membranes usually not present in those diseases; when present, easily removed and not associated with bleeding of underlying mucosa

MANAGEMENT

- If diagnosis considered, strict respiratory isolation required
- Careful monitoring in ICU for cardiac and respiratory complications
- Watch for superimposed bacterial pneumonia.

SPECIFIC THERAPY

- Antitoxin – hyperimmune equine antitoxin given as soon as presumptive diagnosis made; dose depends on severity of disease (details in package insert); skin testing required prior to administration of full dose; if skin test positive, desensitization needed
- Penicillin or erythromycin is the drug of choice for total duration of 14 d; IV administration until patient can swallow, then oral medication to complete therapy

FOLLOW-UP

- Patient should stay in isolation until therapy completed and should have two negative cultures 24 h apart before isolation terminated.

■ Patients should be immunized with diphtheria toxoid, since toxin is so potent that disease itself may not be immunizing.

■ Close contacts should receive therapy with erythromycin for 7 d and have cultures 2 wks after completion of therapy to ensure eradication of the carrier state; close contacts should also be immunized if immunization status unclear or immunizations not up to date.

COMPLICATIONS AND PROGNOSIS

■ Prognosis depends on immunization status and prompt institution of therapy.

■ Full or partial immunization associated with improved outcome

■ Early administration of antitoxin improves outcome.

■ Cardiac disease associated with higher mortality

■ Neuropathy may be slow to resolve, but recovery usually complete.

■ Prevention depends on adequate immunization; following primary immunization in childhood, adults should receive booster doses of Td, tetanus and diphtheria toxoid (dose of diphtheria toxoid lower in the adult than the pediatric preparation) every 10 y.

DISORDERS OF NEUTROPHIL FUNCTION

NANCY BERLINER, MD

HISTORY & PHYSICAL

■ Severe bacterial and fungal infections from early childhood

■ Family history of the disorder: usually X-linked, but autosomal recessive inheritance also occurs

■ Examine for evidence of infection. Most common infections: pneumonia, lymphadenitis, cutaneous infections, hepatic abscesses, osteomyelitis, aphthous ulcers, perirectal abscesses

TESTS

■ Diagnosis confirmed by tests of neutrophil oxidative metabolism: nitroblue tetrazolium (NBT) slide test or measurements of superoxide or peroxide production.

DIFFERENTIAL DIAGNOSIS

■ Heterogeneous group of rare disorders

■ Defective production of superoxide (O_2^-) by neutrophils, monocytes, and eosinophils

■ Caused by mutations in any of four genes encoding the respiratory burst oxidase.

- Also evaluate for other immunodeficiency syndromes and neutrophil functional defects

MANAGEMENT
- Aggressive prophylaxis with prophylactic trimethoprim-sulfamethoxazole or dicloxacillin
- Prompt treatment of infection with parenteral antibiotics
- Surgical interventions including drainage of abscesses and resection of infected tissue

SPECIFIC THERAPY
- Prophylaxis with interferon-gamma helps decreases infections in some patients
- Stem cell transplantation

FOLLOW-UP
n/a

COMPLICATIONS AND PROGNOSIS
- Life-threatening infections shortens life expectancy

DISSEMINATED INTRAVASCULAR COAGULATION, THROMBOTIC THROMBOCYTOPENIC PURPURA, HEMOLYTIC UREMIC SYNDROME (DIC/TTP/HUS)

PETER W. MARKS, MD, PhD

HISTORY & PHYSICAL

Associated with the Development of Disseminated Intravascular Coagulation
- Infections: Gram-negative bacteria, encapsulated gram-positive bacteria, viruses (varicella, Rocky Mountain spotted fever)
- Malignancies: Myeloid leukemia, lymphoma, solid tumors (esp. adenocarcinoma)
- Obstetric complications: Placental abruption, amniotic fluid embolus, retained products of conception, eclampsia
- Miscellaneous: Trauma, burns, snakebites, hemangiomas

Associated with the Development of TTP/HUS
- Infections: E. coli 0157:H7, Shigella (verotoxin-producing), HIV
- Drugs: clopidogrel, ticlopidine, quinine, cyclosporin, tacrolimus, gemcitabine, mitomycin C

- Pregnancy (distinguish from HELLP syndrome = hemolysis, elevated liver function tests and low platelets)
- Family history: Autosomal dominant and recessive
- Many cases without obvious inciting cause (idiopathic)

Signs & Symptoms
- DIC/TTP/HUS may present with mucosal bleeding, petechiae, and/or purpura.
- DIC manifests with bleeding in the setting of abnormal laboratory parameters involving coagulation factors and platelets; signs and symptoms may be suggestive of an underlying disorder.
- DIC more commonly presents with hemorrhage, but can also present with thrombotic complications such as embolic phenomena – purpuric lesions may be manifest on the digits.
- TTP/HUS is of rapid onset, although the disease may become chronic in nature; DIC may be either acute or chronic.
- TTP pentad consists of fever, neurologic manifestations, microangiopathy, thrombocytopenia and renal failure.
- All five features need not be present in order to make the diagnosis.
- HUS may present with symptoms of a diarrheal illness.

Distinction of TTP from HUS
- TTP: Fever and neurologic manifestations
- HUS: Renal insufficiency prominent
  - ➤ Clinical distinction is often difficult or impossible – may simply need to make diagnosis as TTP/HUS.

TESTS
- When suspected, diagnosis of TTP/HUS should be expedited and can be based on historical features and basic laboratory studies.
- TTP/HUS is distinguished from DIC as microangiopathic hemolytic anemia with normal coagulation parameters.

Basic Tests
- CBC, including platelet count: define degree of anemia, thrombocytopenia
- Review of peripheral smear
  - ➤ Schistocytes indicative of microangiopathy: should see at least a few per high-power field
  - ➤ Presence of toxic granulation, vacuoles, or Döhle bodies (light bluish cytoplasmic inclusions) in neutrophils suggests infection potentially associated with DIC.

- Reticulocytes may be assessed on peripheral smear as large bluish red cells without central clearing; often present in increased numbers in TTP/HUS.
- Lactate dehydrogenase (LDH) level is generally elevated.
- Creatinine may be elevated in any of these disorders, but elevation is most prominently a feature of HUS.
- Prothrombin time (PT) and partial thromboplastin time (PTT) are normal in uncomplicated TTP/HUS; may be elevated in DIC.
- Fibrinogen level is normal in TTP/HUS; low or normal in DIC.
- Fibrin split products are elevated in DIC and normal or only slightly elevated in TTP/HUS in the absence of liver disease or injury.

Additional Studies
- For DIC: blood cultures if appropriate; consider CT scan to search for underlying malignancy in chronic DIC
- For suspected HUS: If diarrhea is present send stool for culture; consider HIV test

DIFFERENTIAL DIAGNOSIS
- Since microangiopathic changes may be seen with malignant hypertension or with leaks around mechanical valves, these possibilities should routinely be excluded when a diagnosis of DIC/TTP/HUS is being considered.

MANAGEMENT

What to Do First
- On the basis of history, symptoms and signs, and basic laboratories, decide whether DIC or TTP/HUS is present.
- If DIC is suspected, be sure that the elevation in PT/PTT is not spurious (heparin contamination).

General Measures
- Avoid platelet transfusion until the distinction between DIC and TTP/HUS is established, as it is generally contraindicated in TTP/HUS.
- Packed red blood cell transfusion may be administered as deemed appropriate.

SPECIFIC THERAPY

DIC
- Define the underlying cause and provide appropriate therapy.
- While treating the underlying cause, decide if blood product support is indicated:

- Asymptomatic individuals need not be treated.
- Bleeding patients should be treated with as appropriate:
  - Fresh frozen plasma provides all coagulation factors – use for elevated PT/PTT.
  - Cryoprecipitate provides a concentrated source of fibrinogen – strongly consider its use when fibrinogen level falls below 100 mg/dL – such low levels are not uncommon in amniotic fluid embolism, and repletion of fibrinogen may go far toward normalizing the PT/PTT.
  - Platelets should be transfused judiciously – in patients with major bleeding try to keep >50,000/mm3, for minor bleeding >20,000/mm3
  - Use of heparin is not routinely indicated. Consider in patients with DIC and thrombosis: dose at 500-1500 U/hr without regard to PTT.
- For overt DIC in sepsis, consider treatment with recombinant human activated protein C (drotrecogin alfa, activated) or treatment with antithrombin without heparin – either of these may reduce mortality.
  - Overt DIC is defined as a combination of thrombocytopenia, elevated D-dimer, increased PT, and decreased fibrinogen, though all need not be present.

HUS in a Child with a History of a Diarrheal Illness
- HUS occurring as part of a diarrheal illness is usually self-limited. Supportive care only is indicated.

TTP/HUS
- Once the diagnosis is established:
  - Discontinue any offending agents (i.e., clopidogrel, cyclosporin).
  - Plasma exchange is the treatment of choice – usually performed daily with one plasma volume exchanged with FFP until the platelet count and LDH have been in the normal range for a few days. Alternatively, FFP infusion may be used.
  - TTP/HUS that does not respond to one volume plasma exchange may respond to larger volume exchange – alternatively, cryo-poor plasma may be of utility.
- Routine use of corticosteroids is not indicated and may increase the risk of infectious complications.
- Renal failure may require dialysis.
- Splenectomy or treatment with rituximab may be considered in relapsing TTP.

FOLLOW-UP

DIC

■ Follow hematocrit and serial coagulation tests: PT, PTT, fibrinogen, platelets.

■ Support with blood products as necessary if patient is bleeding or it is otherwise indicated (trauma/surgery)

TTP/HUS

■ Follow hematocrit, platelet count, LDH, and creatinine levels.

■ Transfuse with packed red blood cells as necessary.

COMPLICATIONS AND PROGNOSIS

DIC

■ Complications in DIC are often related to the underlying illness.

■ DIC with thrombosis can cause complications related to embolic phenomena.

■ Depending on the underlying cause, DIC can be mild and self-limited (as in some infections) or severe and life-threatening (amniotic fluid emboli which have a high mortality rate).

HUS in a Child with a History of a Diarrheal Illness

■ Children with HUS due to verocytotoxin-producing E. coli or Shigella generally recover spontaneously with supportive care and rarely require plasmapheresis.

TTP/HUS

■ With plasma exchange, 90% of patients with TTP respond to treatment, 30% will subsequently relapse within weeks after this treatment is stopped – plasma infusion may be of utility for these individuals.

■ Renal failure or neurologic deficits may be long-lasting or permanent.

DIVERTICULITIS AND DIVERTICULAR DISEASE

JOHN P. CELLO, MD

HISTORY & PHYSICAL

■ Note proper nomenclature:

➤ diverticulum (singular)

- diverticula (plural)
- diverticulosis (presence of diverticula)
- diverticulitis (inflammation caused by micro perforation of a diverticulum)

■ Diverticula develop in the bowel at sites of potential weakness where other structures penetrate circular smooth muscle

■ Most diverticula occur in colon related to low residue diets, decreased stool volume, increased intraluminal pressure, increased colonic wall tension

■ Colonic diverticula are mostly acquired starting at age 30–40 years

■ Colonic diverticula always form on mesenteric side of antimesenteric teniae (bands of longitudinal smooth muscle) at sites of passage of neurovascular bundle to submucosa

■ Other diverticula – descending duodenum at site of penetration of wall by bile and pancreatic ducts at papilla of Vater

■ Some diverticula are congenital – most importantly, Meckel's diverticula in preterminal ileum – usually presents with hemorrhage in teenage years

■ Rare diverticula – congenital giant colonic or duodenal diverticula (usually present with hemorrhage).

■ Associated diseases – very rare – scleroderma

■ Usual presentations – note: diverticulitis and diverticular hemorrhage rarely occur simultaneously

■ Diverticulitis – usually pain, typically left lower quadrant, occasionally palpable mass and rebound (rare)

■ Diverticular hemorrhage – painless bleeding without other signs or symptoms

■ Diverticula are never the cause of persistently guaiac positive stools and/or chronic anemia; other causes must be considered

TESTS

Diverticulitis

■ Basic tests
  - Elevated WBC common but sepsis rare
■ Imaging tests
  - CT scan of abdomen usually shows focal colonic wall thickening, stranding of mesenteric fat, and occasionally an abscess.
  - CT is the most helpful – use IV, PO and rectal contrast if colonic diverticulitis is suspected
  - Plain abdominal radiographs – essentially useless but inexpensive

Colonoscopy
- Not essential but helpful – difficult to perform in setting of acute diverticulitis – very edematous bowel with narrow lumen.

Diverticular Hemorrhage, see GI Bleeding Section

Laboratory Tests
- Decreased Hg/Hct: can occasionally have exsanguinating bleed from diverticulosis
- Colonoscopy
  - Helpful when bleeding stops, otherwise need to localize site of hemorrhage by RBC nuclear scans and/or angiography

DIFFERENTIAL DIAGNOSIS
- Differential diagnosis for diverticulitis:
  - Appendicitis – always in consideration unless previously removed
  - Perforating colonic cancer – very difficult to differentiate early
  - Foreign body perforation – don't ask, don't tell, just consider it
  - Ischemic colitis – the great masquerader
  - Adhesions – very common
  - Acute infectious, idiopathic ulcerative colitis or Crohn's disease
- Differential diagnosis for diverticular hemorrhage:
  - Colonic neoplasms – most have chronic anemia indices
  - Vascular ectasias – usually older patients
  - Colitis, infectious or idiopathic – WBC's in stool
  - Hemorrhoids – look for them, don't pass the buck
  - Rectal laceration/ fissure
  - Colonic varices – not only in alcoholics

MANAGEMENT
What to Do First
- Resuscitate
- Stools for WBCs, C&S, O&P
- Early testing
  - CT for suspected diverticulitis
  - Sigmoidoscopy then RBC scan if bleeding

General Management
- Get GI and Surgical consultations
- Follow closely – repeat examinations essential, document your findings in chart

SPECIFIC THERAPY
- Prevention is the best – rarely in time
  - Need to increase bulk in diet – particularly with bran – should have 10 grams of nonabsorbable fiber per day (read the cereal boxes – the best way)
- If acute diverticulitis – need NPO status, fluids and IV antibiotics;
  - usually mixed colonic flora – remember – diverticulitis is a colonic microperforation
- If diverticular hemorrhage – usually stops spontaneously
  - Some data for using somatostatin analogues (octreotide IV infusion)
- Some patients need intervention – colonoscopic therapy (clips, coagulation possible)
  - Diverticular abscesses usually drained by interventional radiologic techniques; occasionally surgical resection
  - Persistent hemorrhage requires surgical resection – need to localize site of bleed – do not assume it is from left sided diverticula

FOLLOW-UP
- For presumed diverticulitis or diverticular bleeding
  - Elective colonoscopy essential to exclude neoplasm – best done when acute inflammation subsides – several weeks or when bleeding subsides (several days)

COMPLICATIONS AND PROGNOSIS
- Most patients do not have recurrent bleeding diverticula or diverticulitis
- Colectomy – rarely needed acutely – usually can stabilize patient with antibiotics and interventional radiology drainage of abscesses; surgical procedure can be scheduled electively
- No good controlled trials of high-residue diet after the onset of complications from diverticula – but easy to institute; no rationale for dietary restrictions on nuts, seeds, grains etc.
- Remember: prevention is best, and easily achievable

DRUG ALLERGY

SHAUN RUDDY, MD

HISTORY & PHYSICAL

History
- Penicillins, sulfonamides, barbiturates, ACE inhibitors are common offenders, but almost any drug may be responsible

Risk Factors

- Concomitant medication (eg, allopurinol w/ aminopenicillins)
- Concomitant disease (e.g., AIDS & sulfonamides, EB virus & aminopenicillins, renal disease & allopurinol)
- Requirement for repeated treatment (eg, chronic sinusitis, immunodeficiency disease, cystic fibrosis)
- Hospitalized pts receive an average of 10 different drugs, have ~10% risk of drug reaction overall, increasing w/ the number of agents to which they are exposed

Types of Reactions

- Systemic
  - ➤ Anaphylaxis (hypotension or, rarely, bronchospasm)
  - ➤ Serum sickness: arthritis, skin rash (including vasculitis), glomerulonephritis, cerebritis
- Cutaneous
  - ➤ Maculopapular, pruritic, resembling viral exanthem, onset ~1 week after beginning treatment
  - ➤ Urticaria: intensely pruritic raised hives, coming in crops, ± subcutaneous swelling of hands, face, oropharynx
  - ➤ Eczematous dermatitis: chronic scaling on erythematous base
    - Photosensitive dermatitis: pruritic, erythematous, scaling in sun-exposed areas
    - Erythema nodosum: indurated, tender nodular lesions on extremities, heal w/ ecchymosis
    - Mucocutaneous eruptions (Stevens-Johnson syndrome): bullae, target lesions, mucous membrane lesions
    - Toxic epidermal necrolysis: widespread skin exfoliation, potentially fatal
    - Vasculitis: palpable purpuric lesions, lasting several days, often ulcerating
- Lupus-like syndrome: rash, arthralgia, positive ANA (internal organ involvement unusual)
  - ➤ Procainamide, hyralazine, phenytoin, thiouracil, quinidine
- Hematologic
  - ➤ Eosinophilia
  - ➤ Hemolytic anemia
  - ➤ Leukopenia
  - ➤ Thrombocytopenia
  - ➤ Pancytopenia (marrow aplasia)
- Renal
  - ➤ Interstitial nephritis

- Pulmonary
  - Cough, infiltrates on radiograph, fever
- Hepatic
  - Cholestasis, hepatocellular damage

TESTS
- Blood: eosinophilia in <10%
- Serum tryptase to detect mast cell degranulation in suspected anaphylaxis
- Complement levels in serum sickness, other suspected immune complex-mediated reactions
- Skin biopsy if vasculitis suspected
- Specific identification of responsible drug by skin testing if possible
  - Standardized reagents available only for penicillin & derivatives
  - Positive reaction to intradermal test w/ non-toxic dose of other drugs may have value

DIFFERENTIAL DIAGNOSIS
- Increased sensitivity to known pharmacologic action of the drug common in elderly
- Nonallergic adverse reactions to drugs
  - Flushing, hypotension w/ radiocontrast media; less frequent w/ isotonic contrast media
  - Aspirin-induced asthma
  - Assoc w/ rhinosinusitis
  - Virtual complete cross-reactivity w/ other NSAIDs implicates pharmacologic action of these drugs
  - Hemolytic anemia w/ G6PD deficiency
  - Primaquine, other antioxidants
  - Opiate-related urticaria
  - Hepatitis caused by reactive drug metabolites (eg, isoniazid)
  - Syncope, usually vasovagal, mimicking anaphylactic reaction to local anesthetics in dentistry

MANAGEMENT
What to Do First
- Recognize that symptoms & signs are cause by drug allergy, identify the offending agent, discontinue it.

General Measures
- Support blood pressure, maintain airway in anaphylaxis
- Maintain skin integrity w/ local treatment in cutaneous disease

SPECIFIC THERAPY

- Anaphylaxis: epinephrine, subcutaneous or if necessary IV H1 & H2 blockers; corticosteroids of marginal benefit
- Serum sickness: H1 & H2 blockers, NSAIDs, oral corticosteroids in severe cases
- Cutaneous reactions: H1 & H2 blockers; systemic corticosteroids often required in mucocutaneous disease, erythema nodosum, vasculitis
- Hospitalization & intensive care for toxic epidermal necrolysis
- Hematologic reactions often require systemic corticosteroids, sometimes immunosuppressive agents (eg, cyclophosphamide)
- Lupus-like syndrome: NSAIDs, hydroxychloroquine, occasionally brief course of low-dose oral corticosteroids
- Renal & pulmonary involvement usually abates w/ discontinuation of responsible agent, may require corticosteroids

FOLLOW-UP

- Daily, during treatment of anaphylaxis, severe cutaneous disease, to assess response to therapy
- Weekly or monthly in lupus-like syndrome, other prolonged disease

COMPLICATIONS & PROGNOSIS

- The majority of allergic reactions to drugs are reversible & w/out serious sequelae, provided they are promptly diagnosed & the offending agent discontinued.
- Maintenance of the allergic state to a particular drug is unpredictable. The majority fades w/ time (years).
- Re-challenging w/ the offending drug to document the allergic state is unwise.
- If re-administration of the drug is absolutely required for effective therapy (eg, penicillin in enterococcal endocarditis, allopurinol in tophaceous gout w/ renal failure), consultation w/ an allergist for skin testing & desensitization to the agent is recommended.

DRUG AND TOXIN-INDUCED LIVER DISEASES

MINDIE H. NGUYEN, MD

HISTORY & PHYSICAL

History

- acetaminophen: intake >15 g in 80% of serious cases; toxic dose 5–10 g in alcoholics; acute GI symptoms in first 24 hr, followed by about 48 hours of well-being and then rising LFTs; FHF in up to 30%; renal failure in up to 20%

- nonsteroidal anti-inflammatory (NSAIDS): mild to severe; usually idiosyncratic
- antibiotics: usually self-limited and idiosyncratic: carbenicillin (necroinflammatory), oxacillin (cholestatic), Augmentin (cholestatic) ceftriaxone (biliary sludge), erythromycin (cholestasis), sulfonamide (mixed)
- antifungals: ketoconazole, fluconazole (necroinflammatory): mild to fulminant
- antituberculous agents: isoniazid (INH): jaundice in 1% of all patients; affects 2% of patients older than 50; female and alcoholics: greatest risk; FHF associated with high mortality. Rifampin: rarely hepatotoxic when taken alone; clinical hepatitis in 5–8% when taken with INH
- antiviral agents: zidovudine (AZT): sporadic cases of biochemical hepatitis, can lead to fatal syndrome of hepatomegaly, lactic acidosis, and steatosis in AIDS patients; didanosine (DDI)
- oral contraceptives: cholestasis, hepatic adenoma, Budd-Chiari syndrome; HCC and focal nodular hyperplasia
- anabolic, androgenic steroids: cholestasis, hepatic adenoma, HCC
- antilipids: niacin – infrequent injury (cholestatic and hepatocellular) at doses >3 g/day; mild to FHF; 50–75% dose reduction required for sustained-release form. HMG-CoA reductase inhibitors – asymptomatic elevated AST and ALT, usually in the first year of therapy
- neurologic/antipsychotic agents: chlorpromazine (cholestasis), carbamazepine, phenytoin, valproic acid
- cardiovascular agents: amiodarone (acute liver failure and chronic hepatitis/steatosis/fibrosis), alpha-methyldopa (chronic hepatitis to FHF), ACE-inhibitors-captopril (cholestatic), enalapril (hepatocellular), lisinopril (mixed pattern), calcium channel blockers-verapamil (hepatocellular), diltiazem (cholestatic), nifedipine (mixed)
- chemotherapeutic/immunosuppressive agents: methotrexate (steatosis, fibrosis, cirrhosis), 5-FU, azathioprine (asymptomatic elevated AST/ALT, cholestasis, peliosis hepatitis, venoocclusive disease, nodular regenerative hyperplasia), cyclosporine (cholestasis)
- total parenteral nutrition (TPN): steatosis, steatohepatitis, cholestasis-usually reversible with cessation of TPN
- herbal medicine/remedies: many hepatotoxic, should be part of history in evaluation of abnormal LFTs

- Amanita mushroom poisoning: most cases in U.S. occur in the Pacific Northwest; ingestion of one mushroom can be fatal; toxin not destroyed by cooking; OLT frequently necessary
- Aflatoxins: HCC
- arsenic: acute exposure – hepatocellular necrosis; chronic – hepatic angiosarcoma
- carbon tetrachloride (in cleaning solvents, propellant, fire extinguisher): potent hepatotoxin with death from liver failure in first week
- vinyl chloride (in solvents): may result in hepatic fibrosis, noncirrhotic portal hypertension, and angiosarcoma

Signs & Symptoms
- systemic features of drug hypersensitivity: fever, rash, eosinophilia, lymphadenopathy, mononucleosis-like syndrome
- temporal pattern of disease evolution and specific exposure
- presentation generally similar to those of chronic, acute, or fulminant hepatitis of other etiologies

TESTS

Basic Tests
- CBC, LFTs, INR, PTT; pH if FHF
- drug levels when available (acetaminophen level)

Imaging
- ultrasound: useful to evaluate hepatic vasculature, hepatic echotexture, signs of portal hypertension

Specific Diagnostic Tests:
- primarily to rule out other causes of liver diseases
- liver biopsy: in general, not useful

DIFFERENTIAL DIAGNOSIS
- chronic liver disease: viral, autoimmune, metabolic, vascular, inherited, cholestatic liver diseases
- acute, subfulminant, fulminant liver disease: other drug reaction, acute viral hepatitis, acute Wilson's disease, ischemic hepatitis, autoimmune hepatitis.

MANAGEMENT

What to Do First
- recognition and immediate removal/discontinuation of possible offending drugs and toxins

General Measures
- general supportive measures for acute liver failure

SPECIFIC THERAPY

■ acetaminophen: N-acetylcysteine (Mucomyst): 140 mg/kg orally followed by 70 mg/kg orally every 4 hours for an additional 17 doses
■ liver transplantation:
➤ indications for FHF due to acetaminophen:
  • pH <7.3 irrespective of stage of encephalopathy, or
  • INR >6.5 and serum Cr >3.4 mg/dL in patients with stage 3 or 4 encephalopathy
➤ indications for FHF due to other drug reaction (or viral hepatitis):
  • INR >6.5, or
  • any 3 or the following:
    • etiology: drug reaction or non-A, non-B hepatitis
    • age: <10 or >40 years
    • duration of jaundice before encephalopathy >7 days
    • serum bilirubin >17.6 mg/dL
    • INR > 3.5

FOLLOW-UP

■ surveillance for abnormal liver tests: important in chronic use of therapeutic agents with known and/or dose-dependent hepatotoxicity
■ methotrexate: a cumulative dose of 1.5 g is associated with significant liver disease; liver biopsy every 2 g is performed by some although its benefit is uncertain

COMPLICATIONS AND PROGNOSIS

■ wide spectrum of hepatotoxicity: subclinical liver disease with mildly abnormal liver function tests to fulminant hepatic failure requiring liver transplantation
■ acetaminophen: usually has good prognosis in the absence of underlying liver disease, chronic alcoholism, delayed administration of antidote, extremes of age
■ with the excepton of acetaminophen, drug and toxin-induced fulminant liver failure seldom recovers spontaneously

DRUG ERUPTIONS

NEIL H. SHEAR, MD, FRCPC, FACP and JOHN R. SULLIVAN, MB, BS, FACD
REVISED BY NEIL H. SHEAR, MD, FRCPC, FACP

HISTORY & PHYSICAL

History

■ Drugs can induce, aggravate or cause eruptions that mimic a broad range of skin disorders. Always consider, "Could this rash be drug-related?"

- Intake of prescribed medications, herbal and naturopathic remedies, over-the-counter products
- Timing of drug intake in relation to rash onset
- Onset varies with reaction pattern (see below) and previous exposure to the same or a cross-reacting drug. Eruptions following re-exposure occur more rapidly (minutes for IgE mediated urticaria, hours-2 days for most other eruptions).
- Past reactions (drugs and topical preparations)
- Conditions increasing risk: HIV/AIDS, chronic lymphocytic leukemia, renal failure, active viral infection (CMV, EBV), collagen vascular disease, atopy, corticosteroids, and family history of similar reaction to medications

Signs & Symptoms
- Clinical assessment: MORPHOLOGY, DISTRIBUTION and EXTENT +/− SYSTEMIC INVOLVEMENT
- Examine: skin including perineum and genitals, mucous membranes (eyes, mouth, pharynx), lymphoreticular system, and any other symptomatic organ
- **MORPHOLOGY**
    - **Exanthematous** – viral exanthem-like, include morbilliform and maculopapular; spotty erythematous symmetrical eruption, blanches with pressure, may be minimally palpable or occasionally purpuric, extends over hours – days; onset usually 5–14 days, range 5 days to 3 months.
    - **Urticaria / angioedema** – raised pruritic wheals that move every few hours, produce bizarre shaped lesions (usually intensely itchy). Onset is minutes in previously sensitized when IgE mediated (penicillin, sulfonamide antibiotics, cephalosporins) and anaphylactoid reactions (intravenous radiocontrast media, vancomycin, narcotics). Onset 1–7 days for aspirin, NSAIDs, codeine, acetaminophen, and opiate intolerance; and weeks to months for ACEI-induced angioedema. Serum sickness-like reaction (urticarial with more fixed lesions that may last days in the same location plus fever, arthralgia, lymphadenopathy) 7–21 days.
    - **Pustular** – Acute Generalized Exanthematous Pustulosis (AGEP) – usually starts groin or head and neck, rapidly evolves to widespread erythematous eruption containing numerous sterile pustules +/− fever and leukocytosis; onset 2–14 days, range 4 weeks. Acneiform drug eruption – monomorphic acneiform

lesions especially pustules, papules and whiteheads, often worse on trunk, onset weeks. Toxic pustuloderma as part of the drug hypersensitivity syndrome (see below). 5 days – 6 weeks, range 3+ months.

➤ **Erythrodermic** – widespread skin involvement with erythema, scaling, and serous exudates; onset usually gradual starting at 1–6 weeks, range to 3+ months.

➤ **Eczematous/Dermatitic** – erythematous and scaling; onset 5 days – 3+ months.

➤ **Blistering** – fluid-filled lesions >5 mm, epidermal shedding. Include Stevens-Johnson syndrome/toxic epidermal necrolysis, which involve mucous membranes (mouth, eyes) +/− atypical target lesions (dusky center with erythematous surrounds, may blister centrally); onset 5–21 days, range 6+ weeks. Other causes of drug-induced blistering: porphyria, pseudoporphyria, linear IgA disease, and pemphigus.

➤ **Fixed Drug Eruption** – single or multiple round to oval lesions, dusky red +/− edematous or central blister; resolves with hyperpigmentation; classic sites periorificial, genital, and perianal areas, onset 30 minutes – 2 days, range minutes – 4 days.

➤ **Vasculitic** – palpable purpura, urticarial plaques, hemorrhagic bullae, ulcers, dermal nodules, Raynaud's disease, and digital necrosis; onset 5 – 21 days, range 3+ months.

▧ DISTRIBUTION and EXTENT – e.g., sharply demarcated photodistributed eruption; involvement of dependent regions (legs and buttocks) in cutaneous vasculitis

▧ SYSTEMIC INVOLVEMENT: Commonly affected internal organs – liver, kidneys, lungs, and hematological system. Features suggestive of severe drug reaction +/− internal organ involvement:

➤ Fever, pharyngitis, anorexia, and malaise or signs and symptoms of internal organ involvement

➤ Erythroderma

➤ Prominent facial involvement +/− edema or swelling

➤ Mucous membrane involvement (particularly if erosive or involving conjunctiva)

➤ Lymphadenopathy

➤ Skin tenderness, blistering or shedding

➤ Purpura

➤ Drug Hypersensitivity Syndrome = Rash + Fever + Internal Organ Involvement

TESTS
- Skin Biopsy + histopathology – more useful and important if skin changes pustular, blistering, purpuric or erythrodermic, or diagnosis uncertain. Do immunofluorescence in blistering eruptions.
- If severe or possible internal organ involvement:
  - ➤ CBC – looking for neutrophilia, atypical lymphocytosis, eosinophilia, cytopenias (platelets, RBCs, WBCs), hemolytic anemia
  - ➤ LFTs (looking for hepatitis)
  - ➤ Urea, creatinine and urine analysis (looking for nephritis)
  - ➤ Investigate other symptomatic organs as needed – e.g., CXR, LP

DIFFERENTIAL DIAGNOSIS
- Depends on reaction morphology
- Exanthematous – infections (viral, bacterial, rickettsial), collagen vascular disease, miliaria
- **Dermatitic** – see Dermatitis chapter
- **Uriticarial** – see Urticaria chapter
- **Pustular** – pustular psoriasis, folliculitits, steroid acne
- **Erythrodermic** – Eczema, psoriasis, seborrheic dermatitis, lymphoma, mycosis fungoides, idiopathic, pityriasis rubra pilaris, hypereosinophilic syndrome
- **Blistering** – bullous pemphigoid, pemphigus, other immune-mediated blistering disorders
- **Purpuric** – vasculitis, coagulopathy

More Common Drug Associations
- **Exanthematous** – antibiotics, antiepileptics, gold
- **Dermatitic** – gold, beta-blockers, "statins", tricyclic antidepressants
- **AGEP** – macrolide antibiotics, penicillins, cephalosporins, calcium antagonists, terbinafine, itraconazole, Chinese herbal remedies
- **Toxic Epidermal Necrolysis** (and Stevens-Johnson syndrome) – sulfonamide antibiotics, phenytoin, phenobarbital, carbamazepine, lamotrigine, NSAIDs, allopurinol, quinolones, Chinese herbal remedies
- **Internal organ involvement** – Phenytoin, phenobarbital, carbamazepine, lamotrigine, sulfonamide antibiotics, dapsone, allopurinol, minocycline, metronidazole, trimethoprim, abacavir
- **Fixed Drug Eruption** – Acetaminophen, sulfonamide antibiotics, tetracyclines, phenobarbital, phenolphthalein
- **Erythroderma** – Gold, penicillin, phenytoin, phenobarbital, carbamazepine, lamotrigine, allopurinol

MANAGEMENT

General Measures
- Diagnosis of reaction type
- Analysis of drug exposure
- Stop associated and potentially associated (non-essential) drugs.
- Assess and monitor for internal involvement.
- Investigate for differential diagnosis +/– associations.
- Avoid cross-reacting drugs.
- Admit – blistering eruptions (other than fixed drug), and other severe reactions
- Literature search/drug information services/references

SPECIFIC THERAPY
- Simple (no internal organ involvement) exanthematous/dermatitic/urticarial eruptions – consider topical moderate potency corticosteroid cream, non-sedating sedating or antihistamine
- Urticaria/angioedema associated with anaphylaxis (i.e., bronchospasm, hypotension) – subcutaneous epinephrine/adrenaline stat and PRN, then antihistamines and prednisone to minimize late-phase reaction
- Erythroderma – biopsy, investigate and monitor for internal involvement and complications, cortisone creams, emollients
- Toxic Epidermal Necrolysis (SJS) – see chapter on EM Major
- AGEP – usually self-limited, rare fatalities, settles over 10 days. Topical cortisone creams for symptomatic relief.
- Drug-induced vasculitis is a diagnosis of exclusion – see chapter on Cutaneous Vasculitis
- Systemic organ involvement (hepatitis, nephritis, pneumonitis) – consider immunosuppression – e.g., prednisone weaned over several weeks. May flare with corticosteroid withdrawal and up to 2–3 months to fully settle. Check for delayed hypothyroidism at 2 months.

Confirmation of Drug Cause
- Effect of drug rechallenge (resolution in expected time frame) – e.g., 10–14 days for exanthematic eruption
- For possible IgE-mediated reactions – skin prick testing or RAST at 6–12 weeks
- Rechallenge should be avoided in serious or potentially severe drug reactions.
- Other tests of uncertain sensitivity and specificity:

- Patch testing 1–2% in PET for erythroderma, eczematous, pustular, blistering, and fixed drug eruptions (over area of fixed eruption)
- In vitro testing (lymphocyte transformation and lymphocyte toxicity test)

Advice to Patient & Family
- Which drug(s) was the most likely cause, potentially cross-reacting drugs, what drugs are safe, increased risk to first-degree relatives in hypersensitivity syndrome

Report
- Report potentially severe or unusual reactions to regulatory authorities/drug manufacturer.

FOLLOW-UP
n/a

COMPLICATIONS AND PROGNOSIS
n/a

DUBIN-JOHNSON SYNDROME

WILLIAM E. BERQUIST, MD

HISTORY & PHYSICAL
- incidence: uncommon
- inheritance: autosomal recessive
- occasional mild jaundice, normal exam
- increased bilirubin noted with estrogens, oral contraceptive use, trauma, pregnancy or surgery

TESTS

Basic Tests
- total bilirubin varies from 1–25 mg/dl and about 60% conjugated
- normal liver enzymes

Specific Diagnostic
- BSP clearance slow (>20% retention at 45 min); late rise at 1.5–2 hours
- urine corproporphyrin pattern: reversed ratio of coproporphyrin III to coproporphyrin I from 3:1 (normal) to 1:4
- normal total urinary corproporphyrins
- liver biopsy histology: melanin-like hepatocyte pigmentation

- absent multiple drug-resistant protein (MRP2) function, an ATP dependent hepatocyte canilicular transporter of multiple anions and conjugated bilirubin
- gene probe: mutations in MRP2

Other Diagnostic
- oral cholecystogram: poor gallbladder visualization

Treatment
- none

DIFFERENTIAL DIAGNOSIS
n/a

MANAGEMENT
n/a

SPECIFIC THERAPY
n/a

FOLLOW-UP
n/a

COMPLICATIONS AND PROGNOSIS
- hepatic adenomas reported rarely; excellent prognosis

DYSPEPSIA

M. BRIAN E. FENNERTY, MD

HISTORY & PHYSICAL

Signs & Symptoms
- epigastric pain
- belching/bloating
- nausea/vomiting
- weight change
- early satiety
- pain may be relieved with acid reduction
- food may make better or worse
- epigastric tenderness
- abdominal distension
- succusion splash in those with gastric outlet obstruction
- weight loss in those with malignancy
- melena in those with bleeding

TESTS

Specific Diagnostic Tests
- upper GI barium study (ulcers, neoplasms, gastroparesis)
- endoscopy (esophagitis, ulcers, neoplasms, gastroparesis)
- ultrasonography (cholelithiasis)
- nuclear medicine gastric emptying studies (gastroparesis)
- electrogastrography (gastroparesis)

Indirect Tests
- antibody, urea breath tests, fecal antigen tests for H. pylori

DIFFERENTIAL DIAGNOSIS
- peptic ulcer (diagnosis best made by endoscopy or UGI barium radiography)
- gastric neoplasia (diagnosis best made by endoscopy or UGI barium radiography)
- non-ulcer dyspepsia (diagnosed made by a negative imaging study)
- gastroesophageal reflux (diagnosis best made by endoscopy, pH study, or response too empirical trial of therapy)
- cholelithiasis (diagnosis best made by ultrasound or CT imaging)
- gastroparesis (diagnosis best made by nuclear medicine gastric imaging)
- medication or food-induced (diagnosis best made by withdrawing suspected agent)

MANAGEMENT

What to Do First
- empiric treatment vs or making a definitive diagnosis?
- this is a philosophical issue and should be decided in conjunction with the patient's needs
- empirical trial of therapy
  - H2RA or PPI as an anti-secretory, acid lowering agent
  - *Helicobacter pylori* treatment
  - prokinetic agent, i.e. metoclopramide
- diagnostic tests for definitive diagnosis
  - endoscopy for ulcers, esophagitis, neoplasms; more accurate than UGI but more expensive and invasive
  - UGI for ulcers, neoplasms; less accurate than endoscopy but cheaper and less invasive
- ultrasound/CT for cholelithiasis; accurate, widely available
- nuclear medicine gastric emptying study for gastroparesis; accurate, but current therapies for this disorder largely ineffective

General Measures
- stop smoking, coffee, alcohol or other offending agents
- stop NSAIDs or other agents associated with dyspepsia
- use acid lower drugs for persistent symptoms

SPECIFIC THERAPY

Indications
- confirmed or suspected specific diagnosis

Treatment Options
- anti-*Helicobacter pylori* therapy if positive (see section on H. pylori)
- anti-secretory therapy with H2-receptor antagonists or proton pump inhibitors for 4–6 weeks for suspected or proven ulcer, GERD, non-ulcer dyspepsia
- prokinetics for gastroparesis
- cholecystectomy for gallstones

Side Effects
- dyspepsia, nausea, vomiting, metallic taste with *Helicobacter pylori* treatments (usually mild)
- side-effects rare with H2RAs or PPIs
- diarrhea, neuropyschiatric symptoms with prokinetics

Contraindications
- absolute: allergy to drug

FOLLOW-UP

Routine
- complicated peptic ulcer
- suspected malignant ulcer
- worried patient
- recurrent symptoms

COMPLICATIONS AND PROGNOSIS

Complications
- peptic ulcer
  - bleeding
  - perforation
  - obstruction
  - symptomatic ulcer
- cholelithiasis
  - cholecysitis

➤ cholangitis
➤ pancreatitis
■ GERD
  ➤ Barrett's esophagus
  ➤ stricture
  ➤ ulceration/erosions
  ➤ bleeding
■ Gastroparesis
  ➤ weight loss/nutritional complications

Prognosis
■ 80% of individuals with peptic ulcer will relapse within one year once anti-secretory therapy is discontinued
■ maintenance therapy with an H2RA or PPI decreases relapse to 10–15%
■ of those infected with and cured of their *H. pylori* 20% will still have an ulcer relapse
■ patients with NUD have chronic intermittent symptoms

DYSPHAGIA

ROY SOETIKNO, MD and MONA LIN, MD

HISTORY & PHYSICAL

Signs & Symptoms
■ Difficult initiation of swallow
■ Sticking sensation during swallow
■ Cough with swallow
■ Gradual vs. sudden onset
■ Solids vs. liquids
■ Persistent vs. intermittent
■ Weight loss may suggest malignancy
■ Neuromuscular diseases (stroke, polio, Parkinson's, myasthenia): may be associated with speech deficits, weakness, muscle atrophy, and sleep apnea
■ Systemic sclerosis (calcinosis, Raynaud's, sclerodactyly, telangiectasias)
■ Goiter, lymphadenopathy (extrinsic compression)

TESTS
■ Radiology (video or barium swallow)

➤ useful for evaluation of oropharyngeal, extrinsic or intrinsic anatomic causes, or in some cases motility causes of symptoms
■ Endoscopy
➤ evaluation of mucosa, biopsy strictures/masses, and dilate/stent strictures.
■ Manometry
➤ evaluation of motility disorders
■ Endoscopic ultrasound or CT scan
➤ staging malignancy

DIFFERENTIAL DIAGNOSIS
■ Oropharyngeal dysphagia
➤ Inability to initiate swallow, worse with liquids
➤ Difficult transfer of food to upper esophagus.
➤ Associated with nasal regurgitation, coughing, nasal speech due to palate weakness, neuromuscular diseases
■ Esophageal dysphagia
➤ Sticking sensation with swallow
➤ Progressive symptoms (obstruction) vs. intermittent (motility disorder or ring/web)
➤ Solid (mechanical obstruction) vs. solids/liquids (motility or severe mechanical obstruction)
➤ Constant: extrinsic compression (vascular anomalies, thoracic aortic aneurysm compression, cervical hypertrophic osteo-arthropathy, lymphadenopathy, goiter)

MANAGEMENT
What to Do First
■ thorough symptom survey to direct tests seeking either anatomic or functional abnormalities

General Measures
■ smaller meals, changing food consistency, drinking liquids during meals
■ antireflux medications
■ specific treatment according to diagnosis
■ gastrostomy tube may be required when calorie intake is inadequate

SPECIFIC THERAPY
Oropharyngeal causes
■ thickened fluids; gastrostomy tube

Stricture
- benign: endoscopic dilation, proton pump inhibitor for peptic stricture
- malignant: surgery for early staging, endoscopic stent placement, laser

Spasm
- nitrates, calcium-channel blocker

Achalasia
- pneumatic dilation, botulinum toxin injections (short acting), myotomy surgery

FOLLOW-UP
- Periodic visits for symptom survey to determine effectiveness of therapy and need for additional treatment strategies

COMPLICATIONS AND PROGNOSIS

Prognosis
- good if diagnosis confirmed and therapy effective

Complications
- aspiration pneumonia
- weight loss

DYSPNEA

THOMAS J. NUCKTON, MD

HISTORY & PHYSICAL
- Dyspnea: subjective difficulty or distress in breathing
- Orthopnea: dyspnea when supine; characteristic of CHF; may occur with asthma, other obstructive lung diseases, diaphragmatic paralysis
- Trepopnea: dyspnea only in the lateral decubitus position; seen with heart disease, unilateral pulmonary or pleural disease, unilateral pleural effusion
- Platypnea: dyspnea only when upright; seen in pulmonary disease that affects lung bases, also congenital heart disease with right-to-left shunting on standing
- Paroxysmal nocturnal dyspnea: attacks of dyspnea at night; "cardiac asthma" with CHF and valvular heart disease; patients with pulmonary disease may also experience sudden onset dyspnea at night

History
- Acute vs gradual onset (gives clues to diagnosis)

Signs & Symptoms
- General: observe for cyanosis, kyphoscoliosis, pectus excavatum, spondylitis
- Cardiac: displaced PMI, S3, irregular rhythm, murmurs suggest CHF or other heart disease
- Chest:
  - Coarse basilar crackles: pulmonary edema
  - Fine crackles: interstitial lung disease
  - Decreased breath sounds: pneumothorax, atelectasis, emphysema
  - Wheeze: asthma, COPD, cardiac disease
  - Stridor: laryngeal or tracheal narrowing, tumor, foreign body
  - Dullness: pleural effusion
- Other:
  - Obesity may cause restriction
  - Clubbing suggests malignancy or bronchiectasis
  - Peripheral edema seen in right-sided heart failure

TESTS
Basic Studies
- Oxygen saturation (SaO_2), CXR

Specific Diagnostic Tests
- PFTs: define obstruction or restriction; decreased DLCO suggests pulmonary vascular involvement
- V/Q lung scan, spiral CT, pulmonary angiogram: for possible pulmonary embolism
- HRCT: evaluation of possible interstitial lung disease
- ECG, echo, exercise testing: may elicit ischemia; echo and catheterization useful for pulmonary hypertenson
- Pulmonary exercise testing: to distinguish cardiac from pulmonary disease, true cardiopulmonary disease from deconditioning; particularly helpful in subtle cases

DIFFERENTIAL DIAGNOSIS
- Distinguish pulmonary from cardiac disease and acute from gradual onset:

➤ Acute onset: bronchospasm, pulmonary embolus, pneumothorax, pulmonary edema, angina, myocardial infarction, dysrhythmia

➤ Gradual onset:
  • Cardiac: coronary artery disease; CHF, valvular disease; dysrhythmia; pericardial tamponade
  • Pulmonary:
  • Obstructive lung disease (asthma, COPD, bronchiectasis):
  • often with wheeze or cough, smoking associated with COPD, exertional dyspnea progressing gradually to dyspnea at rest, PFT to quantify degree of obstruction (spirometry) and diffusion abnormality (DLCO)

■ Diffuse parenchymal/ILD (idiopathic pulmonary fibrosis, sarcoidosis, pneumoconioses): gradually progressive dyspnea on exertion, restriction on PFTs (decreased TLC, normal or elevated FEV1/FVC), HRCT often useful

➤ Pulmonary infection (pneumonia, bronchitis): dyspnea may precede CXR findings

➤ Atelectasis: secondary to tumor, mucus plug, foreign body, breathing patternPleural disease: malignancy (mesothelioma), infection (including TB), collagen vascular disease, nephrotic syndrome, liver disease

➤ Pulmonary vascular disease: pulmonary embolism, vasculitis (SLE, polyarteritis nodosa, rheumatoid arthritis), venoocclusive disease, primary pulmonary hypertension, schistosomiasis; CXR may be normal with pulmonary embolus and pulmonary hypertension; decreased DLCO without obstruction or restriction suggests pulmonary vascular disease

➤ Diseases of chest wall/respiratory muscle weakness: cause restriction, resulting in dyspnea; neurologic disease can cause respiratory muscle weakness

Other

■ Malignancy/anemia: fatigue and/or effusions contribute to dyspnea

■ Anxiety: difficult to evaluate; hyperventilation; history of stress; no relation to activity; variability minute-to-minute; not during sleep

MANAGEMENT

What to Do First

■ Assess cause; determine if acute or gradual; SaO_2, CXR, ECG, ABG; treat emergent conditions as warranted

General Measures
- Additional tests based on clinical suspicion, pulmonary function testing

SPECIFIC THERAPY
- Aimed at treatable etiologies (see specific diseases)
- Severe dyspnea (eg, end-stage lung disease) may require oxygen, noninvasive ventilation (BiPAP), and opiates

FOLLOW-UP
- Careful coordination of care may be needed during extensive work-up

COMPLICATIONS AND PROGNOSIS
- Depends on underlying cause

ECHINOCOCCOSIS

J. GORDON FRIERSON, MD

HISTORY & PHYSICAL

History
- Disease due to *Echinococcus granulosis* and *Echinococcus multilocularis*
  - Life cycle: *E. granulosis*: eggs shed by sheep dog are ingested by sheep or man, develop into larval cysts, mainly in the liver; cysts are eaten by dogs and larvae develop into tapeworm, which gives off eggs
    - *E. multilocularis*: same cycle except hosts are foxes, wolves, other carnivores, and intermediate hosts are voles, shrews, mice. Arctic and alpine disease.
- Exposure: ingestion of eggs of either cestode through dirty hands, food

Signs & Symptoms
- *E. granulosis*: usually silent until cyst in liver reaches 5 or more cm. Then RUQ pain, or pain elsewhere, depending on where cyst is (most are in liver or lung). Rupture or leak causes allergic reactions, occasionally anaphylaxis.
- *E. multilocularis*: grows rapidly, pain is more frequent, generally in liver

TESTS
- Basic tests: blood: sometimes eosinophilia (both diseases)
- Basic tests: urine: normal
- Specific tests:
  - ➤ *E. granulosis*: ultrasound and/or CT scan locates cysts and is sometimes diagnostic, depending on internal morphology. Serology, using immunoelectrotransfer blot (EITB, done at CDC), is sensitive and specific. Double diffusion test (a gel diffusion test) also very good. Lung cysts often have negative serology (any method).
  - ➤ *E. multilocularis*: Ultrasound and CT scans locate cysts and suggest diagnosis. Serology, using the em2 ELISA, is sensitive and specific.
- Other tests: Chest X-ray locates lung cysts but is not usually diagnostic. CT scanning locates cysts in bone, brain, etc. Antigen tests available, but only present in 50% cases. PCR currently research only.

DIFFERENTIAL DIAGNOSIS
- *E. granulosis*: simple liver cysts, amebic abscess, other abscesses in liver. In lung: tuberculosis, abscess, bronchogenic cysts, tumors.
- *E. multilocularis*: carcinoma or sarcoma in liver

MANAGEMENT
What to Do First
- *E. granulosis*: assess entire patient for cysts, and their size. If possible, an estimate of age of cyst(s).
- *E. multilocularis*: assess for possibility of resection.

General Measures
- Instructions on how to avoid rupture. Screen others in area suspect for disease, using serology and/or ultrasound.

SPECIFIC THERAPY
Indications
- Both diseases: All patients with viable or possibly viable cysts

Treatment Options
- *E. granulosis*:
  - ➤ Chemotherapy: for nonresectable disease or small hepatic cysts (<7 cm). Use albendazole for 3–6 months.

> Needle aspiration: for larger cysts where needle can pass through liver to cyst. Hypertonic saline then injected to kill remaining organisms.
> Surgical resection: for larger hepatic cysts, cysts elsewhere. Give albendazole during and 1 month after aspiration or surgery to prevent new disease in case of leakage.

- *E. multilocularis*:
  > Primary resection of cyst when possible is treatment of choice. Liver transplant occasionally done.
  > Albendazole long-term (years), or:
  > Mebendazole long-term. Albendazole gives higher blood and cyst levels.

Side Effects & Complications

- Surgery: rupture and leakage of cyst, other surgical complications
- Albendazole: Hepatic toxicity, such as jaundice, elevated enzymes. Also alopecia, leukopenia, fever.
- Mebendazole: same
- Contraindications to treatment: absolute:
  > *E. granulosis*: dead cysts
  > *E. multilocularis*: none
- Contraindications to treatment: relative:
  > *E. granulosis*: Very small deep cysts. Elderly or debilitated patients.
  > *E. multilocularis*: relative contraindications are same as in a patient with a malignancy.

FOLLOW-UP

During Treatment

- Follow liver function, CBC, and ultrasound or CT. In E. multilocularis, serology follow-up is useful.

Routine

- Continued ultrasound follow-up

COMPLICATIONS AND PROGNOSIS

- *E. granulosis*: Rupture of cyst can produce new cysts in area of rupture, or anaphylaxis. Covering with chemotherapy can usually prevent this. Otherwise good prognosis.
- *E. multilocularis*: Behaves somewhat like a malignancy. If resected, curative. If chemotherapy used, some regress well, some progress to fatal outcome, but 10-year survival rate on therapy is 90%.

EHLERS-DANLOS SYNDROME

MICHAEL WARD, MD

HISTORY & PHYSICAL

History
- Hyperextensible joints
- Soft, velvety, hyperextensible skin
- Easy bruising
- Dystrophic scarring after surgery or minor trauma
- Family history of same (some types autosomal dominant)

Signs & Symptoms
- Type I (gravis): hyperextensible joints and skin, easy bruising, thin "cigarette paper" scars, varicose veins, mitral valve prolapse, pes planus deformity, premature osteoarthritis, prematurity at birth
- Type II (mitis): same as type I, but less severe, no prematurity
- Type III (familial hypermobility): hyperextensible joints, joint dislocations, mildly hyperextensible skin, normal scarring
- Type IV (vascular): thin translucent skin with prominent venous pattern, marked bruising, thin nose and lips, spontaneous arterial rupture with massive hematoma, stroke, or death, spontaneous bowel rupture, uterine rupture during pregnancy, mitral valve prolapse, hypermobility limited to distal interphalangeal joints, friable tissues at surgery
- Type V (X-linked): similar to Type II, males only
- Type VI (ocular): corneal fragility, blue sclerae, retinal detachment, glaucoma, hyperextensible skin and joints, severe scoliosis
- Type VII (arthrochalasis multiplex congenita): hyperextensible skin and joints, congenital hip dislocations, recurrent joint dislocations, moderate bruisability
- Type VIII (periodontal): severe periodontitis with loss of teeth, moderate skin fragility and joint hyperextensibility
- Type IX: occipital horns, short humerus, short broad clavicles, chronic diarrhea, bladder diverticuli and rupture, mild skin hyperextensibility. X-linked (males only).
- Type X: mild joint hyperextensibility, easy bruising, abnormal platelet aggregation

TESTS

Basic Tests
- Radiographs of painful joints, and of spine to detect scoliosis

Specific Diagnostic Tests
- No specific diagnostic tests available clinically
- Ultrastructural abnormalities in collagen detectable on electron microscopy, and biochemical abnormalities in fibroblast collagen in some types
- Mutations in various collagen genes, specific for some types, used as research tool
- Type VI has decreased hydroxylysine content in skin Type I collagen
- Type IX has low serum copper and ceruloplasmin

DIFFERENTIAL DIAGNOSIS
- Marfanoid hypermobility syndrome lacks skin hyperextensibility, bruising, and abnormal scarring
- Osteogenesis imperfecta has osteoporosis, susceptibility to fractures, specific bony abnormalities, blue sclerae, hearing loss

MANAGEMENT
General Measures
- Physical therapy to build muscle mass to stabilize joints
- Avoidance of sports that stress joints
- Braces or surgical correction of scoliosis
- Orthopedic surgery to prevent recurrent dislocations
- Analgesics or nonsteroidal anti-inflammatory drugs for arthralgias or osteoarthritis
- Delay surgical suture removal to decrease scarring
- Diligent investigation and close observation of vascular and visceral symptoms in patients with Type IV
- Elective cesarean section to decrease risk of uterine rupture and vaginal tears
- Genetic counseling

SPECIFIC THERAPY
- None
- High doses of vitamin C may help in Type VI

FOLLOW-UP
- Assess joint symptoms, posture, scarring

COMPLICATIONS AND PROGNOSIS
Complications
- Recurrent dislocations may cause joint effusions or hemarthrosis
- Premature osteoarthritis

- Life-threatening spontaneous arterial rupture, bowel rupture, or uterine rupture in type IV

Prognosis
- Normal life expectancy, except type IV (few live past age 40)

ENCEPHALITIS

CAROL A. GLASER, MD

HISTORY & PHYSICAL

History
- Definition: inflammation of the brain parenchyma
- Many individuals also with meningeal involvement ("meningoencephalitis")
- Significant morbidity and mortality
- 2 entities:
  - ➤ acute/infections – often gray matter
  - ➤ postinfections: often white matter involvement, primarily demyelinating process
  - ➤ overlap in clinical manifestations of infectious vs. postinfectious

Signs & Symptoms
- Altered mental status is hallmark of encephalitis.
- Fever and headache
- Often with lethargy and confusion that may progress to stupor and coma
- Seizures and focal neurologic findings also seen
  - ➤ Bizarre behavior, hallucination, aphasia is characteristic of herpes but can be seen with many other agents

Causative Agent
- Most cases presumed viral, though many bacteria and fungi have been associated
  - ➤ Viral agents include but not limited to:
  - ➤ Herpesviruses (HSV1, HSV2, VZ*, CMV, EBV*, HHV6)
- Enteroviruses
- Arboviruses (e.g. SLE, WEE, EEE, VEE, West Nile)
- Measles*
- Mumps*
- Respiratory viruses; Influenza A/B*, Parainfluenza*, adenovirus

- Rabies
- HIV
- Bacterial agents include but not limited to:
  - Rickettsia; RMSF, Ehrlichia chaffensis
  - Brucella sp.
  - Leptospirosis sp.
  - Bartonella henselae (CSD)
  - Mycobacteria tuberculosis
    - Borrelia burgdorferi (Lyme)
    - Mycoplasma pneumonia
- Fungal agents include but not limited to:
  - Cryptococcus neoformans
  - Histoplasma capsulatum
- Parasitic agents include but not limited to:
  - Naegleria fowleri
  - Acanthoemeoba
  - Toxoplasma gondii
- Unknown – etiology often remains unknown

*often postinfectious

TESTS

Nonspecific:
- CSF – often with lymphocytic pleocytosis and mild protein elevation normal glucose usually
- MRI – may be normal or abnormal
- If infectious etiology not found, consider tests for above differential

Specific:
- testing should be directed by good exposure history (e.g., travel history, mosquito/tick exposure, outdoor exposure, rash illness, respiratory prodrome, ill contacts, etc). Note that in many cases agent is never identified. Important to consider and rule out treatable agents.
- PCR for HSV-1 on spinal fluid – note that false pos/neg occur
- Culture CSF – often low yield
- PCR for specific agent (as above)
  - Serology* for various agents as above – e.g., arboviruses, Lyme, Rickettsia sp, Mycoplasma pneumonia etc. (*for serology extremely important to obtain acute and convalescent bloods)
  - Respiratory and Stool viral cultures

Brain biopsy as last resort

DIFFERENTIAL DIAGNOSIS
- Drug reaction
- Neoplastic; tumors/limbic encephalitis
- Strokes
- Autoimmune

MANAGEMENT
- Vigorous support
  - Respiratory support
  - Monitor electrolytes and glucose
  - Control seizures
  - Monitor and control cerebral edema

SPECIFIC THERAPY
- Acyclovir often started empirically, especially if focal temporal lobe involvement
- Specific therapy depends on agent diagnosed or highly suspected – e.g., if TB suspected, start anti-TB drugs; for Rickettsia, doxycycline, etc.
- Steroids and/or IVIG are often used in post-infectious cases.

FOLLOW-UP
n/a

COMPLICATIONS AND PROGNOSIS
n/a

ENTERAL AND PARENTERAL NUTRITION

PATSY OBAYASHI, MS, RN, CNSD, CDE

HISTORY & PHYSICAL

History
- inability to meet nutrition needs orally

Signs & Symptoms
- hypermetabolism
  - major surgery
  - sepsis
  - trauma
  - burns
  - organ transplantation
  - AIDS

- neurologic disease
  - CVA
  - dysphagia
  - head trauma
  - demyelinating Disease
- gastrointestinal disease
  - short-bowel syndrome (enteral support >100 cm jejunum and 150 cm ileum with ileocecal valve intact)
  - inflammatory bowel disease
  - GI tract fistula output (enteral support: <500 ml/day)
  - pancreatitis (parenteral: abdominal pain, elevated serum amylase or increased pancreatic fistula drainage with oral feedings)
  - esophageal obstruction
- oncologic disease
  - chemotherapy
  - radiotherapy
  - neoplasm
- psychiatric disease
  - anorexia nervosa (parenteral if severe malnutrition and intolerance to enteral feedings)
  - severe depression
- critical care
  - respiratory, renal, cardiac, or hepatic failure
  - parenteral if GI tract nonfunctional or NPO >4 to 5 days

TESTS

Basic Tests: Blood
- glucose sodium potassium
- albumin/pre-albumin blood urea nitrogen creatinine
- hemaglobin hematocrit total lymphocyte count
- transferrin acetone

Basic Tests: Urine
- 24 hour urine urea nitrogen for nitrogen balance

Other Tests:
- height
- weight (actual, usual, ideal)
- weight changes
- chest x-ray
- clinical signs of malnutrition
- intake and output

DIFFERENTIAL DIAGNOSIS
n/a

MANAGEMENT

General Measures

- calories
  - ➤ measureed BEE (using metabolic cart)
  - ➤ calculated:
    - using Harris-Benedict equation:
      - men: $(5 \times \text{Ht cm}) + (13.8 \times \text{Wt kg}) - (6.8 \times \text{age}) + 66.5$
      - women: $(1.8 \times \text{Ht cm}) + (9.6 \times \text{Wt kg}) - (4.7 \times \text{age}) + 66.5$
  - ➤ >30–35 kcal/kg body weight or adjusted weight if morbidly obese (BMI >30 mg/k2)
  - ➤ add stress factors 1.2–1.5 for wound healing, fever, sepsis
- protein
  - ➤ 0.9–1.2 gm/kg (stable)
  - ➤ 1.2–1.5 gm/kg (critically ill)
  - ➤ 2–2.5 gm/kg (burns, trauma, sepsis)
- carbohydrate
  - ➤ starting at 50% total calories, parenteral dextrose 4–5 mg/kg/minute
- fluid
  - ➤ 30–35 ml/kg dry weight; 1 ml/kcal
- fats
  - ➤ >20% total calories, < 4% total calories prevents EFA deficiency
- vitamins/minerals
  - ➤ 100% RDA
- electrolytes
  - ➤ based on needs

SPECIFIC THERAPY

Treatment Options

- enteral access
  - ➤ nasogastric
    - intact gag reflex
    - normal gastric motility and outlet
    - <6 weeks duration
    - inexpensive
  - ➤ nasoduodenal or nasojejunal
    - GERD/aspiration risks reduced
    - impaired gastric emptying
    - less nosocomial pneumonias

➣ gastrostomy
  • >6 weeks duration
  • normal gastric function
  • surgical, radiological, or percutaneous placement
  • large bore tube, medication administration or gastric decompression possible
➣ jejunostomy
  • >6 week duration
  • impaired gastric motility or access
  • GERD/aspiration risk decreased
  • bolus poorly tolerated
  • laparoscopic, fluoroscopic or endoscopic placement
➣ combined gastrostomy/jejunostomy
  • gastric decompression with otherwise intact GI tract
➣ medications via gastric port decrease risk of clogging jejunal port
➣ continuous feedings (16–24 hours)
➣ cyclic feedings (6–8 hours)
➣ bolus (<15 minutes duration, 4–6 times daily)
➣ formula options:
  • polymeric (1–2 kcal/ml, lactose/gluten free, +/−residue)
  • elemental (minimal residue, low viscosity, lactose-free, often hypertonic)
  • disease specific
    • modular components
▇ parenteral access
➣ peripheral
  • standard venipuncture method
  • <600–900 mOsm/L to avoid phlebitis
➣ central
  • centrally placed multilumen catheter placed surgically
➣ composition options:
  • dextrose concentrations 5–70%
  • amino acid concentrations 3–15%
  • lipid concentrations 10–30%
  • electrolytes, vitamins, minerals

Side Effects & Complications
▇ enteral
  ➣ high gastric residuals
  ➣ nasopharyngeal, nasolabial, ostomy site irritation
    • esophageal/laryngeal ulceration/stenosis

- ➤ tube displacement/obstruction
- ➤ hypertonic dehydration
- ➤ overhydration
- ➤ hyper/hypo:
  - kalemia
  - phosphatemia
  - glycemia
- ➤ hypercapnia
- ➤ hypozincemia
- ➤ essential fatty acid deficiency
  - constipation/diarrhea
  - nausea/vomiting
- ■ parenteral
  - ➤ peripheral
    - >60% total energy as lipids, potential immunocompromise
    - peripheral vein thrombosis
    - limited volume/concentration, calorie goals unmet
  - ➤ central
    - catheter related sepsis
    - hyper/hypo;
      - volemia
      - natremia
      - kalemia
      - glycemia
      - magnesemia
      - calcemia
      - phosphatemia
    - hypertriglyceridemia
    - prerenal azotemia
  - ➤ overfeeding
  - ➤ essential fatty acid deficiency
  - ➤ abnormal LFT's

Contraindications
- ■ absolute
  - ➤ enteral
    - nonfunctioning GI tract
    - severe diarrhea/vomiting
    - high output enteric fistula (>500 ml/day)
    - aggressive nutrition support not desired

> parenteral
  - aggressive nutrition support not desired
- relative
  > enteral
    - Intrinsic small bowel disease
    - severe short-bowel syndrome
    - cardiorespiratory insufficiency impairinf hemodynamics
  > parenteral
    - functioning GI tract
    - patient's prognosis
    - risks outweigh benefits

FOLLOW-UP
parenteral (initial 72 hours/critically ill):
- serum Ca, Mg, LFT's, P (2–3/week)
- electrolytes, BUN, Cr (daily)
- serum TG (weekly)
- CBC with differential (weekly)
- PT, PTT (weekly)
- capillary glucose (TID)
- weight (daily)
- intake and output (daily)
- nitrogen balance (as needed)
enteral:
- weight (daily)
- intake and output (daily)
- serum glucose (daily)
- gastric residuals < = every 4 hours (gastric feeding)
- bowel movements/consistency
- electrolytes, BUN, creatinine (daily then, 2–3/week)
- phosphorus, calcium, magnesium, CBC (weekly)
- feeding tube site care (daily)

COMPLICATIONS AND PROGNOSIS
- mechanical, gastrointestinal, metabolic complications
  > corrected with close monitoring
  > hospital-based nutrition support complications associated with medical treatment, procedures, medications rather than solely nutrition support
    - lowest complications with home nutrition support

- short-term enteral/parenteral nutrition supports wound healing and
  - ➤ stabilization until transition back to oral nutrition possible
- if lifelong nutrition support necessary, 100% nutrient needs can be met with careful technique and monitoring

---

ENTEROBIASIS (PINWORM)

J. GORDON FRIERSON, MD

HISTORY & PHYSICAL

History
- Life cycle: Eggs of Enterobius vermicularis are laid by females at night in anal and perianal area, are reingested by original or other host, hatch and develop in small intestine, mate and mature in colon. Generally 3–4 weeks to complete cycle.
- Exposure is by fecal-oral route, either auto-infection after scratching anus, or eggs transmitted by host's fingers or fomites. Eggs may be in dust, on sheets, clothing. Found worldwide.

Signs & Symptoms
- Children most often affected. Complaints are anal pruritus, or small "thread-like" worms coming from anus. In heavy infections may have irritability, restlessness. Rarely eggs or worms found in fallopian tubes or appendix, with corresponding pain, inflammation.

TESTS
- Basic tests: blood: normal
- Basic tests: urine: normal
- Specific tests: Scotch tape test: piece of clear tape pressed against the anus early in AM before washing or defecation, then placed on slide and examined. Eggs should be visible. Kits available as "pinworm kits."
  - ➤ Seeing or capturing adult worm, thin, white, 0.8 to 1.3 cm, is diagnostic. Occasionally seen on sigmoidoscopy.
- Other tests: Stool O&P examination often negative, not recommended

DIFFERENTIAL DIAGNOSIS
- Other causes of pruritus ani, such as anal pruritus, candidiasis, hemorrhoids, and strongyloidiasis

- Other worms that may emerge: occasionally trichuris (whipworm), which is 3 to 5 cm long

MANAGEMENT

What to Do First
- Assess other family members for infestation (or can treat all members empirically).

General Measures
- Teach good hygiene, such as hand washing after defecation, washing of clothes and pajamas, trimming fingernails, vacuuming. These measures help prevent reinfection.

SPECIFIC THERAPY

Indications
- Treat symptomatic patients, and most asymptomatic ones since they can infect others (though their own health is not impaired). In a household, test all children or treat them presumptively.

Treatment Options
- Mebendazole, repeat in 2 weeks (treatment of choice)
  - ➤ pyrantel pamoate, repeat in 2 weeks
  - ➤ albendazole, repeat in 2 weeks for patients >2 yo

Side Effects & Complications
- Rare. All 3 drugs may cause mild intestinal symptoms in small minority, and pyrantel pamoate rarely causes headache, dizziness, or rash.
- Contraindications to treatment: absolute: none
- Contraindications to treatment: relative: asymptomatic adult not with children

FOLLOW-UP

Routine
- No tests necessary after treatment. If symptoms or visible worms return, retreat entire household and enforce general hygienic measures.

COMPLICATIONS AND PROGNOSIS
- If eggs or worms get into fallopian tubes or appendix, abdominal pain and tenderness can occur and mimic other conditions, like appendicitis. Complications from intestinal disease are nil. Prognosis is good.

ENTEROVIRUSES

CAROL A. GLASER, MD

HISTORY & PHYSICAL

History
- Picornaviridae virus family
- Includes:
  - 23 group A coxsackie viruses
  - 3 serotypes of Polioviruses
  - 6 group B coxsackie viruses
  - 31 serotypes of Echoviruses (echo 22, 23 atypical)
  - 4 enterovirus (types 68–71)
  - untyped entroviruses
- Humans only natural host
- Spread fecal-oral primarily, respiratory routes, mother/infant (peripartum) and contaminated fomites
- Incubation: variable depending on specific enterovirus types; generally 1–2 weeks but varies from 2–35 days
- fecal shedding 6–12 weeks, respiratory <1 week
- more common summer and early fall in temperate climates, year-round in tropical and subtropical areas

Signs & Symptoms
- wide range of illness ranging from asymptomatic to serious disease and fatalities. Individual serotypes may be most frequently associated with particular syndromes but considerable overlap in clinical manifestations.
  - Most common: nonspecific febrile illness
  - Respiratory: common cold, pharyngitis, herpangina (sore throat with papulovesicular pharyngeal lesions on erythematous base), pneumonia, pleurodynia
  - Hand, Foot and Mouth; often associated with coxsackie A16 but other serotypes can be involved, mild illness associated with sore throat, fever, scattered vesicular lesions on pharynx/lips and grayish vesicles on hands and feet
  - Gastrointestinal: vomiting, diarrhea, abdominal pain, occasionally hepatitis
  - Acute hemorrhagic conjunctivitis
  - Cardiac: myocarditis; clinical symptoms dependent on region and extent of cardiac involvement, often with palpitations, chest

pain, and have history of preceding illness. Arrhythmia and sudden death can occur when conducting system involved. Pericardial friction rub indicates myopericarditis.

➤ Neonatal Sepsis: fever, nonspecific signs such as vomiting, anorexia, rash and URI

➤ Severe cases: hepatic necrosis, myocarditis, necrotizing enterocolitis and encephalitis

➤ Nervous system: paralytic poliomyelitis, aseptic meningitis, rarely encephalitis

Poliomyelitis (caused by poliovirus serotypes)

➤ 90+% wild-type poliovirus are asymptomatic

➤ remaining 10% develop fever, fatigue, HA, anorexia ×2–3 days

- Small % of these cases develop aseptic meningitis (indistinguishable from nonpolio enteroviruses) and some then develop paralysis

➤ Aseptic Meningitis (many different serotypes cause):

- nuchal rigidity
- headache, photophobia
- vomiting, anorexia, rash, diarrhea, cough, URI, diarrhea, myalgias
- occasionally SIADH
- some with skin rash (hand, foot and mouth)

➤ Encephalitis:

- Generalized encephalitis
  - Less commonly focal encephalitis
  - Chronic enteroviral meningoencephalitis occurs in individuals with defects immunoglobulin production (e.g., hypogammaglobulinemia)

TESTS

Nonspecific:

■ Aseptic meningitis:

➤ CSF: monocytic pleocytosis (100–1,000 cell/mm3)

- normal glucose
- normal to slight increase protein
- Myocarditis
  - myocardial enzymes elevation

Specific:

■ Isolation from affected site: respiratory secretions, stool, conjunctival swab, CSF, and myocardial tissues (note: cell culture isolation is possible with most enteroviruses except group A coxsackievirus, which do not grow in cell culture, only grow in suckling mice. Most enteroviruses grow rapidily. The body site where enterovirus is detected is important for interpretation to differentiate enterovirus colonization versus enterovirus-associated disease. Note that enterovirus is present in stool for weeks (and sometimes months) after initial infection.

■ Nucleic acid detection: available in some settings, specimen best from affected site; CSF, respiratory secretions, conjunctival swab, CSF, and myocardial tissues. Stool possible but as above may persist for weeks.

■ Serology: difficult due to large number of serotypes. Recently developed IgM tests have been developed and have variable success.

DIFFERENTIAL DIAGNOSIS
■ Respiratory illnesses: other respiratory viruses
■ Nervous system: Aseptic meningitis; large number of other viral and bacterial causes
■ Polio-like illness: important to distinguish poliovirus versus other enterovirus (especially enterovirus 71)
■ Cardiac: myocarditis – herpesviruses, adenovirus, parvovirus

MANAGEMENT
■ Supportive

SPECIFIC THERAPY
■ None widely available
  ➤ Chronic enteroviral encephalitis -IVIG has been used successfully

FOLLOW-UP
n/a

COMPLICATIONS AND PROGNOSIS
■ Aseptic meningitis: outcome is excellent (except in neonates)
  ➤ Encephalitis; may have profound acute disease and long-term sequelae, case-dependent
  ➤ Poliomyelitis; long-term outcome determined first 6 months after onset; absence of improvement suggests permanent paralysis with concomitant limb atrophy + deformity. If improvement occurs – gradual, continues 9–18 months. Overall morality spinal poliomyelitis ~5%
  ➤ Myocarditis: most patients recover but some will have residual EKG/ECHO abnormalities for months to years after infection.

Small % develop congestive heart failure, chronic myocarditis, or dilated cardiomyopathy.
- Neonatal sepsis: up to 10% mortality
  - Diabetes mellitus: an association has been suggested with enterovirus, but this remains unproven

EPIDIDYMITIS AND ORCHITIS

ARTHUR I. SAGALOWSKY, MD

HISTORY & PHYSICAL
- acute severe pain; secondary acute infection vs dull chronic pain from infections or trauma
- fever, dyuria common
- painful, fleshy swelling of epididymus or entire testis
- secondary reactive hydrocele common and obscures P.E.
- scrotal skin may be inflamed

TESTS
- urinalysis – pyuria, bactiuria common
- urine culture and sensitivity
- elevated WBC
- fever common
- ultrasound and/or nuclear scan reveal characteristic epididymal enlargement, increased blood flow

DIFFERENTIAL DIAGNOSIS
- must exclude torsion (see below)
- primary (infection, trauma) vs secondary (testis tumor, chronic infection, ascites)

MANAGEMENT
n/a

SPECIFIC THERAPY
- analgesics
- anti-inflammatories
- antibiotics

FOLLOW-UP
n/a

COMPLICATIONS AND PROGNOSIS
n/a

EPILEPSIES

MICHAEL J. AMINOFF, MD, DSc

HISTORY & PHYSICAL

- History of recurrent seizures (ie, stereotyped episodes of motor, sensory or behavioral disturbance or LOC)
- Seizures occur unpredictably but may be precipitated by certain situations (eg, stress, sleep deprivation, flickering lights)
- Pt may be unaware of seizure occurrence
- Seizures may be followed by headache, confusion, drowsiness or focal deficits
- May be history of preceding CNS injury or infection, drug or alcohol abuse
- May be family history of epilepsy
- May be no abnormal finding
- Focal abnormalities in pts w/ underlying structural disorder
- Cognitive deficits or multifocal or generalized deficits if seizures secondary to diffuse cerebral pathology
- Dysmorphic features or cutaneous abnormalities in certain epileptic syndromes

TESTS

- Lab tests: CBC, differential count, FBS, Ca, liver & kidney function tests, VDRL
- EEG to support diagnosis & to characterize, localize & determine prognosis of seizures
- Cranial CT scan or MRI: to detect underlying structural lesion (especially w/ focal seizures or seizure onset after age 20 yr)

DIFFERENTIAL DIAGNOSIS

- TIAs distinguished from focal seizures by their lack of spread & negative symptomatology (loss of motor or sensory function)
- Panic attacks usually relate to external circumstances; may be evidence of psychopathology btwn attacks
- Rage attacks consist of goal-directed aggressive behavior
- Syncopal attacks preceded by sweating, nausea, malaise, pallor; LOC assoc w/ little (if any) motor activity, recovers rapidly w/ recumbency, no postictal confusion
- Cardiac arrhythmia: may be history of cardiac disease, heart murmur or arrhythmia; attacks may relate to physical activity

■ Psychogenic attacks: may simulate convulsions but may relate to external circumstances or stress, in company of others, & after preparation; despite apparent LOC, may be goal-directed or other atypical behavior; no postictal changes; EEG unchanged in attacks; may occur in pts also having seizures

MANAGEMENT
■ Do not restrain during seizures
■ Maintain airway during status epilepticus

SPECIFIC THERAPY
■ Antiepileptic medication, selected based on seizure type; monotherapy preferable to polytherapy; continue treatment until seizure-free for 2 yr; discontinue medication gradually; monitor for compliance clinically & by blood drug measurements; poor compliance predisposes to status epilepticus; side effects depend on anticonvulsant
■ Advise about lifestyle: avoid situations that could be dangerous or life-threatening if a further seizure occurs or that may precipitate further seizures
■ Follow requirements concerning reporting of patients to state authorities

FOLLOW-UP
■ Depends on underlying cause
■ Pts with well-controlled idiopathic seizures should be followed at least once annually

COMPLICATIONS AND PROGNOSIS
■ Delay in initiating effective treatment may lead to greater difficulty in obtaining seizure control

EPISCLERITIS AND SCLERITIS

C. STEPHEN FOSTER, MD

HISTORY & PHYSICAL

History
■ Red eye, usually but not always without change in vision, no discharge
■ Pain/tenderness to touch = scleritis

Signs & Symptoms
■ Conjunctival injection

- Engorgement of superficial and deep episcleral venus plexes
- Tenderness to palpation = scleritis
- Areas of nodule formation and tenderness = nodular scleritis

TESTS

Laboratory
- Basic blood tests:
  - ➤ CBC, ESR, CRP, uric acid, BLN, creatinine
- Basic urine tests:
  - ➤ Urinary sediment and urine analysis
- Specific diagnostic tests:
  - ➤ ANCA, RFs (IgG, IgA, IgM), ANAs (on RAT liver and Hep2 cells), hepatitis B antigen, anti Type II collagen antibody, HLA-1327, FTA-Abs

Imaging
- Chest x-ray and sinus films; B scan ultrasonography

Biopsy
- For histopathology, culture, and PCR studies

DIFFERENTIAL DIAGNOSIS
- Rheumatoid arthritis
- Ankylosing spondylitis
- Wegener granulornatosis
- SLE
- Relapsing polychondritis
- Mixed connective tissue disease
- Polyarteritis nodosa
- Herpes simplex herpes zoster syphilis Hyperuricemia atopy

MANAGEMENT

What to Do First
- Assess whether episcleritis or scleritis, whether or not work-up appropriate, whether or not treatment needed; episcleritis rarely needs work-up or therapy; scleritis always does

General Measures
- Cold compresses
- Rest

SPECIFIC THERAPY

Indications
- Scleritis: always
- Episcleritis that significantly interferes with daily life (eg, someone in public eye)

Treatment Options
- Oral NSAIDs: OTC for episcleritis, Cox-2 specific NSAID, nonspecific NSAID
- Steroid: systemic
- Immunomodulators: methotrexate, azathioprine, mycophenolate mofteil,cyclophosphamide
- N.B. disease-specific to some extent: eg, cyclophosphamide treatment of choice for polyarteritis nodosa, Wegener granulomatosis, and necrotizing scleritis secondary to rheumatoid arthritis or relapsing polychondritis

FOLLOW-UP

During Treatment
- Every 1 to 4 weeks, depending upon response and drug employed

Routine
- For episcleritis: yearly
- For scleritis: every 3 months

COMPLICATIONS AND PROGNOSIS
- Episcleritis
  - transition to true scleritis (10%)
  - Scleritis peripheral keratitis 25% peripheral ulcerative keratitis 15%
  - uveitis 42%
  - cataract 17%
  - loss of vision 37%

ERECTILE DYSFUNCTION

SHAHRAM S. GHOLAMI, MD; WILLIAM O. BRANT, MD;
ANTHONY J. BELLA, MD; MAURICE M. GARCIA, MD; and TOM F. LUE, MD

HISTORY & PHYSICAL
Definition: Inability to achieve and maintain an erection sufficient for satisfactory sexual intercourse

■ A thorough medical and psychosexual history
■ A focused physical exam to rule out gynecomastia, testicular atrophy or penile abnormalities such as Peyronie's disease

TESTS

Laboratory
■ CBC, urinalysis, fasting glucose, creatinine, lipid profile, and testosterone
■ If testosterone low, check free testosterone, prolactin and luteinizing hormone
■ Injection and stimulation test to assess erectile function
■ Doppler ultrasound to assess penile blood flow if necessary
　Arteriography to examine for vascular occlusion
　Cavernosometry/cavernosography to assess venous leakage

DIFFERENTIAL DIAGNOSIS

Distinguish from Erectile Dysfunction
■ Congenital penile curvature or Peyronie's disease – curvature of penis with erection that may interfere with penetration
■ Premature ejaculation – able to get erection but loses it after ejaculation
■ Painful erection – interrupting ability to have intercourse
■ Micropenis – small phallus inhibiting successful intercourse

Classification of Erectile Dysfunction (ED)
■ Organic ED (neurogenic, hormonal, drug-induced, vascular)
　➤ Neurogenic
　　• Failure to initiate or conduct nerve impulse results in difficulty in achieving and maintaining erections
　　• Includes stroke, cerebral trauma, spinal cord injury, radical pelvic surgery, neuropathy, pelvic trauma, Parkinson's and Alzheimer's diseases
　➤ Hormonal
　　• Hypogonadism: low testosterone due to testicular failure or pituitary insufficiency
　　• Hyperprolactinemia may be due to pituitary tumor or drugs
　　• Androgen deficiency may affect nocturnal erections and libido
　➤ Drug-induced
　　• Antipsychotics, antidepressants and centrally acting antihypertensive

- Beta-blockers, thiazides, spironolactone, as well as anti-androgenic drugs (cimetidine, ketoconazole, cyproterone, and estrogens)
- Cigarette smoking via vasoconstriction and penile venous leakage
- Exogenous steroids
- Chronic alcoholism: hypogonadism and polyneuropathy
➤ Vasculogenic ED
- Atherosclerosis, hypertension, hyperlipidemia, cigarette smoking, diabetes mellitus, and pelvic irradiation, degenerative changes (Peyronie's disease, old age, diabetes mellitus), traumatic injury (penile fracture or surgery)
- Inadequate arterial inflow and impaired venous occlusion
■ Psychogenic
➤ Performance anxiety, strained relationship, lack of sexual arousability, and psychiatric disorders (depression and schizophrenia)
➤ Secondary to loss of libido, overinhibition, or impaired nitric oxide release
■ Age-related – increased latent period between sexual stimulation and erection
➤ Erections less turgid
➤ Ejaculation less forceful, with decreased volume
➤ Lengthened refractory period

MANAGEMENT
■ Occasionally, change in lifestyle or medications all that is needed to restore potency
■ Treat underlying medical condition

SPECIFIC THERAPY

Medical
■ Androgen therapy offered to men with ED secondary to hypogonadism only
➤ Testosterone therapy may increase libido and desire but may not improve erections
➤ Side effects: hepatotoxicity, skin irritation, dermatitis, possible stimulation of prostate growth (BPH or cancer)
➤ Avoid in men with normal hormonal levels and men with prostate cancer or enlarged prostate with obstructive voiding symptoms
■ First-line therapy
➤ Oral therapy with phosphodiesterase-5 inhibitor (sildenafil, vardenafil, tadalafil) considered first line

- Contraindicated in men taking nitrates
- Consultation with a cardiologist in men with severe cardiovascular disease
- Side effects include dyspepsia, nasal congestion, headache, and visual changes
- ➤ Yohimbine – alpha-2-adrenergic receptor antagonist acts at the adrenergic receptors in brain
  - Marginal effects on ED
  - Side effects include palpitation, fine tremor, elevation of blood pressure, and anxiety
- ➤ Apomorphine – sublingual medication
  - Acts at the central dopaminergic (D1/D2) receptors
  - Released in Europe, not approved in United States
  - Major side effects are nausea and vomiting.
- ■ Second-line therapy
  - ➤ Need appropriate training and education by medical personnel before beginning
  - ➤ Vacuum constriction device (VCD)
    - Advantages: no drug interactions, very reliable and effective when used properly
    - Disadvantages: Cumbersome and gives an unnatural erection
    - Side effects include petechiae, numbness and a trapped ejaculate.
  - ➤ Transurethral therapy
    - Advantages: locally acting medication, low risk of priapism, avoids needles
    - Major disadvantages: penile pain, urethral bleeding and burning, and moderate response rate
  - ➤ Intracavernous injection therapy (ICI)
    - Advantages: very effective
    - Most common medications used: alprostadil, phentolamine, papaverine, or combinations (only alprostadil is FDA-approved)
    - Disadvantages: requires injection, high dropout rate, and can cause priapism/fibrosis

Surgical
- ■ Patients who fail or are dissatisfied with medical management
- ■ Curative surgery
  - ➤ Patients with congenital or traumatically acquired erectile dysfunction

➤ Arterial bypass surgery for patients with abnormal arterial flow to the penis: usually anastomose inferior epigastric artery to dorsal penile artery or vein
  - Only used in congenital or traumatically induced arterial insufficiency
  - Major complication: glans hyperemia (in arteriovenous bypass)
➤ Venous outflow surgery for patients with congenital or traumatic venous leak: ligate abnormally draining veins
  - Major complication: recurrence of venous leak
■ Prosthesis surgery
  ➤ Patients with generalized disease or older patients
  ➤ Highly effective and reliable
  ➤ Risks associated with infection and device malfunction
  ➤ Multiple varieties including semi-rigid, malleable, and two- or three-piece inflatable

FOLLOW-UP
■ Each 6 months to 1 year routinely to evaluate erectile function and response to treatment

COMPLICATIONS AND PROGNOSIS
n/a

ERYSIPELAS AND CELLULITIS

JEFFREY P. CALLEN, MD

HISTORY & PHYSICAL

History
■ Acute, rapidly spreading non-suppurative infection of the skin and underlying soft tissue
  ➤ Usually streptococcal
  ➤ Occasionally staphylococcal
■ Erysipelas is more superficial than cellulitis.
■ Preceding trauma is frequent.
■ Fever and chills are common.

Signs & Symptoms
■ Erysipelas
  ➤ Usually facial

> Sharply marginated warm, tender, erythematous, edematous, indurated plaque
> Fever, often to 102 degrees F
> Vesicles or bullae may occur on the surface.
- Cellulitis
  > Most often on the extremities
  > Evidence of onychomycosis is frequent and may represent the site of entry for the bacteria.
  > Less well demarcated than erysipelas, but otherwise the findings are identical
- Perianal cellulites
  > Usually in young children
  > May precede a flare of guttate psoriasis

TESTS

Laboratory
- Basic blood studies:
  > Leukocytosis is frequent.
  > Streptozyme (ASO) titer is frequently elevated.
- Biopsy is not necessary, but reveals edema, dilated capillaries, and diffuse neutrophilic infiltration.
- Cultures
  > may be obtained by needle aspiration or biopsy
  > blood cultures may reveal pathologic bacteria

Confirmatory Tests
- Diagnosis is clinical.

Imaging
- Not needed

DIFFERENTIAL DIAGNOSIS
- Thrombophlebitis
- Necrotizing fasciitis
- Gout
- Sweet's syndrome
- Scurvy

MANAGEMENT

What to Do First
- Assess the need for intravenous antibiotic therapy.

General Measures
- Elevation of the inflamed area
- Cool, moist compresses

SPECIFIC THERAPY
- Administer antibiotics
  - ➤ Penicillin
  - ➤ Cephalosporin
  - ➤ Other – erythromycin, vancomycin, clindamycin
- Consider drainage if the area is fluctuant
- Treat associated onychomycosis if present to prevent recurrent disease

FOLLOW-UP

During Rx
- Patients are often hospitalized; if not, they should be re-evaluated daily.

COMPLICATIONS AND PROGNOSIS
- Recurrent cellulitis (or erysipelas) may occur due to disruption of the lymphatic flow.
- Good prognosis, if treated early

ERYTHEMA MULTIFORME MAJOR; AKA STEVENS JOHNSON SYNDROME (SEE ALSO DRUG ERUPTIONS)

RAJANI KATTA, MD and JEFFREY P. CALLEN, MD

HISTORY & PHYSICAL

History
- Most cases related to drug ingestion
- Major offenders: antibiotics (penicillins, sulfonamides, cephalosporins), anticonvulsants (phenytoin, carbamazepine, phenobarbital, lamotrigine), NSAIDS, allopurinol
- Minority of cases may be infection-related (mycoplasma pneumoniae, herpes simplex).

Signs & Symptoms
- Nonspecific prodrome precedes rash (1–14 days) in majority of patients.
  - ➤ Fever, malaise, myalgias, arthralgias, headache, sore throat, cough, rhinitis, diarrhea
- Pain, burning of mucous membranes
- Pain, tenderness of skin

- Initially, diffuse erythematous morbilliform eruption on face, trunk, and then extremities
- Mimics exanthematous drug rash in early stages
- Rapid progression of skin findings
- Atypical targetoid lesions – individual lesions somewhat resemble a target, with a central dusky region
- Purpuric quality to rash
- Flaccid or tense blisters may arise in involved areas
- Mucosal involvement key criteria for diagnosis – may precede or parallel skin involvement
- Involvement typically of 2 or more mucosal surfaces (oral, ocular, genital, gastrointestinal)
- Severe hemorrhagic crusting and erosions of lips
- Extensive erosions and pseudomembranes on buccal mucosa, palate, other oral mucosa
- Erythema and erosions of ocular mucosa
- Toxic epidermal necrolysis (TEN) considered part of SJS spectrum; more severe and extensive involvement (>30% skin involved)

TESTS
- Diagnosis usually made by typical clinical appearance of widespread rash, mucosal erosions, and systemic symptoms
- In questionable cases, punch biopsy of involved area of skin – epidermal necrosis with limited inflammation; degree varies with stage of disease
- No test available to determine causative medication

Laboratory
- Rule out systemic involvement or systemic infection, and monitor fluid and electrolyte status.
- CBC, electrolytes, albumin, liver function tests, renal function, urinalysis
- Blood cultures, skin cultures, other, as clinically indicated

Imaging
- Only needed if internal organ involvement suspected – chest x-ray

DIFFERENTIAL DIAGNOSIS
- Drug rash
  - ➣ Presence of mucosal erosions, targetoid lesions, purpuric areas, and blisters indicates progression to SJS.
- Erythema multiforme minor

➤ Patient does not appear ill (no systemic involvement); targetoid lesions present, but are classic targets and typically on extremities; only one mucosal surface sometimes affected (oral)

■ Staphylococcal scalded skin syndrome
➤ Occurs primarily in children
➤ Rash associated with nasopharyngeal infection, generalized large, flaccid superficial bullae, sparing of mucous membranes

■ Viral exanthem
➤ Morbilliform eruption; no target lesions

■ Vasculitis

■ Acute generalized exanthematous pustulosis

MANAGEMENT

What to Do First

■ Discontinue any possible causative agents.

■ Assess severity of skin involvement – surface area involved, degree of rash/erosions/necrosis.

■ Assess severity of mucosal involvement – oral intake possible, degree of pain.

■ Assess systemic involvement.

■ Evaluate for secondary infection.

General Measures

■ Supportive therapy as indicated by severity of involvement

■ Fluid, electrolyte management

■ Precautions to decrease risk of sepsis

■ Aggressive treatment if any signs of secondary infection

■ Early ophthalmologic evaluation

SPECIFIC THERAPY

■ Systemic corticosteroids or other immunosuppressives as treatment for SJS remains controversial; no controlled trials available

■ Intravenous immune globulin 0.75 g/kg/day for 4 days appears to stop progression and improve prognosis.

FOLLOW-UP

■ Depending on severity, patients are generally hospitalized and cared for in an experienced intensive care unit.

COMPLICATIONS AND PROGNOSIS

Complications

■ Fluid and electrolyte abnormalities

■ Secondary infection, due to breakdown of skin barrier
■ Dehydration and malnutrition, due to pain from oral involvement
■ Ocular sequelae in severe cases – symblepharon, ectropion, corneal scarring, rarely blindness
■ Strictures of mucosal surfaces – esophagus, urethral, anal
■ Cutaneous dyspigmentation
■ Permanent scarring of skin uncommon

Prognosis
■ Estimates of mortality vary widely in published studies
  ➤ SJS 5–15% mortality
  ➤ TEN up to 50% mortality
■ Sepsis is most common cause of death.

ERYTHEMA NODOSUM

JAMES SEWARD, MD and JEFFREY P. CALLEN, MD
REVISED BY JEFFREY P. CALLEN, MD

HISTORY & PHYSICAL

History
■ An acute, inflammatory reaction pattern triggered by wide range of disease processes
■ Commonly associated with streptococcal infections
■ Other etiologic associations:
  ➤ Yersinia, salmonella, shigella, systemic fungal infections (coccidioidomycosis, histoplasmosis, and blastomycosis), sporotrichosis, toxoplasmosis, tuberculosis, inflammatory bowel disease, pregnancy, drugs (bromides, iodides, sulfonamides, and oral contraceptives)
■ Also seen with sarcoidosis (the combination of anterior uveitis, arthritis, bilateral hilar lymphadenopathy, and EN is known as Lofgren's syndrome. These patients may also have fever and malaise. This process is a self-limited form of sarcoidosis.)
■ Inflammatory bowel disease – EN reflects activity of the bowel disease
■ Frequently no underlying disease is found (40%)
■ Most commonly seen in young women
■ Peak incidence 20–30 years old

Signs & Symptoms
- Bilateral, red, tender nodules on the anterior shins
- Other sites: upper legs, extensor aspects of arms, and neck
- Lesions slowly flatten, leaving purple or blue-green color resembling a bruise
- Often accompanied by fever, chills, malaise, arthritis or arthralgia, and leukocytosis
- Usually resolves spontaneously in 3 to 6 weeks

TESTS
- Blood: Elevated ESR is common
  - ➤ CBC indicated in all patients
- Imaging: CXR to rule out sarcoidosis

Other Tests
- Deep skin biopsy including the subcutaneous fat is needed only when the diagnosis is in question or the patient has a recurrent or chronic course.
- Search for underlying disease: based on geographic location, age, history, and physical; a throat culture, ASO (Streptozyme) titer, bacteriologic, virologic or Yersinia titer, and tuberculin or fungal antigen skin test
  Diagnosis: Based on typical clinical appearance and biopsy

DIFFERENTIAL DIAGNOSIS
- other forms of panniculitis
  - ➤ erythema induratum – often on the posterior calf
  - ➤ subcutaneous fat necrosis associated with pancreatitis – associated abdominal pain
- syphilitic gumma
- nodular vasculitis

MANAGEMENT
What to Do First
- Assess the patient for underlying disease.
- Any underlying abnormality should be treated.
- Bed rest, elevation, support hose for mild cases

SPECIFIC THERAPY
- Aspirin, NSAIDS often helpful
- Potassium iodide is frequently effective.
- Intralesional injection of triamcinolone acetonide

- Predinsone for severe cases
- Immunosuppressives may be used for recurrent or chronic, severe disease.

FOLLOW-UP
n/a

COMPLICATIONS AND PROGNOSIS
- Good – Spontaneous resolution often occurs
- Usually runs course in 3 to 6 weeks
- Resolves without atrophy or scarring
- Chronic lesions should suggest alternative diagnosis.
- When using KI, must monitor for induction of hypothyroidism

ESOPHAGEAL CANCER

ROY SOETIKNO, MD, MS and MONA LIN, MD

HISTORY & PHYSICAL

History
- increasing incidence in recent years
- adenocarcinoma and squamous carcinoma comprised more than 90% of cases (adenocarcinoma is more common than squamous)
- benign tumors rare
  - common types: fibrovascular polyp, lipoma, granular cell tumor, leiomyoma

Signs & Symptoms
- asymptomatic until advanced
- dysphagia typically progress from solids to solids and liquids
- anemia
- cough from tracheobronchial fistulas
- weight loss

TESTS
- barium esophagogram
  - confirm presence and extent of tumor
- endoscopy
  - localize and biopsy for pathology
- endoscopic ultrasonography and CT scan
  - determine local and distant staging, respectively

DIFFERENTIAL DIAGNOSIS
- Benign vs malignant (biopsy required)

MANAGEMENT

What to Do First
- stage extent of disease:
- TNM based
- CT scans of chest and abdomen to rule out distant disease
- endoscopic ultrasound most accurate to determine depth of tumor and nodal involvement

General Measures
- assess comorbities and suitability of patient for surgery

SPECIFIC THERAPY
- surgery
  - ➤ curative if not metastatic
- endoscopy
  - ➤ curative for early superficial disease
  - ➤ palliative for obstruction by stent placement
- chemoradiotherapy
  - ➤ unclear if useful as neoadjuvant

FOLLOW-UP
- No specific protocol: recurrence is usually not treatable
- Regular blood tests q 3 months, and CT scans q 12 months

COMPLICATIONS AND PROGNOSIS
- Median survival
  - ➤ Stage I – 63 months
  - ➤ Stage II – 26 months
  - ➤ Stage IIB – 13 months
  - ➤ Stage III – 10 months
  - ➤ Stage IV – 9 months

ESOPHAGEAL INFECTIONS AND INFLAMMATION

LAUREN B. GERSON, MD, MSc

HISTORY & PHYSICAL

History
- immunodeficiency states, AIDS, solid organ transplantation, diabetes mellitus, recent or current antibiotic usage, disorders of

esophageal motility such as achalasia, presence of malignancy such as leukemia or lymphoma, current radiation therapy
- use of immunosuppressive medications including corticosteroids, azathioprine, methotrexate, or medications administered after solid organ transplantation
- medications associated with pill-induced esophagitis: antibiotics including doxycycline, tetracycline, clindamycin, trimethoprim-sulfamethoxazole, quinidine, potassium chloride pills, zalcitabine, zidovudine, alendronate and risedronate, iron, vitamin C
- Hospitalized or bed-bound patients are at greatest risk of pill-induced esophagitis since injury is more likely if pills are swallowed when supine or without water.
- History of accidental (usually in children) or deliberate (suicidal) ingestion of liquid or crystalline alkali (drain cleaners, etc.) or acid causing caustic injury to the esophagus
- History of radiation for lung or thyroid cancer; odynophagia usually occurs after 25–30 Gy and lasts until completion of radiation therapy

Signs & Symptoms
- sudden onset of retrosternal pain, exacerbated by swallowing, can occur hours after pill ingestion. Elderly patients may report less pain.
- odynophagia
- dysphagia
- oral thrush may be a sign of underlying esophageal candidiasis; presence of herpetic vesicles might suggest HSV esophagitis
- rare signs include upper GI hemorrhage, tracheoesophageal fistula or food impaction, unexplained nausea
- Post-radiation patients complain of both odynophagia and dysphagia to solids; pain is constant and exacerbated by swallowing attempts

TESTS

Laboratory

Basic Studies: Blood
- check blood cultures
- WBC and positive blood cultures
- CMV PCR if CMV suspected

Upper Endoscopy
- if no response to empiric antifungal therapy after 3 days
- obtain brushings for candidiasis if suspected

- biopsy any esophageal ulcers and send for viral culture
- endoscopic appearance
  - Candida esophagitis – small, yellow-white raised plaques with surrounding erythema in mild disease; confluent linear and nodular plaques reflect extensive disease
  - HSV esophagitis – vesicles and small, discrete, punched-out ("volcano-like") superficial ulcerations with or without a fibrinous exudate. In later stages, a diffuse erosive esophagitis develops from enlargement and coalescence of the ulcers
  - CMV esophagitis – serpiginous ulcers in an otherwise normal mucosa that may coalesce to form giant ulcers, particularly in the distal esophagus
  - endoscopy is not helpful in patients post-radiation and will increase patient discomfort

Imaging
- not recommended as initial test
  - inability to perform biopsies
  - odynophagia limits ability to drink barium
- findings on barium esophagram:
  - candidiasis: diffuse plaque-like lesions, linear configuration
  - HSV: stellate focal ulcers on background of normal mucosa
  - CMV: linear vertical ulcerations with central umbilication; large (>2 cm) and deep in AIDS patients
  - idiopathic HIV-associated ulcer: large, isolated, deep ulcers

DIFFERENTIAL DIAGNOSIS
- infectious etiologies: Candida, CMV, HSV, varicella zoster, HIV, TB
- differential diagnosis dependent on underlying condition:
  - normal host: HSV or candidiasis in the elderly
  - post-transplantation patients: Candida, CMV, HSV, or VZ
  - malnutrition, corticosteroid usage, diabetes mellitus: candidiasis
- idiopathic esophageal ulcer associated with HIV infection
- pill-induced esophagitis: one or more discrete ulcers in junction of proximal and middle third of the esophagus
- gastroesophageal reflux disease
- esophageal motility disorder, such as achalasia
- esophageal cancer
- rare: Crohn's disease, histoplasmosis, syphilis, sarcoidosis, bacterial esophagitis

MANAGEMENT

What to Do First:

- if candidiasis suspected, empiric treatment with fluconazole for 3 days; reserve endoscopy with biopsy for patients who do not respond to therapy
- in cases of caustic injury, endoscopy should be performed within 24 hours to determine extent of injury and allow for psychiatric referral if no injury is demonstrated

General Measures

- topical analgesics (2% viscous lidocaine swish and swallow 15 cc orally q3–4h or sucralfate slurry 1 g orally QID) for patient discomfort
- liquid diet and consideration for parenteral or nasogastric feeding if oral intake compromised
- identify predisposing conditions
- withdrawal of immunosuppressive medications if possible
- adequate control of concomitant gastroesophageal reflux disease, if present; concomitant acid suppression is recommended for patients with infectious esophagitis

SPECIFIC THERAPY

- esophageal candidiasis
  - topical therapy for patients with normal immune system: Nystatin, 500,000 units "swish and swallow" five times daily or clotrimazole troches, 10 mg dissolved in mouth five times daily) for 7–14 days
  - for immunocompromised hosts:
  - fluconazole 100 mg/day for 14–21 days
  - itraconazole 200 mg/day for 14–21 days
  - refractory cases: amphotericin B IV 0.3–0.5 mg/kg/day
- cytomegalovirus infection
  - in patients with HIV infection, restoration of the immune system with highly active antiretroviral therapy (HAART) is the most effective way of controlling CMV disease
  - ganciclovir 5 mg/kg q12h for 3–6 weeks
  - foscarnet 90 mg/kg IV q12h for 3–6 weeks
- herpes simplex esophagitis
  - in immunocompetent hosts, no treatment may be indicated, but antiviral therapy may result in quicker symptom resolution
  - acyclovir 400–800 mg five times per day for 14–21 days or 5 mg/kg IV q8h for 7–14 days

➤ famciclovir 250 mg three times daily, and valacyclovir, 1 g twice daily
➤ For nonresponders: foscarnet 40 mg/kg IV q8h for 21 days
■ varicella zoster: same treatment as HSV
■ esophageal tuberculosis
➤ 9-month course of multidrug therapy
➤ therapy guided by drug sensitivities to anti-TB therapy
■ idiopathic ulcer or ulceration due to HIV infection
➤ prednisone 40 mg daily for 2 weeks
➤ thalidomide
■ pill-induced esophagitis
➤ withdrawal of offending pill if pill-induced esophagitis suspected
➤ drink at least 4 oz of fluid with pills and stay upright for at least 30 minutes after ingestion
➤ proton-pump inhibitor therapy for 4–6 weeks to heal inflammation
■ caustic-induced injury
➤ patients with mild esophageal injury on endoscopy (edema, erythema, or exudative esophagitis) may be advanced from liquids to a regular diet over 24–48 hours
➤ if signs of severe esophageal injury are present, such as deep or circumferential ulcers or necrosis (black discoloration), patients should be kept fasting with placement of a nasoenteric feeding tube after 24 h. Oral feedings of liquids may be initiated after 2–3 days if the patient is able to tolerate secretions. Neither steroids nor antibiotics are recommended.

FOLLOW-UP
■ repeat endoscopy not indicated unless lack of symptomatic improvement after specific treatment
■ After caustic ingestion, esophageal strictures develop in approximately 70% of patients weeks to months after initial injury, requiring recurrent esophageal dilations. Caustic strictures are usually long and rigid. Endoscopic injection of intralesional corticosteroids (triamcinolone 40 mg) increases the interval between dilations.

COMPLICATIONS AND PROGNOSIS
Complications
■ rare occurrence
■ can include hemorrhage presenting as hematemesis or melena, fistula, fevers, dissemination

- patients with pill-induced esophagitis rarely develop perforation, mediastinitis, or stricture formation requiring surgical correction or repeated endoscopic dilation
- in patients with caustic esophageal injury, there is a high risk (up to 65%) of acute complications, including perforation with mediastinitis or peritonitis, bleeding, stricture, or esophageal-tracheal fistulas. These patients should be monitored closely for signs of deterioration that warrant emergency surgery with possible esophagectomy and colonic or jejunal interposition.

Prognosis
- related to underlying condition
- life span not affected in pill-induced esophagitis
- after caustic injury there is an increased risk of esophageal squamous cancer of approximately 2–3% per year, and endoscopic surveillance is recommended starting approximately 15 years after ingestion.
- 10–15% of patients with chronic GERD may have a precancerous condition called Barrett's esophagus (BE) that can be detected on upper endoscopy. Once BE is detected, the annual risk of esophageal adenocarcinoma is approximately 0.5% per year. Society guidelines recommend endoscopic surveillance every 3 years or more frequently if dysplasia is present. Some case-control studies have suggested improved survival if esophageal adenocarcinoma is detected via a surveillance program.

ESOPHAGEAL MOTOR DISORDERS

GEORGE TRIADAFILOPOULOS, MD

HISTORY & PHYSICAL
- Esophageal motor disorders: functional abnormalities associated with increased or decreased esophageal contractility or uncoordinated esophageal peristalsis that result in dysphagia or chest pain

History
- Patients with generalized intestinal dysmotility, Chagas' disease, collagen vascular disease or infiltrative disorder (ie. amyloidosis)
- Patients with gastric cardia cancer: secondary achalasia
- Chronic GERD: may be complicated by esophageal motor dysfunction

Signs & Symptoms
- Dysphagia and/or chest pain main symptoms
- Both symptoms intermittent, non-progressive and worse with cold liquid ingestion
- Dysphagia noted with either solids or liquids
- Odynophagia suggests superinfection by Candida
- Heartburn, if present, raises the suspicion of secondary dysmotility, due to GERD
- Regurgitation of undigested food is mostly a feature of achalasia and it may lead to aspiration or weight loss

TESTS

Basic Tests
- Chest X-ray shows widening of the mediastinum in achalasia due to the dilated esophagus, and absence of the normal gastric air bubble.
- Barium swallow may reveal tertiary contractions (described as "rosary bead" or "corkscrew" esophagus); however, radiographic studies may be entirely normal.
  - In achalasia, barium swallow shows a dilated, sigmoid-shaped esophagus and in a beak-like narrowing caused by the poorly relaxing, hypertensive LES

Specific Diagnostic Tests
- Esophageal motility study
  - Characteristic manometric features of achalasia: 1) Elevated resting LES pressure, usually above 45 mmHg; 2) Incomplete LES relaxation; and 3) aperistalsis.
  - In cases of vigorous achalasia, the simultaneous esophageal contractions have higher amplitudes.
  - Diffuse esophageal spasm: characterized by high amplitude (>300 mmHg), simultaneous contractions
  - Nutcracker esophagus: distal esophageal peristaltic contractions of >180 mmHg
  - Hypertensive lower esophageal sphincter: pressure >45 mmHg
  - Nonspecific dysmotility: frequent incoordinated contractions of normal amplitude and duration

Other Tests
- Endoscopy
  - Recommended for all patients with achalasia to exclude malignancy (pseudoachalasia)

➤ Typically, the mucosa appears normal, but stasis inflammation or secondary Candidiasis may occur

➤ The gastroesophageal junction usually can be crossed easily with gentle pressure on the endoscope

■ CT scan

➤ May suggest malignancy if there is marked and asymmetric esophageal wall thickening

DIFFERENTIAL DIAGNOSIS

■ Severe GERD complicating scleroderma may simulate achalasia but in such cases the LES is hypotensive and relaxes normally

■ Cancer with secondary achalasia is usually associated with rapid and severe weight loss

■ Myocardial ischemia, GERD, dissecting aortic aneurysm may cause chest pain similar to the esophageal motor disorders

MANAGEMENT

What to Do First

■ Define the diagnosis and exclude malignancy as an underlying cause

General Measures

■ Evaluate the risk for aspiration and prevent it

SPECIFIC THERAPY

Indications for treatment

■ All symptomatic patients with dysphagia, regurgitation or chest pain require therapy.

Treatment Options

■ Calcium channel blockers: relieve chest pain and dysphagia

■ Two tricyclic antidepressants, trazodone and imipramine also effective in relieving chest pain; sublingual or oral nitrates, and anticholinergics may also be used

■ Hot water improves esophageal clearance and decreases the amplitude and duration of esophageal body contractions.

■ In severe cases, pneumatic dilatation, or an extended myotomy should be considered.

■ Pharmacologic therapy is usually ineffective in achalasia and endoscopic or surgical therapy is needed; endoscopically-applied botulinum injection is safe and effective but the results rarely last longer than 18 months

- Pneumatic dilation under fluoroscopic control improves dysphagia, regurgitation and chest pain in the majority of cases but carries the risk for perforation
- Laparoscopic myotomy with or without concomitant partial fundoplication is increasingly used because of its high efficacy and low morbidity

FOLLOW-UP

During Treatment

- Efficacy of therapy needs to be objectively assessed because of the intermittent nature of the symptoms

Routine

- Endoscopic surveillance for cancer in patients with achalasia is not cost-effective and thus not recommended

COMPLICATIONS AND PROGNOSIS

- Patients with achalasia are at an increased risk for developing squamous esophageal cancer
- Generally good prognosis for patients with esophageal motor disorders and most patients manage with medical therapy alone
- In patients with achalasia, botulinum toxin injection provides symptom relief but needs to be repeated
- Both pneumatic dilation and surgery, if successful initially, have long-lasting results

---

ESSENTIAL TREMOR

CHAD CHRISTINE, MD

HISTORY & PHYSICAL

- Tremor of 1 or both hands, head and/or voice
- Family history common
- Tremor may become more prominent over decades
- May improve w/ alcohol or rest
- Worse w/ stress
- Fine, high-frequency postural or kinetic tremor
- May be head tremor (nodding or no-no)

TESTS

- Diagnosis made clinically

- Blood & urine tests normal
- Brain imaging normal

DIFFERENTIAL DIAGNOSIS
- Drug-induced tremor (esp. beta-adrenergic agonists, caffeine, steroids, tamoxifen, antiarrhythmics, valproic acid, cyclosporine, tacrolimus) excluded by history
- Metabolic (eg, hyperthyroidism, electrolyte disturbance, hepatic or renal disorders) differentiated clinically
- Degenerative disorders: Parkinson's disease or atypical parkinsonism excluded clinically
- Structural & hypoxic ischemic injury: excluded by history & brain imaging

MANAGEMENT
- Limit caffeine intake
- Reassure pt that symptoms do not reflect anxiety disorder

SPECIFIC THERAPY

Indications
- Tremor that significantly interferes w/ lifestyle
  - ➤ Propranolol
  - ➤ Primidone
  - ➤ Alprazolam
- For pts refractory to above treatments
  - ➤ Thalamotomy: stereotactic ventrolateral thalamotomy
  - ➤ Thalamic deep brain stimulator

FOLLOW-UP
- Routine follow-up if undergoing therapy

COMPLICATIONS AND PROGNOSIS
- Symptoms progress gradually over decades

EXCESSIVE DAYTIME SLEEPINESS

CHAD CHRISTINE, MD

HISTORY & PHYSICAL
- Excessive daytime sleepiness
- Loud snoring, apneic episodes may occur during sleep (suggestive of sleep apnea)
- Obesity is common in sleep apnea

TESTS
- Lab testing unremarkable
- Brain imaging normal
- Sleep lab studies helpful if sleep apnea or restless legs syndrome suspected

DIFFERENTIAL DIAGNOSIS
- Sleep deprivation excluded by history
- Sleep apnea & narcolepsy diagnosed by history & sleep study
- Meds or drugs (esp benzodiazepines, antidepressants, narcotics, antihistamines, some antihypertensives, anticonvulsants, alcohol) excluded clinically
- Hypothyroidism, anemia, renal or hepatic failure, diabetes, pulmonary insufficiency excluded clinically
- Periodic limb movements in sleep (assoc w/ restless legs syndrome) excluded by history & sleep study
- Anxiety disorders & depression excluded clinically

MANAGEMENT
- Depends on cause

SPECIFIC THERAPY
- Narcolepsy: see "Narcolepsy" section
- Sleep apnea
  - ➤ Avoid alcohol & other CNS depressant drugs
  - ➤ CPAP-assisted ventilation at night
  - ➤ Uvulopalatopharyngoplasty

FOLLOW-UP
- Depends on severity & cause

COMPLICATIONS AND PROGNOSIS
- Depend on cause

EXFOLIATIVE DERMATITIS

J. MARK JACKSON, MD

HISTORY & PHYSICAL
- History – pruritic eruption, patient may consider contact as a possibility

- Physical – usually dermatitis is diffuse with involvement over many areas, up to 100% body surface area
- Generalized erythroderma with desquamation
   May be related to recent medication, viral exanthema, or other infection

TESTS
- Skin biopsy to assess cause

DIFFERENTIAL DIAGNOSIS
- Dermatitis
- Psoriasis
- Cutaneous lymphoma
- Internal malignancy
- Lichen planus or other papulosquamous disease
   Pityriasis rubra pilaris

MANAGEMENT
- Assess cause and remove.
- Assess possible high–output cardiac failure.

SPECIFIC THERAPY
Based on cause, but management of skin usually requires aggressive topical therapy as well as systemic therapy

FOLLOW-UP
Based on cause. It is important that biopsies are occasionally repeated to rule out cutaneous lymphoma, even if they are initially inconclusive.

COMPLICATIONS AND PROGNOSIS
Based on cause. If related to medication, withdrawal and therapy with appropriate measures usually leads to resolution. If T-cell lymphoma, condition may be lifelong.

EYELID LESIONS

DEVRON H. CHAR, MD

HISTORY & PHYSICAL
- Prior basal cell carcinoma (BCC) at any site, mandates a biopsy of new lid lesions.
- Lash loss, a pearly, cavitated border, or a unilateral chronic ulceration requires biopsy.

- Sebacious gland carcinomas (SGC) account for 2–4% of eyelid malignancies.
- A "recurrent stye or chalazoin" in the same eyelid location is possibly a SGC.

TESTS
- All such lesions require a biopsy with a histologic evaluation.

DIFFERENTIAL DIAGNOSIS
- BCC is the most common eyelid malignancy (>90%).
- Much less commonly: sebaceous carcinoma, squamous cell carcinoma, melanoma,
- Kaposi's sarcoma, and rarer malignancies.

MANAGEMENT
- Most eyelid tumors managed surgically with excellent cosmetics.
- In selected cases, radiation or cryotherapy.
- Metastatic patterns of eyelid malignancies similar to other head/neck sites.

SPECIFIC THERAPY
n/a

FOLLOW-UP
n/a

COMPLICATIONS AND PROGNOSIS
n/a

FANCONI SYNDROME

MICHEL BAUM, MD

HISTORY & PHYSICAL
- Presentation varies with underlying etiology.
- Polydipsia and polyuria
- Children present with failure to thrive, short stature and rickets.
- Adults develop osteomalacia.

TESTS
- Hyperchloremic metabolic acidosis, hypophosphatemia, hypokalemia
- Glucosuria, generalized aminoaciduria, phosphaturia (fractional excretion >20%)

DIFFERENTIAL DIAGNOSIS

- Autosomal recessive disorders – cystinosis, galactosemia, glycogen storage
  - ➤ disease type I, tyrosinemia, Wilson's disease, Lowe's syndrome, and hereditary fructose intolerance
- Toxins – ifosfamide, heavy metals, outdated tetracycline, aminoglycoside, valproic acid
- Dysproteinemias such as multiple myeloma

MANAGEMENT

n/a

SPECIFIC THERAPY

- Therapy of underlying cause
- Vitamin D and phosphate
- Potassium and bicarbonate supplements
- May need to decrease GFR (to decrease filtered load) with indomethacin

FOLLOW-UP

- To determine response to therapy and monitor serum electrolytes and growth in children

COMPLICATIONS AND PROGNOSIS

- Electrolyte disorders and volume depletion
- Prognosis dependent on the cause of Fanconi syndrome

FEVER OF UNKNOWN ORIGIN

RICHARD A. JACOBS, MD, PhD

HISTORY & PHYSICAL

History

- Definition – patient with illness lasting at least 3 wks, with fever >38.3C (101F) on several occasions, who remains undiagnosed after 3 outpatient visits or 3 days in the hospital
- Definition arbitrary, but designed to exclude patients with prolonged, self-limited viral illnesses, and to allow adequate time for a cultural, serologic and radiographic evaluation
- Classification of causes:
  - ➤ Infectious (25%–40%): systemic infections: tuberculosis (usually disseminated) and endocarditis most common, but many

others can cause FUO such as brucellosis, Q fever, salmonella, malaria, Whipple's disease, cat-scratch disease and other Bartonella infections, viral infections (especially cytomegalovirus, Epstein-Barr), fungal infections such as coccidioidomycosis, histoplasmosis (usually disseminated), toxoplasmosis; localized infections: osteomyelitis, cholecystitis, occult abscess (hepatic, subdiaphragmatic, intra-renal or perinephric, splenic, pelvic, dental)

➤ Neoplastic (20%–35%) – Hodgkin's and non-Hodgkin's lymphoma, acute leukemia, renal cell carcinoma, primary and metastatic tumors of the liver, atrial myxoma; chronic lymphocytic leukemia and myeloma usually not associated with fever unless there is concomitant infection

➤ Autoimmune or Rheumatologic (10%–20%) – polyarteritis nodosa, polymyalgia rheumatica, systemic lupus, temporal arteritis, cryoglobulinemia, Still's disease, Wegener's granulomatosis

➤ Miscellaneous – granulomatous hepatitis, sarcoidosis, inflammatory bowel disease, familial Mediterranean fever, hyperthyroidism, recurrent pulmonary emboli, alcoholic hepatitis, drug fever, factitious fever

➤ Undiagnosed (10%–15%)

▪ Certain general principles helpful in determining etiology:

➤ Most cases due to common diseases with unusual manifestations, not rare or exotic diseases (tuberculosis, endocarditis, and cholecystitis more common causes than familial Mediterranean fever or Whipple's disease)

➤ Duration of fever – infection, malignancy and autoimmune diseases etiology of FUO in only 20% of patients with prolonged fever (6 months or longer); granulomatous diseases (Crohn's disease, sarcoidosis, granulomatous hepatitis) and factitious fever more common etiologies; 25%-30% have no fever or underlying disease at all – the normal circadian rhythm (temperature 1–2 degrees higher in afternoon than morning) interpreted as abnormal

➤ Episodic or recurrent fever (FUO with periods of 2 wks or longer without fever) – similar in etiology to prolonged fever; familial Mediterranean fever, recurrent embolic disease also considerations

➤ Immunologic status – neutropenic patients often have occult bacterial or fungal infections; organ transplant recipients on immunosuppressive medications prone to viral infections

(CMV, herpes simplex and zoster), fungal infections, nocardia, mycobacterial infections, Pneumocystis carinii and other opportunistic infections

■ Careful history may reveal important clues to diagnosis: family history, social history (drug use, sexual exposures), travel, dietary habits (unpasteurized products, uncooked meats, raw eggs), recreational or vocational exposures (animals, ticks, chemicals), household pets

Signs & Symptoms
■ Etiologies so varied, any organ system potentially could be involved
■ Careful and repeated exams crucial to detect transient, subtle findings that may lead to diagnosis such as rash, conjunctivitis, adenopathy

TESTS
■ Routine blood tests (CBC, electrolytes, liver function studies)
■ Blood cultures should be done off antibiotics; ask laboratory to hold for 2 weeks to detect slow-growing, fastidious organisms (HACEK organisms, Brucella spp) and request special media if considering legionella, nutritionally deficient streptococci or bartonella
■ Cultures of other fluids (urine, sputum, stool, cerebrospinal fluid, pleural fluid) done if clinically indicated
■ Serologic tests done if specific diagnosis considered; "screening" serologic tests not cost-effective or helpful; a single elevated microbiologic titer rarely confirms diagnosis – a 4-fold rise or fall in titer required to make diagnosis
■ Chest radiograph standard; radiographic evaluation of gallbladder, intestines, sinuses low yield as routine tests, but done if clinically indicated; CT scan of abdomen, pelvis and chest often done and helpful – abnormalities require tissue confirmation to make specific diagnosis; MRI more sensitive than CT for detecting CNS lesions; ultrasound sensitive for lesions of hepatobiliary system and kidney; echocardiography if considering endocarditis or myxoma – transesophageal more sensitive than surface echocardiogram; role of radionuclide scans unclear – plagued by high rate of false-positive and -negative results and rarely add to findings of CT or MRI
■ Abnormalities should be pursued; sample pleural or peritoneal fluid (infection/malignancy); biopsy rashes (collagen vascular diseases/infection) and enlarged lymph nodes (malignancy/infection); bone marrow biopsy has low yield (except in HIV disease, where yield is high for mycobacterial infection), but risk is low and procedure

often done; liver biopsy helpful in 5–10% of patients with abnormal LFTs

■ Role of laparoscopy and laparotomy unclear, but should be considered in rapidly deteriorating patient with negative evaluation

DIFFERENTIAL DIAGNOSIS
■ As indicated above

MANAGEMENT
■ Documentation of fever critical initial step as evaluation long, costly and potentially invasive

■ If suspect factitious fever, observe patient while taking temperature

■ Have patient record temperature 3 or 4 times a day for several days to assess frequency, height and periodicity.

SPECIFIC THERAPY
■ If specific diagnosis made, therapy directed at underlying cause

■ Empiric therapy indicated if a specific diagnosis strongly suspected; before therapy started, all relevant cultures should be obtained; endpoints should be set prior to therapy – if no clinical response after several weeks, therapy should be discontinued and re-evaluation undertaken

■ In the rapidly deteriorating patient, empiric therapy indicated: antituberculous therapy (particularly in the elderly or those from endemic areas) and broad-spectrum antibiotics reasonable

■ Steroids to suppress fever not indicated; infection the most common cause of FUO, and steroids may allow infections to become more aggressive or disseminate

FOLLOW-UP
■ In undiagnosed patients, careful and frequent (weekly) follow-up indicated to assess any new signs or symptoms that may lead to a diagnosis

COMPLICATIONS AND PROGNOSIS
■ Prognosis depends on underlying disease; the elderly and those with malignancy have less favorable outcome

■ Of those undiagnosed after extensive evaluation, 75% eventually have resolution of symptoms and etiology remains unknown; in the remainder, more classic signs and symptoms of underlying disease appear, allowing a specific diagnosis to be made

■ Death from FUO is uncommon, occurring in less than 5%.

FIBROMAS

SOL SILVERMAN JR, MD

HISTORY & PHYSICAL
- common soft, sessile, pedunculated benign mucosal growths
- usually painless and slow growing
- mucosal response to acute or chronic irritation; often cause not identified

TESTS
- observe; usually self-limiting growth
- excisional biopsy

DIFFERENTIAL DIAGNOSIS
- benign tumors

MANAGEMENT
- remove irritants (e.g. cheek biting, appliances); observe for growth

SPECIFIC THERAPY
- surgical removal

FOLLOW-UP
- observe for recurrence

COMPLICATIONS AND PROGNOSIS
- usually none

FIBROMYALGIA

DANIEL J. CLAUW, MD

HISTORY & PHYSICAL

History
- Hallmark symptom: chronic widespread pain, above & below the waist
- Pain may be migratory, waxing & waning in intensity
- May involve both peripheral & visceral structures
- 60–80% females
- Associated symptoms
- Fatigue, non-restorative sleep, memory difficulties, headaches, paresthesias, irritable bowel or bladder

- Symptoms that mimic inflammatory disorders, including Raynaud's-like symptoms, livedo reticularis, malar flushing, morning stiffness, subjective swelling of hands & feet, may confound diagnosis
- Symptoms often begin or worsen after exposure to a "stressor" such as trauma, infection, emotional stress

Signs & Symptoms
- Normal except for findings of tenderness present anywhere in body, not just confined to areas of typical "tender points"
- Formal American College of Rheumatology criteria require 11 of 18 tender points present, but in clinical practice at least half of pts w/ fibromyalgia will not have 11 of 18 tender points

TESTS
- Pts w/ acute or subacute symptoms may require an extensive workup, whereas in those w/ chronic symptoms minimal workup is necessary

Lab Tests
- Used to exclude other diseases
- CBC, routine chemistries, creatine kinase, TSH, urinalysis, ESR should be normal
- Rheumatoid factor, antinuclear antibody should only be ordered if there is high suspicion of autoimmune disorder (eg, abnormal physical exam or abnormal screening labs)

Imaging
- Not warranted unless dictated by history & physical findings

DIFFERENTIAL DIAGNOSIS
- Hypothyroidism (high TSH)
- Polymyalgia rheumatica (>50 yrs old, high ESR)
- Hepatitis C
- Drug-induced myopathies (esp. statin drugs)
- Chiari malformation or cervical spinal stenosis
- Early rheumatoid arthritis or SLE may simulate fibromyalgia
- Osteomalacia

MANAGEMENT
What to Do First
- Educate pt

➤ Emphasize that pain is occurring because of disturbance in how nervous system senses pain (ie, "volume control is turned up too high on nervous system"), not because of damage or inflammation in peripheral structures

➤ Emphasize that fibromyalgia cannot be cured (like most chronic illnesses)

➤ Pts do best if they take an active approach to mgt, rather than adopting "victim" mentality, helplessness

■ Explore whether there are stressors that are worsening symptoms

■ Refer patients to high-quality sources of information (eg, Arthritis Foundation, www.fms-cfs.org)

General Measures

■ Most pts require multimodal therapy consisting of symptom-based pharmacologic therapy, exercise, structured education or cognitive-behavioral therapy

■ For all therapy (drugs, exercise), "start low, go slow"

SPECIFIC THERAPY

■ Pharmacologic

➤ If pain is only symptom, non-narcotic analgesic (eg, tramadol or NSAID) may be effective

➤ For pts w/ other symptoms (eg, insomnia, fatigue, etc) initiate a tricyclic agent (eg, amitriptyline, beginning at 10 mg 2–3 hours prior to bedtime). Increase by 10 mg every 1–2 weeks to maximum of 70 mg amitriptyline. Morning sedation, weight gain, dry mouth, constipation are most common side effects. For pts intolerant of tricyclics or where there is incomplete response, SSRIs (fluoxetine or citalopram) may be added.

➤ Other possibilities are trazodone or zolpidem for sleep, gabapentin for pain, bupropion for fatigue

■ Exercise

➤ Low-impact, aerobic-type exercise is of greatest benefit

➤ May be better tolerated once pharmacotherapy has begun

• Start w/ 5–10 minutes 3×/week, increasing to 20–30 minutes 5× or more per week

➤ Strength training may be better late in treatment course

■ Cognitive-behavioral therapy (CBT)

➤ Teaches pts techniques they can use to manage their symptoms better

➤ Most accessible are Arthritis Foundation self-help courses

> Pain-based formal CBT programs can be very useful but are not widely available
> Biofeedback, hypnosis, relaxation techniques may be used w/ CBT or alone

Other Therapies
- Physical therapy can be helpful to educate pts on a range-of-motion exercise program to be used at home
- Trigger point injections w/ depot steroids may be useful for regional pain
- Alternative therapies (eg, acupuncture, chiropractic manipulation) may also be of benefit in some instances

FOLLOW-UP
- Scheduling routine follow-up appointments is preferable to pts presenting w/ crises
- Focus on improving function, rather than specific symptoms
- Reinforce need for exercise, CBT-type program
- Identify & treat comorbid psychiatric diagnoses if present

COMPLICATIONS & PROGNOSIS

Complications
- Most significant complications are decreased function, disability
- May be preventable by early intervention

Prognosis
- Likely to have chronic symptoms for life, but these can be managed
- No decrease in long-term survival

FILARIASIS

J. GORDON FRIERSON, MD

HISTORY & PHYSICAL

History
- Exposure: Wuchereria bancrofti (causes lymphatic filariasis), transmitted by mosquito. Found in Africa, Brazil, India, China, S.E. Asia, Haiti.
- Brugia malayi (causes lymphatic filariasis), transmitted by mosquito. Found in China, S.E. Asia.
- Loa loa (causes loaiasis), transmitted by Chrysops (deer) fly. Found in W. and central Africa.

■ Onchocerca volvulus (causes onchocerciasis, or "river blindness"), transmitted by Simulium flies (black flies). Found in tropical Africa, Guatemala, Ecuador, Venezuela.

Signs & Symptoms
■ Lymphatic filariasis: Many patients have no symptoms
  ➤ Recurrent lymphadenitis with retrograde lymphangitis, generally from groin down thigh or to scrotum, or from axillary nodes down arm
  ➤ Hydrocele
  ➤ In late stages, chronic edema of leg, arm or scrotum, chyluria
■ Loa loa: early stage (usually seen in expatriates): arthralgias, myalgias, mild fatigue, urticaria or other migratory rash, recurrent edematous non-tender swellings on extremities (Calabar swellings), migration of worm across conjunctiva or eyelid, or found in small removed nodule
■ Late, chronic stage: same as above but with less arthralgia, myalgia, and fatigue. In Africans with chronic infections, symptoms are mainly migrating worms and Calabar swellings.
■ Onchocerciasis: light infections: no symptoms
■ Moderate to heavy infections: varying degrees of rash, pruritus, nodules around pelvic girdle and waist (in Africa) or head and neck (W. Hemisphere), keratitis, anterior (and later posterior) uveitis. Later one sees blindness (corneal scarring), enlarged inguinal nodes, and loss of elasticity of skin.

TESTS
■ Basic tests: blood: CBC shows eosinophilia, often high, in all clinical types.
■ Basic tests: urine: may see microfilaria in all clinical types
■ Specific tests:
■ Lymphatic filariasis: Draw blood sample at 11–12 PM. Either run 5cc through micropore filter to see microfilariae, or mix with formalin, spin and examine for microfilariae (Knott concentration test). Somewhat more sensitive is the ICT Filariasis Card Test (from ICI Diagnostics), which detects W. bancrofti antigen in serum by monoclonal antibody.

Circulating filarial antigen (CFA) test available for W. bancrofti only; advantage: no diurnal variability

- Loa-loa: Draw blood at noon, examine in same fashion as above for microfilariae. In light cases, microfilariae often absent.
- Identify adult worm removed from conjunctiva or SQ nodule.
  - Onchocerciasis: remove nodule and examine for adult worms
  - Examine small punch biopsy of skin (using a scleral punch, or scalpel to remove small shaving that includes the dermal papillae) from calves and upper buttocks in African cases, and shoulders and scapular areas in W. Hemisphere cases.
  - Other tests: Lymphatic filariasis: ultrasound of hydrocele or dilated lymph channels in groin may show motile adult worms.
  - Serology: available in some labs but not very sensitive or specific. PCR available on research basis.

DIFFERENTIAL DIAGNOSIS
- Lymphatic filariasis: In acute attacks, streptococcal lymphangitis, thrombophlebitis. In chronic stage, any cause of chronic edema (Milroy's disease, previous lymphatic dissection, etc.).
- Loa loa: In light cases: other causes of urticaria, arthralgias, collagen vascular diseases
- Onchocerciasis: Almost any cause of itching and nonspecific rash. Nodules can resemble enlarged glands, cysts, tumors.

MANAGEMENT

What to Do First
- Assess severity of infection.
- In onchocerciasis, do ophthalmologic exam.

General Measures
- Symptomatic treatment of pruritus, edema, cellulitis, if present

SPECIFIC THERAPY

Indications
- Treatment of light infections in any filariasis is optional. If symptomatic, treatment recommended for all.

Treatment Options
- Lymphatic filariasis: diethylcarbamazine
- Ivermectin single dose (kills microfilariae only)

- Loa loa: diethylcarbamazine
- Onchocerciasis: ivermectin single dose, repeat every 6–12 months for lifetime of adult worms (3–4 years in children, 10–12 years in adults)

Side Effects & Complications

- Diethycarbamazine: at onset of therapy can get allergic reactions due to parasite death: urticaria, intense itching, edema, hypotension. Using graduated dose generally avoids this. Steroids reduce the reaction. Drug otherwise well tolerated.
- Ivermectin: allergic reactions (due to parasite death) are frequent early in treatment, but generally not severe, and respond to steroids. Otherwise drug well tolerated.
- Contraindications to treatment: absolute: diethlycarbamazine should never be used in onchocerciasis where there is eye involvement. First trimester treatment should be avoided.
- Contraindications to treatment: relative. Pregnancy, if no urgency about treatment.

FOLLOW-UP

During Treatment

- Watch for allergic reactions (all filariases), treat with steroids if severe. Patients with heavy loa loa should receive even more cautious gradations of dosage.

Routine

- Lymphatic filariasis and loa loa: clinical follow-up, as well as following eosinophil count and blood examinations. Retreatment may be needed, sometimes several times, to achieve cure.
- Onchocerciasis: needs ivermectin every 6–12 months for 1–2 years, then once yearly. Ophthalmologic follow-up if eyes involved.

COMPLICATIONS AND PROGNOSIS

- Lymphatic disease: lymph nodes can suppurate during treatment. Lymph channel damage prior to treatment will have limited improvement and edema may persist. Streptococcal infections may recur, and sometimes chronic penicillin coverage is needed.
- Loa loa: heavily infected patients can get an encephalitis during treatment; they need to be treated slowly and watched.
- Onchocerciasis: Eye disease may improve some, but corneal scarring will not reverse.

FOLIC ACID/COBALAMIN (VITAMIN B12) DEFICIENCY

ASOK C. ANTONY, MD

HISTORY & PHYSICAL

■ **Three-stage approach**:

> Recognize megaloblastic/neuropathologic manifestations of folate/cobalamin deficiency.

> Distinguish between isolated folate, cobalamin or combined deficiency.

> Define underlying disease/mechanism.

■ Clinical manifestations of Folate/cobalamin deficiency are similar (with notable exceptions).

■ History and physical examination depend on etiology of deficiency. Cobalamin deficiency develops insidiously (∼5–10 years to manifest clinically); folate deficiency manifests within 6 months of onset.

■ **Clinical Presentations**: Pancytopenia with megaloblastic marrow; congestive heart failure; beefy-red tongue; melanin pigmentation, premature graying; infertility/sterility

> Neuropsychiatric presentation (subacute combined degeneration involving posterior, pyramidal, spinocerebellar, and spinothalamic tracts and secondarily peripheral nerves) unique to cobalamin deficiency. Dorsal tract involved earliest in >70% with paresthesias/ataxia, diminished vibration (256 cps) and proprioception sense. Neuropathic involvement of legs precedes arms. Clinical findings can include positive Romberg's and Lhermitte's sign, loss of sphincter and bowel control, cranial nerve palsy, optic neuritis, and cortical dysfunction (dementia, psychoses, mood disturbances).

> Note: In the USA, cobalamin deficiency-related neurologic impairment is often not associated with hematologic manifestations, and vice versa. In developing countries, however, cobalamin deficiency can present with florid pancytopenia, mild hepatosplenomegaly, fever, and thrombocytopenia, with the neuropsychiatric syndrome manifesting later.

■ **Cobalamin Deficiency: General Mechanisms**

> ➤ Nutritional

> ➤ Inadequate dissociation food-cobalamin complex

> ➤ Absent intrinsic factor (IF) secretion or interaction with cobalamin

➤ Usurpation of luminal cobalamin
➤ Inadequate/Diseased ileal absorptive surface
➤ Inactivation of cobalamin by nitrous oxide
➤ **Common Causes**
  • Vegetarians (dietary cobalamin deficiency may be most common cause in developing countries). Note: Nonvegetarians who eat small portions of meat infrequently can have low cobalamin intakes comparable to vegetarians/vegans.
  • Atrophic/partial gastritis with hypochlorhydria, proton-pump inhibitors
  • Total/partial gastrectomy, pernicious anemia (PA)
  • Pancreatic insufficiency, Zollinger-Ellison syndrome
  • Bacterial overgrowth syndromes (blind loops, diverticulosis, strictures, fistulas, anastomoses, scleroderma, hypogammaglobulinemia, fish-tapeworm)
  • Ileal bypass/resection/fistula
  • Tropical/nontropical sprue, Crohn's disease, TB-ileitis, amyloidosis
  • Drugs (slow-K, biguanides, cholestyramine, colchicine, neomycin)
  • Nitrous oxide inhalation

Pernicious anemia (PA): most common cause of cobalamin deficiency in the West; caused by autoimmune destruction of gastric parietal cells leading to intrinsic factor (IF) deficiency. Undiagnosed PA in USA >60-years age group (~1.5% men, ~4% African-American/Caucasian women). Anti-IF antibodies are highly specific for PA (60% of PA have anti-IF antibodies in serum). Positive family history (in 30%). PA is associated with autoimmune diseases (i.e., the polyglandular autoimmune syndrome, Graves' disease, Hashimoto's thyroiditis, vitiligo, Addison's disease, idiopathic hypoparathyroidism, primary ovarian failure, myasthenia gravis, type I diabetes, and adult hypogammaglobulinemia).

■ **Folate Deficiency – General Mechanisms**
■ (multiple causes in same patient)
  ➤ Decreased intake/absorption
  ➤ Increased requirement/destruction/excretion
  ➤ Common Causes
    • Poverty, famine, institutionalized individuals (psychiatric/nursing homes/chronic debilitating disease), ethnic cooking techniques, dieting

- Pregnancy, lactation, prematurity/infancy; increased hematopoietic turnover, malignancy, psoriasis
- Tropical/nontropical sprue, regional enteritis
- Drugs: antifolates, alcohol, sulfasalazine, triamterene, pyrimethamine, trimethoprim-sulfamethoxazole, carbamazepine, diphenylhydantoin, barbiturates

TESTS

Macrocytosis and the evaluation of macrocytic anemia

Anemia is macrocytic if MCV >100 fl. If MCV <110 fl and corrected reticulocyte is >2%, rule out response to acute blood loss or hemolysis (immune hemolytic anemia, infectious or mechanical causes, glucose 6-phosphate dehydrogenase deficiency, or paroxysmal nocturnal hemoglobinuria).

If corrected reticulocyte count is normal or <0.5%, then differentiate between macroovalocytes (central pallor occupies less than one third of cell) and thin macrocytes (central pallor occupies more than one third of cell).

Thin macrocytes (MCV 100–110 fl) are found in the post-splenectomy state, liver disease with or without alcoholism, aplastic/hypoplastic anemia, myelodysplastic (esp. 5q-) syndrome, myelopthisic anemia, hypothyroidism, smoking, chronic lung disease, severe hyperglycemia, and leukocytosis).

Macroovalocytes with MCV >110 fl and low reticulocyte counts (<0.5%) are usually induced by an intrinsic interference with DNA synthesis leading to megaloblastic anemia (e.g., deficiency of cobalamin or folate, or by antineoplastic and immunosuppressive agents [antimetabolites, alkylating agents, topoisomerase inhibitors], and anti-retroviral therapy).

- Morphologic manifestations of megaloblastosis from cobalamin and folate deficiency are similar: Peripheral smear = Increased MCV with macroovalocytes, hypersegmented PMNs, thrombocytopenia (mild). Bone marrow aspirate = classic megaloblastosis (trilineal hyperplasia, orthochromatic megaloblasts, giant metamyelocytes, hypersegmented PMNs, megakaryocytic pseudohyperdiploidy)
- Other supporting tests: reticulocytopenia, hyperbilirubinemia, decreased haptoglobin, increased LDH
- Masked megaloblastosis when inadequate hemoglobinization (iron deficiency/defects in globin synthesis), but hypersegmented PMNs present

DIFFERENTIAL DIAGNOSIS

- Algorithm based on evidence for megaloblastic anemia or neurologic-psychiatric manifestations c/w cobalamin deficiency PLUS test results on serum cobalamin and serum folate
- If cobalamin >300 pg/ml and folate >4 ng/ml, cobalamin and folate deficiency unlikely
- If cobalamin <200 pg/ml and folate >4 ng/ml, c/w cobalamin deficiency
- If cobalamin 200–300 pg/ml and folate >4 ng/ml, cobalamin deficiency still possible in ~15% (go to MMA + HCYS)
- If cobalamin >300 pg/ml and folate <2 ng/ml, c/w folate deficiency
- If cobalamin <200 pg/ml and folate <2 ng/ml, c/w either combined cobalamin plus folate deficiency or isolated folate deficiency (go to MMA + HCYS)
- If cobalamin >300 pg/ml and folate 2–4 ng/ml, c/w either folate deficiency or anemia unrelated to vitamin deficiency (go to MMA = HCYS)
- Note: The test for RBC folate is insufficiently standardized and validated for clinical use; avoid.
- **Interpretation Serum HCYS and Serum MMA tests**
- Normal MMA = <270 nM; Normal HCYS = <14 mcM
- If both MMA + HCYS increased, c/w cobalamin deficiency or combined cobalamin and folate deficiency
- If MMA normal but HCYS increased, folate deficiency likely
- If MMA and HCYS normal, cobalamin and folate deficiency excluded
- Schilling Test identifies locus for cobalamin malabsorption (then further GI workup as indicated)
- Note: Delay test for >2 months after cobalamin replacement to ensure normalization of intestinal morphology/function.
- Stage I test result, >8% of orally absorbed (crystalline) [57Co] cobalamin excreted in urine in 24 hours. In PA, <8% excreted.
- Stage II test (oral IF given with [57Co] cobalamin; if >8% is excreted, result c/w PA; if <8% still excreted, proceed to stage III test – i.e., oral antibiotics using either amoxicillin-clavulanate (875 mg bid), cephalexin (250 mg qid) plus metronidazole (250 mg tid), or norfloxacin 800 mg qd ×10 days – and repeat stage I test. If >8% excretion, result c/w bacterial usurpation; if still <8% excretion, cobalamin malabsorption localized to ileal cause.
- Note: Patients with cobalamin deficiency from inability to break down food protein-bound cobalamin (e.g., hypo/achlorhydria) have

normal stage I test because they can absorb crystalline [57Co] cobalamin normally.

MANAGEMENT

- If patient decompensating from congestive heart failure, give 1 unit of packed cells slowly plus dual vitamin replacement (1 mg cobalamin and 1 mg folic acid) stat. Also for suspected cobalamin-deficient neurologic disease, give cobalamin and folic acid immediately after drawing blood tests.
- With less urgent clinical picture, await confirmatory diagnostic tests before initiating therapy.

SPECIFIC THERAPY

The recommended daily allowance (RDA) of vitamin B12 (cobalamin) for men and nonpregnant women is 2.4 mcg; pregnant women, 2.6 mcg; lactating women, 2.8 mcg; and children 9–18 years, ~1.5–2 mcg. The RDA of folate for adult men and nonpregnant women is 400 mcg; pregnant women, 600 mcg; lactating women, 500 mcg; children 9 to 18 years, 300–400 mcg.

- For PA-related cobalamin deficiency: Intramuscular cobalamin 1 mg daily ×1 week, then 1 mg biweekly for 4 weeks, then monthly injections for life
- Alternatively, oral cobalamin 2 mg orally for life (1% passively absorbed sufficient for daily replacement) after acute replenishment of depleted cobalamin stores using IM regimen above
- Folate deficiency: Oral folic acid 1 mg PO daily, all cases

Modified Therapeutic Trials.

Indication: When clinical suspicion is against folate/cobalamin deficiency but other clinical, morphologic, and/or biochemical abnormalities are inconclusive (e.g., megaloblastic bone marrow that could be secondary to chemotherapy, myelodysplastic syndromes, or acute myeloid leukemia; or in pregnancy, AIDS, or alcoholism, when anemia is likely to be multifactorial). Documenting failure to respond to combination of folic acid 1 mg orally ×10 days and cobalamin 1 mg IM daily ×10 days rules out folate/cobalamin deficiency. After all such negative trials, a bone marrow evaluation is indicated to identify another primary hematologic disease.

FOLLOW-UP

- Note: Folic acid alone cures megaloblastosis of folate/cobalamin deficiency but aggravates neuropathology of cobalamin deficiency.

Beware of hyperuricemia and/or hypokalemia ~3–4 days after initiating therapy.
- Nonresponsiveness to cobalamin or folate:
  - ➤ Wrong diagnosis
  - ➤ Combined folate + cobalamin deficiency treated with 1 vitamin
  - ➤ Unrecognized associated disease (iron deficiency, hemoglobinopathy, chronic disease, hypothyroidism)

COMPLICATIONS AND PROGNOSIS
- Patients with PA can develop subsequent iron deficiency anemia, osteoporosis with fractures of the proximal femur and vertebrae, gastric cancer, and cancer of the buccal cavity and pharynx. Posttreatment endoscopic survey to identify early gastric cancer/carcinoids every ~5 years.
- Indications for prophylaxis with cobalamin/folate
  Cobalamin: Vegetarians/vegans (50 mcg/day); post-total gastrectomy w/ achlorhydria (full doses as for PA + iron); in food-cobalamin malabsorption (i.e., inability to cleave food-cobalamin by acid and pepsin); patients on long-term therapy (>5 years) with histamine-2 blockers or proton pump inhibitors, replace with cobalamin tablets (~100-mcg tablets) per day orally. In all other conditions involving cobalamin malabsorption, give cobalamin 2,000 mcg/day orally.
  - ➤ Folic acid: All women contemplating pregnancy (400 mcg/day), pregnancy/lactation, premature infants, mothers at risk for second neural-tube-defect baby (4 mg/day). For women in the childbearing age with epilepsy on anticonvulsants (diphenylhydantoin, phenobarbitone, carbamazepine, valproate), give folic acid 1 mg/day. For patients with hemolytic anemias/hyperproliferative states and rheumatoid arthritis/psoriasis being treated with methotrexate, give folic acid 1 mg/day.

FOLLICULITIS AND FURUNCULOSIS

SHANNON MCALLISTER, MD and JEFFREY P. CALLEN, MD
REVISED BY JEFFREY P. CALLEN, MD

HISTORY & PHYSICAL
- History – Medical problems such as obesity, diabetes mellitus, corticosteroid use, blood dyscrasia, HIV infection
  - ➤ Friction, perspiration, trauma

➤ Gram-negative folliculitis occurs following exposure to a poorly cleaned or chlorinated pool
➤ Poor hygiene
➤ Staphylococcus and streptococcus are the most common bacterial causes.
➤ Recent hot tub use is associated with Pseudomonas infection and is self-limited.

Signs & Symptoms
- Itching, tenderness, purulent drainage, possibly fever
- Follicularly based pustules (folliculitis)
- Hot tub folliculitis – usually follicular pustules on the back
- A furuncle is a red tender nodule(s).
- A carbuncle is often larger, multilocular and studded with pustules; associated with fever, malaise, and leukocytosis.

TESTS
- Complete blood count
- Gram stain of the exudates or contents
- Cultures are not always necessary.
- Blood sugar determination and/or HIV testing with recurrent disease

DIFFERENTIAL DIAGNOSIS
- Cutaneous candiasis
- Blastomycosis, cryptococcus or other deep fungi
- Inflammatory variant of a dermatophyte infection (Majocchi's granuloma)
- Acute febrile neutrophilic dermatosis (Sweet's syndrome)

MANAGEMENT
What to Do First
- Assess area involved.
- Check status of immune function.

General Measures
- Counsel regarding hygiene.
- Antibacterial soaps if the process is associated with a folliculitis

SPECIFIC THERAPY
- Oral antibiotics with good coverage of Staphylococcus and Streptococcus for furuncles or carbuncles
- Incision and drainage of fluctuant areas

■ Clean hot tub when appropriate

Recurrent lesions

■ Culture nares to exclude the possibly of nasal carriage.
■ Treat nasal carriers with intranasal mupuricin ointment BID for 5 days.
■ Consider the addition of oral rifampin.
■ Culture and sensitivity results dictate therapy.

Side Effects

■ Inappropriate use of antibiotics may lead to antimicrobial resistance.
■ Candidiasis – vaginal, oral or intertriginous

FOLLOW-UP
■ Assess resolution after completing a 10-day course of antibiotic therapy.
■ Assess improvement in hygiene.
■ For patients with recurrent disease – look for the source; nasal carriage of Staphylococcus aureus or a family member may be the carrier

COMPLICATIONS AND PROGNOSIS
■ Bacteremia or sepsis, particularly in an immunocompromised patient
■ Reactions to antibiotics – e.g., psuedomembranous colitis, Stevens-Johnson syndrome

---

FOOD ALLERGIES

JAYSHREE MATADIAL, MD and SUZANNE M. MATSUI, MD

HISTORY & PHYSICAL

History
■ True food allergy estimated to occur in 4–5% of young children and 1–2% of adults
■ History of exposure to common food allergens: cow's milk, eggs, nuts, shellfish soybeans, wheat, fruits, vegetables (glycoproteins) shellfish soybeans, wheat, fruits, vegetables (glycoproteins)
■ History of previous food intolerance: note type of food, quantity of suspected food ingested, time between ingestion and onset of symptoms, type and duration of symptoms
■ History of atopy or allergy: e.g. oral allergy syndrome in patients with pollen induced rhinitis, GI anaphylaxis in patients with skin

and/or respiratory tract allergy, allergic eosinophilic gastroenteritis in patients with asthma or allergic rhinitis
- History of improvement of symptoms after exclusion diet
- History of negative GI diagnostic work-up

Signs & Symptoms
- Immediate – Type I IgE mediated hypersensitivity reaction (within minutes after ingestion)
- Anaphylaxis (generalized systemic shock)
- Postprandial exercise-induced anaphylaxis
- Itching, eczema, urticaria, dermatitis (skin)
- Rhinitis, laryngeal edema, bronchospasm, nasal congestion (respiratory)
- Angioedema of lips, tongue, palate, throat, pruritis, rapid onset and resolution (oral allergy syndrome)
- Vomiting, abdominal pain and cramping, bloating, GI bleed, abdominal distention, diarrhea, onset within minutes to 1 hour of ingesting suspected food allergen (gastrointestinal anaphylaxis)
- Postprandial nausea, vomiting, abdominal pain, diarrhea, steatorrhea, weight loss (allergic eosinophilic gastroenteritis -mucosal form)
- Delayed – Type IV cell-mediated reaction (can occur hours to days post ingestion of suspected food allergen)
- Non IgE mediated syndromes: celiac disease, dermatitis herpetiformis, most cases of cow's milk allergy

TESTS
Basic Studies:
- Serum – IgE, eosinophils
- Stool – IgE, eosinophils

Specific diagnostic Tests: if IgE-mediated disorder is suspected
- Skin test (prick/puncture) with fresh food or commercial extract; (+) test = wheal >3 mm in diameter than control
- In vitro test (RAST = radioallergosorbent test) – used if substantial risk of anaphylaxis exists, semiquantitative measure of allergen specific
- IgE in serum : Elisa or basophil histamine release assay
- Elimination diet for 1–2 weeks
- Food challenge: open single blinded vs double blinded placebo controlled oral food challenge (gold standard)
- Endoscopic biopsy helps document allergic eosinophilic gastroenteritis (eosinophilic infiltrate) vs non IgE-mediated celiac sprue

(complete villous atrophy, extensive cellular infiltrate) and dermatitis herpetiformis (less marked changes than celiac sprue)

DIFFERENTIAL DIAGNOSIS
- IgE-mediated hypersensitivity
- Oral allergy syndrome
- GI anaphylaxis
- Allergic eosinophilic gastroenteritis
- Non IgE-mediated hypersensitivity
- Celiac disease
- Dermatitis herpetiformis
- Food intolerance
- Metabolic disorders: idiosyncratic, non-immunologically mediated-disaccharidase deficiency, G6PD deficiency, hypo- or abetalipoproteinemia, acrodermatitis enteropathica
- Toxin induced reaction from mushrooms, botulism, aflatoxins
- Infections: bacterial enterotoxins, postinfectious malabsorption
- Contaminants: antibiotics, pesticides, dyes, flavorings, preservatives, vasoactive amines
- Other gastrointestinal disorders
  - Allergic eosinophilic gastroenteritis (non-mucosal form)
  - Peptic ulcer disease
  - Cholelithiasis
  - IBD
  - IBS
  - Pancreatic disease
- Psychological illness: phobias, avoidances
- Anatomic abnormalities: Hirschsprung's disease, ileal stenosis, short bowel syndrome, intestinal lymphangiectasia
- Tumors: ZE syndrome, neuroblastoma (catecholamines or VIP)

MANAGEMENT

What to Do First
- Assess severity of reaction, spectrum from urticaria to shock
- Avoidance of offending food if known
- Use of antihistamines
- Possible use of steroids
- Epinephrine for anaphylaxis

General Measures
- Consider non-immunologic causes for symptoms
- Perform diagnostic test, chosen based on severity of reaction/food diary
- Referral to allergist or nutritionist for more advanced workup and education about avoidance of particular groups of foods

SPECIFIC THERAPY
- Based on recognition of disorder, cause and avoidance of offending agent, use of antihistamines, steroids and/or epinephrine
- Side Effects & Contraindications
  - Glucocorticoids: Cushing's syndrome, hyperglycemia, infections, psych disorders, insomnia, HPA axis suppression, glaucoma, cataracts, hypertension, myopathy, osteoporosis, peptic ulcer, electrolyte disorders
    - Contraindications: infection
  - Antihistamines: Drowsiness, anticholinergic effects, paradoxical excitement, blood dyscrasias, hypotension
  - Epinephrine: hypertenison, headache, palpitations, cerebral hemorrhage, tachycardia, pulmonary edema, anxiety
    - Contraindications: cardiac disease, organic brain damage
  - Elimination diet: maluntrition, eating disorders (solid diagnostic criteria must be met before prescribing a strict elimination diet)

FOLLOW-UP
- Proper education of patient and family members of what agents to avoid, signs and symptoms to be watchful for, and emergency treatments such as self-administered epinephrine

COMPLICATIONS AND PROGNOSIS

Complications
- Rash/pruritus
- Gastrointestinal bleed
- Weight loss
- Malabsorption
- Anemia
- Anaphylaxis: Cardiovascular and respiratory collapse
- Death

Prognosis
- Prognosis is good if serious reactions are recognized and treated early
- No alteration in lifespan of mild reactions

FOOD POISONING

JAYSHREE MATADIAL, MD and SUZABBE M. MATSUI, MD

HISTORY & PHYSICAL
- Acute illness with gastrointestinal and/or neurologic features: vomiting, abdominal pain, diarrhea, headache, parasthesias systemic symptoms of cholinergic excess, histamine excess, blisters
- Similar symptoms in others who may have shared suspect meal
- Incubation period usually <24 hr
- History of exposure to possibly contaminated food including roasted, boiled, stewed, steamed, or canned meats, poultry, dairy products, raw or undercooked foods, seafood, unrefrigerated foods, water exposure or food that may have been improperly stored or handled

TESTS

Basic tests:
- Stool for C&S, O&P (patients with prolonged or inflammatory symptoms)
- Blood cultures (if febrile)
- Stool for fecal leukocytes
- Serum for electrolytes to monitor imbalances
- CBC with differential

Specific Diagnostic Tests:
- Endoscopy with biopsy
- Rectal swab (C. perfringens, V. parahaemolyticus, L. monocytogenes, C. jejuni, E. coli, Salmonella, Shigella)
- Food for bacterial culture (S. aureus, Salmonella, C. botulinum, Shigella, C. jejuni, E. coli O157:H7, V. parahaemolyticus, V. cholerae)
- Toxin assays of stool and food (C. botulinum)
- Darkfield microscopy of stool (V. cholerae)
- Serotyping (E. coli)

DIFFERENTIAL DIAGNOSIS
- Incubation period <2 hr
  - Predominantly UGI symptoms, nausea, vomiting
  - Heavy metals
  - Chemicals
  - Mushrooms (usually benign: 6–12 hr incubation for amitoxin or m onomethylhydrazine containing mushrooms)

- Predominantly extra-GI and neurologic symptoms
  - Insecticides
  - Mushrooms and plant toxins
  - Monosodium glutamate
  - Shellfish
  - Scromboid
- Incubation period 1–7 hours
  - Predominantly UGI symptoms, nausea, vomiting
  - S. aureus
  - B. cerus
  - Acute gastric anisakiasis (up to 12 hr after ingestion)
- Predominantly extra-GI and neurologic symptoms
  - Shellfish Ciguatera
    - Incubation period 8–14 hours
- Noninflammatory diarrhea
  - C. perfringens
  - B. ceueus
    - Incubation period >14 hours
- Predominantly UGI symptoms, nausea, vomiting
  - Norwalk virus
- Noninflammatory diarrhea
  - ETEC
  - V. cholerae
  - G. lamblia
  - Norwalk virus
- Inflammatory diarrhea
  - Salmonella
  - Shigella
  - Campylobacter
  - Invasive E. coli
  - V. parahaemolyticus
  - E. histolytica
- Predominantly extra-GI and neurologic symptoms
  - Botulism

MANAGEMENT

What to Do First

- Recognize high-risk patients: neuromuscular symptoms, seizures, immunocompromised, cirrhotic
- Recognize high-risk ingestion: mushrooms, seafood
- Assess severity of disease and administer supportive care

- Rehydration
- Correction of electrolyte disorders
- Avoidance of contaminated food/water

General Measures
- Obtain blood and stool studies prior to specific treatment
- Consider abdominal x-ray or endoscopy for further information

SPECIFIC THERAPY
- Indicated for patients with moderate to severe diarrhea or complicating circumstances such as electrolyte disorders, dehydration, anemia,
- cardiovascular instability etc.
- Antibiotics – specific for agent involved; most cases resolve within 12–24 hr and do not require antibiotics; consider empiric therapy for patients with febrile dysentery
- Antitoxins – specific for agent involved (C. botulinum)
- Avoid antimotility and anti-emetic agents
- Side effects of antibiotic treatment
  - Worsening diarrhea
  - Allergic reactions
  - C. difficile colitis
- Prolonged fecal excretion of certain microorganisms
- Side effects of antimotility agents
  - Toxic megacolon
  - Perforation
  - Contraindicated in certain infectious conditions
- Side effects of anti-emetic agents
  - Further systemic absorption of toxin

FOLLOW-UP
- During treatment or monitoring, assess potential complications of therapy or worsening of disease requiring more aggressive therapy
- Make attempts to recognize outbreak potential/epidemics
- Inform health department of outbreaks
- Patient education with proper handling, storage, selection and preparation of food

COMPLICATIONS AND PROGNOSIS
Complications
- Electrolyte disorders – metabolic alkalosis (V. cholerae)
- Bacteremia (L. monocytogenes, Salmonella)

- Meningitis (L. monocytogenes Y. enterocolitica)
- Endocarditis (L. monocytogenes)
- Guillain-Barre Syndrome (C. jejuni)
- Hemolytic uremic syndrome (E. coli, Shigella)
- Thrombotic thrombocytopenia purpura (E. coli)
- Pharyngitis (Y. enterocolitica)
- Arthritis, Reiter's syndrome (C. jejuni, Y. enterocolitica, Shigella)
- Rashes (Y. enterocolitica)
- Toxic megacolon (E. coli)
- Hypotension, shock
- Bowel perforation
- Necrotizing enterocolitis
- Death

Prognosis
- Prognosis is good in mild disease, poor with serious sequelae

---

FOREIGN BODIES AND BEZOARS

MARTA L. DAVILA, MD

HISTORY & PHYSICAL
- Symptoms from foreign bodies depend on area of lodgment; typical anatomic points of narrowing: cervical, mid and distal esophagus, pylorus, duodenum, ileocecal valve and anus
- Adults may recall in detail the time and type of foreign body ingested
- If a rectal foreign body suspected, patient may be evasive due to embarrassment
- In children, the mentally ill or those ingesting objects for secondary gain, complications related to the foreign body often the presenting symptoms
- Foreign bodies in the esophagus may cause pain, discomfort on swallowing or dysphagia
- Physical findings unremarkable unless a perforation has occurred, in which case fever, pain and tenderness seen
- In the case of inserted rectal foreign bodies, object may be palpable on digital rectal exam
- Patients with gastric bezoars may present with epigastric pain, pyrexia, nausea, vomiting, bleeding gastric ulcers, obstruction, perforation and peritonitis
- Gastric bezoars may present as epigastric palpable mass

TESTS

■ For foreign bodies: a plain radiograph (anteroposterior and lateral views) for localization

■ For bezoars: endoscopy most effective diagnostic test, followed by barium or gastrografin studies

DIFFERENTIAL DIAGNOSIS

n/a

MANAGEMENT

What to Do First

■ Locate the position of the foreign body or bezoar

General Measures

■ If an ingested foreign object has advanced beyond the reach of an endoscope:
  ➤ Passage should be documented with daily radiographs
  ➤ Add bulk-forming agents to facilitate passage
  ➤ If it remains in the same place for more than 2–3 days, surgical removal should be considered

SPECIFIC THERAPY

Indications for Treatment

■ Endoscopy is indicated for:
  ➤ Meat impaction
  ➤ Sharp objects that may result in perforation
  ➤ Button batteries lodged in the esophagus
  ➤ Any kind of object impacted in the alimentary tract and causing symptoms

Treatment

■ Endoscopic removal of a foreign body in the upper gastrointestinal tract requires:
  ➤ Use of a number of devices such as snares, baskets, or forceps
  ➤ Use of an overtube to protect the airway and reduce the number of times the esophagus must be intubated, or alternatively,
  ➤ Use of a latex hood fitted on to the distal end of the endoscope, particularly for sharp or pointed objects

■ For an inserted foreign body in the rectum (low-lying):
  ➤ Intravenous sedation necessary to relax the pelvic musculature
  ➤ Topical anesthesia is added to relax the sphincter

- ➤ Endoscopic extraction if the object is narrow, and can be grasped with a snare or forceps
- ➤ Extraction of large objects require general or spinal anesthesia and larger instruments such as obstetrics forceps
- For a foreign body proximal to the recto-sigmoid junction (high-lying):
    - ➤ Goal is to move object to a low-lying position in the rectum
        - Consider sedation and a 12-hour observation period followed by radiographs
        - If there is no spontaneous descent: anesthesia, bimanual manipulation and possible laparotomy to move object to a more distal position where it can removed endoscopically
- For bezoars treatment varies depending on their composition and size
- Phytobezoars (plant bezoars):
    - ➤ Endoscopic treatment:
        - Mechanical fragmentation using
            - Jet water through the scope
            - Nd-YAG laser
            - Electrohydraulic lithotripsy
            - Endoscopic lithotriptor
        - Saline lavage through a large overtube and suctioning
    - ➤ Enzymatic therapy with cellulase or N-acetylcysteine
- Trichobezoars (hair balls):
    - ➤ Surgery is the standard approach
    - ➤ Endoscopic treatment with Nd-YAG laser is less successful
- Concretions of medicines
    - ➤ Can be removed by lavage or by endoscopy
    - ➤ If these methods fail, surgery is necessary

Complications
- Endoscopic removal of a foreign body or a bezoar can result in perforation, peritonitis, bleeding, mucosal damage, and death

Contraindications
- Known perforation

FOLLOW-UP
- Following removal of a foreign body, the patient should be observed for the possibility of perforation
- Removal of objects from the rectum require immediate rigid or flexible sigmoidoscopy to check for lacerations

- After an episode of esophageal impaction, a complete endoscopy should be performed within 1–2 weeks to determine the cause of narrowing and to perform dilation if necessary
- To prevent recurrence of bezoars
  - Treat with enzyme therapy (cellulase) and pro-motility agents
  - Patients with trichobezoars should undergo counseling

COMPLICATIONS AND PROGNOSIS

- A foreign body can result in perforation, obstruction, infection, aspiration, and death
- Prognosis is good for those patients without an underlying psychiatric disorder

---

FULMINANT HEPATIC FAILURE

GABRIEL GARCIA, MD

HISTORY & PHYSICAL

- Fulminant hepatic failure: acute severe liver injury occurring with no prior history of liver disease and leading to coagulopathy and encephalopathy within 8 weeks of the onset of illness, or within 2 weeks after the onset of jaundice
- Subfulminant hepatic failure: acute liver failure with encephalopathy developing 2 to 12 weeks after the onset of jaundice
- Viral hepatitis:
  - family history
  - injection drug use
  - transfusion
  - dialysis
  - high-risk sexual activity
  - nasal drug use
- Acetaminophen toxicity
  - overdose with suicide intention
  - excessive therapeutic use with chronic alcohol use
- Drug-induced liver disease
  - prescription
  - over the counter
  - herbal drugs
- Toxins
  - occupational exposure, hobbies
- Fatty liver of pregnancy/HELLP syndrome

- ➤ pregnancy
- ■ Wilson's disease
  - ➤ family history
  - ➤ neuropsychiatric symptoms
- ■ Environmental heat illness
  - ➤ heat stroke
- ■ Mushroom poisoning
  - ➤ mushroom ingestion, usually Amanita phalloides
- ■ Malignant infiltration of liver
  - ➤ known primary cancer

Signs & Symptoms
- ■ Jaundice
- ■ Ascites
- ■ Stigmata of chronic liver disease
- ■ Encephalopathy
- ■ Irritability

TESTS

Basic Tests
- ■ elevated aminotransferases, often >1000 U/L
- ■ elevated serum bilirubin
- ■ elevated INR
- ■ possible decreased pH
- ■ possible increased serum creatinine

Special Tests
- ■ Viral hepatitis:
  - ➤ anti-HAV IgM
  - ➤ HBsAg, anti-HBs IgM
  - ➤ anti-HDV, if HBsAg positive
  - ➤ anti-HCV (delayed appearance), HCV RNA (early appearance)
- ■ Acetaminophen
  - ➤ acetaminophen level
- ■ Pregnancy
  - ➤ serum beta-HCG
- ■ Wilson's disease
  - ➤ serum ceruloplasmin
  - ➤ 24-hr urine copper
  - ➤ slit lamp for Kayser-Fleischer rings
- ■ Autoimmune hepatitis

➤ hypergammaglobulinemia
➤ positive ANA

DIFFERENTIAL DIAGNOSIS

■ Acute liver failure superimposed on previously unrecognized chronic liver disease, e.g. exacerbation of chronic hepatitis B

MANAGEMENT

What to Do First

■ Confirm diagnosis
■ Assess severity of disease and need for ICU monitoring and care
■ Assess possible liver transplant

General Measures

■ Full hemodynamic monitoring (arterial line, pulmonary artery catheter)
■ Endotracheal intubation and intracranial pressure monitoring for stage 3 encephalopathy
■ Parenteral glucose (D10–20) to prevent hypoglycemia
■ Correct electrolyte and acid base disorders
■ Parenteral H2 blocker infusion to minimize chance of GI bleeding
■ Treat elevated intracranial pressure with mannitol
■ Treat fever with broad spectrum antibiotics after cultures, and consider antifungal therapy

SPECIFIC THERAPY

■ Acetaminophen poisoning
➤ gastric lavage with large bore tube to remove any pills still present
➤ N-acetylcysteine per nasogastric tube
■ Cerebral edema:
➤ treat to maintain the cerebral perfusion pressure (MAP minus ICP) gradient >50 mm Hg
➤ general measures
  • decrease tactile stimulation
  • raise head of bed 20–30 degrees
  • avoid hypotension, hypoxia, and hypercarbia
➤ specific measures
  • mannitol q hr until effect; ineffective in patient with renal failure unless coupled with CVVH or ultrafiltration, or in patients with osmolarity >310 mosm
  • hyperventilation (consider in stage 4 encephalopathy). Liver transplantation

- King's College prognostic indicators indicate patients who will have a mortality >90% and should be listed for transplant FHF secondary to acetaminophen overdose
- pH <7.30, or
- INR >6.5 and serum creatinine >3.4 mg/dL in patients with grade III or IV encephalopathy

FHF secondary to other causes

- INR >6.5, or any 3 of the following variables:
- etiology non-A, non-B hepatitis or drug reaction
- age <10 and >40 years
- duration of jaundice before encephalopathy >7 days
- serum bilirubin >17.6 mg/dL
- INR >3.5

FOLLOW-UP

- Daily monitoring during acute event
- Outpatient monitoring if liver disease begins to resolve
  - clinical assessment
  - liver tests

COMPLICATIONS AND PROGNOSIS

Complications

- Encephalopathy – risk of multi-organ failure and death is highest
- Cerebral edema – most common cause of death
- Renal failure
- Metabolic disorders:
  - Hypoglycemia
  - Acidosis
  - Alkalosis
  - Hypoxemia
- Coagulopathy
- Infections

Prognosis

- Better with a more rapid onset of encephalopathy; one series showed survival of 36% in patients with encephalopathy within 1 week of the onset of jaundice, and 14% in the remainder

GALACTOSEMIA

GREGORY M. ENNS, MD

HISTORY & PHYSICAL

History
- history of parental consanguinity or previously affected sibling (autosomal recessive inheritance)
- newborn screen positive (most states, many countries screen for galactosemia, incidence ~1/40,000)

Signs & Symptoms
- Neonatal: poor feeding, lethargy, vomiting, diarrhea, jaundice, hepatomegaly, 'neonatal hepatitis', cataracts, sepsis (esp. *E. coli* or other Gram negative organisms), full fontanel
- later features: failure to thrive, mental retardation, ovarian failure
- rare features: seizures, ataxia

TESTS

Laboratory
- basic blood studies:
  - ➤ newborn screen positive (e.g. Beutler fluorescent spot test)
  - ➤ elevated AST/ALT, bilirubin (unconjugated or combined conjugated/unconjugated), prothrombin time, metabolic acidosis (renal tubular dysfunction)
- basic urine studies:
  - ➤ reducing substances positive (after galactose ingestion) – poor sensitivity/specificity
  - ➤ proteinuria, glycosuria, aminoaciduria (renal Fanconi syndrome)

Screening
- newborn screen: prenatal diagnosis is possible (CVS or amniocyte or DNA analysis)
- CT/MRI: usually normal, abnormal white matter, cortical and cerebellar atrophy, basal ganglia and brainstem abnormalities may be present in patients with neurologic disease

Confirmatory Tests
- elevated erythrocyte galactose-1-phosphate (still elevated after transfusion)
- decreased erythrocyte galactose-1-phosphate uridyl transferase (GALT) activity in quantitative assay (NB: test invalid after

transfusion; wait 3 months to perform confirmatory enzymology if transfused)
- GALT immunoelectrophoresis determines genotype (G/G = classic galactosemia, D/G = Duarte variant)

Other Tests
- serum amino acids (esp. phenylalanine, tyrosine, methionine) may be elevated when liver disease is present; elevated phenylalanine may lead to false positive newborn screen for phenylketonuria
- viral serology negative
- liver biopsy: non-specific 'neonatal hepatitis'
- DNA analysis not routine, but may be available in some centers
- prenatal diagnosis by GALT activity or mutation analysis in amniocytes or chorionic villi possible

Imaging
- abdominal ultrasound: non-specific

DIFFERENTIAL DIAGNOSIS
- Duarte/Galactosemia heterozygosity, Duarte allele 50% normal activity, D/G heterozygotes ~25% normal activity, not at risk for classic galactosemia complications, some treat in infancy with galactose restriction (controversial)
- galactokinase deficiency: cataracts, pseudotumor cerebri (rare), no liver disease, urine reducing substances positive (after galactose ingestion), blood & urine with increased galactose, decreased erythrocyte galactokinase, normal erythrocyte GALT activity
- uridyl diphosphate:galactose epimerase deficiency: signs & symptoms similar to galactosemia, increased erythrocyte galactose-1-phosphate, decreased erythrocyte epimerase activity, normal erythrocyte GALT activity
- other causes of 'neonatal hepatitis': alpha$_1$ antitrypsin deficiency, cystic fibrosis, tyrosinemia, neonatal hemochromatosis, glycogen storage disease type IV, bile acid disorders, fatty acid oxidation defects, congenital disorders of glycosylation, peroxisomal disorders, Niemann-Pick disease type C, hereditary fructose intolerance

MANAGEMENT
What to Do First
- monitor closely for neonatal sepsis
- evaluate severity of liver, renal, CNS disease

- immediate exclusion of galactose from diet (use casein hydrolysate or soy formulas) while awaiting results of confirmatory testing
- confirm diagnosis

General Measures
- intravenous fluids, plasma, vitamin K may be needed in sick neonate
- referral to biochemical genetics specialist center
- life-long exclusion of galactose from diet (NB: many medicines contain galactose – avoid if possible)
- adequate calcium intake to aid in osteoporosis prevention

SPECIFIC THERAPY
- above treatment for all confirmed classic galactosemia patients
- galactose restrict D/G heterozygotes for 4–12 months, then start regular diet if galactose-1-phosphate levels normal after galactose challenge (controversial – some centers do not galactose restrict)
- hormone replacement therapy in premature ovarian failure (from ~ age 12 years) – monitor growth, bone age, BP during initiation of therapy

Side Effects & Contraindications
- galactose restricted diet is well-tolerated

FOLLOW-UP

During Treatment
- monitor liver function, renal function and response to antibiotics (if septic)

Routine
- biochemical geneticist/nutritionist evaluation, diet education for family of affected child, genetic counseling
- regular galactose-1-phosphate levels
- annual ophthalmology evaluation for cataracts
- regular developmental assessment (esp. to screen for speech impairment)
- refer girls to pediatric endocrinologist at ~ age 10 years

COMPLICATIONS AND PROGNOSIS

Complications
- cirrhosis, renal dysfunction, cataracts if untreated or noncompliant with diet

- mental retardation, speech abnormalities, ovarian failure may occur despite therapy, ovarian failure common despite therapy

Prognosis
- Hepatic, renal disease reversible with therapy (usually resolve within 1–2 weeks)
- cataracts reversible if therapy started <3 months of age
- mean IQ 70–90 if treated early, treatment does not guarantee normal IQ
- speech and language problems occurs frequently
- ataxia, intention tremor may occur in older children, adults despite therapy
- hypergonadotrophic hypogonadism in most girls >14 years, most women infertile (normal puberty, fertility in males)
- NB: D/G heterozygotes do not have classic galactosemia, normal outcomes without developmental, liver, kidney, ophthalmologic complications

GALLBLADDER CANCERS

SUSAN A. CUMMINGS, MD

HISTORY & PHYSICAL
- adenocarcinoma – 80%
- squamous cell carcinoma, cystadenocarcinoma – 20%

Risk Factors
- chronic cholecystitis
- 80% have gallstones
- polyps when greater than 1cm
- porcelain gallbladder (calcification of gallbladder wall)
- carcinogens (rubber and petroleum products)

History
- abdominal pain, jaundice and fever
- weight loss and pruritus
- palpable mass in area of gallbladder

TESTS

Routine Tests
- elevated alkaline phosphatase and bilirubin but usually not as high as in
- bile duct or ampullary cancers

Special Tests
- Ultrasound
  - ➤ gallstones and gallbladder mass
- CT
  - ➤ mass in the gallbladder or liver, may occlude bile ducts
- ERCP
  - ➤ cutoff of the cystic duct
  - ➤ stricture of the common duct

DIFFERENTIAL DIAGNOSIS
n/a

MANAGEMENT
What to Do First
- suspect diagnosis
- ERCP for support of diagnosis

General Measures
- assess patient's ability to undergo attempted resection

SPECIFIC THERAPY
- surgery
- poor response to chemo or radiation
- stenting via ERCP if biliary obstruction

FOLLOW-UP
- serial visits with physical examination, liver chemistries

COMPLICATIONS AND PROGNOSIS
- depends on whether or not incidental
- if incidental (10%): surgery curative
- remaining 90%: 5% 5-yr survival

GALLSTONE DISEASE

AIJAZ AHMED, MD

HISTORY & PHYSICAL
History
- types of gallstones: cholesterol/mixed stones (90%) and pigmented (10%)

- mechanism promoting gallstones formation include bile supersaturation, nucleation factors (mucin, glycoproteins and calcium) and bile stasis
- common bile duct (CBD) stones (choledocholithiasis) may form de novo in bile ducts (primary) or migrate to the CBD from the gallbladder (secondary)
- risk factors for cholesterol gallstone formation:
  - Fat: obesity, type IV hyperlipidemia, rapid weight loss, diabetes mellitus
  - Female gender
  - Family: maternal family history and Hispanic/Native American/Scandinavian
  - Fetus: pregnancy
  - Forties/Fifties: increasing age
  - Fasting: TPN
  - Fat malabsorption after biliopancreatic bypass surgery, with celiac disease due to impaired CCK release, and in Crohn's disease
  - Fibric acid derivatives (lipid lowering agents) and other medications such as contraceptive steroids/postmenopausal estrogens, octreotide, ceftriaxone
- diabetics are prone to obesity, hypertriglyceridemia and gallbladder hypomotility; no data to prove diabetes as an independent risk factor
- Asians are predisposed to primary CBD stones due to higher prevalence of
- flukes/parasitic infections

Signs & Symptoms
- biliary colic main complaint in 70%–80% of symptomatic patients; onset of pain sudden followed by rapid increase in intensity over next 10–15-min to steady plateau which can last up to 3 hours
- pain >3 hr indicates onset of acute cholecystitis
- older patients may present with minimal symptoms
- vomiting and sweating are not uncommon
- Murphy's sign: direct palpation of the RUQ results in abrupt arrest of breathing during inspiration due to pain (acute cholecystitis)
- acute suppurative cholangitis can present with pain, jaundice, and chills/rigors (Charcot's triad); refractory sepsis characterized by altered mentation, hypotension and Charcot's triad constitutes Raynold's pentad

TESTS

Laboratory

- uncomplicated biliary colic: no changes in hematological/biochemical tests
- acute cholecystitis: leukocytosis with a "left shift"
- liver enzymes, bilirubin and amylase

Imaging

- ultrasound: high sensitivity (>95%) and specificity (>95%) for the diagnosis of gallstones greater than 2 mm in diameter; ultrasound less sensitive for the diagnosis of choledocholithiasis and may only document half of CBD stones
- ERCP is the gold standard for the diagnosis of choledocholithiasis; additional benefit of providing therapeutic options
- CT and MRI now approach the diagnostic accuracy of ERCP
- hepatobiliary scintigraphy can confirm or exclude acute cholecystitis
- bile microscopy (idiopathic pancreatitis)

DIFFERENTIAL DIAGNOSIS

What to Do First

- management varies with the extent, severity and type of gallstone-induced complications

General Measures

- blood cultures, intravenous broad-spectrum antibiotics and transfer to intensive care unit in patients with cholangitis

MANAGEMENT

Asymptomatic Gallstones

- adult patients with silent or incidental gallstones can be managed expectantly;
- exceptions include asymptomatic individuals with a calcified gallbladder (porcelain gallbladder), large gallstones (>2.5 cm), gallbladder polyp greater than 10 mm in diameter, and certain Native Americans (Pima Indians) at higher risk for developing gallbladder cancer

Symptomatic Gallstones

- after an episode of biliary colic, up to 70% of patients will have recurrence of biliary colic (risk of developing gallstone-induced complications at a rate of 1% to 2% per year); decision to perform cholecystectomy individualized based on surgical candidacy and patient's preference

Acute Cholecystitis & Choledocholithiasis
- emergent biliary decompression with ERCP in patients with obstructive cholangitis
- prompt surgery indicated once the diagnosis of acute cholecystitis is made
- concomitant choledocholithiasis may need a preoperative ERCP for stone extraction; alternatively, intraoperative cholangiography can be performed to confirm choledocholithiasis followed by laparoscopic or open CBD exploration or a postoperative ERCP

SPECIFIC THERAPY
Special Situations
- acalculous cholecystitis occurs in 5%–10% of patients with acute cholecystitis; predisposing factors to acalculous cholecystitis include TPN, major surgery, critical illness, extensive trauma, or burn-related injury
- cytomegalovirus and cryptosporidia can result in cholecystitis in severely immunocompromised patients

FOLLOW-UP
n/a

COMPLICATIONS AND PROGNOSIS
Complications
- Biliary colic
- Acute cholecystitis
- Chronic cholecystitis
- Emphysematous cholecystitis
- Hydrops of the gallbladder
- Small bowel obstruction (gallstone ileus)
- Gastric outlet obstruction (Bouveret's syndrome)
- Acute biliary pancreatitis
- Acute suppurative/obstructive cholangitis
- Empyema and/or gangrene
- Perforation of the gallbladder
- Gallbladder cancer

■ Mirizzi's syndrome: edema and swelling (inflammation) secondary to the impacted stone in the cystic duct leads to the compression of common hepatic duct or CBD

Prognosis
■ excellent after cholecystectomy, except for small minority with residual symptoms due to retained CBD stones (1 to 8% post-cholecystectomy), biliary strictures, and postcholecystectomy syndrome

---

GASTRIC ADENOCARCINOMA

LYN SUE KAHNG, MD and ROY SOETIKNO, MD, MS

HISTORY & PHYSICAL

History
■ uncommon in western countries. decreasing incidence
■ older age; male: female = 2:1.
■ increased risk in H. *pylori* infection, post-gastrectomy state, gastric adenomas, chronic atrophic gastritis, intestinal metaplasia, pernicious anemia, FAP, HNPCC, diet containing high nitrates

Signs & Symptoms
■ asymptomatic until advanced
■ nonspecific: anorexia, epigastric pain, early satiety, nausea and vomiting, weight loss, anemia, or overt GI bleeding.
■ palpable mass, hepatomegaly, ascites, succussion splash, and adenopathy in advanced disease

TESTS
■ CBC: anemia. LFT: abnormalities suggesting liver metastasis
■ endoscopy
  ➤ localize and biopsy for pathology (intestinal versus diffuse (signet-ring)-type).
■ double-contrast UGI is useful in more advanced disease

DIFFERENTIAL DIAGNOSIS
■ Menetrier's disease, hypertrophic gastropathy, thickened gastric folds due to infections, lymphoid hyperplasia, lymphoma, and metastatic cancer

MANAGEMENT

What to Do First

- stage disease:
  - ➤ CXR and CT scans to rule out distant disease
  - ➤ endoscopic ultrasound is most accurate to stage for local disease

General Management

- assess candidacy for surgery

SPECIFIC THERAPY

Indications

- surgery:
  - ➤ to cure if non-metastatic (fewer than 40% are candidates)
  - ➤ to palliate bleeding or obstruction
- endoscopy:
  - ➤ to cure early superficial disease
  - ➤ to palliate obstruction (stent placement)
- chemotherapy
  - ➤ 30% response rate but minimal survival benefit
- radiation
  - ➤ often insensitive

Side Effects & Contraindications

- gastrectomy or gastrojejunostomy have significant morbidity and mortality

FOLLOW-UP

- B12 replacement; may develop Fe deficiency
- no specific protocol: recurrence is usually untreatable
  - ➤ regular blood tests q3mos, and endoscopy and CT scans q12mos

COMPLICATIONS AND PROGNOSIS

- 5-yr. survival: Stage I – 80%; Stage II – 50%; Stage III – 20%
- signet cell type has poorer prognosis

GASTRIC CARCINOIDS

LYN SUE KAHNG, MD and ROY SOETIKNO, MD, MS

HISTORY & PHYSICAL

- asymptomatic; can cause abdominal pain, dyspepsia, bleeding.
- carcinoid syndrome (flushing, facial edema, wheezing) with hepatic metastasis

- sporadic carcinoid: often large, solitary, aggressive, metastasize early
- also occur in multiple endocrine neoplasia type I, atrophic gastritis (often small and multiple, with better prognosis, in hypergastrinemic states)

TESTS
- serum gastrin if multiple lesions
- endoscopy with biopsy for diagnosis
- endoscopic ultrasonography with biopsy for subepithelial lesion
- octreotide and CAT scans to assess for metastasis
- foregut carcinoids only rarely have elevated serotonin, so 5-HIAA not so useful

DIFFERENTIAL DIAGNOSIS
n/a

MANAGEMENT
- surgery with lymph node dissection for sporadic carcinoid.
- with hypergastrinemia: resect gastrinoma or the antrum in atrophic gastritis
- medical therapy for metastatic disease with or without surgery to reduce tumor burden.
- poor response to chemotherapy.

SPECIFIC THERAPY
n/a

FOLLOW-UP
- no specific protocol. periodic CAT scans and endoscopy

COMPLICATIONS AND PROGNOSIS
- 50% 5-year survival in metastatic disease

GASTRIC LYMPHOMA

LYN SUE KAHNG, MD and ROY SOETIKNO, MD, MS

HISTORY & PHYSICAL
- nonspecific: abdominal, pain, anorexia, weight loss, bleeding, nausea and vomiting
- adenopathy, hepatospenomegaly

TESTS
- CBC: anemia. LDH may be elevated. LFT: abnormalities suggesting liver metastasis

- endoscopy: localize and biopsy for pathology (low-grade B-cell MALT lymphoma (associated with H. pylori) versus diffuse large B-cell lymphoma)

DIFFERENTIAL DIAGNOSIS

- adenocarcinoma, Menetrier's disease, hypertrophic gastropathy, thickened gastric folds due to infections, reactive lymphoid hyperplasia (immunohistochemistry will establish monoclonality of lymphocytes)

MANAGEMENT

What to Do First

- Stage disease:
- CXR and CT scans: determine distant metastasis
- endoscopic ultrasonography: determine depth and local involvement

SPECIFIC THERAPY

- low-grade MALT lymphomas which are H. pylori positive: antibiotic therapy directed toward H.pylori in early disease; chemotherapy in advanced disease
- diffuse large-cell B-cell lymphoma: surgery may be useful in early disease. chemotherapy and radiation therapy in advanced disease

Side Effects & Contraindications

- related to surgery and chemotherapy or radiation.

FOLLOW-UP

- No standard protocol; similar to gastric adenocarcinoma.

COMPLICATIONS AND PROGNOSIS

- Better for MALT (5-year survival 90%) than large-cell lymphoma (65%).
- Depends on stage and grade

GASTRIC STROMAL TUMOR

LYN SUE KAHNG, MD and ROY SOETIKNO, MD, MS

HISTORY & PHYSICAL

- previously called leiomyoma/leiomyosarcoma

Signs & Symptoms

- often asymptomatic especially if less than 2 cm

- indolent
- bleeding, pain, obstruction or palpable mass in advanced tumor
- Carney's triad: leiomyosarcoma, pulmonary chondroma, and functioning extra-adrenal paraganglioma

TESTS
- CBC: anemia. LFT: liver metastasis is common.
- endoscopy: subepithelial lesion with normal overlying mucosa with or without central umbilication or ulceration. Biopsy of mucosa is usually normal
- endoscopic ultrasonography to confirm diagnosis and to assess likelihood of malignancy (large lesion, mostly extraluminal with irregular border, regional lymph node involvement).

DIFFERENTIAL DIAGNOSIS
- lipoma, pancreatic rest, carcinoid, neuroma, extrinsic compression

MANAGEMENT
- endoscopic ultrasound to confirm diagnosis.
- CXR, CT scan
- Tests
- surgery for suspected malignant lesions
- serial ultrasound may be a useful medium to follow progression

SPECIFIC THERAPY
n/a

FOLLOW-UP
- no specific guidelines.

COMPLICATIONS AND PROGNOSIS
- if malignant, 5-year survival with curative surgery: 60%. In incomplete
- resection: 25%

GASTROENTERITIS

SUZANNE M. MATSUI, MD and JAYSHREE MATADIAL, MD

HISTORY & PHYSICAL

History
- travel: foreign, or to mountainous regions
  ➢ also consider exposure to contaminated water

- eating suspect food
  - ➤ shellfish, fried rice, unrefrigerated milk or meat, undercooked poultry or eggs, fermented canned food, imported food
  - ➤ eating food at events where others also became ill
- recent antibiotic use

Signs & Symptoms
- nausea, vomiting
- crampy abdominal pain
- diarrhea, watery to dysentery
- headache, fever, myalgia to varying degrees
- symptoms usually last 1–4 days

TESTS
- start with stool for culture and O&P in select patients:
  - ➤ extremes of age
  - ➤ immunocompromised host
  - ➤ involved in outbreak (including institutional)
  - ➤ invasive infection suspected
  - ➤ hyposplenism (invasive salmonellosis)

DIFFERENTIAL DIAGNOSIS
- viruses (most common)
  - ➤ Norwalk and related caliciviruses
  - ➤ rotavirus (especially in young children)
  - ➤ astrovirus
  - ➤ enteric adenovirus
- bacteria
  - ➤ agents listed in food poisoning and infectious diarrhea chapters
- microbial and other toxins
  - ➤ listed in food poisoning chapter
- other agents
  - ➤ *G. lamblia, Cryptosporidium, I. belli*
  - ➤ alcohol
  - ➤ heavy metals
- other conditions
  - ➤ eosinophilic gastroenteritis
  - ➤ IBD

MANAGEMENT

What to Do First
- assess hydration status and administer fluids as appropriate
- obtain samples for further testing from high risk patients or those involved in outbreaks

General Measures
- handwashing and other hygienic measures
- avoid antimotility agents, if invasive infection suspected
- avoid anti-emetic agents, if toxin ingestion suspected
- notify health department, if foodborne outbreak suspected

SPECIFIC THERAPY
- antimicrobial agents (see food poisoning and infectious diarrhea chapters)

FOLLOW-UP
- most gastroenteritis (especially viral) is self-limiting: rehydration and general measures sufficient
- if symptoms persist:
  - reevaluate patient
  - assess severity and need for hospitalization
  - repeat stool studies
  - consider endoscopy with biopsy

COMPLICATIONS AND PROGNOSIS
- uncommon to develop sequelae
- post-infectious irritable bowel syndrome
- persistent infection (G. lamblia, immunocompromised host)
- unmasked underlying disease (IBD, celiac disease)
- see infectious diarrhea and food poisoning chapters

GASTROESOPHAGEAL REFLUX DISEASE

GEORGE TRIADAFILOPOULOS, MD

HISTORY & PHYSICAL
- GERD = spectrum ranging from heartburn or acid regurgitation alone (non-erosive reflux disease, NERD) to reflux esophagitis and its complications, including esophageal ulcers, strictures and Barrett's esophagus

Risk Factors
- lower esophageal sphincter (LES) = key mechanism responsible for GERD
- Transient lower esophageal sphincter relaxations (tLESRs) account for the majority of physiologic and pathologic reflux

- >80% of patients with esophagitis have hiatal hernia that dissociates the LES from the crural diaphragm
- Large hiatal hernias (>3cm) are associated with weak LES, poor esophageal peristalsis, severe acid reflux and esophagitis

Symptoms
- Heartburn
- Acid regurgitation
- Dysphagia
- Extra-esophageal symptoms: asthma, recurrent pneumonia, chronic cough, angina-like chest pain, laryngitis (hoarseness), dental erosions, chronic hiccups

Physical Signs
- Usually absent

TESTS
Basic Tests
- CBC: rule out anemia from blood loss

Specific Diagnostic Tests
- **Endoscopy with biopsy**
  - ➤ Best diagnostic study for evaluating mucosal injury and identifying hiatal hernia, peptic strictures, and Barrett's esophagus; it allows dilation of peptic strictures and surveillance for dysplasia and cancer in Barrett's esophagus
- **Esophageal manometry**
  - ➤ Used to assess LES pressure and peristalsis; performed before anti-reflux surgery to identify patients with poor esophageal body peristalsis
- **Ambulatory esophageal pH monitoring**
  - ➤ Evaluation of patients with atypical reflux symptoms or failed antireflux therapy; % time with pH <4 most useful measure to discriminate between physiologic and pathologic esophageal acid exposure

Other Tests
- Barium swallow/UGI
  - ➤ May identify hiatal hernia, strictures and dysmotility
- Barium tablet study
  - ➤ Useful in identifying areas of subtle stenosis and explain dysphagia

DIFFERENTIAL DIAGNOSIS

- Esophageal motor disorders, angina pectoris, asthma, dyspepsia, peptic ulcer disease, cholelithiasis

MANAGEMENT

What to Do First

- Stepwise approach to GERD: lifestyle modification, antacids and OTC H2 antagonists; proton pump inhibitors; surgery

General Measures

- Lifestyle modifications: diet changes, elevation of the head of the bed, avoidance of early recumbency after meals, discontinuation of smoking, alcohol and irritant medications

SPECIFIC THERAPY

Indications for Treatment

- Goals of therapy: relieve symptoms, heal esophageal mucosa, prevent and manage complications, maintain remission

Treatment Options

- Antacids: beneficial in patients with mild reflux without erosive esophagitis who do not require daily medication; ineffective in healing esophagitis
- Promotility drugs (metoclopramide): enhance esophageal peristaltic clearance and gastric emptying; potent antiemetic; does not heal esophagitis
- H2 receptor antagonists (cimetidine, ranitidine, famotidine, and nizatidine): equally effective when used at the proper doses: cimetidine, 400 mg bid; ranitidine and nizatidine 150 mg bid and famotidine, 20 mg bid; therapy for 6–12 wk relieves symptoms in 50%, heals esophagitis in 50% and maintains remission in 25%; efficacy in severe esophagitis
- Proton pump inhibitors (omeprazole, lansoprazole, rabeprazole, and pantoprazole): faster symptom relief; rapid and complete mucosal healing; more effective than H2 receptor antagonists; achieve healing rates of 80–100% within 8 wk; also improves dysphagia and decreases the need for dilation of strictures
- New endoscopic therapies (radiofrequency therapy, endoscopic ligation): recently become available; they both achieve symptom control in 70% of cases
- Antireflux surgery: used for severe, intractable GERD and its complications; laparoscopic Nissen fundoplication most frequently

performed; preoperative 24-hour pH monitoring and esophageal manometry necessary, as abnormal esophageal motility may affect outcome; heals esophagitis in about 90% of patients; complications prevented and remission maintained 80%

Side Effects and Complications
- Antacids: diarrhea or constipation; metoclopramide: drowsiness, agitation, dystonic reactions and tremor; H2 receptor antagonists are generally very well tolerated; proton pump inhibitors: abdominal pain, diarrhea, headache, nausea, and weight gain

FOLLOW-UP
During Treatment
- Maintenance therapy is necessary to prevent recurrence of symptoms and complications; proton pump inhibitors in standard doses are effective in maintaining remission

Routine
- "Once in a lifetime endoscopy" for patients with chronic, intermittent reflux complaints who respond to medical therapy but have frequent relapses to rule out Barrett's esophagus

COMPLICATIONS AND PROGNOSIS
- Unexplained chest pain
- Chronic unexplained cough
- Chronic laryngitis and hoarseness
- Peptic strictures (in 10% of untreated cases)
- Barrett's esophagus (30-fold – risk of adenocarcinoma)
- Adenocarcinoma or high grade dysplasia

GASTROINTESTINAL BLEEDING

JOHN P. CELLO, MD

HISTORY & PHYSICAL
- Upper GI bleeding (i.e., bleeding from esophagus, stomach and proximal small bowel)

History
- Vomiting of grossly bloody (hematemesis) or "coffee grounds" (melenemesis) material
  - ➤ Melena, dark liquid black (tar-like) stools

- Dyspepsia may or may not be present
  - ~50% of patients >60 years have dyspepsia with bleeding
  - ~35% of patient <60 years have dyspepsia with bleeding
- More specific features for some entities: reflux/heartburn – esophagitis; forceful emesis – Mallory-Weiss tear of GE junction; dyspepsia – peptic ulcers; weight loss/early satiety – neoplasms; NSAID use – ulcers; known or suspected cirrhosis – varices
- Occasionally just symptoms of anemia – weakness, pallor, dyspnea

Physical Findings
- occasionally, epigastric tenderness (for ulcer disease), rarely epigastric mass or hepatomegaly for neoplasms or cirrhosis
- Lower GI bleeding (usually bleeding from distal small bowel or colon)

History
- Grossly bloody stools (note: this may occasionally be from brisk upper GI bleed) or normal stools mixed with blood
- Occasionally melena (especially from distal small bowel or right colon)
- Weight loss, constipation, diarrhea, anorexia – with colon cancer
- Abdominal pain, cramps, diarrhea, fevers and arthralgias – with idiopathic inflammatory bowel disease
- Occasionally symptoms of anemia alone

Physical Findings
- palpable mass (colon cancer primary or hepatomegaly from metastases) or tenderness in lower quadrants (colitis); remember that diverticular bleeding is painless
- Occult GI bleeding
- No hematemesis, melena, hematochezia – the most common presentation
- Occasionally, episodes of hematemesis, melena &/or hematochezia with repetitively negative evaluations
- Chronic iron deficiency anemia &/or stools (+) for occult blood
- Usually no symptoms other than those of anemia

Tests

Laboratory Tests: Anemia
- acute blood loss: associated with normal MCV and MCHC, and normal iron and ferritin stores

■ chronic bleeding from ulcer or neoplasm: hypochromic, microcytic anemia with low serum iron and ferritin and elevated transferrin levels

Upper GI Endoscopy
■ routine first step for symptoms/signs of upper GI bleeding; if first exam is unclear then repeat evaluations helpful; occasionally, superficial atypical lesions are missed (i.e., vascular ectasias, gastric varices)

Colonoscopy
■ test of choice for lower GI bleeding; cannot perform exam in patient actively bleeding – requires adequate bowel preparation – prep can be done in 4–6 hours

Other Tests:
■ Red blood cell technetium scan – sensitive for bleeding at rates of 1 unit RBC every 2–4 hours
■ Enteroscopy – uses 3-meter-long endoscope – reaches 1 meter beyond ligament of Treitz
■ Angiography – requires brisk bleeding at rates of 1–2 units/hr
■ Exploratory laparotomy – not useful unless combined with intraoperative panenteroscopy (scope passed directly into small bowel and guided proximally and distally)
■ Capsule video enteroscopy: relatively new technique, extremely useful when endoscopy and colonoscopy are reliably negative

DIFFERENTIAL DIAGNOSIS
■ Major sources of bleeding – upper GI tract
  ➤ Esophagitis
  ➤ Mallory-Weiss tears
  ➤ Varices
  ➤ Gastric ulcer
  ➤ Gastritis
  ➤ Gastric varices
  ➤ Pyloric channel ulcer
  ➤ Duodenal ulcer
  ➤ Duodenitis
    • Gastric or esophageal cancer
    • Dieulafoy's lesions (single superficial blood vessel)
■ Major sources of bleeding – lower GI tract
  ➤ Hemorrhoids
  ➤ Ulcerative proctitis/colitis

- ➤ Colonic diverticula
- ➤ Colonic polyps
- ➤ Colonic cancer
- ➤ Vascular ectasias (also called "angiodysplasia" or "AVMs")
- ■ Major sources of "occult" GI bleeding
  - ➤ Nasopharyngeal bleeding
  - ➤ Gingival bleeding
  - ➤ Tracheobronchial tree
  - ➤ Occult gastric or duodenal varices
  - ➤ Vascular ectasias – "watermelon stomach"
  - ➤ Mesenteric varices
  - ➤ Dieulafoy lesions (large vascular AVMs)
  - ➤ Small bowel neoplasms or diverticula
  - ➤ Meckel's diverticulum
  - ➤ Occult small bowel Crohn's disease
  - ➤ Small bowel tuberculosis
  - ➤ Aorto-enteric fistulae (usually aortoduodenal)
    - Trauma-associated bleeding into bile duct (hemobilia) or pancreatic duct (hemosuccus pancreaticus)

MANAGEMENT

What to Do First

- ■ Resuscitate with adequate fluid and red cells
- ■ Evaluate for cardiopulmonary compromise due to hypovolemia
- ■ Correct any coagulopathy

General Management

- ■ Seek surgical and GI consultation – early for acute bleeders
- ■ Be persistent but appropriately aggressive

SPECIFIC THERAPY

- ■ Intravenous or oral proton pump inhibitors possibly helpful for acid-peptic bleeding
- ■ Antibiotic therapy for H. pylori-associated ulcers possibly decreases early rebleeding
- ■ Endoscopic therapy – heater probe, bipolar electrode, clip fixation, injection of epinephrine decreases rebleeding, transfusions, costs, hospital stay

FOLLOW-UP

- ■ For benign gastric and duodenal ulcers without NSAID use – treat empirically for H. pylori or review gastric biopsies for H. pylori and treat appropriately

- For atypical ulcers (distal duodenum, occurrence while on therapy, etc) – consider Zollinger-Ellison syndrome – draw fasting serum gastric levels
- For patients not biopsied for H. pylori, consider C14 or C13 urea breath test to confirm presence of H. pylori
- Gastric ulcers should be re-examined by endoscopy after 10–12 weeks; patients with other non-variceal bleeding lesions need not be re-endoscoped
- Proton pump or H2 blockers therapy will likely be necessary indefinitely for patients with reflux esophagitis

COMPLICATIONS AND PROGNOSIS
- Upper GI bleeding – major problem is rebleeding – more common with patients in whom "visible vessel" noted on initial endoscopy; rebleeding also more common for gastric ulcers, vascular ectasias
- Marked reduction in recurrent ulcers if H. pylori detected and treated
- Lower GI bleeding – repeat hemorrhage common from diverticula and colitis; neoplasms and vascular ectasias require definitive therapy – polypectomy, surgical resection or coagulation

GASTROPATHY

LAUREN B. GERSON, MD, MSc

HISTORY & PHYSICAL

Risk Factors
- Usage of aspirin or nonsteroidal anti-inflammatory drugs (NSAIDs)
- Excessive alcohol usage and/or underlying cirrhosis
- Associated peptic ulcer disease
- Presence of other infectious diseases (ie, tuberculosis)

Signs and Symptoms
- Dyspepsia
- Weight loss, anorexia
- Nausea and emesis
- Occult GI bleeding
- Upper GI bleeding with hematemesis and/or melena
- May be asymptomatic and detected at time of endoscopy for other reasons
- Hypoalbuminemia and peripheral edema

TESTS

Basic Studies: Blood
- CBC
- If elevated MCV:
  - ➤ Vitamin B12 level
  - ➤ Schilling test or anti-parietal antibody levels
- Serum gastrin level to exclude Zollinger-Ellison syndrome
- H. pylori antibody useful in the setting of suspected peptic ulcer disease or documented lymphoma
- Hypoalbuminemia and low serum protein in Menetrier's disease

Upper Endoscopy with Biopsy
- Mucosal biopsies or urease testing for H. pylori
- False negative urease test can be seen with proton pump inhibitor usage or high dose H2-receptor antagonist therapy
- Endoscopic appearance can be non-specific
- Histologic evidence of gastritis necessary to establish diagnosis
- Tissue for culture if clinically indicated
- In the setting of suspected Menetrier's disease, perform endoscopic mucosal resection to achieve depth required to confirm diagnosis
- Consider endoscopic ultrasound to exclude malignancy

Imaging
- Thickened gastric folds can be demonstrated and are nonspecific
- Small bowel study may be useful to exclude Crohn's disease with gastric involvement

DIFFERENTIAL DIAGNOSIS

Erosive/hemorrhagic gastritis
- Stress lesions in intensive care unit or burn patients
- Drugs: NSAIDS, potassium chloride, iron, chemotherapy, cocaine
- Alcohol
  - ➤ Gastritis
  - ➤ Portal hypertensive gastropathy in setting of cirrhosis
- Localized gastric trauma
  - ➤ Interventional, caustic, radiation, foreign body ingestion
- Reflux injury
  - ➤ Postgastrectomy, duodenogastric reflux
- Ischemia
- Graft-versus-host disease
- Prolapse gastropathy

- Idiopathic
  - ➤ Diffuse varioform (chronic erosive) gastritis
- Nonerosive gastritis
  - ➤ Healthy aging
  - ➤ Associated with *H. pylori* infection
  - ➤ Lymphocytic gastritis
  - ➤ Atrophic gastritis with or without pernicious anemia
  - ➤ Associated with peptic ulcer or gastric adenocarcinoma
- Specific Types of Gastritis
  - ➤ Hypertrophic gastropathy
    - Menetrier's disease
    - Zollinger-Ellison syndrome
    - Multiple gastric polyps
    - Localized hypertrophic gastropathy
  - ➤ Infectious gastritis
    - Syphilis, tuberculosis, candidiasis, aspergillosis, histoplasmosis, giardiasis, cryptosporidiosis, strongyloides, CMV
  - ➤ Other conditions associated with granulomas:
    - Crohn's disease, Whipple's disease, chronic granulomatous disease, allergic granulomatosis, sarcoidosis
- Eosinophilic gastroenteritis

MANAGEMENT

What to Do First

- Upper endoscopy with biopsy

General Measures

- Removal of offending agent: alcohol, NSAIDs, aspirin
- Blood and stool cultures in setting of infection

SPECIFIC THERAPY

- Infectious gastritis
  - ➤ *H. pylori* is nonpathogenic in most infected individuals
  - ➤ Treat for *H. pylori* in the setting of suspected or confirmed peptic
    - ulcer disease, lymphoma, gastric cancer
  - ➤ Specific treatment if other infectious etiologies identified
- Lymphocytic gastritis
  - ➤ Cause is unknown
  - ➤ Exclude lymphoma or other forms of gastritis
  - ➤ Consider treatment with proton pump inhibitors, misoprostol, or corticosteroid therapy

- Esosinophilic gastritis
  - ➤ Corticosteroids
- NSAID-induced gastritis
  - ➤ May be asymptomatic
  - ➤ Treat with withdrawal of offending agent if possible
  - ➤ In patients at increased risk for ulcer formation or those who could not withstand the development of an ulcer, prophylaxis with PPIs or misoprostol
- Ethanol-induced injury
  - ➤ Poor correlation with symptoms
  - ➤ Resolves with alcohol abstention
  - ➤ In setting of portal hypertensive gastropathy, beta-blockers, TIPS or liver transplantation if refractory to treatment
- Stress-related mucosal injury
  - ➤ Improve underlying condition
  - ➤ Prophylaxis with intravenous H2-blocker decreases bleeding rate
- Pernicious anemia
  - ➤ Monthly injections of vitamin B12
- Menetrier's disease
  - ➤ Eradication of *H. pylori* if detected
  - ➤ No treatment if minimal symptoms and borderline low albumin
    - Consider proton pump inhibitor therapy, corticosteroids, and/or octreotide when diarrhea present
  - ➤ Partial gastric resection if persistent symptoms and low albumin

Side Effects of Specific Treatments
- Prednisone
  - ➤ Side Effects: Adrenal insufficiency, psychosis, immunosuppression, peptic ulcer, osteoporosis, appetite change, mood swings, hyperglycemia, hypertension
  - ➤ Contraindications
    - Absolute: Systemic fungal infection
    - Relative: Congestive heart failure, seizure disorder, diabetes, hypertension, osteoporosis, impaired hepatic function
- Vitamin B12
  - ➤ Side Effects: Pruritus, diarrhea, urticaria, peripheral vascular thrombosis
- Misoprostol
  - ➤ Side effects: Miscarriage, diarrhea, abdominal pain, nausea, vomiting, headache, menstrual irregularities
  - ➤ Contraindications

- Absolute: Pregnancy or lactating patients
- Relative: None

FOLLOW-UP
- *H. pylori* infection
  - Antibody titers decline slowly over many months
  - Need to wait 6–12 months to witness significant decline and/or regression in lymphoma
  - Serology positive in up to 40% of successfully treated patients
  - Use urea breath test or upper endoscopy with biopsy to confirm eradication
- Surveillance for gastric cancer in pernicious anemia
  - Endoscopy with biopsy initially
  - No endoscopic surveillance if no dysplasia detected
  - Endoscopy with biopsy every 2 years if dysplasia detected
- Surveillance for gastric cancer in postgastrectomy patients
  - Consider intial screening 10 years post-resection
  - Screening frequency not established
- Role of screening for early gastric cancer in Menetrier's disease
  - True incidence of cancer unclear: ?related to postgastrectomy state
  - Difficult to perform adequate tissue sampling of thickened folds

COMPLICATIONS AND PROGNOSIS
- Gastric cancer in minority of patients
  - Postgastrectomy
  - Pernicious anemia
  - ?Menetrier's disease
- Upper GI bleeding

Prognosis
- Lifespan normal in the absence of gastric cancer development
- Most patients with Menetrier's disease, most do well after partial gastric resection without recurrence

---

GEOGRAPHIC TONGUE

SOL SILVERMAN Jr, DDS

HISTORY & PHYSICAL
- onset at any age
- no known etiology; rarely associated with medications or allergies

- probably occurs in 10% of the population
- depapillated areas of tongue dorsum in variable sizes and shapes, often with keratotic border (elongation of filliform papillae)
- not contagious
- often symptomatic
- chronic or cyclical signs/symptoms

TESTS
- biopsy if in doubt
- CBC to rule out anemia (extremely rare)

DIFFERENTIAL DIAGNOSIS
- candidiasis (antifungal trial-systemic or topical)
- allergic response (corticosteroid trial-systemic or topical)

MANAGEMENT
- rule out potential causative/related conditions
- only treat if symptomatic (empirical use of analgesics, antidepressants, mouth rinses)

SPECIFIC THERAPY
- none

FOLLOW-UP
- only as necessary for flares, symptoms

COMPLICATIONS AND PROGNOSIS
- pain is only complication (chronic life-long condition)

GIANT CELL ARTERITIS

ERIC L. MATTESON, MD

HISTORY & PHYSICAL

History
- Age always > 50 years
- Female:male 2:1
- Associated with polymyalgia rheumatica
- Affects the aorta and branches, including temporal artery

Signs & Symptoms
- New onset headache, often unilateral (80%)
- Jaw claudication (40%)

- Visual changes or loss (20%)
- TIAs or stroke (5%)
- Fever, systemic symptoms (30%)
- Polymyalgia rheumatica (40%)
- Tender temporal artery (50%)

TESTS
n/a

DIFFERENTIAL DIAGNOSIS
n/a

MANAGEMENT
n/a

SPECIFIC THERAPY
n/a

FOLLOW-UP
n/a

COMPLICATIONS AND PROGNOSIS
n/a

GIARDIASIS

J. GORDON FRIERSON, MD

HISTORY & PHYSICAL

History

- Exposure: Ingestion of food or water contaminated with cysts. Water borne outbreaks occur. Contaminated fingers are vehicles and cysts recoverable under fingernails. Spread in day care centers is common; family members are infected when child comes home.

Signs & Symptoms

- Incubation period of 1–2 weeks. Diarrhea, bloating, belching, flatulence are common. Sometimes weight loss and signs of malabsorption. May or may not resolve spontaneously. No specific physical signs.

TESTS

- Basic tests: blood: usually normal CBC, chemistries

- Basic tests: urine: normal
- Specific tests: Stool exam for O&P. A little more sensitive is ELISA-based exam of stool for Giardia antigen.
- Other tests: Serology is available, but many false negatives, and positive could mean old disease. UGI may show dilation of upper small bowel and thickened folds. Duodenal aspirate or biopsy useful when less invasive tests indeterminate.

DIFFERENTIAL DIAGNOSIS
- Infectious diarrheas, other causes of malabsorption, amebiasis, strongyloidiasis, isosporiasis

MANAGEMENT
What to Do First
- Assess severity, evidence of malabsorption.

General Measures
- Determine source of infection, check others exposed.

SPECIFIC THERAPY
Indications
- All symptomatic patients; asymptomatic patients who may transmit infection

Treatment Options
- Metronidazole for 7 days
- Tinadazole single dose
- Paromomycin for 7 days
- Furazolidine for 10 days

Side Effects & Complications
- Metronidazole: metallic taste in mouth, mild GI complaints, dizziness. Antabuse-like reaction with alcohol.
- Paromomycin: nausea, vomiting, diarrhea
- Furazolidine: nausea, occasional allergic reactions, urticaria
- Contraindications to treatment: absolute: none
- Contraindications to treatment: relative: asymptomatic children in day care centers. Treatment of asymptomatic persons in hygienic settings is optional.

FOLLOW-UP
During Treatment
- See that symptoms subside.

Routine
- Obtain follow-up stool exam (preferably with ELISA-based test) 2 weeks after therapy.

COMPLICATIONS AND PROGNOSIS
- Malabsorption, weight loss. IGA deficiency predisposes to more severe and persistent disease.

GILBERT'S SYNDROME

WILLIAM E. BERQUIST, MD

HISTORY & PHYSICAL
- incidence: 7–10% of population
- autosomal dominant inheritance
- presentation: prolonged neonatal jaundice or incidental laboratory detection
- normal physical exam

TESTS

Basic Tests
- plasma bilirubin <3 mg/dl in non-fasting, non-hemolytic state; nearly all unconjugated
- normal liver enzymes

Special Diagnostic Tests
- phenobarbital therapy (5mg/kg/d): decreased bilirubin in 7–10 days
- DNA insertional mutation of the UGT1A1 gene that conjugates bilirubin

Other Tests
- liver biopsy: normal histology
- oral cholecystography: normal

DIFFERENTIAL DIAGNOSIS
- hemolysis
  - ➤ Crigler-Najjer syndrome type 2: much higher degree of jaundice

MANAGEMENT
- hydration and avoid fasting; no other therapy or liver biopsy necessary

SPECIFIC THERAPY
n/a

FOLLOW-UP
■ none required after diagnosis

COMPLICATIONS AND PROGNOSIS
■ no complications expected
■ excellent prognosis

GITELMAN'S SYNDROME

MICHEL BAUM, MD

HISTORY & PHYSICAL
■ Salt craving, muscle cramps, tetany, constipation

TESTS
■ Hypokalemia, metabolic alkalosis, hypomagnesemia
■ Fractional excretion of Na and Cl >1%, UCa/UCr <0.10

DIFFERENTIAL DIAGNOSIS
■ Autosomal recessive defect in distal convoluted tubule NaCl cotransporter
■ Distinguish from other causes of salt wasting

MANAGEMENT
n/a

SPECIFIC THERAPY
■ KCl and Mg supplements

FOLLOW-UP
■ To follow serum electrolytes and determine response to therapy

COMPLICATIONS AND PROGNOSIS
■ Prognosis usually excellent

GLAUCOMA

A. SYDNEY WILLIAMS, MD

HISTORY & PHYSICAL

History
■ Hereditary, family history often positive
■ any adult age but usually over age 60

- prevalence increases 5 times in African-Americans
- nearsightedness is a risk for open angle
- farsightedness is a risk for closed angle
- main risk is high intraocular pressure (usually over 20)
- glucocorticoid use also a risk factor (usually topically or intranasal)

Signs & Symptoms

- Open angle glaucoma is without symptoms
- Closed angle glaucoma preceded by periodic misty vision or rainbow colored haloes
- Acute closed angle causes sudden, severe trigeminal pain, blurring and often associated nausea
- intraocular pressure (IOP) is usually elevated
- optic nerve cup is expanded – loss of rim tissue
- A thin cornea (<555 microns) triples risk of glaucoma
- visual acuity is usually normal in chronic glaucomas
- secondary glaucomas may mimic primary disease, angle recession, exfoliation, pigmentary, steroid induced

TESTS

- Tonometry to check IOP-tonopen or Applanation
- Visual field testing-automated
- Optic nerve visualization
- Gonioscopy to visualize open and normal angle

DIFFERENTIAL DIAGNOSIS

- Ocular hypertension
- Inaccurate pressure readings
- Physiologic cupping of the optic nerve
- Angle closure glaucoma
- Acute glaucomas mimic other causes of painful red eye: corneal ulcers, keratitis, iritis

MANAGEMENT

General Measures

- Obtain accurate pressure data
- Determine degree of damage by nerve appearance and field testing
- Photography of optic nerve
- Optic nerve analysis with HRT, OCT or GDX
- Baseline threshold visual field
- Determine target pressure level (depends on damaging pressure level and presenting degree of damage)

- Lower intraocular pressure to "safe" level
- Stabilize – vision loss from glaucoma cannot be cured or repaired

SPECIFIC THERAPY
- Indicated in most glaucomas where risk of progression is high
- Medications, laser or surgery are all options
- 80% with open angles receive only eyedrop therapy
- Laser iridotomy is initial therapy if angle closure
- Therapy is increased step-wise to obtain target pressure and ideally stop disease progression
- Because target pressure is arbitrary and the disease progression often slow, long follow-up is required to assess efficacy of treatment.

Medical Therapy
- *Prostaglandin derivatives (bimatoprost, latanaprost, travaprost and unoprostone)*
  - ➢ Strongest once-daily therapy (bimatoprost, latanaprost, travaprost)
  - ➢ Outflow agent
  - ➢ *Side effects & contraindications*
    - Red eyes, keratitis, rarely myalgias
    - Increased iris pigmentation in hazel eye
    - Increased lash growth
    - Relatively contraindicated in postoperative glaucomas and H. simplex keratitis patients
- *Beta-blockers (timolol, Betaxolol, levobunolol, etc.)*
  - ➢ Once or twice daily, inflow agent and strong
  - ➢ Many more serious potential side effects
  - ➢ *Side effects & contraindications*
    - Contraindicated in asthma and 2d-3d degree heart block
    - fatigue, impotence, depression, confusion and memory loss
  - ➢ Betaxolol is only beta-I selective and can be used in asthmatics and COPD; not as strong as non-selectives and is BID
- *Alpha-agonists (apraclonidine, iopidine)*
  - ➢ Good pressure lowering affecting outflow and inflow
  - ➢ Favorable toxicity profile
  - ➢ *Side effects & contraindications*
    - Contraindicated in babies and children
    - Dry mouth and hypotension
    - Fatigue syndrome prominent but rare
    - Allergic reactions 10–30% with this medication

■ *Carbonic-anhydrase inhibitors (dorzolamide, brinzolamide, acetazolamide, methazolantide)*
  ➤ Newer agents are topical (dorzolamide and brinzolamide)
  ➤ Medium-strength pressure reduction as drops, strong as pills
  ➤ Inflow agents
  ➤ *Side effects & contraindications*
    • Contraindicated in patients with proven sulfa allergy
    • Few side effects with topical
    • Systemic agents rarely useful for chronic therapy
    • Dysgustia occasional
    • May worsen corneal edema if pre-existing
    • Systemic agents are quite toxic, causing fatigue, disorientation, somnolence, diarrhea, anorexia, weight loss, kidney stones and rarely an idiosyncratic aplastic anemia

■ *Cholinergic agents (pilocarpine, acetylcholine)*
  ➤ Strong pressure reduction by improving outflow
  ➤ Many ocular side effects
  ➤ Pilocarpine is best tolerated but QID dosing
  ➤ Best used in angle closure and pseudophalda
  ➤ *Side effects & contraindications*
    • Miosis and accommodation
    • Retinal tears or vitreous hemorrhage
    • Increased cataract and ocular inflammation

■ *Epinephrine derivatives (epinephrine and dipivefrin)*
  ➤ Rarely used today
  ➤ Ineffective in combination with other newer agent

Laser Therapy
■ *Selective Laser Trabeculoplasty*
■ For open angle glaucomas including pigmentary and exfoliation glaucomas
  ➤ Office procedure, 75% effective, 2–3 year duration
  ➤ Complements medical therapy, doesn't replace it
  ➤ Can be repeated and is very safe and simple
  ➤ *Side effects & contraindications*
  ➤ mild iritis, rarely severe
  ➤ contraindicated if angle closed or in angle recession and uveitic glaucomas

Surgical Therapy
■ *Trabeculectomy or Tube-shunt procedures*

- Outpatient surgeries
- Extremely effective for many glaucomas
- Risk is higher than with medication or laser
- As close to a cure possible, over 90% effective, 50% for 10 years or longer
- Useful in severe glaucomas or progressive glaucomas despite medical therapy
- Tube-shunts are useful in eyes likely to scar or those that have failed multiple trabeculectomies

FOLLOW-UP
- Medically treated stable eyes
- IOP check every 3–6 months
- Visual field annually
- Stereo disc photos every 2–4 years

COMPLICATIONS AND PROGNOSIS
- Depends on initial disease severity and age at presentation
- Earlier, severe disease most risky
- Careful follow-up and treatment to lower pressure dramatically
- 2–3% of glaucoma patients become blind
- 5 times greater blindness in African-Americans

GLOMERULAR DISEASES

GERALD B. APPEL, MD, FACP

HISTORY & PHYSICAL
- Swelling of extremities and especially around the eyes in AM, weight gain, foamy or bubbly urine, decreased urine output, fatigue, weakness.
- History of systemic condition associated with glomerulonephritis (diabetes, lupus, amyloidosis), use of medications (e.g. NSAIDs, lithium, gold salts), hx of infections (Hep C, Hep B, streptococcal, HIV), family history (Alport's).
- Ankle and leg edema, periorbital edema in the A.M., if excessive systemic fluid retention anasarca, ascites, pleural effusions.

TESTS
- **Blood:** BUN/ creatinine, serum albumin, serum cholesterol. FBS and HgBA1C.

- **Urine:** Urinalysis, 24 hr urine for protein and creatinine, in select cases UPEP.
- **Specific Diagnostic Tests:**
- ANA, serum complement, in select cases VDRL, SPEP, ANCA, ASLO, Hepatitis B and C serology, anti-GBM antibodies.
- **Other Tests:** renal ultrasound, renal biopsy in select cases.

DIFFERENTIAL DIAGNOSIS
- **Distinguish from other fluid retaining states:** CHF, liver disease (only NS has periorbital edema), hyperlipidemic states, conditions with proteinuria but less than nephrotic levels (HBP).

Determine which syndrome best fits the patient
- Nephrotic syndrome (NS) characterized by: proteinuria, edema, hypoalbuminemia, and hyperlipidemia.
- Minimal change disease: most common in children, up to 5–10% adults with idiopathic NS; rarely seen with NSAIDs, lithium use, Hodgkin's disease-Leukemias; sudden onset severe edema
- Focal segmental glomerulosclerosis: Up to 25% of idiopathic nephrotic syndrome; Most common pattern in Blacks with idiopathic NS. Secondary forms seen with HIV, obesity, remnant kidneys, reflux, sickle cell disease, heroin nephropathy
- Membranous Nephropathy: Most common pattern idiopathic NS in Caucasians; Secondary forms with gold salts, NSAIDs, syphilis, Hepatitis B and rarely C, SLE
- Membranoproliferative GN (MPGN): Most patients have Hepatitis C MPGN or cryoglobulinemia; young females r/o SLE
- Glomerulonephritis characterized by edema, hypertension, oliguria and urine sediment with rbc and rbc casts
- IgA Nephropathy: Most common form of idiopathic GN in world. Presents in young persons with gross hematuria (dark or Coca Cola urine) after exercise or upper resp infection. Presents in older persons as asymptomatic microhematuria and proteinuria. 10% present with severe nephritis and rapid renal failure or NS. Small overlap with Henoch Schoenlein purpura (HSP) (IgA vasculitis with skin, GI tract, arthritis, and more severe kidney disease)
- Post-Streptococcal GN: Follows certain strains of ß-hemolytic streptococcal throat, skin and other infections; Onset 10 days to 2 wks post infection with dark urine (Coca Cola color), edema, HBP, oliguria, and renal dysfunction. Most have low C3 during acute phase. Only few percent of adults have severe course with renal failure or heavy proteinuria

- Rapidly progressive glomerulonephritis: Proliferative GN progressing to renal failure in weeks to months; Sudden onset of oliguria, dark urine, HBP, and renal dysfunction. Biopsy with proliferation in Bowman's space i.e. crescents. Three patterns based on pathogenesis and Course:
  - ➤ Type I: Anti-GBM disease
  - ➤ Type II: Immune Complex
  - ➤ Type III: Pauci-immune (ANCA positive)
- May be associated with systemic symptoms
- Anti-GBM disease with pulmonary disease and hemorrhage (Goodpasture's)
  - ➤ Pauci-immune with vasculitis, upper and lower respiratory (Wegener's)
  - ➤ Immune Complex associated with Henoch Schoenlein Purpura (see above) SLE, post-streptococcal disease (see above)
- Asymptomatic urinary findings: isolated microscopic hematuria and/or proteinuria. In hereditary GN due to Alport's synd hearing defects, lens defects eye. Biopsy often deferred if normal Ccr and <1 gm proteinuria/day. Due to:
  - ➤ hereditary nephritis (Alport's, thin basement membrane dis),
  - ➤ early stage of a progressive GN
- Glomerular Disease associated with systemic diseases
- See sections on DM, SLE, Amyloidosis, Hepatitis B and C, HIV disease

MANAGEMENT
- Control edema: loop diuretics (start with low dose BID, increase progressively)
  - ➤ add second diuretic – metolozone
  - ➤ low salt diet
  - ➤ rarely albumin infusion with diuretics
- Control lipids: Low cholesterol, low saturated fat diet
  - ➤ HMG Co-A reductase (statin) therapy
  - ➤ Try to reduce cholesterol to 200 mg/dl and LDL to <160 mg/dl
- Control hypertension: ACE inhibitors and ARBs first line since reduce proteinuria
  - ➤ (watch K+ and BUN/ creatinine)
- Watch for hypercoagulable state (pulmonary emboli and renal vein thrombosis)
  - ➤ Especially if serum albumin <2 g/dl or pt has membranous NS
- Dialysis for renal failure

SPECIFIC THERAPY

- Minimal Change Disease: Prednisone for 2 months and then taper. Second line therapies cyclosporine, cyclophosphamide, other immunosuppressives.
- Focal glomerulosclerosis: Primary-Idiopathic Disease- Only treat patients with >3 g proteinuria/Day; Prednisone at a high starting dose and then taper for at least 6 months. Prednisone failures Rx with cyclosporine for 6 mo; Alternate therapy cyclophosphamide or other immunosuppression.
- Membranous Nephropathy: Only treat patients at high risk for renal failure (heavy proteinuria, increased age, male sex, elevated plasma creatinine). Possible treatments: 1) monthly steroids alternating with monthly cyclophosphamide or chlorambucil for 6 mo. 2) 6 months QOD prednisone in tapering dose. 3) cyclosporine
- MPGN: None proven
- IgA Nephropathy: Control of HBP with ACE inhibitor or ARB; Low protein diet; Even if BP normal use ACE inhibitor or ARB to decrease progressive disease. In higher risk patients (males, heavy proteinuria, high creatinine, etc) may try alternate day steroids for 6 mo, fish oils, other immunosuppressives
- Poststreptococcal glomerulonephritis: Antibiotics to treat acute infection; No specific therapy; in most cases renal failure and sxs resolve spontaneously
- Rapidly Progressive GN
- Anti-GBM disease – steroids, cyclophosphamide and plasmapheresis (to remove anti-GBM antibody)
- ANCA+ disease – cyclophosphamide and prednisone
- Immune complex RPGN – treat basic disease (SLE: cyclophosphamide and steroids, post-strep: no immunosuppressive)
- Asymptomatic urinary findings: No specific therapy

FOLLOW-UP

- Follow for remission of proteinuria
- Minimal Change Disease: Relapses in many patients – retreat with steroids for first and second relapse; Frequent relapses or steroid resistant use cyclosporine or cyclophosphamide.
- Asymptomatic urinary findings: Biopsy if systemic sx or decrease Ccr or increase proteinuria >1 g/day

COMPLICATIONS AND PROGNOSIS

- In general persistent heavier proteinuria predicts worse outcome.

- Minimal Change Disease: Patients remaining in remission of NS never develop renal failure; Up to 10% adults develop episodes acute renal failure of hemodynamic nature responding to volume removal.
- Focal glomerulosclerosis: If remain with NS most over 5–10 years develop renal failure.
- IgA Nephropathy: Excellent for patients without risk factors for progression. Progression to renal failure in 10% at 10 yrs, >30% at 20 yrs.
- Poststreptococcal glomerulonephritis: Most adults have good prognosis, some residual HBP or proteinuria, renal failure rare.
- Rapidly Progressive GN:
  - Anti-GBM: responds well if renal function is not greatly reduced at the start of Rx
  - ANCA +: responds well to Rx often even if patients present with severe renal failure
  - Immune Complex patients follow prognosis of the basic disease.

GLUCOCORTICOID-REMEDIABLE ALDOSTERONISM

MICHEL BAUM, MD

HISTORY & PHYSICAL
- Hypertension with family history of hypertension

TESTS
- Hypokalemic alkalosis
- Elevated plasma aldosterone

DIFFERENTIAL DIAGNOSIS
- Autosomal dominant disease due to translocation resulting in hybrid mutant gene where aldosterone synthase is regulated by ACTH
- Distinguish from other causes of hypertension.

MANAGEMENT
- Low-salt diet
- Control hypertension.

SPECIFIC THERAPY
- Glucocorticoid therapy to suppress ACTH

FOLLOW-UP
- To follow blood pressure

COMPLICATIONS AND PROGNOSIS
- Dependent on blood pressure control

GLYCOGEN STORAGE DISEASE

RANDOLPH B. LINDE, MD

HISTORY & PHYSICAL

History

■ Inherited and uncommon enzyme deficiencies that vary by:
  ➤ Age of presentation: from infancy to senior citizen
  ➤ Whether defect is in synthesis or degradation of glycogen
  ➤ Involvement of muscle, liver, or both, with or without other tissues
  ➤ Whether muscle involvement is limited to exercise intolerance or progresses to a fatal outcome
  ➤ Whether cardiac muscle is involved
  ➤ Severity of liver disease, including risk of cirrhosis or cancer
  ➤ Presence or absence of fasting hypoglycemia

Signs & Symptoms

■ Vary per missing enzyme (Types 0, I–VII) and organ system involved
  ➤ Most severe
    • A fatal form in infancy with cardiomegaly and hypotonia (II: Pompe disease from lysosomal acid alpha-glucosidase deficiency)
    • Another form can cause neuromuscular disease with neonatal death, or fatal liver disease in childhood (IV: Andersen disease from branching enzyme deficiency)
  ➤ Most mild
    • Asymptomatic siblings of affected children have been described (0: from glycogen synthase deficiency)
  ➤ Most common presentations
    • Infant with failure to thrive, hypoglycemia as feeding time intervals increase, and a protuberant abdomen from hepatomegaly (I: Von Gierke disease from glucose-6-phosphatase deficiency)
    • Infant or child with growth retardation, hepatomegaly, less prominent hypoglycemia with ketosis (III: Cori or Forbes disease from debranching enzyme deficiency) (VI: Hers disease from liver phosphorylase deficiency) (VIa: phosphorylase kinase deficiency)
    • Child with exertional muscle cramping which can be severe with nausea, vomiting, and passage of burgundy urine from

myoglobinuria (VII: Tarui disease from muscle phosphofructokinase deficiency)

- Adult with weakness and poor exercise tolerance. May present vaguely or with severe cramps and burgundy urine.
- (V: McArdle disease from muscle phosphorylase deficiency)
- Hypertrophic cardiomyopathy (Danon's disease from X-linked lysosome-associated membrane protein [LAMP2] deficiency) (mutations in PRKAG2, the regulatory gamma subunit of AMP-activated protein kinase)

➤ Other findings
- Short stature, gout, steatorrhea, epistaxis, bruising, xanthomas, pancreatitis, kidney stones, osteoporosis, hepatic adenomas (I)
- Bacterial infections, mucosal ulcerations, inflammatory bowel disease (Ib: Von Gierke disease from translocase deficiency)
- Weak muscles of respiration (II, III)
- Splenomegaly (III)
- Hemolysis (VII)

TESTS

Laboratory
■ Basic Blood Studies
➤ Blood genetic analyses (LAMP2, PRKAG2)
➤ Fasting hypoglycemia with low insulin levels and ketosis
- With normal lactate and uric acid (0, III, VI, IX)
- With normal lactate and high uric acid (VII)
- With high lactate and uric acid (I)
➤ Elevated transaminases (III, IV, VI, IX)
- Usually normal in type I
➤ Elevated triglycerides (mild: III, VI, IX; severe: I)
➤ Elevated CPK (II, IV, V, VII)
➤ Renal insufficiency (I)
■ Basic Urine Studies
➤ May show Fanconi's syndrome (I)
➤ Myoglobinuria (V, VI, VII)
■ Specific Diagnostic Tests
➤ Lactate, free fatty acids, ketones and uric acid increase hourly after an oral glucose load of 1.75 g/kg (I)
➤ Minimal glucose response to IM or IV glucagon (30 mcg/kg, maximum 1 mg), while elevated lactate rises further (I)

➤ Exercise fails to increase lactate, but enhances ammonia response (IIIa, V, VII)
➤ Electromyogram may show generalized myopathy (II, IIIa, V, VII)
➤ Electrocardiogram may show ventricular hypertrophy (II, IIIa)
■ *Abdominal imaging*
➤ Liver ultrasound, CT or MRI to assess adenoma size and number, hemorrhage, and malignancy (Type I)
■ *Tissue biopsy*
➤ To evaluate glycogen and fat content
➤ To assess presence and degree of hepatic fibrosis
➤ To assay for putative missing enzyme
  • Liver (Ia, Ib, Ic, IIIa, IIIc, IV, VI, IX)
  • Muscle (II, IV, V, VII)
  • Nerve (IV)
  • Skin (II, VII)

DIFFERENTIAL DIAGNOSIS
■ Other inborn error of metabolism
➤ Weakness, exercise-induced myalgias and cramps
  • Disorders of fatty acid oxidation
    • Carnitine palmitoyltransferase II deficiency
    • Long-chain acyl CoA dehydrogenase deficiency
➤ Muscular weakness and atrophy
  • Charcot-Marie-Tooth disease
➤ Myoglobinuria
  • Familial recurrent myoglobinuria
➤ Liver disease with hypoglycemia
  • Galactosemia
  • Fructose intolerance

MANAGEMENT
What to Do First
■ Prevent hypoglycemia
➤ Nocturnal nasogastric glucose feedings (I, III)
➤ Frequent small meals including uncooked cornstarch (I, III)
➤ Restrict fructose and galactose (I)
➤ Teach home blood glucose monitoring

General Measures
■ Avoid strenuous exercise (V, VII)
■ Genetic counseling

SPECIFIC THERAPY
- Frequently none
  - ➤ Unavailable in most forms of fatal disease
    - Enzyme replacement therapy (II)
  - ➤ Unnecessary in most forms of mild disease
- Allopurinol (I, VII)
- Colony-stimulating factor (Ib)
- Liver transplantation in selected cases (I, IV)

FOLLOW-UP
- Depends on type and severity
  - ➤ Frequent for hypoglycemic forms until stable (0, I, III, VI, IX)
  - ➤ Infrequent when restricted to mild and non-progressive muscle symptoms (adults with V, VII)
  - ➤ Annual imaging and alpha-fetoprotein if multiple hepatic adenomas (I)

COMPLICATIONS AND PROGNOSIS

Complications
- Rarely, acute renal failure from rhabdomyolysis (V)
- Commonly, chronic renal disease from focal segmental glomerulosclerosis (I)

Prognosis
- Some types are fatal (II, IV)
- Some types have a fair prognosis with careful management (I)
- Some types have a good prognosis with little intervention by adulthood (0, III, V–VII)

GOITER

LAWRENCE CRAPO, MD, PhD

HISTORY & PHYSICAL

History
- Personal/family history of goiter
- Medications: lithium, amiodarone, kelp, cough syrup
- Pregnancy
- Residence in region of iodine deficiency

Signs & Symptoms
- Neck enlargement: obtain duration and rate; painful or not
- Compressive symptoms: neck pressure, dyspnea, dysphagia
- Persistent hoarseness
- Goiter: diffuse or nodular, soft or firm, tender or not
- Associated cervical adenopathy
- Pemberton sign: facial congestion with redness or cyanosis when arms raised above head (suggests large substernal goiter)

TESTS

Laboratory
- Basic blood tests: free T4, TSH
- Specific Diagnostic Tests
  - Blood: antithyroid antibodies (anti-TPO, antithyroglobulin), occasional serum thyroglobulin

Imaging
- Thyroid ultrasound to evaluate for cysts, nodules,, and follow growth
- CT of neck and chest PRN to evaluate tracheal and esophageal integrity in large or substernal goiters

DIFFERENTIAL DIAGNOSIS
- Benign goiters:
  - Autoimmune thyroid disease (AITD): Hashimoto or Graves disease
  - Idiopathic diffuse and multinodular goiter
  - Iodine deficiency
  - Goitrogens: lithium, food and water supply
  - Rare: enzyme defects, thyroid hormone resistance
- Malignant goiters:
  - Follicular carcinoma
  - Anaplastic carcinoma
  - Primary lymphoma

MANAGEMENT

What to Do First
- Assess degree of severity using rate of growth, airway integrity, difficulty swallowing

General Measures
- Assess for discomfort from goiter and risk of surgery, including cardiac disease

SPECIFIC THERAPY

■ Levothyroxine: may be useful to suppress small diffuse goiters, esp. if recent onset and TSH slightly elevated or in upper normal range; may prevent further enlargement of multinodular goiters given in dose that completely suppresses the serum TSH level

■ Thyroidectomy: suspected malignancy or large long-standing goiters with compressive symptoms

■ I-131: occasionally useful to shrink goiter, esp. if I-123 uptake increased

■ Iodine repletion: useful only for iodine deficiency

FOLLOW-UP

During Treatment

■ After thyroidectomy: treat with levothyroxine and follow free T4 and TSH; check serum calcium

■ After levothyroxine and I-131: follow free T4, TSH, goiter size

COMPLICATIONS AND PROGNOSIS

Complications

■ Hypothyroidism: after thyroidectomy, I-131

■ Hyperthyroidism: after levothyroxine

■ Hypoparathyroidism: after thyroidectomy (permanent in 5% of cases)

■ Recurrent laryngeal nerve injury: after thyroidectomy (5% of cases)

Prognosis

■ Benign goiter: excellent, may eventually require thyroidectomy

■ Lymphoma: good

■ Anaplastic cancer: poor

GONORRHEA

SARAH STAEDKE, MD

HISTORY & PHYSICAL

History

■ *Neisseria gonorrhoeae* is a gram-negative diplococcus that infects non-cornified epithelial cells of the urogenital tract, rectum, pharynx, and conjunctivae.

■ Risk factors: young age, race/ethnicity (highest reported rates in African-Americans), sexual preference (recent increase in men who

have sex with men [MSM]), unmarried persons, lower socioeconomic status, urban residence, lower education level, illicit drug use, prostitution
- Infected carriers with absent or mild symptoms are primary transmitters.

Signs & Symptoms
- Male urethral infection (symptomatic in <95%)
  - Incubation period 2–5 days, typically ≤14 days
  - Symptoms: urethral discharge (scant to purulent), dysuria
- Female urogenital infection (symptomatic in 60–80%)
  - Incubation period estimated at 10 days
  - Symptoms: vaginal discharge, dysuria, vaginal bleeding
  - Signs: mucopurulent cervical discharge, friable cervix, urethral or accessory gland purulence
- Rectal infection
  - Usually asymptomatic, but severe proctitis occurs
  - Symptoms: anal pruritus, anorectal pain, tenesmus, mucopurulent discharge, rectal bleeding
- Pharyngeal infection
  - Majority asymptomatic but exudative pharyngitis occurs
  - Symptoms: fever, sore throat, lymphadenopathy
- Conjunctivitis
  - Ophthalmia neonatorum in neonates, autoinoculation in adults
  - Symptoms: purulent conjunctival discharge
- Disseminated Gonococcal Infection (DGI)
  - Occurs in 0.5–3% of GC infections, mostly in women
  - Caused by organisms that tend to be more resistant to lysis by complement; AHU auxotype; sensitive to penicillin
  - Symptoms: fever, skin lesions, arthritis, asymptomatic genital infection

TESTS

Basic Tests
- Urogenital infection: urinalysis – pyuria, hematuria

Specific Diagnostic Tests
- Gram-stained smears: positive = gram-negative intracellular diplococci present within leukocytes; specificity of 95–100%; sensitivity 90–95% in males with symptomatic urethritis; lower in females, asymptomatic men; not useful for pharyngeal infection

- Culture: gold standard, requires selective media for non-sterile sites (Thayer-Martin), incubation in high C02 environment, sensitivity 80–95%
- Non-culture assays: EIA, DFA, DNA probe, nucleic acid amplification (SDA, TMA, PCR), sensitivity 85–95%, specificity 95%
- Blood culture: positive in 20–30% of DGI cases

Other Tests
- Genital infection: CT co-infection in 20–30% of GC cases
- DGI: synovial fluid analysis – leukocytosis; synovial fluid culture – rarely positive if synovial WBC is <20,000/mm3

DIFFERENTIAL DIAGNOSIS
- Male urethritis: CT, HSV, trichomoniasis, UTI, prostatitis
- Female urogenital infection: CT, HSV, trichomoniasis, vaginitis, UTI
- DGI: meningococcemia, septic arthritis, Reiter's syndrome

MANAGEMENT
What to Do First
- Obtain specimens from exposed sites for Gram stain and culture.
- Hospitalization recommended for DGI; examine for evidence of endocarditis and meningitis

General Measures
- Test for concomitant STDs: CT, syphilis, HIV
- Treat for possible CT co-infection (including DGI cases)
- Report case to local public health authorities and refer sexual partners for evaluation and treatment.
- Screen for complement deficiency (C5-C9) with recurrent DGI; consider in all DGI cases.

SPECIFIC THERAPY
Indications
- Positive Gram-stained urethral, endocervical, or synovial specimen
- Positive culture from any site
- Sexual contact to GC-infected patient

Treatment Options
- Uncomplicated genital, rectal, pharyngeal infections in adults Cefixime (not currently available)

OR Cefpoxime
> OR Ceftriaxone

- ➤ OR Ciprofloxacin*
- ➤ OR Ofloxacin*
- ➤ PLUS Azithromycin OR Doxycycline
- ▦ Alternative: Spectinomycin (not for pharyngeal infection)
- ▦ In pregnancy: cephalosporin (or Spectinomycin if penicillin allergic) plus Erythomycin or Amoxacillin
- ▦ Gonococcal Conjunctivitis
  - ➤ Ceftriaxone 1 g single IM dose
  - ➤ Lavage infected eye with saline solution once.
- ▦ DGI
  - ➤ Ceftriaxone
  - ➤ Alternatives: Cefotaxime, Ceftizoxime, Ciprofloxacin*, Ofloxacin*, Spectinomycin
  - ➤ Continue parenteral med for 24–48 h after improvement
  - ➤ THEN change to oral therapy with
  - ➤ Cefixime OR Ciprofloxacin OR Ofloxacin to complete 7–10 days
  - ➤ PLUS Azithromycin OR Doxycycline 7 days

*Note: increasing prevalence of fluoroquinolone-resistant GC in the western US states and in MSM (men who have sex with men) nationwide. Must treat with a cephalosporin.

Side Effects & Contraindications

- ▦ Azithromycin: side effects: nausea, diarrhea, abdominal pain; safety in pregnancy not known = B
- ▦ Cefixime: side effects: diarrhea; contraindicated with penicillin allergy; pregnancy − B
- ▦ Ceftriaxone: side effects: pain with IM injection, phlebitis, diarrhea, cholestasis; contraindicated with penicillin allergy; pregnancy = B
- ▦ Ciprofloxacin/Ofloxacin: side effects: GI intolerance, CNS stimulation, dizziness; contraindicated in pregnancy (C) and patients <18 years
- ▦ Doxycycline: side effects: GI distress, photosensitivity, erosive esophagitis; contraindicated in pregnancy (D) and growing children

FOLLOW-UP

- ▦ If symptoms persist or recur, repeat cultures and sensitivities.
- ▦ DGI arthritis may require repeated joint aspirations or closed irrigation; open drainage rarely required.

COMPLICATIONS AND PROGNOSIS

Male urethral infection

- Epididymitis: uncommon; unilateral testicular pain and swelling; consider testicular torsion; treat with Ceftriaxone or Ofloxacin plus Doxycycline
- Other: all uncommon; prostatitis, inguinal lymphadenitis, penile edema lymphangitis or thrombophlebitis, seminal vesiculitis, accessory gland infections, urethral stricture

Female urogenital infection

- PID: in 10–20% of acute infections; lower abdominal pain, cervical motion, uterine and adenexal tenderness; fever, elevated WBC, ESR or C-reactive protein; check pregnancy test to rule out ectopic; treat with broad-spectrum antibiotics; consider hospitalization
- Other: tubo-ovarian abscess, perihepatitis, Bartholin's gland abscess (<10% of urogenital infections)
  - ➤ DGI
  - ➤ Perihepatitis, endocarditis (1–3% of cases), meningitis (rare)

GORDON SYNDROME (PSEUDOHYPOALDOSTERONISM TYPE 2)

MICHEL BAUM, MD

HISTORY & PHYSICAL

- Gordon syndrome (or pseudohypoaldosteronism type 2) is an autosomal dominant cause of hypertension and hyperkalemia.

TESTS

- Hyperkalemia
- Aldosterone levels are normal or low.

DIFFERENTIAL DIAGNOSIS

- Due to mutation in WNK1 or WNK4 kinase resulting in increase in thiazide-sensitive NaCl cotransporter activity and a reduction in potassium channel (ROMK) activity
- Hypertension associated with other causes of hyperkalemia

MANAGEMENT

- Low-sodium diet
- Thiazide diuretics
- Low-potassium diet

SPECIFIC THERAPY

- NA

FOLLOW-UP
- Frequent follow-up to follow blood pressure

COMPLICATIONS AND PROGNOSIS
- Dependent on blood pressure control

GRANULOMA ANNULARE

KAREN GOULD, MD and JEFFERY P. CALLEN, MD

HISTORY & PHYSICAL
- Asymptomatic
- Commonly presents as annular flesh-colored or red plaques
- Subcutaneous nodules are a rare manifestation.
- Lesions are often multiple, and occur more frequently on the extremities.
- Generalized eruptions may occur.
- Children and young adults are typically affected.

TESTS
- Skin biopsy is usually diagnostic but may not always be needed.
- Potassium hydroxide preparation if any scale is present

DIFFERENTIAL DIAGNOSIS
- necrobiosis lipoidica – more often on the anterior legs
- Sarcoidosis – may be difficult, but biopsy should be helpful
- Annular lichen planus – often pigmented lesion, biopsy is helpful
- erythema elevatum diutinum – over bony prominences
- erythema annulare centrifugum – usually has trailing scale
- Hansen's disease (leprosy) – may be anesthetic

MANAGEMENT
Localized disease
- Potent topical corticosteroids or intralesional corticosteroids
- Cryosurgery

SPECIFIC THERAPY
- Treatment for generalized granuloma annulare includes dapsone, oral psoralen and ultraviolet A light, hydroxychloroquine, chloroquine, niacinamide, cyclosporine, pentoxyfylline, and isotretinoin.

FOLLOW-UP
- Patient should be seen on a regular basis until lesions resolve.

COMPLICATIONS AND PROGNOSIS
- Spontaneous resolution occurs within 2 years in 50% of affected persons.

GRANULOMATOUS LIVER DISEASE

AIJAZ AHMED, MD

HISTORY & PHYSICAL

History
- Major causes: TB, sarcoidosis, PBC, Crohn disease, foreign body, drugs, neoplasms (Hodgkin lymphoma), misc infections
- Cause unknown in 50% of cases

Signs & Symptoms
- Abdominal pain, weight loss, fatigue, fever of unknown origin, hepatomegaly, splenomegaly

TESTS

Basic Blood Tests
- Alkaline phosphatase; normal to mildly – AST & ALT

Specific Diagnostic Test
- Liver biopsy

DIFFERENTIAL DIAGNOSIS
- Various causes of hepatic granulomas vs idiopathic granulomatous hepatitis

MANAGEMENT

What to Do First
- Avoid/discontinue causative agent if known (drug), treat underlying infections, steroids in sarcoidosis

SPECIFIC THERAPY
- No proven therapy for idiopathic granulomatous hepatitis; may improve/resolve spontaneously & w/ steroid or methotrexate use

FOLLOW-UP
- Clinical & lab

COMPLICATIONS AND PROGNOSIS
- Rarely progresses to cirrhosis & portal hypertension

GRANULOMATOUS VASCULITIS

ERIC L. MATTESON, MD

HISTORY & PHYSICAL
Wegener's Granulomatosis (WG)
- Constitutional symptoms
- "Prolonged sinus infection" w/ oral-nasal bloody discharge
- Male:female 1:1

Signs & Symptoms
- Sinusitis, cough; nasal or oral ulcerations (90%)
- Hemoptysis, pleuritis, lower airways disease (85%)
- Arthritis (65%)
- Vasculitic skin lesions (45%)
- Peripheral or central neuropathy (25%)
- Peripheral edema (renal disease)(65%)
- Proptosis, eye pain (50%)

Giant Cell Arteritis (GCA)
- Age always >50 yrs
- Female:male 2:1
- Assoc w/ polymyalgia rheumatica
- Affects the aorta & branches, including temporal artery

Signs & Symptoms
- New-onset headache, often unilateral (80%)
- Jaw claudication (40%)
- Visual changes or loss (20%)
- TIAs or stroke (5%)
- Fever, systemic symptoms (30%)
- Polymyalgia rheumatica (40%)
- Tender temporal artery (50%)

Takayasu Arteritis (TA)
- Female:male 10:1; <40 yrs of age

Signs & Symptoms
- Dizziness, syncope, upper or lower extremity
- Claudication
- Vascular bruits & pulse deficits
- Hypertension more common than in GCA

Churg-Strauss Disease (CS)
- Similar to Wegener's, w/ asthma
- History of atopy, allergic rhinitis
- After 5-lipoxygenase inhibitors in asthma
- GI complaints more common, renal disease less so

TESTS

Lab Tests
- CBC for anemia, thrombocytosis (marked eosinophilia in CS $1,000/mm^3$)
- ESR and/or C-reactive protein elevated
- Urinalysis
- Anti-neutrophil anti-cytoplasmic antibody (c-ANCA) positive in >90% of pts w/ WG & many w/ CS

Other Tests
- Biopsy
  - GCA: Temporal artery shows mononuclear cell infiltration & multinucleated giant cells, intimal proliferation. Histology in TA is similar.
  - WG, CS: noncaseating granuloma, vasculitis in mucosal, dermal, retroocular, pulmonary lesions; rapidly progressive or focal segmental glomerulonephritis in kidney

Imaging
- Chest radiography & CT: pulmonary nodules, pleural effusions in WG; fleeting infiltrates more common in CS
- Arteriogram required for diagnosis & follow-up of TA, may be needed in GCA for symptomatic stenosis
- Echocardiography in TA or GCA may reveal aortic aneurysm

DIFFERENTIAL DIAGNOSIS
- GCA, TA
  - Migraine, especially ophthalmoplegic migraine
  - Cluster headache
  - Viral syndromes
  - Polymyalgia rheumatica in patients >50 yrs of age
  - Occult infection or malignancy
  - Myocardial ischemia

- ➤ Wegener's granulomatosis & polyarteritis nodosa
- ➤ Central retinal artery occlusion, retinal detachment, glaucoma
- ➤ Thyroid disease
- ➤ Polymyositis, SLE, rheumatoid arthritis
- ➤ Arterial fibrodysplasia
- ■ WG, CS
  - ➤ Chronic sinusitis
  - ➤ Polyarteritis nodosa; microscopic polyangiitis
  - ➤ Fungal, bacterial diseases; syphilis
  - ➤ SLE

MANAGEMENT

What to Do First

- ■ Assess extent & severity of vascular disease by history & physical exam; angiography especially in suspected TA
- ■ Control blood pressure
- ■ W/ impending organ damage (eg, visual loss, evolving stroke), begin immediate "pulse" steroids (methylprednisolone, 1 g/d qd × 3).
- ■ Ophthalmologic consultation in GCA (eye disease often unilateral initially, but may soon involve the other eye)
- ■ ENT consultation in WG

SPECIFIC THERAPY

- ■ GCA
  - ➤ Prednisone is usually dramatically effective w/in 2–3 days. Taper slowly.
- ■ TA, WG, CS
  - ➤ Prednisone, tapering slowly over months, usually sufficient for TA or CS
  - ➤ Cyclophosphamide IV to induce remission in WG, then orally
  - ➤ Methotrexate may suffice for remission induction in milder or controlled WG
  - ➤ Trimethoprim-sulfamethoxazole may suffice in pts w/ WG confined to the upper airways; should be considered even in systemic disease
  - ➤ Other options include mycophenolate mofetil, azathioprine

Side Effects & Contraindications

- ■ As in nongranulomatous vasculitis

FOLLOW-UP

During Treatment
■ Regularly assess disease activity by history & physical exam, including bilateral blood pressures & heart exam
  ➤ GCA
    • After 1 month, taper corticosteroid dose by about 5 mg every 2 weeks to 10–15 mg/day, & more slowly thereafter. Most relapses occur in the first 18 months of treatment. Average duration of therapy is about 2–3 years.
  ➤ TA
    • Therapy may be protracted; one-fourth of pts will require years of immunosuppression
    • Subclavian involvement is common (90%), & blood pressure readings may not reflect aortic root pressure. Angiography & echocardiography may help
    • Follow-up vascular imaging required
    • Surgical intervention for critical stenosis or aneurysms
  ➤ WG, CS
    • Monitor urinalysis, chest radiograph, clinical status
    • Long-term immunosuppression is usually required
    • c-ANCA roughly correlates w/ disease activity

COMPLICATIONS & PROGNOSIS
■ Side effects of high-dose steroids: glaucoma, osteoporosis, infection, hyperglycemia, hyperlipidemia
■ GCA
  ➤ Thoracic aortic aneurysms 17 times, abdominal aneurysms 2.5 times more likely than in age-matched controls
  ➤ Vision loss (6–10%)
  ➤ Stroke
  ➤ Pts w/ GCA have a normal life expectancy
■ TA
  ➤ Aortic root involvement w/ valvular insufficiency & congestive heart failure in 20%
  ➤ Stroke
  ➤ Progressive arterial & aorta lesions may require surgery
  ➤ 5-year survival 83%; 10-year survival 58% in pts w/ severe disease
■ WS, CS
  ➤ Renal failure, stroke, mononeuritis, vision loss; tracheal stenosis, nasal deformity, infection
  ➤ 5-year survival >80%

HAEMOPHILUS INFECTIONS

RICHARD A. JACOBS, MD, PhD

HISTORY & PHYSICAL

History

- Haemophilus spp. are fastidious (require hemin or NADPH for aerobic growth) Gram-negative coccobacilli that grow in both aerobic and anaerobic conditions.
- Presence of a polysaccharide capsule is virulence factor responsible for the invasive disease of H influenzae type B (Hib); strains without polysaccharide capsule are nontypable and usually associated with local disease
- Humans are only known host and are colonized in the nasopharynx; 75% colonized with nontypable strains; less than 5% colonized with Hib; spread is by droplets or direct contact with secretions
- In addition to nontypable H influenzae and Hib, other less common human pathogens include H parainfluenzae, H aphrophilus, H paraphrophilus and H ducreyi (see sexually transmitted diseases and chancroid)

Signs & Symptoms

- Hib causes meningitis (fever, headache, mental status changes, nuchal rigidity indistinguishable from other causes of bacterial meningitis), epiglottitis (sore throat, fever, dysphagia, dyspnea, difficulty handling secretions), pneumonia (fever, chills, productive cough similar to other causes of bacterial pneumonia), bacteremia with metastatic seeding (arthritis, pericarditis, endocarditis)
- Infections with nontypable strains cause sinusitis, otitis media, acute exacerbations of chronic bronchitis, conjunctivitis and community acquired pneumonia in the adult
- Haemophilus spp other than H influenzae produce disease similar to nontypable H influenzae; also cause about 5% of cases of endocarditis

TESTS

- Diagnosis confirmed by positive culture of normally sterile body fluid (blood, cerebral spinal fluid, pleural fluid); confirming infection with nontypable strains (sinusitis, bronchitis, pneumonia) difficult since these organisms are part of normal flora

DIFFERENTIAL DIAGNOSIS

- Must distinguish syndromes from those caused by other bacteria (can only do by culture) or viruses; no clinical criteria allow reliable determination of specific microbial etiology

MANAGEMENT

- General supportive measures for syndromes as needed: meningitis – decrease intracranial pressure if >20 mmHg with mannitol or hyperventilation, support blood pressure; epiglottitis – maintain airway patency; pneumonia – supplemental oxygen, drain empyema; bacteremia – support blood pressure; septic arthritis – drain joint

SPECIFIC THERAPY

- Invasive Hib infection can be rapidly progressive and life-threatening; meningitis treated with third-generation cephalosporin (ceftriaxone IV or cefotaxime IV) for 7–10 days; epiglottitis and bacteremia treated similarly, but ceftriaxone every 24 hours; endocarditis treated with ceftriaxone for 4 weeks; up to one third of strains produce beta-lactamase, thus making ampicillin an inappropriate drug for therapy of serious, life-threatening infections; in severely penicillin-allergic patient (anaphylaxis) alternatives include desensitization or use of chloramphenicol, fluoroquinolones or aztreonam
- Infections due to nontypable strains (sinusitis, otitis, exacerbations of chronic bronchitis) usually treated with oral drugs; doxycycline, amoxicillin, trimethoprim-sulfamethoxazole commonly used; other agents with activity include amoxicillin-clavulanate, fluoroquinolones, newer macrolides (azithromycin, clarithromycin), extended spectrum cephalosporins (cefuroxime, cefpodoxime, cefprozil)

FOLLOW-UP

- Follow-up as for the syndrome treated

COMPLICATIONS AND PROGNOSIS

- See specific syndromes for complications and prognosis.
- Conjugate vaccines against invasive type B disease very effective in infants and children; not studied in adults, but immunization of highly susceptible adults (asplenia, hypogammaglobulinemia) should be considered
- Chemoprophylaxis with rifampin is recommended for all household contacts, including adults, if there is a case of invasive Haemophilus type B disease and immunization of children <4 y of age living in

the house is incomplete; chemoprophylaxis is indicated in daycare settings if there is an outbreak (2 cases of invasive disease within 60 d) and unvaccinated or incompletely vaccinated children attend the center.

HAIRY CELL LEUKEMIA

KANTI R. RAI, MD

HISTORY & PHYSICAL

Clinical features
- Rare lymphoproliferative disorder
- Median age at diagnosis is 52 years
- Male:female – 4:1
- Usually has an indolent course

Signs & Symptoms
- Patients may be asymptomatic
- May have "B" symptoms and abdominal fullness (secondary to splenomegaly)
- May have any or all of the following
- Pallor, lymphadenopathy, splenomegaly, skin involvement (pyoderma gangrenosum, scleroderma)

TESTS
Splenomegaly

Blood
- Pancytopenia (50% of the patients)
- Characteristic large lymphocytes with
- hairy projections on peripheral blood smear

Bone Marrow
- Inaspirable marrow ("Dry tap") is common
- Hypercellular, occasionally hypocellular
- Diffuse or focal infiltration with hairy cells
- Residual hematopoietic cells are decreased
- TRAP (tartrate resistant acid phosphatase) positive
- Flow Cytometry: CD5 (−), CD19, CD20, CD11c, CD25 and CD103 (+)

DIFFERENTIAL DIAGNOSIS
- Lymphoproliferative disorders (see table under CLL)

■ Agnogenic myeloid metaplasia
■ Systemic mastocytosis

MANAGEMENT

What to Do First
■ To decide when to initiate treatment

Indications for Treatment
■ Constitutional symptoms
■ Symptomatic organomegaly
■ Significant cytopenias (ANC <1,000/mm3, Hb <11 g/dl, Plt <100,000/mm3)

SPECIFIC THERAPY
■ Cladribine (2-CdA): 0.1 mg/kg/day continuous iv
  ➤ infusion × 7 days × 1 dose or
■ Pentostatin 4 mg/m2 i.v. q 2 wks for 2–4 mths or
■ Interferon 2 million U SQ TIW for 12–18 mths

Surgery
■ Splenectomy

FOLLOW-UP
n/a

COMPLICATIONS AND PROGNOSIS

Complications
■ Pancytopenia
■ Recurrent infection

Prognosis
■ 90% of the patients respond to 2-CdA
■ 4-year survival is about 85–95%

HANTAVIRUS PULMONARY SYNDROME

CAROL A. GLASER, MD

HISTORY & PHYSICAL

History
■ Bunyaviridae family
■ Many hantaviruses worldwide; this section will cover only HPS, which is clinically important hantavirus in the U.S.

- Hantavirus pulmonary syndrome first identified 1993 in humans in the U.S.
- Primarily Sin Nombre virus (aka "Four Corners virus") in U.S.
- Reservoir is deer mouse, Peromyscus maniculatus (widespread in U.S.)
- Humans accidental host
- Aerosol transmission from rodent excreta
- Incubation approximately 2 wks (with range: few days-6 wks)
- Almost all cases occur in adults.
- Risk factors; handling or trapping rodents, cleaning or entering closed rodent-infested structures, cleaning feed storage or animal shelter areas
  - ➤ Or living in home with increased density of mice
- Risk groups: Mammal workers, utility company staff, agricultural and forestry employees

Signs & Symptoms
- Prodrome lasts 3–7 days: myalgias/chills/fever (pharyngitis and rhinorrhea are rare), sometimes GI complaints
- Later non-productive cough that progresses to dyspnea
- Level of dyspnea is variable.
- Profound capillary leak syndrome often occurs, which results in pulmonary edema and pleural effusions
- Respiratory failure, myocardial depression and shock seen in severe cases
- Milder cases (without severe pulmonary edema) have been described.

TESTS

Nonspecific
- CXR: may be normal early on, later interstitial pulmonary infiltrates, pleural effusions
- Low albumin
- Hemoconcentration, hypoproteinemia common
- LDH may be increased
- Thrombocytopenia (around 40,000 is common)
- Leukocytosis with left shift
- Severe cases: immunoblastic lymphocytes

Specific
- Best method of diagnosis is serologic

- IgG/IgM tests excellent (ELISA/ strip immunoblot/Western blot) almost always positive at time of hospitalization
- PCR/sequencing good for epidemiology, available in research settings

DIFFERENTIAL DIAGNOSIS
n/a

MANAGEMENT
- Ribavarin was initially thought to be effective, but no longer.
- Good supportive care
- In severe cases, extracorporeal membrane oxygenation (ECMO) should be considered.
- Clinical consultation available from the staff at the University of New Mexico – call 1-888-UNMPALS.
- Some experts believe early transfer to a tertiary care center (particularly those with experience in treating HPS) is beneficial.
- No person-to-person transmission in the U.S.

SPECIFIC THERAPY
n/a

FOLLOW-UP
n/a

COMPLICATIONS AND PROGNOSIS

Complications
- Mortality rate for patients with cardiopulmonary disease 40–45%
- If patient survives pulmonary capillary leak phase, permanent sequelae are uncommon.

Prevention
- Prevention is main way to decrease morbidity and mortality.
- Avoid exposure to wild rodents and excreta, especially indoor exposure in closed, poorly ventilated spaces.

HARTNUP'S DISEASE

MICHEL BAUM, MD

HISTORY & PHYSICAL
- Pellagra-like skin rash, ataxia and behavioral disturbances

TESTS
- Niacin deficiency, low plasma levels of neutral amino acids

DIFFERENTIAL DIAGNOSIS
■ Autosomal recessive defect in intestinal and kidney neutral amino acid transport

MANAGEMENT
n/a

SPECIFIC THERAPY
■ Nicotinamide

FOLLOW-UP
n/a

COMPLICATIONS AND PROGNOSIS
Symptoms are variable but worse on low-protein diet.

HEAD AND NECK CANCER

MICHAEL KAPLAN, MD

HISTORY & PHYSICAL

History
■ alcohol &/or tobacco abuse in >95%
■ for nasopharynx carcinoma (NPC) southern Chinese ancestry
■ prior head and neck (H&N) squamous cell carcinoma (SCC): rate of second SCC
■ as much as 4–5% per year (i.e. 20–25% at 5 years)

Signs & Symptoms
■ any 1%:
  ➢ new neck mass, bleeding
  ➢ referred otalgia (via CN X) or local pain
  ➢ weight loss
■ OP/HP/larynx:
  ➢ persistent change in voice quality ("hoarseness")
  ➢ airway compromise may occur if large
■ NPC:
  ➢ middle ear effusion (MEE) common
  ➢ epistaxis and/or nasal obstruction if large
  ➢ cranial nerve deficits if skull base erosion
    • Full head & neck exam mandatory, including inspection of larynx & hypopharynx (HP), nasopharynx (NP), & oropharynx

(OP) using mirror or fiberoptic endoscopy. Palpation of base of tongue (BOT) and inspection & palpation of neck also essential. Check for MEE.
- 95% of time visible or palpable primary detectable
- 5% "unknown" primary: confirmed neck disease by fine needle aspiration (FNA) . . . see below, but no obvious primary

TESTS

Laboratory
- EBV IgA viral capsid antigen (VCA) often elevated in NPC; otherwise no specific tests indicated. However metastatic evaluation (AST/ALT and CXR) appropriate

Imaging
- MRI
  - almost always superior to CT for soft-tissue imaging: aids in evaluating
  - extent of primary & extent of neck nodes
  - may assist subsequent radiation therapy planning and in followup
- CT and MRI
  - fail to detect small involved neck nodes 20–30% of time
- Role of PET:
  - not fully established, but high-resolution PET scanning may aid in identifying unknown primary, additional second lung carcinoma, or metastatic disease in neck/chest/liver. Post-treatment, may assist in cancer surveillance.

Biopsy
- FNA of neck mass may confirm SCC when primary inapparent. FNA may not be necessary if primary is biopsy-proven (or soon will be)
- Prior to planning treatment, biopsy of primary usually indicated. May be done at time of "panendoscopy" (direct laryngoscopy, fiberoptic bronchoscopy, and esophagoscopy under general anesthesia): assesses extent of primary, evaluates for second malignancy, affords biopsy opportunity

DIFFERENTIAL DIAGNOSIS
- When primary apparent, biopsy is diagnostic:
  - SCC by far most common (lymphomas, salivary gland

malignancies, neuroendocrine carcinoma, sarcomas all much less frequent)

■ If only a neck mass:

➤ Ddx depends on age of patient, duration of mass (present how long), inflammatory signs (fever, erythema, tenderness), and prior history of malignancy. In an adult, includes branchial cleft cyst, lymphadenitis, lymphoma, parotid tumor (if at tail of parotid), and metastases from non head and neck sites as well as rare primary sarcomas. In a HIV (−) adult, 80% of neck masses are malignant and 80% of these are metastases from a head and neck site In a child, lymphadenitis is common (including bacterial and viral, Cat Scratch, and tuberculous etiology), with the others all possible.

MANAGEMENT

What to Do First

■ Referral to a physician or otolaryngologist, for Dx and coordination of care.

General Measures

■ General assessment of health, especially cardiopulmonary, to assess surgical risk

■ Metastatic evaluation: at least CXR, AST/ALT; possible chest CT

■ If primary site inapparent, not unreasonable to obtain FNA of neck mass (though recommend referral: he/she will do FNA, etc.)

SPECIFIC THERAPY

Treatment Alternatives

■ Complex: dependent on numerous factors

■ Treatment strategies include:

➤ EBRT (external beam radiation therapy) or surgical resection for limited disease; Organ preservation approaches (initial EBRT with concomitant cisplatin as a radiosensitizer) or combined treatment (surgery and EBRT) for advanced disease. Complex radiation planning, including hyperfractionation and brachytherapy, often play a role.

■ For NPC, treatment includes cisplatin and RT concomitantly followed by three cycles of chemotherapy with cisplatin and 5-fluorouracil.

- Role of chemotherapy alone generally is limited for palliation in unresectable tumor. Radiation also often plays a role in palliation of unreseectable tumor, as may other modalities.
- For recurrent cancer in previously irradiated areas: if resectable, intraoperative radiation therapy (IORT) is being used in a number of centers with some encouraging results. If unresectable, then palliative approaches Early disease (T1 N0)-designed to minimize long-term side effects. For example, EBRT for larynx and BOT, but surgical resection for lateral tongue Management of neck when apparently N0: dependent on management of primary site
- Selective neck dissection may be indicated when Rx of primary is surgical
- Clinical followup without treatment indicated for T1-2 larynx EBRT to both neck as well as primary often indicated if EBRT is most appropriate for primary.
- Advanced resectable disease: organ preservation approaches often best initial choice; combined treatment often necessary
- Recurrent disease: IORT may be useful when surgically resectable; otherwise palliative chemotherapy and pain management likely best options

Side Effects & Complications
- Radiation:
  - dry mouth (xerostomia) is permanent and always occurs. sometimes mildly improved with the use of artifical saliva wetting agents and/or with pilocarpine altered taste-degree of recovery variable
  - transient mucositis and skin reaction: recovers in 4–8 wks
  - dysphagia, dependent on primary site, may be severe enough to require nasogastric (or percutaneous gastrostomy) tube for weeks, months, or permanently
- Chemotherapy:
  - cisplatin: peripheral neuropathy, ototoxicity, renal toxicity, nausea on day of administration
  - 5-fluorouracil: marrow toxicity, mucositis
  - carboplatin: marrow toxicity
- Surgery:
  - dependent on site and extent, & underlying medical health
  - requiring speech/swallowing therapy: may include dysarthria, dysphagia, need for soft diet, aphonia following total laryngectomy usually managed successfully with Blom-Singer device

➤ donor site issues in reconstruction usually mild and transient (e.g. rehabilatation following fibula free flap; shoulder physical therapy following pectoralis major myocutaneous flap)

➤ wound healing: infection, fitula, delay in post-operative RT

➤ medical: aspiration & pneumonia, MI, numbness, scars generally esthetically acceptable, DVT/embolus, etc

FOLLOW-UP

During Radiation

■ Regularly assess potential side effects of radiotherapy and chemotherapy: low WBC, low RBC, low platelelets, mucositis

Perioperative

■ Monitor for infection, wound healing issues, and medical complications

■ associated with surgery

Long-Term Routine Follow-Up

■ Essential because of risk for second tumors and for management of side effects and complications of treatment, as well as coordination of other medical problems.

■ Clinical exam

➤ monthly 1st year, every other month in year 2, every 3rd month year 3,

➤ every 4th month year 4, every 6 months thereafter

■ Radiologic exam

➤ Baseline post-treatment MRI 2 months after completion of all Rx

➤ Annual CXR (if no PET)

➤ Consider annual PET as cancer surveillance, especially in younger

➤ patients under 60 and those without usual risk factors

■ Laboratory tests

➤ TSH every 6 months for 3 yrs (30% incidence of hypothyroidism in irradiated necks)

➤ AST/ALT annually (if no PET)

COMPLICATIONS AND PROGNOSIS

Complications

■ Radiation

➤ dysphagia (see side effects) may be permanent, incidence depends in part on extent of pharyngeal tumor

➤ osteoradionecrosis of mandible (2–5%) minimized by pre-treatment dental evaluation, extractions as needed, and subsequent rigorous long-term attention to periodontal care including extra fluoride treatments

➤ prior radiation severely restricts the ability to subsequently irradiate the same anatomic area

➤ radiation-induced malignancy: incidence estimated to be between 0.01% and as high as 1%; 7–30 years later

➤ 1% incidence of tracheotomy dependence following successful glottic irradiation for T1–2 tumors

■ Chemotherapy

➤ cisplatin: peripheral neuropathy, ototoxicity, renal toxicity

Prognosis

■ Strongly dependent on TNM staging of primary site as well as numerous other factors; N (+) neck generally halves survival statistics; of all H&N SCC, about 65% is cured

■ Examples:

➤ T1 N0 glottic SCC is cured by EBRT in >95%, and the rare failure frequently salvaged with surgery

➤ T1 N0 lateral tongue SCC cured by surgery 80–90%

➤ T3 N0 BOT 60% by EBRT

➤ T3 N2 hypopharynx <20–35% with combined therapy

■ Rate of 2nd tumors 4–5%/year (20–25% at 5 yrs)

■ IORT, data suggests, improves prognosis for resectable recurrent neck disease from <15–20% 2-year survival to 70% 2-year survival and 50% 2-yr NED survival.

■ Overall patient survival affected by nondisease comorbidities associated with alcohol and tobacco

HEAD TRAUMA

MICHAEL J. AMINOFF, MD, DSc

HISTORY & PHYSICAL

■ Head injury w/ or w/o LOC

■ May be headache, confusion, personality change, drowsiness

■ Seizures may occur in 1st week

■ Findings may be normal

■ Coma or obtundation may be present

■ Focal deficits sometimes present; depend on location & severity of injury

■ Signs of increased ICP or meningeal irritation may be present

TESTS

- CT scan of head and neck: may reveal intracranial hemorrhage, cerebral edema, cervical fracture-dislocation

DIFFERENTIAL DIAGNOSIS
N/A

MANAGEMENT

- Maintain airway; support vital functions
- Specific therapy as suggested by clinical & CT scan assessment of severity of head injury

SPECIFIC THERAPY

- If no LOC, no neurologic abnormality & normal CT scan, pt can go home w/ supervising adult to check level of arousal & pupillary responses periodically for 24 hrs
- If LOC for >5 min, focal deficit, obtundation, signs of increased ICP or skull fracture present, observe in hospital even if no hematoma present on CT scan
- If CT scan shows small subdural or intracerebral hematoma, observe in hospital
- If CT scan shows large subdural hematoma, evacuate surgically

FOLLOW-UP
N/A

COMPLICATIONS AND PROGNOSIS

- Subarachnoid hemorrhage: no specific action needed
- Acute hydrocephalus: consider shunt
- Subdural hygroma: may require evacuation
- CSF leak: close surgically if persists or leads to meningitis
- Post-traumatic seizure disorder (beyond 1st week): anticonvulsants
- Postconcussion syndrome of headache, personality change, poor attention span, dysequilibrium, visual disturbances: antidepressant medication; typically settles spontaneously after weeks or months

HEARING LOSS

ANIL K. LALWANI, MD

HISTORY & PHYSICAL
History
Conductive hearing loss (CHL)

- Usually due to pathology in the external or middle ear

- Acute otitis media (AOM) and serous otitis media (SOM) most common cause in children
- Otosclerosis, associated with fixation of stapes, may present in pregnancy
- Trauma may lead to perforation of tympanic membrane or ossicular discontinuity

Sensorineural hearing loss (SNHL)

- Usually due to problems within the cochlea or central auditory pathway
- Aging is the most common cause of SNHL
- Exposure to ototoxic medication may lead to high frequency hearing loss
- Trauma can result in temporal bone fracture and SNHL
- Vestibular schwannoma (or its more famous misnomer, acoustic neuroma), the most common tumor of the cerebellopontine angle, is associated with asymmetric hearing loss
- 1 in 1000 infants are born with profound hearing loss
- This risk is 20× higher in the NICU
- 10% of the elderly have significant SNHL

Signs & Symptoms

- Most common complaint is reduced hearing
- With SNHL, patients also complain of decreased clarity, specially in background noise
- Tinnitus can be present in CHL and SNHL and can be greatly bothersome
- Pulsatile tinnitus is more common in CHL
- Neurological symptoms or signs are ominous and may reflect the presence of cerebellopontine angle tumors

TESTS

- Audiological Evaluation for CHL and SNHL: pure tone audiometry, speech audiometry, immittance testing, acoustic reflexes
- Auditory Brainsterm Response (ABR) testing to exclude retrocochlear pathology when asymmetric SNHL is present
- Laboratory test including CBC, Platelets, ESR, ANA, RF, TSH, Cholesterol, glucose, FTA, BUN, Creatinine, UA for evaluation of progressive or premature SNHL
- CT scan of the temporal bone (1.0 min fine cuts, axial and direct coronal images) to evaluate CHL (external ear canal and ossicular chain) and SNHL (inner ear malformations)
- MRI of the internal auditory canal and brain with gadolinium contrast enhancement to evaluate asymmetric or progressive SNHL

DIFFERENTIAL DIAGNOSIS

- Audiologic evaluation should establish CHL, SNHL, or mixed hearing loss when both are present.
- CHL: external auditory canal atresia, microtia, cerumen impaction, tympanic membrane perforation, ossicular discontinuity, otosclerosis, otitis media, trauma
- SNHL: cochlear hearing loss, vestibular schwannoma, trauma, multiple sclerosis, aging, ototoxicity

MANAGEMENT

- Amplification with hearing aids for SNHL and CHL
- Cochlear implantation when HA are inadequate
- Ventilation tube for AOM or SOM
- Stapedectomy for otosclerosis will successfully restore hearing in 95%.
- Surgery or radiation therapy for tumors of the cerebellopontine angle (eg vestibular schwannoma)

Side Effects

- Hearing aids, while making things louder, may not help with clarity
- Surgical risks are present with cochlear implantation, placement of ventilation tubes or resection of cerebellopontine angle tumors

SPECIFIC THERAPY

n/a

FOLLOW-UP

- Audiological evaluation every 2 to 3 years once hearing loss has been identified
- Hearing aid checks as necessary

COMPLICATIONS AND PROGNOSIS

- CHL: medical or surgical intervention usually corrects the underlying problem or provides excellent rehabilitation
- SNHL: Hearing loss usually progresses at a variable rate. Hearing aids may provide adequate rehabilitation.

HELICOBACTER PYLORI

M. BRIAN FENNERTY, MD

HISTORY & PHYSICAL

Risk Factors for Infection

- Age (cohort effect):

➤ Prevalence has decreased dramatically over past 50 years; high prevalence in those >60 years of age

➤ Low lifetime risk in current children/young adults

- Country of birth:
  ➤ Developed countries – infection now infrequent
  ➤ Developing countries – infection still frequent
- Socioeconomic status in childhood: Infection related to sanitation, crowding, etc.

Transmission

- Infection usually acquired in early childhood
- Adult infection or reinfection rare
- Transmitted human-to-human
- Oral-oral transmission more common in developed countries
- Fecal-oral transmission more common in developing areas
- No likely natural animal reservoir

Signs and Symptoms

- Most infected individuals (>80%) will never develop associated disease/symptoms
- Symptoms related to associated disease, not infection
- No physical findings associated with infection
- Physical findings of peptic ulcer are epigastric tenderness
- Physical findings of gastric neoplasm are weight loss, abdominal mass, etc.

TESTS

Specific Diagnostic Tests

- Blood: whole blood or serum antibody tests (qualitative and quantitative)
- Stool: fecal antigen test
- Breath: C13 and C14 urea breath tests
- Endoscopic:
  ➤ Biopsy urease test
  ➤ Histology with or without special stains
  ➤ Culture
- Antibody tests may remain positive after eradication of infection and should not be used as a follow-up test
- Antibody tests are not accurate enough for clinical use in low-prevalence populations.

Imaging

- Necessary only to diagnose *H. pylori*-related disease
- Endoscopy/barium studies used to diagnose peptic ulcer, gastric neoplasia

DIFFERENTIAL DIAGNOSIS

- Established *H. pylori*-associated diseases
  - ➤ Peptic ulcer
  - ➤ Gastric cancer
  - ➤ Gastric lymphoma
- Differential diagnosis of dyspepsia not strongly associated with *H. pylori*
  - ➤ Non-ulcer dyspepsia
  - ➤ Gastroesophageal reflux
  - ➤ Cholelithiasis
  - ➤ Gastroparesis

MANAGEMENT

What to Do First

- Decide whether to test for infection
  - ➤ *H. pylori* a class I carcinogen
  - ➤ Lifetime risk of ulcer disease 10–15% in those infected
  - ➤ thus, in those testing positive, treatment should be presumed; otherwise, why test and how do you explain decision not to treat?
- Testing should occur only if treatment will be beneficial (those with ulcers, gastric MALT lymphoma, and possibly uninvestigated dyspepsia)

SPECIFIC THERAPY

Indications

- Patients testing positive for *H. pylori*

Treatment Options

- First line: A proton pump inhibitor (PPI) twice daily plus two of the following antibiotics for 7–14 days (clarithromycin, amoxicillin or metronidazole D)
- cure rates 75–80% in U.S.
- Option: A BID PPI combined with Pepto-Bismol 2 tabs QID, metronidazole and tetracycline for 14 days
- cure rates 70–80% in U.S. studies

- Retreatment: A BID PPI along with Pepto-Bismol, clarithromycin and either amoxicillin, tetracycline or metronidazole (if they haven't been used previously) for 14 days
- cure rates unknown in U.S.

Side Effects
- Dyspepsia, nausea, vomiting, metallic taste with all of the above treatments (usually mild)

Contraindications
- Absolute
  - Allergy to drug in regimen
- Relative
  - *H. pylori* status unknown
  - Eradication of organism of little or no benefit in those with non-ulcer dyspepsia and no benefit in those with GERD, or the asymptomatic patient

FOLLOW-UP

Routine
- Complicated peptic ulcer
- Worried patient

Optional
- All treated patients given failure rate of 20–30%

COMPLICATIONS AND PROGNOSIS

Complications
- Peptic ulcer
  - Bleeding
  - Perforation
  - Obstruction
  - Symptomatic ulcer
- Gastric neoplasm
  - Bleeding
  - Obstruction
  - Weight loss
  - Death

Prognosis
- 80% of infected individuals will never develop *H. pylori*-related disease

- 80% of untreated peptic ulcer patients infected with *H. pylori* will relapse
- 20% of peptic ulcer patients treated for and cured of *H. pylori* will still relapse

---

HEMIBALLISMUS

CHAD CHRISTINE, MD

HISTORY & PHYSICAL
- Unilateral chorea of acute to subacute onset
- Continuous movement that pt may attempt to restrain
- Proximal muscle involvement causes particularly violent movements
- May involve face, arm, leg or both extremities on one side of body
- Cognitive, motor, sensory deficits may be present

TESTS
- Diagnosis made clinically
- Lab tests: CBC, sed rate, HIV test, toxicology screen
- Imaging may demonstrate lesion of contralateral subthalamic nucleus

DIFFERENTIAL DIAGNOSIS
- Stroke & mass lesion (eg, tumor, abscess, AVM) excluded by brain MRI
- Inflammatory disorders (SLE, antiphospholipid antibody syndrome) & metabolic disorders (hyper-/hypoglycemia) excluded by serum studies
- Infections excluded by blood & CSF studies

MANAGEMENT
- What to do first: evaluate for stroke or mass lesion
- General measures: comfortable setting, restrain limb, pad bedside

SPECIFIC THERAPY
- Depends on underlying disorder
- Indications: intractable violent movements
- Treatment options
  - Medical treatment
    - Haloperidol
    - Chlorpromazine
  - Surgical treatment

FOLLOW-UP
- Depends on cause

COMPLICATIONS AND PROGNOSIS
- Typically resolves in weeks to months

HEMOCHROMATOSIS

ERIC LEONG, MD, FRCPC

HISTORY & PHYSICAL

Risk Factors for Iron Overload
- Hereditary *HFE*-associated hemochromatosis
- Hereditary non-*HFE*-associated hemochromatosis
- Multiple blood transfusions
- Multiple doses of parenteral iron
- Thalassemia major
- Acquired sideroblastic anemias
- Alcoholic liver disease (mild hepatic iron overload)
- Porphyria cutanea tarda (mild hepatic iron overload)

Symptoms and Signs
- Many patients asymptomatic
- Symptomatic stage: fatigue, arthralgia, RUQ pain, hepatomegaly, increased skin pigmentation, loss of libido, impotence, amenorrhea, symptoms related to diabetes mellitus, dyspnea and/or cardiac arrhythmias
- Advanced disease: decompensated cirrhosis with liver failure, HCC

TESTS

Basic Tests: Blood
- Early disease:
  - Transferrin saturation >45%; warrants further testing
  - Serum ferritin increases linearly with total body iron stores
  - AST and ALT may rise with significant hepatic iron overload
- Advanced disease:
  - Low serum albumin, elevated bilirubin and INR

Specific Diagnostic Test
- *HFE*

- Genotyping identifies individuals at risk for hereditary hemochromatosis; 85% are C282Y/C282Y homozygotes &
- 3% are C282Y/H63D compound heterozygotes

Imaging
- Ultrasound or CT scan: not diagnostic and usually normal in early disease; may show hepatomegaly or evidence of advanced disease (cirrhosis with splenomegaly, HCC)

Liver Biopsy
- Definitive test for determining severity of hepatic iron overload and liver damage; consider when ferritin >1,000 mcg/L or when AST and ALT elevated; may not need to perform in patients <30 years of age, with normal AST and ALT, and serum ferritin < 500 mcg/L, as cirrhosis is unlikely
- Hepatic iron concentration (HIC) >80 mcmol per gram of dry liver tissue associated with increased risk of hepatic fibrosis and cirrhosis; HIC >400 mcmol/g associated with increased risk of HCC and death
- Hepatic iron index (HIC divided by patient's age in years) typically >1.9 in patients with homozygous hereditary hemochromatosis and expressed iron overload

DIFFERENTIAL DIAGNOSIS
- Exclude causes of secondary iron overload by history and appropriate laboratory tests
- Consider other causes of chronic liver disease (e.g., hepatitis B, hepatitis C, alcohol)

MANAGEMENT
What to Do First
- Assess severity of liver disease and complications
- Determine need for liver biopsy and patient's candidacy for therapy

General Measures
- Adjust or avoid potentially hepatotoxic medications; avoid alcohol and high doses of vitamin C
- Evaluate liver disease by history, physical examination, transferrin saturation, ferritin, liver biochemistry ± liver biopsy
- Consider HFE genotyping; if patient is homozygous for C282Y, consider screening first-degree relatives

SPECIFIC THERAPY

Indications for Treatment
- Remove excess iron if serum ferritin >300 μg/L

Treatment Options
- Phlebotomy (treatment of choice): remove 500 mL of blood per week until ferritin < 50 mcg/L; thereafter, every 3–4 months
- Deferoxamine: with severe cardiac disease or significant anemia, consider parenteral deferoxamine; inconvenient, expensive, and removes only 60–80 mg of iron per day.

Side Effects and Contraindications
- Phlebotomy
  - Side effects: anemia
  - Contraindications
    - Absolute: severe cardiac disease, severe anemia
    - Relative: hemoglobin <11 g/dL or hematocrit <35%
- Deferoxamine
  - Side effects: flushing, urticaria, hypotension, and shock may occur. High doses may cause visual disturbances, hearing loss, respiratory distress syndrome, and death.
  - Contraindications
    - Absolute: known hypersensitivity
    - Relative: severe renal failure

FOLLOW-UP

During Treatment
- Symptoms & hematocrit weekly
- Aim for transferrin saturation <30% and ferritin <50 mcg/L, with checks every 1–3 months

Routine
- Transferrin saturation and ferritin every 12 months

COMPLICATIONS AND PROGNOSIS
- Cirrhosis: seen in 50–70% of patients with symptoms; screen for HCC and treat as per liver failure due to other causes; consider liver transplantation for end-stage liver disease
- HCC: risk increased 200-fold in cirrhotic patients; occurs in 25–30% of cirrhotic individuals; can screen with serum alpha-fetoprotein and ultrasound every 6 months, but no data proves this improves outcome

- Abnormal skin pigmentation: occurs in up to 98% of symptomatic patients; frequently improves with phlebotomy
- Diabetes mellitus: occurs in 30–60% of patients with advanced disease; sometimes improves with phlebotomy
- Anterior pituitary dysfunction: deficiency in gonadotropin and pro-lactin secretion in 50% of patients; rarely improves
- Arthropathy: reported in 20–70% with symptoms; rarely improves with phlebotomy; pseudogout may occur and require nonsteroidal anti-inflammatory drug therapy
- Cardiac: presenting manifestation in 5–15% with symptoms of CHF most commonly seen; frequently improves with phlebotomy.

Prognosis
- Normal life span in noncirrhotic patients
- 60% 10-year survival in cirrhotic patients

HEMOPHILIA A AND B

KATHERINE A. HIGH, MD

HISTORY & PHYSICAL
- Bleeding diathesis due to deficiency of factor VIII (hemophilia A) or factor IX (hemophilia B)
- Disease occurs in all populations, ~1 in 5000 births. X-linked, males are affected, women are carriers.
- Disease symptoms correlate with circulating levels of factor, <1% = severe, 1–5% moderate, >5% mild
- Major morbidity of disease is spontaneous recurrent painful joint and soft tissue bleeds; chronic arthropathy commonly results
- Bleeding into intracranial space can be rapidly fatal
- Patients do not bleed from minor cuts and abrasions. Platelet function is intact.
- 2/3 cases occur in kindreds known to carry the disease; 1/3 in kindreds not previously suspected.
- Male infants often diagnosed at circumcision.

TESTS
- Screening test- aPTT prolonged in both hemophilia A and B
- 1:1 mix with normal plasma fully corrects aPTT in uncomplicated hemophilia

- Specific factor assays (FVIII or FIX) show reduced level
- Bethesda assay positive in patients with inhibitory antibodies

DIFFERENTIAL DIAGNOSIS

- For FVIII deficiency
  - ➤ R/O von Willebrand's disease (vWD). Bleeding time is long in vWD, normal in hemophilia A. Symptoms in vWD suggest mucosal bleeding, not joint and soft tissue. Autosomal dominant, not X-linked inheritance. FVIII level low, but so are ristocetin cofactor (RCF) and vW antigen.
- For FVIII or FIX deficiency
  - ➤ Acquired FVIII or FIX inhibitor. No family hx of bleeding. Patient's symptoms are recent in onset, not lifelong. APTT prolonged, does not correct with mix, factor level low, Bethesda assay positive.

MANAGEMENT

- Be certain that correct factor deficiency has been identified.
- For serious or life-threatening bleeds (e.g., symptoms that suggest intracranial or retropharyngeal bleeds), infuse factor to 100%, then undertake diagnostic studies.
- Early infusion of factor after any bleed reduces morbidity.
- Joint bleeds do not require aspiration unless pain and swelling are severe or unless sepsis is suspected.

SPECIFIC THERAPY

- Management of acute bleeding episodes in severe hemophilia
  - ➤ Assess whether bleed is life-threatening (intracranial, retroperitoneal. retropharyngeal with compromise of airway, major trauma, major surgery), major (severe joint or soft tissue bleed, severe trauma without evidence of bleed, GI bleeding), or minor (most joint and soft tissue bleeds, epistaxis, dental bleeding).
  - ➤ Life-threatening bleeds, replace to 80–100%; major, replace to 50%; minor, to 30%
  - ➤ Clotting factor concentrates dosed in units (U) with 1 U defined as amount of Factor VIII or Factor IX in 1 ml of normal plasma. To calculate FVIII dose, assume that 1 U/kg raises circulating level by 2%. To dose 70-kg man to 100% level will require 70 (kg) × 50 = 3500 U, and to dose him to 30% will require 70 × 15 = 1050 U. To calculate FIX dose, assume that 1 U/kg raises circulating level by 1%, so to dose 70-kg man to 100% requires 70 × 100 = 7,000 U. Doses for recombinant FIX (Benefix) require

an increase of 20–30% because of reduced recovery. CRITICAL TO CHECK FVIII/FIX LEVELS AFTER DOSING AND TO ADJUST DOSE ACCORDINGLY!

➤ Duration of treatment. For uncomplicated minor bleeds, 2–3 doses given q12h suffice. For major or life-threatening bleeds, treatment must be continued for 7–10 days.

➤ Both plasma-derived and recombinant products are available. With current viral inactivation techniques, plasma-derived products are generally safe from HIV and hepatitis, but avoid infusing plasma-derived product into patients who have previously been treated only with recombinant product.

➤ FOR MILD HEMOPHILIA, MAY BE POSSIBLE TO MANAGE BLEEDS WITH DDAVP, SYNTHETIC ANALOGUE OF VASO-PRESSIN. CONSULT A HEMATOLOGIST BEFORE GIVING CLOT-TING FACTOR CONCENTRATES TO A PATIENT WHO HAS NEVER RECEIVED THEM.

■ Long-term management of disease

➤ Multiple studies demonstrate that 3× weekly prophylactic infusion of 25–40 U/kg of FVIII concentrate, begun at 1–2 yrs of age, prevents life-threatening bleeds and greatly improves joint disease in children with hemophilia. Many patients now maintained on such a regimen.

➤ For those still treated in response to bleeds, not prophylactically, early factor infusion in response to bleeds is critical for best outcome.

➤ For chronic synovitis/anthropathy, options include intensive physical therapy, surgical or radioactive synovectomy, or joint replacement.

Side Effects and Complications

■ Failure to infuse adequate dose of factor leads to poor control of bleeding and resulting tissue damage.

■ Current major complication of therapy is development of inhibitory antibodies; occurs in 25% of hemophilia A pts and ~3% of hemophilia B. In this setting infused factor is rapidly neutralized by antibodies and bleeding is uncontrolled (vide infra).

■ Plasma-derived concentrates are now manufactured using viral inactivation techniques, but these are less effective for non-enveloped viruses. Also unclear whether they inactivate prions. Thus, some concern remains about risk of viral blood-borne disease transmission.

Contraindications

- Occasional patients with severe hemophilia B develop anaphylactic type reactions to FIX infusions.
- For patients with inhibitors, factor infusion is not harmful but is expensive and non-efficacious and should be avoided as a strategy for controlling bleeding except in cases of low titer inhibitor (vide infra).

FOLLOW-UP

- For uncomplicated joint bleeds, range of motion should improve over course of few days.
- For minor bleeds, check factor levels only if clinical response is sub-therapeutic or if questions arise about dosing. For major or life-threatening bleeds, important to follow factor levels during treatment.

COMPLICATIONS AND PROGNOSIS

- Most common causes of mortality in severe hemophilia in US are HIV-related complications; hepatitis-related complications; bleeding complications.
- Current life expectancy for severe hemophiliac not infected with HIV or hepatitis is 63 years of age. Most individuals <22 years of age are free of HIV and hepatitis, many >22 yrs have been exposed.
- HIV disease: >80% of those with severe hemophilia A infected in late 1970s through early 1980s from plasma-derived concentrates.% was slightly less for those with hemophilia B.
- Many now on standard HAART regimens. A few reports have suggested greater frequency of bleeding episodes on protease inhibitors; treaters should be alert for this problem.
- Hepatitis C: >90% of those with severe hemophilia infected during 1970s and 80s. Natural history of disease in hemophilia population similar to that seen in other affected groups. Co-infection with HIV may accelerate progression of liver disease.
- Inhibitory antibody formation is now major complication of treatment – occurs in 25% of hemophilia A, 3% of hemophilia B.
  - ➤ Inhibitors prevent successful treatment with clotting factor concentrates.
  - ➤ Diagnosis: clinically patient fails to respond to infused concentrate; laboratory: 1:1 mix does not correct, inhibitor is quantitated using Bethesda assay.
  - ➤ Inhibitors can be transient or long-lasting, and low or high titer.

➤ Acute management of bleeding episodes in inhibitor patients
- Low titer inhibitor (<5 Bethesda units [BU]), infuse high doses of concentrate to overcome inhibitor. Other options as below.
- High titer inhibitor (>5 BU). Best option is recombinant FVIIa, activates FX directly. Other options include activated prothrombin complex concentrates.

➤ Long-term management of inhibitors
- Immune tolerance regimen, daily infusion of high doses of FVIII results in disappearance of inhibitor in 70–90% of inhibitor patients, but therapy may be required for up to 2 yrs. Success rate lower with FIX inhibitors.

HEPATIC ENCEPHALOPATHY

ANDY S. YU, MD and EMMET B. KEEFFE, MD

HISTORY & PHYSICAL

History

- risk factors for liver disease: excessive alcohol use, injection drug use, blood transfusion, multiple sexual partners, Asian country of origin, family history
- risk factors for portal hypertension: cirrhosis

Physical Signs

- stigmata of chronic liver disease: gynecomastia, jaundice, spider nevi, firm liver, splenomegaly, ascites, testicular atrophy, palmar erythema,
- fetor hepaticus, altered consciousness, wide range of neuropsychiatric presentations
- staging of HE
  ➤ Stage 1: impaired attention, personality change, sleep reversal
  ➤ Stage 2: drowsiness, disorientation, confusion
  ➤ Stage 3: stupor, somnolence, but arousable
  ➤ Stage 4: unresponsiveness, coma
- movement disorders nonspecific for HE, including asterixis, hyperreflexia, hypertonia, extensor plantar response, slow monotonous speech

TESTS

- diagnosis of HE is clinical and is based on (1) identifying significant liver dysfunction, and (2) excluding other causes of CNS dysfunction

- elevated blood ammonia level
  - arterial specimen is the only accurate assay
  - diagnosis or treatment response should not be based on ammonia
- psychometric tests: sensitive for subclinical HE when neurological examination is otherwise normal, e.g., Reitan or trail-making tests
- electroencephalogram (not used routinely): high-frequency, low-voltage waves
- cerebrospinal fluid (not used routinely): elevated glutamine level

DIFFERENTIAL DIAGNOSIS
- subcategories of HE
- Type A: acute liver failure-associated hepatic encephalopathy
- Type B: major portosystemic shunting without cirrhosis
- Type C: cirrhosis, with 5 major subtypes of presentations
  - subclinical HE
  - single or recurrent episodes of overt HE
  - chronic overt HE
  - acquired hepatocerebral degeneration
  - spastic paresis
- non-hepatic causes of encephalopathy or CNS dysfunction: hypoxia, hypoglycemia, electrolytic disturbances, uremia, diabetic coma, drugs, infection, CNS structural lesion
- combined hepatic and non-hepatic encephalopathy

MANAGEMENT
What to Do First
- systematic neurologic and mini-mental examination
- panculture, including diagnostic paracentesis
- digital rectal exam to exclude gastrointestinal bleed

General Measures
- altered mental status in a patient with known or suspected cirrhosis should be considered HE until proven otherwise
- four-pronged simultaneous approach:
  - supportive measures for a patient with altered mental status
    - aspiration precaution, pressure sore prevention, toilet care; maintenance of fluid, electrolyte, and nutrition
  - exclude other causes of encephalopathy
  - identify and treat correctable precipitating factors
  - initiate empirical treatment

SPECIFIC THERAPY

Indication

■ clinical HE (uncertain if treating subclinical HE is beneficial)

Treatment Options

■ lactulose: via nasogastric tube for comatose patients until loose bowel movements are achieved; retention enema is a less effective route for patients in coma; orally if patient is sufficiently conscious, titrated to 3 bowel movements daily

■ neomycin

■ metronidazole: orally; only short-term use recommended because of adverse effects

■ dietary protein restriction: <40 g daily

■ flumazenil (benzodiazepine antagonist), given intravenously as boluses; costly; short duration of action; clinical utility limited to overt HE

■ promising medications not yet approved in the United States
  ➤ lactitol: nonabsorbable synthetic disaccharide with efficacy equivalent to that of lactulose; absence of sweet taste enhances compliance
  ➤ rifaximin: poorly absorbed macrolide; shows great promise
  ➤ sodium benzoate: may cause dyspepsia and fluid retention;

Side Effects and Contraindications

■ lactulose
  ➤ side effects: dehydration, hypernatremia, flatulence, and abdominal cramps

■ neomycin
  ➤ side effects: ototoxicity, nephrotoxicity, peripheral neuropathy
  ➤ contraindications
    • absolute: tinnitus, renal failure
    • relative: serum creatinine >1.5 mg/dL

■ metronidazole
  ➤ side effects: peripheral neuropathy, carcinogenicity, metallic taste, disulfiram-like reaction

■ dietary protein restriction
  ➤ side effects: protein-calorie malnutrition (negative nitrogen balance and obligatory endogenous protein breakdown)

FOLLOW-UP

During Treatment

■ monitor neurologic status

■ titrate medications according to therapeutic response and side effects of the medications

Routine
■ lactulose titrated to 2–3 loose bowel movements per day
■ alternative or additional therapy may include
  ➤ neomycin q.i.d. orally
  ➤ vegetable-based protein diet
■ therapeutic options for refractory HE
  ➤ TIPS shunt reduction or obliteration
  ➤ liver transplantation

COMPLICATIONS AND PROGNOSIS
■ 60–85% 1-year survival with refractory hepatic encephalopathy

---

HEPATIC VENO-OCCLUSIVE DISEASE

MINDIE H. NGUYEN

HISTORY & PHYSICAL

History
■ acute form: following bone marrow transplantation (BMT) with high-dose cytoreductive chemotherapy with or without hepatic irradiation

Risk Factors:
■ pretransplant fever or elevation of AST or ALT
■ fever before cytoreductive therapy not responsive to broad-spectrum antibiotics or fever occurring after cytoreductive therapy
■ history of abdominal radiation, history of viral or drug-induced hepatitis
■ radiation dose >12 Gy
■ cytoreductive regimens of cyclophosphamide plus busulfan, or cyclophosphamide plus BCNU and etoposide
■ chronic form: secondary to toxicity of pyrrolizidine alkaloids from plants of the Crotalatia, Senecio, Heliotropium genera found in herbal teas (Jamaican bush tea disease)

Signs & Symptoms
■ 2 or more of the following criteria within 20 days after BMT (Seattle criteria):
■ painful hepatomegaly

- sudden weight gain >2% of baseline body weight
- total serum bilirubin >2.0 mg/dL
- may correlate with subsequent development of renal insufficiency, pleural effusion, cardiac failure, pulmonary infiltrates, bleeding.
- chronic form: similar to those of chronic BCS

TESTS

Laboratory
- basic studies: nonspecific elevation of aminotransferases, alkaline phosphatase bilirubin, prothrombin time

Imaging
- Doppler flow studies: usually normal
- ultrasound: signs of portal hypertension (splenomegaly, ascites)
- hepatic venous pressure (measured by transjugular approach): very specific for VOD if >10 mmHg

Liver Biopsy
- histologic features:
- nonthrombotic obliteration of small intrahepatic veins
- concentric subendothelial thickening
- thrombosis secondary to sclerosis
- perivenular and sinusoidal fibrosis
- centrilobar hepatocyte necrosis
- no single histologic feature pathognomonic

DIFFERENTIAL DIAGNOSIS
- graft-versus-host disease: rarely occurs before day 15 post-BMT
- drug toxicity: rarely causes ascites and hepatomegaly
- sepsis
- post-transfusion hepatitis: usually occurs later in the course

MANAGEMENT

What to Do First
- evaluate pulmonary status and possible need for ventilatory support
- assess patient's fluid status, possible bleeding and infection
- recognition of possible multiple organ failure

General Measures
- diuresis for fluid overload, platelet and RBCs as necessary
- broad-spectrum antibiotics to treat presumptive infection

SPECIFIC THERAPY
- treatment is largely supportive
- prophylactic heparin for high-risk BMT patients is controversial
- various antithrombotic and thrombolytic agents have been used
- liver transplantation: usually required for chronic VOD
- TIPS and surgical shunts: options for chronic portal hypertension

FOLLOW-UP
- acute VOD: careful inpatient monitoring as above
- chronic VOD: similar follow-up as in chronic Budd-Chiari syndrome:
- periodic surveillance for TIPS or portosystemic shunt patency
- periodic monitoring for progressive chronic liver disease

COMPLICATIONS AND PROGNOSIS

Complications
- same as for treatment of Budd-Chiari syndrom

Prognosis
- incidence of VOD in BMT patients: 50%
- mortality: 20–40%

HEPATITIS A AND E

EMMET B. KEEFFE, MD

HISTORY & PHYSICAL

History
- HAV and HEV enterically transmitted viruses; shed in feces
- HAV and HEV not associated with chronic viremia or chronic liver disease
- HAV worldwide distribution; highly endemic in developing countries; decreasing incidence in U.S.
- HEV widely distributed; rare in U.S. (seen in travelers returning from endemic areas)
- HAV risk factors: day care centers, institutions for developmentally disadvantaged, international travel, homosexual contact, injection drug use
- HEV risk factors: largely waterborne epidemic disease; contaminateded water supply; most common type of sporadic hepatitis in developing countries
- Anti-HAV seroprevalance rate in U.S. – 33%

Signs & Symptoms

- Spectrum of acute HAV and HEV infection: asymptomatic to FHF (rare; 0.1%)
- Typical symptoms in acute infection: malaise, anorexia, nausea, vomiting
- Onset of symptoms abrupt in HAV and HEV infection
- Cholestatic hepatitis may complicate HAV infection
- Relapsing or biphasic HAV infection may occur

Physical

- Liver mildly enlarged and tender

TESTS

Basic Tests: Blood

- Mild disease: increased AST/ALT (vary from 500 to 5000 IU); normal or mild decreased WBC, with or without lymphocytosis
- Severe disease: increased bilirubin (usually <10 mg/dl) and INR; decreased albumin
- Cholestatic disease: bilirubin may be >20 mg/dl; AST/ALT decline toward normal even though bilirubin high; variable increased alkaline phosphatase

Specific Tests
- **Serology**
- Acute HAV infection:
- Positive IgM anti-HAV confirms acute infection; disappears in convalescence
- Positive IgG anti-HAV also present; persists indefinitely
- Acute HEV infection:
- IgM anti-HEV confirms acute infection; IgG anti-HEV may also be present; HEV RNA in stool; tests not yet licensed in U.S.
- Positive IgG anti-HEV in convalescence; IgM anti-HEV and HEV RNA disappears

Imaging
- Ultrasound: nondiagnostic

Biopsy
- Not routinely performed; diagnosis of acute HAV and HEV infection based on serology
- Biopsy findings: focal hepatocyte necrosis with cell dropout; Councilman bodies; diffuse mononuclear cell infiltrate

DIFFERENTIAL DIAGNOSIS

- Nonspecific symptoms (malaise, anorexia, nausea, vomiting): many other causes, including EBV infection, flu syndromes, depression
- Other acute liver diseases: acute HBV or HCV infection; drug-induced hepatitis, especially acetaminophen hepatotoxicity; auto-immune hepatitis; alcoholic hepatitis

MANAGEMENT

What to Do First

- Confirm diagnosis
- Assess severity of acute liver disease

General Measures

- Outpatient care unless persistent vomiting, severe anorexia or dehydration
- Maintenance of adequate calorie and fluid intake
- No specific dietary recommendations
- All nonessential drugs discontinued
- Limitation of daily activities and rest periods as needed

SPECIFIC THERAPY

- No specific therapy for usual acute HAV and HEV infection
- Corticosteroids of no value
- Liver transplantation for FHF

FOLLOW-UP

- Serial LFTs to confirm early peak of illness and improvement
- Serial visits to ensure adequate nutrition and hydration
- Urgent visits or hospitalization for mental status changes, raising concern for FHF

COMPLICATIONS AND PROGNOSIS

Complications

- Vomiting with dehydration
- Severe anorexia with inadequate nutrition
- FHF

Prognosis

- Complete clinical, histologic, and biochemical recovery within 3–6 months
- Occasional FHF, with greatest mortality in individuals >40 years of age
- Increased risk of FHF in pregnant women with HEV infection

HEPATITIS B

JEFFREY S. GLENN, MD, PhD

HISTORY & PHYSICAL

History
- maternal HBV infection
- sexual exposure
- exposure to blood/blood products (IVDA, tattoos, piercings, hemophiliacs)
- occupational exposure
- non-endemic areas, ~1/3 patients deny known risk factors

Signs and Symptoms
- most asymptomatic
- when present, symptoms = anorexia, fatigue, myalgias, nausea
- jaundice < 50% 1–2 weeks after onset of symptoms
- less frequent findings = arthritis, rash, glomerulonephritis, and vasculitis
- advanced disease: cirrhosis with liver failure, HCC

TESTS

Laboratory
- characteristic (but nonspecific):
- acute: elevated ALT/AST; elevated bilirubin and INR in severe disease
- chronic: elevated bilirubin and INR; decreased albumin

Serology and Virology
- confirmation of infection
- in chronological sequence of appearance:
- HBsAg-first marker to appear; if present for >6 mo, indicates chronic infection
- anti-HBc IgM – indicates acute, recent infection
- anti-HBs – detectable after resolution; may decrease with time; also induced by active vaccination
- HBV DNA – hybridization, PCR or branched-DNA based assays
- HBeAg – associated with active viral replication; marker of high infectivity
- Anti-HBe – signals decreased (but not absent) viral replication and infectivity

Imaging
■ Ultrasound or CT: nondiagnostic; abnormal with advanced disease–revealing cirrhosis and portal hypertension

Liver Biopsy
■ May be used for staging, or to exclude co-existing liver disease

DIFFERENTIAL DIAGNOSIS
■ Other viral infections (e.g., HAV, HCV, EBV, etc.), gallstone disease
■ Other chronic liver diseases: alcohol, HCV, autoimmune, genetic diseases

MANAGEMENT

What to Do First
■ Evaluate the virological status and severity of the liver disease, including complications and suitability for therapies.

General Measures
■ Minimize hepatotoxins (alcohol, potentially hepatotoxic medications)
■ Care of acute infection mainly supportive
■ HAV vaccination if susceptible

SPECIFIC THERAPY

Indications
■ Positive HBeAg, elevated HBV DNA, elevated ALT

Treatment Options
■ Interferon (alpha-2b or pegylated alpha-2a)
  ➤ Favorable factors: high ALT and low HBV DNA
  ➤ Loss of viral markers of replication and ALT normalization 20% more often in treated vs. controls.
■ Lamivudine (Epvirir-HBV)
  ➤ Rapid suppression of serum viral DNA, but no clearance of HBsAg
  ➤ May have favorable outcome on progression of fibrosis
  ➤ Viral resistance mutants emerge by first year of therapy in 20% of patients
  ➤ Optimal duration of therapy currently uncertain
■ Adefovir dipivoxil
  ➤ Optimal duration of therapy currently uncertain; generally until HBeAg seroconversion
  ➤ initial resistance rate lower than lamivudine, but rising

- Entecavir
  - ➤ better HBV DNA suppression than lamivudine; similar HBeAg seroconversion rate

Side Effects & Contraindications
- Interferon
  - ➤ side effects:
    - include flu-like syndrome, decreased WBC and platelet counts, autoimmune disease, depression
  - ➤ contraindications:
    - absolute: decompensated cirrhosis, neutropenia, thrombocytopenia, s/p organ transplant, psychosis, uncontrolled seizures, severe heart disease
    - relative: uncontrolled diabetes, autoimmune disease
- Lamivudine
  - ➤ side effects:
    - none
  - ➤ contraindications:
    - relative: concern re: development of resistance mutants
- Adefovir
  - ➤ side effects:
    - similar to placebo
  - ➤ contraindications:
    - concern re nephrotoxicity in post-OLT patients and decompensated cirrhotics
- Entecavir
  - ➤ side effects:
    - similar to lamivudine

Special Situations
- Severe, decompensated liver disease
  - ➤ Oral agents preferable option
- Precore mutant infections
  - ➤ Represent subset of anti-HBe-negative patients with good response to above agents, but relapse common; long-term therapy required. If oral agent used, ones with lower initial rates of resistance mutations (adefovir or entecavir) are favored.
- HIV co-infections
  - ➤ Represent potential for combined treatment with oral agent such as lamivudine (higher doses) as part of multi-drug anti-HIV regimen

- During chemotherapy
  - Risk of HBV flare; consider pre-emptive lamivudine for expected limited (through 3–6 months post chemotherapy) course

Prevention
- Passive immunization: with HBIG (used alone only in post-OLT setting)
- Active immunization: recombinant vaccine (required component of all other immunization protocols)

FOLLOW-UP
During Treatment
- Monitor for potential complications (check CBC, TSH during interferon), and efficacy (ALT, HBeAg, HBV quantitative DNA)

Routine
- Monitor ALT, albumin, prothrombin time, bilirubin, CBC
- Screen for HCC with ultrasound and AFP every 6 months

COMPLICATIONS AND PROGNOSIS
- if adult:
  - 90–95% uneventful recovery
  - ~1% fulminant hepatic failure
  - 5–10% become chronic carriers
- if child <5 yr:
  - 25–50% develop chronic infection
- if acquired perinatally:
  - 70–90% become chronically infected
- All chronic carriers at risk for:
  - cirrhosis
  - HCC (~200-fold relative risk)

HEPATITIS C

BRUCE F. SCHARSCHMIDT, MD

HISTORY & PHYSICAL
History of Exposure
- IV drug use, body piercing, hemodialysis, hemophiliacs, high-risk sexual exposure

- risk from blood transfusion <<0.01% per transfusion (>5% from transfusions before 1990)
- risk to unborn child of infected mother ~5%, may be higher if mother HIV-co-infected < 5% of sexual partners of affected patients get HCV
- 10–40% of cases without obvious exposure history

Signs & Symptoms

- acute infection usually asymptomatic
- chronic infection: ~70% of patients develop chronic disease
- often detected when patient is asymptomatic
- early symptoms mild and nonspecific: malaise, fatigue, musculoskeletal
- advanced disease: liver failure (jaundice, ascites, edema, encephalopathy, GI bleeding); 2–4% annual risk of hepatocellular carcinoma if cirrhosis present
- less common manifestations: renal disease, essential mixed cryoglobulinemia

TESTS

Laboratory

- basic studies: blood
  - ➤ early disease: elevated AST/ALT
  - ➤ advanced disease: elevated bilirubin and prothrombin time,
  - ➤ decreased albumin
- basic studies: urine
  - ➤ early disease: normal
  - ➤ advanced disease: bilirubinuria

Screening

- anti-HCV antibody: positive 2–3 months after infection

Confirmatory Tests

- recombinant immunoblot assay: largely replaced by next test
- qualitative HCV RNA test: positive within days of infection

Other Tests

- HCV genotype: used to assess duration of therapy
- quantitative HCV RNA test: measures viral load; used to assess response to therapy

Imaging

- abdominal ultrasound or CT scan: not diagnostic
- early disease: usually normal

■ advanced disease: small shrunken cirrhotic liver, collaterals suggestive of portal hypertension

Liver Biopsy
■ usually performed before therapy to assess severity of liver disease, although not a prerequisite for treatment
■ particularly useful in patients without clinical evidence of cirrhosis/advanced liver disease
■ early disease: variable inflammation and stage 1–2 fibrosis
■ advanced disease: stage 3 (bridging) fibrosis, stage 4 fibrosis (cirrhosis)

DIFFERENTIAL DIAGNOSIS
■ HCV-specific lab tests will confirm HCV infection
■ fatigue, malaise, other subjective Sx may be due to many causes (e.g., EBV infection, depression)
■ chronic liver disease may result from alcohol, other infections(e.g., HBV), other disorders (e.g., hemochromatosis), or a
■ combination of factors (e.g., HCV plus alcohol)

MANAGEMENT
What to Do First
■ assess severity of liver disease, candidacy for therapy

General Measures
■ adjust or avoid potentially hepatotoxic medications
■ assess for immunity to hepatitis A and B; immunize those without protection
■ history, physical, LFTs, consider liver biopsy, ultrasound to assess liver disease
■ check HCV genotype: predicts chance of successful therapy, defined as sustained virological response (SVR); i.e., loss of circulating HCV RNA by PCR or TMA assay 24 weeks after stopping therapy
  ➤ 1a, 1b: 70% of U.S. infections
  ➤ 2a, 2b, 3: 25% of U.S. infections
  ➤ 4 (Egypt and Middle East), 5 (Africa), and 6 (Vietnam) uncommon

SPECIFIC THERAPY
■ indicated for adult patients with chronic infection and liver injury, but not with severe, decompensated liver disease

Rx Options
- peginterferon plus ribavirin (Rx of choice)
  - peginterferon: once weekly
  - ribavirin:
  - treat 12 months for genotypes 1a and 1b and viral load >2 mIU; 6 months for other genotypes
  - response rate (loss of HCV RNA): <50% for genotypes 1a and 1b, >70% for other genotypes
  - response rate less for black patients and obese patients
- peginterferon monotherapy
  - 1 year Rx, regimen same as above
  - preferred only for patients who cannot take ribavirin
  - response rate 25–40% overall, less for genotypes 1a and 1b and for black patients

Side Effects & Contraindications
- interferon
  - side effects: flu-like symptoms (e.g., myalgia, fever), thrombocytopenia, depression
  - contraindications
    - absolute: decompensated cirrhosis, psychosis, organ transplant (except liver), neutropenia thrombocytopenia, uncontrolled seizures, severe heart disease
    - relative: uncontrolled diabetes, autoimmune disease, active alcohol or substance abuse
- Ribavirin
  - side effects: teratogenic, hemolysis
  - contraindications:
    - absolute: pregnancy or potential to conceive or father a child and no reliable contraception, end-stage renal disease, hemoglobinopathies, anemia
    - relative: uncontrolled hypertension, active alcohol or substance abuse

Special Situations
- Children with chronic infection: same protocols as for adults
- HIV-positive patients with chronic infection: same protocols, but treat only if HIV is well-controlled
- Decompensated cirrhosis: lower response rate and higher risk of anemia and thrombocytopenia. Rx may be warranted in

selected circumstances. Gradual dose escalation may be helpful, adjunct/supportive therapy (e.g., erythropoietin for anemia) often necessary.

■ Non-responders: No approved "salvage" Rx. Chronic suppressive Rx with peginterferon being explored in ongoing clinical studies but not yet approved or established to confer clinical benefit.

■ Acute infection: Rx with peginterferon lowers risk of chronic infection and should be initiated within 12 weeks; ribavirin not shown to be of benefit with acute infection

FOLLOW-UP

During Rx

■ Regularly assess potential complications of therapy; hemolysis, thrombocytopenia, hypothyroidism

■ peginterferon/ribavirin: CBC at 2–4 weeks;
  ➢ CBC, hepatic panel monthly
  ➢ TSH every 3–6 months
  ➢ quantitative HCV RNA at week 12 (if <2 log drop in HCV-RNA, likelihood of SVR low, strongly consider stopping therapy)

■ peginterferon mono Rx: Same as for combination therapy

■ ALT, albumin, PT, bilirubin, CBC every 6–12 months

■ follow-up liver biopsy is discretionary; may be considered every 3–5 years in patients with mild disease

COMPLICATIONS AND PROGNOSIS

■ Cirrhosis: develops in 10–30% of patients 10 to 40 years after infection

■ treat as per liver failure due to other causes (see liver transplantation)

■ consider liver transplantation for end-stage

■ cirrhosis; HCV infection usually recurs in the transplanted organ; transplant is beneficial only for highly selected patients with hepatocellular cancer (e.g., small/early cancer)

■ Hepatocellular carcinoma: annual incidence in 2–4% of patients with cirrhosis; screening with alpha-fetoprotein plus ultrasound every 6 months standard

■ Membranoproliferative glomerulonephritis: rare; consider interferon and ribavirin

■ Essential mixed cryoglobulinemia: rare; consider interferon and ribavirin

Prognosis

■ Good in the absence of cirrhosis or liver cancer

■ a minority of patients develop life-threatening complications

HEPATITIS DELTA VIRUS

JEFFREY S. GLENN, MD, PhD

HISTORY & PHYSICAL
- "Parasite virus" of HBV
- HDV has own genome and coat protein; requires HBV to provide envelope; therefore, always found in association with HBV infection

History
- same as for HBV (although different areas of predominant endemicity)
- two clinical scenarios (requires high index of suspicion for diagnosis):
- coinfection-simultaneous with acute HBV infection-of previously uninfected patient
- superinfection-HDV infection of chronically-infected HBV patient-manifested by sudden worsening/ "flare" of previously stable chronic HBV carrier
- clinical course characteristically more severe than for HBV infection alone

TESTS

Laboratory
- same as for HBV
- in addition, anti-HD IgM-best for diagnosis of acute infection
- anti-HD IgG develops late; often transiently; low titer in acute infection
- HDV RNA-reliable marker for acute and chronic infection
- HDAg–reliable marker for acute and chronic infection in serum and liver biopsy
- HBV markers of replication often suppressed upon acute HDV infection

DIFFERENTIAL DIAGNOSIS
- Same as for HBV

MANAGEMENT
- Same as for HBV

SPECIFIC THERAPY
- No proven effective specific anti-HDV therapy

- Treatments which fail to eradicate HBsAg (e.g. lamivudine) unlikely to be of benefit long-term
- Prenylation inhibitors hold great promise (investigational at present)
- Outcome post-liver transplant good

FOLLOW-UP
- Same as for HBV

COMPLICATIONS AND PROGNOSIS
- Same as for HBV except:
  - ➤ course generally more severe
  - ➤ HDV increases likelihood of, and rate of progression to, cirrhosis

---

HEPATORENAL SYNDROME

GABRIEL GARCIA, MD

HISTORY & PHYSICAL
- After onset of cirrhotic ascites, 20% develop HRS in 2 years and 40% in 5 years
- Two patterns of presentation:
- Type 1 HRS – doubling of serum creatinine or 50% reduction in creatinine clearance within 2 weeks of onset; usually associated with decompensated liver disease such as variceal bleeding, jaundice, peritonitis, bacteremia, or encephalopathy
- Type 2 HRS – renal function slowly deteriorates over many weeks to months in a more stable patient

Major Criteria
- Chronic or acute liver disease with liver failure and portal hypertension
- Low GFR (serum creatinine >1.5 mg/dL or creatinine clearance <40 ml/min)
- Absence of shock, bacterial infection or recent treatment with nephrotoxic drugs
- Absence of excessive fluid losses (gastrointestinal, extensive burn)
- No improvement following volume expansion with at least 1.5 liters of saline
- No significant proteinuria (<500 mg/day)
- No ultrasound evidence of intrinsic renal

Minor Criteria
- Urine volume <500 mL/day
- Urine sodium <10 mmol/day
- Urine osmolality < plasma osmolality
- Urine RBC <50 per high power field
- Serum sodium <130 mmol/L

Potential Precipitating Factors
- Infection, particularly spontaneous bacterial peritonitis
- Rapid diuresis, particularly large volume paracentesis without volume expansion
- Excessive gastrointestinal fluid loss due to vomiting or diarrhea (lactulose)
- GI bleeding
- NSAID use

TESTS
- To establish the diagnosis (i.e., major criteria):
  - Serum electrolytes and creatinine
  - Creatinine clearance and 24 hour urine protein excretion
  - Abdominal ultrasound
  - Routine urinalysis and microscopic exam
  - Spot urine sodium and osmolality
- Additional tests to look for potential precipitants
  - Diagnostic paracentesis with WBC count and bedside culture
  - Blood cultures

DIFFERENTIAL DIAGNOSIS
- Acute tubular necrosis (ATN)
- Intrinsic kidney disease
- Obstructed urinary tract
- Recent treatment with nephrotoxic drugs
- Volume depletion from excessive fluid losses, e.g., vomiting, diarrhea, diuretics

MANAGEMENT

What to Do First
- Confirm diagnosis, using major criteria
- Look for precipitating factors in type 1 HRS

General Measures
- Expand the plasma volume, ideally in an ICU with a pulmonary artery catheter in place to guide the volume therapy.

- Diagnose and treat infection aggressively
- Discontinue any potential nephrotoxic therapy
- Avoid large volume paracentesis, as it may precipitate further reduction of the central blood volume; use only for tense ascites if the rupture of an umbilical hernia seems likely

SPECIFIC THERAPY
- No specific proven medical therapy is available (terlipressin effective, but not yet licensed in U.S.)
- Catecholamines (midodrine alone, or with octreotide infusion, may be beneficial based on limited studies; dose range of midodrine is 2.5 to 7.5 mg/d, increased up to 12.5 mg/d; octreotide may be administered 100 ug subcutaneously three times daily, and increased to 200 ug if needed; treatment course is 1–2 weeks
- Albumin infusion (1 g/kg) on the first day, followed by 25–50 g/d, should be considered in all patients
- Evaluate for liver transplantation – the treatment of choice
- Dialysis is ineffective in the long-term management but may provide support until a transplant is possible

FOLLOW-UP
- Daily monitoring of renal function, central venous pressures, urine output in type 1 HRS
- Serial monitoring of renal function in outpatient with type 2 HRS

COMPLICATIONS AND PROGNOSIS

Complications
- Renal failure with associated electrolyte and metabolic complications
- Death

Prognosis
- Survival in type 1 HRS is less than 20% 4 weeks after the diagnosis is made, and less than 5% at 10 weeks.

HEREDITARY ELLIPTOCYTOSIS (HE) AND HEREDITARY PYROPOIKILOCYTOSIS (HPP)

PATRICK G. GALLAGHER, MD

HISTORY & PHYSICAL

History
- history of anemia, jaundice, gallstones, splenectomy

- family history of anemia, jaundice, gallstones, splenectomy
- HE: dominant inheritance; Hemolytic HE and HPP: recessive inheritance
- common in people of African and Mediterranean ancestry

Signs & Symptoms

- most HE patients are asymptomatic
- most hemolytic HE and HPP patients have well-compensated anemia
- hemolysis and anemia are exaggerated in infancy
- diagnosed incidentally during testing for unrelated conditions
- splenomegaly, jaundice, pallor in hemolytic HE and HPP

TESTS

Laboratory

- HE: Peripheral blood smear with normocytic, normochromic elliptocytes, few to 100%
- HPP: elliptocytes, bizarre-shaped cells with fragmentation or budding, poikilocytes, pyknocytes, microspherocytes
- elliptocytes rare on blood smear before 6 months of age
- anemia - mild or none in HE, mild to moderate in hemolytic HE and HPP
- decreased MCV (50-70 fl) in HPP
- markers of hemolysis - increased reticulocyte count, serum bilirubin, urinary urobilinogen, lactate dehydrogenase and decreased haptoglobin if significant hemolysis
- negative antiglobulin (Coombs') test
- increased incubated osmotic fragility in HPP (not HE)

Imaging

- splenomegaly on abdominal ultrasound or radionuclide scanning
- cholelithiasis on abdominal ultrasound

DIFFERENTIAL DIAGNOSIS

- elliptocytes seen in megaloblastic anemias, hypochromic microcytic anemias (including iron deficiency anemia and thalassemia), myelodysplastic syndromes, and myelodysplasia

MANAGEMENT

What to Do First

- assess degree of anemia, hemolysis, and potential complications
- therapy rarely needed in HE
- RBC transfusion if symptomatic anemia

General Measures
- provide folate supplementation
- counsel/diagnose other family members

SPECIFIC THERAPY
- indications and complications of splenectomy similar to hereditary spherocytosis (above)
- splenectomy is almost always curative

FOLLOW-UP
- monitor for hematologic decompensation during acute illnesses
- interval ultrasounds for cholelithiasis

COMPLICATIONS AND PROGNOSIS
- HE: Complications are uncommon and prognosis is good
- if hemolysis, cholelithiasis possible
- megaloblastic anemia due to folate deficiency
- hemolytic, aplastic, and megaloblastic crises similar to spherocytosis

---

HEREDITARY SPHEROCYTOSIS

PATRICK G. GALLAGHER, MD

HISTORY & PHYSICAL

History
- history of anemia, jaundice, gallstones, splenectomy
- family history of anemia, jaundice, gallstones, splenectomy
- ~two thirds dominant inheritance, ~one third recessive inheritance or de novo mutation

Signs & Symptoms
- anemia, jaundice, pallor, and splenomegaly
- clinically heterogeneous
- typical patient relatively asymptomatic due to marrow compensation
- often identified when complications related to anemia or chronic hemolysis occur or when studied for unrelated disorder
- hemolysis and anemia exaggerated in infancy

TESTS

Laboratory
- peripheral blood smear shows spherocytes lacking central pallor

- hemolytic anemia of varying degree
- mean corpuscular hemoglobin (MCHC) increased >35%
- mean cell volume (MCV) normal or slightly decreased
  - red cell distribution width (RDW) increased >14
  - hyperchromic, dense cells on RBC histogram
- if significant hemolysis – increased reticulocyte count, serum bilirubin, urinary and fecal urobilinogen, lactate dehydrogenase and decreased haptoglobin
- negative antiglobulin (Coombs') test
- increased osmotic fragility with "tail" of conditioned cells seen before splenectomy

Imaging
- splenomegaly on abdominal ultrasound or radionuclide scanning
- cholelithiasis on abdominal ultrasound

DIFFERENTIAL DIAGNOSIS
- spherocytes seen in autoimmune hemolytic anemia, liver disease, thermal injury, micro and macroangiopathic hemolytic anemias, Clostridial sepsis, transfusion reaction with hemolysis, severe hypophosphatemia, ABO incompatibility, poisoning with certain snake, spider, and hymenoptera venoms
- may be confused with rare Rh deficiency and intermediate hereditary stomatocytosis syndromes

MANAGEMENT
What to Do First
- assess degree of anemia, hemolysis, and potential complications
- RBC transfusion if symptomatic anemia

General Measures
- provide folate supplementation
- counsel/diagnose other family members

SPECIFIC THERAPY
- splenectomy alleviates anemia and eliminates RBC transfusion
- indications for splenectomy are controversial; consider degree of anemia and hemolysis, transfusion dependence, recurrent crises, failure to thrive, signs of extramedullary erythropoiesis
- immunize with Streptococcus pneumoniae, Meningococcus, and Haemophilus influenzae vaccines prior to splenectomy
- overwhelming post-splenectomy infection risk unknown

- splenectomy "failure" due to accessory spleens missed at surgery or another superimposed RBC disorder
- limited follow-up data available for partial splenectomy

FOLLOW-UP
- follow for symptomatic anemia (exercise tolerance, dyspnea, tachycardia)
- monitor growth and development
- observe for hematologic decompensation during acute illnesses
- interval ultrasounds for cholelithiasis

COMPLICATIONS AND PROGNOSIS
- symptomatic hemolytic anemia
- megaloblastic anemia due to folate deficiency
- cholelithiasis – ~50% patients, presents in adolescents and young adults
- hemolytic crisis – jaundice, splenomegaly, and decreased hematocrit, associated with viral infection,
- aplastic crisis – fever, lethargy, nausea, vomiting, abdominal pain, due to parvovirus B19 infection; Severe anemia may be life-threatening; may be first manifestation of HS.
- megaloblastic crisis – patients with increased folate demands – e.g. pregnant patient, growing child, recovering from aplastic crisis, or elderly
- Rare: Chronic leg dermatitis/ulceration, gout, cardiomyopathy, neuromuscular abnormalities, "tumors" due to extramedullary erythropoiesis

---

HERNIA

ARTHUR I. SAGALOWSKY, MD

HISTORY & PHYSICAL
- bulge in scrotum; may extend into inguinal canal
- size may change with activity
- asymptomatic or vague pressure, pain on exertion
- possible acute pain if incarcerated (non-reducible) or strangulated

TESTS
- Physical exam alone usually diagnostic
- acute tenderness, fever, elevated WBC suggest acute incarceration, strangulation, impending infarction, and is a surgical emergency

DIFFERENTIAL DIAGNOSIS
n/a

MANAGEMENT
n/a

SPECIFIC THERAPY
- surgery in most cases
- support or binder for non-surgical cases

FOLLOW-UP
n/a

COMPLICATIONS AND PROGNOSIS
n/a

HERPES LABIALIS

SOL SILVERMAN JR, DDS

HISTORY & PHYSICAL
- recurrent lip ulcers
- vary in size, frequency, duration
- due to reactivation of herpes simplex virus I (rarely HSV 2)
- spontaneous; aggravated by sunlight, cold, irritation/trauma

TESTS
- characteristic recurrent, crusted lesion on vermilion border of the lip
- biopsy or culture if in doubt; virus sheds for first 3–5 days

DIFFERENTIAL DIAGNOSIS
- benign cheilitis; actinic cheilitis
- squamous cell carcinoma (biopsy if persists more than 3 weeks)

MANAGEMENT
- palliative

SPECIFIC THERAPY
- antiviral drugs if severe, e.g. acyclovir
- topical antivirals, e.g. penciclovir 1% cream
- antiinflammatory topical steroids after 5 days (avoid eye contact)

FOLLOW-UP
- as needed

COMPLICATIONS AND PROGNOSIS
- chronic recurrences
- avoid irritating associated factors
- contagious from viral shedding first 3 to 5 days

HERPES SIMPLEX

JEFFREY P. CALLEN, MD

HISTORY & PHYSICAL

History
- Primary disease is often clinically unapparent and asymptomatic.
- Recurrent disease is frequently preceded by symptoms of itching or burning.
- Herpes simplex virus has two distinct variants – HSV 1 and HSV 2.
- Although either variant can affect any surface on the body, HSV 1 is more common on the lips and HSV 2 is more common on the genitalia or buttocks.
- Recurrences are often triggered by trauma, fever, sunburn or stress.
- Primary disease on the fingers and subsequent recurrences are more frequent in dentists, dental assistants, and respiratory therapists and are termed herpetic whitlow (this is less common with the use of universal precautions and gloves).
- Atypical clinical appearances are more frequent in patients who are immunosuppressed either due to disease (cancer, HIV, etc.) or to immunosuppressive medications.

Signs & Symptoms
- Classic presentation includes grouped vesicles on the affected site.
- Often patients present with crusting that follows the resolution of the vesicular lesions.
- Chronic scalloped ulceration is possible in patients who are immunosuppressed.

TESTS
- Tzanck smears are frequently positive.
- Culture for the virus from a fresh lesion
- Biopsy may reveal characteristic viral changes, but is usually not necessary.

DIFFERENTIAL DIAGNOSIS

- Impetigo
- Herpes zoster
- Eczema

MANAGEMENT

What to Do First

- The disease is self-limited, and it is not clear that treatment with either topically or systemically administered antiviral agents alters the course.
- This is an infectious disease that can spread from person to person by contact with viral particles that are shed most during vesiculation, but can even be shed between episodes.

General Measures

- Prevention of spread may be possible with continuous oral antiviral therapies.
- Recurrences can be prevented with continuous antiviral therapy.

SPECIFIC THERAPY

- Famciclovir 125 mg bid, valacyclovir 1000 mg bid, acyclovir 200 mg 5X/d for 5 days for acute infection
- Famciclovir 250 mg bid, valacyclovir 1000 mg/d, acyclovir 400 mg tid: effective suppressive therapies

FOLLOW-UP

- None is generally needed.

COMPLICATIONS AND PROGNOSIS

- Secondary impetigo is possible.
- Rarely scarring may occur.

HERPES TYPE 1/TYPE 2

CAROL A. GLASER, MD

HISTORY & PHYSICAL

History

- DNA virus in herpes family (herpes 1 and 2)
- Occurs worldwide without seasonal variation
- Human only known reservoir

- Transmission via close contact or sexual activity, subclinical shedding HSV occurs frequently
- Primary mechanism of transmission HSV-1 in saliva, HSV-2 is usually by sexual contact
- Both HSV-1 and HSV-2 can be transmitted to sites via oral-genital, oral-anal or anal-genital contact.
- Transmission to neonate usually via birth canal
- Health care personnel can acquire infection from patients.
- Incubation period (non-neonatal): 2 days-2 weeks
- HSV-1 is extremely common infection, often acquired in childhood
- HSV-1 seroprevalence in US ~70% adult population
- HSV-1 accounts for most of oral herpes, sometimes due to HSV-2
- HSV-1 as cause of genital herpes likely increasing (20–24% cases), while remainder HSV2
- HSV-2 infection rarely occurs before onset of sexual activity.
- ~20% of adults infected with HSV-2
- Herpes encephalitis usually due to HSV-1

Signs & Symptoms

Oral Herpes
- Primary infection:
  - Approximately one-third of cases develop gingivostomatitis/pharyngitis.
  - Lesions on hard and soft palate, gingival surfaces, tongue and lip
  - May also have fever, difficulty swallowing and painful cervical lymphadenopathy
  - Occasional features (esp in pediatrics):
    - malaise
    - irritability
    - earache/otitis media (serous effusion)
    - coryza
- Reactivation:
  - often prodrome of tingling, pain and/or itching
  - small cluster of vesicles usually on lips (not as extensive as primary

Genital
- First episode, broad spectrum of disease:
  - bilateral vesiculopustular lesions
  - tender inguinal adenopathy
  - fever
  - headache

- malaise
- itching
- dysuria
- vaginal/urethral discharge
- genital and/or anorectal pain
- some asymptomatic (get numbers)

■ Recurrent episodes;
  - ~50% of patients will have prodrome of:
    - genital or rectal itching
    - tingling
    - pain

TESTS

Genital Herpes

■ Often clinical diagnosis
  - Culture lesion – easy to isolate
  - DFA/Tzank smear of lesion – quick, often available
  - HSV-1 vs. HSV-2
  - Antibodies to gG develop late in course – 3–6 months. Routine serology does not distinguish HSV 1 vs. HSV 2.
  - Type specific serology: type-specific protein gG can differentiate

Oral Herpes

■ Often clinical diagnosis
  - Culture lesion
  - DFA/Tzank

Encephalitis

■ Virus isolation low yield
■ Spinal fluid PCR fairly sensitive

DIFFERENTIAL DIAGNOSIS

n/a

MANAGEMENT

Condoms and daily suppressive therapy decrease risk of genital herpes transmission to a susceptible partner.

SPECIFIC THERAPY

Several antiviral drugs widely available to treat oral, genital, ocular, neonatal herpes, herpes encephalitis. These include:

■ Acyclovir
■ Valacyclovir – advantage: twice/day (vs. 5× day)
■ Famciclovir – given 2–3× day, comparable to acyclovir for acute herpes, also used to suppress infections

- Forscarnet – more toxicity than acyclovir, sometimes used for acyclovir-resistant infections
- Trifluridine/Idoxuridine – ophthalmic solution for keratoconjunctivitis

Penciclovir – cream for orolabial herpes

Consider suppressive therapy when frequent recurrences.

FOLLOW-UP

n/a

COMPLICATIONS AND PROGNOSIS

Herpes Proctitis
- pain
- anal discharge
- tenesmus
- constipation

Central Nervous System
- usually involves focal area of brain – temporal lobe
- often with behavior changes and altered consciousness
- severe condition
- untreated – 70% mortality

Aseptic Meningitis
- common complication of primary genital herpes
- 30% of females, 10% of males
- headache, fever, photophobia
- lymphocytic pleocytosis

Autonomic and Peripheral Neuropathies
- associated with rectal and less frequently genital infection
- transverse myelitis
- Bell's Palsy may be associated with HSV-1 reactivation

Herpetic Whitlow
- Most HSV-1, occasionally HSV-2
  - Painful infection on finger
  - Cutaneous vesicle
  - May have fever
  - May have lymphadenitis; epitrochlear and axillary sites

Herpes Gladiatorum
- Cutaneous herpes in areas of close contact during wrestling

Eye infections (usually HSV-1)
- Uni- or bilateral conjunctivitis
- Blepharitis
- Pain
- Photophobia
- Blurred vision
- Tearing
- Preauricular adenopathy

Neonatal
- Potential fatal, very serious with high risk of neurologic disease
- 3 main categories:
  - Skin, eye and mouth
  - CNS
  - disseminated

Special Hosts
- Immunosuppressed pts (malignancy, organ transplant, HIV) often develop severe complications from herpes infection – e.g.:
  - Esophagitis
  - Hepatitis
  - Anogenital ulceration
  - Interstitial pneumonia
  - Focal necrotizing pneumonia

HERPES ZOSTER

JEFFREY P. CALLEN, MD

HISTORY & PHYSICAL

History
- Recurrence of chickenpox (varicella zoster virus)
- Usually there is a prodrome of several days.
- Physical findings are often preceded by severe dermatomal pain.

Signs & Symptoms
- Initial lesions are erythematous papules followed shortly by vesicles.
- Dermatomal distribution

TESTS
- Tzanck smear
- Culture is possible, but varicella zoster virus is more difficult to culture than herpes simplex.
- Biopsy is rarely needed.

DIFFERENTIAL DIAGNOSIS
- Herpes simplex can simulate zoster in rare patients.
- Insect bites
- Cellulitis

MANAGEMENT

What to Do First
- Assess the timing of the eruption, as intervention with therapy is effective only in patients with early diagnosis (~72 hours).
- Assess whether the patient is immunosuppressed.
  - ➤ Consider testing for HIV infection.

General Measures
- Pain management
- Local soaks
- Although this is an infection, it is spread only by contact with vesicles and for people who are naive to the virus (non-immunized or not previously infected with varicella).

SPECIFIC THERAPY
- Valacyclovir 1000 mg tid for 10 days (contraindicated in patients who are immunosuppressed)
- Famciclovir 500 mg tid for 7 days
- Acyclovir 800 mg five times per day for 5–7 days
- Oral prednisone has been advocated by some in conjunction with antiviral therapy in a 2-week tapering dose (60 to 0 mg).

FOLLOW-UP
- Persistent pain is a problem, and its likelihood correlates with the age of the patient.

COMPLICATIONS AND PROGNOSIS
- Post-herpetic neuralgia
- Secondary infection

HIDRADENITIS SUPPURATIVA

JEFFREY P. CALLEN, MD

HISTORY & PHYSICAL

History
- Tender, red lesions that may drain serosangineous or suppurative material in the axilla, genital, perianal areas and under breasts

- Location in areas with apocrine glands
- Women are more frequently affected.
- Flares are intermittent.

Signs & Symptoms
- Erythematous, fluctuant nodules in areas with apocrine glands
- Multiple patulous follicles may mimic comedones.
- Sinus tracts are common.
- Drainage of serosangineous material and pus

TESTS
- HS is a clinical diagnosis; there are no confirmatory tests

DIFFERENTIAL DIAGNOSIS
- Includes furunculosis, Crohn's disease, deep mycoses, scrofulo-derma, lymphogranuloma venereum, pilonidal sinus

MANAGEMENT
What to Do First
- Culture to exclude a treatable infection

General Measures
- Cleansers with antibacterial activity
- Oral antibiotics – generally tetracycline derivatives
- Intralesional injection of triamcinolone acetonide
- Intravenous infliximab or subcutaneous adalimumab have been reported to be helpful.
- Oral isotretinoin might be useful.
- Other therapies include intralesional botulinum toxin and oral finasteride.
- Excision is the only assured method of inducing remission.

SPECIFIC THERAPY
- See above

FOLLOW-UP
- Repeated incision and drainage
- Aggressive surgical exoneration is the only definitive method or eradicating the disease.

COMPLICATIONS AND PROGNOSIS
- Pain and scarring
- Chronic inflammation due to sinus tract formation
- With time, the inflammatory reaction subsides.

HIGH-OXYGEN-AFFINITY HEMOGLOBINS

AKIKO SHIMAMURA, MD, PhD

HISTORY & PHYSICAL

History
- Positive family history (autosomal dominant inheritance) though may also occur sporadically
- Patients often asymptomatic

Signs & Symptoms
- Splenomegaly is uncommon

TESTS

Blood
- Polycythemia with erythrocytosis (hb ranges between 17–22 g/dl)
- No evidence of hemolysis
- Normal rbc morphology on peripheral smear
- Only 50% are detectable by hemoglobin electrophoresis

Specific Diagnostic Tests
- Low P50 and hemoglobin oxygen dissociation curve shifted to the left (decreased oxygen availability)
- Sequence analysis of alpha or beta globin genes

DIFFERENTIAL DIAGNOSIS
- Polycythemia vera
- Mutations in the erythropoietin receptor
- Increased erythropoietin production
- Some unstable hemoglobins have abnormal oxygen dissociation curves

MANAGEMENT
- No treatment generally required
- Hyperviscosity-related symptoms are rare
- Generally no adverse effect on fetus of mother with high oxygen affinity hemoglobin

SPECIFIC THERAPY
n/a

FOLLOW-UP
n/a

COMPLICATIONS AND PROGNOSIS
n/a

HIRSUTISM (DERMATOLOGY)

LEE CARSON, MD and MICHAEL J. WHITE, MD

HISTORY & PHYSICAL

History
- Normally a complaint of female patients, except for medication effects (below)
- **Previous Diagnoses**: Cushing's, acromegaly or other endocrine disorders
- **Medications**: Androgens, cyclosporine, dizoxide, glucocorticoids, and minoxidil
- **Racial predilection**: Middle Eastern, Russian, and Southern European countries
- **Related history**: Family history of hirsutism, menstrual irregularities, infertility, diabetes, rate of progression of clinical hirsutism

Signs & Symptoms
- **Hirsutism:**
  - ➤ Subjective judgment that excess hair exists. Hair may be in unwanted places or terminal hair replacing vellus hair.
  - ➤ Excess of terminal hair growth involving the upper lip, cheeks, chin, central chest, breasts, lower abdomen, or groin
- **Other related findings:** Temporal/androgenic balding, masculine body habitus, acne, obesity, acanthosis nigricans, galactorrhea, deepening of voice, and clitoral hypertrophy; in general "masculinization" features

TESTS

Laboratory
- If problem is mild, gradual onset, with regular menses – none
- Moderate to more severe, with other signs and symptoms: serum testosterone + DHEAS
- Suspected polycystic ovarian syndrome (PCOS): fasting blood sugar

- Suspected Cushing's: dexamethasone suppression test
- Suspected congenital adrenal hyperplasia: test for 17-hydroxypro-gesterone
- With galactorrhea: prolactin corticotropin stimulation

Imaging
- Rapid onset of virilization: Look for tumor
  - CT of adrenals
  - Pelvic ultrasound
- Suspected PCOS: Pelvic ultrasound
- **Consultation request:** Endocrine or OB/GYN as needed

DIFFERENTIAL DIAGNOSIS
- Increased skin sensitivity to androgens (ISSA) – most common
- Racial variation (ethnicity, family history)
- Congenital adrenal hyperplasia (CAH)
- Polycystic ovarian syndrome
- Ovarian/adrenal androgen-secreting tumors
- Adrenal or ovarian enzyme deficiency
  - Late-onset CAH (21-hydroxylase deficiency with elevated 17-hydroxyprogesterone)
  - Serum testosterone of >2 ng/ml and DHEAS >7000 ng/ml suggests a neoplasm.
- Cushing's syndrome
- Acromegaly
- Elevated testosterone
  - Most commonly secondary to PCOS
- Hyperprolactinemia – adrenal or ovarian source
- Increased growth hormone
- Hypothyroidism (rare)

MANAGEMENT
- Careful history and PE, rule out more serious causes (above)
- General measures
  - Most cases are ISSA, mild to moderate symptoms
  - Major workup not indicated

SPECIFIC THERAPY
- Workup for gradual onset of mild to moderate hirsutism rarely influences treatment – i.e., no specific treatable underlying cause is found.
- Shave
- Wax/depilatories

- Hair bleach
- Laser hair removal
- Electrolysis
- Oral contraception: helps 75% of cases with ovarian or adrenal etiology
- Glucocorticoids as needed for CAH
- Eflornithine cream (Vaniqa) – 13.9% applied BID
  - Not a hair remover – slows growth and lengthens normal hair cycle
- Antiandrogens
  - Cimetidine – weak
  - Cyproterone acetate – FDA orphan drug
    - Generic Name: Cyproterone acetate; Trade Name: Androcur
    - Orphan Indication: Treatment of severe hirsutism
    - Sponsor: Berlex Laboratories, Inc. Contact: Dr. Suzanne Hampton, Wayne, NJ; (973) 694–4100
  - Spironolactone: 75–200 mg/day, start at 50 mg BID
  - Finasteride: 5-alpha-reductase inhibitor, 5 mg/day
  - GnRH (gonadatropin releasing hormone)
- Surgical treatment of any neoplasm

Side Effects & Complication
- Systemic Rx: all require strict contraception – possible feminization of male fetus
- Spironolactone: contraindicated in renal insufficiency
- Laser: post-inflammatory pigmentation changes, hypertrophic scarring

FOLLOW-UP
- Depends on treatment modality
- Rule out any serious underlying disorder.
- OB/GYN or Endocrine consults for severe or rapid-onset cases, or where underlying disease diagnosis warrants

COMPLICATIONS AND PROGNOSIS
Complications
- Feminization of male fetus
- Side effects of individual treatments

Prognosis
- Treatable underlying disorder (e.g., neoplasm): varies with etiology
  - Hirsutism may resolve.

- Majority of cases: mild to moderate severity, no treatable underlying disorder
  - ➤ Will require treatment indefinitely

HIRSUTISM (ENDOCRINOLOGY)

RANDOLPH B. LINDE, MD

HISTORY & PHYSICAL

History

- Excessive growth of nonscalp hair in women common; highly subjective
- Hair distribution mainly genetic
- Irregular menstruation, acne, and scalp hair loss
- Etiology
  - ➤ Common:
    - Postmenopausal: physiologic
    - Adolescent or young adult
    - With irregular menses: polycystic ovary syndrome (PCOS), defined as hyperandrogenism, anovulation without other cause (5% of women)
    - With regular menses: idiopathic; late-onset congenital adrenal hyperplasia (CAH), esp in some ethnic groups (Ashkenazi Jews)

Signs & Symptoms

- Use modified Ferriman-Gallwey score of 9 body areas to assess excess terminal hair: values from 0 to 4 for none to extensive; significant if cumulative score >7 (upper 5% of population)
- Differentiate vellus from terminal hair:
- Vellus hair excess: ethnic (Whites with dark hair and skin, Asians, African Americans); familial; secondary to glucocorticoids or drugs (phenytoin, cyclosporine)
- Terminal hair excess: thicker, darker, male distribution (face, neck, sternum, low back)
- Obesity in 50% with PCOS
- Uncommon: androgenic body habitus (pseudoacromegaly); acanthosis nigricans (axillary, inguinal and posterior neck skin folds)
- Rare: Cushing syndrome; hypothyroidism; acromegaly; galactorrhea

TESTS

Laboratory
- Basic blood tests:
  - ➤ None if mild and nonprogressive
  - ➤ Testosterone, >2 ng/mL (7 nmol/L) characteristic of ovarian tumor
  - ➤ DHEAS: adrenal source:
    - >8 mcg/mL (22 mcmol/L): tumor
    - Modest elevation: consider 17-hydroxyprogesterone for CAH
- Specific Diagnostic Tests
  - ➤ Fasting insulin:
    - Glucose/insulin <4.5: insulin resistance
    - C-peptide level
    - Free testosterone may be elevated when total testosterone normal, but rarely helpful

Imaging
- Ovarian US usually unnecessary
- CT or MRI of the adrenals and ovaries when neoplasm suspected

DIFFERENTIAL DIAGNOSIS

Differential Diagnosis
- Rare:
  - ➤ Children: CAH or tumor, especially adrenal carcinoma
  - ➤ With rapid onset or virilization (deep voice, male musculature, temporal balding, clitoromegaly): Ovarian (>80%) or adrenal tumor
- PCOS
- Idiopathic hirsutism (diagnosis of exclusion)
- Medication effect
- Late-onset CAH (21-hydroxylase, 11-hydroxylase, or 3-beta-hydroxysteroid dehydrogenase deficiency)
- Ovarian or adrenal androgen-producing tumor (ovarian tumors often large, adrenal adenomas usually small, large virilizing adrenal tumor may be malignant)
- Cushing syndrome
- Hypothyroidism, acromegaly, or hyperprolactinemia

MANAGEMENT

What to Do First
- Establish cause

General Measures

■ Discuss potential problems, treatments, implications, follow-up

SPECIFIC THERAPY

■ Indications for Treatment
  ➤ Hirsutism cosmetic problem
  ➤ Modified Ferriman-Gallwey score >7
  ➤ Mild hirsutism better candidate for drug treatment if family history of moderate to severe hirsutism
  ➤ Do not restrict medication to women with high androgens

Treatment Options

■ Nonpharmacologic, esp when mild:
  ➤ Tweezing, bleaching, waxing, shaving, depilatories: do not accelerate hair growth
  ➤ Electrolysis, laser epilation: outcome operator-dependent
  ➤ Bilateral oophorectomy: hyperthecosis unresponsive to medical therapy, fertility no longer desired
■ Pharmacologic: no systemic drug FDA-approved for hirsutism
  ➤ Androgen suppression:
    • Oral contraceptives (OCs): norethindrone, norgestrel, and levonorgestrel androgenic; norgestimate, desogestrel least androgenic; drospirenone antiandrogenic
    • If side effects with OCs, GnRH analogue with low doses of estrogen (and progestin)
    • Glucocorticoids in selected patients with CAH
  ➤ Androgen inhibition:
    • Spironolactone: alone or coadminister with OC
    • Flutamide: as effective as spironolactone, but risk of hepatotoxicity
    • Finasteride: costly, less effective, but works additively with spironolactone
  ➤ Modulation of hair follicle:
    • Eflornithine cream: topical to facial hair twice daily
■ Psychological evaluation/counseling when problem of body image

Side Effects and Contraindications

■ Oral contraceptives:
  ➤ Side effects: migraine headaches, depression, breast tenderness, thrombophlebitis
  ➤ Contraindications:

- Absolute: pregnancy; breast, ovarian or uterine cancer; clotting disorders; previous thrombophlebitis
- Relative: migraine headaches

■ Spironolactone:
  - Side effects: common: irregular menses; infrequent: polyuria, dry skin, hypotension, fatigue, hyperkalemia, hepatotoxicity, dyspepsia, breast tenderness
  - Contraindications:
  - Absolute: pregnancy, renal insufficiency, hyperkalemia, abnormal uterine bleeding
  - Relative: drugs that elevate potassium; family history of breast cancer

■ Flutamide:
  - Side effects: amenorrhea, increased appetite, dry skin, green-hued urine, hepatotoxicity
  - Contraindications: pregnancy (absolute)

■ Finasteride:
  - Side effects: none
  - Contraindications: pregnancy (absolute)

■ Eflornithine:
  - Side effects: dysesthesias at application sites
  - Contraindications: pregnancy (absolute)

FOLLOW-UP

During Treatment

■ At 3–6 mo intervals: related acne usually responds in 1–3 mo
■ Slow response, mechanical means needed for existing hair
■ Establish 1 or more objective measures to follow:
  - Time spent on hair removal
  - Frequency of mechanical interventions
  - Photographs after using no cosmetic measures for arbitrary time q 3 mo
  - Weigh shaven hair q 3 mo
  - Periodically repeat Ferriman-Gallwey score

Routine

■ Quarterly to annual office visit for 1 or 2 y, periodically thereafter, depending on severity and associated problems
■ Add medicine if no improvement in 6 mo
■ Reduce dose of antiandrogen if benefit stable

COMPLICATIONS AND PROGNOSIS

- PCOS increased risk of uterine, ovarian cancer, type 2 diabetes, dyslipidemia, hypertension, atherosclerosis
- Unrecognized, tumor can grow, and malignancy can spread
- Cushing syndrome can be subtle, worsening if not diagnosed and cured
- Hirsutism can be psychologically scarring

HISTOPLASMA CAPSULATUM

RICHARD A. JACOBS, MD, PhD

HISTORY & PHYSICAL

History

- Inhalation of mycelial fragments and microconidia
- Endemic in Ohio and Mississippi River valleys, soil-based fungus
- Strong association between bird and bat guano and presence of histoplasma
- Disruption of soil by excavation or construction is associated with organism release.
- People exposed to disrupted soil through recreation or work activities are most at risk.
- Disease develops in men > women by 4:1 ratio.
- No differences in racial or ethnic groups

Signs & Symptoms

- Acute Primary Infection:
  - \>90% unrecognized
  - Asymptomatic or mild influenza-like illness
  - In those ill, incubation 7–21 days. Fever (up to 42C), HA, nonproductive cough, chills, chest pain
  - Arthralgias, E. nodosum, E. multiforme 6% pts, mostly women
  - Physical findings minimal – rales, rarely organomegaly
  - 6% acute pericarditis – precordial chest pain, fever – pericardial friction rub, pulsus paradoxus, enlarged cardiac silhouette
- Acute Reinfection: milder influenza-like illness
- Histoplasmoma: mass lesion resembling fibroma, can enlarge over years to form calcified mass
- Mediastinal Granuloma: massive enlargement of mediastinal lymph nodes by granulomatous inflammation. Asymptomatic or can affect major airways; fibrosis in healing can cause retraction.

- Mediastinal Fibrosis: rare but grave consequence of mediastinal involvement – massive fibrotic deposition within mediastinum – can cause hypoxemia, SVC syndrome, dysphagia, can encroach on all major structures
- Chronic Pulmonary Histoplasmosis
  - ➤ Cavitary pulmonary histoplasmosis
  - ➤ Cavitary lesions in upper lobes in >90% of cases
  - ➤ Males >50 years old, preexisting chronic lung disease (emphysema), unusual in <40 group
  - ➤ Symptoms: low-grade fever, productive cough, dyspnea, weight loss; night sweats, chest pain, hemoptysis, malaise less common
- Progressive Disseminated Histoplasmosis (PDH)
  - ➤ Relentless growth in multiple organ systems
  - ➤ Acute form: severely immunosuppressed (AIDS, Hodgkins, NHL), infants/young children. Abrupt onset, fever/malaise, hepatosplenomegaly, lymphadenopathy, rales.
  - ➤ HIV: CD4 <200, exposure to chicken coops. Fever, weight loss, rales, hepatosplenomegaly, lymphadenopathy. Cutaneous: maculopapular eruption, petechiae, ecchymosis.
  - ➤ Subacute: more prolonged nature of symptoms, hepatosplenomegaly and oropharyngeal ulcers (deeper), focal lesions of various organ systems (GI, CNS, adrenal glands), endocarditis. CNS: chronic meningitis, mass lesions, cerebritis.
  - ➤ Chronic: Chronic, mild symptoms, almost all in adults. Malaise and lethargy most frequent, fever less common and low-grade. Most common finding (50%) is deep and painless oropharyngeal ulcer. Hepatosplenomegaly in 1/3, absence of other organ involvement.
  - ➤ Ocular: Uveitis or panophthalmitis in association with active histo; also ocular histoplasmosis syndrome – posterior uveitis or choroiditis in skin-test positive individuals

TESTS

Laboratory

- Acute Pulmonary: WBC nl, 30% leukocytosis or leukopenia, transient increase in serum alkaline phosphatase
- Chronic Pulmonary: leukocytosis and elevated alk phos in 1/3, anemia in 1/2
- Acute PDH: anemia 90% (often <20), leukopenia, thrombocytopenia, ALT and alk phos elevation
- Subacute PDH: less striking than in acute PDH

- Massively elevated serum ferritin levels may indicate disease, especially in HIV/AIDS patients
- CSF (with meningitis):
  - ➤ Pleocytosis: cell counts 10–100, lymphocyte predominance
  - ➤ Hypoglycorrhachia, elevated protein 80%

Specific Tests
- Cultures:
  - ➤ Sputum – 10–15% acute, 60% of cavitary disease, yield increases with number of specimens
  - ➤ AIDS with pulmonary disease – 90% of bronchoscopy specimens positive, BM and Blood cx 50% positive
  - ➤ Meningitis – 20–65% recovery
  - ➤ Pericardial/pleural disease – fluid low recovery, tissue better
- Antigen detection – urine (occ. serum): mainstay of diagnosis, 90% of patients with PDH will be positive, 40% with cavitary disease, 20% with acute disease. Excellent test for immunosuppressed
- Serology: Comp-fix (CF) 1:8 positive, 1:32 strongly suggests active infection; four-fold rise in titer indicative of infection. False-positive rate 15%, commonly observed with coccidioidomycosis or blastomycosis.

Imaging (CXR)
- Acute: patchy pneumonitis that calcifies and hilar LAN (heavy exposure leads to "buckshot" appearance). Ghon complex and pulmonary calcifications with healed disease.
- Acute reinfection: numerous small nodules that are diffusely scattered throughout both lung fields.
- Histoplasmoma: central core of calcium, rings of calcium, clusters ("mulberry" calcifications)
- Cavitary disease: cavitary lesions in upper lobes, distinguish from preexisting bullae
- Acute Progressive Disseminated Histo: patchy pneumonitis with hilar node enlargement

DIFFERENTIAL DIAGNOSIS
- Acute pulmonary histo: distinguish influenza, other forms of community-acquired pneumonia
- Mediastinal lymphadenopathy: often considered hematologic malignancy when actually is histo
- Sarcoidosis difficult to distinguish

■ Distinguish from other fungal lung infections (Cocci, Cryptococcus), other chronic pneumonias (including mycobacterial disease, PCP)

MANAGEMENT

What to Do first
■ Establish diagnosis.

General Measures
■ Consider category of disease and category of host before deciding on treatment plan.

SPECIFIC THERAPY
■ *Acute Pulmonary Histoplasmosis*
  ➤ Majority of cases do not require therapy (normal hosts) – bed rest and antipyretics
  ➤ High inoculum or fevers >1 wk with respiratory compromise, anorexia, malaise: treat
  ➤ Itraconazole (oral suspension) 4–6 wks (can also consider IV form)
  ➤ Ketoconazole – more side effects
  ➤ Amphotericin B for intolerance to oral meds or progressive disease
  ➤ Fluconazole not as active
■ *Mediastinal Granuloma, Fibrosis, Histoplasmoma*
  ➤ Enlarged lymph nodes – only treat if mass effect, itra vs. Ampho B
  ➤ Fibrosis – no consensus, very difficult
  ➤ Histoplasmoma – surgical resection vs. watchful waiting, consider azole for 2–3 mo after surgery
■ *Cavitary Pulmonary Histoplasmosis*
  ➤ Thin-walled cavities: no intervention necessary
  ➤ Thick-walled, progressive infiltrates, persistent cavities: Itraconazole or Ketoconazole for 6 mo
  ➤ Amphotericin B for progression or severely immunocompromised, total dose 2 g
■ *Acute Progressive Disseminated Histoplasmosis*
  ➤ Life-threatening: Amphotericin B, can change to itraconazole when symptoms improve
  ➤ Less severe illness: Itraconazole; AIDS: lifelong suppression with itra

No role for caspofungin; posaconazole may be useful as salvage

- *Subacute and Chronic PDH*
  - ➤ Itraconazole
  - ➤ Amphotericin

Side Effects & Complications
- Itraconazole – absorption issues related to acidity, IV form not approved for severely impaired renal function. Interferes with P450 metabolism, multiple drug interactions, possible hepatitis
- Ketoconazole – more drug-drug interactions, GI side effects, hepatitis
- Amphotericin B – nephrotoxicity, infusion-related side effects, hypokalemia, hypomagnesemia

FOLLOW-UP

During Treatment
- Clinical follow-up
- Periodic CXR with cavitary disease
- Document negative cultures from normally sterile site (blood, CSF, pleural/pericardial)

Routine
- Lifelong suppression for AIDS or post-transplant/severely immunocompromised

COMPLICATIONS AND PROGNOSIS
- Disseminated disease (see above) – meningitis, endocarditis, pericarditis
- Progressive disease (see above)
- Prognosis – Good for acute disease, chronic disease in non-immunosuppressed individuals; poor for acute disseminated disease, especially if continued immunosuppression

---

HOMOCYSTINURIA

GREGORY M. ENNS, MD

HISTORY & PHYSICAL

History
- history of parental consanguinity or previously affected sibling (autosomal recessive inheritance)
- newborn screening in some states, countries (incidence ~1/250,000)

Signs & Symptoms

- mental retardation (not invariable), lens dislocation (usually downwards), myopia, glaucoma, cataracts, retinal detachment, Marfanoid body habitus (true arachnodactyly rare), osteoporosis, genu valgum, scoliosis, pectus deformity, vascular occlusive disease, strokes, malar flush, livido reticularis, mental retardation (not invariable), psychiatric abnormalities
- less common features: optic atrophy, failure to thrive, hypopigmentation, spontaneous pneumothorax, short stature, dystonia, seizures (20%)

TESTS

Laboratory

- basic blood studies:
  - ➤ routine studies normal
- basic urine studies:
  - ➤ routine studies normal

Screening

- serum amino acid analysis (increased methionine, cystine, cystine-homocystine disulfide)
- increased serum total homocyst(e)ine
- positive urine cyanide nitroprusside test
- increased urine homocystine

Confirmatory Tests

- assay cystathionine beta-synthetase activity in cultured fibroblasts, lymphoblasts, or hepatocytes

Other Tests

- DNA mutation analysis available in some centers
- prenatal diagnosis possible by enzyme assay (amniocytes, fetal liver biopsy after 2nd trimester), direct DNA analysis of informative markers (chorionic villi, amniocytes), or direct DNA if mutation known

Imaging

- X-rays: skeletal abnormalities common (osteoporosis, platyspondyly, kyphoscoliosis)
- head CT/MRI: normal until appearance of cerebrovascular disease (venous and dural sinus thrombosis)
- angiography: may reveal narrow arteries

DIFFERENTIAL DIAGNOSIS

■ Marfan syndrome (normal homocystine levels, aortic root dilatation, lens dislocation usually upwards)
■ other causes of homocystinuria: 5,10-methylene tetrahydrofolate reductase (MTHFR) deficiency (normal or decreased serum methionine), functional methionine synthetase deficiency (cobalamin G or E disease) – diagnosed by fibroblast complementation analysis, functional combined methylmalonyl-CoA mutase/methionine synthetase deficiency (cobalamin C, D, or F disease) – these disorders also have elevated blood and urine methylmalonic acid, diagnosed by fibroblast complementation analysis

MANAGEMENT

What to Do First

■ trial of vitamin B6 (pyridoxine); treat concomitantly with folate
■ assess severity of eye, vascular, bone disease

General Measures

■ referral to biochemical genetics specialist center
■ avoid folate/vitamin B12 deficiency

SPECIFIC THERAPY

■ indicated for all patients for life
■ *Treatment options*
■ pyridoxine titrated to individual response in vitamin B6-responsive patients
■ low methionine diet in vitamin B6-unresponsive patients (may not be tolerated by many patients diagnosed after infancy)
■ supplement with vitamins (esp. folate and vitamin B12), minerals, trace elements
■ betaine may decrease homocystine in vitamin B6-unresponsive patients
■ consider use of platelet function inhibitors and/or aspirin to decrease risk of thromboembolism

Side Effects & Complications

■ large doses of vitamin B6 (>500 mg/day) may cause peripheral neuropathy with ataxia

FOLLOW-UP

During Treatment

■ monitor blood methionine, total homocyst(e)ine, urine homocystine to assess vitamin B6 responsiveness

Routine
- genetic counseling
- regular ophthalmology, orthopedics evaluations (as needed on an individual basis)
- psychiatric evaluation if needed

COMPLICATIONS AND PROGNOSIS

Complications
- dietary non-compliance results in increased complications
- osteoporosis in 50% by age 20 years
- ectopia lentis nearly universal by age 40 years
- mental retardation common, but more severe in vitamin B6-unresponsive patients
- psychiatric abnormalities in >50%
- cerebrovascular disease in 1/3 of patients (surgery is especially associated with thromboembolism – increase IV hydration pre- and post-operatively)

Prognosis
- progressive disease in patients with severe B6-unresponsive patients
- better prognosis in vitamin B6-responsive patients (IQ 82 in patients diagnosed after infancy)
- early treated patients detected by newborn screening may result in good outcome (median IQ 100 v. 58 in patients diagnosed after infancy)
- vascular complications rare with therapy

HOOKWORM

J. GORDON FRIERSON, MD

HISTORY & PHYSICAL

History
- Life cycle: Eggs of either Ancylostoma duodenale or Necatur americanus are passed in stool, hatch in soil. Larvae penetrate skin of human, pass in circulation to lungs, cross to alveolae, migrate up respiratory tract, and are swallowed. Upon reaching the intestine, they attach with teeth to upper small intestine, feed on blood, and mate, and new eggs are laid. Eggs appear 5 weeks after larvae penetrate skin.

■ Exposure: walking barefoot or other contact of skin with contaminated soil

Signs & Symptoms
■ Penetration stage: local dermatitis and itching
■ Migratory phase: cough, wheeze, eosinophilia, and sometimes shadows on chest x-ray (Loeffler's syndrome)
■ Intestinal phase: no symptoms in light infection. In heavier infections, epigastric or midabdominal pain, dyspepsia, and/or diarrhea, and in severe infections, abdominal protuberance.

TESTS
■ Basic tests: blood: Migration phase: eosinophilia
■ Intestinal phase: Sometimes eosinophilia. In heavy infection there is microcytic hypochromic anemia, low serum iron and ferritin.
■ Basic tests: urine: normal
■ Specific tests: Stool O&P shows eggs and is diagnostic.
■ Other tests: Barium study may show irritable upper small bowel, where worms attached.

DIFFERENTIAL DIAGNOSIS
■ Migratory phase: mimics migratory phase of ascariasis, strongyloidiasis, schistosomiasis
■ Intestinal phase: mimics many causes of dyspepsia, diarrhea. Most important in differential are strongyloides and schistosomiasis.

MANAGEMENT
What to Do First
■ Assess severity, nutritional state, degree of anemia. Administer iron if needed. Anemia responds to iron even if worms not treated.

General measures
■ Determine source of infection.

SPECIFIC THERAPY
Indications
■ All symptomatic or anemic patients. Light infections are treated optionally.

Treatment Options
■ Mebendazole for 3 days
■ Pyrantel pamoate
■ Albendazole

Side Effects & Complications
- Mebendazole: rarely mild intestinal complaints
- Pyrantel pamoate: occasional mild intestinal complaints, headache, dizziness
- Albendazole: occasional mild intestinal complaints

  Contraindications: First trimester of pregnancy. If mild infection, no treatment at any time; if severe, treat with pyrantel pamoate after first trimester. Iron will correct anemia even if worms not treated.

  Complications of treatment: None beyond side effects listed.

FOLLOW-UP

Routine
- See that anemia and hypoproteinemia is corrected. No need to eradicate all worms, so follow-up stool examinations are optional.

COMPLICATIONS AND PROGNOSIS
- Prognosis good. Proper instruction in wearing shoes, care in handling soil, and proper disposal of excrement will prevent new infection.

HORNER'S SYNDROME

MICHAEL J. AMINOFF, MD, DSc

HISTORY & PHYSICAL
- Typically found incidentally
- Occasional pts note unequal pupils
- Ipsilateral small (meiotic) pupil & ptosis
- Normal pupillary response to light & accommodation
- Ipsilateral sweating impairment may be present depending on site of lesion

TESTS
- Cocaine (4%) instillation dilates a normal pupil but has no effect on pupil of Horner's syndrome

DIFFERENTIAL DIAGNOSIS
- Physiologic anisocoria is not accompanied by ptosis or sweating abnormality, and the pupil dilates in response to 4% cocaine
- Pupillary responses to light & accommodation distinguish other causes of pupillary inequality

- Cause of syndrome may be central lesion or lesion of preganglionic or postganglionic sympathetic neuron; associated clinical context & findings & results of chest x-ray or CT scan will help to localize lesion & distinguish brain stem or cervical cord lesion, thoracic or neck tumor, cervical trauma, carotid artery lesion, intracranial disease

MANAGEMENT
- Evaluate underlying cause

SPECIFIC THERAPY
- Treat underlying cause

FOLLOW-UP
- Depends on underlying cause

COMPLICATIONS AND PROGNOSIS
- Depend on underlying cause

HUMAN HERPES 6

CAROL A. GLASER, MD

HISTORY & PHYSICAL

History
- HHV6 member herpesvirus family (herpesvirus 6) (aka "sixth disease")
- Humans only host
- Transmission; via respiratory secretions
- Incubation period: Around 9–10 days
- Attack rate highest 6–24 months
- Ubiquitous agent
- Lifelong persistent infection – intermittent asymptomatic shedding
- reactivation can occur

Signs & Symptoms
- "roseola" (exanthem subitum)
- high fever (>39.5) × 3–7 days followed by erythematous maculopapular rash
- seizures can occur in primary infection encephalitis in immunocompetent pt
- cervical/posterior occipital lymphadenopathy
- gastrointestinal symptoms

- respiratory symptoms
- inflamed tympanic membranes

Immunocompromised pt – can be associated with encephalitis, pneumonitis, graft rejection

TESTS
- PCR HHV6 available research settings
- Viral antigen isolation from blood and tissue

Paired serology can be helpful.

DIFFERENTIAL DIAGNOSIS
n/a

MANAGEMENT
- Supportive

SPECIFIC THERAPY
- For immunocompromised pt (limited data); ganciclovir or foscarnet

FOLLOW-UP
n/a

COMPLICATIONS AND PROGNOSIS
- HHV6 can reactivate and cause fever, hepatitis, bone marrow suppression, pneumonia and encephalitis.

HUMAN IMMUNODEFICIENCY VIRUS TYPE 1 (HIV-1)

MALCOLM D.V. JOHN, MD, MPH

HISTORY & PHYSICAL

History

- High-risk sexual practices, esp. unprotected receptive anal/vaginal sex (average risk 0.1–0.3%, as high as 3% in highest-risk situations); cofactors for sexual transmission include STDs, esp. ulcerative genital diseases, traumatic intercourse, and uncircumcised males
- IV drug use esp. sharing uncleaned needles
- Blood transfusion between 1978–1985; current risk from blood transfusion 1:450,000–1:660,000 units of blood
- Perinatal from HIV+ mother to infant; risk varies from 15% to 60% (about 25% in the U.S.)
- Occupational exposure esp. deep parenteral injection with a hollow-bore needle with blood from HIV+ patient with high viremia; average

risk is about 0.3% per percutaneous exposure and 0.09% per mucocutaneous exposure
- Other modes of transmission such as orogenital sex are infrequent routes of transmission; organ transplants and sports contact are exceedingly rare modes of transmission; in about 7% of HIV+ cases the risk group is either unidentified or not reported.

Signs & Symptoms
- Acute antiretroviral syndrome (reported rates vary greatly, 20% vs. 50%-90%) seen in some individuals at time of seroconversion (6–12 wks); consists of non-specific mononucleosis-like syndrome of fever, skin rashes, headaches, meningismus, myalgias, arthralgias, lymphadenopathy, pharyngitis, oral ulcers, abdominal complaints, genital ulcers, other constitutional complaints and other less common findings.
- Often asymptomatic until develop AIDS (CD4 count <200 or AIDS defining opportunistic infections, OI); often thrush, oral hairy leukoplakia, intermittent fevers, weight loss, skin rashes, and other systemic symptoms

TESTS
Laboratory
- Basic blood studies:
  - acute seroconversion: low CD4 count, extremely high HIV-1 viral load (100,000's)
  - early-intermediate chronic stage: variably low CD4 count, detectable but variable levels of HIV-1 viral load (different 'set points' for each patient that lasts for years)
  - advanced/late stage: CD4 <200, high viral load
- Basic urine studies:
  - may be abnormal if HIV nephropathy present (proteinuria, hematuria)

Screening
- Anti-HIV antibody (Ab) positive 2 months after infection in most; positive by EIA in 95% by 6 months

Confirmatory Tests
- Blood
  - Enzyme immunoassay (EIA) followed by Western Blot (WB) is standard; 99.9% sensitive, 99.9% specific

- ➤ Home Test Kits require blood on a filter strip that is then tested by EIA and WB; 100% sensitive, 99.95% specific
- ➤ Rapid Detection Kits (< 30 minutes) requires confirmation by standard serology due to decreased specificity (98.9%–100%)
- Other secretions
  - ➤ Oral secretion kit detects Abs in oral secretions and requires WB confirmation on oral secretions; 99.9% sensitive and specific
  - ➤ Urine kits detect Abs in urine and require urine WB confirmation; 99.7% sensitive, 100% specific

Other Tests

- HIV-1 p24 Antigen (Ag) used to screen all donated blood; can be used to diagnose acute HIV syndrome though becomes negative with appearance of high levels of anti-p24 Abs thus nucleic acid-based diagnosis preferred in such cases
- Qualitative PCR on circulating cells/plasma can be used in early disease e.g. acute HIV infection, newborns; also used to resolve indeterminate Western blots; detects >99% HIV-1 variants from US and Europe (subtype B); limited use as expensive and not generally available
- Quantitative measurement of HIV nucleic acid sequences in plasma ('viral loads (VL)/viral burdens) most widely used test to diagnose acute HIV infection, initiate antiretroviral Rx, predict disease prognosis, monitor response to treatment, predict likelihood of perinatal transmission from HIV+ mother to infant
- At least 3 competing methods exist:
- 1. DNA PCR Amplification with Reverse transcriptase (RT-PCR)
- 2. Nucleic acid sequence-based amplification (NASBA)
- 3. Signal amplification by DNA branched-chain technique (bDNA)
- For a given assay, need a change of > 0.5 log to be a significant change
- Tests for HIV-1 Antiretroviral Drug Resistance used to aid Rx changes and initiation of Rx during acute infection, pregnancy, etc.
- Two types of in vitro resistance tests:
- 1. genotypic resistance-detects gene mutation, use to predict phenotypic resistance.
- 2. Phenotypic resistance-assess ability of HIV to grow in vitro in presence of HIV antiretroviral drugs.

Imaging

- None needed unless evidence of possible acute opportunistic infection; CXR for those who are PPD+; CXR for TB screening advocated by some irregardless of PPD result

DIFFERENTIAL DIAGNOSIS

- HIV-specific lab tests will confirm HIV infection
- Differential diagnosis (DDx) of acute retroviral syndrome (fatigue, malaise, other subjective symptoms) include EBV, CMV, HSV, viral hepatitis, rubella, toxoplasmosis, drug reaction, secondary syphilis, measles, disseminated gonococcemia, pityriasis rosea, and acute rheumatologic syndrome
- DDx of persistent CD4 decline includes idiopathic CD4 lymphopenia

MANAGEMENT

What to Do First

- Thorough history and physical (including pap smear if needed) with emphasis on conditions and behaviors relevant to HIV; laboratory tests should include confirmatory HIV serology, CBC with CD4 count, viral load (VL), renal function tests, liver function tests (LFTs), toxoplasma serology, RPR/VDRL, hepatitis serologies (HAV, HBV, HCV), baseline lipids and glucose if to start antiretrovirals, PPD ± CXR, G6PD (optional)
- Assess severity of injury to immune system (CD4 and VL)
- Assess need for antiretroviral therapy (acute infection or severe immunosuppression)
- Provide secondary prevention counseling to decrease risk of acquiring opportunistic infection and decrease risk of further HIV transmission.

General Measures

- Use history, physical exam, CD4, VL, LFT's, renal function tests to assess changes in immune status and possible need to initiate antiretroviral treatment (Rx) or in preparation to start Rx; CD4 count and HIV viral load independently predict prognosis and indicate response to Rx; rate of CD4 decline also correlates with disease progression
- Check HIV genotype or phenotype when changing Rx b/c drug failure. Guidelines suggest resistance testing may be helpful during acute HIV infection or during pregnancy and also in chronically infected prior to starting HAART.
- Vaccinate as needed with: Pneumovax, influenza vaccine, HBV vaccine, HAV vaccine, tetanus booster

SPECIFIC THERAPY

- Indications for highly active antiretroviral treatment (HAART): pregnancy, symptomatic HIV infection (AIDS, thrush, fever of unknown origin), asymptomatic chronic infection with severe immunosuppression or high viral loads

■ General indications during asymptomatic chronic infection include:

➤ IAS:
- CD4 <350: recommend
- CD4 350–500: consider if VL <5000, recommend in all other cases
- CD4 >500: defer if VL <5000, consider if VL 5000–3000, recommend if VL >30,000

➤ DHHS:
- CD4 <350: recommend (some controversy for CD4 = 200–350)
- CD4 >350: recommend if VL>30,000

Treatment Options

■ 3 major drug classes:

➤ Nucleotide reverse transcriptase inhibitors (NRTIs) – AZT, 3TC, d4T, ddI, ddC,abacavir, tenofovir, FTC

➤ Non-Nucleotide reverse transcriptase inhibitors (NNRTIs) – efavirenz, nevirapine, delavirdine

➤ Protease inhibitors (PIs) – indinavir, ritonvir, nelfinavir, saquinavir, amprenavir, fosamprenavirlopinavir-ritonavir, atazanavir, tipranavir

Entry inhibitors – enfuvirtide

■ Recommended: PI + 2NRTIs, NNRTI + 2NRTIs, or 2PIs + 2NRTIs

■ Alternatives: 3NRTIs (3TC +AZT+ ABC), PI + NNRTI + NRTI, low dose ritonavir + PI (crixivan, amprenavir, lopinavir) as a PI component of a regiment

■ Avoid: d4T +AZT, ddC + 3TC, ddC + d4T, ddC + ddI

Fixed combination drugs (NRTIs) available and decrease pill burden

Side Effects & Contraindications

■ NRTIs: bone marrow suppression, subjective complaints, GI intolerance, headache, insomnia, asthenia, pancreatitis, peripheral neuropathy, abacavir hypersensitivity

■ NNRTIs: rash; nevirapine liver disease in settings of hepatitis; efavirenz associated disconnectedness, intense dreams, and teratogenicity

■ PIs: GI intolerance, nephrolithiasis or nephrotoxicity, diarrhea, drug interactions, lipodystrophy (fat redistribution, hypertriglyceridemia, insulin resistance)

Special Situations
- Efavirenz contraindicated during pregnancy; nevirapine should be avoid in liver disease esp. HCV coinfected individuals

FOLLOW-UP

During Treatment
- CD4, VL, LFTs every 4 weeks for first 6 months to assess Rx success and need for intensification (addition of another antiretroviral) or treatment changes; adherence should be emphasized; evaluation for adverse events important; baseline lipids and at 3 months and 12 months on HAART

Routine
- CD4, VL at baseline with confirmatory test 2–4 weeks later then q3months if stable (all major changes require confirmatory testing); annual PPD, annual pap smear (some indicate anal pap smear for all q 1–2 years), baseline lipids

COMPLICATIONS AND PROGNOSIS

Complications
- Possible complications correlate with degree of immunosuppression
- CD4>500: acute HIV syndrome, candida vaginitis, persistent generalized lymphadenopathy (PGL), polymyositis, aseptic meningitis, Guillain-Barre syndrome
- CD4 200–500: pneumococcal and other bacterial pneumonias, pulmonary TB, Kaposi sarcoma, herpes zoster, thrush, cryptosporidiosis, oral hairy leukoplakia, cervical cancer, anal cancer, lymphocytic interstitial pneumonitis, mononeural multiplex, anemia, idiopathic thrombocytopenic purpura
- CD4<200: Pneumocystis carinii pneumonia, candida esophagitis, disseminated/chronic herpes simplex, toxoplasmosis, cryptococcosis, disseminated coccidioidomyocosis, cryptosporidiosis, chronic, progressive multifocal leukoencephalopathy, microsporidiosis, miliary/extrapulmonary TB, CMV disease, disseminated M. avium complex, wasting, B-cell lymphoma, cardiomyopathy, peripheral neuropathy, HIV-associated dementia, CNS lymphoma, HIV-associated nephropathy

Prognosis
- Median incubation time (HIV to AIDS) is 7–11 years.
- Median survival (HIV to death) without HAART is 8–12 years.

- CD4 and viral load help predict prognosis.
- Age, genetics, and physician's experience with HIV care were only population-based variables affecting natural history (older age at HIV infection and less physician experience associated with worse outcomes)
- Since introduction of HAART, 2-year AIDS survival increased from 34% to 70% in 1997; African-Americans and Latinos not benefiting as much as others

HUNTINGTON'S DISEASE

CHAD CHRISTINE, MD

HISTORY & PHYSICAL
- Gradual onset of chorea, dementia or both
- Family history (autosomal dominant inheritance)
- Onset at any age, typically btwn 30–50 years of age
- Early cognitive changes of moodiness, antisocial behavior & later dementia
- Movement disorder
  - Restlessness or frank chorea
  - In childhood-onset cases, progressive rigidity & akinesia predominate

TESTS
- Laboratory: blood & urine testing is normal; genetic testing is available
- Imaging: CT or MRI may show atrophy of cerebral cortex & caudate nucleus

DIFFERENTIAL DIAGNOSIS
- Drug-induced chorea (stimulants, estrogen, neuroleptics, dopaminergics, anticonvulsants, opiates, antihistamines), benign hereditary chorea, chorea-acanthocytosis, paroxysmal choreoathetosis differentiated by history
- Wilson's disease excluded clinically & if necessary by slit-lamp examination of cornea & by testing for serum ceruloplasmin & 24-hour urine for copper
- Stroke, brain tumor, cerebral vasculitis excluded by history & brain imaging

MANAGEMENT

What to Do First

■ Genetic counseling & genetic testing should be considered in most cases

General Measures

■ Psychiatric, physical therapy & neurologic consultations are helpful
  ➤ Support groups are helpful

SPECIFIC THERAPY

■ No definitive treatment available

Indications

■ Chorea
  ➤ D2 receptor blocking drugs: haloperidol or chlorpromazine
  ➤ Dopamine-depleting agents: reserpine or tetrabenazine (not available in U.S.)
  ➤ Benzodiazipines: clonazepam
■ Depression
  ➤ Tricyclics, SSRIs, other novel antidepressants are effective

FOLLOW-UP

N/A

COMPLICATIONS AND PROGNOSIS

■ Chronic progressive condition over 10–20 years
  ➤ Depression & suicide common

HYDATID CYST DISEASE

AIJAZ AHMED, MD

HISTORY & PHYSICAL

History

■ Endemic in sheep & cattle rearing regions

Signs & Symptoms

■ Many cysts asymptomatic; can become symptomatic after decades of slow growth w/ abdominal pain, fever, jaundice anorexia, weight loss, vomiting, pruritus; symptoms may follow rupture, leakage, or secondary bacterial infection
■ Examination: tender mass, fever, jaundice

TESTS

Basic Blood Tests
- Serum alkaline phosphatase, rarely hyperbilirubinemia; CT/US can be diagnostic

Specific Diagnostic Tests
- IHA: 75–94% sensitivity; specificity lower, requiring PCR

DIFFERENTIAL DIAGNOSIS
- Amebic abscess, pygenic abscess

MANAGEMENT

What to Do First
- History, physical exam, imaging

General Measures
- Admit to hospital if ill or unstable

SPECIFIC THERAPY

Treatment Options
- Drug therapy: albendazole, mebendazole, or praziquantel employed first to minimize risk of dissemination
- Surgery: radical cystpericystectomy +/− cyst evacuation & local instillation of scolicidal agents; treatment of choice
- Recent reports of successful radiologic cyst aspiration & scolicide instillation; avoid diagnostic cyst aspiration in suspected cases of hydatid cyst disease

FOLLOW-UP
n/a

COMPLICATIONS AND PROGNOSIS

Complications
- Allergic reaction, incl anaphylaxis, dissemination, & cholangitis

Prognosis
- May remain asymptomatic for life; cyst infection/rupture increases mortality

HYDROCELE

ARTHUR I. SAGALOWSKY, MD

HISTORY & PHYSICAL
- simple fluid-filled mass in tunica vaginalis
- confined to scrotum most often; may extend to spermatic cord or peritoneum (communicating type)
- congenital (patent processus vaginalis), spontaneous, or secondary to inflammation, infection, trauma
- smooth, round, cystic, non-tender scrotal mass

TESTS
- transilluminates
- ultrasound helpful

DIFFERENTIAL DIAGNOSIS
n/a

MANAGEMENT
n/a

SPECIFIC THERAPY
- observation if small, asymptomatic
- surgery if symptomatic

FOLLOW-UP
n/a

COMPLICATIONS AND PROGNOSIS
n/a

HYPERCALCEMIA

DOLORES SHOBACK, MD

HISTORY & PHYSICAL
History
- Nausea, constipation, abdominal pain, decreased mentation, lassitude, thirst, dehydration, reduced urine flow, nocturia, polyuria

- Short duration of hypercalcemia (weeks to months) in malignancy-associated hypercalcemia (MAH)
- Longer duration in primary hyperparathyroidism (HPTH)
- 90% with MAH dead in 3 mo
- Pancreatitis, fractures, renal stones – seen in HPTH
- Family history of hypercalcemia – present in MEN-1, familial benign hypercalcemia (FBH)
- Drugs: thiazides, lithium, vitamin D or A
- Granulomatous disease: sarcoid, TB, coccidioidomycosis, histoplasmosis, cryptococcosis
- Thyrotoxicosis: weight loss, tremor, palpitations, thyroid enlargement

Signs & Symptoms
- General – hypercalcemia: if severe, dehydration, tachycardia, hypotension; abdominal pain; poor memory and concentration, depression, stupor, coma
- HPTH: band keratopathy, hypertension, itching, fractures, osteitis fibrosa cystica (rare)
- Cancer: dehydration, clinically evident tumor burden, bone lesions and pain (especially myeloma, osseous metastases)
- Granulomatous disease: dyspnea, cough, abnormal chest exam, lymphadenopathy

TESTS

Laboratory
- Blood
  - HPTH: elevated Ca, low or normal P, elevated intact PTH
  - Cancer (majority-humoral): elevated Ca, low or normal P, suppressed PTH, elevated PTH-rP
  - Cancer (minority-bone metastases): elevated Ca, suppressed intact PTH and PTHrP
  - Lymphoma (rare): elevated Ca, P, and $1,25\text{-}(OH)_2$ vitamin D; suppressed PTH and PTHrP
  - Myeloma: anemia, elevated Ca, suppressed PTH, low PTHrP (most cases) monoclonal spike in SPEP
  - Thyrotoxicosis: elevated Ca, high normal P, suppressed PTH and TSH, elevated T4 and/or T3
  - Granulomatous disease: elevated Ca, P, and $1,25\text{-}(OH)_2$ vitamin D, suppressed PTH and PTHrP

- ➤ FBH: elevated Ca, elevated or normal Mg, low or normal P, inappropriately normal (85%) or slightly elevated (15%) PTH
- ➤ Vitamin D toxicity: elevated Ca, P, 25-OH vitamin D, suppressed PTH and PTHrP
- ➤ Lithium: elevated Ca and intact PTH
- ■ Urine
  - ➤ Cancer and HPTH: elevated Ca excretion
  - ➤ Myeloma: Bence Jones protein or M-spike
  - ➤ FBH: reduced Ca excretion (<100 mg/24 hours); Ca/creatinine clearance (<0.01)
  - ➤ Vitamin D toxicity, granulomatous disease: marked hypercalciuria

Specific Diagnostic Tests
- ■ Skeletal lesions and bone marrow plasmacytosis in myeloma
- ■ Elevated ACE levels in sarcoidosis
- ■ Mutations in 1, calcium-sensing receptor (FBH), menin (MEN 1), and ret oncogene (MEN 2)

DIFFERENTIAL DIAGNOSIS
- ■ Common cancers: lung, renal, breast, squamous cell, myeloma; rarely non-Hodgkin's lymphoma
- ■ Primary HPTH
- ■ Family history of hypercalcemia – FBH or MEN syndromes
- ■ Granulomatous disease: sarcoidosis, tbc, coccidioidomycosis, histoplasmosis, cryptococcosis
- ■ Thyrotoxicosis
- ■ Drugs: thiazides, lithium, vitamin A and D
- ■ Rare: milk-alkali syndrome, immobilization

MANAGEMENT

What to Do First
- ■ Assess severity of hypercalcemia, dehydration, mental status changes, cardiovascular status; monitor urine output
- ■ Hydration with normal saline (200–500 ml/hour) to restore intravascular volume, loop diuretics (Lasix 20 to 40 mg IV every 2 to 4 hours) to induce natriuresis after volume repletion

General Measures

- IV Pamidronate 60 to 90 mg or Zoledronic acid 4 mg IV repeated every 2–4 wks
- Calcitonin (IM or SQ) 4–8 IU/kg q 12

SPECIFIC THERAPY

- Primary HPTH – consider parathyroidectomy
- Cancer – treat underlying tumor (radiation, surgery, chemotherapy)
- Vitamin D toxicity, granulomatous disease, myeloma – 40 to 60 mg prednisone /day
- FBH – avoid surgical referral
- Thyrotoxicosis- antithyroid drugs, beta blockers, 131I ablation

Side-Effects & Complications

- Pamidronate or zoledronic acid – leukopenia; small percentage of patients – flu-like syndrome (fever, arthralgias myalgias); rare complication – jaw necrosis
- Calcitonin – itching, rash, nausea, vomiting, dizziness

Contraindications

- Absolute
  - ➤ Pamidronate or zoledronic acid – renal failure, creat >2.5 mg/dl
  - ➤ Calcitonin – allergy to salmon
- Relative
  - ➤ Active periodontal disease

FOLLOW-UP

- Slow response to pamidronate or zoledronic acid (3 to 7 days) may persist 4 to 6 weeks before need to re-treat
- More rapid response to calcitonin (1 to 2 days), tachyphylaxis common with prolonged administration
- Gradual response to steroids

COMPLICATIONS AND PROGNOSIS

- General: renal failure, dehydration, hypotension, vascular collapse, delirium, stupor, coma, death
- Primary HPTH: stones, renal insufficiency, fractures, psychiatric disturbances, depression
- Cancer: unremitting hypercalcemia, bone pain, pathologic fractures, cachexia, death
- Glucocorticoids: glucose intolerance, osteoporosis, infection

HYPERCHOLESTEROLEMIA

FREDRIC B. KRAEMER, MD

HISTORY & PHYSICAL

History
- diabetes
- obesity
- myocardial infarction
- stroke
- peripheral vascular disease
- hypertension
- smoking
- alcohol use
- estrogen or steroid use
- family history of diabetes
- family history of hypertriglyceridemia or hypercholesterolemia
- family history of myocardial infarction
- family history of stroke
- family history of peripheral vascular disease

Signs & Symptoms
- may be asymptomatic
- presentation:
  - symptoms: angina, myocardial infarction, stroke, claudication
  - signs:
    - tendinous or tuberous xanthoma, xanthelasma, arterial bruits, decreased pulses

TESTS

Laboratory
- basic blood studies:
  - fasting lipid panel: elevated total cholesterol, LDL cholesterol elevated, triglyceride normal or elevated, HDL cholesterol low, normal or elevated
  - glucose, HgbA1c
  - thyroid function tests
- basic urine studies:
  - proteinuria
    - ECG

Specific Diagnostic Tests

■ Apolipoprotcin B
■ Apolipoprotein E genotype

Imaging

■ none

DIFFERENTIAL DIAGNOSIS

■ Familial hypercholesterolemia
■ Polygenic hypercholesterolemia
  ➤ Secondary causes:
    • Hypothyroidism
    • Nephrotic syndrome
    • Dysglobulinemia
    • Glucocorticoid excess
    • Hepatic cholestasis
    • Anorexia nervosa
■ Familial combined hyperlipidemia (elevated cholesterol and triglyceride in patient or in various family members)
■ Dysbetalipoproteinemia (elevated cholesterol and triglyceride with apolipoprotein E2 genotype)
■ Hyperalphalipoproteinemia (isolated elevated HDL cholesterol)

MANAGEMENT

What to Do First

■ Establish whether secondary causes and treat those
■ Assess cardiovascular risk factors
  ➤ Men >45 years
  ➤ Women >55 years
  ➤ Family history of premature cardiovascular disease (<55 in male or <65 in female first-degree relative)
  ➤ Current smoking
  ➤ Hypertension
  ➤ Diabetes mellitus
  ➤ HDL cholesterol <40 mg/dl ($\geq$60 mg/dl is a negative risk factor)

General Measures

■ Diet: reduce saturated fat (<10%), total fat intake <30% of calories, weight loss if indicated
■ Regular exercise
■ Treatment goals
  ➤ Primary Prevention

- Men <35 and premenopausal women:
  - LDL cholesterol <190 mg/dl
- Men > 35 and women >45 with <2 other cardiovascular risk factors:
  - LDL cholesterol <160 mg/dl
- Adults with ≥2 other cardiovascular risk factors:
  - LDL cholesterol <130 mg/dl
- Diabetes mellitus or family history of early cardiovascular disease:
  - LDL cholesterol <100 mg/dl
- Secondary prevention:
  - LDL cholesterol <100 mg/dl

SPECIFIC THERAPY

- Statins
  - currently first line agents
  - several available: lovastatin, pravastatin, simvastatin, fluvastatin, atorvastatin, and rosuvastatin
  - 15–45% reduction in total cholesterol, 20–60% reduction in LDL cholesterol
  - 25–40% reduction in cardiovascular mortality
  - 20–30% reduction in all cause mortality
- Cholesterol absorption inhibitor
  - ezetimibe
  - add to statin or use if statin not tolerated
  - 15–20% reduction in total and LDL cholesterol
  - no outcomes studies yet
- Bile acid sequestrants
  - colestipol, cholestyramine
  - should be given with meals
  - add to statin or use if statin not tolerated
  - 15–25% reduction in total and LDL cholesterol
  - up to 20% reduction in cardiovascular events
  - no significant effects on cardiovascular or all cause mortality
- Niacin
  - crystalline, time-released
  - start at low dose and titrate weekly up to therapeutic level
  - can add to statin or bile acid sequestrant
  - more effective for hypertriglyceridemia
  - 10–15% reduction in total and LDL cholesterol, increase HDL cholesterol
  - 20–25% reduction in cardiovascular events

➤ unclear whether any significant effects on cardiovascular or all cause mortality
■ Fibrates
➤ clofibrate, gemfibrozil, fenofibrate, gemfibrozil and fenofibrate preferred
➤ can add to statin, bile acid sequestrant, or niacin
➤ more effective for hypertriglyceridemia
➤ 10% reduction in total cholesterol, LDL cholesterol may increase, not change or decrease, increase HDL cholesterol
➤ 20–30% reduction in cardiovascular events
➤ unclear whether any significant effects on cardiovascular or all cause mortality

Side Effects & Contraindications
■ Statins
➤ side effects: elevated AST, ALT, myositis
➤ contraindications: pregnancy, breast feeding
■ Cholesterol absorption inhibitor
➤ side effects: none
➤ contraindications: hypersensitivity
■ Bile acid sequestrants
➤ side effects: constipation, flatulence, abdominal discomfort, fat malabsorption and fat soluble vitamin deficiency at highest doses only
➤ contraindications: marked hypertriglyceridemia
■ Niacin
➤ side effects: cutaneous flush, hepatic dysfunction, glucose intolerance, hyperuricemia, skin changes with hyperpigmentation and acanthosis nigracans, increased risk of myositis when combined with statins
➤ contraindications:
➤ relative: peptic ulcer disease, gout, diabetes mellitus
■ Fibrates
➤ side effects: abdominal pain, nausea, vomiting, cholelithiasis, hepatic dysfunction, myositis (risk increased when combined with statins), potentiate action of oral anticoagulants
➤ contraindications:
➤ relative: renal insufficiency, pregnancy, breast feeding

FOLLOW-UP
■ Well controlled, stable patients every 6 months
➤ Obtain lipid panel, ALT, AST

- Uncontrolled patients every 3 months
  - ➤ Obtain lipid panel, ALT, AST

COMPLICATIONS AND PROGNOSIS
- Coronary artery disease
- Peripheral vascular disease
- Cerebrovascular disease

HYPEREMESIS GRAVIDARUM

CAROLINE A. RIELY, MD

HISTORY & PHYSICAL

History
- Intractable nausea and vomiting in the first trimester

Signs and Symptoms
- Intractable vomiting, sensitive to food smells, hyperptyalism (excessive spitting)

TESTS

Laboratory
- Elevated AST/ALT in 50% of cases, may be > 1,000
- Ketones in the urine

Liver Biopsy
- Normal, rarely hepatocyte dropout. Usually not indicated as diagnosis based on clinical findings

DIFFERENTIAL DIAGNOSIS
- Other causes of vomiting, such as gastric outlet obstruction from ulcer (EGD may be indicated in severe cases)
- Viral hepatitis (+ serologies, risk factors)

MANAGEMENT

What to Do First
- Gut rest, IV rehydration

General Measures
- Antiemetics, including promethazine, odansetron, droperidol

SPECIFIC THERAPY
- Enteral feeding if not resolved on gut rest, of if persistent
- Rarely, parenteral feeding

FOLLOW-UP
- Recovery with resolution of nausea by week 20 of gestation
- Rarely persists into second trimester
- Jaundice only in untreated, severe cases that in previous eras lead to death
- Successful outcome to the pregnancy

COMPLICATIONS AND PROGNOSIS
- Associated hyperthyroidism that resolves with resolution in nausea

---

HYPERKALEMIA

BIFF F. PALMER, MD

HISTORY & PHYSICAL
- clinical setting helpful in determining etiology
- does patient have leukocytosis (>100,000) or thrombocytosis (>500,000), hemolysis during process of phlebotomy
- intravenous or oral K load in setting of chronic renal failure
- uncontrolled diabetes
- acute oligo-anuric or end-stage renal disease
- History of drugs such as K sparing diuretics, cyclosporine, nonsteroidal antiinflammatory agents, heparin, ketoconazol

TESTS
- check EKG
  - ➤ severe hyperkalemia and a normal EKG suggests pseudohyperkalemia
  - ➤ EKG changes of hyperkalemia warrant urgent treatment is required (see below)
- serum creatinine, BUN, HCO3, creatinine clearance
- measure glucose to screen for diabetes
- other testing is based on clinical setting

DIFFERENTIAL DIAGNOSIS
- pseudohyperkalemia
  - ➤ WBC count >100,000 or platelet count >500,000

- excess intake
  - intravenous fluids containing K
  - increased dietary K important only with defect in renal K excretion
- cell shift
  - cell damage: rhabdomyolysis, tumor lysis, tissue ischemia, massive hemolysis
  - insulin deficiency: diabetic ketoacidosis
  - hyperosmolality: diabetic ketoacidosis, nonketotic hyperosmolar coma
  - metabolic acidosis: only with mineral acidosis (hyperchloremic acidosis) and not organic acidosis
    - increased K in diabetic ketoacidosis due to insulin deficiency and hyperosmolality, not metabolic acidosis
    - increased K in lactic acidosis due to inhibition of Na/K ATPase and cell leakage from injury or ischemia
  - drugs: beta blockers in setting of exercise, neuromuscular blockade with succinylcholine
  - toxin: digoxin overdose
  - familial hyperkalemic periodic paralysis: recurrent episodes of flaccid paralysis precipitated by cold or exercise; mutation in voltage activated Na channel decreased renal K excretion responsible for sustained hyperkalemia
  - often accompanied by normal gap metabolic acidosis (type IV RTA)
  - due to one or more of several abnormalities: renal insufficiency, decreased mineralocorticoid activity, or a distal tubular defect
    - renal insufficiency
      - GFR <10 ml/min: end stage renal disease from any cause
      - GFR >10 ml/min: tubulointerstitial renal disease
    - decreased mineralocorticoid activity
      - decreased renin, decreased aldosterone
        - mild to moderate diabetic nephropathy
        - drugs
          - nonsteroidal antiinflammatory agents
          - beta-blockers
          - cyclosporine
      - increased renin, decreased aldosterone
        - adrenal destruction (Addison's disease)
        - angiotensin converting enzyme inhibitors
        - angiotensin receptor blockers

- heparin
- azol-antifungal agents (ketoconozol)
- distal tubular defect (increased renin, increased aldosterone)
  - tubulointerstitial renal disease
  - drug
    - spironolacton
    - triamterene
    - amiloride
    - high dose trimethoprim, intravenous pentamidine

MANAGEMENT
- obtain EKG to exclude pseudohyperkalemia and to detect presence of EKG changes that require urgent treatment
- renal failure is responsible in setting of acute oligo-anuric renal failure or end stage renal failure with GFR <10 ml/min
- with mild to moderate renal failure (GFR >10 ml/min)
  - look for evidence of tubulointerstitial renal disease: sterile pyuria, WBC casts, low grade proteinuria, eosinophiluria
  - determine if drugs that impair renal K excretion are present
  - if diabetic, consider hyporeninemic hypoaldosteronism
  - measure renin and aldosterone if indicated

SPECIFIC THERAPY
- level of serum K and presence or absence of EKG changes determine therapy
- hyperkalemia in setting of diabetic ketoacidosis responds to insulin and fluids (with therapy anticipate development of hypokalemia)
- Acute treatment: EKG changes or symptoms of muscle weakness
  - Reverse effects on heart
    - calcium
  - Shift K into cells
    - glucose and insulin NaHCO3
    - beta2- adrenergic agonist: albuterol inhaler
  - Remove K from body
    - hemodialysis
    - cation exchange resin: sodium polystyrene sulfonate
- Chronic treatment: asymptomatic hyperkalemia without EKG changes
  - low K diet
  - loop diuretics
  - NaHCO3 tablets
  - fludrocortisone if patient not hypertensive

FOLLOW-UP

- frequent monitoring of K is required to ensure that hyperkalemia has been successfully treated
- avoid foods high in K
- avoid medications that impair renal K excretion

COMPLICATIONS AND PROGNOSIS

- complications of hyperkalemia are cardiac and muscular
  - ➤ musculoskeletal: severe weakness
  - ➤ cardiac: peaked T waves, increased P-R interval, QRS widening, Sine wave and ventricular fibrillation
- during treatment avoid development of hypokalemia
- use of insulin can be associated with hypoglycemia
- administration of glucose without insulin in type I diabetes can lead to worsening of hyperkalemia
- NaHCO3 tablets can lead to volume overload in renal failure patients
- sodium polystyrene sulfonate with sorbitol can lead to intestinal necrosis in post-surgical patients
- use 0-K bath in hemodialysis for no >1 hour to avoid precipitating arrhythmias
- hyperkalemia is readily treatable, ultimate prognosis dependent upon underlying cause

HYPERMAGNESEMIA

STANLEY GOLDFARB, MD

HISTORY & PHYSICAL

History

- Usually is iatrogenic and occurs in patients who have impaired renal function and ingest magnesium as either laxatives or antacids.
- Acute magnesium intoxication may occur in women who are treated for toxemia of pregnancy with intravenous magnesium salts that are administered at an excessive rate. Muscular paralysis can develop at serum magnesium levels of 10 mg/dl.

Signs & Symptoms

- Magnesium level > 4 mEq per liter.
  - ➤ Inhibition of neuromuscular transmission
  - ➤ Deep tendon reflexes are abolished

- Magnesium level >7 mEq per liter
  - Lethargy
- Magnesium level 5 to 10 mEq per liter
  - Hypotension and prolongation of the PR and QT intervals as well as QRS duration.
- Magnesium level >10 mEq per liter
  - Paralysis of voluntary muscles and respiratory failure
- Magnesium level >15 mEq per liter
  - Complete heart block or asystole

TESTS
n/a

DIFFERENTIAL DIAGNOSIS
n/a

MANAGEMENT
n/a

SPECIFIC THERAPY
- Calcium ion is a direct antagonist of magnesium and should be given to patients who are seriously ill with magnesium intoxication. Hemodialysis may be required following cessation of magnesium therapy.

FOLLOW-UP
n/a

COMPLICATIONS AND PROGNOSIS
n/a

HYPERNATREMIA

CHIRAG PARIKH, MD, PhD and TOMAS BERL, MD

HISTORY & PHYSICAL
- Polyuria, polydipsia
- Vomiting, diarrhea
- Drugs – loop diuretics

Signs & Symptoms
- Volume status: Important guide to diagnosis and treatment
  - Edema, orthostasis, skin turgor and axillary sweat

- Hypernatremia
  - Seen more with acute hypernatremia
  - Nonspecific CNS symptoms due to cellular dehydration
  - Subcortical and subarachnoid bleeding have been described due to tearing of cerebral blood vessels.

TESTS
- Basic metabolic profile
- Other tests in differential diagnosis of hypernatremia
  - Serum osmolality
  - Urine sodium
  - Urine osmolality
  - ADH measurement is expensive and unnecessary.

DIFFERENTIAL DIAGNOSIS
- Central diabetes insipidus vs. nephrogenic diabetes insipidus
- Do a water deprivation test followed by a DDAVP challenge. In both setting the urine remains hypotonic (<300 mOsm/Kg) or isotonic (~300 mOsm/Kg) with water deprivation, but in central diabetes insipidus only, the urine osmolality increases with DDAVP.

Approach to Hypernatremia
- Based on the volume status and Urine Na, it can be divided into following categories:
- Hypovolemic hypernatremia and Urine Na <10 mEq/L
  - Urine is hypertonic (>300 mOsm/Kg)
  - Extrarenal hypoosmolar losses – i.e., sweating, febrile states, burns, diarrhea, fistulas
- Hypovolemic hypernatremia and Urine Na >20 mEq/L
  - Urine is hypotonic or isotonic
  - Renal hypo-osmolar losses: diuretic use, osmotic diuresis, renal disease, post obstruction
- Hypervolemic hypernatremia (Urine Na is usually >20 mEq/L)
  - Urine is hypertonic or isotonic
  - Hypertonic Na (usually Na bicarbonate) administration, primary hyperaldosteronism, Cushing's syndrome
- Euvolemic hypernatremia (Urine Na and osmolality variable)
  - Renal losses of water due to the deficiency or resistance of ADH secretion
  - Central diabetes insipidus – defect in ADH production
    - Idiopathic or secondary to malignancies, infections or granulomatous diseases of the pituitary gland

- Can be complete or partial
- Treated with DDAVP
➤ Nephrogenic diabetes insipidus – resistance to ADH action
  - Congenital – X-linked and autosomal recessive
  - Acquired – secondary to renal diseases, hypokalemia, hypercalcemia, drugs (lithium, amphotericin)
  - Does not respond to DDAVP
➤ Diabetes insipidus secondary to vasopressinase
  - Seen during pregnancy or early post-partum states – uncommon condition
  - Due to degradation of endogenous ADH (vasopressin) by placental vasopressinase
  - Treated with DDAVP, which is not lysed by this enzyme

MANAGEMENT
n/a

SPECIFIC THERAPY
- Involves judicious administration of water and hypotonic fluids
- Depends on two factors: ECF volume status and rate of development of hypernatremia
- Correction of ECF volume depletion
  ➤ Normal saline used until euvolemia is restored
  ➤ Neck veins, orthostasis can be used to guide therapy if CVP monitoring not available
  ➤ Hypotonic fluids (0.45% saline, 5% dextrose) used to correct hypernatremia once volume status is restored
- Correction of ECF volume expansion:
  ➤ Diuretics mainstay of therapy
  ➤ Dialysis may be needed if renal failure is advanced
- Water Replacement
  ➤ Water replacement done orally, via NG tube or parenterally
  ➤ Hypotonic fluids like 5% dextrose and 0.45% saline should be used.
  ➤ Fluid deficit should be calculated as follows:
    - Total body water (TBW) = current body weight $\times$ 0.6
    - Fluid deficit = TBW (Current plasma sodium$/140 - 1$)
      - Ongoing losses (e.g., diarrhea) should be added to the fluid deficit.
      - The rate of correction depends on the rate of development of hypernatremia. Acute hypernatremia with symptoms

should be corrected rapidly. Chronic hypernatremia should be corrected slowly.
- The general rule for chronic hypernatremia is to correct half the fluid deficit in 12 h and the remaining half in next 24 h.
- Frequent measurement of electrolytes is essential to guide the therapy.

FOLLOW-UP
n/a

COMPLICATIONS AND PROGNOSIS
- Subarachnoid bleed, subcortical bleed and irreversible neurologic damage known to occur
- 75% mortality reported in adults with acute hypernatremia (Na >160 mEq/L) – death is due to underlying disorder and not hypernatremia per se.

HYPEROXALURIA

GREGORY M. ENNS, MD

HISTORY & PHYSICAL
- Primary hyperoxaluria type I (PHI):
  - alanine:glyoxalate aminotransferase (AGT) deficiency
- Primary hyperoxaluria type II (PHII):
  - D-glycerate dehydrogenase deficiency

History
- history of parental consanguinity or affected siblings (autosomal recessive inheritance)

Signs & Symptoms
- renal colic, UTI, recurrent calcium oxalate lithiasis
- failure to thrive, short stature
- asymptomatic hematuria
- systemic oxalosis in advanced disease: renal failure, compromised circulation (Raynaud disease, livedo reticularis, gangrene), retinopathy, optic atrophy, heart block, stroke, hypothyroidism, arthropathy, peripheral neuropathy, hepatosplenomegaly, pancytopenia
- PHI: presents in first decade (median age 9 years) with variable features from relatively mild form to severe, rapidly progressive neonatal form with end-stage renal disease (54%)

■ PHII: longer survival than type I despite similar urinary oxalate excretion, median onset 16 years, clinical heterogeneity (siblings with mutations may be asymptomatic), end-stage renal disease may still occur (12%), <30 documented cases

TESTS

Laboratory
■ basic blood studies:
  ➤ BUN, creatinine, Ca2+, PO4 2-, PTH may be normal or elevated
■ basic urine studies:
  ➤ urinalysis may show hematuria, calcium oxalate crystals

Screening
■ elevated urine oxalate (>0.5 mmol/24 h/1.72 m2, but may be normal in impaired renal function), glycolate (>1 mmol/24 h/1.72 m2, but may be normal in ~1/3 PHI patients) in PHI, L-glycerate (> 0.2 mmol/24 h/1.72 m2) in PHII. NB: oxalate excretion in children increases linearly with age and reaches adult levels at ~14 years
■ elevated urine oxalate:creatinine ratio (>0.10 mmol/mmol)
■ elevated blood oxalate (>30 mcM/liter), glycolate (>2500 mcM/liter)

Confirmatory Tests
■ liver biopsy (PHI, PHII) or leukocytes (PHII) for enzymatic assay
■ AGT immunoblotting by Western analysis (PHI)
■ DNA analysis may be available in some centers (G170R and I144T mutations account for up to 40% of mutant alleles in PHI)

Prenatal Diagnosis
■ possible on chorionic villi or amniocytes by direct DNA for PHI (genetic counseling must stress lack of genotype-phenotype correlation in PHI)
■ enzymatic on fetal liver for PHI

Imaging
■ abdominal X-ray: calcified arteries (calcium oxalate crystals)
■ renal ultrasound: nephrolithiasis
■ skeletal X-rays: dense bone, 'bone-in-bone' phenomenon, radiolucent metaphyseal bands, pathologic fractures

DIFFERENTIAL DIAGNOSIS
■ causes of secondary oxalosis: renal failure from any cause, gastrointestinal disorders (Crohn's disease, cystic fibrosis, pancreatic

insufficiency, intestinal surgery, alteration in intestinal flora), increased dietary oxalate (e.g., chocolate, TPN in SGA neonates)

MANAGEMENT

What to Do First
- EKG
- assess severity of renal disease
- trial of vitamin B6 (pyridoxine): PHI may respond to pharmacologic doses of vitamin B6
- consider administration of magnesium and citrate (100 mg/kg/d in 4 divided doses) to prevent further crystal formation

General Measures
- high fluid intake (>2 liters/m2/day)
- decrease dietary oxalate
- monitor cardiac function for heart block
- lithotripsy for urolithiasis
- ophthalmology evaluation
- reduce calcium oxalate crystal formation: sodium or potassium citrate 100–150 mg/kg/d

SPECIFIC THERAPY
- vitamin B6 (pyridoxine) in responsive PHI patients (10–40%): start with 3–5 mg/kg with stepwise increase up to 15 mg/kg
- hemodialysis or peritoneal dialysis in anuric patients (temporary measure: dialysis unable to keep pace with endogenous oxalate production)
- liver transplantation +/− kidney transplantation in patients with end-stage renal disease
- kidney transplantation: temporary measure (25% graft 3 year survival)
- liver + kidney transplantation: definitive correction

Side Effects & Contraindications
- operative morbidity and mortality
- immunosuppressive therapy complications

FOLLOW-UP

During Treatment
- monitor blood/urine oxalate during vitamin B6 administration to check responsiveness (NB: response may be gradual and take weeks)

Routine

- monitor renal function regularly (frequency determined on individual basis)

COMPLICATIONS AND PROGNOSIS

Complications

- PHI: recurrent urolithiasis
- end-stage renal disease in nearly all if untreated (50% by age 15 years, 80% by age 30 years)
- recurrent disease in 100% if renal transplant alone (15–25% 3-year graft survival)
- systemic oxalate deposition (e.g., liver, brain not affected)
- pathologic fractures
- cardiac conduction defect: sudden death
- PHII: may have recurrent urolithiasis
- may be asymptomatic

Prognosis

- PHI: end-stage renal disease in 50% by 15 years
- 80% 5 year survival with combined liver/kidney transplant, 70% at 10 years
- 15–25% 3 year survival of graft if kidney only transplant
- reversal of systemic storage in bone, heart, vessels, nerve after liver transplant
- PHII: considered more benign that PHI, but end-stage renal disease may develop (12% of patients 23–50 years)
- outcome of organ transplantation unknown

HYPERPHOSPHATEMIA

SHARON M. MOE, MD

HISTORY & PHYSICAL

History

- Renal failure
- Tumor lysis syndrome
- Rhabdomyolysis

Signs & Symptoms

- Asymptomatic unless hypocalcemia occurs leading to tetany, or with metastatic calcification due to precipitation of insoluble calcium phosphorus complexes and decreased calcitrol synthesis

■ Chronic hyperphosphatemia in renal failure is associated with vascular calcification and increased mortality

TESTS
■ *Basic blood tests*: Serum phosphorus, creatinine

DIFFERENTIAL DIAGNOSIS
■ Renal failure: Hyperphosphatemia occurs almost exclusively with impaired GFR
■ Other rare causes:
  ➤ Increased renal reabsorption: hypoparathyroidism, acromegaly, thyrotoxicosis
  ➤ Massive release from intracellular stores in tumor lysis syndrome, rhabdomyolysis
■ Overdose of vitamin D derivatives, phosphate containing enemas

MANAGEMENT
What to Do First
■ Assess renal function and normalize if possible.

SPECIFIC THERAPY
Indications
■ All hyperphosphatemia should be treated, but treatment is limited.

Treatment options:
■ Acute hyperphosphatemia: intravenous volume repletion with normal saline will enhance renal excretion, add 10 U insulin and 1 ampule D50 to enhance cellular uptake. Best removal is obtained with dialysis but this is limited due to non-extracellular location of phosphorus.
■ Chronic hyperphosphatemia: dietary restriction to 800 mg/day (although very difficult to maintain this diet), phosphate binders with each meal, calcium acetate or carbonate with each meal, sevelamer HCL with each meal, lanthanum carbonate with each meal. Choice of binder is dependent on serum calcium level and tolerability of agent. Number of pills needs to be titrated to oral intake of phosphorus and serum levels. For severe hyperphosphatemia, short-term administration (ideally <1 month) of aluminum hydroxide with each meal may be necessary.
Side effects of phosphate binders include constipation, diarrhea, bloating, nausea, anorexia due to taste of binders. Side effect of

aluminum hydroxide is osteomalacia, and CNS disturbances with long-term use.

FOLLOW-UP

- Serial assessments are required. If due to acute renal failure, patients may become hypophosphatemic with post-obstructive or resolving ATN diuresis.

COMPLICATIONS AND PROGNOSIS

- The primary complication of hyperphosphatemia is extraskeletal calcification, including coronary artery and other vascular calcification with resultant hemodynamic changes. In addition, recent data indicate that hyperphosphatemia (>5.5 mg/dl) is associated with increased mortality in dialysis patients.

HYPERSENSITIVE CAROTID SYNDROME AND SYNCOPE

EDMUND C. KEUNG, MD

HISTORY & PHYSICAL

History

- More commonly in men and in elderly.
- Syncope or presyncope caused by a hypersensitive reflex response to carotid sinus stimulation.
- Tight collar, shaving and sudden head turning.
- Often associated with neck pathology, sinus and AV node dysfunction and coronary artery disease.

Signs & Symptoms

- Near or frank syncope with carotid stimulation.
- Three types of response:
  - cardioinhibitory, 34 to 78% (ventricular asystole from sinus arrest of block)
  - vasodepressor with hypotension, 5–10%
  - mixed type.

TESTS

- Basic Tests
  - 12-lead ECG during carotid sinus massage:
  - Defined as > 3 s asystole for abnormal cardioinhibitory response and a decrease in 30 (with symptoms) or 50 mm Hg (without

symptoms) in systolic pressure for abnormal vasodepressor response.

➤ Abnormal response may occur in normal subjects.

■ Specific Diagnostic Test

  ➤ see above.

DIFFERENTIAL DIAGNOSIS

■ Syncope from other causes

MANAGEMENT

What to Do First

■ No acute intervention.

General Measures

■ Avoidance of maneuvers leading to carotid stimulation.

SPECIFIC THERAPY

■ Dual chamber or ventricular pacemaker implantation, most effective for cardioinhibitory response.

■ Elastic support hose and sodium retaining drugs have some but limited effect for vasodepressor response.

Side Effects & Contraindications

■ Excessive fluid retention with sodium retaining drugs

FOLLOW-UP

■ Monitoring of recurrence of syncope. Pacemaker follow-up after implantation

COMPLICATIONS AND PROGNOSIS

■ Survival related to underlying diseases, not altered by pacemaker implantation.

HYPERTENSION

JOHN R. TEERLINK, MD

HISTORY & PHYSICAL

[see also Chobanian AV, et al. The Seventh Report of the Joint National Committee on Prevention, Detection, Evaluation, and Treatment of High Blood Pressure: the JNC 7 report. JAMA. 2003 May 21;289(19):2560–72; European Society of Hypertension – European Society of Cardiology Guidelines Committee. 2003 European Society of

Hypertension – European Society of Cardiology guidelines for the management of arterial hypertension. J Hypertens. 2003 Jun;21(6):1011–53.]

History

- Over 50 million in US have hypertension (HTN; SBP >140 or DBP >90); 70% aware of disease, 59% treated for HTN, 34% treated to goal of BP < 140/90
- 59 million in US have pre-hypertension (SBP 120–139 or DBP 80–89)
- Incidence increases with age, blacks > whites
- Usual age of onset 25–55 years of age
- Family history of HTN
- Salt intake in context of genetic predisposition
- Patients with HTN at early age or new onset >50 y more likely to have secondary HTN
- Estrogen use (5% women on estrogen have BP > 140/90; more common in women >35 y, = 5 y use, or obese)
- Renal disease

Signs & Symptoms

- Most commonly asymptomatic
- Headache (suboccipital, pulsating)
- Accelerated HTN: somnolence, confusion, visual disturbances, nausea/ vomiting
- Pheochromocytoma: occasional attacks last minutes-hours with nausea/ vomiting, excessive perspiration, palpitations, pallor, tremor, anxiety.
- Primary hyperaldosteronism: generalized weakness, paralysis, paresthesias, polyuria/ nocturia
- Other symptoms related to end organ damage from HTN (i.e. dyspnea, edema with CHF or renal failure)
- Blood pressure (BP): examine both arms (legs, if lower extremity pulses decreased; consider aortic coarctation); orthostasis (pheochromocytoma)
- Osler's sign: palpable brachial/ radial artery with BP cuff above systolic BP
- Retinas: K-W Class = II (poor prognosis; arteriolar narrowing, copper/ silver wire appearance, exudates, hemorrhage, papilledema)
- Heart: loud aortic S2, early systolic ejection click, LV heave, systolic ejection murmur, S4
- Pulses: check timing between upper and lower extremities (aortic coarctation)

TESTS

Basic Blood Tests

- Hemoglobin/ hematocrit
- BUN/ creatinine
- Potassium (hyperaldosteronism)
- Fasting blood sugar (diabetes mellitus, pheochromocytoma)
- Calcium
- Lipids (stratifies risk for atherosclerosis)

Basic Urine Tests

- Urinalysis: hematuria, proteinuria, casts for possible renal disease, urinary albumin excretion or albumin/creatinine ratio

Specific Diagnostic Tests

- Blood pressure measurement: Office, portable, ambulatory
  - Cuff with bladder >80% arm circumference
  - Measure 5 minutes after resting comfortably in chair, >30 minutes after smoking or coffee ingestion
  - Obtain ≥2 BP measurements.
  - Ambulatory BP measurement (ABPM) for patients with variable BP or to address specific management problems, including therapy or "white coat" HTN; correlates better with end-organ injury; awake ABPM >135/85 or asleep >120/75 consistent with HTN
  - Arterial BP monitoring in emergent hypertension (inpatient)
- JNC VII classification (when systolic or diastolic differ, select the greater relative value)
  - Normal <120 and <80
  - Pre-hypertension SBP 120–139 or DBP 80–89
  - HTN-Stage 1 SBP 140–159 or DBP 90–99
  - HTN-Stage 2 SBP ≥160 or DBP ≥100

Other Tests as Appropriate

- ECG: highly specific, less sensitive for LVH; "strain-pattern" associated with poor prognosis
- Echocardiogram: to assess structural heart disease and LV mass
- Renal ultrasound, renal angiography (invasive or non-invasive), abdominal CT/ MRI for secondary HTN
- Plasma renin activity: rarely clinically useful

DIFFERENTIAL DIAGNOSIS

- Essential (or idiopathic) HTN: 95% cases

- "White-coat" HTN: ambulatory or portable BP measurements may assist
- Sleep apnea
- Drug-induced: NSAIDs, COX-2 inhibitors, oral contraceptives, cocaine, amphetamines, sympathomimetics, adrenal steroids, cyclosporine, tacrolimus, erythropoietin, licorice and some chewing tobacco, selected over-the-counter supplements/medications
- Renal disease (especially related to diabetes mellitus)
- Renal vascular HTN: 1–2% of cases
- Primary hyperaldosteronism
- Cushing's syndrome or chronic steroid therapy
- Pheochromocytoma
- Coarctation of the aorta
- Pregnancy-associated
- Acromegaly
- Thyroid or parathyroid disease

MANAGEMENT

What to Do First

- Initial therapy as per JNC VII by classification (without compelling indications; for therapy with compelling indications, see Specific Therapy below):
  - Normal: encourage lifestyle modifications; no antihypertensive drug indicated
  - Prehypertension: treat with lifestyle modifications; no antihypertensive drug indicated
  - HTN-Stage 1: treat with lifestyle modifications; start with single-agent antihypertensive therapy (often thiazide diuretic)
  - HTN-Stage 2: treat with lifestyle modifications; most will require at least two drugs in combination (usually thiazide diuretic and ACE inhibitor or ARB or beta blocker or calcium channel blocker)

General Measures

- Lifestyle modifications important to preventing/reversing HTN and limiting complications
  - Lose weight
  - Dietary Approaches to Stop Hypertension (DASH) eating plan: diet rich in fruits, vegetables, low-fat dairy products; reduce intake of dietary saturated fats and cholesterol
  - Increase aerobic physical activity
  - Reduce sodium intake ($\leq$6 g NaCl/d)

➤ Limit alcohol intake (≤2 drinks/d for men; ≤1 drink/day for women and lighter-weight persons)

➤ Maintain adequate potassium (~90 mmol/d), calcium and magnesium intake

➤ Stop smoking

SPECIFIC THERAPY

■ Initial single-drug therapy: six agent classes recommended (including compelling indications for preferential selection of specific class if not specifically contraindicated):

➤ Diuretics, usually thiazides (heart failure – loop diuretics, isolated systolic hypertension of the elderly – thiazides; high coronary disease risk, diabetes, recurrent stroke prevention)

➤ Beta-blockers (heart failure, post-myocardial infarction, high coronary disease risk, diabetes)

➤ ACE inhibitors (heart failure, post-myocardial infarction, diabetes, chronic kidney disease, recurrent stroke prevention)

➤ Calcium channel blockers (possibly preferred in blacks and elderly; high coronary disease risk, diabetes)

➤ Angiotensin II receptor blockers (heart failure, diabetes, chronic kidney disease)

➤ Aldosterone antagonist (heart failure, post-myocardial infarction)

■ Second-line agents:

➤ Alpha-adrenoreceptor antagonists (ALLHAT discontinued due to increased CHF and stroke in patients treated with doxazosin; may consider in men with prostatism)

➤ Central sympatholytic agents (i.e., clonidine, methyldopa)

➤ Arteriolar vasodilators (i.e., hydralazine, minoxidil)

➤ Peripheral sympatholytic agents (i.e., reserspine)

Indications for Treatment

■ Selection of therapy based on JNC classification and presence of compelling indications, as above

Treatment Options

■ Initiate therapy at low dose unless severe HTN.

■ If the first-line therapy does not meet goals, consider increasing dose or adding low dose of a complementary agent.

■ If no discernable effect of agent at reasonable dose, consider switching to another agent.

■ Multi-drug regimens are often necessary, especially in patients with diabetes or higher SBP.

- Treatment goal generally to BP <140/<90, except in patients at high risk for cardiovascular complications (<130/<85)

Side Effects and Contraindications:
- General info on drug classes, check for more complete prescribing information
- Diuretics: Volume depletion, hypokalemia (hyperkalemia for potassium-sparing agents), hypomagnesemia, gout, worsening blood sugar and lipid profile, rash and erectile dysfunction
  - ➤ Absolute Contraindications: Anuria
  - ➤ Relative Contraindications: Gout, renal insufficiency (potassium-sparing), dyslipidemia (high dose)
- Beta-blockers: use acutely worsens bronchospasm and LV dysfunction (though indicated for CHF), sinus/AV node depression, CNS symptoms (depression, nightmares, excitement, confusion), fatigue, lethargy, impotence, hypotension, increased triglycerides (depression of HDL)
  - ➤ Absolute Contraindications: Severe peripheral vascular disease, severe bronchospastic disease, liver disease (labetalol)
  - ➤ Relative Contraindications: Types I and II diabetes, depression, dyslipidemia, peripheral vascular disease
- ACE inhibitors: Hyperkalemia (especially with Type IV RTA), hypotension, chronic dry cough (causes ~5% to discontinue in blinded trials; should rechallenge later to establish diagnosis), angioedema, dizziness, skin rash, dysgusia (captopril; often resolves spontaneously)
  - ➤ Absolute Contraindications: Any prior angioedema, pregnancy, hyperkalemia, renovascular disease
  - ➤ Relative Contraindications: Renal failure (although ACE inhibitors may improve renal dysfunction)
- Calcium channel blockers: Hypotension, headache, flushing, congestive heart failure, peripheral edema, bradycardia with sinus/AV node depression (especially verapamil and diltiazem), palpitations/reflex tachycardia, constipation (especially verapamil in elderly), GI distress, exacerbate heart failure in patients with systolic dysfunction, possible increase in myocardial infarction in diabetics with renal disease (nisoldipine, amlodipine)
  - ➤ Absolute Contraindications: 2nd/3rd-degree AV block, sick sinus syndrome, systolic dysfunction (perhaps except amlodipine), post-myocardial infarction, hypotension, pulmonary congestion
  - ➤ Relative Contraindications: Impaired liver or renal function

- Angiotensin II receptor blockers: Hyperkalemia (especially with Type IV RTA), hypotension, angioedema (less frequent than ACE inhibitor), dizziness, skin rash (less frequent than ACE inhibitor), hepatotoxicity
  - Absolute Contraindications: Any prior angioedema, pregnancy, hyperkalemia, renovascular disease
  - Relative Contraindications: Renal failure, volume depletion
- Alpha-adrenoreceptor antagonists: Marked hypotension, orthostasis, syncope, palpitations, headache, agitation, somnolence, arrhythmias, ALLHAT discontinued due to increased CHF and stroke in patients treated with doxazosin
  - Absolute Contraindications: Hypotension
  - Relative Contraindications: Impaired liver function
- Central sympatholytic agents: sedation, dry mouth, fatigue, postural hypotension, impotence; rebound hypertension with withdrawal
  - Absolute Contraindications: Depression, liver disease (methyldopa)
  - Relative Contraindications: Coronary artery disease, impaired renal or liver function
- Arteriolar vasodilators: headache, palpitations, reflex tachycardia, fluid retention, GI distress, rash, neutropenia, agranulocytosis, SLE-like syndrome (hydralazine), pericardial effusion and hirsutism (minoxidil)
  - Absolute Contraindications: Pheochromocytoma, pericardial effusion (minoxidil); stenotic valvular disease
  - Relative Contraindications: Impaired renal function, acute MI
- Peripheral sympatholytic agents: mental depression, orthostatic hypotension (especially with guanethedine and guanadrel), sedation, sleep disturbances, fluid retention, nasal congestion, peptic ulcers, diarrhea
  - Absolute Contraindications: Depression, orthostatic hypotension
  - Relative Contraindications: Impaired liver or renal function

FOLLOW-UP

During Treatment
- Every 4–6 weeks during dose titration and regimen adjustment

Routine
- Recommended follow-up as per JNC VII by classification
  - Normal: Recheck in 2 years
  - Pre-hypertension: Recheck in 1 year
  - HTN Stage 1–2: Every 6–12 months, when stable

- Lipid profile: every 12 months
- ECG every 2–4 years depending on baseline abnormalities
- Consider reducing therapy ("step down"), especially in patients with significant improvements in lifestyle

COMPLICATIONS AND PROGNOSIS

- Cardiovascular disease: Left ventricular hypertrophy (2–15% by ECG), Left ventricular systolic dysfunction, heart failure due to systolic and/or diastolic dysfunction, ischemic heart disease and myocardial infarction
- Cerebrovascular disease: Stroke, dementia
- Renal disease: nephrosclerosis, renal failure
- Aortic dissection
- Atherosclerosis and related complications: Myocardial ischemia/infarction, TIAs/stroke, peripheral vascular disease

HYPERTHERMIA

DAVID C. MCGEE, MD and STEPHEN J. RUOSS, MD

HISTORY & PHYSICAL

History

- Excessive heat production: exercise in heat by unacclimatized individuals, drug abuse (cocaine, amphetamines), salicylate intoxication, malignant hyperthermia of anesthesia, neuroleptic malignant syndrome, endocrine disorders (thyrotoxicosis, pheochromocytoma), status epilepticus, generalized tetanus
- Diminished heat dissipation: heat exposure and inappropriate homeostasis (chronic illness, old age, dementia, high humidity, obesity, lack of air-conditioning, no access to fluids); anticholinergic agents, dehydration, autonomic dysfunction, and neuroleptic malignant syndrome
- Disordered temperature regulation: neuroleptic malignant syndrome, CVA, encephalitis, sarcoidosis, granulomatous infections, and trauma
- Infection can accompany any of the above

Signs & Symptoms

- Hyperthermia = core body temperature > 38.5°C; need rectal probe or tympanic membrane thermometer
- Mild to moderate hyperthermia (38.6–40°C): headache, nausea, vomiting, dizziness, weakness, irritability, muscle cramps, diaphoresis

- Severe hyperthermia (>40°C): confusion, delirium, stupor, or coma; hyperpnea and hyperventilation; petechiae from DIC; red urine from rhabdomyolysis
- Heat stroke: temperature >40.6°C with altered mental status and anhidrosis
- Malignant hyperthermia of anesthesia, neuroleptic malignant syndrome: temp often >41°C, muscle rigidity, hypotension, arrhythmias, hypoxia, extrapyramidal abnormalities, altered consciousness
- Heart rate increases by 8 bpm/1°C increase in temperature in young healthy individuals
- Intravascular volume contraction very common

TESTS

Diagnostic Tests
- Check CBC with differential, electrolytes, renal panel, glucose, calcium, coagulation profile, DIC panel, creatinine kinase, LFTs, arterial blood gas, urinalysis, and ECG
- Azotemia, elevated liver, muscle enzymes, hemoconcentration, leukocytosis, thrombocytosis common with temperature 38.6–40°C
- Hypoxia, respiratory alkalosis, metabolic acidosis, hypokalemia, hypernatremia, hypophosphatemia, hypomagnesemia and hypoglycemia occur with temperature >40°C; renal failure, hepatic failure, rhabdomyolysis, and DIC less frequent; rhabdomyolysis more common in exertional hyperthermia
- Lactate elevated in exertional heat stroke; often normal in classical heat stroke

Other Tests as Appropriate
- Screen for drugs of abuse
- Cultures, esp in older patients with preexisting medical conditions
- Malignant hyperthermia of anesthesia: caffeine-halothane contracture test useful for susceptibility screening; formal diagnosis requires muscle biopsy

DIFFERENTIAL DIAGNOSIS
n/a

MANAGEMENT

What to Do First
- Confirm hyperthermia.

■ Move patient to cool environment and promptly initiate treatment; outcome related to time of hyperthermia; improved survival if temperature <38.9°C within 30 min

General Measures

■ Intubate if comatose or depressed protective airway reflexes
■ Rapidly cool patient until <38.9°C, then slow cooling to prevent iatrogenic hypothermia
■ Obtain IV access and place urinary catheter to monitor urine output
■ Volume resuscitation: most patients significantly volume depleted; adequate intravascular volume needed for good peripheral perfusion and success of convective or evaporative cooling
■ Identify predisposing conditions and determine duration and severity of exposure

SPECIFIC THERAPY

Indications

■ Core body temperature >38.5°C, esp in patients with neurologic deficits

Treatment Options

■ Fluid resuscitation:
  ➤ Oral salt-containing solutions for mild hyperthermia only
  ➤ IV fluids for moderate to severe hyperthermia
  ➤ Urine alkalinization for rhabdomyolysis

Cooling Methods

■ Electric fan cooling: for mild hyperthermia only
■ Maximal evaporative cooling: for moderate to severe hyperthermia; mist patient with tepid (helps prevent shivering) water; use electric fan to blow warm air across patient
■ Ice packs at points of major heat transfer (groin, axilla, chest): may speed cooling when combined with maximal evaporative cooling
■ Ice water lavage (gastric and rectal) and cold peritoneal lavage: for severely elevated core temperature; may speed cooling when combined with maximal evaporative cooling
■ Correct hemodynamic and metabolic derangements: oxygen for hypoxemia; mechanical ventilation and PEEP for ARDS; crystalloids and vasopressors for hypotension (focus on fluid resuscitation since alpha-adrenergic agents may slow cooling by exacerbating peripheral vasoconstriction).
■ Diazepam and phenytoin for seizures

- Dantrolene sodium: For malignant hyperthermia of anesthesia or neuroleptic malignant syndrome: repeat dose until symptoms subside or max dose reached, immediate interruption of anesthesia or discontinuation of neuroleptic indicated
- Bromocriptine may be useful in neuroleptic malignant syndrome

Side Effects & Complications
- Shivering and vasoconstriction common: treat with chlorpromazine IM or diazepam IV
- Chlorpromazine can lower seizure threshold
- Dantrolene sodium may cause generalized muscle weakness, sedation and hepatitis
- Aggressive IV fluid replacement can result in pulmonary edema, esp in patients who develop myoglobinuria-induced renal failure or myocardial infarction

Contraindications
- Relative: dantrolene sodium not effective for heat stroke

FOLLOW-UP

During Treatment
- Monitor core temperature continuously; changes in rectal temperature may lag changes in actual core temperature
- Cool as rapidly as possible until temperature <38.9°C

COMPLICATIONS AND PROGNOSIS
- Time to correction of temperature correlates with severity of neurologic injury and residual deficits.
- Febrile seizure in 2 to 4% of children
- Renal failure in 5–25% of patients with severe hyperthermia
- Mortality from severe hyperthermia 10% with treatment and increases to 76% in patients with temperature >41.0°C
- Mortality from malignant hyperthermia of anesthesia and neuroleptic malignant syndrome 8–20% with treatment

---

HYPERTHYROIDISM

LAWRENCE CRAPO, MD, PhD

HISTORY & PHYSICAL

History
- Personal or family history of thyroid disease
- Recent viral illness

- Medications: levothyroxine, triiodothyronine, amiodarone, contrast dye
- Current or recent pregnancy

Signs & Symptoms
- Weight loss, fatigue, heat intolerance
- Anxiety, insomnia, nervousness
- Palpitations, dyspnea at rest or on exertion
- Diarrhea, loose stools, hyperdefecation
- Proptosis, diplopia, eye inflammation, decreased visual acuity
- Neck pain, neck swelling
- Anxiousness, weakness, insomnia
- Tachycardia: regular or irregular, bounding pulses
- Stare, lid lag, exophthalmos, chemosis
- Goiter: diffuse, nodular, tenderness
- Hands: tremor, warm, sweaty, erythema, onycholysis
- Skin: warm, sweaty, smooth, pretibial dermopathy
- BP: increased systolic or pulse pressure
- Hyperreflexia, restlessness

TESTS
- Basic Blood Tests
  - Free T4, TSH
- Specific Diagnostic Tests
  - Total T3, free T3, thyroid antibodies
- Imaging
  - Radioiodine-123 uptake and scan

DIFFERENTIAL DIAGNOSIS
- I-123 uptake increased:
  - Scan diffuse: Graves disease (GD), inappropriate TSH secretion, molar pregnancy
  - Scan patchy: multinodular toxic goiter (MNTG), toxic adenoma (TA)
- I-123 uptake decreased:
  - Subacute thyroiditis: viral (DeQuervain's), lymphocytic (silent, postpartum)
  - Levothyroxine excess:
    - Exogenous: iatrogenic, inadvertent, surreptitious
    - Endogenous: struma ovariae
  - Iodine excess: amiodarone, contrast, miscellaneous
- Other: bulky or metastatic well-differentiated thyroid cancer

MANAGEMENT

What to Do First
- Assess severity by clinical toxicity, extent of free T4 and T3 elevation

General Measures
- Assess for associated disorders such as cardiovascular disease, infections

SPECIFIC THERAPY
- Beta-blockade: propranolol, metoprolol, atenolol: for all causes of symptomatic hyperthyroidism; dose depends on degree of severity
- I-131: useful for uncomplicated GD, MNTG, toxic adenoma of mild to moderate severity
- Propylthiouracil (PTU) or methimazole (MTZ): useful for GD, MNTG, toxic adenoma, esp when complicated by pregnancy, heart disease, or severe illness
- Thyroid surgery: in pregnancy, toxic adenoma, amiodarone-induced hyperthyroidism when other therapies fail
- NSAIDs: for treatment of DeQuervain's thyroiditis, prednisone in severe cases
- Saturated potassium iodide (SSKI): in GD when mild or as adjunct after I-131 treatment, in thyroid storm
- Side Effects
- I-131: hypothyroidism, infrequent radiation thyroiditis, rare thyroid storm
- PTU or MTZ: common allergic reactions such as rash, infrequent agranulocytosis, rare liver toxicity
- Thyroid surgery: hypoparathyroidism, recurrent laryngeal nerve injury, thyroid storm if not euthyroid at time of surgery

FOLLOW-UP

During Treatment
- Initially: assessment of thyroid status q 1–2 mo by clinical exam and serum free T4 or total T3
- Eventually: assessment by exam and serum TSH with free T4

Routine
- Ultimately: annual assessment of thyroid status; if taking PTU or MTZ, obtain CBC if patient develops sore throat or fever to rule out agranulocytosis

COMPLICATIONS AND PROGNOSIS

Complications
- Thyroid storm: rare; requires intensive care
- Hypothyroidism: treated with levothyroxine and occurs in most GD patients treated with I-131
- Agranulocytosis: occurs in 0.3% of patients treated with PTU or MTZ; discontinue drug; treat patient with antibiotics, isolation, and IV G-CSF

Prognosis
- GD: I-131 usually causes hypothyroidism, requiring life-long levothyroxine; permanent cure uncommon (~20%) in U. S. after antithyroid drugs; ~80% require life-long MTZ or PTU
- MNTG and toxic adenoma: usually cured by I-131 or surgery
- Subacute thyroiditis: resolves spontaneously within 3–12 mo

---

HYPERTRIGLYCERIDEMIA

FREDRIC B. KRAEMER, MD

HISTORY & PHYSICAL

History
- diabetes
- obesity
- pancreatitis
- myocardial infarction
- stroke
- peripheral vascular disease
- hypertension
- smoking
- alcohol use
- estrogen or steroid use
- family history of diabetes
- family history of hypertriglyceridemia or hypercholesterolemia
- family history of myocardial infarction
- family history of stroke
- family history of peripheral vascular disease

Signs & Symptoms
- may be asymptomatic

- presentation: nausea, vomiting, abdominal pain
  - ➤ additional symptoms:
    - angina, myocardial infarction, stroke, claudication
  - ➤ signs:
    - eruptive xanthoma, lipemia retinalis, hepatosplenomegaly

TESTS

Laboratory
- basic blood studies:
  - ➤ fasting lipid panel: elevated triglyceride, total cholesterol normal or elevated, HDL cholesterol usually low, LDL cholesterol low, normal or elevated
  - ➤ glucose, HgbA1c
  - ➤ thyroid function tests
- basic urine studies:
  - ➤ proteinuria
- ECG

Specific Diagnostic Tests
- Apolipoprotein E genotype

Imaging
- none

DIFFERENTIAL DIAGNOSIS
- Chylomicronemia (present when triglycerides >1,000 mg/dl)
- Dysbetalipoproteinemia (elevated cholesterol and triglyceride with apolipoprotein E2 genotype)
- Familial combined hyperlipidemia (elevated cholesterol and triglyceride in patient or in various family members)
- Familial hypertriglyceridemia
  - ➤ Secondary causes:
    - Diabetes mellitus
    - Uremia
    - Nephrotic syndrome
    - Alcohol abuse
    - Estrogen use
    - Pregnancy
    - Metabolic stress
    - Glycogen storage disease
    - Dysglobulinemia
    - Lipodystrophy

MANAGEMENT

What to Do First

- Establish whether secondary causes
- Assess cardiovascular risk factors
  - Men ≥45 years
  - Women ≥55 years
  - Family history of premature cardiovascular disease (≤55 in male or ≤65 in female first-degree relative)
  - Current smoking
  - Hypertension
  - Diabetes mellitus
  - HDL cholesterol <40 mg/dl (≥60 mg/dl is a negative risk factor)

General Measures

- Diet: reduce saturated fat (<10%), total fat intake <30% of calories
  - if triglycerides >>1,000 mg/dl reduce total fat intake to 5–15% of calories
- weight loss if indicated
- Regular exercise
- If diabetes mellitus, aggressively manage glucose control
- If alcohol, reduce intake
- If estrogen, reduce dose
- If pancreatitis, NPO and intravenous glucose
- Treatment goals
  - Primary prevention
    - No other cardiovascular risk factors:
      - Triglycerides <500 mg/dl
    - Adults with = 2 other cardiovascular risk factors
- Triglycerides <150 mg/dl
  - Secondary prevention or diabetes mellitus or family history of early cardiovascular disease
    - Triglycerides = <150 mg/dl

SPECIFIC THERAPY

- Fibrates
  - clofibrate, gemfibrozil, fenofibrate, gemfibrozil and fenofibrate preferred
  - usually first line agents due to high incidence of adverse effects with niacin
  - 25–60% reduction in triglycerides, 10% reduction in total cholesterol, LDL cholesterol may increase, not change or decrease, increase HDL cholesterol

➤ 20–30% reduction in cardiovascular events
➤ unclear whether any significant effects on cardiovascular or all cause mortality
■ Niacin
➤ crystalline, time-released
➤ start at low dose and titrate weekly up to therapeutic level
➤ can combine with fibrate
➤ 20–80% reduction in triglycerides, 10–15% reduction in total and LDL cholesterol, increase HDL cholesterol
➤ 20–25% reduction in cardiovascular events
➤ unclear whether any significant effects on cardiovascular or all cause mortality
■ Statins
➤ several available: lovastatin, pravastatin, simvastatin, fluvastatin, atorvastatin, and rosuvastatin
➤ more effective when cholesterol and apolipoprotein B elevated
➤ 10–30% reduction in triglycerides, 15–45% reduction in total cholesterol, 20–60% reduction in LDL cholesterol
➤ 25–40% reduction in cardiovascular mortality
➤ 20–30% reduction in all cause mortality

Side Effects & Contraindications
■ Fibrates
➤ side effects: abdominal pain, nausea, vomiting, cholelithiasis, hepatic dysfunction, myositis (risk increased when combined with statins), potentiate action of oral anticoagulants
➤ contraindications:
➤ relative: renal insufficiency, pregnancy (can be used), breast feeding
■ Niacin
➤ side effects: cutaneous flush, hepatic dysfunction, glucose intolerance, hyperuricemia, skin changes with hyperpigmentation and acanthosis nigracans, increased risk of myositis when combined with statins
➤ contraindications:
➤ relative: peptic ulcer disease, gout, diabetes mellitus
■ Statins
➤ side effects: elevated AST, ALT, myositis
➤ contraindications: pregnancy, breast feeding

FOLLOW-UP
■ Well controlled, stable patients every 6 months
➤ Obtain lipid panel, ALT, AST

■ Uncontrolled patients every 3 months
  ➤ Obtain lipid panel, ALT, AST

COMPLICATIONS AND PROGNOSIS
■ Pancreatitis when triglycerides $\geq$ 1,000 mg/dl
■ Coronary artery disease
■ Peripheral vascular disease
■ Cerebrovascular disease

HYPOCALCEMIA

DOLORES SHOBACK, MD

HISTORY & PHYSICAL
History
■ Previous thyroid, parathyroid, or neck surgery
■ Other autoimmune disorders: adrenal insufficiency, mucocutaneous candidiasis
■ Chronic renal failure
■ Diarrhea, steatorrhea
■ Previous bowel surgery
■ Muscle cramps, tetany, weakness
■ Numbness, circumoral tingling
■ Shortness of breath
■ Laryngospasm
■ Wheezing
■ Seizures
■ Rickets
■ Bone pain
■ Delayed growth, mental retardation, short neck, shortened digits
■ Lack of sunlight
■ Low dietary Ca and vitamin D

Signs & Symptoms
■ Neck scar, + Chvostek's, + Trousseau's signs
■ Carpal-pedal spasm
■ Tetany
■ Dyspnea, stridor, wheezing
■ Seizures
■ Bone pain
■ Muscle weakness
■ Cataracts

- Rachitic deformities
- Albright's hereditary osteodystrophy:
  - Shortened 4th and 5th metacarpal bones
  - Obesity
  - Short stature
  - Round facies

TESTS

Laboratory
- Blood
  - Measure Ca, albumin, ionized Ca, P, PTH, 25-OH vitamin D
  - Hypoparathyroidism: low Ca, high normal or high P, low PTH
  - Vitamin D deficiency: low Ca, low or normal P, high PTH, low 25-OH vitamin D
  - Magnesium depletion: low Mg, low Ca, low PTH, normal P
  - Pseudohypoparathyroidism: low Ca, high or normal P, increased PTH
- Urine
  - Measure Ca and creatinine
  - Vitamin D deficiency: low urine Ca
    - Ellsworth-Howard test
    - Reduced urinary P and cyclic AMP excretion with infusion of PTH in pseudohypoparathyroidism

DIFFERENTIAL DIAGNOSIS
- Hypoparathyroidism: post-surgical, post-radiation, congenital, autoimmune, autosomal dominant hypoparathyroidism (ADH) due to activating calcium receptor mutations
- Vitamin D deficiency: renal failure, poor nutrition, malabsorption, short bowel, cirrhosis
- Pancreatitis
- Pseudohypoparathyroidism
- Hypomagnesemia
- Rhabdomyolysis
- "Hungry bone" syndrome
- Tumor lysis
- Hyperphosphatemia

MANAGEMENT

What to Do First
- Assess severity of symptoms

- Assess integrity of airway
- Parenteral Ca salts for severe or life-threatening symptoms
  - Ca gluconate (90 mg Ca/10 ml)
  - Infuse 2 ampules over 10 to 20 minutes
  - IV Ca infusion: 60 ml in 500 ml D5W (1 mg/ml) – infuse at 0.5–2.0 mg/kg/hr to control symptoms
  - Measure serum total and ionized Ca every 4–6 hours
  - Maintain serum Ca 8–9 mg/dl or ionized Ca approximately 1.0 mM
  - Begin oral Ca supplements and vitamin D as soon as feasible
- If Mg – depleted, replete with Mg salts first

General Measures
- Treat symptoms, not number
- Maintain serum Ca 8.5–9 mg/dl
- Maintain urine Ca ≤300 mg/24 hours

SPECIFIC THERAPY
- Oral Ca supplements
- Add vitamin D metabolites depending on severity and titrate:
  - Ergocalciferol either daily or several times weekly
  - Calcitriol
- Thiazide diuretics as adjunctive therapy to increase Ca reabsorption
- For ADH, only treat if clinical symptoms

FOLLOW-UP
- Monitor symptoms
- Monitor serum Ca frequently during initial titration
- Monitor serum and urine Ca and renal function every 6 months when stable
- In vitamin D deficiency – monitor 25-OH D and PTH levels
- Annual eye exam for cataracts
- Consider abdominal x-ray for nephrocalcinosis in chronic therapy
- Assess bone density if needed

COMPLICATIONS AND PROGNOSIS
- General: hypercalcemia, vitamin D toxicity, renal failure (usually reversible)
- In chronic therapy: cataracts, nephrocalcinosis, and renal stones
- Hypoparathyroidism: lifelong treatment usually indicated
- Vitamin D deficiency: curable but may require lifelong treatment

- Mg depletion: treatment often self-limited
- Pseudohypoparathyroidism: lifelong treatment, may lose bone mass over time

HYPOGLYCEMIA

FREDRIC B. KRAEMER, MD

HISTORY & PHYSICAL

History
- Diabetes or chronic illness, such as liver or renal failure, currently hospitalized, medication use, alcohol, psychiatric problems, history of GI surgery

Signs & Symptoms
- Generally nonspecific, but may include lightheadedness, dizziness, sweating, palpitations, headache, inability to concentrate, confusion, loss of consciousness, seizures
- Occurrence of symptoms in relation to meals often not helpful

TESTS

Laboratory
- Basic blood studies:
  - ➤ low glucose
- Specific Diagnostic Tests
  - ➤ 72-h fast with glucose, insulin, C-peptide, proinsulin values; fast should be halted when patient becomes symptomatic and glucose falls below 55 mg/dL
- Blood for sulfonylureas
- Glucose tolerance tests should not be performed to try to diagnose postprandial hypoglycemia; likewise, glucose meters for nondiabetic patients to monitor glucose levels at home should generally be avoided because of inaccuracy at low glucose values and the high frequency of falsely low readings due to poor technique

Imaging
- Generally not useful for localization of insulinomas, but CT, MRI, endoscopic ultrasound, or selective arteriography can be used

DIFFERENTIAL DIAGNOSIS

- Healthy appearing patient:
  - Drugs (ethanol, salicylates, quinine, insulin or sulfonylureas in diabetic patients)
  - Factitious from insulin or sulfonylureas
  - Alimentary
  - Functional
  - Insulinoma
  - Islet hyperplasia/nesidioblastosis
  - Ketotic hypoglycemia
- Ill-appearing patient:
  - Liver failure
  - Renal failure
  - Sepsis
  - Shock
  - Lactic acidosis
  - Iatrogenic
  - Drugs: pentamidine, quinine; drug-dispensing error
  - Parenteral nutrition and insulin therapy
  - Infant of diabetic mother
  - Glycogen storage disease
  - Galactosemia
  - Hereditary fructose intolerance
  - Carnitine deficiency
  - Defects in amino acid and fatty acid metabolism
  - Reye's syndrome
  - Starvation
  - Anorexia nervosa
  - Hypopituitarism
  - Growth hormone deficiency in infants and children
  - Adrenal insufficiency
  - Large, non-beta cell tumor
  - Autoimmune diseases

MANAGEMENT

What to Do First

- Verify that symptoms occur at a time when hypoglycemia is present and document that the symptoms resolve with correction of the low glucose level
- If a normal glucose is found at the time of symptoms, no further evaluation for hypoglycemia generally is needed

General Measures
- Use history to establish the clinical setting in which symptoms occur, then use diagnostic tests to establish cause
- Occurrence of hypoglycemia in a patient with a known underlying disease known to be associated with hypoglycemia generally requires no further evaluation
- Drugs, including insulin, most common cause in hospitalized patients

SPECIFIC THERAPY
- Symptomatic patient: give oral or IV glucose
- Hypoglycemia secondary to drugs or alcohol: remove inciting agent or adjust dose of insulin or sulfonylurea in diabetic; patients with hypoglycemia due to sulfonylureas may require hospitalization and prolonged IV glucose ($D_{10}W$)
- Factitious hypoglycemia: refer for psychiatric evaluation/care
- Alimentary hypoglycemia: try frequent small meals, avoiding large carbohydrate loads; if persists, oral Dilantin, oral diazoxide, or SC octreotide
- Functional hypoglycemia: try frequent small meals, avoiding large carbohydrate loads; psychiatric counseling/treatment for depression
- Insulinoma: surgical resection; 10% malignant; for nonsurgical cures, oral diazoxide or SC octreotide for control of hypoglycemia, chemotherapy for treatment of tumor
- Ill/hospitalized patients: treatment of underlying condition and supportive care with oral and/or parenteral nutrition
- Hormone deficiencies: replacement of glucocorticoids and/or growth hormone
- Large, non-beta cell tumor: surgical resection and chemotherapy, SC octreotide or growth hormone for control of hypoglycemia
- Autoimmune diseases: glucocorticoids and immunosuppressive agents

Side Effects & Contraindications
- Diazoxide:
  - ➤ Side effects: edema, lanugo hair growth
  - ➤ Contraindications: none
- Octreotide:
  - ➤ Side effects: nausea, vomiting, diarrhea
  - ➤ Contraindications: none

FOLLOW-UP
- Depends on underlying cause
- None usually required for functional hypoglycemia
- For other causes, document correction of hypoglycemia and symptoms, follow-up dictated by underlying disorder

COMPLICATIONS AND PROGNOSIS
- Severe, recurrent hypoglycemia associated with loss of mental function
- Most insulinomas are cured following surgical resection

HYPOGONADISM IN MEN

SHALENDER BHASIN, MD

HISTORY & PHYSICAL

History
- General health problems
- Eating disorder
- Excessive exercise
- Medications: glucocorticoids, ketoconazole, GnRH agonist, cancer chemotherapy, neuroleptics
- Abuse of drugs such as marijuana, cocaine, alcohol, opiates
- Pubertal development
- Frequency of shaving
- Energy and mood
- Sexual desire and activity

Signs & Symptoms
- Height and span, weight
- Hair growth on face, axillae, pubic region
- Escutcheon
- Breast enlargement
- Testicular volume
- Phallic size and location of meatus
- Prostate size
- Sense of smell
- Dysmorphic features (polydactyly, hearing deficit)

TESTS

Laboratory
- CBC, chemistry panel for general evaluation

- Total testosterone level; if <200 ng/dL, androgen deficiency likely; if >400 ng/dL, androgen deficiency unlikely
- Free testosterone by equilibrium dialysis, or bioavailable testosterone by ammonium sulfate precipitation, if total testosterone level is between 200 and 400 ng/dL, particularly in obese or older men and in chronic illness
- Elevated serum LH indicates primary testicular dysfunction; obtain karyotype to rule out Klinefelter syndrome (XXY)
- Prolactin if low testosterone but low or normal LH

Imaging
- MRI of hypothalamic-pituitary region if low testosterone but normal or low LH (hypogonadotropic hypogonadism)
- Bone age in children with delayed pubertal development

Other Tests
- Evaluation of other pituitary hormones in hypogonadotropic hypogonadism

DIFFERENTIAL DIAGNOSIS
- Normal aging
- Obesity
- Erectile dysfunction
- Systemic illness

MANAGEMENT
What to Do First
- High index of suspicion
- Exclude systemic illness, eating disorders, excessive exercise, drug abuse, or medication-induced androgen deficiency
- Confirm diagnosis by proper tests

General Measures
- Diagnose underlying cause
- Counsel patient and partner about risks and benefits
- Evaluate patient for possible contraindications
- Must diagnose and treat androgen deficiency because untreated, it can contribute to osteoporosis, loss of muscle mass and function, impaired sexual function, lowered mood and energy level, increased fat mass, insulin resistance

- Hypogonadism may be manifestation of serious underlying disease: pituitary tumor or HIV infection

SPECIFIC THERAPY

- All testosterone formulations can correct androgen deficiency; various formulations differ in pharmacokinetics
- Initiate testosterone replacement therapy:
  - IM testosterone enanthate or cypionate: inexpensive and effective; results in fluctuating testosterone levels and need for frequent injections
  - Nongenital transdermal systems: easy to use, mimic diurnal rhythm of testosterone secretion; causes skin reactions
  - Scrotal testosterone patch: must shave scrotal skin for good adhesion
  - Testosterone gel: easy to apply; dosing flexibility; potential for transfer of testosterone to female partner or child
- 17-alpha-methyl testosterone should not be used for androgen replacement because of risk of liver toxicity
  - Androgen supplementation contraindications:
    - Prostate or breast cancer
    - Baseline PSA ≥4 ng/mL or a palpable abnormality in prostate without urologic evaluation to rule out prostate cancer
    - Benign prostatic hypertrophy with severe symptoms
    - Baseline hematocrit >52%
    - Severe sleep apnea
- Side Effects
  - Acne, oiliness of skin, breast tenderness, gynecomastia, erythrocytosis, induction or worsening of sleep apnea

FOLLOW-UP

- During testosterone replacement:
  - Measure PSA, perform digital rectal exam, evaluate symptoms of benign prostatic hypertrophy using IPSS or AUA questionnaires at baseline, 3, 6, & 12 mo, then annually
  - Inquire about symptoms of sleep apnea and measure hemoglobin at baseline, 3, 6, & 12 mo, then annually
  - General health evaluation at baseline, then annually

COMPLICATIONS AND PROGNOSIS

- Patients with androgen deficiency need lifelong replacement and monitoring
- Replacement therapy does not adversely affect serum lipids

HYPOKALEMIA

BIFF F. PALMER, MD

HISTORY & PHYSICAL
- clinical setting often helpful in determining etiology
- does patient have significant leukocytosis (>100,000)
- recurrent sudden weakness precipitated by high carbohydrate meal or exercise, symptoms of hyperthyroidism in Asian or Mexican patient
- chronic alcoholic, anorexia nervosa
- diarrhea, laxative abuse
- vomiting/nasogastric suction, diuretic use
- presence or absence of hypertension

TESTS
- measure 24 hour urinary K excretion to determine renal versus extrarenal loss
- if urine K <20 mEq/24h, check stool phenolphthalein to screen for surreptitious laxative abuse
- if hypertensive measure plasma renin and aldosterone
- measure plasma HCO3, Mg++

DIFFERENTIAL DIAGNOSIS
- pseudohypokalemia (WBC >100,000)
- redistribution (can account for transient not chronic hypokalemia)
  - insulin use
  - alkalosis (can only explain minimal declines in plasma K)
  - beta-2 adrenergic stimulants (epinephrine, albuterol inhaler)
  - post-vitamin B(12) for megaloblastic anemia
  - hypothermia
  - familial hypokalemic periodic paralysis (mutation in voltage activated Ca channel)
  - Acquired hypokalemic periodic paralysis with thyrotoxicosis
- extrarenal loss
  - diarrhea, surreptitious laxative use, villous adenoma, excessive sweating (unusual)
- renal loss
  - primary increase in distal Na delivery (normal or low EABV) (UNa >20 mEq/L)
    - increased serum HCO3, increased urine Cl (>20 mEq/L)

- loop or thiazide diuretics, not K sparing diuretics
- Mg++ deficiency
- Bartter's syndrome
- Gitelman's syndrome
- increased serum HCO3, decreased Cl (<20 mEq/L)
  - active vomiting/nasogastric suction
  - penicillins (ticarcillin, carbenicillin)
- decreased serum HCO3, increased urine Cl (>20 mEq/L)
  - metabolic acidosis
  - type I and II RTA
- decreased serum HCO3, decreased urine Cl (<20 mEq/L)
  - ketoacid excretion
- primary increase in mineralocorticoid or mineralocorticoid effect (high EABV, high BP)
  - increased renin, increased aldosterone
    - renal artery stenosis
    - malignant hypertension
    - renin secreting tumor
  - decreased renin, increased aldosterone
    - adrenal adenoma
    - bilateral adrenal hyperplasia
    - glucocorticoid remediable hyperaldosteronism
  - decreased renin, decreased aldosterone
    - Cushing syndrome
    - carbenoxolone
    - licorice or chewing tobacco containing glycyrrhetinic acid
    - 11 beta-hydroxysteroid dehydrogenase deficiency
    - Liddle's syndrome

MANAGEMENT

- history and physical and routine laboratory evaluation will establish etiology in most cases
- initial management depends on etiology and severity of hypokalemia
- redistribution hypokalemia does not require K administration
- poor correlation between serum K and total deficit
  - in general 200–400 mEq K deficit will lower the serum K by 1 mEq/L

SPECIFIC THERAPY

- oral K supplements are indicated for serum K concentrations between 2.5–3.5 mEq/L

- KCl is preferred when hypokalemia is accompanied by metabolic alkalosis
- K citrate or KHCO3 is preferred when accompanied by metabolic acidosis
- intravenous K may be preferred with symptomatic hypokalemia, EKG changes, current use of digoxin, or when the patient cannot take PO
  - K concentration in intravenous solutions should not be >40 mEq/L
  - ECG monitoring is recommended with intravenous K administration
- with more life threatening hypokalemia such as paralysis or ventricular arrhythmias
  - concentration >40 mEq/l and infusion of >40 mEq/L may be indicated
  - such concentrations require access to a central vein,
  - cardiac monitoring absolutely required
- in setting of Mg++ deficiency, correction of Mg++ deficit is required to correct K
- redistribution – self limited
- periodic paralysis – acetazolamide
- type I distal renal tubular acidosis – K citrate
- Bartter's syndrome – KCl, MgCl2, amiloride
- aldosterone producing tumor – surgical removal or spironolactone
- bilateral adrenal hyperplasia – spironolactone
- Liddle's syndrome – amiloride or triamterene
- glucocorticoid remedial hyperaldosteronism – glucocorticoids

FOLLOW-UP
- measure K to ensure replacement therapy is effective
- treat hypertension aggressively when present
  - use caution when using angiotensin converting enzyme inhibitor or angiotensin receptor blocker in setting of oral K or K sparing diuretics

COMPLICATIONS AND PROGNOSIS
- clinical manifestations of hypokalemia often subtle
- hypokalemia can be complicated by:
  - neuromuscular: weakness, fatigue, paralysis
  - gastrointestinal: constipation
  - renal: polyuria, polydipsia (nephrogenic diabetes insipidus)
  - endocrine: glucose intolerance

➤ cardiac: palpitations secondary to ventricular arrhythmia
  • EKG changes: U waves, ST-segment depression, widening, flattening, or inversion of T waves
➤ hypokalemia is generally readily treatable and has good prognosis
➤ some causes of hypokalemia require chronic therapy with oral K and K sparing diuretics
  • spironolactone in high doses can cause gynecomastia

HYPOMAGNESEMIA

STANLEY GOLDFARB, MD

HISTORY & PHYSICAL

History
■ Usually diagnosed with screening lab tests. Symptoms include apathy, depression, some or all facets of delirium, seizures, paresthesias.

Signs & Symptoms
■ Tremor of extremities and tongue, myoclonic jerks, Chvostek sign (common), Trousseau sign (rarely), tetany (rarely unless concomitant hypocalcemia), general muscular weakness (particularly respiratory muscles), coma, vertigo, nystagmus and movement disorders (rarely).

TESTS
Laboratory
Blood Tests:
■ Determining Magnesium Deficiency
■ Only parameter to consistently predict magnesium depletion is retention of >75% of magnesium after a magnesium infusion.
■ A low serum magnesium level is the parameter that prompts therapy.
■ A very low serum value (<1 mg/dl) always indicates significant deficits that require therapy.
■ Other findings:
■ Refractory hypocalcemia responsive only to magnesium therapy
■ Refractory hypokalemia responsive only to magnesium therapy
ECG
■ Increased susceptibility to digoxin-related ventricular arrhythmias: premature ventricular contractions, ventricular tachycardia, torsades de pointes, ventricular fibrillation

DIFFERENTIAL DIAGNOSIS

- Redistribution from extracellular to intracellular fluids:
  - ➤ Insulin administration post therapy of diabetic ketoacidosis, hungry bone syndrome post parathyroidectomy, catecholamine excess states such as ETOH withdrawal syndrome, acute pancreatitis, excessive lactation
- Reduced intake:
  - ➤ Starvation, alcoholism, prolonged postoperative state
- Reduced absorption
  - ➤ Specific GI magnesium malabsorption, generalized malabsorption syndrome, post extensive bowel resections, diffuse bowel disease or injury, chronic diarrhea, laxative abuse
- Extra-renal factors that increase magnesuria
  - ➤ Drug-induced losses: Diuretics, aminoglycosides, digoxin, cisplatinum and cyclosporine.

Hormone-induced magnesuria: Aldosteronism, hypoparathyroidism, hyperthyroidism.

Ion or nutrient-induced tubular losses: Hypercalcemia, extracellular fluid volume expansion.

Miscellaneous causes: Phosphate depletion syndrome, alcohol ingestion.

Hereditary causes of renal losses: Bartter's and Gitelman's syndrome; familial hypomagnesemia with hypercalciuria/nephrocalcinosis (secondary to abnormalities in paracellin)

MANAGEMENT
n/a

SPECIFIC THERAPY

- Calcium ion is a direct antagonist of magnesium and should be given to patients who are seriously ill with life-threatening magnesium intoxication. Administer IV calcium as 100–200 mg of elemental calcium over 5–10 min.
- Hemodialysis may be required following cessation of magnesium therapy.

FOLLOW-UP
n/a

COMPLICATIONS AND PROGNOSIS
n/a

HYPONATREMIA

CHIRAG PARIKH, MD, PhD and TOMAS BERL, MD

HISTORY & PHYSICAL

History
- For etiology of hyponatremia:
  - Assessment of fluid intake
  - Drugs
  - Psychiatric history
  - Nausea, vomiting, diarrhea
  - Heart, liver or kidney disease
  - Hypothyroidism
  - Adrenal insufficiency hypopituitarism

Signs & Symptoms
- Assess volume status
  - Edema, orthostasis, skin turgor, axillary sweat
  - Hyponatremia (seen with acute hyponatremia and Na <125 mEq/L
  - Primarily CNS – lethargy, disorientation, muscle cramps, abnormal sensorium, depressed tendon reflexes, seizures and coma

TESTS
Basic Metabolic Profile, including glucose
- 3 most important tests for differential diagnosis of hyponatremia:
  - Serum osmolality
  - Urine sodium
  - Urine osmolality

Other blood tests for etiology
- TSH
- Serum cortisol
- Serum triglycerides
- Total serum proteins

DIFFERENTIAL DIAGNOSIS
- First, ensure that hyponatremia is not pseudohyponatremia or translocational, which requires no treatment.
- Pseudohyponatremia
  - Associated with normal or high serum osmolality
  - Seen with severe hyperproteinemias and hypertriglyceridemias

➤ Due to flame photometry methods used in many laboratories
➤ Direct (undiluted) ion-specific electrodes are accurate for Na measurements.

■ Translocational Hyponatremia
➤ Associated with high serum osmolality
➤ The osmotically active substance draws the water out of the cells and lowers the serum sodium.
➤ Common causes are uncontrolled diabetes, glycine intoxication (endometrial and prostatic surgeries) and mannitol therapy.
➤ With hyperglycemia, serum sodium falls approximately by 1.6 mEq/L for each 100-mg/dL rise in blood glucose.

■ Hypoosmolar Hyponatremia
➤ Assessment of volume status and urinary Na provides a useful classification.
➤ Hypovolemic hyponatremia and Urine Na <10 mEq/L
  • Vomiting, diarrhea, third-space losses (pancreatitis)
➤ Hypovolemic hyponatremia and Urine Na >20 mEq/L
  • Diuretic, mineralocorticoid deficiency, osmotic diuresis
➤ Euvolemic hyponatremia (Urine Na >20 mEq/L usually)
  • Glucocorticoid deficiency, hypothyroidism, physical or emotional stress, drugs (morphine, nicotine), syndrome of inappropriate antidiuretic hormone secretion (SIADH)
  • SIADH:
  • Associated with hypo-osmolality, a urine osmolality >100 mOsmol/kg, urine sodium concentration that is usually >40 mEq/L, normal acid-base and potassium balance, and frequently a low plasma uric acid concentration
  • Diagnosis of exclusion
  • Some important causes include carcinomas, pulmonary disorders, CNS disorders, AIDS and geriatric patients (idiopathic).
➤ Hypervolemic hyponatremia and Urine Na >20 mEq/L
  • Acute and chronic renal failure
➤ Hypervolemic hyponatremia and Urine Na <10 mEq/L
  • Nephrotic syndrome, cirrhosis, cardiac failure

MANAGEMENT
n/a

SPECIFIC THERAPY
■ Depends on 2 factors: symptoms and duration
■ Acute Symptomatic Hyponatremia
➤ Goal: Increase serum Na until symptoms resolve

➤ Hypertonic saline (3% NaCl)

➤ Furosemide may be used to increase free water excretion.

➤ Frequent monitoring of serum electrolytes is essential.

■ Chronic Symptomatic Hyponatremia

➤ Slow correction

➤ Hypertonic saline (for seizures only) or normal saline with furosemide is used.

➤ Replace sodium, potassium and water losses if excessive.

■ Chronic Asymptomatic Hyponatremia – Euvolemic or unknown cause

➤ a) Treat underlying cause: hypothyroidism, adrenal insufficiency, drugs causing SIADH

➤ If etiology is unclear, the following general measures are recommended:

• Fluid restriction to 0.5–1 L/day (all fluids)

• Increase solute excretion: This will improve free water excretion – Urea (30–60 g/day), NaCl (2–3 g/day) with furosemide are options to increase solute excretion.

• Drugs: Demeclocycline agent of choice. Lithium not used.

• Newer agents: V2 receptor antagonists increase selective water excretion in cirrhosis, heart failure and SIADH

■ Hypovolemic Hyponatremia

➤ Restore ECF volume (crystalloids and colloids).

➤ Replace potassium.

➤ Stop diuretics.

■ Hypervolemic hyponatremia:

➤ Marker of poor prognosis

➤ Needs attention to underlying disorder

➤ Difficult to treat

➤ V2 antagonist may be helpful.

➤ Fluid and Na restriction is the mainstay of therapy.

➤ Loop diuretics (or change from HCTZ to loop diuretic) usually needed

➤ ACE inhibitors required in cardiac failure and nephrotic syndrome

FOLLOW-UP

n/a

COMPLICATIONS AND PROGNOSIS

■ Due to hyponatremia

➤ Cerebral edema caused by acute severe fall in serum Na
➤ Patient may develop seizures or go into coma.
➤ Usually seen in postoperative patients
➤ Premenopausal women are particularly susceptible.
➤ Rapid treatment of hyponatremia is needed.
■ Due to therapy
➤ Osmotic demyelination (also known as central pontine myelinolysis)
➤ Seen with excessive correction of Na (>12 mEq /24 hrs) in chronic hyponatremia
➤ Alcoholics, burn victims and severely hypokalemic patients are very susceptible to this syndrome.
➤ Prevented by gentle correction of serum Na (up to 12 mEq/L/day) in chronic hyponatremia

---

HYPOPHOSPHATEMIA

SHARON M. MOE, MD

HISTORY & PHYSICAL

History

■ Observed in 10% of hospitalized alcoholics
■ Gastrointestinal disorders, diarrhea, recent severe illness, weight change
■ Diabetic ketoacidosis
■ Critical illness/ventilated – observed in 3% of all hospitalized patients, up to 70% of ICU patients on TPN
■ New medications, renal transplant

Signs & Symptoms

■ Usually only present if phosphorus <1 mg/dl, or occasionally <2.5 mg/dl if chronic loss
■ Skeletal muscle: weakness, respiratory failure, rhabdomyolysis
■ CNS: seizures, delirium, coma, paresthesias, encephalopathy
■ Cardiac: cardiomyopathy, CHF
■ Hematopoeitic: RBC hemolysis, thrombocytopenia, hemorrhage, WBC dysfunction
■ Bone: osteomalacia/rickets
■ Renal: decreased GFR, tubular abnormalities, insulin resistance

TESTS

- Low serum phosphorus does not necessarily indicate total body depletion as only 1% of body phosphorus is in blood.
- *Basic blood tests*: Serum phosphorus: (moderate = serum phosph <2.5 mg/dl; severe <1.0 mg/dl)
- *Basic urine tests*: Diagnosis based on history, trend in phosphorus values and blood pH (to distinguish acute shift), and urine phosphorus (<100 mg/day = GI loss or shift)
- *Other tests*: If urine phosphorus >100 mg/day, measure 24-h urine for glucose, amino acids for Fanconi's syndrome, and serum calcium (high in primary hyperparathyroidism, low in vitamin D-resistant rickets)

DIFFERENTIAL DIAGNOSIS

- Hypophosphatemia occurs because of 1) decreased intestinal absorption, 2) increased urinary losses, and/or 3) extracellular to intracellular shift. Severe hypophosphatemia is usually due to combination of factors.
- Decreased intestinal absorption: antacid abuse, malabsorption, chronic diarrhea, vitamin D deficiency, starvation, anorexia, alcoholism
- Increased urinary losses: primary hyperparathyroidism, post renal transplant, extracellular fluid volume expansion, glucosuria (after treating DKA), post obstructive or resolving ATN diuresis, acetazolamide, Fanconi's syndrome, X-linked and vitamin D-dependent rickets, oncogenic osteomalacia due to circulating phosphatonins
- Redistribution: respiratory alkalosis, alcohol withdrawal, severe burns, TPN, recovery from malnutrition when inadequate phosph is provided (post feeding syndrome), leukemic blast crisis

MANAGEMENT

What to Do First

- Assess severity and symptoms so as not to overtreat hypophosphatemia due to cellular shifts.

General Measures

- If possible, treat orally to avoid metastatic calcification.

SPECIFIC THERAPY

- *Indications*: Only treat symptomatic severe hypophosphatemia with intravenous agents. Otherwise choose oral agent. Phosph comes as

Naphosph or Kphosph; choice dictated by other illnesses such as heart or renal failure.

- *Goal of therapy*: provide 1,000 mg (32 mM)/day of elemental phosphorus with max of 3,000 mg/day
- *Oral*: skim milk (1,000 mg/quart), whole milk (850 mg/quart), Neutraphosph K capsules, Neutraphosph solution
- *Intravenous*: Kphosphate, Na phosphate. Do not exceed 2 mg phosphorus/kg body weight q6h to avoid metastatic calcification.
- *In hyperalimentation:* To avoid refeeding syndrome, make sure have 450 mg phosphorus for each 1,000 kcal infused
- *Side effects* include diarrhea, hyperphosphatemia, hypocalcemia, and hyperkalemia (with Kphosph preparations)

FOLLOW-UP

- Measure phosphorus levels as trough values for oral replacement. Frequent measurement of phosphorus and calcium levels should be done with IV therapy to avoid toxicity, but peak levels may be false-positive indicator of actual body stores.

COMPLICATIONS AND PROGNOSIS

- Prognosis is good with therapy.

HYPOPITUITARISM

ANDREW R. HOFFMAN, MD

HISTORY & PHYSICAL

History

- Weakness, weight loss
- Infertility
- Amenorrhea or oligoamenorrhea
- Postpartum hemorrhage, recent pregnancy
- Autoimmune disease
- History of pituitary tumor, surgery, apoplexy, or irradiation
- History of traumatic brain injury
- CNS irradiation
- Head trauma
- Craniopharyngioma, dysgerminoma
- Metastatic breast and lung cancer
- Histiocytosis X, sarcoidosis, TB
- Absent or delayed puberty

Signs & Symptoms
- Fatigue, lethargy
- Headache, cachexia
- Altered mental status, coma
- Cold intolerance
- Constipation
- Diminished pubic, axillary hair
- Inability to lactate
- Increased adiposity, decreased lean tissue
- Orthostatic hypotension
- Polydipsia, polyuria, nocturia
- Impotence
- Decreased libido
- Hypoglycemia
- Dry, pale, wrinkled skin
- Visual field defect

TESTS

Laboratory
- Basic blood studies:
  - LH, FSH, prolactin, free T4, TSH, testosterone
  - Cortisol after Cosyntropin or insulin tolerance test
  - Electrolytes, glucose
  - Urinalysis
  - Insulin-like growth factor-I (IGF-I)
  - Growth hormone (GH)
- Ancillary blood test: estradiol

Imaging
- MRI of pituitary and brain

DIFFERENTIAL DIAGNOSIS
- Pituitary tumor: nonsecretory, prolactinoma, acromegaly, Cushing syndrome;
  - Usually causes partial or complete anterior pituitary insufficiency
  - Most common deficiencies: GH > LH, FSH > TSH, ACTH
- Pituitary apoplexy
- Hypothalamic mass: craniopharyngioma, dysgerminoma, metastases
  - Usually causes diabetes insipidus

- Granulomatous disease and histiocytosis: may cause anterior and posterior pituitary deficiency

MANAGEMENT

What to Do First

- Determine hormone deficiencies (partial or panhypopituitarism) and excesses
- Assess size/resectability of tumor
- Rule out apoplexy

SPECIFIC THERAPY

- Hormone replacement therapy:
  - ➤ Cortisol
  - ➤ Thyroid hormone
  - ➤ DDAVP
  - ➤ Testosterone
  - ➤ Estrogen/progestin
  - ➤ Growth hormone
  - ➤ Gonadotropins for fertility only
  - ➤ Restoration of libido and potency
- Normalize prolactin, ACTH, or GH hypersecretion
- Surgical resection of tumor
- Medical therapy for prolactinoma and acromegaly
- Radiation therapy
- Treat granulomatous diseases
- Observation with repeated pituitary MRI to determine if tumor is growing

Treatment Goals

- Treat hormone deficiencies and excesses
- Resect or diminish size of pituitary or CNS mass

Side Effects & Contraindications

- Surgery and radiation: panhypopituitarism, CNS injury

FOLLOW-UP

- Assess adequacy of hormone replacement therapy every 6–12 months
- Repeat pituitary MRI in 3–6 mo to assess tumor growth

COMPLICATIONS AND PROGNOSIS

- Pituitary apoplexy
- Visual field changes
- Patients require lifelong observation

HYPOTHERMIA

DAVID C. McGEE, MD and STEPHEN J. RUOSS, MD

HISTORY & PHYSICAL

History

- Exposure to cold; wind chill magnifies thermal losses
- Debilitated, elderly, young, alcoholism, psychiatric illness
- Trauma, overdose, and CVAs may mask or amplify hypothermia

Signs & Symptoms

- Hypothermia = core temperature 35°C; need low-reading rectal probe or esophageal thermometer
- Mild hypothermia (34–35°C): apathy, uncooperative, flat affect, shivers, chills, stiff joints, dizziness, nausea, hunger, pruritus; tachycardia secondary to catecholamine release
- Moderate hypothermia (30–33°C): slurred speech, loss of coordination, ataxia, progressively depressed level of consciousness, coma; no shivering <32°C; high urine output secondary to cold diuresis
- Severe hypothermia (<30°C): bradycardia, dilated, sluggish pupils, stiffness and rigor mortis; high urine output secondary to cold diuresis; loss of plantar responses (<25°C)

TESTS

Diagnostic Tests

- CBC with differential, electrolytes, renal panel, glucose, calcium, magnesium, amylase, lipase, coagulation profile, arterial blood gas, ECG, toxicology screen, CXR
- Acidosis, hypokalemia, and hyperkalemia common; hypoglycemia (depletion of glycogen stores) and hyperglycemia (inactivation of insulin) occur. Do NOT treat hyperglycemia because rebound hypoglycemia common during rewarming
- ECG shows sinus bradycardia and QT prolongation; Osborn waves (J-point elevation) seen best in leads II and V6; arrhythmia risk increases at <32°C; asystole or silent ECG can occur at temperature <30°C
- EEG flat at temperature <18°C

Other Tests as Appropriate

- Cultures, esp in older patients with preexisting medical conditions
- Cervical spine series when trauma suspected

DIFFERENTIAL DIAGNOSIS

n/a

MANAGEMENT

What to Do First

■ Confirm hypothermia

■ Move patient to warm environment; replace wet clothing with clean, dry insulating material

■ Asystole NOT equivalent to death in cold patient; aggressive treatment indicated

General Measures

■ Avoid rough handling; do not place pulmonary artery catheters because myocardium very irritable; high risk for ventricular fibrillation

■ Intubate if comatose or depressed protective airway reflexes

■ Obtain IV access, monitor on telemetry, and place urinary catheter to monitor output

■ Resuscitate with D-5 normal saline; most patients volume depleted from cold-induced diuresis and third spacing

■ Identify predisposing conditions and determine duration and severity of exposure

SPECIFIC THERAPY

Treatment Options

■ Altered mental status: D-50, naloxone, thiamine

■ Passive external rewarming (for mild hypothermia that developed over days): cover patient with insulating material (eg, aluminized coverings) to prevent further heat loss; rate of temperature rise 0.3–2.0°C/h

■ Active external rewarming (for mild hypothermia that developed acutely: apply heat (hot packs, warm blankets, plumed garments, or radiant heaters with temperature 40–45°C) to skin on patient's trunk; immersion in 40°C water bath another option; usually combined with active core rewarming

■ Active core rewarming (for moderate to severe hypothermia):
  ➢ First-line treatment: heated oxygen (45°C) delivered through a cascade humidifier; raises temperature 1–2°C/h

■ Cardiopulmonary bypass most effective technique, esp in patients with cardiac arrest or unstable arrhythmias; raises temperature 1°C q 5 to 10 min

- Heated IV fluids (40–43°C) usually not effective, but helps prevent further cooling
- Heated GI and bladder irrigation not very effective because of limited surface area; reserved for patients with cardiovascular collapse
- Peritoneal dialysis with heated (40–45°C) dialysate effective; leave fluid in place for 15 min then drain off; raises temperature 2°C/h; reserved for patients with cardiovascular collapse
- Open and closed thoracic lavage effective, but invasive; requires two chest tubes; infuse heated (40–42°C) normal saline into one and remove through other
- Hemodialysis useful if IV access and equipment available
- Cardiac arrest requires CPR AND rapid rewarming; defibrillation not reliable at core temperature <32°C; defibrillate ×1 while patient hypothermic; if unsuccessful, continue CPR and resuscitation until patient rewarmed, then attempt defibrillation
- Bretylium IV: only antiarrhythmic drug effective for ventricular fibrillation in setting of hypothermia
- Consider antibiotics

Side Effects and Complications
- Active external rewarming may cause peripheral vasodilation and core temperature drop when cold blood from peripheries returns to central circulation; can cause acidosis and shock
- In severe hypothermia, rigor mortis, lividity, or fixed dilated pupils are NOT reliable indicators of death; CPR should NOT be withheld; delay in instituting CPR in field NOT contraindication to full resuscitation
- Peritoneal dialysis can result in DIC and intraabdominal hemorrhage and can exacerbate hypokalemia
- Open and closed thoracic lavage can induce ventricular fibrillation
- Cardiopulmonary bypass can cause bleeding, air embolization, pulmonary edema, and DIC; third spacing common and requires aggressive volume replacement

Contraindications
- Avoid procainamide, which increases temperature necessary to defibrillate successfully and may precipitate ventricular fibrillation
- Avoid pulmonary artery catheterization, which may precipitate ventricular fibrillation
- Avoid Ringer's lactate solution because cold liver metabolizes lactate poorly

FOLLOW-UP

During Treatment
- Monitor core temperature continuously
- Monitor for electrolyte abnormalities and hypoglycemia
- Goal for rewarming is 0.5–2.0°C/h

COMPLICATIONS AND PROGNOSIS

- Assess for frostbite and other cold injuries
- Prognosis good if rewarming achieved
- Neurologic deficits can be long-standing, but degree of deficit NOT predicted by degree of hypothermia

HYPOTHYROIDISM

LAWRENCE CRAPO MD, PhD

HISTORY & PHYSICAL

History
- Thyroid surgery
- Family history of thyroid disease
- I-131 treatment
- Therapeutic irradiation of the neck or thorax (mantle)
- Iodine excess: amiodarone, contrast, kelp, cough syrup
- Medications: lithium
- Iodine deficiency
- Pregnancy: recent, complicated

Signs & Symptoms
- Weight gain, cold intolerance, tiredness, fatigue, depression
- Neck enlargement
- Dry, puffy, yellowish skin
- Thin, brittle hair; alopecia
- Constipation, abdominal pain
- Sluggish, tiredness
- Bradycardia, hypothermia
- Delayed deep tendon reflexes, proximal muscle weakness, myalgias, cramps
- Puffiness of face and extremities
- Goiter

TESTS

Laboratory
- Basic blood tests: free T4, TSH
- Specific Diagnostic Tests
  - Anti-TPO antibody, antithyroglobulin antibody, lipid panel, CPK, sodium

Imaging
- MRI of pituitary region if free T4 low and TSH low or normal
- I-123 uptake and scan not needed

DIFFERENTIAL DIAGNOSIS
- Primary hypothyroidism (low T4, high TSH):
  - Hashimoto disease
  - Subacute thyroiditis: viral, silent, postpartum
  - Status postthyroidectomy or I-131 therapy
  - Goitrogen induced: lithium, PTU, MTZ
  - Iodine induced: amiodarone, contrast, kelp
  - Rare causes: iodine deficiency, Riedel struma, enzyme defect
- Secondary hypothyroidism (low T4, low or normal TSH):
  - Pituitary or hypothalamic tumors
  - Status postpituitary or hypothalamic surgery
  - Granulomatous diseases
  - Postpartum necrosis
  - Other pituitary and hypothalamic disorders

MANAGEMENT

What to Do First
- Assess degree of severity using clinical presentation, extent of free T4 lowering or TSH elevation

General Measures
- Assess for associated disorders, hypothermia, hyponatremia, mental status, hypoventilation

SPECIFIC THERAPY
- Levothyroxine: full dose of 1.6 mcg/kg in myxedema coma and young patients without ischemic heart disease; low dose in elderly patients and those with ischemic heart disease; take fasting, because absorption inhibited by food and drugs (iron, calcium, fiber); increased dose usually required during pregnancy

- Hydrocortisone: use if secondary hypothyroidism or myxedema coma present
- Avoid excessive sedative drugs and fluids to decrease possibility of hyponatremia and coma
- Passive warming if hypothermia present

FOLLOW-UP

During Treatment

- Assess thyroid status q 6–8 wks by clinical exam and serum free T4 or TSH

Routine

- Annual assessment of thyroid status with free T4 or TSH

COMPLICATIONS AND PROGNOSIS

Complications

- Myxedema coma: rare and requires intensive care
- Ischemic heart disease may be worsened by levothyroxine
- Levothyroxine alone may precipitate adrenal crisis in secondary hypothyroidism if concomitant secondary hypoadrenalism present
- Hyponatremia may result from poor free water clearance

Prognosis

- Myxedema coma: up to 50% mortality
- Euthyroid state easily achieved except when ischemic heart disease present

ICHTHYOSIS

MOISE L. LEVY, MD

HISTORY & PHYSICAL

History

- Onset in adulthood – ichthyosis with onset in childhood is generally an entirely different disorder (see differential diagnosis)
- Acquired ichthyosis is commonly a cutaneous marker for various chronic and malignant diseases, so history of concomitant disorder should be elicited
  - ➢ Common malignancies associated with acquired ichthyosis

- Hodgkin's disease (MOST COMMON), other lymphoproliferative disorders
- Leukemia
- Kaposi's sarcoma
- Carcinoma of breast, lung, or cervix
- Common systemic diseases associated with ichthyosis
  - AIDS (MOST COMMON)
  - Sarcoidosis
  - Endocrinopathies – hyperparathyroidism, hypothyroidism, hypopituitarism
  - Chronic renal disease
- Acquired ichthyosis may also be caused by several drugs:
  - Cimetidine
  - Allopurinol
  - Niacin
  - Clofazamine

Signs & Symptoms

- Mild generalized hyperkeratosis characterized by small white to brown scales with free edges
- Usually found on the trunk and extensor surfaces of the limbs
- Palms and soles are usually spared
- Affected skin may be pruritic
- Skin tends to be worse in cold, dry weather and better in warm, humid areas.

TESTS

- The diagnosis of ichthyosis is generally made by clinical findings; however, skin biopsy may prove useful; genetic testing is available for some of the inherited forms of ichthyosis.

DIFFERENTIAL DIAGNOSIS

- Xerosis (normally distinguished from ichthyosis by clinical findings – e.g., patchy distribution, lack of ichthyotic scale)
- Asteatotic dermatitis (normally distinguished from ichthyosis by clinical findings – e.g., patchy distribution of inflammation)
- Widespread epidermal dermatophytosis (distinguished from ichthyosis by visualization of hyphae in KOH preparation and positive culture)
- Hereditary ichthyosiform dermatoses

> These ichthyoses generally manifest themselves at birth or very shortly thereafter (except ichthyosis vulgaris, which has an age of onset at 3–12 months).
  • Ichthyosis vulgaris
■ MOST COMMON form of inherited ichthyosis
■ autosomal dominant disorder that appears similar to acquired ichthyosis
■ diagnosis made by clinical findings
  > Recessive X-linked ichthyosis
■ involves flexural surfaces as well as trunk and extremities
■ associated with corneal opacities in adults
■ tests of steroid sulfatase activity and levels of cholesterol sulfate aid in diagnosis
  > Epidermolytic hyperkeratosis
■ autosomal dominant disorder characterized by erythematous, scaly plaques, thick ichthyotic scale, and bullae
■ blistering with secondary infection is common
■ skin biopsy and keratin gene studies will confirm diagnosis
  > Lamellar ichthyosis
■ autosomal recessive disorder that presents as large plate-like scales over the entire body
■ presents at birth as collodion baby (i.e., child is born encased in transparent, parchment-like membrane)
■ diagnosis usually made by clinical findings, though testing for keratinocyte transglutaminase-1 (TGM-1) mutations is available
  > Congenital ichthyosiform erythroderma
    • autosomal recessive disorder that presents at birth with collodion membrane
    • clinically presents with widespread varying erythroderma and fine white scale
    • diagnosis made by clinical appearance; testing for TGM-1 mutations (seen in some cases), as well as ALOX12B or ALOXE3 (lipoxygenase genes) mutations may be pursued

MANAGEMENT

What to Do First

■ Determine the underlying disorder. Acquired ichthyosis normally appears after the manifestations of the disease associated with it; therefore, acquired ichthyosis is rarely the sole manifestation of a significant underlying disease.

- If inherited ichthyosis is considered, careful family history is required.

General Measures
- Several treatments may improve the patient's symptoms, but therapy of the underlying disorder is essential.

SPECIFIC THERAPY

Treatment Options
- Emollients (e.g., hydrated petrolatum) are the mainstay of therapy; these agents should be applied liberally and frequently during the day.
  - ➤ Long baths followed by application of emollients are recommended to hydrate the skin and prevent subsequent transepidermal water loss.
- Keratolytic agents may be used in addition to emollients.
  - ➤ 40–60% propylene glycol in water applied h.s. after bath with occlusion can be performed weekly to enhance removal of excess scale.
  - ➤ Alpha hydroxy acids (lactic, citric, glycolic) can also be used.
  - ➤ Salicylic acid 5–10% in petrolatum
- Retinoids
  - ➤ Topical retinoids
  - ➤ Systemic retinoids may be useful for severe congenital forms of ichthyosis.
- Humidifying the home can improve symptoms as well.

FOLLOW-UP
- Frequency of follow-up and studies to be done are generally dictated by the underlying disease.

COMPLICATIONS AND PROGNOSIS

Complications
- Complications of acquired ichthyosis are infrequent; extremely vigorous scratching may lead to erosions and/or ulcerations and risk of secondary infection; dehydration and electrolyte abnormalities can occur in neonates with inherited forms of ichthyosis.

Prognosis
- Treatment of acquired ichthyosis can significantly improve symptoms but will not cure the disorder.
- Long-term prognosis is directly related to underlying disorder.
- Congenital ichthyoses are life-long disorders.

IDIOPATHIC (IMMUNE) THROMBOCYTOPENIC PURPURA (ITP)

MORTIMER PONCZ, MD and MICHELE LAMBERT, MD

HISTORY & PHYSICAL

- Peak age: 2–4 years old; >10 years old more likely to have chronic ITP.
- Males and females equally affected in childhood ITP; females predominate 3:1 in adult ITP.
- Sudden onset of bruising, petechiae, epistaxis, oral mucosal bleeding
- More rarely, menorrhagia, hematuria, GI bleed, intracranial hemorrhage in an otherwise healthy child
- Often preceding viral illness (could be diarrheal) or immunization 1–3 weeks prior to presentation
- Can complicate HIV infection
- Medication history: aspirin, sulfonamides, heparin, quinidine, anticonvulsants
- Hemolytic anemia: jaundice, dark brown urine, pallor (if blood lost or Evan's syndrome and not ITP)

TESTS

- CBC, reticulocyte count, PT, PTT
- Review peripheral smear for platelet size and number, WBC morphology, RBC fragments, spherocytes.
- Coombs/direct antiglobulin test: rule out hemolytic anemia component associated with Evan's syndrome
- ANA in the older child, especially girls; can be presentation for SLE
- Blood type if intravenous anti-Rh(D) immunoglobulin treatment considered
- Bone marrow aspiration: not required for diagnosis but may be done prior to steroid use. Many now feel if there is good initial response to immune modulation (IVIG or anti-Rh(D), this is sufficient for diagnosis; normal or increased numbers of megakaryocytes in ITP; increased erythropoiesis if hemolytic component present; no leukemia or tumor clumps.
- Low thrombopoietin levels (not measured in straightforward cases)
- Elevated platelet-associated IgG (not measured in straightforward cases)
- Iron deficiency possible if prolonged bleeding

DIFFERENTIAL DIAGNOSIS

- Leukemia, tumor infiltration of bone marrow, aplastic anemia, but ITP is the most likely diagnosis if platelets <20,000/mm^3 and all other cell lines are normal.
- Drug-induced thrombocytopenia
- HIV
- Evan's syndrome with positive Coombs
- TTP, HUS: microangiopathic changes on peripheral smear
- Congenital quantitative platelet disorder. TAR (thrombocytopenia with absent radii) syndrome or, more likely if moderate thrombocytopenia, MHY9-associated thrombocytopenia (May-Hegglin anomaly)
- Wiskott-Aldrich syndrome: male infant with isolated thrombocytopenia, microplatelets, eczema, recurrent infections

MANAGEMENT

- No aspirin
- Avoid intramuscular injections.
- Head injury precautions, no contact sports, parental education on controlling nosebleeds
- Hospitalization if mucocutaneous bleeding, life-threatening bleeding, parents unable to restrict child's activity
- Consider no therapy in platelet count >10,000/mm^3 and only minor bruising with emphasis on education about head trauma.
- Treatment for patients with extensive mucocutaneous bleeding, life-threatening bleeding (treatment does NOT decrease the duration of the disease)
    - ➤ IVIG: side effects include severe headache, aseptic meningitis, anaphylaxis (especially in IgA deficiency)
    - ➤ Corticosteroids: orally (for 1–2 weeks); some experts recommend bone marrow examination prior to steroid use, especially in the setting of poor response to initial therapy
    - ➤ IV anti-Rh(D) immunoglobulin if patient's blood type is Rh(D) – positive. Rarely, renal failure secondary to severe intravascular hemolysis and hemoglobinuria can occur. Also, recent reports in adults have associated life-threatening DIC after treatment with IV anti-Rh(D) for ITP.
    - ➤ Splenectomy for patients with life-threatening bleeding or chronic ITP. Pneumovax and penicillin coverage post-operatively.
    - ➤ Vinca alkaloids: vincristine, vinblastine IV weekly for 4 weeks. Side effects include peripheral neuropathy and abdominal and jaw pain.

➤ Danazol androgen: orally for 2–3 months; side effects include acne, hirsutism, weight gain, liver toxicity

➤ Azathioprine: used in other autoimmune disorders; side effects include neutropenia

➤ Cyclophosphamide: orally for 2–10 weeks or IV q 3 weeks; side effects include bone marrow suppression, alopecia, liver toxicity, hemorrhagic cystitis, secondary leukemia

- Rituximab: weekly for 3–6 weeks in steroid-dependent cases instead of splenectomy in more chronic ITP or in Evan's syndrome. Monoclonal anti-CD20 antibody. Side effects include anaphylaxis, life-threatening mucocutaneous syndrome. Give only by slow iv infusion.

- Thrombopoietin mimetics may become a therapeutic option in the near future as clinical trials support efficacy in ITP.

SPECIFIC THERAPY
n/a

FOLLOW-UP
n/a

COMPLICATIONS AND PROGNOSIS
■ Acute ITP: about 90% of children recover within 6 months with or without therapy; <1% intracranial hemorrhage
■ Chronic ITP: thrombocytopenia of >6 months; accounts for 10% of childhood ITP; may later develop other chronic autoimmune disorder (e.g., SLE)

IMMUNE HEMOLYTIC ANEMIA

CHRISTINE CSERTI, MD; FRANK J. STROBL, MD; and LESLIE SILBERSTEIN, MD

HISTORY & PHYSICAL

Etiology
■ encompasses several autoantibody- and alloantibody-mediated disorders that result in accelerated red blood cell destruction
■ autoantibodies: warm autoimmune hemolytic anemia (WAHA), cold autoimmune hemolytic anemia (CAHA), paroxysmal cold hemoglobinuria (PCH), mixed-type (warm and cold reactive antibody induced) autoimmune hemolytic anemia (MTHA), drug-induced hemolytic anemia (DIHA)

- alloantibodies: acute and delayed hemolytic transfusion reactions, post-transplant hemolysis, and hemolytic disease of the newborn
- generation of autoantibodies is either a primary/idiopathic event or secondary to lymphoproliferative disorders (e.g., chronic lymphocytic leukemia, non-Hodgkin's and Hodgkin's lymphoma), connective tissue disorders (e.g., SLE), infections (e.g., Mycoplasma pneumonia, infectious mononucleosis, tertiary syphilis), or drugs
- generation of alloantibodies is naturally occurring or secondary to transfusion, pregnancy, or hematopoietic/solid-organ transplants
- binding of antibodies to endogenous red blood cells or to transfused red blood cells results in extravascular and/or intravascular hemolysis
- extravascular hemolysis: antibody (IgG)-coated or complement (c3b/c3bi) – coated red blood cells are phagocytosed by splenic/hepatic macrophages; predominates in WAHA, DIHA, delayed hemolytic transfusion reactions, post-transplant hemolysis and hemolytic disease of the newborn
- intravascular hemolysis: antibody (IgM/IgG)-induced complement fixation leads to phagocyte-independent lysis; predominates in CAHA and acute hemolytic transfusion reactions

History
- WAHA
- incidence 1 to 2 per 100,000 population; most common (65%) autoimmune hemolytic anemia
- more common in elderly and females
- associated with connective tissue and lymphoproliferative disorders
- CAHA
- accounts for approximately 25% of autoimmune hemolytic anemias
- acute form seen in adolescents/adults following Mycoplasma pneumoniae infection or infectious mononucleosis
- chronic form seen in elderly idiopathically or associated with lymphoproliferative disorders
- PCH
- rarest form of autoimmune hemolytic anemia
- in children a self-limited, non-recurring disorder which develops following viral infection; idiopathic chronic form in adults
- in the past, associated with congenital or tertiary syphilis
- recurrent episodes of acute intravascular hemolysis following exposure to cold ambient temperatures
- MTHA

- accounts for approximately 8% of all autoimmune hemolytic anemias
- idiopathic or associated with connective tissue and lymphoproliferative disorders
- DIHA
- exposure to drugs (e.g., penicillins, cephalosporins, quinidine, phenacetin, chlorpropamide, sulfonylureas, alpha-methyldopa, and procainamide)
- can result from one of three different mechanisms:
- hapten: drug binds to red blood cell membrane forming neoantigen to which antibodies develop; direct antiglobulin (Coombs) test (DAT) positive for IgG; extravascular hemolysis; penicillins and cephalosporins
- immune complex: drug binds to plasma proteins eliciting antibodies that form circulating immune complexes and activate complement; DAT positive for complement; intravascular or extravascular hemolysis; sulfonamides, phenothiazines, quinidine, isoniazid
- autoantibody: drug directly stimulates production of autoantibody to antigens on red cell membrane; DAT positive for IgG; extravascular hemolysis; alpha-methyldopa, levodopa, procainamide, mefenamic acid
  - ➤ Drugs inducing T-cell dysregulation and increasing the likelihood of disease-mediated AIHA: fludarabine in CLL, cladribine, etc.

Signs & Symptoms
- General
- fatigue, fever, tachycardia, dyspnea, angina, pallor, jaundice, CHF (pulmonary edema, jugular venous distention, peripheral edema), splenomegaly
- intravascular hemolysis may additionally present with hemoglobinemia, hemoglobinuria, DIC (petechiae, purpura, bleeding, thrombosis) and acute renal failure
- WAHA
- severity of extravascular hemolyis ranges from indolent to life threatening
- mildest form: DAT is positive; no hemolysis
- symptomatic form: anemia (Hgb <8 g/dl), jaundice, splenomegaly
- severest form: fulminant hemolysis, progressive anemia, congestive heart failure, respiratory distress, and neurologic abnormalities
- Evan's syndrome: accompanied by immune thrombocytopenia

- CAHA
- general signs and symptoms; intravscular/extravascular hemolysis; red cell agglutination leads to acrocyanosis in the cooler distal areas of the body
- severity depends on the titer and thermal amplitude of the autoantibody
- PCH
- general signs and symptoms; intravascular hemolysis; accompanied by cold urticaria and abdominal pain
- MTHA
- general signs and symptoms; extravascular hemolysis is often severe and chronic with intermittent exacerbations
- DIHA
- general signs and symptoms; extravascular or intravascular hemolysis

TESTS

Basic Blood Tests

- General
  - ➤ anemia, decreased haptoglobin, increased LDH, increased unconjugated bilirubin, increased reticulocyte count, increased free hemoglobin

Basic Urine Tests

- General
  - ➤ hemoglobinuria, hemosiderinuria, increased urobilinogen

Other Tests

- General
  - ➤ peripheral smear: macrocytosis, polychromasia, spherocytosis, schistocytosis, nucleated red blood cells, red blood cell agglutination
  - ➤ bone marrow: erythroid hyperplasia, infiltration by neoplasm

Specific Diagnostic Tests

- WAHA
- DAT: positive for IgG; false positive rate up to 15% of hospitalized patients; negative result does not rule out WAHA
- indirect antiglobulin (Coombs) test (IAT): performed on serum and/or red blood cell eluate; positive for IgG panagglutinin; approximately 50% of warm-reactive autoantibodies have specificities within the Rh antigen system

- CAHA
- peripheral smear may demonstrate red blood cell agglutination
- DAT positive for complement, negative for IgG; Donath-Landsteiner test negative
- autoantibodies are most commonly IgM; rare examples of IgG and IgA cold-reactive autoantibodies
- cold agglutinin titers > 1:1000; high thermal range reacting at 30oC or above
- autoantibody specificity against oligosaccharide red blood cell antigens of the I/i antigen system;
- polyclonal anti-I following Mycoplasma pneumoniae infection; polyclonal anti-i following infectious mononucleosis; monoclonal anti-I (IgM) in chronic CAHA
- PCH
- DAT infrequently positive for complement, negative for IgG; Donath-Landsteiner test positive
- non-agglutinating, complement-fixing IgG autoantibody (Donath-Landsteiner antibody); specificity against the P blood group antigen; titer <1:64; moderate thermal range reacting at <20oC
- MTHA
- DAT positive for IgG and complement; IAT positive for warm-reactive IgG autoantibodies and cold-reactive, hemagglutinating IgM autoantibodies
- cold-reactive autoantibody component typically has low titer (<1:64) and high thermal range reacting at 30oC or above
- DIHA
- DAT positive for IgG and/or complement; IAT positive for IgG or IgM autoantibodies
- hapten or immune complex autoantibodies in serum or from a red blood cell eluate react only with red blood cells pre-incubated with suspected drug
- autoantibodies formed through the "autoantibody mechanism" react with red blood cells in the absence of the drug and are similar to autoantibodies found in WAHA

DIFFERENTIAL DIAGNOSIS

- acute hemolytic transfusion reaction (see chapter on Transfusion Reactions): naturally occurring anti-A and anti-B isohemagglutinins react with transfused ABO-incompatible red blood cells, which may lead to intravascular hemolysis, fever, nausea, vomiting, hypotension, respiratory distress, hemoglobinuria, chest/flank/infusion site pain, acute renal failure, DIC, and death; STOP TRANSFUSION

IMMEDIATELY; aggressive treatment for or to prevent renal failure with iv fluids and diuretics (furosemide); pressor support if needed (low-dose dopamine has also been thought to promote renal blood flow) (but there is progressively *less* convincing evidence from critical care medicine clinical trials that this is indeed the case!); treat DIC with platelets and plasma or cyroprecipitate as needed for life-threatening bleeding; heparin for thrombosis

- delayed hemolytic transfusion reaction (see chapter on Transfusion Reactions): alloantibodies to non-ABO red blood cell antigens (e.g., Rhesus, Kidd, Kell, Duffy, MNSs) react with transfused incompatible red blood cells, often resulting in extravascular hemolysis, fever, jaundice and inadequate hemoglobin responses to transfusion; DAT positive for IgG; IAT positive for IgG alloantibody; supportive care and transfusion with antigen-negative red blood cells

- post-transplant hemolysis: extravascular hemolysis infrequently seen following hematopoietic or solid organ transplants; donor lymphocytes contained within graft produce alloantibodies against ABO or other red blood cell antigens absent in the donor but present in the recipient; fever, jaundice, progressive anemia; DAT positive for IgG; IAT positive for IgG alloantibody; self-limiting; supportive care and transfusion with antigen-negative red blood cells

- hemolytic disease of the newborn: IgG alloantibodies to non-ABO red cell antigens and naturally occurring anti-A,B IgG antibodies in the mother cross the placenta and bind to corresponding antigens present on the fetal red blood cells; extravascular hemolysis; severity ranges greatly from asymptomatic with a positive DAT to severe anemia and jaundice resulting in kernicterus, mental retardation, hydrops fetalis, stillbirth, or death shortly after birth. Prevention and treatment include prenatal screening (maternal ABO/Rh typing, antibody screen, antibody titers; paternal red cell antigen typing), RhoGAM administration, ultrasonography, amniocentesis, PUBS and intrauterine transfusion, Kleihauer-Betke test, phototherapy, exchange transfusion, newborn screening (ABO/Rh typing, DAT, hemoglobin levels and bilirubin levels)

MANAGEMENT

What to Do First/General Measures

- WAHA
- transfuse symptomatic patients with ABO/Rh compatible cross-match least incompatible red blood cells
- patients with accompanying clinically significant alloantibody or warm-reactive autoantibody with a definite specificity should

be transfused with red blood cells that lack the corresponding antigen

■ transfusions in life-threatening situations (severe anemia with hemoglobin <7 g/dl) with high-output cardiac failure or cerebral compromise should never be delayed

■ CAHA

■ supportive care; avoidance of cold temperatures to prevent recurrent attacks; transfuse red blood cells for life-threatening anemia; transfusing through a blood warmer is advocated.

■ PCH

■ supportive care for most post-infectious cases; avoidance of cold temperatures to prevent recurrent attacks; transfuse red blood cells for life-threatening anemia; transfusing through a blood warmer is advocated.

■ MTHA

■ blood transfusions should adhere to guidelines outlined earlier for WAHA; transfusing through a blood warmer is advocated.

■ DIHA

■ supportive care; transfuse red blood cells for clinically significant anemia; attempt to identify and withdraw offending medication

SPECIFIC THERAPY

Indications

■ Severe hemolysis and life-threatening anemia; acrocyanosis

Treatment Options

■ WAHA
  ➤ Steroids
    • primary therapy; acutely diminish extravascular hemolysis by blocking macrophage Fc receptor activity; inhibit antibody production
    • prednisone 1 to 2 mg/kg/day PO until hemoglobin levels stabilize then gradually taper at a rate of 5 to 10 mg per week; some patients may require a more gradual tapering schedule.
    • methylprednisolone 2 to 4 mg/kg/day IV in divided doses for critically ill patients
  ➤ Splenectomy
    • steroid-refractory patients or patients requiring unacceptably high (>15 mg/day) doses of prednisone to maintain remission
  ➤ Azathioprine
    • 1.5 mg/kg/day PO for patients unfit for surgery or patients who failed steroids and splenectomy; should not be used for extended periods due to side effects.

➤ Cyclophosphamide
  • 2 mg/kg/day PO for patients unfit for surgery or patients who failed steroids and splenectomy; should not be used for extended periods due to side effects
➤ Other
  • IVIG, danazol, plasma exchange, anti-B cell monoclonal antibodies
➤ CAHA
➤ Oral alkylating agents (chlorambucil and cyclophosphamide) for severe disease secondary to lymphoproliferative disorders; plasma exchange in critically ill patients unresponsive to transfusions; steroids for rare IgG cold agglutinins, anti-B cell monoclonal antibodies
➤ PCH
➤ no specific therapy; transfuse rare P-antigen negative red blood cells to patients who do not respond to random donor red blood cells; consider steroids for episodes of severe hemolysis
➤ MTHA
➤ therapy should follow guidelines outlined above for WAHA
➤ DIHA
➤ no specific therapy other than withdrawing implicated medication; consider steroids for severe hemolysis

Side Effects & Complications
■ doses of prednisone greater than 1 to 2 mg/kg/day provide little additional benefit and increase the number and severity of side effects; side effects of chronic steroid administration are reduced by alternate-day schedules
■ splenectomy requires immunization with pneumococcal/meningococcal vaccines to prevent sepsis secondary to encapsulated bacteria
■ azathioprine and cyclophosphamide have been associated with bone marrow suppression, increased risk of infection and malignancy, and decreased fertility
■ in patients with cold-reactive autoantibodies hypothermia must be avoided during surgery in particular procedures involving extracorporeal circuits

FOLLOW-UP
■ regularly assess degree of hemolysis and anemia – CBC, LDH level, unconjugated bilirubin, DAT, IAT, cold agglutinin titers, cold agglutinin thermal range
■ assess potential complications of ongoing therapy

■ surveillance for neoplastic process as cause of chronic hemolysis or as a side-effect of therapy

COMPLICATIONS AND PROGNOSIS

Complications
■ severe anemia, cardiac failure, renal failure, DIC (thrombosis and bleeding) neurologic abnormalities, and death

Prognosis
■ WAHA
■ 25% of steroid-treated patients will experience complete remission; remaining patients will have either partial or no response at all; response rate also depends on treatment of underlying disorder.
■ splenectomy produces partial or complete remission in 50% of cases
■ CAHA
■ post-infectious CAHA may be very severe and life threatening requiring aggressive supportive care in hospital. However, the majority of cases are self-limited with full recovery within one month
■ chronic idiopathic CAHA is characterized by prolonged survival with spontaneous remissions and exacerbations
■ in CAHA associated with malignancy the hemolysis often parallels the activity of the neoplasm
■ PCH
■ post-infectious PCH is self-limited with full recovery within one month; primary PCH has a natural history that extends over many years punctuated by episodes of severe hemolysis
■ MTHA
■ steroids usually effective; disorder often persistent with intermittent episodes of hemolysis
■ DIHA
■ positive DAT and hemolysis may persist for weeks to months following discontinuation of drug

IMMUNODEFICIENCY DISORDERS, CONGENITAL

ANNE-MARIE IRANI, MD

HISTORY & PHYSICAL

History
■ Otitis media, sinusitis, pneumonia, meningitis: B-cell deficiency; X-linked or autosomal recessive

- Gingivitis, skin infections, organ abscesses, lymphadenitis: neutrophil/phagocyte defect
- Viruses (herpes, varicella, CMV): T-cell deficiency
- Fungi
  - Candida: T-cell deficiency
  - Aspergillus: T-cell/phagocyte defects
- Parasites
  - Giardia lamblia: B-cell deficiency
  - Pneumocystis carinii: T-cell deficiency
- Bacteria
  - Encapsulated organisms: B-cell or complement deficiency
  - Low-virulence organisms: neutrophil/phagocyte defects
- Diarrhea, malabsorption: T- or B-cell deficiency

Signs & Symptoms
- Eczema: Wiskott-Aldrich syndrome, hyper-IgE syndrome
- Abscesses: neutrophil/phagocyte defects
- Telangiectasia: ataxia-telangiectasia
- Partial oculocutaneous albinism: Chediak-Higashi syndrome
- Candidiasis: T-cell deficiency
- Digital clubbing, rales: B-cell, T-cell deficiency
- Diffuse lymphadenopathy: neutrophil/phagocyte defects
- Lupus-like syndrome: complement deficiencies
- Ataxia: ataxia-telangiectasia

TESTS

Lab Tests
- Evaluation of B-cell immunity
  - Quantitative serum immunoglobulins: IgG, IgM, IgA
  - IgG subclasses are usually not helpful; test results vary among different labs
- Specific antibody titers
  - Isohemagglutinins (IgM antibodies to A & B blood groups)
  - Antibodies to protein antigens (tetanus, diphtheria): IgG1 subclass
  - Antibodies to polysaccharide antigens (Pneumococcus, Haemophilus influenzae): IgG2 subclass
- B-cell enumeration
  - CD19 surface marker
- Evaluation of T-cell immunity
  - T-cell enumeration

- Absolute peripheral blood lymphocyte count
- T-cell numbers: CD2, CD3
- T-cell subsets: CD4, CD8
■ Delayed-type hypersensitivity (DTH) skin reaction
  ➤ Candida, mumps
■ In vitro proliferative responses
  ➤ Nonspecific: phytohemagglutinin (PHA), concanavalin A (CON A)
  ➤ Specific: tetanus, Candida
■ Evaluation of phagocytic function
  ➤ Enumeration of neutrophils
  ➤ Absolute neutrophil count
■ Oxidative burst assays
  ➤ Nitroblue tetrazolium reduction test (NBT)
  ➤ Dihydrorhodamine reductase assay (DHR), more sensitive
■ Enzyme determination
  ➤ Myeloperoxidase
  ➤ Glucose-6-phosphate dehydrogenase
■ Chemotaxis assay
  ➤ Defective in Chediak-Higashi syndrome, hyper-IgE syndrome
■ Adhesion molecules
  ➤ Determination of CD18 surface marker: absent in leukocyte adhesion deficiency type 1 (LAD 1)
■ Evaluation of complement system
  ➤ Determination of complement proteins, C3 & C4
  ➤ Total hemolytic complement CH 50, screening test, extremely low or nondetectable in complement deficiencies
  ➤ Individual complement components determined in specialized labs

DIFFERENTIAL DIAGNOSIS

Antibody Deficiency Disorders
■ IgA deficiency
  ➤ Most common: 1/700 of the general population
  ➤ IgA low or decreased w/ normal IgG & IgM
  ➤ Variable clinical features
    - Asymptomatic
    - Assoc w/ respiratory infections (sinusitis)
    - Assoc w/ autoimmune disorders
■ Selective IgG subclass deficiency
  ➤ Variable decreases in IgG2, IgG3 or IgG4; normal total IgG

➤ Variable clinical manifestations
➤ Functional defect in antibody responses to polysaccharide antigens usually assoc w/ recurrent respiratory infections
■ Common variable immunodeficiency
➤ Low IgG, absent specific antibodies
➤ Clinically heterogeneous group of disorders
➤ Peak incidence in the 2nd or 3rd decade of life
➤ Often assoc. w/ autoimmune disorders (inflammatory bowel disease, arthritis)
➤ Increased incidence of lymphoid malignancies
■ Hyper-IgM syndrome
➤ X-linked mutation of the gene for CD40 ligand: inability of B cells to switch from IgM to other isotypes
➤ Absent IgG & IgA, normal or elevated IgM
➤ Increased incidence of autoimmune neutropenia, anemia, thrombocytopenia
■ Bruton's disease
➤ X-linked agammaglobulinemia w/ absent B cells
➤ Mutation in the gene for Bruton's tyrosine kinase interferes w/ normal B-cell development
➤ May develop echovirus encephalitis if untreated

T-Cell Deficiency Disorders
■ DiGeorge syndrome: deletions of 22q11
➤ Thymic hypoplasia (partial) or aplasia (complete), hypocalcemia, congenital heart disease
➤ Complete DiGeorge: absent T cells or immunoglobulins
➤ Partial DiGeorge: low but functional T cells w/out significant infections
■ Chronic Mucocutaneous Candidiasis
➤ May be associated w/ other disorders (polyendocrinopathies, autoimmune disorders, thymoma)
➤ Absent DTH responses to Candida albicans only
➤ Requires chronic antifungal therapy

Phagocytic Defects
■ Chronic granulomatous disease (CGD)
➤ Defects in NADPH-oxidase, X-linked or autosomal recessive
➤ Recurrent bacterial or fungal infections
➤ Granulomas w/ GU or GI obstruction
■ Complement deficiencies

➤ Early component (C1, C4, C2) deficiency associated w/ SLE
➤ Late components: C5–C9; recurrent Neisseria infections

MANAGEMENT

What to Do First

■ Determine presence & type of immunodeficiency disorder

General Measures

■ Appropriate antibiotic therapy for infections

SPECIFIC THERAPY

■ IVIg replacement therapy
  ➤ Treatment of choice for common variable, hyper-IgM syndrome, Bruton's disease
    • NOT indicated in IgA or IgG subclass deficiency
    • Maintain trough IgG level >600 mg/dL
  ➤ Side effects: chills, fever, nausea, vomiting, headache, aseptic meningitis (related to rate of infusion)
    • No risk of HIV; small risk of hepatitis
■ Stem cell transplantation (bone marrow, cord blood)
  ➤ Treatment of choice for hyper-IgM, complete DiGeorge, Wiskott-Aldrich, leukocyte adhesion deficiency
■ Replacement of specific proteins
  ➤ IFN ?subcutaneously for CGD

FOLLOW-UP

■ IgG trough levels, blood count & differential, liver enzymes every 3–6 months
■ Blood & urine culture when febrile

COMPLICATIONS & PROGNOSIS

■ Echovirus encephalitis in agammaglobulinemia
■ Autoimmune diseases: neutropenia, inflammatory bowel disease, arthritis
■ Chronic lung disease if not treated early
■ Lymphoid malignancies

IMPETIGO

ALFRED L. KNABLE, MD

HISTORY & PHYSICAL

History

■ Seen in all age groups, but MOST common in infants and children

- Risk from exposure to other infected individuals, pets, spas, swimming pools, dirty fingernails
- Risk increased with superficial cutaneous trauma. Recent epidemics have been reported in football players at all levels and wrestlers.
- Often seen as a secondary complication in individuals with atopic dermatitis, pediculosis capitis, herpes simplex (or zoster), scabies, insect bites or contact dermatitis
- More frequent in temperate zones, summer months because of increased heat and humidity

Signs and Symptoms
- may involve any body area, but most common one exposed surfaces (i.e., face, hands, neck, extremities)
- begins as 1–2 mm red macules
- rapidly develops into either thin-roofed vesicles or bullae
- bullous variant from phage group II staphylococci; NOTE: Community-acquired methicillin-resistant organisms have become increasingly prevalent.
- vesiculopustular variant from beta-hemolytic streptococci (often in combination with staphylococci)
- either variant prone to rupture of lesion with discharge of cloudy fluid – subsequent formation of thick, honey-colored crust is hallmark of disease
- autoinoculation via scratching or fomites can lead to development of satellite lesions
- mature lesions may clear centrally while remaining peripherally active, giving an annular appearance
- fever and lymphadenopathy may develop in widespread disease

TESTS

Laboratory
- Basic studies: surface cultures can be useful if diagnosis in doubt, also helpful when considering methicillin-resistant organisms
- Other tests: nares culture to determine Staph aureus
- carriage in recurrent cases
- Urinalysis: perform if nephritogenic strains of streptococci are endemic in patient's area

DIFFERENTIAL DIAGNOSIS
- Annular lesions may mimic tinea corporis (i.e., ringworm). KOH preparation can be done if necessary.

- Annular and crusted lesions may be seen in syphilis. Serologic tests (RPR, etc) can be performed.
- Crusted lesions may be seen with ecthyma or varicella.

MANAGEMENT

What to Do First

- Assess percentage of body surface area involved.

General Measures

- Gentle cleansing with soap and water at least daily
- Larger or draining lesions may be covered with an absorptive dressing.

SPECIFIC THERAPY

- Localized (<1% BSA) will usually respond to topical therapy.
- Effective topical agents include mupirocin, bacitracin, polymyxin, erythromycin and gramicidin.
- More extensive involvement will require oral antibiotics for 7–14 days.
- Staphylococcal disease should respond to dicloxacillin or a cephalosporin (erythromycin resistance has become common).

FOLLOW-UP

- If lesions continue to spread after 24–48 hours of therapy
- If fever or lymphadenopathy continue or develop after 24–48 hours of therapy
- If signs or symptoms of glomerulonephritis develop

COMPLICATIONS AND PROGNOSIS

Complications

- Glomerulonephritis: uncommon, but is high (12–28%) following skin infection with a nephritogenic strain of streptococcus
- More common in children
- Patients should be watched for signs of glomerulonephritis for at least 7 weeks after cutaneous infection clears in endemic areas for nephritogenic M strains of streptococci
- Scarring: uncommon, best prevention is early therapeutic intervention

Prognosis

- Generally excellent, with complete recovery the rule
- Recurrence because of staph nasal carriage can occur
- Glomerulonephritis a rare complication

INFECTIOUS DIARRHEAS

SUZANNE M. MATSUI, MD and JEFFREY W. KWAN, MD, MS

HISTORY & PHYSICAL

History

- most episodes self-limiting (nearly half last <1 day); evaluate those with more severe illness
- character of fecal output: >6 unformed stools/24 h, blood or mucus in stools
- presence of fever, vomiting, dysentery, abdominal pain, tenesmus
- duration of illness (>48 h)
- male homosexual
- history of immunocompromise
- setting in which patient became ill: travel, institutional/day care/family exposure, recent antibiotic use
- age of patient
- comorbid conditions: vascular disease, IBD, radiation therapy

Signs and Symptoms

- noninflammatory (less likely to require extensive evaluation):
  - ➤ profuse watery diarrhea may precipitate dehydration
  - ➤ minimal or no fever
- inflammatory (usually associated with specific pathogen and treatment):
  - ➤ dysentery
  - ➤ many small-volume stools with blood and mucus
  - ➤ fever >38.5°C (101.3°F) suggests invasive pathogen/inflammation
- enteric fever
  - ➤ constipation early in course: S. typhi, C. fetus, some Yersinia
  - ➤ systemic infection
  - ➤ infection returns to gut via biliary tract

TESTS

- moderate to severe acute infectious diarrhea: screen with fecal leukocytes or lactoferrin (leukocyte marker) or fecal occult blood
- severe diarrhea: stool culture; O & P, if parasitic/protozoal infection suspected (>10 d duration, consumption of untreated water, homosexual/AIDS patients); C. difficile toxins A & B, if suspected; endoscopy (to distinguish between IBD and infectious diarrhea, to

detect opportunistic infections such as CMV in immunocompromised pts, and rarely to diagnose C. difficile with pseudomembranes while toxin assays are pending)

DIFFERENTIAL DIAGNOSIS

- nausea, vomiting, watery diarrhea: viral gastroenteritis (e.g., noroviruses in families and outbreaks; rotaviruses in young children) or preformed toxin (e.g., *S. aureus, B. cereus*)
- dehydration: cholera, ETEC (in very young & very old), EPEC (infants), rotavirus, rarely Salmonella
- large volume diarrhea, upper abdominal pain/cramps: small intestinal pathogen ± colonic involvement
- many small frequent stools, urgency, tenesmus, dysentery:
  - ➤ colitis – Campylobacter most common; IBD
  - ➤ proctitis – N. gonorrhoeae
- persistent diarrhea (≥14 days): parasites (e.g., *Giardia, Cryptosporidium, Cyclospora, Microspidium, Isospora*), bacterial infection or overgrowth, malabsorption
- recent travel to: developing countries (bacteria); mountainous areas/recreational waters with wildlife (*Giardia*); Russia (*Cryptosporidium, Giardia*)
- recent antibiotic treatment (≤2 mo) or recent hospitalization: C. difficile
- day care center contact: any agent spread by fecal-oral route
- food- or water-borne outbreak: Norwalk virus, *S. aureus, B. cereus, V. parahaemolyticus, V. cholerae, Aeromonas, Plesiomonas, L. monocytogenes, Cyclospora, Giardia*

MANAGEMENT

What To Do First
- assess hydration
- prompt fluid and electrolyte therapy

General Measures
- nondehydrated, otherwise healthy: sport drinks, diluted fruit juices, soft drinks and saltine crackers/broths/soups, avoidance of milk products, use of "BRAT" diet (bananas, rice, applesauce, and toast)
- elderly and/or immunosuppressed: Pedialyte or Rehydrolyte solutions (containing 45–75 mEq Na per liter)
- dehydrating, cholera-like: WHO oral rehydration solution or homemade recipe (1/2 tsp table salt, 1/2 tsp baking soda, 4 tbsp sugar, 1 liter clean water)
- severe dehydration, hypovolemic shock: IV hydration

SPECIFIC THERAPY

- empiric antimicrobial therapy without additional evaluation:
  - ➤ moderate-to-severe travelers' diarrhea
  - ➤ 8 stools/d, with blood or pus, fever
  - ➤ if bacterial diarrhea suspected by clinical features and/or positive fecal occult blood or fecal leukocytes; not for Shiga toxin-producing E. coli or C. difficile
  - ➤ if Giardia suspected and ≥2 wk duration (metronidazole)
- nonspecific (not for patients with febrile dysentery or Shiga toxin-producing E. coli):
  - ➤ opiates and derivatives (decrease intestinal motility)
    - loperamide (Imodium) – reduces number of stools
    - diphenoxylate-atropine (Lomotil) – less expensive, but has central opiate and adverse cholinergic effects
  - ➤ bismuth subsalicylate for vomiting and mild to moderate acute diarrhea
  - ➤ specific antimicrobial therapy (treatment of choice listed):
    - *Campylobacter jejuni* (most common pathogen in immuno-competent patients with bacterial diarrhea)
      - fluoroquinolones
    - *Campylobacter fetus* (immunocompromised patients)
      - ampicillin + gentamicin IV
    - *Shigella* (treat all moderate and severe dysentery)
      - fluoroquinolones
    - *Salmonella* gastroenteritis, uncomplicated
      - no antibiotics
    - *Salmonella* gastroenteritis, severe, or in immunocompromised or elderly
      - trimethoprim-sulfamethoxazole (if susceptible) or ciprofloxacin
    - enteric (typhoid) fever
      - fluoroquinolones
      - if shock or deteriorating mental status – dexamethasone (before antibiotic)
    - Shiga toxin-producing E. coli (including O157:H7)
      - antimotility agents and antibiotics should be avoided
    - enterotoxigenic *E. coli* (traveler's diarrhea)
      - consider empiric therapy with fluoroquinolones, or rifaximin
    - enteropathogenic E. coli
      - fluoroquinolones
    - *Clostridium difficile*

- discontinue inciting antibiotic(s), if possible
- avoid antimotility agents
- metronidazole (first line) or oral vancomycin
- for severe disease or unable to take po:
  - metronidazole IV
  - vancomycin (NG, enema, intracecal)
- *Vibrio cholerae*
  - rehydration
  - doxycycline, tetracycline, or fluoroquinolones
- *Vibrio parahaemolyticus*
  - antibiotics do not shorten course
- *Yersinia enterocolitica*
  - antibiotics usually not needed
  - if severe: doxycycline + aminoglycoside (in combination), trimethoprim-sulfamethoxazole, or fluoroquinolones

FOLLOW-UP
n/a

COMPLICATIONS AND PROGNOSIS
- ▨ most cases resolve spontaneously or with appropriate antimicrobial treatment
- ▨ toxic megacolon, intestinal perforation
  - ➤ *Shigella*
  - ➤ rarely: Shiga toxin-producing E. coli, *C. difficile, Campylobacter, Yersinia, Salmonella*
- ▨ hemolytic-uremic syndrome, thrombotic thrombocytopenic purpura
  - ➤ Shiga toxin-producing E. coli (10%, with 5–10% mortality among afflicted), Shigella, rarely Campylobacter
- ▨ reactive arthritis
  - ➤ *Shigella, Salmonella, Yersinia, Campylobacter*
- ▨ metastatic infection
  - ➤ *Salmonella*
  - ➤ rarely: *Yersinia, Campylobacter*
- ▨ malnutrition, weight loss
  - ➤ *Giardia*
- ▨ Guillain-Barré syndrome
  - ➤ rarely: *C. jejuni*
- ▨ relapses (not antibiotic resistance)
  - ➤ *C. difficile* diarrhea and colitis: reinfection with same strain, 1 wk (usual) to 2 months (less common) after stopping treatment

INFECTIVE ENDOCARDITIS

RICHARD A. JACOBS, MD, PhD

HISTORY & PHYSICAL

History

- Usually, but not always (ie, IV drug users), an underlying abnormality predisposing to infection – valvular disease (rheumatic heart disease, mitral valve prolapse), damage to endothelium from regurgitant jet flow or congenital abnormalities (VSD, patent ductus)
- Etiology depends on clinical setting: Native valve endocarditis due to viridans streptococci, S. aureus and enterococci; prosthetic valve endocarditis within 2 months of surgery (early infection) due to S. epidermidis (and other coagulase-negative staphylococci), S. aureus, Gram negative bacilli; late infections (greater than 2 months post-operatively) similar to native valve endocarditis; endocarditis in IV drug users caused predominantly by S. aureus; culture negative endocarditis due to previous administration of antibiotics, fungi (blood cultures positive in only 50% of cases), slow growing organisms such as the HACEK organisms and Brucella, organisms that require special media for growth such as Legionella, Bartonella, and nutritionally variant streptococci, and organisms that do not grow on conventional media such as Coxiella burnetii (Q fever)

Signs & Symptoms

- Virulent organisms (S. aureus) usually present acutely with rapidly progressive infection, tissue destruction and systemic emboli, although more indolent presentation (especially IV drug users with tricuspid infection) can occur; less virulent organisms (streptococci, enterococci, fungi, HACEK organisms) present most often with a subacute course
- Presenting symptoms often nonspecific – fever, chills, malaise, arthralgias, back pain; peripheral embolization manifest as stroke or abdominal pain (splenic embolization); fever (90%), heart murmur (80–90%), splenomegaly (40%) and peripheral manifestations such as petechiae, splinter hemorrhages, Osler nodes, Janeway lesions and Roth spots occur in 10–40%

TESTS

- Elevated WBCs in acute disease; anemia with subacute disease; hematuria from embolization to kidneys or immune-mediated glomerulonephritis; pulmonary infiltrates on CXR with right-sided endocarditis and embolization to the lungs; conduction abnormalities on EKG suggest myocardial abscess

- Definitive diagnosis made by blood culture; 3 blood cultures obtained over 24 hours (in acutely ill, 3 blood cultures at least 1 hour apart) positive in over 95%; negative cultures due causes listed above

    If culture negative: serology, valve tissue PCR, or histopathology (if early surgery) may aid diagnosis.

- Echocardiography helpful in establishing diagnosis and defining valve involved; transthoracic echo positive in 60%; transesophageal echo positive in 90% (especially good for pulmonic valve and prosthetic valve endocarditis and detecting myocardial abscesses

- Duke criteria for clinical diagnosis; probable endocarditis (80% likelihood) if 2 major criteria, 1 major and 3 minor criteria or 5 minor criteria; possible endocarditis if 1 major and 1 minor criteria or 3 minor criteria; major criteria = (1) two separate positive blood culture for organisms that typically cause endocarditis (2) evidence of endocardial involvement pathologically or by echo (vegetation, abscess or dehiscence of prosthetic valve) (3) new regurgitant murmur; minor criteria = (1) predisposing heart disease or IV drug use (2) fever greater than 38 (3) vascular phenomenon (systemic or pulmonary embolization (4) immunologic phenomenon (glomerulonephritis, Osler node, Roth spot) and (5) positive blood cultures, but not meeting the major criteria

DIFFERENTIAL DIAGNOSIS

- Nonspecific clinical manifestations similar to many febrile illnesses including other infections, collagen vascular disease, cancer; consider in anyone with fever and heart murmur, a prosthetic valve and fever, any young person with an unexplained neurologic event and in IV drug users with fever

MANAGEMENT

- Establish diagnosis with blood cultures; in acutely ill, do not delay therapy to obtain multiple blood cultures; in nonacute patients on antibiotics, reasonable to withhold antibiotics 3–4 days to obtain cultures off therapy

- Anticoagulation contraindicated in native valve endocarditis; in prosthetic valve endocarditis, anticoagulation continued unless there has been an intracerebral bleed

- Surgical intervention indicated if heart failure fails to respond to medical management, if blood cultures remain positive 7–10 days despite appropriate antibiotic therapy, in fungal endocarditis, in many cases of Gram-negative endocarditis, myocardial or valve ring abscesses and if recurrent embolic events occur

SPECIFIC THERAPY

- Empirical therapy while awaiting the results of cultures directed against streptococci, enterococci and S. aureus – nafcillin or oxacillin plus penicillin or ampicillin plus gentamicin; in the penicillin-allergic patient, vancomycin used instead of the penicillins
- Viridans streptococci – for susceptible strains (minimum inhibitory concentration or MIC ≤0.1 micrograms/mL) penicillin or ceftriaxone or vancomycin (in penicillin allergic patient) for 4 weeks; duration of therapy shortened to 2 weeks if gentamicin added to the penicillin regimen; 2-week regimen not indicated if symptoms present for greater than 3 months, if complications present, in renal failure or the elderly; prosthetic valve endocarditis treated 6 weeks with penicillin and 2 weeks with gentamicin; if MIC >0.1 micrograms/mL and ≤0.5 micrograms/mL, penicillin for 4 weeks and gentamicin for the first 2 weeks; in the penicillin-allergic patient, vancomycin for 4 weeks; for nutritionally variant streptococci and viridans streptococci with MIC's >0.5 micrograms/mL, therapy as for enterococci
- Enterococci – penicillin or ampicillin or vancomycin (in the penicillin-allergic patient) plus gentamicin for 4–6 weeks (6 weeks for prosthetic valves and if symptoms >3 months); no established regimens if high-level resistance to aminoglycosides (MIC >500–2000 micrograms/mL), but 8–12 weeks of intermittent or continuous infusion of high-dose penicillin or ampicillin may be curative in 50%; surgery may be only other therapeutic option
- Staphylococci – for methicillin-susceptible strains, nafcillin or oxacillin or cefazolin (in the penicillin-allergic patient without IgE hypersensitivity) for 4–6 weeks; addition of gentamicin for 3–5 days shortens duration of bacteremia; in patients with anaphylaxis to penicillin with methicillin-sensitive S. aureus, or those with methicillin-resistant strains, only therapy is vancomycin for 4–6 weeks; tricuspid valve endocarditis in IV drug users can be treated for 2 weeks if gentamicin and anti-staphylococcal drug used in combination; coagulase-negative staphylococci usually cause prosthetic valve endocarditis and are treated with vancomycin plus rifampin for 6 weeks plus gentamicin for the first 2 weeks

- HACEK organisms treated with ceftriaxone for 4 weeks (6 weeks for prosthetic valves); therapy in the allergic patient not established, but trimethoprim-sulfamethoxazole, fluoroquinolones and aztreonam have in vitro activity

FOLLOW-UP

- Blood cultures usually negative in 3–5 days; fever may persist 10–12 days; persistent fever should prompt evaluation for myocardial abscess, infected or sterile systemic emboli with or without infarction, superinfection or drug reaction
- Most relapses occur within 1–2 months of completion of therapy; careful clinical follow-up and blood cultures every other week to detect early relapses
- Progressive valvular dysfunction after successful antibiotic therapy may require valve replacement, especially in the first year.

COMPLICATIONS AND PROGNOSIS

- Major complications include valvular destruction with heart failure requiring valve replacement, myocardial abscess, systemic embolization with infarction (kidney, spleen), mycotic aneurysms that can rupture (great vessels or intracerebral vessels) and pulmonary emboli resulting in infarcts or abscesses.
- Use of prophylactic antibiotics indicated in high-risk patients (prosthetic valves, previous endocarditis) or moderate-risk patients (congenital abnormalities other than atrial septal defects, rheumatic heart disease with valvular dysfunction, mitral valve prolapse with regurgitation) undergoing procedures likely to result in bacteremia (dental procedures associated with significant bleeding, periodontal procedures, implant placement; respiratory procedures that breach the mucosa such as tonsillectomy; invasive gastrointestinal procedures such as ERCP, sclerotherapy; invasive genitourinary procedures, prostatic surgery); for dental, respiratory or esophageal procedures, amoxicillin (clindamycin if penicillin allergic) 1 hour before; for gastrointestinal procedures (other than esophageal) and genitourinary procedures in high-risk patients ampicillin plus gentamicin parenterally 30 minutes before and either ampicillin g IV or IM or amoxicillin orally, 6 hours after (vancomycin instead of ampicillin in the penicillin-allergic patient); in moderate-risk patients amoxicillin 1 hour before (vancomycin as above for the penicillin-allergic patient)

INFLUENZA

CAROL A. GLASER, MD

HISTORY & PHYSICAL

History

- 3 types of flu virus recognized: A, B, C
  - A includes 3 subtypes: H1N1, H2N2, H3N2
  - A subtypes – classified by antigenic properties of surface glycoprotein – hemagglutinin (H), neuraminidase (N)
  - Type A associated with widespread epidemics/pandemics
  - Emergence of completely new subtypes occurs at irregular intervals, only with A responsible for pandemics
  - Type B – infrequently associated with regional or widespread epidemics
  - Type C – usually sporadic cases, minor localized cases
- Human host
- Transmitted airborne (especially enclosed spaces) and direct contact
- Short incubation period (1–3 days)
- Highly contagious
- Highest incidence in winter

Signs & Symptoms

- Sudden onset of fever, frequently with headache, myalgia, prostration, coryza, sore throat and cough
- Cough often severe
- Occasionally GI tract manifestations (nausea, vomiting, diarrhea), especially in children
- Manifestations other than cough usually limited 2–7 days

TESTS

During Early Febrile Stages:

- Antigen detection (DFA or ELISA) in respiratory secretions sensitive, widely available
- Isolation of virus in respiratory secretions is also good test
- Nucleic acid methods (e.g., PCR) available in some settings
- Serology of limited utility in acute setting, confirm infection with acute and convalescent bloods

DIFFERENTIAL DIAGNOSIS

- Common cold – generally influenza has higher fever/sicker with influenza
- Croup
- Bronchiolitis
- Viral pneumonia

MANAGEMENT

- Influenza vaccine should be given to high-risk individuals before influenza season starts.
- Yearly vaccine needed
- High risk
- Antiviral drugs may play role in outbreak settings

SPECIFIC THERAPY

- Amantadine/Rimantadine – **Note: CDC recommends against using currently due to documented resistance**
  - ➤ Decreases severity if administered within 48 hours of illness
  - ➤ Not active against influenza B
  - ➤ Generally amantadine has more side effects than rimantadine (lightheadedness, insomnia, loss of balance, especially in elderly)
- Neuraminidase inhibitors: Zanamivir (Relenza): inhalation drug; Oseltamivir (Tamiflu): oral drug
  - ➤ if started within 30 hours after onset, can shorten duration of symptoms and decrease incidence of complications
  - ➤ effective against both A and B

FOLLOW-UP

n/a

COMPLICATIONS AND PROGNOSIS

- Reyes syndrome in children, particularly in children given salicylates
- Fatal viral pneumonia
- Secondary bacterial pneumonia
- Exacerbation of respiratory and cardiac conditions such as asthma, heart failure, and COPD

INFLUENZA, AVIAN

SUSAN PHILIP, MD, MPH

HISTORY & PHYSICAL

Note: Please refer to the CDC website for the most current epidemiology and management. www.CDC.gov

- No travel advisories at time of writing (check CDC website for updates)
- Travelers to areas of bird or human disease advised to avoid contact with domestic birds, avoid consuming undercooked poultry meat, blood, or eggs. Practice frequent handwashing with soap and water or alcohol-based hand rub.
- No licensed vaccine currently, but ongoing human trials in multiple countries

History
Subtype of Influenza A (H5N1)

- Usually infects wild birds, but has caused large outbreaks of severe disease in domestic poultry in a growing number of countries. Initially was in SE Asia, but recently also reported in birds in Europe, India and Africa.
- First documented human case in 1997, re-emerged in 2003 coinciding with extensive outbreaks in birds throughout Asia. Current virus in human cases antigenically distinct from earlier cases.

    Transmission – animal to human, environment to human and human to human (nonsustained)

    Most cases report handling or close contact with secretions of infected poultry (sick or dying birds). Ingesting uncooked poultry meat or blood has also been associated and contaminated surfaces may transmit virus. Human-to-human transmission reported in a family cluster with close contact. No airborne transmission yet reported.
- Unlike seasonal influenza, attack rate is highest in children and young adults.
- Incubation period up to 8 days

Signs & Symptoms
- Fever, lower respiratory symptoms, diarrhea may be present.
- May also present with encephalopathy without pulmonary disease

TESTS
- Blood: lymphopenia, elevated LFTs

During Early Febrile Stages:
- Limit testing based on appropriate clinical presentation and history of travel to area with documented H5N1 in birds or humans.

    Lab must be alerted to follow biosafety precautions. Send specimens (throat and nasal) as quickly as possible.

    Culture: Viral culture (require biosafety 3+ facility)

Molecular: H5N1 PCR – most sensitive test

Immunofluorescence antigen – less sensitive and specific than PCR

Paired serology – ELISA, Western blot. Not useful in the clinical setting, but needed for epidemiology.

DIFFERENTIAL DIAGNOSIS
- Other causes of atypical pneumonia and respiratory viruses, including SARS

MANAGEMENT
- For hospitalized patients, full isolation measures as in SARS: standard and contact precautions, eye protection, airborne precautions, including use of N95 masks
- Supportive care

SPECIFIC THERAPY
- Neuraminidase inhibitors: Zanamivir (Relenza): inhalation drug; Oseltamivir (Tamiflu): oral drug
  - ➤ Note that some resistance has been reported.
- No role for amantadine or rimantadine (virus resistant)

COMPLICATIONS AND PROGNOSIS
- High mortality rate of nearly 50%

INGUINOFEMORAL HERNIA

BASSEM SAFADI, MD and ROY SOETIKNO, MD, MS

HISTORY & PHYSICAL

Risk Factors
- male
- increased intra-abdominal pressure (COPD, ascites, chronic constipation or urinary retention)

Types
- indirect: through internal ring due to patent processus vaginalis.
- direct: through transversalis fascia in the area of Hasselbach's triangle.
- femoral: through femoral canal (less frequent than inguinal hernias; more common in women)

Symptoms & Signs
- groin pain or discomfort
- bulge/mass associated with straining, coughing, or valsalva

- incarceration: when hernia cannot be reduced, may present with bowel obstruction
- strangulation: when contents of an incarcerated hernia become ischemic/gangrenous (more common in femoral hernias)

TESTS
- usually not necessary; diagnosis based on physical examination
- CT scan or ultrasound may be helpful in obese patients

DIFFERENTIAL DIAGNOSIS
- Testicular cancer; inguinal lymphadenopathy

MANAGEMENT
What to Do First
- Watchful waiting: acceptable in asymptomatic or patients with significant comorbidities

General Management
- Determine if incarcerated or strangulated vs reducible

SPECIFIC THERAPY
Surgery
- anterior repair with or without prosthetic mesh; usually performed using local/regional anesthesia
- posterior repair with mesh: laparoscopic or open

FOLLOW-UP
- Periodic examinations for symptoms if nonoperative approach taken
- Usual postoperative visits to confirm healing and absence of recurrence

COMPLICATIONS AND PROGNOSIS
- Recurrence with prosthetic mesh 1–3% and higher if mesh not used

INNER EAR DISORDERS PRODUCING VERTIGO

ANIL K. LALWANI, MD

HISTORY & PHYSICAL

History
- Define symptom: vertigo (illusion of movement); imbalance or disequilibrium (postural instability or difficulty with gait), lightheaded

(feeling of faintness with change in position); dizzy (often used for vertigo, imbalance, disequilibrium or lightheadedness)

■ Duration of vertigo important in differential diagnosis

■ Association of auditory symptoms, such as hearing loss, tinnitus and aural fullness, usually implicates peripheral ear dysfunction

■ Neurological symptoms suggest central pathology

■ History of prior trauma, viral infection, ototoxic exposure, otologic surgery may provide important clues to the underlying pathology

■ Physical examination should include a complete otologic, neurotologic, cerebellar, gait and cranial nerve examination

Signs & Symptoms

■ Rotatory vertigo or sensation of environmental movement lasting seconds, minutes, hours, or days

■ Hearing loss may be present and may increase in severity with episodes

■ Tinnitus is often present, and in absence of hearing loss, may provide a clue to which ear is affected

■ Aural pressure that does not clear with opening of the Eustachian tube could be a clue to the diagnosis of Meniere's disease

■ Meniere's Disease: episodic vertigo lasting several hours, fluctuate hearing loss, tinnitus, aural fullness

■ Labyrinthitis: acute vertigo for hour to days, hearing loss, fever, nausea, vomiting

■ Vestibular neuronitis: vertigo lasting days, severe nausea and vomiting, antecedent viral infection, and absence of hearing loss

■ Ototoxic vestibulopathy: usually associated with imbalance or disequilibrium, oscillopsia in sever cases, high frequency hearing loss

■ Benign Paroxysmal Positioning Vertigo (BPPV): vertigo lasting minutes with turning of head to side, fatigable, no hearing loss, history of past trauma, vestibular neuronitis, or otologic surgery

■ Positional Vertigo: persistent vertigo that comes on with specific position

■ Superior semicircular canal dehiscence syndrome: vertigo with positive pressure on the ear, loud noise, running or valsalva

■ Migraine associated vertigo: unilateral headache, visual symptoms

■ Multiple sclerosis: muscle weakness, neurologic symptoms

TESTS

■ Audiological Evaluation to rule out hearing loss: pure tone audiometry, speech audiometry, immittance testing, acoustic reflexes

- Auditory Brainstem Response (ABR) testing to exclude retrocochlear pathology when asymmetric SNHL is present
- Laboratory test including CBC, Platelets, ESR, ANA, RF, TSI I, Cholesterol, glucose, FTA, BUN, Creatinine, UA for evaluation of progressive or premature SNHL
- Electronystagmography to test for nystagmus and peripheral labyrinth function
- CT scan of the temporal bone (1.0 mm fine cuts, axial and direct coronal images) to evaluate for inner ear malformation and superior semicircular canal dehiscence syndrome
- MRI of the internal auditory canal and brain with gadolinium contrast enhancement to exclude cerebellopontine angle or brain tumors and multiple sclerosis

DIFFERENTIAL DIAGNOSIS

- Goal is to establish the tissue/organ responsible for vestibular symptoms: peripheral labyrinth, visual system, proprioception or cerebellar/central nervous system.

MANAGEMENT

- Initially, supportive care to control acute vertigo is crucial – usually with valium and compazine
- Vestibular physical therapy for persistent imbalance or disequilibrium
- Meniere's Disease:
  - ➤ low salt diet (2 gram Na/day), diuretics, intratympanic gentamicin if medical therapy fails
- Labyrinthitis:
  - ➤ antibiotics
- BPPV:
  - ➤ Epley maneuver
- Positional vertigo:
  - ➤ Cawthorne head exercises
- Superior semicircular canal dehiscence syndrome: observation or surgery

SPECIFIC THERAPY

n/a

FOLLOW-UP

- Vestibular physical therapy for persistent imbalance or disequilibrium

■ Surgery should be considered for persistent vertigo. Labyrithectomy is curative but results in complete hearing loss. Vestibular neurectomy is curative when patients have hearing

COMPLICATIONS AND PROGNOSIS
■ Most patients improve with little or no balance dysfunction.

INSOMNIA

CHAD CHRISTINE, MD

HISTORY & PHYSICAL
■ Difficulty initiating sleep
■ Difficulty maintaining sleep
■ Early awakening
■ May be notable for anxiety or depression

TESTS
■ Lab tests unremarkable
■ Brain imaging unremarkable
■ Sleep lab studies helpful if sleep apnea or restless legs syndrome suspected

DIFFERENTIAL DIAGNOSIS
■ Meds: steroids, beta-blockers, excessive thyroid hormone, decongestants, herbs, stimulants (pemoline, methylphenidate, etc), diuretics causing nocturia
■ Stimulants (caffeine, nicotine, alcohol, cocaine, amphetamine) excluded clinically
■ Periodic limb movements in sleep (often described as limb discomfort by pt & observed as rhythmic flexion movement of one or both legs) is excluded by history & sleep study (see "Restless Legs Syndrome" for treatment)
■ Medical disorders such as hyperthyroidism, gastroesophageal reflux, congestive heart failure (orthopnea), nocturia excluded clinically
■ Anxiety disorders & depression excluded clinically
■ Neurodegenerative disorders (Parkinson's disease, Alzheimer's disease/sundowning, etc) excluded clinically

MANAGEMENT
■ Depends on cause
■ General measures

➤ Maintain regular sleep/wake schedule; avoid naps
➤ Avoid caffeine, alcohol, heavy meals before sleep
➤ Stop or replace potentially offending meds
➤ Sleeping area should be cool, quiet, dark

SPECIFIC THERAPY
■ Depends on cause
■ Pts w/ sleep apnea benefit from continuous positive airway pressure
■ See treatment of restless leg syndrome for periodic limb movements in sleep

FOLLOW-UP
■ Depends on cause

COMPLICATIONS AND PROGNOSIS
■ Depend on cause

INTERSTITIAL LUNG DISEASES

JEFFREY A. GOLDEN, MD

HISTORY & PHYSICAL

History
■ Dyspnea and diffusely abnormal radiograph in context of chronic process exclusive of infection & malignancy
■ Shortness of breath with exertion; progressing to dyspnea at rest
■ Nonproductive cough, esp with a deep breath
■ Etiologic exposure &/or associated systemic diseases:
➤ work/environment (asbestos; organic materials/dusts, moldy wood, birds)
➤ Medication with lung toxicity
➤ Rheumatologic symptoms and signs
■ Associated systemic illness: rheumatologic disease

Signs & Symptoms
■ Rapid shallow breathing
■ Inspiratory dry ("Velcro") crackles

TESTS

Laboratory
■ ESR, ANA, rheumatoid factor, other serologies

Imaging

- CXR: normal in 10%; diffuse interstitial patterns: reticulation (lines/lace), ground glass, nodules, honeycombing, adenopathy
- CT:
  - Interstitial abnormalities, patterns as above
  - Dynamic exhalation demonstrates peripheral airway disease (air-trapping/mosaic perfusion)

PFTs

- Lung volumes (reduced TLC, VC)
- Diffusing capacity (reduced)
- Spirometry (may show increased flow rates)
- ABG
- Exercise testing: to detect equivocal disease or establish baseline:
  - SaO2 during walking
  - Formal incremental exercise test with arterial line and exhaled gas analysis

Lung Biopsy

- If history and imaging insufficient
- Bronchoscopic transbronchial biopsy:
  - Sarcoid, lymphangiitic carcinoma
  - Special studies:
    - Alveolar proteinosis: PAS stain
    - Eosinophilic granuloma:
      - EM – Langerhans cells
      - Stains: CD1A or S100
    - Lymphangioleiomyomatosis (LAM): smooth muscle stains including HMB45
    - Eosinophilic pneumonia: BAL eosinophil >40%
- Open lung biopsy/video-assisted thoracoscopic (VAT) biopsy for idiopathic interstitial pneumonia (IPF)

DIFFERENTIAL DIAGNOSIS

- Connective tissue diseases
- Medication-induced lung disease (furantoin, amiodarone, bleomycin)
- Environmental lung disease:
  - Inorganic: asbestos, silica, beryllium, coal
  - Organic: bird breeder's lung, farmer's lung
- Idiopathic interstitial lung diseases require biopsy:
  - Idiopathic pulmonary fibrosis (IPF)

- Pathology usual interstitial pneumonia (UIP)
- Patchy lung involvement (subpleural, basilar)
- Familial form (autosomal dominant)
➤ Nonspecific interstitial pneumonia (NSIP): uniform cellular alveolar wall infiltration
➤ Acute interstitial pneumonia (Hamman-Rich syndrome: rapid onset and death in months; uniform fibrosis
➤ Respiratory bronchiolitis and ILD:
- Desquamative interstitial pneumonitis (DIP)
- Cigarette abuse
- Intraalveolar macrophages
➤ Unclassified (primary) disease:
- Diagnosis: clinical or imaging may avoid biopsy:
- Sarcoid
- Eosinophilic granuloma
- Lymphangioleiomyomatosis (LAM)
- Tuberous sclerosis
- Amyloid
- Eosinophilic pneumonia
- Alveolar proteinosis
➤ Autoimmune lung fibrosis:
- IBD
- Primary biliary cirrhosis
- Thyroiditis
➤ Other:
- Bronchiolitis obliterans organizing pneumonia (BOOP)
- Lymphocytic interstitial pneumonia (LIP) (AIDS, connective tissue disease, thyroiditis)
- HIV: nonspecific interstitial pneumonia
- Pulmonary hemorrhage syndromes; hemoptysis may be absent

MANAGEMENT

What to Do First
- Establish diagnosis
- Clinical, radiographic &/or biopsy

General Measures
- Eliminate relevant exposures:
  ➤ Cigarettes in DIP, eosinophilic granuloma
  ➤ Antigen in hypersensitivity pneumonitis

- Baseline PFTs, CXR, CT
- Treat intercurrent infection
- Avoid aspiration; asymptomatic acid reflux common

SPECIFIC THERAPY

Indications

- Presence of disease unless extremely end-stage

Treatment Options

- Antiinflammatory therapy:
  - prednisone
  - azathioprine, cyclophosphamide: usually added as second agent to spare steroid adverse effects
  - Colchicine: may be antifibrotic; efficacy unclear
- Referral for lung transplantation

Side Effects & Contraindications

- Prednisone:
  - Systemic effects of steroids
  - If used with azathioprine or cyclophosphamide, give PCP prophylaxis
  - Contraindications:
    - Absolute: prior severe adverse reactions
    - Relative: mild diabetes, past history of ulcers, anxiety and irritability
- Azathioprine:
  - Side Effects: bone marrow suppression, liver toxicity, nausea, future malignancy
  - Contraindications
    - Absolute: liver disease, low blood counts
    - Relative: mildly low blood counts
- Cyclophosphamide:
  - Side effects: bone marrow suppression, esp leukopenia (adjust dose), bladder hemorrhage (take with large volume of water early in day), bladder tumors, azoospermia and amenorrhea, nausea, future malignancy
  - Contraindications
    - Absolute: preexisting hematologic abnormalities
    - Relative: mild hematologic abnormalities
- Colchicine:
  - Side effects: diarrhea, muscle weakness
  - Contraindications:

- Absolute: diarrhea
- Relative: prior allergic reaction or diarrhea

FOLLOW-UP

During Treatment

■ Assess complications and benefits:
  - ➤ CBC and LFT monthly (azathioprine)
  - ➤ UA monthly (cyclophosphamide)
  - ➤ BP, weight, glucose, bone density (prednisone)
  - ➤ Symptoms, 6-min walk test
  - ➤ Radiograph and CT
  - ➤ Pulmonary function including lung volume and diffusing capacity
  - ➤ Prednisone benefit usually apparent in 1–3 mo; azathioprine or cyclophosphamide usually require 3–6 mo

COMPLICATIONS AND PROGNOSIS

Complications

■ Acute exacerbation after prior insidious course
■ Progressive respiratory impairment and death
■ Cor pulmonale
■ Pulmonary embolism
■ Lung cancer in up to 10% of IPF patients, independent of smoking risk
■ Pulmonary infection

Prognosis

■ Depends on disease and reversible features such as exposure cessation
■ IPF invariably progressive: 50% mortality 2.8 y after diagnosis; objective improvement in less than 20%
■ Better prognosis for nonspecific interstitial pneumonia and respiratory bronchiolitis/ILD

INTERTRIGO

JEFFREY P. CALLEN, MD

HISTORY & PHYSICAL

History

■ Irritant dermatitis of intertriginous folds
■ Caused by maceration and rubbing

- Excessive moisture may predispose.
- Obesity is a predisposing factor.
- Candida is frequently involved.
- Diabetes mellitus may predispose.

Signs & Symptoms
- Inflammation characterized by erythema, maceration and pustules in the folds, primarily the inguinal folds

TESTS
- Basic tests: Potassium hydroxide preparation

Specific Diagnostic Tests
- Fungal culture
- Imaging studies – none

DIFFERENTIAL DIAGNOSIS
- Inverse psoriasis
- Dermatophyte infection
- Seborrheic dermatitis
- Benign familial pemphigus (Hailey-Hailey disease)
- Necrolytic migratory erythema
- Nutritional deficiencies (e.g., zinc)
- Extramammary Paget's disease (particularly if unilateral)

MANAGEMENT
What to Do First
- Assess the risk factors, such as trauma, exposure to excess moisture, diabetes.

General Measures
- Keep area dry.
- Assess the need for systemic therapy vs. local therapy.

SPECIFIC THERAPY
- Drying techniques
- Topical antifungal cream (e.g., clotrimazole, ketoconazole) combined with a low-potency corticosteroid cream (e.g., desonide, hydrocortisone). Avoid using existing mixtures that contain

higher-potency corticosteroids such as betamethasone diproprion-ate or triamcinolone, as they frequently cause atrophy and striae.

FOLLOW-UP

During Treatment
■ Re-evaluate patient 1–2 weeks after initiating therapy.

COMPLICATIONS AND PROGNOSIS
n/a

INTERVERTEBRAL DISC DISEASE

MICHAEL J. AMINOFF, MD, DSc

HISTORY & PHYSICAL
■ Pain in neck or back
■ Radicular pain
■ Aggravation of pain by increased intraspinal pressure (eg, cough) or stretch of compressed roots
■ Weakness, numbness or paresthesias in a radicular distribution may occur
■ Sphincter or sexual disturbances may occur
■ Spasm of paraspinal muscle & restriction of spinal movements
■ Spinal tenderness may be present
■ Weakness, sensory changes or both in radicular distribution some-times found
■ Reduced or absent tendon reflex subserved by affected root
■ Pain reproduced by root stretch (eg, passive straight leg raising; femoral stretch test)
■ May be bilateral radicular deficits w/ central disc prolapse affecting cauda equina or associated spinal stenosis
■ May be signs of cord compression w/ central disc protrusion above L1 level

TESTS
■ MRI to define nature & extent of root compression & exclude other causes of compression
■ EMG to define extent & severity of root involvement & likely prognosis

DIFFERENTIAL DIAGNOSIS
- Other spinal diseases & causes of root compression (eg, metastatic disease) will generally be recognized by the MRI findings

MANAGEMENT
- Bed rest for 2 or 3 days, followed by mobilization
- Simple analgesics or NSAIDs

SPECIFIC THERAPY
- Brief course of oral steroids sometimes used but of uncertain benefit
- Epidural or subarachnoid injections of steroids are sometimes given but are not advised (risk of infection or inflammation)
- Surgical decompression, especially for central disc protrusion, sphincter involvement, cord compression, pain unresponsive to other measures or progressive neurologic deficit

FOLLOW-UP
- Depends on severity of symptoms

COMPLICATIONS AND PROGNOSIS
- Delay in diagnosis of central disc prolapse may lead to sphincter impairment
- Recurrence of pain common after medical or surgical treatment

---

INTESTINAL FLUKES

J. GORDON FRIERSON, MD

HISTORY & PHYSICAL

History
- Life cycle: All these flukes live in upper small bowel, pass eggs into stool. In fresh water they go to snails. New larvae are released (cercariae), which attach to freshwater plants (fasciolopsis) or penetrate fish (heterophyes, metagonimus), which are then eaten. Larvae develop in small bowel, mate, and produce eggs.
  - ➤ Exposure: ingestion of undercooked freshwater plants or fish that are infested. The flukes are found in the Far East.

Signs & Symptoms
- Usually none, but can have abdominal pains, nausea, bloating in heavier infections

TESTS
- Basic tests: blood: may see eosinophilia
- Basic tests: urine: normal
- Specific tests: Stool O&P exam, finds eggs. It is difficult to distinguish various fluke eggs; expert help may be needed.
- Other tests: Barium study may show irritability, edema of upper small bowel.

DIFFERENTIAL DIAGNOSIS
- Peptic ulcer disease, gastritis, giardiasis, other bowel infections

MANAGEMENT

What to Do First
- Assess severity.

General Measures
- Determine source of infection, educate patient.

SPECIFIC THERAPY

Indications
- All infected patients

Treatment Options
- All 3 flukes: Praziquantel. Cure rate is high.

Side Effects & Complications
- Abdominal pain, diarrhea, probably relating to worm death
- Contraindications to treatment: absolute: Allergy to medication
- Contraindications to treatment: relative: light or asymptomatic infections due to Fasciolopsis buski. They die off in about 1 year without treatment.

FOLLOW-UP

During Treatment
- Monitor side effects.

Routine
- Repeat stool O&P exam 2 or more weeks after treatment.

COMPLICATIONS AND PROGNOSIS
- Metagonimus and Heterophyes worms become encapsulated in bowel wall, and eggs can enter circulation and embolize to the heart,

causing a myocarditis, or the brain, causing focal problems. In the absence of these complications, prognosis for all 3 flukes is good.

INTESTINAL MOTOR DISORDERS

GEORGE TRIADAFILOPOULOS, MD

HISTORY & PHYSICAL

■ Chronic intestinal pseudo-obstruction: syndrome that suggests mechanical bowel obstruction in the absence of anatomic obstruction

Risk Factors

■ Neuropathic damage:
  ➤ Amyloidosis, diabetes mellitus, multiple sclerosis, collagen vascular disease and paraneoplastic syndromes
■ Neurological intestinal dysfunction:
  ➤ Brainstem tumors, cerebrovascular accidents, spinal cord injury, Parkinson's disease or autonomic system degeneration
  ➤ Drugs: anticholinergics, antidepressants, calcium channel blockers, and alpha-2 adrenergic agonists
■ Early neuropathic damage but later myopathy:
  ➤ Scleroderma

Symptoms

■ Acute, recurrent, or chronic nausea and vomiting
■ Abdominal distension and pain
■ Constipation or diarrhea
■ Early satiety, anorexia, and weight loss
■ Occasionally urinary symptoms, such frequency and incontinence

Physical Signs

■ Abdominal distention
■ Succussion splash
■ Clinical signs suggestive of collagen vascular or neuromuscular disease

TESTS

Basic Tests

■ Serum electrolytes and albumin: hypokalemia and metabolic acidosis or alkalosis due to diarrhea or vomiting
■ Hypoalbuminemia: suggests malnutrition

- Occasionally intestinal bacterial overgrowth: decreased vitamin B12 levels or a positive Schilling's test
- Plain abdominal films: air-fluid levels and/or distended loops of small bowel

Specific Diagnostic Tests

- Upper gastrointestinal series:
  - ➤ exclusion of mechanical obstruction such as adhesions or Crohn's disease; dilated intestinal loops, poor motility, or diverticula
- Gastric and intestinal scintigraphy:
  - ➤ assessment of the presence of a disturbed intestinal and/or colonic transit; breath tests, such as breath hydrogen excretion, inaccurate in intestinal pseudo-obstruction since the substrate can be metabolized by bacterial overgrowth
- Gastroduodenal manometry:
  - ➤ measurement of the pressure profile of the stomach and small intestine over several hours during fasting and after a standard meal
  - ➤ manometric tracing may reveal: 1) simultaneous, prolonged contractions suggestive of mechanical intestinal obstruction; 2) low amplitude contractions suggestive of a myopathic process; and 3) abnormal organization and coordination of contractions typically associated with neuropathy
- Autonomic tests:
  - ➤ assessment of the sympathetic adrenergic, sympathetic cholinergic, and vagal innervation and to differentiate a preganglionic or central nervous system lesion from peripheral neuropathy associated with autonomic dysfunction
- Brain and spinal cord MRI
  - ➤ important to rule out a central lesion; screening for a toxic, metabolic, or paraneoplastic process should be done when peripheral dysautonomia is found
- Laparoscopy:
  - ➤ may be performed if mechanical obstruction suspected, or if a venting or feeding tube needed; full-thickness intestinal biopsy may be obtained

Other Tests

- Patients with steatorrhea, or vitamin B12 malabsorption, may benefit from a quantitative small bowel aspiration culture to rule out small bowel bacterial overgrowth

DIFFERENTIAL DIAGNOSIS
- Mechanical bowel obstruction (strictures, tumors, adhesions)

MANAGEMENT

What to Do First
- Rule out mechanical obstruction by radiologic or endoscopic means

General Measures
- Early institution of enteral nutrition for neuropathic disorders
- Parenteral nutrition may be necessary for patients with severe myopathic pseudo-obstruction

SPECIFIC THERAPY

Indications for Treatment
- Nausea, vomiting, constipation and diarrhea require symptomatic therapy Weight loss requires nutritional support

Treatment Options
- Intermittent courses of antibiotics, such as ciprofloxacin, doxycycline, and metronidazole in patients with small bowel bacterial overgrowth.
- Intravenous erythromycin effective during acute exacerbations of intestinal pseudo-obstruction, acting as a motilin receptor stimulant; not very effective as chronic therapy; IV metoclopramide may also be used during acute exacerbations
- Octreotide partly recovers the migratory motor complex and may improve motility in patients with scleroderma or idiopathic intestinal pseudo-obstruction
- Neostigmine, an acetylcholinesterase inhibitor, effective acutely but not for patients with chronic pseudoobstruction
- Serotonin (5HT) receptor agonists currently under investigation.
- Surgical resection of the small bowel or colon or bypass of dilated intestinal segments may be needed
- Laparoscopy also used to place venting and/or feeding tubes and to obtain a full-thickness biopsy of the intestinal wall for histologic examination
- Intestinal pacing and transplantation still experimental

Side Effects and Complications
- Metabolic and electrolyte abnormalities are due to uncontrolled disease Extrapyramidal signs with metoclopramide administration

Contraindications to Treatment
- Octreotide: not used in patients with bacterial overgrowth since it delays small bowel transit time

FOLLOW-UP

During Treatment
- Monitoring of electrolytes, hydration status and for drug side effects

Routine
- Periodic clinical and laboratory evaluations and nutritional assessment are needed

COMPLICATIONS AND PROGNOSIS

Complications
- Malnutrition to be avoided by all means

Prognosis
- Variable
- Hospitalizations for rehydration and nutritional support frequently needed

---

INTRACRANIAL HYPERTENSION

MICHAEL J. AMINOFF, MD, DSc

HISTORY & PHYSICAL
- Headache, often worse in the morning or on straining
- Visual blurring, obscurations, sometimes diplopia
- Reduced level of consciousness w/ increasing ICP
- No other neurologic complaints unless from herniation syndrome or from cause of increased ICP (eg, hematoma, tumor, venous sinus thrombosis)
- Bilateral papilledema
- 6th nerve palsy sometimes found
- Mild neck stiffness common
- Other neurologic deficits depend on underlying structural lesion

TESTS
- MRI or CT scan reveals underlying structural lesion, extent of mass effect; in pseudotumor cerebri, ventricles are small, slitlike; MRI provides better resolution of soft tissues & of posterior fossa than CT

- Spinal tap should not be undertaken prior to imaging study; reveals increased ICP & may suggest cause (eg, SAH, meningitis) if not evident on MRI

DIFFERENTIAL DIAGNOSIS
- All causes of increased ICP must be considered & excluded by tests
- MRI identifies, localizes & often characterizes structural lesions
- For pseudotumor cerebri, search for causes such as venous sinus thrombosis (imaging studies), hormonal disorder (oral contraceptive use, Cushing's or Addison's disease, steroid withdrawal, hypoparathyroidism), iatrogenic cause (hypervitaminosis A, tetracycline therapy in infants), chronic meningitis

MANAGEMENT
- Lower ICP acutely if herniation threatened from structural lesion; give mannitol

SPECIFIC THERAPY
- Depends on cause
- Reduce ICP by hyperventilation & w/ mannitol when caused by acute intracranial lesions; consider surgical decompression of cerebellar hematomas or superficial cerebral hematoma exerting mass effect
- For pseudotumor, give acetazolamide, diuretics or both; prednisone daily; repeated spinal taps, shunt placement or optic nerve sheath fenestration may be needed to lower ICP or protect optic nerve; treat any identified cause of pseudotumor

FOLLOW-UP
- Depends on cause
- For pseudotumor, measure CSF pressure weekly, then monthly, until control ensured; monitor visual fields & size of blind spot monthly thereafter

COMPLICATIONS AND PROGNOSIS
- Depends on cause of increased ICP
- Optic atrophy w/ resultant blindness is the consequence of untreated pseudotumor; idiopathic pseudotumor is self-limited & treatment can typically be reduced and discontinued after several months

---

INTRACRANIAL HYPOTENSION

MICHAEL J. AMINOFF, MD, DSc

HISTORY & PHYSICAL
- Headache, relieved by recumbency & worsened by upright position; worsened by Valsalva maneuver

- Nausea, vomiting, uni- or bilateral 6th nerve palsy occur commonly; tinnitus, hyperacusis sometimes occur
- May be history of lumbar puncture (LP) in previous week, or of trauma
- No neurologic deficit

TESTS
- None required unless symptoms occur in absence of history of LP; gadolinium-enhanced MRI may then show dural enhancement or associated subdural hematoma

DIFFERENTIAL DIAGNOSIS
- Absence of fever, other neurologic symptoms & signs of meningeal irritation makes meningitis unlikely
- History of trauma suggests cranial CSF fistula (eg, otorrhea or rhinorrhea)
- MRI will detect subdural hematoma or pituitary tumor, which may erode sella to cause CSF leak
- Absence of overt cause suggests CSF leak from arachnoid cyst related to spinal root sleeve

MANAGEMENT
- Bed rest may alleviate headache

SPECIFIC THERAPY
- Symptoms occasionally respond to caffeine, sodium benzoate
- Persistent symptoms may respond to epidural blood patch or epidural or intrathecal saline infusion
- Surgical closure of spontaneous dural leak is required in rare instances
- Surgery may be required for subdural hematoma or fistula related to trauma or tumor

FOLLOW-UP
- None needed once symptoms settle

COMPLICATIONS AND PROGNOSIS
- Symptoms eventually settle spontaneously

INTRAOCULAR INFECTION

TODD P. MARGOLIS, MD, PhD

HISTORY & PHYSICAL

History
- Decreased vision

- Pain, redness, light sensitivity
- Recent ocular trauma (bacillus), ocular surgery (staph epi or P acnes), or external herpes virus infection (HSV or VZV)
- Immunosuppression, either iatrogenic or secondary to systemic disease
- Disseminated infection (TB, fungi, bacteria, syphilis)
- Prolonged history of indwelling catheter (candida)

Signs & Symptoms
- Redness (ciliary flush), cell & flare, keratic precipitates (type and distribution), hypopyon
- Increasing (rather than decreasing) postop pain and redness
- Fine white plaque on lens capsule (suggests postop infection with P. acnes)
- IOP may be elevated with HSV, VZV and toxo
- Inflammatory cells in vitreous
  - "String of pearls" sign suggests fungus
- Retinal inflammation
  - Unifocal – toxoplasmosis and most CMV
  - Multifocal – VZV, HSV, endogenous bacterial or fungal endophthalmitis
  - No view – bacterial endophthalmitis
  - Old retinal scar with adjacent inflammation suggests toxoplasmosis.

TESTS

Laboratory
- Specific:
  - Corneal sensation if considering HSV or VZV
  - Serology for HSV, VZV, T. gondii rarely of value
  - PPD, FTA, Lyme and Bartonella serology as dictated by exam
  - Blood cultures for suspected endogenous endophthalmitis
  - Vitreous biopsy for bacterial/fungal culture and PCR (for HSV, VZV, CMV and T. gondii)
  - Note: aqueous tap may be as sensitive for PCR detection of viral DNA, but not for PCR detection of T. gondii. Aqueous also rarely of value in determining local elevated antibody titers (Goldmann-Witmer coefficent).

Imaging
- CXR to rule out systemic TB

■ B-scan ultrasound to confirm vitreal/retinal inflammation if view of posterior pole is poor

DIFFERENTIAL DIAGNOSIS

■ Immune-mediated uveitis: history, exam and absence of risk factors for ocular infection will help
■ Tumor: rule these out by age, history, exam and cytology of vitreous fluid
  ➣ Primary: melanoma, retinoblastoma, large cell lymphoma
  ➣ Metastatic: primarily to choroid

MANAGEMENT

What to Do First

■ Assess likelihood of postop or endogenous endophthalmitis, since these will require immediate vitreous biopsy and intravitreal antimicrobial therapy.
■ Determine if visual acuity is hand motions or worse. Postop endophthalmitis with hand motions or worse will require emergency vitrectomy for best visual outcome.
■ Determine if ocular inflammation fits pattern of acute retinal necrosis syndrome (rapidly progressive necrotizing peripheral retinitis, mid-peripheral vasculitis and vitiritis), since this will require immediate, intravitreal injection of foscarnet.

General Measures

■ Topical prednisolone acetate (1%) to control anterior segment inflammation after specific therapy is instituted
■ Cycloplegia (e.g., cyclopentolate 1%) to reduce development of posterior synechiae

SPECIFIC THERAPY

■ Depends on diagnosis:
  ➣ Bacterial endophthalmitis – intravitreal vancomycin & ceftazidime. Intravitreal dexamethasone may also be used. Consider amikacin or gentamicin as alterantives for gram-negative coverage and cefazolin as alternative for gram-positive coverage. Vitrectomy indicated for visual acuity of hand motions or worse. Intravitreal aminoglycosides are potentially toxic to retina.
■ Fungal endophthalmitis
  ➣ Intravitreal amphotericin and oral flucytosine. Check electrolytes and renal function before starting flucytosine.
■ Acute retinal necrosis

> Intravitreal foscamet and intravenous acyclovir. May also use intravitreal ganciclovir. Adjust acyclovir dose for reduced renal function.

■ Ocular toxoplasmosis

> Bactrim DS BID. Add pyrimethamine, clindamycin, and prednisone for recurrences threatening optic nerve or macula or for marked vitreal inflammation. Folinic acid twice weekly to reduce complications of pyrimethamine. Bactrim contraindicted in patients with sulfa allergy.

■ CMV

> systemic ganciclovir, foscarnet or valganciclovir. Consider ganciclovir implant. Reduce systemic immunosuppression.

> Bone marrow suppression is major complication of ganciclovir.

> Renal toxicity is major complication of foscamet.

■ Systemic therapy of TB, Bartonella and Lyme as indicated

FOLLOW-UP

■ Bacterial & fungal endophthalmitis:

> Daily for first 3–7 days, reduced frequency thereafter depending on response

■ Acute retinal necrosis:

> Two or three times a week initially, weekly for next month

■ Ocular toxoplasmosis:

> Every 2–3 weeks

■ CMV:

> 2 weeks after induction therapy, every 4–8 weeks thereafter, depending on response to therapy and CD4 count

COMPLICATIONS AND PROGNOSIS

■ Prognosis is guarded for bacterial and fungal endophthalmitis, but rapid recognition and response will usually result in visual acuity better than 20/80. Complications include cataract, glaucoma and retinal detachment.

Prognosis for acute retinal necrosis syndrome is also guarded. Most cases treated solely with systemic antivirals end up with vision worse than 20/400. However, treatment with intravitreal antivirals can significantly improve results. Complications include retinal detachment (common), cataract, persistent vitreal opacification.

Cases of ocular toxoplasmosis usually do quite well unless there is involvement of the optic nerve or macula. Major complication is retinal scarring.

The prognosis of CMV retinitis depends on location of the disease. Involvement of the optic nerve or macula leads to profound visual loss. Unless the immune system is reconstituted, the ultimate prognosis is very poor. With immune reconstitution, prognosis can be very favorable. Complications include retinal detachment, cataract and immune reconstitution uveitis.

INTRAOCULAR TUMORS

DEVRON H. CHAR, MD

HISTORY & PHYSICAL

■ Asymptomatic; decreased vision; rarely unilateral cataract, or painful red eye.

TESTS

■ Most diagnosed with non-invasive tests
■ Intraocular lymphoma may be diagnosed by vitrectomy cytology.
■ Retinal angioma patients should have a molecular genetic test for VHL.

DIFFERENTIAL DIAGNOSIS

■ Intraocular tumors are rare.
■ An apparent intraocular tumor is more likely hemorrhage associated with an idiopathic age-related macular degeneration or a localized choroidal hemorrhage (hypertension or after recent eye sugery).
■ Other benign conditions including scleritis can simulate an ocular malignancy.
■ Most common primary intraocular neoplasm in ambulatory adults is uveal melanoma (incidence of ~7/1,000,000/year); mainly older Caucasians.
■ <1% of uveal melanomas present simultaneously with detectable metastases.
■ Metastases to the choroid can be the first sign of a systemic malignancy.
■ ~ 10% of breast choroid metastases present before discovery of primary tumor.
■ ~ 90% of renal or lung patients have diagnosis of ocular tumor prior to discovery of primary lesion.
■ Metastases non-pigmented; clinical and ancillary imaging usually diagnostic

- If necessary, intraocular FNAB is definitive in primary and metastatic tumors.

MANAGEMENT

- ~80% of intraocular melanoma eyes can be salvaged, often with good vision.
- Treatments include laser, radiation, (brachytherapy, protons, or IMCT), removal of the tumor with retention of the eye, and enucleation.
- Metastases from uveal melanoma have a predilection for the liver.
- Uveal melanoma patients screened with serum LDH, GGT, CT/PET scan
- Metastases to the eye treated with chemotherapy or radiation; rarely a solitary lesion is amenable to brachytherapy or laser.
- ~33% of metastases to the eye have simultaneous CNS metastases; brain MRI with contrast

SPECIFIC THERAPY
n/a

FOLLOW-UP

- Depending on histology, and potential for effective therapy, metastatic evaluation accordingly.
- Retinoblastoma (Rb) virtually never presents in adults; bilateral Rb survivors pass the disease in an autosomal dominant manner.
- Molecular gene testing, especially in familial Rb disease, is quite accurate.
- More bilateral Rb children die from a second malignancy than Rb in the USA.
- Bilateral Rb survivors require constant vigilance for second tumors.

COMPLICATIONS AND PROGNOSIS
n/a

INTRAVASCULAR, NON-IMMUNE HEMOLYTIC ANEMIA – MICROANGIOPATHIC HEMOLYTIC ANEMIAS

CHRISTINE CSERTI, MD; FRANK J. STROBL, MD; JONATHAN KURTIS, MD, PhD; and LESLIE SILBERSTEIN, MD

HISTORY & PHYSICAL

History

- premature destruction of circulating red blood cells via direct mechanical, lytic, oxidizing, or thermal forces (see Differential Diagnosis)

- Disseminated intravascular coagulation (DIC)
- abnormal consumption of coagulation factors with secondary activation of fibrinolysis
- sepsis (e.g., gram-negative bacteria, encapsulated gram-positive bacteria, viral infections), obstetric complications, trauma, neoplasms, snakebites, burns, heat stroke, shock, hemolytic transfusion reactions, severe liver cirrhosis, malignant hypertension, cavernous hemangiomas
- Thrombotic thrombocytopenic purpura (TTP)
- congenital deficiency or acquired inhibitor to a serum metalloprotease responsible for normal cleavage of unusually large multimers of von Willebrand's factor; uncleaved large von Willebrand's multimers lead to agglutination of platelets
- most cases idiopathic
- associated with infection, pregnancy, transplant, AIDS, and drugs (e.g. mitomycin C, ticlopidine, cyclosporine, and tacrolimus)
- Hemolytic uremic syndrome (HUS)
- primarily a disease of childhood
- may be sporadic or associated with pregnancy (adult), epidemic (pediatric), or endemic
- onset of adult cases often as gastroenteritis or upper respiratory tract infection followed a week later by malaise, fatigue and oliguria
- pediatric cases typically develop following a febrile illness or infections with verotoxin-secreting strains of Escherichia coli (strain O157:H7) or Shigella dysenteriae

Signs & Symptoms
- Disseminated intravascular coagulation (DIC)
- often obscured by clinical features associated with primary initiating illness
- bleeding, thrombosis, fever, pallor
- Thrombotic thrombocytopenic purpura (TTP)
- pentad: fever, thrombocytopenia, microangiopathic hemolytic anemia, neurologic abnormalities, renal dysfunction
- pallor, purpura, petechiae, mucosal bleeding, jaundice, nausea/vomiting, abdominal pain, arthralgias, myalgias, hepatospenomegaly, delirium, seizures, coma, paralysis, aphasia, visual field defects
- Hemolytic uremic syndrome (HUS)
- triad: microangiopathic hemolytic anemia, thrombocytopenia, acute renal failure

- fever, pallor, jaundice, edema, nausea/vomiting, bloody diarrhea, abdominal pain, hypertension, purpura, petechiae, bleeding, hepatosplenomegaly

TESTS

Basic Blood Studies
- anemia, thrombocytopenia, hemoglobinemia, reduced haptoglobin levels, increased lactate dehydrogenase levels, increased unconjugated bilirubin levels, direct and indirect antiglobulin (Coombs') tests negative, increased BUN and creatinine
- DIC
- abnormal PT, PTT, and TT, decreased fibrinogen, increased fibrin degradation products, increased D-dimers, decreased Factor V and Factor VIII
- TTP
- normal PT, PTT, and TT, fibrinogen, coagulation factors
- HUS
- normal PT, PTT, and TT, fibrinogen, coagulation factors

Basic Studies: Peripheral Smear
- thrombocytopenia, schistocytes, microspherocytes, nucleated red blood cells, reticulocytosis (polychromasia and macrocytosis), leukocytosis

Basic Urine Studies
- hemoglobinuria, hemosiderinuria, increased urobilinogen, microscopic hematuria, proteinuria, granular casts

Bone Marrow Biopsy
- erythroid hyperplasia

Tissue Biopsy
- eosinophilic, hyaline thrombi containing fibrin and/or platelet aggregates occlude arterioles and small arteries

DIFFERENTIAL DIAGNOSIS

Infectious Agents
- gram-negative bacteria (e.g., Clostridium welchii) via secretion of proteolytic enzymes
- parasites (e.g., Plasmodium sp., Babesia sp., Bartonella bacilliformis) via direct parasitization of red blood cells

Chemical/Venom

- strong oxidant or proteolytic activity (venom) overwhelm normal reduction mechanisms or physical barriers responsible for protecting the integrity of the red blood cell
- often a metabolite of the chemical/drug is responsible
- fetal/newborn red cells have immature reduction pathways and thus are more sensitive to oxidant activity
- nitrofurantoin, sulfasalazine, p-Aminosalicylic acid, phenazopyridine, phenacetin, paraquat, naphthalene, isobutyl nitrate, amyl nitrite, dapsone, heavy metals (copper, lead, arsenic), cobra venom, brown recluse spider venom

Thermal

- normal red cells undergo lysis when heated to temperatures >49 degrees Celsius
- seen in patients transfused with faulty blood warmers and patients who have experienced extensive burns

Mechanical

- faulty natural valves or foreign material is placed within the vasculature (e.g., artificial valvular prostheses, stents, coils, TIPS, shunts, cardiopulmonary bypass)
- fibrin strands and/or platelet thrombi obstruct small blood vessels (microangiopathic hemolytic anemias – DIC, TTP, HUS)
- direct physical force compresses superficial blood vessels (e.g., marching, jogging, karate, conga drummers)

MANAGEMENT

What to Do First/General Measures

- DIC
- identify and correct underlying etiology; supportive care
- TTP
- initiate plasma exchange with fresh frozen plasma, steroids, and supportive care
- HUS
- supportive care and initiate dialysis for acute renal failure

SPECIFIC THERAPY

Indications

- DIC
- bleeding, thrombosis, anemia

- TTP
- thrombocytopenia, bleeding, anemia, neurologic abnormalities, renal failure
- HUS
- renal failure, hypertension, anemia, bleeding

Treatment options

- DIC
- in bleeding patients replace coagulation factors, platelets and red blood cells by transfusion with fresh frozen plasma, cryoprecipitate, platelets, and packed red blood cells as needed

*the following two bullets are recommending full-dose heparinization for those with thrombotic complications, which is appropriate; however, in cases of DIC wherein frank macrovascular thrombosis is not evident, there is also the option of using lower continuous infusion doses of heparin (not necessarily with a bolus) – i.e., 100–500 u/h (10–50% of the therapeutic dose) rather than the typical 1000 u/h (as per the 18 u/kg/h calculation), the rationale being the provision of an approach that quells the disseminated intravascular coagulation. which is the source of the consumptive coagulopathy.

- heparin therapy for patients with thrombotic complications (typically patients with chronic DIC secondary to neoplasm); 80 U heparin/kg intravenously followed by 18 U/kg/hr infusion; for long-term outpatient therapy give 35,000 U subcutaneously daily in divided doses 12 hours apart
- low-molecular-weight heparin: enoxaparin subcutaneously at 30 mg every 12 hours for prophylaxis against thrombosis or therapeutically 1 mg/kg every 12 hours; dalteparin subcutaneously 2,500 U daily for prophylaxis or therapeutically at 100 U/kg every 12 hours
- TTP
- plasma exchange: daily (1.0 to 1.5 plasma volume) exchanges with fresh frozen plasma, solvent-detergent treated plasma, donor-retested plasma, or cryo-poor supernatant (refractory patients) until platelet count and LDH within normal range for three consecutive days
- oral prednisone 1 to 2 mg/kg/day; taper at rate of 5 to 10 mg per week; iv methylprednisolone in divided doses ranging from 2 to 4 mg/kg/day for critically ill patients
- adjunctive therapies: vincristine, cyclophosphamide, cyclosporine, splenectomy, aspirin, dipyridamole, IVIG, protein A columns
- HUS

- acute renal failure and hematologic abnormalities are the main targets of therapy
- dialysis
- antihypertensive therapy
- plasma exchange is frequently initiated but is often not efficacious
- transfuse packed red blood cells and platelets as needed

Side Effects/Complications/Contraindications

- DIC
- heparin therapy should be avoided in patients with documented CNS bleed or recent surgery
- TTP
- transfuse platelets only to treat life-threatening bleeding; platelet transfusions may exacerbate disease process, and reports of death have consistently occurred in those transfused with platelets *before* treatment has been initiated with the first therapeutic plasma exchange
- anti-platelet drugs may increase the risk of bleeding
- HUS
- plasma exchange, steroids, heparin and anti-platelet drugs have not been helpful or their role has not been clearly defined
  - ➤ Antifibrinolytics, prothrombin complex concentrates, and recombinant activated factor VII are contraindicated in DIC due to risk of precipitating disseminated thrombosis.

FOLLOW-UP

- DIC
- the efficacy of therapy can be monitored by following changes in D-dimers, fibrinogen, and platelets
- the PTT or heparin level should be checked several hours after heparin administration and dosage adjustments made accordingly
- TTP
- the efficacy of therapy can be monitored by following changes in mental status, platelet count, hemoglobin, LDH, schistocyte number, and renal function; platelet counts can be monitored periodically with decreasing frequency as duration of remission lengthens
- HUS
- monitor blood pressure, renal function, platelet count, LDH, hemoglobin levels, schistocyte number

COMPLICATIONS AND PROGNOSIS

Complications
- DIC
- bleeding, thrombosis, death
- TTP
- seizure, coma, stroke, paralysis, myocardial infarction, sudden death
- HUS
- hypertension, renal insufficiency, seizure, coma, death

Prognosis
- DIC
- depends primarily on initiating illness
- TTP
- almost universally fatal if left untreated
- 80 to 90% of patients with primary TTP attain an initial remission; one or more relapses occur in up to 40 % of patients at variable times of weeks to years after initial event
- individuals with drug-induced or transplant-associated disease appear less responsive to therapy
- HUS
- up to 60% of adult patients require dialysis; 50% develop chronic renal insufficiency
- mortality up to 25% in adults
- epidemic cases have best prognosis
- sporadic cases, familial cases, older patients, patients without diarrhea and patients with severe renal dysfunction have poorer prognosis

IRON DEFICIENCY

KENNETH R. BRIDGES, MD

HISTORY & PHYSICAL

History
- Gastrointestinal bleeding
- colon cancer
- peptic ulcer disease
- esophageal or gastric varices
- Meckel's diverticulum

- hemorrhoids
- parasites (e.g., hookworm)
- Menstruation – may or may not be "heavy"
- Small intestinal disease
- Celiac disease (can be mild or even subclinical)
- Crohn's disease
- High gastric pH
- hemigastrectomy
- vagotomy
- pernicious anemia
- calcium-carbonate-based antacids
- histamine H-2 receptor blockers
- Inhibitors of iron absorption
- phytates (wheat and bran)
- tannins (teas)
- soil clay
- laundry starch
- Competitors of iron absorption
- lead
- Urinary tract bleeding
- papillary necrosis
- Pulmonary hemosiderosis
- chronic infection
- idiopathic

Signs & Symptoms
- fatigue
- palpitations
- dyspnea on exertion
- pica (ice, soil clay, laundry starch)
- Pallor
- Koilonychia
- Thinning of hair
- Angular stomatitis
- Glossitis
- Cardiac systolic flow murmur
Blue sclerae

TESTS

Basic Tests:
- **Blood**

➤ complete blood count and mean corpuscular volume (CBC)
➤ reticulocyte count
➤ RDW (iron deficiency – elevated; thalassemia trait – normal)
➤ serum iron
➤ total iron-binding capacity (TIBC)
➤ serum ferritin
➤ erythrocyte sedimentation rate (ESR)
- **Stool**
  ➤ guaiac
- **Urine**
  ➤ hemosiderin
  ➤ hemoglobin

Specific Diagnostic Tests
- Bone marrow aspirate with Perl's Prussian blue iron stain (Zenker's fixative can wash iron out of biopsies).
- Red cell zinc protoporphyrin levels
Reticulocyte hemoglobin concentration

DIFFERENTIAL DIAGNOSIS
n/a

MANAGEMENT

What to Do First
- Determine and interdict the source of blood loss.

General Measures
- Assess hemodynamic stability with acute bleeding superimposed on chronic blood loss.

SPECIFIC THERAPY

Indications for Treatment
- organ hypoxia due to decreased oxygen-carrying capacity
- fatigue, dyspnea
- glossitis, angular stomatitis

Treatment Options
- oral iron replacement. Preferred route on an empty stomach. Vitamin C increases absorption. Delayed-release tablets primarily release below the duodenum, missing the major site of iron absorption. Add meat to diet if meat intake is low.

- parenteral iron replacement. Intramuscular or intravenous. Iron dextran or iron saccharates. Test dose is essential. Methylprednisolone given before iron dextran replacement aborts late side effects (myalgias, arthralgias, fever). IM iron dextran replacement is limited to 100 mg per treatment.
- Red cell transfusion: Life-threatening anemia only

Side Effects and Complications
- oral iron – cramps, constipation, diarrhea. One tablet at bedtime has fewer side effects. Ferrous gluconate better than ferrous sulfate; about the same price. Warn patients of black stools.
- parenteral iron replacement
  - ➤ Iron dextran – Test dose always IV; cessation with first sign of reaction. IM treatment – black discoloration of skin, local irritation with fibrosis, pain. IV iron dextran – myalgias, arthralgias, fever the day after treatment.
  - ➤ Iron saccharates – FDA approved for dialysis patients. Maximum IV dose – 125 mg elemental iron. Very few side effects. An alternative for patients with allergy to iron dextran.
- Red cell transfusion – Pulmonary edema due to plasma volume expansion with rapid RBC replacement; viral infections; hemolytic reactions

Contraindications – Absolute
- oral iron: None
- parenteral iron: History of allergic or anaphylactic reactions to specific IV iron preparations
- red cell transfusions: None

Contraindications – Relative
- oral iron: Gastrointestinal intolerance, low gastric pH, rapid correction needed
- parenteral iron: History of multiple drug allergies (atopic state); History of reactions to dextran plasma expanders; ongoing treatment with high-dose corticosteroids that might mask allergic reaction to test dose
- red cell transfusions
  - ➤ Religion (e.g., Jehovah's Witness)
  - ➤ alloimmunization
  - ➤ plasma volume expansion

FOLLOW-UP

During Treatment
- Monitor hematocrit, MCV.
- Monitor ferritin. IV iron makes serum iron value unreliable.
- Monitor GI symptoms with oral iron.
- Assess systemic symptoms with IV iron dextran replacement.

Routine
- Follow CBC, MCV.
- Monitor iron, TIBC, ferritin.

COMPLICATIONS AND PROGNOSIS

Complications
- Common
  - oral iron: GI symptoms. Change preparation.
  - Iron dextran: arthralgias, myalgias, fever. Pretreat with corticosteroids.
- Rare
  - Iron dextran: anaphylaxis. IV test dose.
  - Iron saccharates: hypotension. Oral hydration, brief recumbence.

Transfusion: Pulmonary edema – slow infusion. Acute hemolytic reaction-good cross-matching. Delayed transfusion reaction. History of alloantibodies to minor RBC antigens.

Prognosis
- Excellent for iron deficiency per se. Overall prognosis depends on cause of iron deficiency.

IRRITABLE BOWEL SYNDROME

MARTA L. DAVILA, MD

HISTORY & PHYSICAL

History
- Abdominal pain
  - Crampy with variable intensity and periodic exacerbations, generally located in the lower abdomen
  - Severity from mild to debilitating
- Altered bowel habits

- ➤ Diarrhea
  - Frequent loose stools of small to moderate volume with or without mucus
  - Occurs during waking hours and very often after meals
  - Accompanied by urgency and a feeling of incomplete evacuation
- ➤ Constipation
  - Hard, pellet shaped stools, with straining and a feeling of incomplete evacuation
- ➤ Alternating diarrhea and constipation
- ■ Other common gastrointestinal symptoms :
  - ➤ Bloating, flatulence, belching, intermittent dyspepsia, nausea, early satiety, gastroesophageal reflux, dysphagia and non-cardiac chest pain
- ■ Other extra-intestinal symptoms:
  - ➤ Impaired sexual function, dysmenorrhea, dsyspareunia, increased urinary frequency and urgency, and fibromyalgia

Physical Signs
- ■ Physical exam usually unremarkable
- ■ Palpable and tender sigmoid colon or discomfort on rectal examination in patients with constipation

TESTS

Diagnostic Criteria
- ■ No biological disease markers to make a diagnosis
- ■ Diagnosis based on identification of symptoms consistent with IBS, and exclusion of organic disorders
- ■ Two sets of diagnostic criteria have been used for definition:
  - ➤ Manning criteria: the likelihood of IBS is proportional to the number of criteria present:
    - Pain relieved with defecation
    - More frequent stools at the onset of pain
    - Looser stools at the onset of pain
    - Visible abdominal distension
    - Passage of mucus
    - Sensation of incomplete evacuation
  - ➤ The Rome criteria developed by an international consensus team:
    - At least three months of continuous or recurrent symptoms of the following:

- Abdominal pain or discomfort
- Relieved with defecation, or
- Associated with a change in frequency of stool, or
- Associated with a change in consistency of stool
- Two or more of the following, at least on one fourth of occasions or days:
  - Altered stool frequency
  - Altered stool form
  - Altered stool passage, or
  - Passage of mucus, or
  - Bloating or feeling of abdominal distension

Diagnostic Approach to Rule Out Organic Disease

- Basic studies:
  - Blood: CBC, chemistry panel, ESR and thyroid function tests
- Basic studies:
  - Stool for blood
  - Stool (if diarrhea predominant) for ova and parasites, fecal leukocytes and qualitative fat
  - Flexible sigmoidoscopy with biopsy in patients with diarrhea or blood in stool, or in any patient over the age of 40

DIFFERENTIAL DIAGNOSIS

- Features not compatible with IBS:
  - Pain associated with anorexia, malnutrition or weight loss
  - Pain that awakens patient from sleep or prevents sleep
  - Gastrointestinal bleeding, anemia, fever
- Differential diagnosis include:
  - Inflammatory bowel disease
  - Gastrointestinal infections
  - Lactose intolerance
  - Endocrine disorders (hypo- or hyperthyroidsm, diabetes)
  - Medication-induced diarrhea or constipation
  - Malabsorption syndromes
  - Colorectal cancer
  - Endocrine tumors
  - Microscopic colitis

MANAGEMENT

What to Do First

- Establish a therapeutic physician-patient relationship
- Educate the patient regarding the possible pathophysiology of the syndrome and involve the patient in treatment decisions

- Reassure the patient regarding the chronic and benign nature of the syndrome

General Measures
- Dietary modification; exclusion of foods that increase flatulence
- Increase dietary fiber

SPECIFIC THERAPY

Pharmacological Therapy
- Medications only an adjunct to treatment
- Pharmacologic therapy depends on patient's symptoms
- Anticholinergic agents
  - ➤ May be beneficial in patients with post-prandial abdominal pain, gas, bloating and fecal urgency
  - ➤ Commonly used:
    - Dicyclomine
    - Hyoscyamine
    - Hyoscyamine
- Anti-diarrheal agents
  - ➤ Beneficial in diarrhea-predominant IBS
  - ➤ Should be used on an as needed basis
  - ➤ Loperamide and cholestyramine have been found to be helpful
- Antidepressants
  - ➤ May be beneficial in patients with neuropathic-type pain
  - ➤ Improvement in pain may occur at lower doses than those needed for the treatment of depression
  - ➤ Tricyclic antidepressants (amitriptyline and imipramine) and selective serotonin re-uptake inhibitors can be used (paroxetine, fluoxetine, or sertraline)
- 5-hydroxytryptamine agonists
  - ➤ May increase colonic motility and improve constipation
  - ➤ First drug of its class undergoing evaluation and may be approved for use in the near future
- Anxiolytics
  - ➤ Limited usefulness due to risk of habituation and withdrawal
  - ➤ May be used in the short-term to reduce anxiety if it is an aggravating factor

Psychosocial therapies
- Cognitive behavioral treatment, hypnosis, psychotherapy, relaxation techniques can help reduce anxiety, improve health promoting behavior and pain tolerance

FOLLOW-UP
- Reevaluate 3–6 weeks after initiation of therapy to assess response
- More extensive evaluation (symptom-dependent) is considered in patients who have had a change or progression of symptoms, or in those who do not respond

COMPLICATIONS AND PROGNOSIS
- Good with normal life span

ISCHEMIC BOWEL DISEASE

JOHN P. CELLO, MD

HISTORY & PHYSICAL
- Variable manifestations ranging from intestinal angina to necrotic bowel; classically, pain out of proportion to the physical finding; must always consider ischemic bowel when a patient at risk for ischemia (age >50, arrhythmia, CHF, diabetes, known coronary artery or general atherosclerosis) has new onset of abdominal pain with or without hematochezia
- Presentation depends upon sit blood flow, collateral circulation present and rapidity of restoration of normal perfusion.
- Large bowel:
  - Transient loss of flow and good collateral circulation (usually a "low flow state" from diminished cardiac output) – minimal abdominal pain and some hematochezia; may be recurrent for weeks
  - Abrupt loss of perfusion (e.g. embolus or acute thrombosis) long lasting ischemia with poor collaterals
    - moderately severe abdominal pain and hematochezia
- Total loss of perfusion – "dead bowel" – severe abdominal pain with cardiovascular collapse and sepsis; a surgical emergency
- Small Bowel:
  - Transient loss of flow and good collaterals – usually stressed by food intake – "intestinal angina" – classically "fear of eating"
    - No classic physical or laboratory findings – weight loss common
- Abrupt loss of perfusion, long lasting with poor collaterals –
  - severe abdominal pain out of proportion to physical exam findings; may actually have normal abdominal exam yet patient looks and acts sick – believe him/her and proceed with rapid evaluation

■ Total loss of perfusion from catastrophic thrombosis or embolus – "dead bowel" – severe abdominal pain with cardiovascular collapse and sepsis; a surgical emergency

TESTS

Laboratory Tests
■ Usually some elevation of WBC and left shift
■ Elevated serum amylase and/or lipase if proximal small bowel ischemia
■ Anion gap acidosis and lactic acidosis late manifestations – often too late to have meaningful impact on outcome
■ Usually hemoconcentrated; not anemic

Radiography
■ Plain radiographs rarely specific – may show "thumbprints" of edematous bowel wall, air in wall of bowel or portal venous air. Rarely show "free air"
■ Contrast radiography – barium enema and UGI series show edematous bowel wall; do not do barium exams prior to CT
■ CT scans – very helpful at suggesting diagnosis – need IV, oral and rectal contrast – show edematous bowel wall (thickened valvulae of small bowel and/or haustra), air in bowel wall and portal venous air

Endoscopy
■ Rarely see actual small bowel ischemia – may rule out other causes of abdominal pain

Colonoscopy
■ Very helpful – classic findings, normal rectum yet submucosal hemorrhages and shallow ulcers beginning in segmental distribution

Angiography:
■ Helpful only for acute emboli/thrombosis or to identify severe
■ ASCVD

DIFFERENTIAL DIAGNOSIS
■ Early clinical manifestations often dismissed as trivial/self-limited
■ Major differential diagnoses:
   ➢ Appendicitis – CT helpful here
   ➢ Peptic ulcer disease – endoscopy helpful to exclude

➤ Pancreatitis – CT helpful
➤ Inflammatory bowel disease – sigmoidoscopy/colonoscopy
  • important to make distinction – NOTE: rectum usually involved in ulcerative colitis but rarely so in ischemia.
■ If any question about diagnosis – early surgery is essential – time is of the essence.

MANAGEMENT

What to Do First
■ Resuscitate quickly
■ CT early in work-up-IV, oral and rectal contrast essential

General Measures
■ Consult GI and Surgery quickly (limited colonoscopy may be helpful)
■ Always have index of suspicion for ischemic bowel disease when pain is "out of proportion" to the physical findings
■ when in doubt – exploratory laparotomy or laparoscopy

SPECIFIC THERAPY
■ For severe ischemia with likely dead bowel – urgent surgery
■ For intestinal angina – evaluate by elective angiography and consider vascular reconstruction, angioplasty, stent, etc.
■ For ischemic colitis – consider cardiology evaluation detect occult may be helpful to look CHF, arrhythmias or valvular disease
■ Elective angiography for treatable stenosis

FOLLOW-UP
■ When self-limited ischemic bowel subsides, evaluate for ASCVD, coagulopathy, valvular heart disease, arrhythmias, occult CHF
■ Small bowel ischemia with resection, common cause of chronic malabsorbtion "short gut syndrome" – may need TPN or supplements

COMPLICATIONS AND PROGNOSIS
■ Major problem is missed diagnosis with subsequent dead bowel and patient death
■ "Short gut" syndrome with malabsorption common following extensive small bowel resections
■ If etiology not discovered and corrected, recurrent episodes common often leading to a fatal outcome

ISOSPORIASIS

J. GORDON FRIERSON, MD

HISTORY & PHYSICAL

History

■ Life cycle: ingested sporozoites of Isospora belli release sporozoites in small bowel, which invade epithelial cells, mature, are re-released to invade new cells. Some produce sporozoites, which mature to sporocysts and pass in stool.

■ Exposure: ingestion of sporocysts through contaminated food and water

Signs & Symptoms

■ Some pts are asymptomatic. Others may develop diarrhea, abdominal cramps, flatulence, anorexia, sometimes low-grade fever. Abdominal exam may show mild tenderness, distention. Usually self-limited infection, lasting a few weeks, occasionally chronic. Immunocompromised patients can have very prolonged symptoms.

TESTS

■ Basic tests: blood: may show eosinophilia
■ Basic tests: urine: normal
■ Specific tests: Stool exam for O&P, which should include acid-fast stain or immunofluorescence assays. May need multiple stools.
■ Other tests: Entero-test (string test) or small bowel drainage and/or biopsy will show organisms.

DIFFERENTIAL DIAGNOSIS

■ Other causes of diarrhea, especially giardiasis, cyclosporiasis, cryptosporidiosis, travelers' diarrhea

MANAGEMENT

What to Do First

■ Assess need for fluids, electrolyte therapy.

General Measures

■ Assess for source of infection.

SPECIFIC THERAPY

Indications

■ All symptomatic patients

Treatment Options

- Trimethoprim-sulfamethoxazole
- Pyrimethamine alone in case of sulfa allergy

Side Effects & Complications

- Usually due to sulfamethoxazole: rash, fever, leukopenia, thrombocytopenia
- Contraindications to treatment: absolute: allergy to medications
- Contraindications to treatment: relative: asymptomatic patient

FOLLOW-UP

During Treatment

- Watch for allergic reactions.

Routine

- Follow-up stool exam 2–3 weeks after treatment finished

COMPLICATIONS AND PROGNOSIS

- Prognosis is good in immunocompetent host. Immunocompromised patients may need chronic therapy.

JAW SWELLING AND MASSES

ANDREW H. MURR, MD, FACS

HISTORY & PHYSICAL

History

- Duration
- Changes in size
- Presence or absence of pain
- Exposure to animals or pets
- Recent travel
- Accompanying cold or upper respiratory infection
- Recent dental work or toothache
- History of immunocompromise
- Fatigue, night sweats, lethargy
- History of chronic cough
- History of cigarette smoking and alcohol use
- Asian ancestry (for nasopharyngeal carcinoma)

Signs & Symptoms

- Size and shape, presence or absence of tenderness or erythema, mobility versus fixation, fluctuance, skin necrosis.

- Exact location: tail of parotid, level I of neck (submandibular triangle) level II of neck (jugulodigastric lymph node chain).
- Purulence expressible from Wharton's or Stensen's duct
- Condition of teeth: presence of caries, tenderness to percussion.
- Facial nerve evaluation and exam.
- Presence of swollen lymph nodes in other parts of the body.
- Presence or absence of fever.
- Complete head and neck examination including examinations of the tympanic membranes, cranial nerves, nose, nasopharynx, oral cavity, oropharynx, hypopharynx, and larynx. Complete neck examination.

TESTS
- Blood:
  - CBC with platelets and differential
- Other:
  - PPD and anergy panel, Anti-Viral Capsid Antigen for Epstein-Barr virus
- Imaging:
  - CT scan with contrast for suspected infectious etiology
  - MRI with Gadolinium for suspected neoplastic or congenital etiology
- Pathology:
  - Fine Needle Aspiration (FNA) for cytological examination and culture
  - Office endoscopic laryngeal examination
  - Open biopsy is contraindicated in most neoplastic situations except where tissue is needed for lymphoma typing. FNA will frequently yield the diagnosis, especially with squamous cell carcinoma and nasopharyngeal carcinoma.
  - Operative laryngoscopy, esophagoscopy, and bronchoscopy sometimes necessary depending on results of above

DIFFERENTIAL DIAGNOSIS

Congenital Masses
- Branchial cleft cysts (Types I, II, III, IV), Hemangioma, Lymphangioma (Cystic Hygroma), Vascular Abnormalities

Neoplastic Masses
- Parotid Tumors (80% benign, 20% malignant): Benign (Warthin's tumor, Benign Mixed Tumors, Benign Lymphoepithelial Cyst of

IRV), Malignant (Mucoepidermoid Carcinoma, Adenoid Cystic Carcinoma, Malignant Mixed Tumors, Adenocarcinoma).
- Submandibular Masses (50% benign, 50% malignant): same pathological types as for parotid tumors.
- Lymphoma
- Squamous Cell Carcinoma
- Nasopharyngeal Carcinoma

Infectious Masses
- Salivary Calculi: duct stones in Stensen's or Wharton's duct
- Dental infection
- Cat-Scratch Disease
- Atypical Mycobacterial infection
- Tuberculosis
- Actinomycosis
- Bacterial Adenitis
- Kikuchi's Disease
- Kawasaki's Disease
- Castleman's Disease
- HIV

MANAGEMENT
- Directed tests such as endoscopy in the office, computerized imaging, and FNA with cultures are usually the studies that will significantly narrow down the diagnosis.
- Patients with infectious masses are often admitted to the hospital for IV antibiotics if the infection is acute, while more chronic infections can usually be treated on an outpatient basis with oral antibiotic coverage as directed by the diagnosis.
- Neoplastic conditions and congenital masses are often worked up on an outpatient basis.

SPECIFIC THERAPY
Congenital Masses
- Branchial cleft cysts are usually excised.

   Hemangiomas often regress at about 18 months of age and regression can occasionally be hastened with steroids.

   Lymphangiomas can be excised and/or sclerosed.

   Low-flow vascular malformations can be sclerosed.

   High-flow lesions can be treated via intra-arterial occlusion with or without excision.

Neoplastic Masses

- All parotid masses should be excised, the exception being known Warthin's tumors and known lymphoepithelial cysts (which can be sclerosed).

    Submandibular tumors should be removed.

    Lymphomas are treated non-surgically, usually with chemotherapeutic regimens when appropriate.

- Squamous cell carcinomas are treated primarily with surgery and/or radiation therapy with chemotherapy sometimes included, especially in neoadjuvant combination with radiation therapy.

- Nasopharyngeal carcinoma is treated with neoadjuvant chemotherapy and radiation therapy, with surgery being reserved when salvage is necessary or when residual disease remains after chemo/radiation intervention.

Infectious Masses

- Stones are treated with antibiotics, sialogogues, hydration, and occasionally with surgical removal of the stone itself or of the gland itself.

    Bacterial adenitis is treated with broad-spectrum antibiotics, which cover anaerobes and aerobes; penicillin derivatives are often preferred. However, abscesses from adenitis are treated with surgical incision and drainage.

    Cat-Scratch can be treated with ciprofloxacin.

    Actinomycosis can be treated with 6 weeks of IV penicillin.

    Atypical Mycobacterial infection can be treated with macrolides, quinolones, or surgical excision or surgical debridement.

    TB is treated with various triple antibiotic regimens.

    Dental infections are treated with antibiotics, often in combination with dental surgery, such as root canal procedures or tooth extraction.

FOLLOW-UP

n/a

COMPLICATIONS AND PROGNOSIS

Complications

- Surgical excision can result in cranial nerve injury and subsequent deficit.

    Medical therapy with antibiotics can result in a myriad of problems related to the specific drug selected for treatment.

- Complications of FNA are minimal, especially with regard to seeding tumor in the needle tract.

Prognosis
- Varies with the diagnosis. Infectious problems usually have a good prognosis, whereas malignancies carry a fair mortality risk, depending on the exact type.
- Congenital lesions like lymphangiomas and vascular malformations can cause a great deal of morbidity and even mortality if extensive.

KELOIDS

DAVID OUTLAND, MD and JEFFREY P. CALLEN, MD
REVISED BY JEFFREY P. CALLEN, MD

HISTORY & PHYSICAL
- Usually a history of trauma or injury at site; however, the injury might have been minor
- Occurs more commonly in dark-skinned individuals
- A genetic predisposition is likely.
- Occurs equally among men and women
- Flesh-colored, pink, purple or hyperpigmented
- Usually painless but can be painful or pruritic
- Extends beyond the site of physical injury
- Most commonly occurs on ears, upper chest, upper back, suprapubic and shoulders

TESTS
- None indicated unless diagnosis is questionable
- Biopsy is diagnostic but is rarely indicated.
- Biopsy shows thickened collagen bundles that are whorled, with occasional increased numbers of mast cells and plasma cells.

DIFFERENTIAL DIAGNOSIS
- Hypertrophic scar

MANAGEMENT
- Mostly surgical; however, injection with intralesional corticosteroids may prove beneficial

SPECIFIC THERAPY
- Generally referred to dermatologist, surgeon and/or radiation therapist
- Intralesional corticosteroids such as triamcinolone acetonide

- ■ Surgical excision
  - ➤ Alone
  - ➤ With immediate and periodic injection of intralesional corticosteroids into site
  - ➤ With postoperative silicone gel dressings
  - ➤ With intralesional interferon alfa-2b
  - ➤ With intralesional injection of 5-fluorouracil
  - ➤ With topical application of imiquimod
  - ➤ With radiotherapy immediately postop
- ■ Possible success with 585-nm flashlamp pumped pulsed dye laser

FOLLOW-UP
- ■ Postop follow-up with adjunctive therapy such as intralesional steroids, silicone gel dressings, pressure dressings, etc.

COMPLICATIONS AND PROGNOSIS
- ■ Most common complication is recurrence.
- ■ Frequent follow-up with adjunctive therapy may decrease risk of recurrence.
- ■ Postop wound infection is rare.

LACERATION OR MYOCARDIAL PERFORATION

JUDITH A. WISNESKI, MD

HISTORY & PHYSICAL
- ■ Hypotension
- ■ Cardiac tamponade
- ■ New heart murmur

TESTS
- ■ Echo/Doppler – location of laceration
- ■ MRI (pending stability of patient) – location of laceration

DIFFERENTIAL DIAGNOSIS
n/a

MANAGEMENT
- ■ Pericardiocentesis for tamponade
- ■ Emergency surgical intervention for laceration repair

SPECIFIC THERAPY
n/a

FOLLOW-UP
n/a

COMPLICATIONS AND PROGNOSIS
- Ventricular aneurysm (true or false)
- Septal perforation with VSD (ventricular septal defect)

LARYNGOTRACHEITIS

CAROL A. GLASER, MD

HISTORY & PHYSICAL

History
Overlap with Croup
Etiologies same as croup

Signs & Symptoms
- Cold symptoms initially
- Later dryness, irritation and coryza
- Fever
- Then 12–48 hours later, upper airway obstructive
- Cough is "croupy" (sounds like a barking seal)
- Then increase in respiratory stridor
- Usually lasts 3–7 days
- Etiologies: usually viral, same as croup above

TESTS
PA CXR; subglottic narrowing; WBC may be increased

DIFFERENTIAL DIAGNOSIS
n/a

MANAGEMENT
n/a

SPECIFIC THERAPY
Close observation
Vaporizers may produce symptomatic relief.

FOLLOW-UP
n/a

COMPLICATIONS AND PROGNOSIS

■ Obstruction can become progressive and lead to severe respiratory distress with hypoxia.
■ May predispose to hyperreactive airways later in life

LAXATIVE ABUSE

MARTA L. DAVILA, MD

HISTORY & PHYSICAL

■ Possible presentations: diarrhea, abdominal discomfort, nausea, vomiting, weight loss, muscle weakness, bone pain, rectal pain and lassitude
■ Laxative abuse present in 4–15% of patients with chronic diarrhea
■ Most patients women with an altered self-image, often with anorexia or bulimia nervosa
■ Other patients with hysteria-like characteristics in the absence of a motive for gain
■ Chronic stimulant laxative abuse (>15 years) may result in cathartic colon, which can present with constipation and vague abdominal discomfort rather than diarrhea
■ Admission of laxative use unusual, unless confronted with evidence
■ Signs: skin pigmentation, cyclic edema, kidney stones, clubbing

TESTS

Basic Tests: Blood
■ Electrolytes (hypokalemia, metabolic alkalosis)

Diagnostic Tests:
■ Stool for osmolarity and electrolytes
  ➢ High fecal sodium with a low fecal chloride concentration suggest sodium sulfate or sodium phosphate ingestion
  ➢ Osmotic diarrhea suggests magnesium laxatives
■ Stool or urine for phenolphtalein
  ➢ 3 ml of stool supernate or urine mixed with one drop of one normal (1N) sodium hydroxide; pink or red color indicates phenolphtalein is present
■ Stool or urine for emetine, bisacodyl and its metabolites, and anthraquinone derivatives

Other Tests:

- Sigmoidoscopy or colonoscopy: may reveal melanosis coli, a benign condition characterized by dark pigmentation of the mucosa caused by anthracene-containing laxatives (senna, cascara, aloe, danthron)
- Barium enema: may reveal a cathartic colon – dilated colon with loss of haustra, and focal areas of transient narrowing or "pseudostrictures", a gaping ileoceal valve and a tubular terminal ileum

DIFFERENTIAL DIAGNOSIS

- Any condition that causes chronic diarrhea (secretory or osmotic)

MANAGEMENT

What to Do First

- Patient should be confronted and laxatives must be stopped

General Measures

- Education re: normal bowel habits

SPECIFIC THERAPY

- Anorexia and bulimia: psychiatric consultation
- Cathartic colon:
  - ➤ High-fiber diet and bulk laxatives
  - ➤ Enemas may help during the bowel retraining period
  - ➤ If medical therapy fails, consideration of surgery (subtotal colectomy)
- Melanosis coli: no need for specific therapy; colonic changes are reversible once laxatives stopped

FOLLOW-UP

- Follow-up to assess response to medical therapy
- Some have reversal of radiographic abnormalities and function within a few months
- Patients with melanosis coli do not need follow-up

COMPLICATIONS AND PROGNOSIS

Complications

- Laxative abuse could lead to severe electrolyte and metabolic disturbances serious enough to cause death
- Laxative abuse has been incriminated as the cause of melanosis coli and cathartic colon

Prognosis

- For those able to stop laxatives, prognosis good since electrolyte and metabolic complications are reversible

- For those with underlying psychological factors or altered self-image, prognosis depends on the success of psychiatric treatment
- For those who progress to cathartic colon, chronic constipation refractory to medical therapy may occur

LEGIONELLA INFECTIONS

RICHARD A. JACOBS, MD, PhD

HISTORY & PHYSICAL

History

- Legionella are small, fastidious (grow on charcoal yeast extract, but not routine culture media), slow-growing (3–5 days for culture to turn positive), aerobic, Gram-negative bacilli.
- Over 40 species and 60 serogroups, but most human infections caused by L. pneumophila serogroups 1, 4, and 6
- Other species that less commonly cause human infection include L. micdadei, L. bozmonii. L. dumoffi, L. longbeachae and L. wadsworthii.
- Natural habitat of Legionella is water; low numbers of organisms in natural bodies of water (lakes, rivers); larger numbers in reservoirs (water towers, water condensers, potable water distribution systems)
- Transmission by aerosolization and inhalation of contaminated water or aspiration after colonization of the upper airways
- Risk factors include immunosuppression, chronic lung disease, smoking and older age.

Signs & Symptoms

- Pneumonia most common clinical syndrome; manifestations similar to other causes of pneumonia; cough productive of small amounts of sputum; fever almost always present (25% with temperatures above 40°C); GI symptoms (abdominal pain, nausea, vomiting) common, with diarrhea in up to 50%; headache and confusion also common; exam frequently reveals rales or consolidation
- Extrapulmonary infection uncommon and results from hematogenous spread from lungs; cardiac involvement (myocarditis, pericarditis, endocarditis) most common extrapulmonary site; other sites (skin, pyelonephritis, peritonitis, dialysis shunts, wounds) described, particularly in the immunosuppressed patient

- Pontiac fever is an acute self-limited disease characterized by fever, malaise, myalgias and headache without pneumonia; complete recovery in 1 week, even without therapy, is the rule.

TESTS

- Chest x-ray abnormalities nonspecific; early infiltrates usually in lower lobes and alveoli, but can be patchy and diffuse and can progress to lobar consolidation; nodular densities with cavitation more common in the immunocompromised, as are interstitial infiltrates; pleural effusions (usually small) in up to one third
- Laboratory abnormalities nonspecific except hyponatremia (sodium <130 mEq/ml), which is more common in Legionella pneumonia than pneumonia caused by other agents; normal or elevated WBC, abnormal liver function tests, hypophosphatemia all described
- Gram stain of sputum or other sterile fluid usually shows many polymorphonuclear leukocytes with few or no Gram-negative organisms (Legionella stain poorly, are small and thus difficult to see on Gram stain)
- Culture of sputum is the gold standard & positive in 80% (slightly higher with bronchoalveolar lavage). Direct fluorescent antibody test on sputum is rapid, but sensitivity only 30–70%. Urinary antigen test rapid, sensitive (70–80%) but only detects L. pneumophila serogroup 1 and can remain positive for months. Serum antibody testing limited by slow rise in antibody titers (6–12 weeks); a single titer of 1:128 suggestive of infection, but 4-fold rise is required to document infection. PCR available, but not more sensitive than culture.

DIFFERENTIAL DIAGNOSIS

- Other causes of pneumonia due to S. pneumoniae, H. influenzae, Mycoplasma pneumoniae, Chlamydia pneumonia, Chlamydia psitiaci, etc.

MANAGEMENT

- General supportive care with supplemental oxygen, fluids and pressors, if indicated

SPECIFIC THERAPY

- Newer macrolides (azithromycin, clarithromycin) or fluoroquinolones (ciprofloxacin IV, levofloxacin) are first-line drugs. Some observational studies suggest that levofloxacin is superior to

macrolides; in severely ill patients, some recommend addition of rifampin to above regimens; anecdotal case reports of success with imipenem, trimethoprim-sulfamethoxazole and clindamycin
- Duration of therapy 10–14 days in immunocompetent patients and 3 weeks in immunosuppressed
- Initial therapy usually parenteral, with switch to oral drugs after clinical improvement

FOLLOW-UP
- Clinical improvement in 3–5 days
- Chest x-ray may worsen initially, even with appropriate therapy and clinical improvement; may take months for complete resolution of infiltrates

COMPLICATIONS AND PROGNOSIS
- Mortality <5% in immunocompetent and up to 30% in immunocompromised
- Superheating water (140°F) eliminates organism.

LEISHMANIASIS, CUTANEOUS

J. GORDON FRIERSON, MD

HISTORY & PHYSICAL

History
- Exposure: bite of phlebotomine fly while in endemic area. The disorder is generally divided into Old World and New World disease. Causative agents of Old World disease are Leishmania tropica (found in Mediterranean countries, Middle East, SW Asia), L major (found in the Middle East, Central Asia, Indian subcontinent, tropical Africa), L aethiopica (found in Ethiopia, Kenya). Causative agents of New World disease are the L mexicana complex (L mexicana, L amazonensis, L venezuelensis), and the L braziliensis complex (L braziliensis, L panamensis, L guyanensis, L peruviana), all found in Central America and tropical parts of South American countries.

Signs & Symptoms
- A papule at the site of the fly bite, sometimes at a site of trauma (puncture wound, etc.) develops and gradually ulcerates. Ulcers are single or multiple, have raised edges, are only mildly painful. Local adenopathy is common; sometimes nodules occur along

lymphatic channels. L braziliensis complex can metastasize to nasal septum and adjacent tissues (known as mucocutaneous leishmaniasis, or espundia), producing erosion of the septum, palate, and other nasopharyngeal tissues.

TESTS

- Basic tests: blood: usually normal
- Basic tests: urine: normal
- Specific tests: Biopsy specimen should include a portion sent for culture (on NNN or similar medium), a portion sent for touch prep, and a portion sent for routine pathology. Kinetoplasts should be noted on path to diagnose leishmaniasis.
- Other tests: PCR available as research tool, also helpful in speciating leishmania. The CDC speciates using monoclonal antibodies. Serology variably positive, not diagnostic.

DIFFERENTIAL DIAGNOSIS

- Most common similar lesion is pyogenic ulcer, usually with less raised border. Other causes of skin ulcer are tuberculosis, cutaneous diphtheria, paracoccidioidomycosis, other fungus diseases, atypical mycobacterial disease, syphilis. Mucocutaneous disease resembles midline granuloma, syphilis, tuberculosis, tumors.

MANAGEMENT

What to Do First

- Treat any secondary infection with antibiotics. In mucocutaneous disease, assess extent of damage, include CT scanning.

General Measures

- Obtain baseline studies, including CBC, renal function (creatinine), liver function tests, pancreatic enzymes, and EKG, in preparation for treatment.

SPECIFIC THERAPY

Indications

- All patients with L braziliensis complex infections, to avoid metastasis
- All patients with mucocutaneous disease should be treated.
- All patients with New World disease that cannot be speciated
- With other species, treat large or multiple lesions, or lesions in functionally important or cosmetically sensitive areas. Treatment for other lesions is optional.

Treatment Options

- Sodium stibogluconate for 20 days for cutaneous disease, 30 days in mucocutaneous disease
- Liposomal amphotericin B over 5 or more days
- Topical paromomycin (15% in soft white paraffin) effective in some Old World disease

Side Effects & Complications

- Sodium stibogluconate: see Leishmaniasis, Visceral
- Liposomal amphotericin B: see Leishmaniasis, Visceral
- Topical paromomycin: local irritation and sometimes pain
- Contraindications to treatment: absolute: allergies to the medication, first trimester of pregnancy
- Contraindications to treatment: relative. Pregnancy, small or single lesions of Old World disease or known mexicana complex (which do not metastasize)

FOLLOW-UP

During Treatment

- See Leishmaniasis, Visceral

Routine

- Relapse can occur, may need retreatment. Mucocutaneous disease not considered cured until 2-year follow-up.

COMPLICATIONS AND PROGNOSIS

- Cutaneous disease leaves a scar. Mucocutaneous disease is destructive and may require plastic surgery after cure. Immunosuppressed patients may develop visceral disease and require prolonged or maintenance therapy. Otherwise prognosis is good.

LEISHMANIASIS, VISCERAL

J. GORDON FRIERSON, MD

HISTORY & PHYSICAL

History

- Exposure: bite of phlebotomine fly. Disease due to Leishmania infantum (found in Mediterranean littoral, middle East, southern Russia, northern China), L. donovani (found in Indian subcontinent, Pakistan, Nepal, China), and L. chagasi (found in Central and South America).

Signs & Symptoms
- Spectrum from asymptomatic to severely ill. Gradual onset, 2–6 months after bite(s), of fever, weight loss, gradual enlargement of liver and spleen, pallor, sometimes darkening of skin. Exam shows pallor, weight loss, enlarged lymph nodes, enlarged liver and spleen, sometimes mucosal ulcerations.

TESTS
- Basic tests: blood: CBC shows anemia, neutropenia. LFTs show mild transaminase elevations, low albumin, high globulin (polyclonal increase in IGG).
- Basic tests: urine: albuminuria sometimes seen.
- Specific tests: Bone marrow aspirate for amastigotes. Splenic puncture for amastigotes (should be done only by experienced personnel). Serologic tests helpful but vary in accuracy and subject to some cross-reactions. Most helpful in screening patient as an FUO. ELISA and IFA are preferred tests (done by the CDC).
- Other tests: none helpful

DIFFERENTIAL DIAGNOSIS
- Malaria, brucellosis, tuberculosis, endocarditis, hematologic and lymphatic malignancies, disseminated histoplasmosis, tropical splenomegaly

MANAGEMENT
What to Do First
- Nutritious diet, look for and treat any complicating infection, transfuse if needed.

General Measures
- Assess renal function, EKG, pancreatic enzymes, in preparation for treatment.

SPECIFIC THERAPY
Indications
- Any symptomatic patient

Treatment Options
- Sodium stibogluconate for 28 days, occasionally longer
- Liposomal amphotericin B (considered drug of choice by some but very expensive)

Side Effects & Complications

■ Sodium stibogluconate: myalgias, arthralgias, nausea, anorexia, malaise are common. EKG changes, pancreatitis, renal impairment, abnormal liver function, anemia, neutropenia, thrombocytopenia may all be seen.

■ Liposomal amphotericin B: fever, chills, cough, wheeze, renal impairment, hypokalemia, all generally less severe than plain amphotericin B.

■ Contraindications to treatment: absolute: asymptomatic patient.

■ Contraindications to treatment: relative: none.

FOLLOW-UP

During Treatment

■ Sodium stibogluconate: CBC, creatinine, EKG, pancreatic enzymes, LFTs must be followed. Interrupt treatment if severe problems.

Routine

■ Clinical follow-up (temperature, weight, liver and spleen size), blood counts, and periodic assessment for parasites (bone marrow or splenic puncture). Retreatment may be needed, and follow-up for relapse is important.

COMPLICATIONS AND PROGNOSIS

■ Many cases from India are resistant to sodium stibogluconate and require amphotericin. Assuming the parasites are eliminated, prognosis is good. Untreated or partly treated cases have a poor prognosis. In immunosuppressed patients the infection is often incurable, and monthly or bimonthly injections of Pentostam or amphotericin may be needed.

LEPTOSPIROSIS, RELAPSING FEVER AND RAT-BITE FEVER

RICHARD A. JACOBS, MD, PhD

HISTORY & PHYSICAL

History

■ Leptospirosis caused by Leptospira interrogans, a Gram-negative spirochete that contains 23 serogroups and >200 serovars; most common human pathogens are L. icterohaemorrhagiae (found in rats), L. canicola (dogs) and L. pomona (cattle and swine).

- Organism is ubiquitous in nature and found in many animals (rodents, cattle, dogs, etc.) that serve as reservoirs by being asymptomatic carriers, excreting the organism in urine and contaminating soil and water. Humans become infected by direct contact with infected animals or by exposure to soil or water that is contaminated. Increased risk seen in abattoir workers, sewer workers (direct contact with rats or material contaminated with infected rat urine), cattle ranchers, the urban homeless (rat exposure). Also identified in adventure travelers (eg, white water rafting).
- Relapsing fever caused by Borrelia recurrentis and other Borrelia species
- Louse-borne disease causes epidemic infection, is due to B. recurrentis and is transmitted to humans by the human body louse (Pediculus humanus); tick-borne disease caused by other Borrelia species and transmitted to humans by soft ticks (Ornithodoros) that usually reside in mountainous areas (1,500–6,000 feet); major reservoir for tick-borne infection is rodents
- Rat-bite fever caused by Spirillium minus, a spirochete found in the mouth of rodents; transmission to humans follows the bite of a colonized animal

Signs & Symptoms
- Leptospirosis is classically a biphasic illness. The first or "septicemic" phase is characterized by acute onset of high fever, chills, severe myalgias and headaches, conjunctival suffusion, abdominal pain with anorexia, nausea, vomiting and diarrhea (severe pain in back and calf muscles, and conjunctival suffusion are characteristic features of disease). A brief (1–3 days) period of improvement is followed by the "immune" phase, characterized by a recurrence of the systemic symptoms seen in the first phase, but in milder form, and the onset of meningitis, uveitis, adenopathy and rash. Second phase persists from several days to several weeks and resolves spontaneously.
- Manifestations of louse-borne and tick-borne relapsing fever similar: a nonspecific illness with abrupt onset of high fever, chills and rigors, headache, myalgias, arthralgias and confusion most common presentation; hepatosplenomegaly, rash, irits, myocarditis and neurologic abnormalities (CN palsy, seizure, meningitis) less common; after 3–10 days, symptoms abate only to be followed by a relapse in 1–2 weeks; 3–10 relapses may occur, each milder and shorter than the previous one, until the disease "burns out"

■ The site of the original bite in rat-bite fever heals initially, but several weeks later the site becomes swollen, painful, and bluish, ulcerates and is associated with lymphangitis, regional adenopathy, fevers, chills, and a diffuse reddish-blue or reddish-brown rash. Symptoms resolve in several days. Without therapy relapses of fever, generally without other manifestations of disease, recur at weekly intervals for several months.

TESTS

■ Leptospirosis – WBC may be normal or high; liver function tests often abnormal; CXR may show nonspecific infiltrates; CSF in meningitis characterized by a lymphocytic pleocytosis and elevated protein; organism can be cultured from blood, urine and CSF in septicemic phase, but special medium required and growth slow; diagnosis usually made serologically. PCR not yet widely available.

■ Relapsing fever – normal or elevated WBC; lymphocytic pleocytosis in CSF in meningitis; diagnosis usually made by observing spirochetes in Giemsa- or Wright-stained smears of peripheral blood during periods of fever; Proteus OXK agglutinins may be positive; false-positive nontreponemal tests for syphilis and false-positive serologic tests for Lyme disease can occur. Animal inoculation and in vitro cultivation possible in select labs. Little evidence for PCR for clinical diagnosis.

■ Spirillium minus cannot be grown on synthetic medium; diagnosis made by observing organism in blood, cutaneous lesion or aspirate of lymph node using Giemsa or Wright stain; false-positive nontreponemal test for syphilis can occur

DIFFERENTIAL DIAGNOSIS

■ Leptospirosis must be differentiated from relapsing fever, rat-bite fever, systemic viral infections, rickettsial infections, bacterial and viral meningitis and other causes of hepatitis in Weil's syndrome (see complications).

■ Relapsing fever may be confused with leptospirosis, rat-bite fever, Colorado tick fever, malaria, dengue.

■ Rat-bite fever must be distinguished from other form of rat-bite infection caused by Streptobacillus moniliformis, which is characterized by severe myalgias and arthritis; other considerations include relapsing fever, malaria, tularemia and Pasteurella moltocida infections.

MANAGEMENT
■ General supportive care

SPECIFIC THERAPY
■ Leptospirosis – doxycycline for 7 days is efficacious in mild to moderate disease if started within 72 hours of onset of symptoms; alternative is amoxicillin
■ Severe disease requiring hospitalization is usually treated with IV penicillin G 1.5 million units IV every 4–6 hours.
■ Relapsing fever – louse-borne disease treated with a single dose of tetracycline or erythromycin or a single dose of procaine penicillin G; tick-borne disease treated with 7–10 days of tetracycline or erythromycin
■ Rat-bite fever – penicillin G for 10–14 days; oral therapy with penicillin or tetracycline appropriate for mild disease

FOLLOW-UP
■ Jarisch-Herxheimer reaction can occur with therapy; usually seen within several hours of first dose, and symptoms may be ameliorated with aspirin or prevented with antibody to tumor necrosis factor; hypotension may occur, requiring supportive therapy

COMPLICATIONS AND PROGNOSIS
■ Weil's syndrome is a severe form of leptospirosis characterized by liver and renal failure and associated with a 20% mortality rate; a severe hemorrhagic pneumonia can also occur.
■ Prophylaxis in endemic areas with doxycycline once weekly is 95% effective in preventing leptospirosis.
■ Mortality of treated relapsing fever is 5%.
■ Major complication of rat-bite fever is endocarditis. It occurs in those with pre-existing heart disease and requires 4–6 weeks of parenteral antibiotic therapy; mortality of untreated disease is about 5%.

LEUKOCYTOSIS: NEUTROPHIL

NANCY BERLINER, MD

HISTORY & PHYSICAL

History
■ Leukocytosis is usually reactive.
■ Careful history, including recent fever, infections, travel history, medication use

Signs & Symptoms
- Vital signs, especially to exclude fever
- Evidence of adenopathy, hepatosplenomegaly
- Peripheral stigmata of infection

TESTS

Peripheral Blood Studies
- Repeat CBC to rule out laboratory error or transient leukocytosis
- Leukocyte alkaline phosphatase (LAP) score: 0 or near zero in CML, elevated in infection
- Examination of the peripheral smear
  - Morphology of the neutrophils-evidence of toxic granulation, immature forms
  - Erythrocyte morphology
    - Leukoerythroblastic picture
    - fragmented erythrocytes, teardrops, and nucleated red cells
    - suggests myclophthysic involvement of the bone marrow
    - suspicious for granulomatous disease, tumor, myeloproliferative disease

Bone Marrow Studies
- Usually unnecessary in evaluation of neutrophilia
- Indicated in setting of leukoerythroblastic changes
- Studies should include
  - cytogenetics, especially for Philadelphia chromosome
  - marrow culture, especially for mycobacteria, fungus
  - stem cell culture for cytokine-independent colony growth (marker of myeloproliferative dx)

DIFFERENTIAL DIAGNOSIS

Hereditary Neutrophilia
- Congenital
  - Hereditary neutrophilia
    - Autosomal dominant
    - Leukocytosis, splenomegaly, and widened diploe of the skull
    - Laboratory evaluation:
      - WBC 20,000–70,000/microliter
      - Elevated LAP
    - Clinical course benign.

➤ Chronic idiopathic neutrophilia
- sporadic condition
- Laboratory evaluation:
  - WBC 11,000–40,000/microliter, neutrophilic predominance
- Clinical course benign.

➤ Leukocyte adhesion deficiency
- Rare autosomal dominant disorder
- Recurrent life-threatening bacterial and fungal infections
  - Cutaneous abscesses, gingivitis, periodontal infections
- Caused by deficient expression CD11b/CD18, failure of chemotaxis
- Treated with antibiotics
- Severe cases: allogeneic stem cell transplantation

Acquired Neutrophilia
- Secondary to other disease process
  - ➤ Infection
    - Acute
      - Most common cause of an elevated leukocyte count is infection.
      - May be accompanied by increased immature precursors ("left shift")
      - More common with bacterial infection, can also occur with viral processes.
      - Morphologic changes in the neutrophil with bacterial infection
        - Toxic granulation, Dohle bodies, and cytoplasmic vacuoles
      - Resolves with treatment or resolution of the infectious process
    - Chronic
      - Increased marrow granulocyte production
      - Sometimes with monocytosis (especially with mycobacteria, fungus)
      - Leukemoid reaction
        - Seen with chronic infections (osteomyelitis, empyema, mycobacteria)
        - WBC markedly elevated (>50,000)
        - Associated with a marked left shift

- Acute Stress
  - Causes demargination of neutrophils, mediated by adrenergic stimulation
  - Common stresses: exercise, surgery, seizure, and myocardial infarction.
- Drugs
  - Steroids
    - Increase marrow release of mature neutrophils
    - Should not cause left shift
  - Beta agonists
    - Induce demargination of neutrophils adherent to endothelium
    - White blood cell count may double
  - Lithium
    - Causes chronic elevation of white count
  - Cytokine stimulation (e.g., G-CSF)
    - Stimulate marrow production of neutrophils
    - Can cause dramatic elevations in the white blood count
    - Majority of cells are neutrophils, often with left shift
- Chronic Inflammation
- Primary hematologic abnormalities
  - Myelophthysis
    - Non-hematologic malignancies (lung and breast common)
    - Tumors metastatic to the marrow may cause leukoerythroblastic changes
  - Marrow hyperstimulation
    - Chronic hemolysis, immune thrombocytopenia
    - May reflect disease activity, steroid therapy, or splenectomy
  - Recovery from marrow suppression
  - Myeloproliferative disease
    - Frequently associated with elevated hematocrit and platlets as well
    - Elevated eosinophil and basophil counts often seen
    - Frequently associated with splenomegaly
    - LAP may be low or undetectable in chronic myelogenous leukemia.
- Altered margination
  - Post-splenectomy
  - Sickle cell disease

MANAGEMENT
- Dependent on the cause of the neutrophilia

SPECIFIC THERAPY
- No specific therapy required for treatment of white count itself
- Managed by treatment of underlying disease

FOLLOW-UP
- Determined by the etiology of the leukocytosis

COMPLICATIONS AND PROGNOSIS
- Dependent on the underlying disorder

LEUKOPENIA

NANCY BERLINER, MD

HISTORY & PHYSICAL
- Comprehensive history
  - Inquire about fever, infection, new drugs, potential toxic exposures, previous blood counts
  - Family history of neutropenia, low blood counts
  - History suggestive of collagen vascular disease
- Physical examination
  - Thorough examination for evidence of infection, lymphoma, collagen vascular disease
  - Look for oral mucosal lesions, pharyngeal exudates
  - Evidence of lymphoma: adenopathy, splenomegaly
  - Evidence of collagen vascular disease: joints, skin

TESTS
CBC, Differential, Platelet Count
- Confirm neutropenia
- In some populations (e.g. Africans and Yemenite Jews), normal ANC is lower (lower limit of normal of 1.2×106/microliter)
- Urgency of evaluation dependent on degree of neutropenia.
  - ANC 1000–1500 Mild neutropenia, no increased infectious risk
  - ANC 500–1000 Moderate neutropenia, slight increased risk of infection
  - ANC <500 Severe neutropenia, markedly increased risk of infection

➤ Low platelets, hematocrit suggestive of primary marrow failure syndrome or hematopoietic malignancy

▣ In patient with fever and ANC<500, evaluation should include cultures of blood and urine, chest xray.

Bone Marrow Examination

▣ Most patients require bone marrow examination

▣ With accompanying anemia, thrombocytopenia: R/O aplasia, leukemia, myelodysplasia, other primary marrow malignancy

▣ Hyperplastic myeloid precursors and a "maturation arrest": suggests peripheral neutrophil destruction, as seen in collagen vascular disease or drug-induced neutropenia

DIFFERENTIAL DIAGNOSIS

Decreased Production of Neutrophils

▣ Congenital syndromes

➤ Congenital agranulocytosis (Kostmann's syndrome)
- Usually autosomal recessive, but also autosomal dominant and sporadic cases
- Early onset, frequent, life-threatening infections with severe neutropenia
- Bone marrow aspirate: maturation arrest at the promyelocyte stage.
- Responds to G CSF
- Responds to hematopoietic cell transplantation
- Increased incidence of AML and MDS
- Linked to mutations in neutrophil elastase, a primary granule protein

➤ Benign cyclic neutropenia (cyclic hematopoiesis)
- Rare dominantly inherited marrow disorder
- Characterized by cyclic fluctuations in neutrophil counts in 21 day cycle
- Episodes of neutropenia severe, ANC $<200\times10^6$/microliter; may be accompanied by fevers, pharyngitis, stomatitis, and other bacterial infections.
- Also linked to the neutrophil elastase gene
- Unlike Kostmann's syndrome, no increased incidence of AML and MDS.

- Acquired syndromes
  - ➤ Postinfectious
    - Commonly seen following viral infections (Varicella, measles, EBV, CMV, influenza, hepatitis, parvovirus, HIV)
    - Also seen with bacterial infections (rickettsial infections, typhoid fever, brucellosis, and tularemia), or sepsis with any bacteria
    - Occurs several days after onset of infection, may last several weeks
    - Resolves spontaneously
  - ➤ Nutritional deficiency
    - Megaloblastic hematopoiesis 2o B_{12}, folate deficiency
    - Copper deficiency: rare nutritional cause of neutropenia in severe malnutrition
    - Mild neutropenia may also occur with anorexia nervosa
  - ➤ Drug-induced
    - Multiple mechanisms of drug-induced neutropenia
      - direct marrow suppression
      - immune destruction with antibody or complement mediated damage of myeloid precursors
      - peripheral destruction of neutrophils.
    - Direct marrow suppression usually dose dependent.
      - Common offending drugs include cancer chemotherapeutic agents, phenothiazines, anticonvulsants, and ganciclovir. Alcohol can also cause neutropenia by marrow suppression.
    - In *dose-dependent* neutropenia, if not possible to stop the drug, drug may be continued with careful monitoring in face of mild neutropenia
    - Drugs that cause immune neutropenia usually cause profound agranulocytosis,
      - Common offending drugs: anti-thyroid medications, sulfonamides, and semi-synthetic penicillins.
      - Bone marrow shows a maturation arrest of myeloid lineage
      - Drug *must* be stopped.
    - Recovery of the neutrophil count can be accelerated by the administration of G-CSF.
  - ➤ Primary marrow failure
    - Aplastic anemia
    - Myelodysplasia
    - Acute leukemia

Increased Peripheral Destruction of Neutrophils

- Overwhelming infection
- Immune destruction
  - ➤ Autoimmune neutropenia:
    - Seen with collagen vascular disorders (SLE, RA), drugs
    - Also seen with immune thrombocytopenia and autoimmune hemolytic anemia
    - Mediated by IgG or IgM antibodies
    - Marrow: hypercellular with a late myeloid maturation arrest.
    - Felty's Syndrome: neutropenia with rheumatoid arthritis and splenomegaly.
  - ➤ Large granular lymphocytosis
    - May cause profound neutropenia accompanied by severe infections.
    - Frequently seen with rheumatoid arthritis
    - Lymphoproliferative maligancy of T cells
    - Variable clinical course
- Hypersplenism/Sequestration
  - ➤ Mild or moderate neutropenia along with anemia and thrombocytopenia.
  - ➤ Normal myeloid maturation in the marrow.
  - ➤ Neutropenia is rarely severe.

MANAGEMENT

Management of Fever and Neutropenia:

- Depends on degree of neutropenia
- Fever in setting of severe neutropenia (ANC $<500 \times 10^6$/microliter): a medical emergency
- Culture blood, bodily fluids
- Empiric broad-spectrum antibiotics to cover gram-negative enteric pathogens
- Duration of therapy dependent on duration of neutropenia
- Prolonged neutropenia: recurrent/persistent fever requires empiric anti-fungal therapy
- Granulocyte transfusions for gram-negative sepsis not responsive to antibiotics

SPECIFIC THERAPY

- Therapy directed at cause of neutropenia.
- Kostmann's syndrome, cyclic hematopoiesis, LGL neutropenia may respond to G-CSF

- Drug induced neutropenia: stop drug, may speed recovery with G-CSF

FOLLOW-UP
- Follow-up dependent on underlying diagnosis

COMPLICATIONS AND PROGNOSIS
- Major risk of severe neutropenia is overwhelming infection
- Prognosis dependent on the recovery of neutrophils, underlying diagnosis

LEUKOPLAKIA

SOL SILVERMAN JR, DDS

HISTORY & PHYSICAL
- white patch on any mucosal surface that cannot be wiped off
- usually soft and asymptomatic
- can be flat or verrucal
- pain and/or red component increases risk for dysplasia, carcinoma
- adult onset; duration variable (months to years)
- often associated with smoking; can be idiopathic

TESTS
- biopsy

DIFFERENTIAL DIAGNOSIS
- epithelial dysplasia, carcinoma, candidiasis, lichen planus

MANAGEMENT
- remove irritants, e.g. tobacco, spicey/hot foods, other irritants

SPECIFIC THERAPY
- surgical excision; laser very effective
- chemoprevention not effective and can be toxic

FOLLOW-UP
- watch for changes in signs, symptoms, pain, extension
- observe for recurrence if excised

COMPLICATIONS AND PROGNOSIS
- moderate risk for spread and/or transformation to carcinoma

LICHEN PLANUS

MARK WALDMAN, MD and JEFFREY P. CALLEN, MD
REVISED BY JEFFREY P. CALLEN, MD

HISTORY & PHYSICAL

History
- Common pruritic inflammatory disease of skin, hair follicles, and mucous membranes
- All races affected
- Occurs in males 20–60 years old
- Occurs in females at increasing rate with increasing age, with peak in 60s

Classification
- Classical lichen planus
- Oral lichen planus – may occur in the absence of cutaneous involvement or in conjunction with it. May be accompanied by disease of other mucous membranes (e.g., vulvo-vaginal).
- Genital lichen planus (frequently pt has accompanying oral disease)
- Inverse lichen planus – intertriginous involvement
- Hypertrophic lichen planus verrucous lesions, often on the legs
- Lichen planopilaris – scarring alopecia
- Lichenoid drug eruption – gold salts, antimalarials, penicillamine are the most common

Signs & Symptoms
- Classic lesion: violaceous, flat-topped, polygonal papule with glistening surface and scant adherent scale; may also see Wickham's striae on surface
- Begin as pinpoint papules and increase to 0.5–1.0 cm plaques
- Predilection for flexor wrists, trunk, medial thighs, dorsal hands and glans penis
- Pruritus often prominent
- Nail changes in 5–10% patients; may result in permanent nail dystrophy
- Mucous membrane frequently affected; seen as reticulated white patch
- Hypertrophic LP – verrucous lesions most often on the anterior legs

TESTS

Blood Tests
- Possibly patients should be tested for hepatitis C infection

Other Tests
- Skin biopsy often shows "wedge-like hypergranulosis," "sawtooth of rete ridges," hyperkeratosis, vacuolization of basal cell layer, and dense bandlike infiltrate that obscures DE junction

DIFFERENTIAL DIAGNOSIS
- Lichenoid drug eruption – history of an associated drug
- Pytiriasis rosea – herald patch, "Christmas tree" pattern
- Psoriasis
- Syphilis – palmar lesions, positive STS
- Scalp lesions
  - lupus erythematosus – typical lesions elsewhere
  - folliculitis decalvans – pustular lesions
- Hypertrophic lesions – warts, hypertrophic lupus erythematosus, squamous cell carcinoma
- Oral lesions – lupus erythematosus, leukoplakia, squamous cell carcinoma

MANAGEMENT
n/a

SPECIFIC THERAPY
- Limited lesions, treat with super-potent topical corticosteroid or intralesional corticosteroids
- If widespread, may use:
  - systemic corticosteroids
  - PUVA
  - Isotretinoin or acitretin
  - Cyclosporine, azathioprine, mycophenolate mofetil may be used for severe cases.

FOLLOW-UP
n/a

COMPLICATIONS AND PROGNOSIS
- Reported risk of oral SCC in oral and genital lesions
- Variable outcomes: 2/3 of pts have LP <1 yr, most clear in 2nd year
  - Recurrence in half of patients
  - Some may require long-term follow-up.

LIDDLE'S SYNDROME

MICHEL BAUM, MD

HISTORY & PHYSICAL
- Hypertension with family history of hypertension
- Autosomal dominant inheritance

TESTS
- Hypokalemic alkalosis with low plasma aldosterone and renin

DIFFERENTIAL DIAGNOSIS
- Distinguish from other causes of hypertension
- Due to mutation in collecting tubule Na channel with an increase in Na channel activity

MANAGEMENT
- Low-salt diet

SPECIFIC THERAPY
- Amiloride or triamterene

FOLLOW-UP
- For management of hypertension

COMPLICATIONS AND PROGNOSIS
- Secondary to hypertension

LIVER FLUKE INFECTIONS

J. GORDON FRIERSON, MD

HISTORY & PHYSICAL

History
- Life cycle: Adults of Chlonorchis sinensis and Opisthorchis viverini live in biliary tree and lay eggs, which pass to fresh water and hatch. The larvae enter snails, multiply, and are released to water as cercariae. They penetrate to muscle of fish and encyst.
  - ➤ Exposure: eating poorly cooked or raw fish. Larvae migrate to biliary tree, mature there.

Signs & Symptoms
- In acute infection, RUQ pain, fever, abdominal swelling, myalgias, rash, lymphadenopathy, urticaria. Examination shows hepatomegaly and tender liver, may be jaundice, rashes. In chronic

infection, no symptoms or findings, or in heavy infections can find chronic abdominal aches, fatigue, urticaria, hepatomegaly.

TESTS
- Basic tests: blood: eosinophilia, may be pronounced
- Basic tests: urine: normal
- Specific tests: Stool for O&P shows eggs. They are hard to distinguish from other small flukes.
- Other tests: Ultrasound or CT may show defects along intrahepatic biliary tree. In obstruction, worms found at surgery. Serology, available in some labs, can be helpful.

DIFFERENTIAL DIAGNOSIS
- Other inflammatory liver diseases, hepatic tumors

MANAGEMENT
What to Do First
- Determine severity.

General Measures
- Assess for source of infection.

SPECIFIC THERAPY
Indications for Treatment
- All patients

Treatment Options
- Praziquantel for 1 day
- Albendazole for 7 days

Side Effects & Complications
- Mild GI upset may occur.
- Contraindications to treatment: absolute: allergy to medications
- Contraindications to treatment: relative: asymptomatic patient with few eggs will do well without treatment.

FOLLOW-UP
Routine
- Stool O&P 2 or more weeks after treatment

COMPLICATIONS AND PROGNOSIS

■ Biliary obstruction, recurrent cholangitis, gallstones, cholangiocarcinoma. Prognosis good in absence of complications. Carcinoma has poor prognosis. Cholangitis responds to antibiotics.

LIVER FLUKES

J. GORDON FRIERSON, MD

HISTORY & PHYSICAL

History

■ Life cycle: Eggs are passed in stool and hatch in water. Organisms enter snails, reproduce, emerge from snail, and encyst on aquatic vegetation. When vegetation is eaten by man or sheep, cysts hatch and larvae penetrate the bowel wall, migrate through the liver to the biliary tree, and mate, and eggs pass again in stool.

➢ Exposure is by ingestion of watercress infected with metacercariae. Exists in most countries in the world.

Signs & Symptoms

■ Acute disease (when flukes are in liver): fever, RUQ pain, diarrhea, nausea, vomiting. Signs include fever, tender RUQ, enlarged liver, urticaria.

■ Chronic phase: Often no symptoms or signs. May have continued RUQ pain, hepatomegaly, jaundice.

TESTS

■ Basic tests: blood: eosinophilia, may be pronounced

■ Basic tests: urine: normal

■ Specific tests: stool for O&P exam. Eggs may not be seen in early phase of disease, and hard to distinguish from Fasciolopsis buski.

■ Other tests: Serology using ELISA is useful. Ultrasound may show flukes in biliary tree, and CT scan may show defects in liver where worm has burrowed.

DIFFERENTIAL DIAGNOSIS

■ Chlonorchis and opisthorchis infections, biliary tract disease, cholangitis

MANAGEMENT

What to Do First

- Assess severity of disease, including possible ectopic flukes.

General Measures

- Determine source of infestation; educate patient on prevention.

SPECIFIC THERAPY

Indications

- All patients

Treatment Options

- Bithional, on alternate days for 10–15 doses (must be obtained from the CDC)
- Triclabendazole once (available only as a veterinary preparation in U.S. Excellent record of efficacy and safety in reports)

Side Effects & Complications

- Bithional: vomiting, diarrhea, abdominal pain, urticaria, photosensitivity. Occasionally hepatitis, leukopenia.
- Triclabendazole: so far well tolerated
- Contraindications to treatment: absolute: allergy to medications
- Contraindications to treatment: relative: light infection, asymptomatic

FOLLOW-UP

During Treatment

- Monitor liver function, clinical course.

Routine

- Repeat stool exams 2–4 weeks after treatment, retreat if needed (bithional cures about 50% in one course).

COMPLICATIONS AND PROGNOSIS

- Biliary obstruction, syndromes due to ectopic worms that migrate to abdominal cavity, heart, brain. Prognosis of hepatic infection is good if treated. Prognosis of ectopic worms depends on location and possible surgical complications.

LIVER TRANSPLANTATION

ANDY S. YU, MD and EMMET B. KEEFFE, MD

HISTORY & PHYSICAL

History

■ decompensated cirrhosis: hepatic encephalopathy, portal hypertensive bleeding, ascites, SBP, intractable pruritus, recurrent biliary sepsis

Physical Signs

■ stigmata of chronic liver disease

TESTS
Pre-OLT Evaluation

Basic Tests: Blood

■ CBC; liver and kidney panel; prothrombin time, PTT
■ virologic test: anti-HAV antibody; HBsAg, anti-HBc, anti-HBs; (HBeAg, anti-HBe and HBV DNA if HBsAg+); anti-HCV (HCV RNA by PCR if anti-HCV+); anti-HDV; CMV antibody; EBV antibody; anti-HIV antibody
■ autoimmune markers: ANA, SMA, AMA
■ metabolic markers: iron studies; serum ceruloplasmin, alpha1–antitrypsin level and phenotype
■ other infectious markers: serum RPR
■ tumor markers: alpha-fetoprotein; carcinoembryonic antigen

Basic Tests: Urine

■ routine urinalysis, culture and sensitivity
■ 24 hour urine collection for creatinine clearance and protein

Additional Noninvasive Tests

■ ultrasound: exclude occlusion of portal vein, hepatic vein, hepatic artery, or inferior vena cava
■ biphasic abdominal CT to rule out liver cancer
■ MRI and MR angiogram (if CT contraindicated)
■ PPD skin test with controls
■ electrocardiogram
■ dobutamine echocardiogram-for patients with cardiac risk factors
■ carotid duplex-for patients older or with cardiovascular disease
■ chest radiograph
■ pulmonary function tests

- mammogram for female over 45 years of age
- pelvic exam with PAP smear for female

Invasive Tests When Indicated
- liver biopsy-if diagnosis of cirrhosis is uncertain
- ERCP-rule out cholangiocarcinoma in primary sclerosing cholangitis
- angiography (if vascular findings equivocal with Doppler)
- bubble echocardiography or radiolabeled albumin macroaggregate study when hepatopulmonary syndrome is suspected

DIFFERENTIAL DIAGNOSIS
- hepatocellular disease, e.g., chronic hepatitis B and hepatitis C, alcoholic cirrhosis
- cholestatic liver disease, e.g., primary biliary cirrhosis, primary sclerosing cholangitis
- inborn errors of metabolism, e.g., hemochromatosis, Wilson's disease, alpha$_1$-antitrypsin deficiency, and diseases not associated with liver injury (e.g., primary hyperoxaluria, familial homozygous hypercholesterolemia)

MANAGEMENT
What to Do First
- early referral to transplant center with first evidence of decompensated cirrhosis, or biochemical impairment of liver function
  - minimal listing criteria for OLT: Child's class B (CTP score ≥7), or any episode of variceal bleeding or SBP

General Measures
- OLT evaluation, including underlying diagnosis and disease severity, status of complications, assessment of comorbid conditions, psychosocial condition, financial and insurance status
- United Network for Organ Sharing organ allocation rules:
  - Status 1: FHF with life expectancy <7 days
  - Model for End-stage Liver Disease (MELD) score (based on bilirubin, INR and creatinine) determines priority for available organs since implementation in 2002; increased MELD points given to patients with stage 2 HCC; exceptions may be made in special circumstances and high MELD score assigned

SPECIFIC THERAPY
Specific Therapy of Liver Failure
Indications for OLT
- hepatocellular liver disease

> severe impairment of quality of life and CTP ≥ 7
  - severe or progressive hepatic encephalopathy
  - refractory ascites
  - recurrent portal hypertensive hemorrhage
  - progressive and incapacitating fatigue
> indicators of poor 1-year survival
  - hepatorenal syndrome
  - recurrent spontaneous bacterial peritonitis
  - prothrombin time >5 seconds prolonged
  - serum bilirubin >5 mg/dL
  - serum albumin <2.5 gm/dL
■ cholestatic liver disease
  > severe impairment of quality of life and CTP ≥ 7
    - intractable pruritus
    - recurrent biliary sepsis
    - metabolic bone disease with fractures
    - xanthomatous neuropathy
  > indicators of poor 1-year survival
    - serum bilirubin >10 mg/dL
    - Mayo risk score for primary biliary cirrhosis or primary sclerosing cholangitis predictive of <90% 1-year survival
■ inborn errors of metabolism (OLT corrects nonhepatic manifestations)

Absolute Contraindications to OLT

■ advanced cardiac disease
■ advanced pulmonary disease
■ multisystem organ failure
■ HIV seropositivity
■ extrahepatic malignancy
■ hemangiosarcomas
■ cholangiocarcinoma
■ active alcoholism or substance abuse
■ medical noncompliance with immunosuppressive protocol
■ anatomic abnormalities precluding OLT surgery

Immunosuppressive Drugs and Side Effects

■ corticosteroids
  > hypertension, hyperglycemia, poor wound healing osteoporosis, cataracts, mental status changes, susceptibility to infection, edema, hirsutism

- cyclosporine
  - ➤ nephrotoxicity, neurotoxicity, hypertension, hyperkalemia, hypercholesterolemia, gingival hyperplasia, hirsutism, lymphoproliferative disorder
- tacrolimus
  - ➤ nephrotoxicity, neurotoxicity, hyperglycemia, diarrhea, allergic reactions, lymphoproliferative disorder
- azathioprine
  - ➤ pancreatitis, bone marrow suppression, hepatotoxicity, cholestasis
- mycophenolate mofetil
  - ➤ neurotoxicity, neutropenia, gastrointestinal ulceration and bleeding, lymphoproliferative disorder
    - sirolimus
      - infection, bone marrow suppression, hepatic artery thrombosis, hyperlipidemia, peripheral edema, hypertension

Immunosuppressive strategies in evolution
- early corticosteroid withdrawal (3–6 months); calcineurin-sparing regiments (mycophenolate, sirolimus) when renal insufficiency present

FOLLOW-UP
Routine Outpatient Management
- outpatient clinic visits weekly initially then less frequently thereafter
- CBC, liver and kidney panel, immunosuppressant levels twice weekly initially, then eventually monthly

COMPLICATIONS AND PROGNOSIS
Complications
- **Early Post-OLT Complications**
  - ➤ primary graft nonfunction (2–23%)
  - ➤ bleeding (10%)
  - ➤ biliary complications (10–25%)
  - ➤ hepatic artery thrombosis (<3% in adults and 10–18% in children)
  - ➤ acute cellular rejection (40–70%)
  - ➤ early infectious complications (67%)
- **Late Post-OLT Complications**
  - ➤ chronic ductopenic rejection
  - ➤ recurrence of hepatitis B (80–90% without prophylaxis; 10–20% with lamivudine and hepatitis B immune globulin)

- recurrence of hepatitis C (100%)
- biliary complications (10–25%)
- opportunistic infections

Prognosis
- 5-year graft and patient survival 80–85%

LOCALIZED SCLERODERMA

RAJANI KATTA, MD

HISTORY & PHYSICAL

Signs & Symptoms
- Limited to skin and soft tissue involvement
- May be asymptomatic, itchy, or painful
- Several clinical variants
    - Localized morphea – single or few lesions, typically on trunk
    - Lesions of morphea may begin as red or violaceous patches
    - Progression to sclerotic, or firm, hypopigmented plaques
    - In active sclerotic lesions, red or violaceous border may be visible
- Generalized morphea – widespread, multiple plaques
- Linear scleroderma – linear unilateral plaques, usually on face or extremities
    - Coup de saber – linear scleroderma on forehead; clinical appearance similar to "blow from a sword"
    - Facial hemiatrophy (Parry-Romberg syndrome) is a variant associated with atrophy of underlying muscle, bone and even brain
- Morphea profunda – subcutaneous bound-down plaques; sclerosis may even affect fascia and muscle

TESTS

Laboratory
- Frequently positive anti-nuclear antibodies, including anti-single stranded DNA and anti-histone antibody may be reflective of disease activity and may be associated with a poorer prognosis, but in most cases do not alter management

Skin Biopsy
- Histology varies according to stage of disease
    - Lymphocytic inflammation in dermis
    - Sclerosis of collagen

DIFFERENTIAL DIAGNOSIS

- Systemic scleroderma – associated with acral sclerosis, Raynaud's phenomenon, and internal organ involvement (pulmonary, renal)
- Acrodermatitis chronica atrophicans – seen in Europe, due to Borrelia burgdorferi transmitted by tick bite; begins on extremity
- Sclerodermatous graft-versus-host disease – manifestation of chronic GVHD in patient with history of transplantation

MANAGEMENT

What to Do First

- Assess stage of disease – early, active, late or "burned out"
- Assess degree of involvement

General Measures

- Physical therapy/education to maintain joint mobility
- Camouflage cosmetics

SPECIFIC THERAPY

Indications

- Early or active disease
- Extensive involvement
- Involvement causing muscle atrophy or joint contractures
- Patient concerns, even if mild disease

Treatment Options

- High potency topical corticosteroids
  - ➤ Apply directly to involved areas twice daily; occlusion may be attempted to increase effect
  - ➤ Recommended for active lesions; avoid in late, sclerotic lesions
  - ➤ More useful for limited involvement; if widespread involvement, may be difficult to apply and may result in systemic absorption of steroids
  - ➤ May rarely lead to atrophy of skin, striae, telangiectasias, although uncommon if used only in involved areas
- Topical calcipotriene (Dovonex)
  - ➤ Use on active lesions with occlusion
  - ➤ May cause irritation
- Intralesional corticosteroids
  - ➤ Triamcinolone acetonide injected directly into lesions
  - ➤ Use only on active lesions
  - ➤ Use only for single or few localized lesions
  - ➤ Side effects include pain, and risk of more pronounced atrophy

- Phototherapy and photochemotherapy
  - ➤ UVA1 therapy, bath PUVA, topical PUVA (psoralen + UVA phototherapy)
  - ➤ Must be administered in specialized centers
  - ➤ Treatments administered 2–4 times/week over months
  - ➤ Risk of burning, secondary skin malignancies
- Methotrexate with or without systemic corticosteroids has been reported to be useful in a limited number of patients

FOLLOW-UP

During Treatment

- Re-evaluate skin lesions every 1–3 months during treatment to monitor efficacy of treatment and to note side effects

COMPLICATIONS AND PROGNOSIS

Complications

- Cosmetic concerns; disfigurement resulting from atrophy and pigmentary changes
- Contractures and limited mobility if involvement extends over a joint
- In severe cases, muscle atrophy

Prognosis

- Good, with spontaneous remission of disease in most
- May remit in few months or years
- Atrophy and pigmentary changes (hypo- or hyper-) may persist

LOW-OXYGEN-AFFINITY HEMOGLOBINS

AKIKO SHIMAMURA, MD, PhD

HISTORY & PHYSICAL

History

- Positive family history (autosomal dominant inheritance)
- Generally asymptomatic (normal tissue oxygen delivery)

Signs & Symptoms

- Cyanosis may be present

TESTS

Blood

- Sometimes associated with mild hemolytic anemia

Specific Diagnostic Tests
- High P50, hemoglobin oxygen dissociation curve shifted to the right
- Some cases may be detected on hemoglobin electrophoresis

DIFFERENTIAL DIAGNOSIS
- Methemoglobinemia
- Cyanosis secondary to cardiac or pulmonary disorders

MANAGEMENT
- No therapy.

SPECIFIC THERAPY
n/a

FOLLOW-UP
n/a

COMPLICATIONS AND PROGNOSIS
- No associated morbidity or mortality.

LUNG ABSCESS

STEVEN R. HAYS, MD

HISTORY & PHYSICAL

History & Risk Factors
- May be associated with infections caused by pyogenic bacteria, mycobacterium, fungi and parasites
- Anaerobic infection most common cause, up to 90% of cases
- Aspiration biggest risk factor, often associated with periodontal disease
- Predisposing conditions (73% of patients have at least one):
  - Loss of cough reflex: alcoholism, seizure disorder, drug overdose, general anesthesia, protracted vomiting
  - Neurologic disorders: cerebrovascular disease, myasthenia gravis, amyotropic lateral sclerosis, other bulbar processes
  - Poor deglutination associated with neurologic disorders or esophageal disease
- May complicate:
  - Primary or metastatic malignancy as postobstructive pneumonia; 8–18% of abscesses have associated malignancy
  - Pulmonary infarctions

- ➤ Septic emboli from bacterial endocarditis
- ➤ Necrotic conglomerate lesions of silicosis and pneumoconiosis

Signs & Symptoms

- Insidious presentation, symptoms usually present for 2–3 wks
- Cough, sputum, fevers, chills, sweats, anorexia, pleuritic chest pain
- Foul-smelling sputum in 50–60%; indicates anaerobic infection
- Acute: symptoms are those of acute pneumonia; nonanaerobic such as *S aureus* or *K pneumonia*
- Chronic: symptoms for more than 2 wks; anaerobic
- Exam: fever, poor dental hygiene, clubbing
- Early: signs are those of pneumonia with egophony, dullness to percussion
- Later: breath sounds become amphoric over involved lung, clubbing may occur

TESTS
Laboratory

Basic blood tests:

- Often marked leukocytosis and reactive thrombocytosis
- Blood cultures can be positive with pyogenic infection
- Basic tests: sputum most often polymicrobic
  - ➤ Gram stain/culture for pyogenic infections: *S aureus, K pneumonia, E coli, P aeruginosa, S pyogenes, H influenza, L pneumophilia, N asteroides, Actinomyces, S pneumonia*

Imaging

- CXR: thick walled cavity with irregular lumen of lucency, or air-fluid level within an area of pneumonia
- Usual location of abscess due to aspiration (85%): superior segment of RLL and LLL and axillary sub-segment of anterior/posterior segments of RUL
- CT of chest can help distinguish abscess from empyema with bronchopleural fistula

DIFFERENTIAL DIAGNOSIS

- Empyema
- Necrotizing squamous cell CA
- Multiple cavitary lesions suggest necrotizing pneumonitis, not anaerobic infection
- Fluid filled bleb or cyst

- If not connected with a bronchus, may have no air-fluid level and appear like consolidation
- Chest CT can usually distinguish parenchymal abscess from pleural fluid/empyema

MANAGEMENT

What to Do First

- Assess hemodynamic status, oxygenation and need for admission

General Measures

- Start IV antibiotics; continue 4–8 d or until afebrile and stable

SPECIFIC THERAPY

Indications

- All pulmonary abscesses require antibiotics
- If abscess fails to respond or is in an unusual location proceed to bronchoscopy to rule out endobronchial lesion

Treatment Options

- Antibiotics: clindamycin preferred because of effectiveness and cost
- Alternative antibiotics:
  - Penicillin and metronidazole in combination
  - Cefoxitin
  - Ticarcillin/clavulanate
  - Piperacillin/tazobactam
- Drainage: important for resolution:
  - Postural drainage generally sufficient
  - Nasal tracheal suctioning sometimes needed for patients without cough
  - Bronchoscopy if patient fails to respond and suspicion of underlying endobronchial lesion or foreign body
  - Percutaneous drainage under CT guidance if not improving and ongoing sepsis
- Surgical resection: reserved for massive hemoptysis, unresponding sepsis or respiratory failure

Side Effects & Complications

- Antibiotics:
  - Side effects: diarrhea
  - Complications: pseudomembranous colitis/ C dificile colitis particularly with clindamycin
  - Contraindications: absolute: hypersensitivity to antibiotic

FOLLOW-UP
- Continue antibiotic therapy until resolution of abscess: usually 6–8 wks
- Serial CXR q 2–4 wks help document improvement and resolution

COMPLICATIONS AND PROGNOSIS

Complications
- Empyema with bronchopleural fistula
- Rupture into uninvolved segments
- Sepsis
- Massive hemoptysis
- Nonresolution
- Residual cavities and fibrosis should be left alone unless they are the source of complications such as recurrent pneumonia or hemoptysis

Prognosis
- Generally abscess resolves in 6–8 wks with antibiotics
- Mortality 5–10%

LUNG CANCER

PAUL G. BRUNETTA, MD

HISTORY & PHYSICAL

History
- Cigarette smoking, asbestos, family history, COPD, radiation exposure (miners), prior cancer (oral, laryngeal or lung), age, pulmonary fibrosis
- Leading cause of cancer death in U.S.
- 85% of cases and all subtypes associated with smoking

Signs & Symptoms
- Pleural effusion, focal crackles or wheezes, palpable lymphadenopathy, clubbing, cachexia, pneumonia (postobstructive)
- 90% present with cough (new or changed), dyspnea, hemoptysis, chest pain; less common are weight loss, clubbing, dysphagia
- Paraneoplastic syndromes more associated with small-cell-lung cancer (SCLC)
  - ➤ Superior vena cava (SVC) syndrome, Pancoast syndrome, or paraneoplastic syndromes and a history of smoking suggest lung cancer

TESTS

Imaging

- Basic studies: CXR and CT (contrast; cuts through upper abdomen and adrenals); lymph nodes >1 cm abnormal
- Advanced: bone scan and/or brain MRI if symptoms/signs present; PET scanning for mediastinal staging

Laboratory

- Suggestive but nondiagnostic:
  - ➤ CBC, platelets, PT, PTT: for anemia, marrow involvement, biopsy risk
- Electrolytes, BUN/CR: assess SIADH, renal function for CT
- LFTs: assess hepatic metastasis.
- Alk phos, Ca^{++}: for bony mets, hypercalcemia
- LDH: some prognostic features

Biopsy

- Bronchoscopy: 60–80% yield for central airway tumors, postobstructive changes or accessible mediastinal nodes
- FNA: 80% yield if lesion ≥ 2 cm and peripheral
- Sputum cytology: low yield (<20%), but useful with bilateral involvement, cavitary disease and/or relative contraindications to bronchoscopy
- Mediastinoscopy: sample mediastinal nodes for staging; normal nodes on chest CT and normal PET reduces need for mediastinoscopy
- Biopsy of suspected metastasis crucial for accurate staging

DIFFERENTIAL DIAGNOSIS

- TB: most cancers occur in upper lobes; cavitary squamous cell can look like TB
- Pneumonia: repeat CXR in 6–8 wks in high-risk patients
- Benign pulmonary tumors (hamartoma)
- Cancer metastatic to lung
- Other cancers (lymphoma, KS)
- Lung inflammatory disorders (sarcoid, Wegener)
- Lymphangitic spread can mimic CHF or ILD

MANAGEMENT

What to Do First

- Assess oxygenation, infection, anemia if hemoptysis present
- Aggressively manage symptoms (wheezing, infection, bone pain)

General Measures
- Thorough, rapid staging:
  - Non-small-cell lung cancer (NSCLC): TNM classification (T1–4, N0-3, M0-1): lesions Ia – IIIa generally considered resectable/curable
  - SCLC: limited vs extensive
    - Limited: confined to 1 hemithorax (radiation port)
    - Extensive: metastatic (majority of cases)
- PFTs if potentially resectable or having pulmonary symptoms

SPECIFIC THERAPY
- Indicated for all patients: curative vs palliative

Treatment Options
- Surgery:
  - 1/3 of patients with symptoms are resectable
  - NSCLC:
    - Indicated for patients Ia–IIIa
    - Neoadjuvant (preoperative) chemotherapy investigational but promising
  - Lobectomy more effective that segmentectomy
  - SCLC: surgery with chemotherapy improves survival with coin lesions
- Radiation therapy:
  - Less effective than surgery: important for patients with limited pulmonary reserve, and preop for Pancoast tumors
  - Chemoradiation mainstay of therapy in limited stage SCLC.
  - Successful palliation for documented bone mets
  - Gamma knife brain irradiation useful in CNS met control
- Chemotherapy:
  - Cis-platinum regimens standard
  - Multiple newer agents (taxol, gemcitibine, navalbine, others) with comparable benefits and varying side effects; survival and cost effectiveness documented for stage IV NSCLC and good performance status
  - Response rates 30–50%
  - Mainstay of treatment in SCLC with good rates response, symptom control but eventual development of resistence
- Stents/laser therapy:
  - For obstructed bronchi, central tumors and collapse; endovascular stents an option in SVC syndrome

Side Effects & Contraindications
- Surgery:
  - Side effects: prolonged pleuritic pain (weeks), infection (wound, pneumonia), arrhythmia, bronchopleural fistula
  - Contraindications:
    - Absolute: active cardiac or cerebrovascular disease
    - Relative: severe pulmonary disease. Patients with apical tumors and bullous disease may tolerate resection/bullectomy without compromise
- Chemotherapy:
  - Side effects: leukopenia, anemia, nausea/emesis, renal dysfunction, fatigue, neuropathy
  - Contraindications:
    - Absolute: infection
    - Relative: renal dysfunction, poor performance status
- Radiation therapy:
  - Side effects: esophagitis, dermatitis, pulmonary fibrosis, radiation pneumonitis
  - Contraindications:
    - Relative: limited pulmonary reserve with high likelihood of pneumonitis
    - Absolute: inability to shield vital structures (spinal cord)
- Special Situations:
  - Carcinoma in situ: treatment options include brachytherapy, photodynamic therapy (PDT), laser or cryotherapy
  - Isolated CNS or adrenal metastasis: aggressive resection of both tumors improves survival
  - Synchronous primaries: stage/treat separately with independent prognoses
  - Malignant pleural effusions: pleurodesis (talc, bleomycin, tetracycline) either tube thoracostomy or video-assisted thoracoscopy (VATS)
  - Progressive hemoptysis: bronchial artery embolization

FOLLOW-UP

During Treatment
- Determined by specialty service (oncology, radiation oncology, surgery or pulmonary)

Routine
- CBC, renal function weekly during chemotherapy
- CXR q 3 mo, annual chest CT

COMPLICATIONS AND PROGNOSIS

Complications

- 1/3 of recurrences occur locally, 2/3 distant
- Postobstructive pneumonia: antibiotics; consider local therapy (stent, laser)
- Radiation pneumonitis: weeks-months after finishing treatment; trial of prednisone
- Hypercalcemia: hydration, etidronate or pamidronate

Prognosis

- 5-y survival for stage I disease >60%
- Overall 5-y survival 13–15%
- Histopathologic response to chemotherapy correlates with survival
- Second malignancies occur at 1–5% per year after treated disease

---

LUNG FLUKE

J. GORDON FRIERSON, MD

HISTORY & PHYSICAL

History

- Life cycle: Adult worms live encysted in lung tissue. Eggs are passed and coughed up into sputum or swallowed and pass in the stool. In fresh water they hatch, larvae invade snails and multiply. New larvae (cercariae) are released and encyst in fresh-water crabs. When eaten, the larvae penetrate gut wall and migrate to the lungs, where they encyst, mate and produce new eggs.
  - ➤ Exposure: Ingestion of undercooked infested fresh-water crabs. Present in Asia, India, Pacific islands, Africa, South and Central America.

Signs & Symptoms

- Acute phase: abdominal pain, diarrhea, fever, urticaria, followed by cough, wheeze, dyspnea
- Chronic phase: cough, sputum, often blood-streaked, wheeze, dyspnea, chest pains

TESTS

- Basic tests: blood: eosinophilia
- Basic tests: urine: normal
- Specific tests: exam of sputum and/or stool for eggs

- Other tests: Chest X-ray often shows scattered opacities in early stage, later cysts, scarring, small effusions. Serology helpful, done by CIE (at CDC).

DIFFERENTIAL DIAGNOSIS
- Pulmonary form: tuberculosis, other chronic infections, COPD, carcinoma
- During migration: other causes of abdominal pain

MANAGEMENT
What to Do First
- Assess severity of infection, and look for ectopic disease (brain, abdomen).

General Measures
- Determine source of infection, educate patient, ensure good nutrition.

SPECIFIC THERAPY
Indications
- All patients

Treatment Options
- Praziquantel for 3 days: generally curative.
  Triclabendazole (compassionate use)

Side Effects & Complications
- May have abdominal pains, wheeze, relating to death of worms
  - ➤ Contraindications to treatment: absolute: allergy to medication
  - ➤ Contraindications to treatment: relative: none

FOLLOW-UP
During Treatment
- Monitor symptoms.

Routine
- Check stools, sputum (if available) for ova 2–4 weeks after treatment. Obtain chest X-ray at intervals.

COMPLICATIONS AND PROGNOSIS
- Main complication is ectopic worms, especially in brain, which can cause seizures, headache, focal neurologic signs, coma. Treatment is with praziquantel with steroid coverage. Abdominal worms can

mimic appendicitis, diverticulitis, etc., and surgery is sometimes indicated to make diagnosis. After treatment, prognosis is good, though residual neurologic signs may exist, and scarring remains in lungs.

LYME DISEASE

RICHARD A. JACOBS, MD, PhD

HISTORY & PHYSICAL

History
- In the US, caused by *Borrelia burgdorferi*, an aerobic Gram-negative bacillus (*B. garinii* and *B. afzelii* agents in Europe and Asia)
- Transmitted by Ixodes ticks (the black-legged tick); Ixodes scapularis vector in New England, mid-Atlantic and upper Midwest; *Ixodes pacificus* vector on West Coast
- Ticks infected by feeding on white-footed mouse or deer, the natural reservoirs for *B. burgdorferi*
- Risk of transmission to humans depends on stage of tick (nymphs and adults more likely to transmit disease than larvae), geographic location (15%–65% of ticks infected in Northeast and Midwest, but only 1%–3% of ticks in Western US infected) and duration of feeding (ticks must feed at least 48 hours to transmit organism)
- Over 90% of cases reported from southern New England, the mid-Atlantic states and the upper Midwest; smaller endemic area exists along northern Pacific coast

Signs & Symptoms
- Early localized disease-80% have erythema migrans, a flat or slightly raised, nontender, erythematous lesion that expands over days to weeks, often but not invariably, with central clearing; begins 7–10 days after bite (range 3–30 days) and clears spontaneously even without therapy; associated fevers, chills myalgias present in about 50%
- Early disseminated disease-usually occurs several weeks to months after tick bite and can involve skin, the nervous system or the heart; multiple erythema migrans lesions develop in 50%; myopericarditis with arrhythmias or heart block seen in 4%–10%; neurologic involvement (10%–20%) usually manifests as aseptic meningitis with mild headache or Bell's palsy, but peripheral neuropathy (sensory or motor) and eye disease (optic neuritis, iritis, keratitis, conjunctivitis)

also reported; systemic symptoms (fatigue, myalgias, joint pain, fever) also common

■ Late disease-occurs months to years after initial exposure; most common manifestation is mono or oligoarthritis of large weight-bearing joints, usually the knees; much less common is encephalopathy (with sleep disturbances, memory and concentration difficulties) and peripheral neuropathy (paresthesias and radicular pain)

■ Congenital transmission of disease has not been documented

TESTS

■ Serologic tests often negative in early disease and diagnosis made clinically

■ Later stages of disease almost always associated with positive serologic tests; two stage antibody testing required: screening test is either by indirect immunofluorescence (IFA) or enzyme-linked immunosorbent assay (ELISA); all positive screening tests must be confirmed by Western blot

■ IgM antibody appears 2–4 weeks after erythema migrans, peaks at 6–8 weeks and declines to low levels by 6 months; IgG appears 6–8 weeks after infection, peaks at 4–6 months and remains positive at low levels indefinitely

■ Lyme urinary antigen test (LUAT) – not standardized and should NOT be used to make diagnosis

■ Neuroborelliosis – associated with abnormal cerebrospinal fluid (pleocytosis, elevated protein or low glucose) and localized antibody production (higher titers in cerebrospinal fluid than serum)

■ Peripheral neuropathy associated with abnormal nerve conduction studies

■ Serologic tests plagued by lack of sensitivity and specificity, inter and intralaboratory reproducibility and absence of national standard; thus, serologic tests must be interpreted in context of clinical presentation and should only be ordered in patients with high likelihood of disease, not in those with nonspecific symptoms of fatigue or malaise

■ Culture of organism not routinely done; PCR for organism not yet standardized

DIFFERENTIAL DIAGNOSIS

■ Local reaction to tick bite, urticaria, cellulitis can be confused with erythema migrans; infectious or inflammatory arthritis; viral or syphilitic meningitis

MANAGEMENT

- If tick available, identify as Ixodes (2–4 mm with black legs and red body); if still attached, remove with fine tweezers by pulling firmly on the mouth where it enters the skin; tick analysis to see if it is infected not indicated
- Prophylactic antibiotics NOT indicated except in highly endemic areas, following bite by nymphal or adult engorged Ixodes tick
- Serologic tests early in disease are often negative and should not be done.

SPECIFIC THERAPY

- Localized erythema migrans or disseminated erythema migrans in the absence of third-degree heart block or neurologic manifestations-doxycycline or amoxicillin for 14–21 days; cefuroxime axetil equally as efficacious, but more costly; macrolides less effective and not recommended as first line therapy
- First and second-degree heart block treated as erythema migrans; third-degree block treated with ceftriaxone for 14–21 days
- Bell's palsy, if not associated with CNS involvement, treated like erythema migrans; if associated with CNS involvement, ceftriaxone for 14–28 days (lumbar puncture may be required to determine if CNS involvement present)
- Meningitis, encephalopathy and peripheral neuropathy treated with ceftriaxone for 14–28 days; cefotaxime or penicillin (18–24 million units in equally divided doses every 4 hours) are alternatives
- Arthritis treated initially with oral regimens of doxycycline or amoxicillin for 28 days; failures or recurrences treated with ceftriaxone for 14–28 days

FOLLOW-UP

- After adequate therapy of early disease, nonspecific symptoms (fatigue, arthralgias, myalgias) may persist for weeks or months; therapy is symptomatic – additional antibiotic therapy NOT indicated
- Symptoms of arthritis slow to resolve; after initial therapy, if symptoms persist, wait several months before retreating; if symptoms persist after second course of antibiotics, treat symptomatically, not with additional or prolonged courses of antibiotics
- Coinfection with Ehrlichia species or Babesia microti, on rare occasions, can cause prolonged symptoms and should be excluded.

COMPLICATIONS AND PROGNOSIS

- Prognosis excellent with complete response in 4–6 weeks; residual synovitis, facial nerve palsy and need for permanent pacemaker all rare occurrences; early treatment almost always prevents later stages of disease
- Prevention includes avoiding tick-infested areas, covering exposed skin, using insect repellants and inspecting and removal of ticks after exposures
- Previous vaccine taken off the market in 2002 due to reports of toxicity. No vaccine currently available.

LYMPHADENITIS AND LYMPHANGITIS

RICHARD A. JACOBS, MD, PhD

HISTORY & PHYSICAL

History

- Lymphadenitis is inflammation of lymph nodes – can be acute, developing over several days, or chronic, developing over weeks
- Lymphangitis is inflammation of lymphatic vessels – can be acute or chronic
- Acute lymphadenitis most commonly due to Staphylococcus aureus or Streptococcus pyogenes (group A streptococcus); anatomic sites most commonly affected include cervical (due to infection of face or scalp, tonsillitis or periodontal infection); axillary (due to infections of hand or arm); epitrochlear (associated with infection of middle, ring or little finger)
- Chronic lymphadenitis due to mycobacterium (atypical mycobacterium such as M. scrofulaceum more common in children and M. tuberculosis more common in adults), fungi (Histoplasma capsulatum, Cryptococcus neoformans, Coccidiodes immitis), Bartonella spp (cat-scratch disease)
- Oculoglandular syndrome (Parinaud's syndrome) – granulomatous conjunctivitis with preauricular adenopathy seen with cat-scratch disease, tularemia (Francisella tularensis), lymphogranuloma venereum (Chlamydia trachomatis) and adenovirus (type 8 and 19)
- Inguinal adenopathy of venereal origin usually bilateral – primary syphilis, lymphogranuloma venereum, chancroid (Haemophilus ducreyi); nonvenereal causes include tularemia and plague (Yersinia

pestis); unilateral inguinal adenopathy due to pyogenic infections (S. aureus or group A streptococcus) or cat-scratch disease

- Generalized adenopathy seen in many diseases, including brucellosis, infectious mononucleosis, toxoplasmosis, CMV, acute HIV, secondary syphilis, disseminated tuberculosis or atypical mycobacterial disease, etc.
- Acute lymphangitis most commonly caused by group A streptococcus and S. aureus; less common causes include other streptocooci, Pasteurella multocida (following a cat or dog bite) and Spirillum minor (rat-bite fever)
- Chronic nodular lymphangitis due to Sporothrix schenckii (sporotichosis), nocardia and Mycobacterium marinum (swimming pool granuloma); other fungi and atypical mycobacteria as well as leishmania also rare causes

Signs & Symptoms

- Acute lymphadenitis associated with swollen, tender, erythematous node; localized cellulitis may be present; systemic symptoms of fever, chills and malaise common
- Chronic lymphadenitis presents insidiously with swollen node that may or may not be tender and usually not associated with systemic symptoms
- Acute lymphangitis presents with a red streak from a primary site of infection that extends to a regional lymph node; fever and chills common; lymph node tender
- Chronic lymphangitis presents with a primary papule or nodule at inoculation site with subcutaneous spread of nodules that follow along lymphatic vessels; systemic symptoms usually absent

TESTS

- Blood cultures in febrile patient; culture of node if draining (culture for bacteria, fungus and mycobacteria)
- Aspiration of node for culture and cytology in chronic cases; excisional biopsy may be needed if aspiration fails to reveal etiology
- Serologic studies (syphilis, cat-scratch disease, toxoplasmosis, acute HIV, mono spot or Epstein-Barr virus antibody titers) or skin test (PPD) if history suggestive of specific disease

DIFFERENTIAL DIAGNOSIS

- Lymphoma, Kawasaki syndrome, Kikuchi Fujimoto's disease (necrotizing histiocytic lymphadenitis), sarcoidosis, systemic lupus, Still's disease, Sjogren syndrome

MANAGEMENT

- Careful exam to detect local site of infection
- Detailed history may reveal clues to underlying etiology: social history (sexual practices, partners), vocational exposures (animals, others with illnesses), recreational history (camping, gardening), dietary habits (unpasteurized dairy products), recent travel

SPECIFIC THERAPY

- Therapy depends on etiologic agent; acute lymphadenitis and lymphangitis due to S. aureus or group A Streptococcus and empiric therapy with cephalexin or dicloxacillin reasonable; if patient fails to respond or chronic disease present, specific etiology should be sought by blood tests (see above), aspiration of node or excisional biopsy for culture and pathologic examination with therapy directed at causative agent

FOLLOW-UP

- Routine to ensure resolution of underlying process

COMPLICATIONS AND PROGNOSIS

- Bacteremia can occur with acute lymphadenitis and lymphangitis, requiring hospitalization and parenteral antibiotic therapy.
- Suppuration may occur, but it usually resolves with appropriate therapy.
- Prognosis depends on underlying etiology but overall is favorable.

LYMPHOMAS

M.A. SHIPP, MD
REVISED BY ARNOLD S. FREEDMAN, MD

HISTORY & PHYSICAL

- Approximately 57,000 new cases will be diagnosed in USA in 2006. From 1992 to 2001, the rate has decreased 1% per year in men, and remained stable in women.
- Associations
  - ➤ HD – EBV (mostly in developing countries, <20% elsewhere)
  - ➤ NHL
    - Inherited or acquired immunodeficiencies (severe combined immunodeficiency, hypogammaglobulinemia, common variable immunodeficiency, Wiskott-Aldrich syndrome, ataxia-telangiectasia)

- Infectious agents (EBV, HTLV-1, HHV-8, hepatitis C virus, Helicobacter pylori, HIV, Camphylobacter)
- Environmental exposures (herbicides, hair dyes, organic solvents [weak evidence])

Signs & Symptoms
- Lymph node enlargement
- Fevers, night sweats, unexplained weight loss (B symptoms)
- Splenomegaly
- Symptoms referable to specific disease sites – i.e., chest pain, shortness of breath (mediastinal mass), abdominal discomfort (mesenteric/retroperitoneal lymphadenopathy, infiltration GI tract), bone pain
- Pruritus, alcohol intolerance (HD)
  - ➢ Most indolent lymphomas are asymptomatic.
    - CNS disease is associated with aggressive NHL; patients with bone marrow, testicular, paranasal sinus, multiple extranodal sites of disease

TESTS

Laboratory
- CBC with differential
- Screening chemistries (renal and hepatic function), calcium, lactate dehydrogenase
- b2 microglobulin (mostly indolent NHL subtypes)

Biopsies
- Lymph node (preferred, nodal architecture necessary to diagnose subtypes of both HD and NHL), excisional biopsy preferred. Fine needle aspirate very limited yield.
- Other disease site if no involved/accessible lymph node
- Unilateral bone marrow (aspirate and biopsy)
- Accurate diagnosis requires review by experienced hematopathologist
- Immunophenotypic analysis via immunohistochemistry and, in certain cases, flow cytometry
- Analysis of antigen receptor gene rearrangement and, in certain cases, disease-specific cytogenetic abnormalities – for example, t(14:18) – follicular lymphoma; t(8;14)– Burkitt's lymphoma

Imaging Studies
- Chest radiograph
- Chest, abdomen, pelvic CT scans

- MRI in selected cases, only useful in identifying bone or CNS involvement
- FDG PET scan
  - provides functional rather than purely anatomic information
  - most useful in monitoring HD and aggressive NHL

Other
- Lumbar puncture (mandatory with certain NHL subtypes, such as Burkitt's, recommended with referable symptoms, or in patients with high risk of CNS disease [see above])

DIFFERENTIAL DIAGNOSIS
- Benign etiologies of lymphadenopathy – infections, autoimmune diseases (rheumatoid arthritis, systemic lupus erythematosus), sarcoid, medications (phenytoin)
- Metastatic carcinomas
- Lymph node biopsy used to differentiate lymphoma from carcinoma or benign lymphadenopathies

MANAGEMENT
- Therapeutic approaches to HD and NHL based on specific subtype, stage of disease, prognosis and physiologic status of the patient
- HD and NHL subtypes identified according to updated WHO pathologic classification
  - HD – classic HD (nodular sclerosis and mixed cellularity) and nodular lymphocyte predominance HD
  - NHL – most common entities include
    - Chronic lymphocytic leukemia (CLL)/small lymphocytic lymphoma (SLL), plasma cell myeloma, follicular lymphoma (FL) – indolent lymphomas with natural histories measured in years
    - Mantle cell lymphoma (MCL), diffuse large B-cell lymphoma (DLBCL), Burkitt's lymphoma, peripheral T-cell lymphomas (PTCL) – aggressive/highly aggressive lymphomas with untreated natural histories measured in months or weeks

Stage (Ann Arbor)
- I – single lymph node
- II – 2 or more lymph nodes, same side of diaphragm
- III – lymph node involvement on both sides of the diaphragm
- IV – disseminated involvement of extranodal sites with or without lymph node involvement
- A – absence of B symptoms (fever, night sweats, or weight loss)

General Measures

■ adequate hydration prior to systemic chemotherapy, allopurinol to reduce risk of tumor lysis syndrome in certain aggressive NHL subtypes

SPECIFIC THERAPY

■ See disease-specific National Cancer Center Network (NCCN) HD and NHL Guidelines for details of initial (induction) therapy and therapy following relapse.

■ Optimal induction therapy dependent upon specific disease subtype

➤ Classic HD – immediate stage-specific treatment (radiation therapy alone used much less frequently)

• combination chemotherapy alone or combined modality therapy

➤ NHL

• Indolent lymphomas (such as CLL/SLL and FL)

• Therapy dictated by symptoms and tumor burden. Options include no therapy with careful follow-up ("watch and wait"), radiotherapy alone for stage I disease or local symptomatic progression in absence of systemic symptomatic disease, single agent chemotherapy (alkylating agents), combination chemotherapy (cyclophosphamide, vincristine, prednisone), aggressive combination chemotherapy (usually only for relapsed and refractory disease), B-cell-specific monoclonal antibodies, specifically the anti-CD20 monoclonal antibody rituximab and treatment with newer experimental agents.

• Aggressive lymphomas (such as DLBCL, PTCL, most MCL) require immediate Adriamycin-containing combination chemotherapy (CHOP: cyclophosphamide, doxorubicin, vincristine, prednisone plus rituximab) with or without radiation therapy (used for some stage I patients). There is no role for any maintenance therapy after complete remission.

• Highly aggressive lymphomas (such as Burkitt's lymphoma) require immediate, very intense acute leukemia-like regimens with CNS prophylaxis.

FOLLOW-UP

■ During therapy – CBC with differential, platelets and routine chemistries

■ Following induction therapy – Complete radiographic and laboratory restaging to assess response, repeat BM and any additional specialized studies (i.e., LP) that were positive at diagnosis

■ Subsequent follow-up – Frequency dependent on disease subtype – usually exam and labs q 3 mos and scans q 6 months × 3 years with increasing/individualized intervals thereafter

COMPLICATIONS AND PROGNOSIS

■ Complications dependent upon specific disease subtype and therapy
  ➤ Most chemotherapeutic regimens associated with reversible dose-dependent drops in normal blood counts (WBC > platelets > hematocrit)
  ➤ Increased risk of febrile neutropenia when absolute neutrophil count <500 – administration of granulocyte colony-stimulating factor (G-CSF) may decrease neutropenic period
  ➤ Age- and treatment-specific reductions in fertility
  ➤ Increased incidence of secondary leukemia and second solid tumors in HD treated with combined modality therapy
■ Prognosis – disease- and stage-specific
■ HD
  ➤ Early-stage classic HD frequently curable in 70–90% with appropriate induction therapy
  ➤ Advanced-stage classic HD curable in 50–65% with appropriate induction therapy
  ➤ Salvage chemotherapy often with autologous stem cell transplantation cures a subset of patients with recurrent disease
■ NHL
  ➤ Clinical risk models such as International Prognostic Index used to predict efficacy of combination chemotherapy in specific NHL subtypes (most useful in DLBCL)
  ➤ "Indolent" lymphomas (such as CLL/SLL, myeloma, FL)
    • Currently incurable with current standard therapies
    • Treatable for years with available alternatives
    • Many new experimental options aimed at increasing curability, response duration
  ➤ "Aggressive and highly aggressive" lymphomas (such as DLBCL, certain PTCLs, Burkitt's lymphoma)
    • Subset curable with standard induction therapy (ranging from 40–90% depending on risk factors)
    • Additional subset of relapsed DLBCLs and certain PTCLs curable with high-dose therapy and stem cell rescue
  ➤ Mantle cell lymphoma treatable, but majority of patients relapse with current options

LYSOSOMAL DISEASES

DONALD M. OLSON, MD

HISTORY & PHYSICAL

- Multi-organ system involvement
- Highly variable between specific diseases
  - ➤ 40 lysosomal diseases known

History

- Neurological (rare in Farber disease, adult-onset Gaucher disease, Niemann-Pick B, Fabry disease, cystinosis): psychomotor regression: dementia, psychiatric, school (Krabbe, metachromatic leukodystophy, GM1 gangliosidosis, Tay-Sachs/Sandhoff disease/GM2 gangliosidosis, Niemann-Pick A), ataxia (Niemann-Pick C, Salla disease, late metachromatic leukodystophy, Tay-Sachs/Sandhoff disease/GM2, neuronal ceroid lipofucinosis/Batten disease), seizures (prominent and early in neuronal ceroid lipofucinosis/Batten disease, late in Tay-Sachs/Sandhoff disease/GM2, Krabbe, myoclonic in neuronal ceroid lipofucinosis/Batten disease), excessive startle (Tay-Sachs/Sandhoff disease/GM2 [esp. with loud sound], Krabbe), vision loss (usually late, Tay-Sachs/Sandhoff disease/GM2, Krabbe, Niemann-Pick A, neuronal ceroid lipofucinosis/Batten disease), peripheral neuropathy (weakness, sensory changes, pain: variable among different diseases), speech changes, dysarthria (GM1, Niemann-Pick, Tay-Sachs/Sandhoff disease/GM2), movement disorder (Niemann-Pick, metachromatic leukodystophy), deafness (sialidosis)
- GI: Vomiting, feeding problems (Krabbe, Farber disease, Niemann-Pick A, Niemann-Pick B, Gaucher disease)
- Skin, skeletal: joint swelling, deformity (Farber disease), subcutaneous nodules (Farber disease), pain crises (Fabry disease, Gaucher disease), easy bruisability (Gaucher disease)
- Pulmonary: dyspnea (Farber disease, Niemann-Pick B)
- Ethnicity: Jewish (Tay-Sachs/Sandhoff disease/GM2, some Niemann-Pick A), Finnish (Salla disease, some neuronal ceroid lipofucinosis/Batten disease)
- Family history: most autosomal recessive, Fabry disease X-linked

Signs & Symptoms

- Appearance: dysmorphic in many, esp. with infancy or childhood onset

- Abdomen: hepatosplenomegaly (Niemann-Pick, Tay-Sachs/Sandhoff disease/GM2, Gaucher disease [esp. spleen])
- Neurological: eye movements (gaze palsies: Gaucher disease, Niemann-Pick, nystagmus: Niemann-Pick, GM1), spasticity, rigidity (Gaucher disease, Krabbe, metachromatic leukodystophy, late Tay-Sachs/Sandhoff disease/GM2, GM1), hypotonia (GM1, Tay-Sachs/Sandhoff disease/GM2), areflexia (Krabbe, Metachromatic leukodystophy, GM1, late-onset Tay-Sachs/Sandhoff disease/GM2), strokes (Fabry disease)
- Skeletal: degenerative changes (Gaucher disease, GM1), limb deformities (Krabbe)
- Eye: optic atrophy, macular changes (cherry red spot: Niemann-Pick, Tay-Sachs/Sandhoff disease/GM2, Krabbe), corneal opacities (Fabry disease), blindness (neuronal ceroid lipofucinosis/Batten disease), gaze palsy (Gaucher disease)
- Skin: telangectasias, hypohydrosis (Fabry disease)
- Genitourinary: renal failure (Fabry disease)

TESTS

Laboratory
- basic blood studies:
  Very long chain fatty acids
  - Specific enzyme tests on WBCs, skin fibroblasts (see "Differential Diagnosis")
  - WBCs for electron microscopy (lysosomal inclusions)
  - increased acid phosphatase (Gaucher disease)
  - CBC (pancytopenia: Gaucher disease, vacuolated lymphocytes: GM1)
- basic urine studies:
  - Sialic acid, oligosaccharides, sulfatides

Other Tests
- Bone marrow: foamy macrophages (Farber disease, Niemann-Pick), sea blue histiocytes (Gaucher disease)
- CSF: increased protein (metachromatic leukodystophy)

Imaging
- MRI: white matter changes (Krabbe, metachromatic leukodystophy)
- Bone survey: bone thinning, diaphyseal splaying, vertebral changes, lytic lesions (Sialidosis, Gaucher disease, GM1)

DIFFERENTIAL DIAGNOSIS
- Examples of lysosomal disorders: "Name [Enzyme defect]"
- Cystinosis [cysteine transporter]

- Fabry disease [alpha-galactosidase A]
- Farber disease [ceramidase]
- Gaucher disease [glucocerebrosidase]
- GM1 gangliosidosis [beta-galactosidase]
- Tay-Sachs/Sandhoff disease/GM2 gangliosidosis [hexosaminidase]
- Krabbe [galactosylceramidase]
- Metachromatic leukodystophy [arylsulfatase]
- Neuronal ceroid lipofucinosis/Batten disease [multiple defects, not all are known. Eight genetic loci designated CLN1-8]
- Niemann-Pick types A, B, C [sphingomyelinase in A and B, cholesterol transport in C]
- Salla disease [sialic acid transporter]
- Sialidosis [alpha-neuraminidase]

MANAGEMENT

What to Do First
- Supportive in most cases

General Measures
- Antiseizure medication (broad-spectrum drugs – e.g., levetiracetam, topiramate, lamotrigine, zonisamide, valproate; if myoclonic seizures consider clonazepam, chlorazepate, diazepam, lorazepam)
- Antispasticity drugs (e.g., diazepam, lioresal, dantrolene)
- Adaptive equipment
- Genetic counseling for family members

SPECIFIC THERAPY
- Bone marrow transplant in some cases, especially presymptomatic
- Future?: Stem cells, gene therapy

FOLLOW-UP
n/a

COMPLICATIONS AND PROGNOSIS
- Rapidly progressive and fatal: Niemann-Pick-A, Tay-Sachs/Sandhoff disease/GM2, Farber disease, infant Neuronal ceroid lipofucinosis/Batten disease, infant and juvenile Gaucher disease, infantile Krabbe
- Slowly progressive over years: Niemann-Pick B, Niemann-Pick C, Fabry disease; late-onset Gaucher disease, Krabbe, metachromatic leukodystophy, neuronal ceroid lipofucinosis/Batten disease

MAGNESIUM DEFICIENCY

ELISABETH RYZEN, MD

HISTORY & PHYSICAL

History

- Clinical deficiency occurs primarily due to renal or gut Mg wasting, often coupled with inadequate intake
  - ➤ Causes include malabsorption syndromes, diarrhea, alcohol abuse, protein-calorie malnutrition, diuretic therapy, diabetes mellitus, cisplatin, aminoglycosides, amphotericin B, hypercalcemia, IV saline therapy, hungry bone syndrome

SIGNS & SYMPTOMS

- Neurologic: weakness, tetany (+Chvostek's or Trousseau's), seizures, fasciculations, psychiatric problems
- Cardiovascular: prolonged QT, ventricular arrhythmias resistant to antiarrhythmic therapy
- Metabolic: hypocalcemia due to impaired release or action of PTH, hypokalemia from renal potassium wasting; hypophosphatemia

TESTS

Laboratory

- basic studies: blood
- serum magnesium <1.5 mEq/L (may be falsely higher if patient is initially dehydrated)
  - ➤ intracellular Mg may be depleted even if serum level is normal; symptoms may occur with normal serum levels (no easy way of measuring intracellular Mg clinically)

DIFFERENTIAL DIAGNOSIS

- Hypocalcemia, hypokalemia may cause some similar symptoms, often coexist (hypocalcemia is resistant to calcium and Vitamin D Rx; hypokalemia resistant to K supplements)

MANAGEMENT

What to Do First

- assess severity of symptoms and renal function (Mg is cleared by the kidney)

General Measures

- Treat underlying cause, adequate diet if possible (vegetables, meats, legumes, nuts)

SPECIFIC TREATMENT

- When symptoms or hypomagnesemia with continued losses
  - ➤ If acute symptoms (seizure, arrhythmia): 2 g 50% MgSO4 solution IV over 5 minutes (16 mEq elemental Mg), followed by 32–48 mEq IV per 24 hours (for several days); monitor renal function and serum Mg (level will normalize before intracellular stores are repleted)
  - ➤ No IV bolus needed if no acute symptoms
- Oral therapy: e.g., Mg oxide 400 mg p.o. tid, Milk of Magnesium 5 cc tid; Mg-chloride and Mg-gluconate therapeutic options

SIDE EFFECTS & CONTRAINDICATIONS

- IV magnesium
- Side effects: uncommon unless excess doses given; with level >4 mEq/L, deep tendon reflexes disappear, PR interval prolongs; further elevations cause hypotension, respiratory depression, coma at 10–12 mEq/L
- Contraindications
- absolute: elevated serum magnesium level, renal failure
- relative: hypotension (replacement doses of IV Mg may drop systolic BP 5 mm Hg)
- Oral magnesium
- side effects: diarrhea (minimize by dividing dose into more frequent intervals, smaller amount)

FOLLOW-UP

During Rx

- Monitor BP, heart rate, DTR, serum creatinine, daily serum Mg level (may need to continue slow IV Mg infusion for several days to replete stores even if level normalizes, if patient not eating)
- Correct cause of Mg deficiency; long-term, potassium-sparing diuretics are also magnesium-sparing (e.g., aldactone, amiloride)

COMPLICATIONS & PROGNOSIS

- If deficiency uncorrected, symptoms can persist – risk of death from untreated seizures, cardiac arrhythmias

Prognosis

- Symptoms of Mg deficiency completely reversible if Mg deficiency is corrected

MALARIA

SARAH STAEDKE, MD

HISTORY & PHYSICAL

History

■ Malaria is caused by one (or more) of the plasmodial species that infect humans: P. falciparum, P. vivax, P. ovale, and P. malariae. P. knowlesi, an agent of malaria in monkeys, has been recently shown to cause human disease.

■ P. falciparum causes >90% of all deaths.

■ Malaria is primarily transmitted by infected female anopheles mosquitoes that bite from dusk to dawn.

■ Other modes of transmission: blood transfusion, needlestick injury, IVDA, organ transplantation, congenital

■ Risk factors: non-immune host (children <5 years); pregnant women; travel to endemic region; mosquito exposure; chemoprophylaxis and compliance. P. knowlesi associated with travel to forested tropical regions with infected monkeys.

■ Drug resistance (particularly P. falciparum) is a major problem.

■ Important features of P. falciparum: infects RBCs of all ages, producing high-level parasitemia; infected RBCs adhere to endothelial cells and sequester in peripheral vasculature, contributing to microvascular disease

■ P. vivax and P. ovale form dormant intrahepatic hypnozoites, which may produce relapses years after initial infection and require specific therapy.

■ Complete immunity does not develop after infection; semi-immunity develops after years of exposure but wanes in the absence of exposure to malaria parasites.

Signs & Symptoms

■ Incubation period usually 7–21 days; onset may be delayed for years

■ Fever is primary symptom; classic malaria paroxysm = chills, high fever, and sweating; cyclical fevers occur only in well-established infections, and fever pattern is usually not helpful; tertian – fever every 48 h = P. vivax and P. ovale; irregular tertian = P. falciparum; quartan – fever every 72 h = P. malariae

■ Other symptoms: headache, malaise, backache, arthralgias, myalgias, nausea and vomiting, abdominal pain, diarrhea, cough

■ Signs: pallor, jaundice, splenomegaly; no rash

■ Severe falciparum malaria: cerebral malaria (altered mental status, seizures, coma), renal failure, pulmonary edema, severe anemia, hypoglycemia, metabolic acidosis

P. knowlesi can also cause severe acute illness with high-grade parasitemia.

TESTS

Basic Tests: Blood
■ WBC typically normal or decreased, thrombocytopenia common, anemia with progressive disease, hemolysis = elevated bilirubin and LDH, decreased haptoglobin, increased reticulocyte count
■ In severe disease: hypoglycemia, elevated BUN and creatinine, metabolic acidosis, elevated liver enzymes, DIC picture (uncommon)

Basic Tests: Other
■ Urinalysis: hemoglobinuria, proteinuria with severe disease
■ CSF in cerebral malaria: usually normal, protein may be slightly elevated

Specific Diagnostic Tests
■ Thick and thin blood smears: diagnostic tests of choice; Giemsa staining (pH 7.2) preferred; increased sensitivity with thick smear; thin smear used for determining parasite species (multiply infected RBCs, parasitemia >1%, banana-shaped gametocytes = P. falciparum; RBC enlargement, circulating schizonts = P. vivax or ovale)
■ To determine level of parasitemia, examine slides on high power under oil immersion; for thick smear, count the number of asexual parasites per 200 WBCs and calculate the number of parasites/mcl assuming a WBC of 8,000/mcl; for thin smear, count the number of parasitized RBCs among 1,000 RBCs and calculate the% infected RBCs
■ Other: acridine orange staining of centrifuged parasites in Quantitative Buffy Coat (QBC), immunochromatographic assay for histidine-rich protein 2 (HRP-2) of P. falciparum (ParaSight F assay, Becton Dickinson); PCR amplification of parasite DNA or mRNA

DIFFERENTIAL DIAGNOSIS
■ Extensive; includes typhoid fever, meningitis, encephalitis, brain abscess, pneumonia, gastroenteritis, bacterial sepsis, hepatitis, dengue fever, yellow fever, leptospirosis, viral hemorrhagic fever

MANAGEMENT

What to Do First

- Evaluate blood smears to confirm diagnosis and parasite species.
- Consider hospitalization for all patients with falciparum malaria.
- Admit patients with severe disease to ICU (abnormal mental status; >3% parasitemia; hematocrit <20%; hypoglycemia; renal, cardiac, pulmonary, or hepatic dysfunction; DIC; prolonged hyperthermia; severe vomiting or diarrhea) and treat with parenteral therapy.

General Measures

- One negative blood smear does not rule out malaria; if initially negative, repeat thick blood smears every 12 h for 48 h.
- If uncertain about parasite species or drug sensitivity, treat for chloroquine-resistant P. falciparum with quinine or quinidine.
- In severe disease, carefully monitor glucose, hemoglobin/hematocrit, fluid, electrolyte, and acid-base balance; give prophylactic anticonvulsants (phenobarbital) to unconscious patients; consider exchange transfusion for severely ill patients with hyperparasitemia (>5–15%); avoid use of corticosteroids in cerebral malaria.
- Check G6PD level before prescribing primaquine.

SPECIFIC THERAPY

Indication

- Positive blood smear or other diagnostic test; empiric treatment indicated if clinical suspicion is high and diagnostic tests are pending
- Consult CDC for current recommendations: www.cdc.gov; malaria hotlines 770-488-7788 (treatment) and 888-232-3228 (prophylaxis)
- Antimalarial drug doses can be expressed either in amounts of base or salt; be specific when ordering medications.
- Uncomplicated Chloroquine-Sensitive Malaria
  - ➤ Chloroquine
  - ➤ PLUS Primaquine (for radical cure of P. vivax and P. ovale only)
- Severe Chloroquine-sensitive Malaria
  - ➤ Chloroquine
- Uncomplicated Chloroquine-Resistant Malaria
  - ➤ Quinine orally PLUS Doxycycline OR Tetracycline OR Clindamycin OR sulfadoxine-pyrimethamine (Fansidar)
  - ➤ OR Mefloquine (Larium)
  - ➤ OR Atovaquone/Proguanil (Malarone)

- ➤ OR Artesuntate* (alone or in combination with longer-acting agent)
- ➤ OR Artemether* (alone or in combination with longer-acting agent)
- ➤ OR Halofantrine

Sulfadoxine-pyrimethamine (Fansidar) single agent – avoid due to widespread resistance

- ■ Severe Chloroquine-Resistant Malaria
  - ➤ Quinine parenterally
  - ➤ OR Quinidine: call Eli Lilly Company (800-821-0538) if rapid shipment of drug is needed
  - ➤ OR Artesunate*
  - ➤ OR Artemether*

*Not available in US

- ■ Chemoprophylaxis
  - ➤ Avoiding mosquito bites is best protective measure; advise patients to use insect repellant (20–35% DEET), suitable clothing, and permethrin-treated bed nets.
  - ➤ Prophylactic regimens should be started 1–2 weeks prior to departure and continued for 4 weeks after return.
  - ➤ Chloroquine: only for chloroquine-sensitive regions
  - ➤ Mefloquine (Larium): for chloroquine-resistant areas
  - ➤ Doxycycline: for mefloquine-resistant areas and as an alternative to mefloquine
  - ➤ Atovaquone/Proguanil (Malarone): adult dosing, one tablet daily; begin 1–2 days before departure and continue for 7 days after return
  - ➤ Chloroquine PLUS Proguanil: no longer recommended by CDC
  - ➤ Self-treatment: consider for patients traveling to chloroquine-resistant areas who may not have immediate access to medical care; advise patients to take medication only if fever develops and to seek medical care at once; sulfadoxine-pyrimethamine (Fansidar)

Side Effects & Contraindications

- ■ Artemisinin derivatives: not available in US; decreased reticulocyte count, mild EKG changes, neurotoxicity in animals (not reported in humans); limited data on use in pregnancy
- ■ Atovaquone/Proguanil: abdominal pain, nausea, vomiting, headache; not recommended for use in pregnant and lactating women, or children <11 kg due to insufficient data

- Chloroquine: bitter taste, blurred vision, nausea, pruritus in dark-skinned patients; with rapid IV infusion or large IM bolus, hypotensive shock, cardiac arrest; with chronic use, retinopathy; safe in pregnancy

- Doxycycline/Tetracycline: gastrointestinal intolerance, photosensitivity, vulvovaginal candidiasis, deposition in growing bones and teeth; contraindicated in pregnant and lactating women, children <8 years

- Halofantrine: not available in the US; diarrhea, PR and QT interval prolongation, cardiac arrhythmias; contraindicated in pregnant and lactating women, cardiac conduction abnormalities, electrolyte imbalance, concurrent QT-prolonging drugs; avoid within 28 d of prior mefloquine; check EKG prior to use

- Mefloquine: nausea, dizziness, insomnia, nightmares, neuropsychiatric reactions (with prophylaxis, moderate in 1:250–500, severe in 1:10,000; with treatment, severe in 1:250–1,700), convulsions; contraindicated in mefloquine allergy, not recommended for patients with history of seizure disorders, severe psychiatric disorders, or cardiac conduction abnormalities; now recommended by CDC for prophylaxis in pregnancy, but avoid (especially during 1st trimester) if possible

- Primaquine: dizziness, nausea, vomiting, abdominal pain; severe hemolysis in G6PD-deficient patients; contraindicated in patients with <10% normal G6PD activity; with 10–20% activity, can treat with adjusted doses (0.6 mg base/kg, max 45 mg, weekly for 8 weeks); contraindicated in pregnancy (for pregnant women with P. vivax or P. ovale infections, after initial treatment continue chloroquine prophylaxis weekly until delivery, then treat with primaquine)

- Quinine/Quinidine: bitter taste, cinchonism (tinnitus, hearing loss, nausea, vomiting, blurred vision), QT interval prolongation, hypoglycemia; with IV infusion, hypotension, cardiac arrhythmias, death; use cautiously if given within 2 weeks of mefloquine (increased risk of cardiac toxicity), and in diabetics; for IV quinidine therapy, cardiac monitoring is required, drug levels should be followed and dose reduction is required after 3 days; can be used to treat severe disease in pregnancy

- Sulfadoxine-pyrimethamine: severe mucocutaneous reactions with prophylactic dosing (1 in 11,000 to 25,000); contraindicated in sulfa-allergic patients, children <1 month, generally considered safe in pregnancy

FOLLOW-UP
- With appropriate treatment, fever should resolve in 48–72 h and parasitemia should be <25% of the original value 48 h after initiating therapy.
- In non-immune patients with uncomplicated disease, repeat blood smears daily until negative; repeat smears if fever recurs >48 h after treatment.
- In severe cases, repeat blood smears frequently (every 6–12 h) until patient stabilizes and then daily until negative.
- In all patients, repeat smears if fever recurs >48 h after treatment.
- Consider treatment failure and need for alternative therapy if evidence of severe disease develops at any time during therapy; parasite count at 48 h is >25% of original value; fever is present ≥72 h and blood smear is still positive; blood smear remains positive 7 days after initiating therapy.

COMPLICATIONS AND PROGNOSIS
- Overall mortality in returning travelers: ~5%
- Cerebral malaria: mortality in 15–20%; neurologic sequelae more common in children (>10%) than adults (<5%)
- Renal failure: multifactorial but resembles acute tubular necrosis; increases mortality risk; may require dialysis
- Pulmonary edema: associated with hyperparasitemia, uncommon but frequently fatal (mortality >80%); resembles ARDS and may require mechanical ventilation
- Hypoglycemia: occurs in 5–30% of patients with cerebral malaria; more common in children, pregnant women, hyperparasitemia, with quinine/quinidine therapy
- Late splenic rupture (P. vivax): uncommon, occurs after 2–3 months
- Immune complex glomerulonephritis (P. malariae): seen with chronic or repeated infections; results in nephrotic syndrome

MALIGNANT TUMORS OF THE LIVER

EMMET B. KEEFFE, MD

HISTORY & PHYSICAL

History
- metastases most common hepatic malignancy
- most frequent origin for hepatic metastases are lung, breast, and gastrointestinal tract

- HCC one of the most common malignancies worldwide
- HCC associated with cirrhosis in the majority of cases, particularly chronic hepatitis B, chronic hepatitis C and hemochromatosis; the rising incidence of HCC can be attributed to chronic HCV infection
- other conditions associated with HCC include hemochromatosis, androgenic steroids, alpha-1-antitrypsin deficiency, etc.

Signs and Symptoms
- presentation is variable
- asymptomatic detection on screening with ultrasound and AFP
- abdominal pain or mass occurs in 60%
- weight loss common
- decompensation of previously-existing cirrhosis occurs in 20%
- perineoplastic manifestations include erythrocytosis, hypoglycemia, and feminization

TESTS

Basic Tests: Blood:
- nonspecific: increased AST, ALT, alkaline phosphatase, bilirubin
- 75% of patients with HCC have increased AFP

Imaging
- ultrasound and CT main imaging studies used for diagnosis
- screening ultrasound: HCC hyperdense lesions as small as 0.5–1 cm
- biphasic CT: useful to confirm the presence of HCC and assess for additional lesions
- CT angiography: may be used as a confirmatory test to detect additional lesions

Biopsy
- liver biopsy may be required to confirm the diagnosis, particularly if AFP level is normal.
- fibrolamellar HCC is a variant of HCC that is usually not associated with cirrhosis and appears to have a better prognosis

DIFFERENTIAL DIAGNOSIS
- benign tumors, including FNH and hepatocellular adenoma
- isolated single metastatic lesion

MANAGEMENT

What to Do First
- assess the security of the diagnosis, i.e., chronic HBV or HCV infection with (incr.) AFP and new lesion on screening ultrasound virtually diagnostic

- if lesion atypical on imaging studies and/or AFP level normal, liver biopsy may be required
- assess the severity of chronic liver disease, i.e., Child-Pugh score

General Measures
- assess candidacy for resection or liver transplantation

SPECIFIC THERAPY

Curative Treatments for HCC
- resection (Child's class A, technically feasible, no advanced portal hypertension, acceptable comorbidities)
- liver transplantation (single lesion <5 cm, or no more than 3 lesions <3 cm; confined to the liver; no portal vein invasion); various palliative treatments used as "bridge" to transplantation

Palliative Treatments for HCC
- transcatheter arterial embolization
- transcatheter arterial chemo-embolization
- percutaneous ethanol injection
- intravenous or intra-arterial chemotherapy
- radiotherapy

Treatment of Metastatic Cancer
- generally palliative, using one or more of the above therapies, with the exception of colorectal cancer where isolated lesions are amenable to resection and potential cure

FOLLOW-UP
- serial imaging studies to detect recurrent or new lesions

COMPLICATIONS AND PROGNOSIS
- natural history of untreated HCC death within 2–6 months
- cause of death usually malignant cachexia, or complications of cirrhosis with liver failure

MARASMUS

PATSY OBAYASHI, MS, RD, CNSD, CDE

HISTORY & PHYSICAL

History
- Chronic deprivation of dietary calories and protein

Physical Signs
- Weight loss

- Severe tissue wasting
- Loss of subcutaneous fat (decreased mid-arm muscle circumference and triceps skinfold)
- Dehydration
- Anorexia
- Diarrhea
- Lassitude
- Glossitis
- Alopecia
- Dry/depigmented hair
- Desquamation of skin
- Weakness, decreased muscle strength
- Decline in functional activities of daily living
- Depressed immune function
- Skin breakdown, pressure ulcers
- Decreased cardiopulmonary function
- Increased morbidity and mortality

TESTS

Basic Studies: Blood
- Sodium, Iron, CBC, Chloride
- Magnesium, Ferritin, Creatinine
- Calcium, Transferrin, T3, T4
- Potassium, Albumin, Copper
- Phosphorus, Cholesterol, B12, chloride

Basic Studies: Urine
- Urinary urea nitrogen
- Urine acetone

Anthropometrics
- Blood pressure
- Mid-arm muscle circumference (MAMC)
- Height
- Triceps skinfold (TSF)
- Weight
- usual
- present
- changes
- Arm muscle circumference (AMC)

Specific Diagnostic Tests
- Pre-albumin
- Creatinine height index (CHI)

- Nitrogen balance
- Cell-mediated immunity (skin test)

DIFFERENTIAL DIAGNOSIS

- Malignancy/cancer cachexia (blood testing, imaging studies, exploratory
- surgeries to differentiate)
- GI tract obstruction (imaging studies to differentiate)
- Malabsorption related to ulcerative colitis, celiac sprue, Crohn's disease, inflammatory bowel disease, chronic liver disease (radiologic exam or biopsy)
- AIDS (HIV blood testing)
- COPD (pulmonary function studies)
- Cystic fibrosis (sweat chloride test, chest x-ray, pancreatic enzyme studies)
- Diabetes mellitus (fasting glucose to differentiate)
- Eating disorders (psychiatric evaluation to differentiate)

MANAGEMENT

- Provide energy immediately
- Hydrate
- Replete electrolytes
- Treat infections
- Replete deficient vitamins and minerals

SPECIFIC THERAPY

Treatment Options

- Oral or IV glucose to start, gradually add lactose-free liquids and
- progress to solids (30 cc/kg actual weight)
- High biological value proteins, 1.0–1.2 gm/kg actual weight
- Avoid over-feeding: 30–35 kcalories/kg actual weight for calculated energy needs
  - ➤ metabolic cart for measured energy needs
- Add vitamin-mineral supplements, including thiamine

Contraindications to Treatment

- Refeeding syndrome
  - ➤ Hypophosphatemia
  - ➤ Hypomagnesemia
  - ➤ Hypokalemia
  - ➤ Hyperglycemia
  - ➤ Congestive heart failure
  - ➤ Sepsis

FOLLOW-UP

During Rx

- Blood pressure
- Serum sodium, chloride, potassium, magnesium, phosphorus, calcium, and glucose

Routine

- Weight
- Albumin or pre-albumin
- Transferrin
- CBC

COMPLICATIONS AND PROGNOSIS

Common Complications

- Progressive weight loss and lethargy: 100% if no intervention
- Delayed physical rehabilitation
- Decubitus ulcers: common, especially in non-ambulatory
- Increased infections
- Impaired wound healing
- Increased pneumonitis and urinary tract infections
- Decreased response to chemotherapy and radiotherapy: common in
- Immunosuppressed patients

Prognosis

- Without nutrition intervention, complications proceed in a cascading manner, resulting in death due to overwhelming infection and/or
- respiratory failure.
- With immediate nutrition support, full recovery is possible.

MARFAN'S SYNDROME

MICHAEL WARD, MD

HISTORY & PHYSICAL

History

- abnormal posture, long limbs, hyperextensible
- myopia
- cardiac murmur, congestive heart failure
- family history of same (autosomal dominant), but 25% are new mutations

Signs and Symptoms

- tall (>95th percentile)

- short upper body (head to pubis:pubis to floor ratio <0.85)
- kyphoscoliosis
- arachnodactyly (long limbs, fingers); arm span to height ratio >1.05; thumb sign (distal thumb extends well beyond margin of hand when placed across palm); wrist sign (thumb and 5th finger overlap around wrist)
- high-arched palate
- pectus excavatum (hollow chest)
- pectus carinatum (pigeon chest)
- joint laxity
- normal skin texture and elasticity
- ectopic lens, myopia, retinal detachment
- aortic insufficiency murmur; congestive failure
- mitral valve prolapse

TESTS
- documentation of mutations in fibrillin-1 (FBN-1) gene for research purposes only
- echocardiography to document aortic insufficiency and monitor aortic root dilatation
- slit-lamp exam
- extrinsic restrictive ventilatory defect with severe kyphoscoliosis

DIFFERENTIAL DIAGNOSIS
- evaluate for other causes of aortic insufficiency or mitral valve prolapse
- homocystinuria has positive urine cyanide-nitroprusside test
- congenital contractural arachnodactyly lacks eye or cardiac problems
- marfanoid hypermobility syndrome lacks eye or cardiac problems and has greater joint hypermobility
- Pts with Ehlers-Danlos types I, II, and III have greater joint hypermobility and normal skeletal proportions

MANAGEMENT

What to Do First
- assess aortic root size and severity of aortic insufficiency

General Measures
- avoid athletics or other strenuous activities
- prophylactic antibiotics before dental work or high-risk operations
- braces or surgical correction of scoliosis

- refraction for myopia
- psychological and genetic counseling

Specific Treatment
- Beta-blockers for all patients to reduce rate of aortic root dilatation and risk of dissection as blood pressure tolerates

Side Effects and Contraindications
- side effects: fatigue, excessive bradycardia or hypotension, bronchospasm, depression, erectile dysfunction, insensitivity to hypoglycemic symptoms
- contraindications:
  - absolute: decompensated congestive heart failure, severe COPD, heart block
  - relative: CHF, COPD, diabetes with frequent hypoglycemia

FOLLOW-UP

During Treatment
- Annual EKG and echocardiogram to monitor aortic root size until aortic root = 45 mm, then more frequently
- Prophylactic aortic valve replacement and ascending aortic conduit surgery if moderate aortic insufficiency, aortic root >50 mm, or aortic root increases >1 cm/year

COMPLICATIONS
- dilated aortic root in 50% of children and 80% of adults
- aortic dissection (usually ascending) in 44% at autopsy
- pregnancy increases risk of dissection; avoid if aortic root >40 mm
- nondissecting aortic aneurysms common

PROGNOSIS
- Mortality from untreated heart disease or aortic dissection
- 20-year survival after aortic valve and root surgery 65%

MEASLES

CAROL A. GLASER, MD

HISTORY & PHYSICAL

History
- RNA virus, morbilliform virus within the Paramyxovirus family
- Humans only host

- Transmission mainly by aerosolized droplets of respiratory secretions, direct contact of respiratory secretions
- Contagious 1–2 days before onset symptoms (3–5 day before rash, 0 to 4 day after rash appears)
- Highly contagious
- Incubation period 8–12 days
- Disease mildest in children, more severe in very young and adults
- Malnourished individuals have a high rate of complications (vitamin A deficiency increases severity).
- Peak incidence winter/spring
- Vaccine has dramatically reduced cases, >99% reduction since introduction of vaccine
- Disease most severe in infants and adults, milder in children

Signs & Symptoms
- URI prodrome 2–4 days, then
- fever (peaks 2–3 days of rash)
- cough – often severe and very "troublesome"
- coryza
- characteristic erythematous maculopapular rash (immunocompetent host may not have characteristic rash)
  - ➤ first appears behind ears and forehead hairline
  - ➤ spreads in centrifugal pattern from head to feet
  - ➤ rash can become confluent, later may desquamate
- pathognomonic enanthem (Koplik spots); bluish-white specks upon a bright red mucosal surface usually involving the buccal and lower labial mucous membranes. Initially few in number, which then progress to high numbers.

Modified Measles
- occurs in partially immune individuals
- clinically similar to measles as above but milder
- Koplik spots may not be present
- Exanthem follows progression of regular measles but usually no confluence

Atypical Measles
- Occurs in previously immunized persons
- Fever
- Headache
- Abdominal pain
- Myalgia

- Dry, nonproductive cough
- Pleuritic chest pain
- 2–3 days after onset
  - rash appears first on distal extremities and progresses in cephalad direction
  - rash most pronounced on wrists/ankles
  - rash may be maculopapular, vesicular, petechial, and/or pruritic
- respiratory symptoms; dyspnea, rales
- hepatosplenomegaly
- marked hyperesthesia
- numbness, paresthesia

TESTS

Nonspecific
- leukopenia

Specific
- most utilized test if measles-specific IgM – usually detectable 3–4 days after onset of rash, no longer detectable 30–60 days after onset
- Measles can be isolated from the nasopharynx, conjunctiva, and/or urine during acute phase
- Atypical measles; high titers
- SSPE: very high titers IgG in serum and CSF

Special Hosts
- immunocompromised individuals are more susceptible to complications of measles and have a higher fatality rate

DIFFERENTIAL DIAGNOSIS
n/a

MANAGEMENT
Report all cases of measles to the local health department.

SPECIFIC THERAPY
- no specific antiviral available
- consider vitamin A supplement in special circumstances

FOLLOW-UP
n/a

COMPLICATIONS AND PROGNOSIS

Complications
- otitis media: 5–15%

- Diarrhea
  - ➤ Pneumonia – either primary viral or secondary bacterial
  - ➤ Laryngotracheobronchitis (croup)
  - ➤ Acute encephalitis – 0.1–0.2% of cases
- SSPE: result of persistent measles, develops years after infection (mean incubation 7 years)
- Myocarditis/pericarditis
- death due to respiratory or neurologic complications: 1–2/1000 cases

Prevention
- acquired immunity after illness is permanent
- in U.S. vaccine recommended at 12–15 months and a 2nd dose at school age
- reportable disease
- measles vaccine recommended in outbreak setting

MEDIASTINAL MASSES

STEPHEN C. LAZARUS, MD

HISTORY & PHYSICAL

History
- Since differential diagnosis is broad, a detailed history is important

Signs & Symptoms
- <50% asymptomatic – 80% of these are benign
- Common symptoms are cough, dyspnea, dysphagia, chest pain, SVC obstruction, hoarseness, stridor; Horner's less common

TESTS

Imaging
- CXR: look for location, teeth
- Chest CT: very sensitive and specific for teratomas, thymolipomas, fat
- MRI: can demonstrate continuity with thymus
- PET: may help identify neoplasm

Specific Tests
- Thyroid function (goiter, thyroid)
- HCG, alphaFP (germ cell tumor)
- Antiacetycholine receptor antibody (myasthenia gravis)
- ^{99M}Technetium-Sestamibi (parathyroid)

DIFFERENTIAL DIAGNOSIS

- Differential diagnosis depends on location
- Anterior Mediastinum
  - ➤ Thymic neoplasms, esp thymoma:
    - most are benign
    - evidence of myasthenia gravis in 10–50% of patients with thymoma
    - require tissue for diagnosis
  - ➤ Germ cell tumors:
    - 10–12% of mediastinal masses; 80% benign
    - Teratoma and teratocarcinoma:
      - 2/3 symptomatic (cough, pain, dyspnea)
      - smooth, rounded
      - may contain teeth, bone
    - Seminoma:
      - men, 20–30 y old
      - SVC obstruction common
      - extend locally, metastasize to bone
    - Embryonal cell carcinoma, choriocarcinoma:
      - often secrete HCG, alphaFP, CEA
  - ➤ Lymphoma:
    - 10–20% of mediastinal masses
  - ➤ Thyroid:
    - ectopic thyroid = 10–20% of masses
    - identifiable by radioactive iodine scanning
  - ➤ Parathyroid:
    - adenomas, cysts, carcinoma
    - 99m Technitium sestamibi
  - ➤ Mesenchymal tumors, tissue:
    - lipomas, fibromas, mesotheliomas, lymphangiomas, lipomatosis
  - ➤ Diaphragmatic hernia (Morgagni)
  - ➤ Primary cancer
- Middle Mediastinum
  - ➤ Lymphadenopathy:
    - >1 cm = abnormal
    - from lymphoma, metastases, granulomatous inflammation
  - ➤ Developmental cysts:
    - 10–20% of mediastinal masses
    - pericardial, bronchogenic, enteric

- ➢ Vascular masses:
  - aneurysms, dilatations
- ➢ Diaphragmatic hernia (hiatal)
- ▪ Posterior Mediastinum
  - ➢ Neural tumors:
    - neurofibroma, neurilemoma, neurosarcoma, ganglioneu-roma, ganglioneuroblastoma, pheochromocytoma
  - ➢ Esophageal carcinoma, diverticuli
  - ➢ Diaphragmatic hernia (Bochdalek)

MANAGEMENT

What to Do First
- ▪ Define location
- ▪ Look for involvement of vital structures
- ▪ Consider systemic effects (myasthenia, Cushing, hypertension)

SPECIFIC THERAPY
- ▪ Resection:
  - ➢ Indicated for all, even benign
  - ➢ Otherwise, may enlarge and compress vital structures, become infected, rupture
- ▪ Radiation therapy, chemotherapy:
  - ➢ Useful adjuncts to resection for some tumors
  - ➢ Seminomas are extremely radio- and chemosensitive

FOLLOW-UP
- ▪ Depends on histopathology of mass
- ▪ Monitor systemic effects where appropriate – these often resolve after resection

COMPLICATIONS AND PROGNOSIS

Complications
- ▪ Goiter – thyrotoxicosis
- ▪ HCG-secreting germ cell tumor – gynecomastia
- ▪ Parathyroid adenoma, lymphoma – hypercalcemia
- ▪ Thymoma, carcinoid – Cushing's
- ▪ Pheochromocytoma – hypertension
- ▪ Thymoma – myasthenia gravis, RBC aplasia, myocarditis, hypogam-maglobulinemia, other autoimmune diseases

Prognosis
- Depends on underlying histopathology
- For benign lesions, survival is normal, unless there is compression of vital structures
- Thymoma:
  - ➤ 30% recur after resection
  - ➤ Encapsulated: Normal survival
  - ➤ Invasive: 50–77% 5-y; 30–55% 10-y
- Germ cell tumors:
  - ➤ Very radio- and chemosensitive
  - ➤ Long-term survival ~80%
- Lymphoma:
  - ➤ Very radio- and chemosensitive

MEGACOLON

GEORGE TRIADAFILOPOULOS, MD

HISTORY & PHYSICAL

Megacolon implies cecal dilation of more than 12 cm or sigmoid colon dilation more than 6.5 cm. Primary megacolon is associated with neurogenic dysfunction. If it is acute (Ogilvie's syndrome) the megacolon is a reflex response to various medical or surgical conditions. Secondary chronic megacolon and megarectum develop later in life as a response to chronic fecal retention. Toxic megacolon is a serious complication of inflammatory bowel disease (IBD) or infectious colitis that is associated with systemic toxicity. Colonic dilatation is also seen with congenital megacolon (Hirshsprung's disease) and chronic intestinal pseudoobstruction, a manifestation of diffuse gastrointestinal dysmotility of various causes.

Risk Factors

- Children or physically and mentally impaired elderly with longstanding constipation or defecatory difficulties and fecal impaction are particularly at risk. Megacolon may also be seen in Hirschsprung's disease, meningomyelocele, or spinal cord lesions. Toxic megacolon often affects patients with IBD early in their disease. C. difficile infection, Salmonella, Shigella, Campylobacter and amebic colitis may also be complicated by toxic megacolon. In patients with HIV infection or AIDS, cytomegalovirus (CMV) colitis is the leading cause of toxic megacolon.

Symptoms

■ In acute megacolon bloating, obstipation and abdominal pain are the main symptoms. In cases of toxic megacolon, signs and symptoms of acute colitis precede the onset of acute dilation. Improvement of diarrhea may herald the onset of megacolon. Chronic megacolon usually presents with constipation and abdominal fullness.

Physical Signs

■ The general physical examination is not helpful in most patients presenting with chronic constipation and megacolon. In acute megacolon (Ogilvie's syndrome) pronounced abdominal distention with generalized abdominal tenderness is noted. In toxic megacolon, physical examination reveals an ill-appearing patient with tachycardia, fever, hypotension, abdominal distension and tenderness, with or without signs of peritonitis.

TESTS

Basic Tests

■ Plain abdominal radiographs are critical for diagnosis and follow-up. Multiple air-fluid levels in the colon are common. The normal colonic haustral pattern is either absent or severely disturbed and significant stool is evident.

Specific Diagnostic Tests

■ Flexible sigmoidoscopy and colonoscopy help identify lesions that narrow or occlude the bowel. Colonoscopy is extremely risky in patients with toxic megacolon. If needed for decompression, only minimal amounts of air should be introduced into the colon to avoid perforation. A guidewire is placed through the colonoscope and a decompression tube is then passed into the right colon.

Other Tests

■ Barium enema is less costly and may be preferable in detecting megacolon and megarectum. Barium radiographs may also show the aganglionic distal bowel with proximal dilatation of the colon in classic Hirschsprung's disease. Although anorectal manometry may provide useful information in patients with severe constipation, it has no value in the assessment of acute megacolon. Colonic transit studies are important for cases of chronic megacolon due to colonic inertia.

- CT scanning may determine the etiology of megacolon as in the case of C. difficile infection, where diffuse colonic thickening is a very sensitive finding
- In toxic megacolon, anemia related to blood loss and leukocytosis with a left shift occur frequently; electrolyte disturbances (metabolic alkalosis and hypokalemia) are extremely common. Hypoalbuminemia is due to protein loss and decreased hepatic synthesis due to chronic inflammation and malnutrition. In other cases of megacolon, the laboratory findings are unremarkable.
- In Hirschprung's disease anorectal manometry demonstrates paradoxical contraction of the internal anal sphincter. Biopsies of the rectal and colonic wall demonstrate the absence of ganglia provide a definitive diagnosis.

DIFFERENTIAL DIAGNOSIS
- Mechanical obstruction, infection and idiopathic inflammatory bowel disease are key diagnostic considerations.

MANAGEMENT
What to Do First
- Plain abdominal films should be obtained immediately. If the patient is toxic or has peripheral leukocytosis, stool specimens should be sent for culture, microscopic analysis, and C. difficile toxin. Decompress the rectum with an indwelling catheter.

General Measures
- Repositioning of the patient results in redistribution of air in the colon. Intravenous fluids and antibiotics (for toxic cases) should be administered. Exclude mechanical obstruction (with a hypaque enema or sigmoidoscopy), discontinue medications that would adversely affect colonic motility and correct metabolic disturbances.

SPECIFIC THERAPY
Indications for Treatment
- In toxic megacolon, aggressive therapy of colitis restores normal colonic motility and decreases the likelihood of perforation. The initial therapy is medical, which is successful in preventing surgery in up to 50 percent of patients. Intravenous neostigmine is effective and safe for acute megacolon.

Treatment Options

- Endoscopic decompression should be performed in patients who do not respond to neostigmine or relapse. Surgical resection and colostomy are indicated if ischemic bowel or perforation are suspected.
- For Hirschprung's disease-related enterocolitis, volume resuscitation and intravenous antibiotics, which should provide broad-spectrum coverage against aerobic and anaerobic organisms. Repeated rectal irrigation with saline decompresses the colon and may decrease the severity of disease. Surgical excision of the aganglionic segment and a decompressing colostomy should be performed as soon as the child is stable and the diagnosis established.

Side Effects and Complications

- Neostigmine causes bradycardia, colic, hypersalivation and nausea.
- Contraindications to treatment
- Neostigmine is contraindicated in true intestinal (mechanical) and urinary obstruction, or bradycardia

FOLLOW-UP

During Treatment

- In all cases of megacolon, surgical consultation should be obtained upon admission, and the patient should be evaluated daily by both the medical and surgical team. Bowel rest, and close monitoring.

Routine

- In chronic megacolon, colonic evacuation with osmotic laxatives and enemas may suffice. A subtotal colectomy with ileorectal anastomosis or a decopressive ileostomy may be needed.

COMPLICATIONS AND PROGNOSIS

- Volvulus is a rare complication of Hirschprung's disease and chronic megacolon. Clinical manifestations include abdominal pain and distension and vomiting. The diagnosis can be confirmed with a contrast enema, which may also detorse the volvulus. Surgery is indicated if detorsion is unsuccessful or if bowel necrosis or perforation is suspected.
- The prognosis in acute megacolon (Ogilvie's syndrome) depends on the underlying disease. Toxic megacolon carries very high mortality.

MELANOMA

TIMOTHY S. BROWN, MD

HISTORY & PHYSICAL

History
- High risk (>50-fold increased risk)
  - Changing mole
  - Atypical moles in a patient with a family history of melanoma
  - >50 nevi ≥2 mm
- Intermediate risk (10 fold)
  - Family history of melanoma
  - Sporadic atypical moles
  - Congenital nevi
  - Personal history of prior melanoma
- Low risk (2–4 fold)
  - Immunosuppression
  - Sun sensitivity or excess sun exposure
  - Light skin color with inability to tan
  - Upper socioeconomic status

Signs & Symptoms
- Clinical presentation (symptoms)
  - Most often asymptomatic
  - Burning, itching, and bleeding have been described
  - Asymmetry
  - Border irregularity
  - Color variability
  - Diameter >6 mm
- Practical tips to assist with diagnosis
  - Perform full body skin exam.
  - Conduct exam with optimal lighting.
  - Magnifying lens/dermoscopy to facilitate exam
  - Wood's lamp accentuates epidermal pigmentation.
- Classification of melanoma types
  - Superficial spreading melanoma 70%
  - Nodular melanoma 15%
  - Lentigo maligna melanoma 5%
  - Acral lentiginous melanoma 5–10%
- Precursor lesions
  - Clark's (dysplastic) melanocytic nevus

> Congenital nevomelanocytic nevus (giant or small)
> Lentigo maligna

TESTS

Biopsy

■ Excisional biopsy with narrow margin of normal skin
■ Incisional or punch biopsy acceptable when total excisional biopsy cannot be performed due to large size or location
■ Provide your dermatopathologist with as much tissue as possible so that an accurate diagnosis can be established.

DIFFERENTIAL DIAGNOSIS

■ Nevi (benign, dysplastic, blue)
■ Seborrheic keratosis
■ Solar lentigo
■ Pigmented basal cell carcinoma
■ Pyogenic granuloma
■ Hemangioma

MANAGEMENT

■ Establish the correct diagnosis with a proper biopsy.
■ Refer to a skin cancer specialist such as a dermatologist or a surgical oncologist.

SPECIFIC THERAPY

Primary Melanoma

■ Standard treatment in primary cutaneous melanoma is the complete excision of the lesion
    > Guidelines for melanoma in situ
        • Surgically excise with 5-mm margins of normal skin extending to subcutaneous layer.
    > Guidelines for stage I melanoma
        • ≤2 mm thick, 1-cm surgical margins extending to fascia
        • >2 mm thick, 2-cm surgical margins extending to fascia
■ Elective lymph node dissection (ELND)
    > Controversial – directed by positive sentinel node
■ Sentinel lymph node biopsy
    > First node draining the lymphatic basin (sentinel node) – predicts the presence or absence of melanoma in the entire basin
    > Lymphoscintigraphy and a radioactive tracer used to locate the sentinel node
    > Sentinel lymph node biopsy is recommended for lesions 1 mm or greater in depth.

Regional Metastases
- Surgery
- Hyperthermic regional limb perfusion
- Adjuvant therapy – interferon alpha-2b
- Adjuvant therapy – experimental melanoma vaccines

Distant Metastases (Stage IV) Melanoma
- Radiation
- Chemotherapy
- Chemoimmunotherapy
- Biologic therapy (interferon, interleukins, monoclonal antibodies, melanoma vaccines)

FOLLOW-UP
Total skin examinations for melanoma and its precursors should be routinely done.
- Localized disease – follow q3 months for the 1st year, then q6 months for the next 5 years, yearly thereafter.
- Locoregional metastasis(nodal metastasis) – follow q3 months for 2 years after the excision, then q6 months
  - Serum LDH and chest x-ray tests at each visit. PET/CT scan at initial staging and then q6 months. Additional studies directed toward symptoms.
- Distant metastases – q3 months for 5 years, then q6 months
  - Radiologic and laboratory investigations dependent upon symptoms and exam (i.e., cervical lymphadenopathy – CT scan)

COMPLICATIONS AND PROGNOSIS

Stage I Melanoma
- Sex – women > men
- Tumor site – *b*ack, posterior *a*rm, posterior *n*eck, *s*calp (BANS) worse prognosis
- Age younger > older
- Tumor thickness – thin > thick
  - <0.76 mm, 96% 5-year survival
  - 0.76–1.49, 87%
  - 1.50–2.49, 75%
  - 2.50–3.99, 66%
  - >4.0, 47%
- Clark's level of invasion
  - Intraepidermal (Level I)
  - In papillary dermis (Level II)
  - Fills papillary dermis (Level III)

> Reticular dermis (Level IV)
> Enters fat (Level V)
- Regression
- Ulceration
- Mitotic rate
- Microscopic satellitosis
- Vascular invasion
- Sentinel lymph node status

Stage II Melanoma
- Presence of vertical growth phase – radial > vertical
- Mitotic rate – lower > higher
- Tumor-infiltrating lymphocytes – absence > presence
- Tumor thickness
- Anatomic site
- Sex
- Regression – presence > absence
- Sentinel lymph node status

Stage III Melanoma
- Number of positive nodes – lower > higher
- Anatomic location
- Age

Stage IV Melanoma
- Number of metastatic sites – lower number > higher number
- Surgical respectability
- Duration of remission – longer > shorter
- Location of metastases

MENOPAUSE

MAXINE H. DORIN, MD
REVISED BY ANDREW R. HOFFMAN, MD; FREDRIC B. KRAEMER, MD; and
THOMAS F. McELRATH, MD, PhD

HISTORY & PHYSICAL

History of Menstrual Pattern
- Menopause: no spontaneous menses for 1 full year
- Perimenopause: transitional years plus 1 y
- Average age of menopause: 51.2 y (>90% by age 55 y)
- Most begin perimenopause about age 47 y

- Perimenopause usually lasts 4–5 y, but may last only 2 y
- On average, nulliparous women and smokers have earlier menopause

Signs & Symptoms
- Perimenopause changes:
  - ➤ Change in menstrual flow & length of cycle
  - ➤ Risk of unintended pregnancy
- Vasomotor symptoms: hot flashes, day/night sweats (80%)
- Vaginal dryness/dyspareunia
- Other symptoms reported by midlife women:
  - ➤ Stiffness/soreness, insomnia/sleep disturbances, depression (esp if prior history), urine leakage, changes in libido, headaches and backaches, forgetfulness, palpitations, UTIs, fatigue
- Not associated with perimenopause/menopause: major depressive disorder

TESTS
FSH levels (preferably several)

DIFFERENTIAL DIAGNOSIS
Premature ovarian senescence

MANAGEMENT

What to Do First
- Topics to cover in counseling:
  - ➤ Hot flashes, day/night sweats
  - ➤ Vaginal dryness/dyspareunia
  - ➤ CHD
  - ➤ Osteoporosis
  - ➤ Estrogen/hormone replacement therapy (HRT):
    - Not indicated for routine therapy
    - Short-term use for hot flashes
    - Increased risk of breast cancer with progestin component of HRT
    - Increased risk of thrombosis

General Measures
- Hot flashes, day/night sweats:
- Nonpharmacologic: dress in layers, identify and avoid triggers, aerobic exercise
- Pharmacologic: short-term estrogen/HRT, clonidine, herbal preparations/dietary supplements
- Vaginal dryness/dyspareunia:

- ➤ Nonpharmacologic: vaginal lubricants/moisturizers, regular sexual stimulation
- ➤ Pharmacologic: short-term estrogen/HRT, vaginal estrogen creams, vaginal estrogen ring, herbal preparations/dietary supplements
- ■ CHD (leading cause of death in women):
  - ➤ CHD increases in older women.
  - ➤ Assessment, counseling about risk factors
  - ➤ Smoking cessation
  - ➤ Exercise, diet, weight loss if overweight
  - ➤ Stress management
  - ➤ Control of BP, diabetes if present
  - ➤ Optimal total serum cholesterol, LDL, HDL, triglycerides
  - ➤ Statins
- ■ Osteoporosis:
  - ➤ Assessment, counseling about risk factors
  - ➤ Dietary calcium and vitamin D
  - ➤ Exercise
  - ➤ Fall prevention
  - ➤ Smoking cessation
  - ➤ Limit alcohol
  - ➤ Bone mineral density (BMD) testing for all postmenopausal women with fractures and consider for:
    - • Postmenopausal women <65 y who have additional osteoporosis risk factors
    - • All women >65 y
    - • All women whose decision to begin treatment would be influenced by BMD result
- ■ Consider osteoporosis treatment for postmenopausal women with vertebral or hip fractures, or BMD T-score −2.0 (or −1.5 if additional risk factors):
  - ➤ Bisphosphonates
  - ➤ SERMs
  - ➤ Calcitonin
  - ➤ PTH analogs
  - ➤ Calcium and vitamin D (supplemental only)

SPECIFIC THERAPY

- ■ None

  Estrogen replacement therapy is of questionable safety for long-term therapy:

    For short-term for hot flashes only, if uterus absent:
- ➤ Oral conjugated estrogens
- ➤ Oral microcronized estradiol
- ➤ Transdermal estradiol
- ■ HRT if uterus present, add progestin to estrogen to prevent endometrial carcinoma: medroxyprogesterone or other progestins daily or for part of cycle
- ■ Clonidine

Side Effects & Contraindications
- ■ Side Effects
  - ➤ Irregular vaginal bleeding/spotting
  - ➤ Breast tenderness
  - ➤ Leg cramps
  - ➤ Endometrial cancer/hyperplasia with unopposed estrogens
  - ➤ Gallbladder disease
  - ➤ Abnormal clotting
  - ➤ Hypertriglyceridemia and pancreatitis
- ■ Contraindications
  - ➤ Personal/family history of breast or endometrial cancer
  - ➤ Abnormal vaginal bleeding
  - ➤ Pain in calf or chest, shortness of breath, or coughing of blood
  - ➤ Severe headache, dizziness, faintness, or changes in vision
  - ➤ Unevaluated breast lumps
  - ➤ Jaundice
  - ➤ Depression

FOLLOW-UP
n/a

COMPLICATIONS AND PROGNOSIS
Osteoporosis

MENSTRUAL CYCLE DISORDERS FOR THE GENERALIST

MAXINE H. DORIN, MD
REVISED BY FREDRIC B. KRAEMER, MD; ANDREW R. HOFFMAN, MD; and
THOMAS F. McELRATH, MD, PhD

HISTORY & PHYSICAL

History
- ■ Premenstrual syndrome (PMS): cyclic appearance of symptoms just prior to menses that adversely affects lifestyle or work, followed by period entirely free of symptoms

Signs & Symptoms
- Most frequent: abdominal bloating, anxiety or tension, breast tenderness, crying spells, dysmenorrhea, depression, fatigue, unprovoked anger or irritability, difficulty concentrating, thirst and appetite changes, edema

TESTS
n/a

DIFFERENTIAL DIAGNOSIS
- Established guidelines for diagnosis:
  - ➤ Criteria for diagnosis of PMS: = 30% increase in severity of symptoms in 5 d prior to menses compared with the 5 d after menses
  - ➤ American Psychiatric Association criteria for premenstrual dysphoric disorder (more severe than PMS):
    - Symptoms begin last wk of luteal phase, remit after onset of menses
    - Diagnosis requires >4 of the following, including 1 of first 4:
      - Affective lability
      - Persistent and marked anger or irritability
      - Anxiety or tension
      - Depressed mood, feelings of hopelessness
      - Decreased interest in usual activities
      - Easy fatigability or marked lack of energy
      - Subjective sense of difficulty concentrating
      - Changes in appetite, overeating, food craving
      - Hypersomnia or insomnia
      - Feelings of being overwhelmed, out of control
      - Physical symptoms, such as breast tenderness, headaches, edema, joint or muscle pain, weight gain
      - Symptoms interfere with work, usual activities or relationships
      - Symptoms not exacerbation of another psychiatric disorder

MANAGEMENT

What to Do First
- Prospective recording (3 mo) to prove problem recurs in luteal phase, followed by periods free of symptoms
- Exploration of lifestyle, relationships, and interactions
- Focus on issues producing conflict, lack of control

General Measures
- Intensive involvement of clinician

- Find changes that allow greater control over their lives: changes in diet, exercise, work, recreation
- Isolate specific symptoms, treat with specific therapy: fluid retention with diuretic therapy, dysmenorrhea with prostaglandin synthesis inhibitors, calcium supplementation

SPECIFIC THERAPY
- Selective serotonin reuptake inhibitors (SSRIs)
- Alprazolam (benzodiazepine) occasionally effective but highly addictive
- GnRH agonists and/or Danazol
- Oral or IM contraceptives

Side Effects
- SSRIs: dry mouth, tremor, dizziness, somnolence, headaches, constipation, nausea, sweating, insomnia, dyspepsia, libido changes (decrease, delayed ejaculation, anorgasmia, impotence), abnormal dreams, weight gain, seizures, anxiety, blurred vision, hyponatremia
- Contraceptives: nausea, vomiting, abdominal cramps, bloating, breakthrough bleeding, altered menstrual flow, breast tenderness, edema, headaches, weight changes, rash, ache, thromboembolism, myocardial infarction, hypertension, hepatic adenoma, stroke, dizziness, increased risk of depression
     GnRH agonists: hot flashes, osteoporosis
     Danazol: hirsutism, acne
- Contraindications
- SSRIs: MAO inhibitor use, seizure disorder
- Oral contraceptives: migraine with aura, pregnancy, undiagnosed vaginal bleeding, breast, endometrial or hepatic cancer, thromboembolic disorders, smokers >35 y, CAD, CVD

Special Situations
- Menstrual headache:
  - Association with menses in 60% of women with migraine
  - Menstrual migraines typically without aura
  - Further evaluation needed for acute onset of severe headache pain, unremitting headaches, vomiting headaches, vision changes
- Management:
  - Menstrually related migraines: oral and SC sumatriptan
  - NSAIDs
  - Oral contraceptives

➤ IM medroxyprogesterone acetate
➤ Estrogen transdermal application during menses
■ Catamenial seizures:
➤ Epileptic seizures more common during menstruation
➤ Seizure frequency increases at midcycle
➤ Induced amenorrhea can decrease seizure frequency
■ Premenstrual asthma:
➤ 30–40% of women with asthma have exacerbation with menses
➤ Estradiol improves symptoms and PFTs
■ Catamenial pneumothorax:
➤ Recurrent pneumothoraces, at time of menses (due to endometriosis)
➤ IM medroxyprogesterone acetate

FOLLOW-UP
n/a

COMPLICATIONS AND PROGNOSIS
■ PMS resolves at menopause in most women but may recur on cyclic HRT

METABOLIC ACIDOSIS

BIFF F. PALMER, MD

HISTORY & PHYSICAL
■ clinical setting helpful in determining etiology
■ history of toxin ingestion, uncontrolled diabetes, cardiovascular collapse, end-stage renal disease
■ history of diarrhea, use of amphotericin B, toluene

TESTS
■ check arterial blood gas to exclude chronic respiratory alkalosis
➤ HCO3 <24 mEq/L with pH <7.40 confirms metabolic acidosis
➤ HCO3 <24 mEq/L with pH >7.40 suggests chronic respiratory alkalosis
■ measure plasma anion gap: Na – (Cl + HCO3), normal value 8–16
■ increased anion gap
➤ calculate osmolar gap to screen for intoxication with methanol or ethylene glycol
• Calculated osmolity = serum Na (mEq/L) $\times$ 2 + glucose (mg/dl)/18 + BUN (mg/dl)/2.0

- measured serum osmolality – calculated osmolality = osmolar gap, normal value <10 mOsm/kg
- urine calcium oxalate crystals is consistent with ethylene glycol poisoning

➤ measure plasma creatinine, BUN, glucose, serum ketones, salicylate level, ethylene glycol, serum L-lactate, consider D-lactate level if clinically indicated

➤ urine dipstick for ketones may underestimate degree of ketosis due to marked increase in the beta-OH butyrate/acetoacetate ratio

- ▦ normal plasma anion gap
  - ➤ calculate urine anion gap (UAG): UAG = urine (Na + K − Cl)
    - negative: extrarenal origin, gastrointestinal loss of HCO3
    - positive: renal origin, RTA's
      - assess proximal tubular function
  - ➤ abnormal (glycosuria, phosphaturia, aminoaciduria): type I proximal RTA
  - ➤ if normal, measure plasma K levels
    - if normal or low K, measure urine pH
      - plasma K <3.5 mEq/L, urine pH >5.5, type I hypokalemic distal RTA, screen for nephrocalcinosis on KUB of abdomen
      - plasma K 3.5–5.0 mEq/L, urine pH <5.5, RTA of renal insufficiency
    - if increased plasma K: type IV hyperkalemic distal RTA, measure urine pH
      - if pH<5.5, suggests low mineralocorticoid secretion
      - if pH >5.5, suggests collecting duct abnormality

DIFFERENTIAL DIAGNOSIS

- ▦ increased plasma anion gap
  - ➤ increased osmolar gap: methanol, ethylene glycol poisoning, alcoholic ketoacidosis
  - ➤ normal osmolar gap: diabetic ketoacidosis, L-lactic acidosis, D-lactic acidosis, alcoholic ketoacidosis (alcohol no longer present), uremic acidosis (GFR <15 ml/min), salicylate poisoning
- ▦ normal plasma anion gap
  - ➤ negative urine anion gap: diarrhea, external loss of pancreatic or biliary secretions, ureterosigmoidoscopy
  - ➤ positive urine anion gap
    - type II proximal RTA: multiple myeloma, cystinosis, chronic mercury and lead poisoning, ifosfamide

- type I hypokalemic distal RTA: hereditary, glue sniffing, amphotericin B, Sjogren's syndrome, primary biliary cirrhosis
- RTA of renal insufficiency: mild to moderate chronic renal failure of any cause (GFR >15 ml/min)
- type IV hyperkalemic distal RTA, urine pH >5.5: tubulointerstitial renal disease, analgesic nephropathy, obstructive uropathy, sickle cell disease
- type IV hyperkalemic distal RTA, urine pH <5.5: syndrome of hyporeninemic hypoaldosteronism, diabetic nephropathy, primary adrenal failure

MANAGEMENT
- first determine cause of metabolic acidosis and treat underlying disorder

SPECIFIC THERAPY
- specific therapy will depend on underlying cause of acidosis
- anion gap metabolic acidosis
  - diabetic ketoacidosis-intravenous fluids, insulin, and potassium, HCO3 therapy only indicated for severe acidemia (pH <7.10 and HCO3 <10 mEq/L)
  - L-lactic acidosis-treat underlying disorder, HCO3 therapy only indicated for severe acidemia (pH <7.10 and HCO (3) <10 mEq/L)
  - alcoholic ketoacidosis-dextrose-containing saline to reverse ketogenesis and correct ECF volume deficit, give thiamine prior to dextrose in order to avoid Wernicke's encephalopathy
  - salicylate intoxication-alkalinization of urine to enhance urinary excretion, dialysis may be required for levels >80 mg/dl with severe clinical toxicity
  - ethylene glycol and methanol intoxication-administer ethanol to impair conversion of parent compounds to toxic metabolites, hemodialysis to remove parent compounds, HCO3 therapy for severe acidemia, 4-methylpyrazol (potent inhibitor of alcohol dehydrogenase) can be used in place of ethanol infusion if available
  - D-lactic acidosis-antibiotics to treat bacterial overgrowth, surgical correction of intestinal abnormality leading to bacterial overgrowth
- normal anion gap metabolic acidosis
  - extrarenal acidosis
    - treat underlying condition

- acidosis due to gastrointestinal-ureteral connections can be improved by minimizing urine contact time and bowel surface area in contact with urine
- oral NaHCO3 tablets
➤ renal acidosis
  - type I hypokalemic distal RTA
    - treat underlying cause
    - administer HCO3 or citrate in an amount to equal daily acid production (1 mEq/kg/d)
    - treat hypokalemia prior to or at same time as $HCO_{3<}$ administration to avoid worsening hypokalemia
    - K citrate corrects acidemia, hypokalemia and lessens long term risk for nephrolithiasis
  - type II proximal RTA
    - treat underlying cause if possible
    - difficult to correct acidosis, administered HCO3 is rapidly lost in urine and contributes to increased renal K loss
    - therapy consists of oral HCO3, thiazide diuretic to induce volume contraction, K sparing diuretic, oral K
    - frequent monitoring of serum electrolytes required
    - vitamin D therapy required to prevent rickets or osteomalacia
  - type IV hyperkalemic distal RTA
    - treatment dependent on underlying cause
    - adrenal failure is treated with appropriate hormone replacement therapy
    - in setting of renal insufficiency treatment dependent upon blood pressure
➤ normotensive: fludrocortisone (complicated by Na retention)
➤ hypertension: K restricted diet, loop diuretics, NaHCO3 tablets
  - RTA of renal insufficiency
    - HCO3 in an amount to equal daily acid production (1 mEq/kg/d) will correct acidosis

FOLLOW-UP
■ high anion gap acidosis
➤ once underlying cause is corrected no specific follow up is needed
■ normal anion gap acidosis
➤ if long term therapy required keep HCO_3 near normal (22–24 mEq/L) to avoid long term complications of acidemia
➤ monitor K closely if receiving K replacement

COMPLICATIONS AND PROGNOSIS
- complications of severe acidemia
  - decreased cardiac contractility
  - venoconstriction with centralization of blood
  - fatigue
  - dyspnea
- complications of long term acidemia
  - short stature in children
  - osteopenia
  - malnutrition, loss of muscle mass
- anion gap acidosis prognosis dependent upon outcome of underlying condition
- normal gap acidosis prognosis generally good with proper correction of electrolytes

METABOLIC ALKALOSIS

BIFF F. PALMER, MD

HISTORY & PHYSICAL
- history and physical directed toward determining volume status of patient
- normal or low blood pressure
  - light-headedness, loop and thiazide diuretics, vomiting/nasogastric suction
- hypertension
  - family history of hypertension

TESTS
- distinguish between primary metabolic alkalosis and compensated respiratory acidosis
  - HCO3 concentration >24 mEq/L and blood pH >7.40 confirms metabolic alkalosis
  - HCO3 concentration >24 mEq/L and blood pH <7.40 suggests compensated respiratory acidosis
- Blood tests:
  - BUN, creatinine, Mg++
  - hemoconcentration of hematocrit and albumin suggest decreased effective arterial volume (EABV)
  - if hypertensive, measure plasma renin and aldosterone

- urine tests:
  - ➤ [Na] and [Cl]

DIFFERENTIAL DIAGNOSIS

- decreased EABV, normal or low blood pressure
  - ➤ decreased urine [Cl] (<20 mEq/L) and decreased urine [Na] (<20 mEq/L)
    - remote use of loop or thiazide diuretics
    - posthypercapneic metabolic alkalosis
    - vomiting (not active)
    - villous adenoma
  - ➤ decreased urine [Cl] (<20 mEq/L) and increased urine [Na] (>20 mEq/L)
    - vomiting (active)
    - excretion of nonreabsorbable anion (ticarcillin, carbenicillin)
  - ➤ increased urine [Cl] (>20 mEq/L) and increased urine [Na] (>20 mEq/L)
    - active diuretic use
    - Bartter's syndrome, Gitelman's syndrome
    - Mg++ deficiency
- increased EABV, hypertension, increased urine [Cl] (>20 mEq/L) and increased urine [Na] (>20 mEq/L)
  - ➤ increased renin, increased aldosterone
    - malignant hypertension
    - renal artery stenosis
    - renin secreting tumor
  - ➤ decreased renin and increased aldosterone
    - adrenal adenoma
    - bilateral adrenal hyperplasia
    - glucocorticoid remediable hyperaldosteronism
  - ➤ decreased renin and decreased aldosterone (syndromes of apparent mineralocorticoid excess)
    - Cushing's syndrome
    - 11 beta hydroxylase deficiency
    - acquired 11 beta hydroxylase deficiency
    - carbenoxolone
      - licorice or chewing tobacco containing glycyrrhetinic acid
  - ➤ Liddle's syndrome

MANAGEMENT

- confirm presence of primary metabolic alkalosis with arterial blood gas

- determine if metabolic alkalosis is in setting of increased EABV or decreased EABV (see differential diagnosis)
- identify and correct factors generating metabolic alkalosis (discontinue diuretics, treat nausea and vomiting, remove source of excess mineralocorticoid if possible)
- identify and correct factors maintaining metabolic alkalosis (volume depletion, hypokalemia)

SPECIFIC THERAPY
- decreased EABV and decreased total body Na
  - ➤ normal saline to replete extracellular fluid volume
  - ➤ replete potassium deficit
  - ➤ use of H2 blockers can minimize generation in nasogastric suction
  - ➤ correct Mg^{++} deficit if present
- decreased EABV and increased total body Na (congestive heart failure, chronic obstructive pulmonary disease with right sided heart failure)
  - ➤ acetazolamide (250–500 mg twice daily)
- increased EABV
  - ➤ treat underlying cause of mineralocorticoid excess if possible
  - ➤ if underlying cause cannot be corrected treat with K sparing diuretic
  - ➤ Liddle's syndrome use amiloride or triamterene, spironolactone is ineffective
  - ➤ for metabolic alkalosis patients who require aggressive treatment and maintenance factors cannot be corrected (critically ill patients with pH > 7.55)
    - 0.15 NaHCl infusion via central vein
    - ammonium chloride infusion: contraindicated in chronic liver disease due to ammonia toxicity
    - frequent monitoring of arterial blood gas and serum electrolytes are required with these therapies

FOLLOW-UP
- monitor serum HCO3 and K to ensure alkalosis and hypokalemia are corrected
- treat hypertension aggressively when present
- avoid hyperkalemia when using angiotensin converting enzyme inhibitors or angiotensin receptor blockers with K sparing diuretics

COMPLICATIONS AND PROGNOSIS

■ prognosis generally related to etiology of metabolic alkalosis

■ metabolic alkalosis can contribute to mortality under certain circumstances

■ increased pH can lead to respiratory depression, vasoconstriction of coronary and cerebral circulation, and cause tissue hypoxia

■ metabolic alkalosis in the setting of low EABV is generally reversible with therapy and has a good prognosis

■ with mineralocorticoid excess syndromes chronic therapy may be required when underlying cause cannot be corrected, correction of hypertension is critical

METHEMOGLOBINEMIA

XYLINA GREGG, MD and JOSEF PRCHAL, MD

HISTORY & PHYSICAL

History

■ Clinical suspicion when cyanosis occurs in presence of normal PaO2

■ Acquired – Acute toxic
  ➤ Most common form
  ➤ Exposure to local anesthetics, oxidants – antifreeze, acetaminophen, many others
    • Persons heterozygous for cytochrome b5 reductase deficiency may develop after exposure to agents harmless to normal individuals in
  ➤ Infants – developmentally decreased cytochrome b5 reductase activity
    • Occurs after diarrheal illness or exposure to nitrate-containing well water
  ➤ Symptoms related to impaired tissue O2 delivery
    • Early – headache, SOB, lethargy
    • Late – respiratory depression, altered consciousness, seizures, death

■ Chronic, congenital
  ➤ Cyanotic, but usually asymptomatic; may develop compensatory polycythemia
  ➤ However, type 2 cytochrome b5 reductase deficiency (defect not restricted to erythrocytes) associated with neurological syndrome/failure to thrive

➤ Inheritance
  • Autosomal recessive – type 1 (erythrocyte restricted) and 2 (ubiquitously expressed) cytochrome b5 reductase deficiency
  • Autosomal dominant – mutant hemoglobin (Hb M)

Signs & Symptoms
- Cyanosis – clinically apparent when methemoglobin exceeds 1.5 gm%
- (10–15% methemoglobin at normal hemoglobin concentration)
- Blood characteristic "chocolate" color

TESTS
- Methemoglobin detection:
  ➤ Co-oximeter analysis at specific absorption spectrum
    • false positive from other substances and medications
  ➤ Evelyn-Malloy assay – specific for methemoglobin
- cytochrome b5 reductase assay and assays for hemoglobin M mutants in congenital cases

DIFFERENTIAL DIAGNOSIS
- Hypoxemia with unsaturated hemoglobin >4 gm% (low PaO2)
- Sulfhemoglobin >0.5 gm% (also has normal PaO2 and may be mistaken for methemoglobin by co-oximeter; distinguish by Evelyn-Malloy assay)

MANAGEMENT
What to Do First
- Withdraw offending agent in acquired (acute toxic)
- No other treatment may be necessary

SPECIFIC THERAPY
Indications
- Symptomatic – usually the case in overdoses or poisoning
- Treatment not needed for chronic asymptomatic – cosmetic purposes only

Treatment Options
- Methylene Blue
- Ascorbic acid
  ➤ If methylene blue is contraindicated
  ➤ May be useful in chronic, congenital b5R deficiency
- Riboflavin – reported use in b5R deficiency (chronic)
- No known beneficial treatment for type 2 b5R deficiency

Side Effects & Complications
- Methylene Blue
  - High doses associated with SOB, chest pain, hemolysis
  - Interferes with measurement of methemoglobin by co-oximetry

Contraindications
- Methylene blue – G6PD deficiency as it induces hemolysis

FOLLOW-UP
During Treatment
- May repeat methylene blue, but generally not necessary
- Cannot use co-oximetry to monitor methemoglobin after methylene blue given

COMPLICATIONS AND PROGNOSIS
- *Most congenital methemoglobinemias*
  - Normal life expectancy
- *Type 2 cytochrome b5 reductase deficiency*
  - Dismal prognosis
  - Prenatal diagnosis possible
  - Hope for gene therapy

MIGRAINE HEADACHE

CHAD CHRISTINE, MD

HISTORY & PHYSICAL
- Recurrent headaches develop over minutes to hours
- Headache often unilateral & pulsatile
- Visual auras (field defects, scotomas, scintillation, etc) in 10% of cases
- Often assoc w/ nausea, photophobia, phonophobia, malaise
- 2–3 times more common in women, onset usually before age 40 yr
- Family history is common
- Headache duration is typically >2 hours & <1 day
- Neurologic deficits occur uncommonly
- Attacks can be precipitated by certain foods, fasting, emotional experiences, menses, drugs, caffeine, alcohol, bright lights
- Usually normal
- Visual disturbance, mild hemiparesis or hemisensory deficit may occur

TESTS

- Diagnosis made clinically
- Lab tests & brain imaging are normal
- Lumbar puncture opening pressure & CSF studies normal

DIFFERENTIAL DIAGNOSIS

- Brain mass lesion or subdural hematoma excluded by history & brain imaging
- Pseudotumor cerebri excluded clinically (& by LP if necessary)
- Postconcussion syndrome & hypothyroidism excluded clinically
- Brain imaging indicated for prominent change in headache quality or frequency

MANAGEMENT

- Depends on severity & prior treatment

General measures

- Headache diary may elucidate precipitants
- Ensure adequate relaxation & exercise
- Reduce caffeine & alcohol use
- Physical therapy, relaxation techniques, hot or cold packs may help
- Hormone replacement may reduce attacks during menopause

SPECIFIC THERAPY

Indications

- Abortive meds indicated for rare headaches (<1 per week); prophylactic meds used for more frequent moderate to severe headaches

Treatment options

- Abortive agents for head pain
  - Acetaminophen
  - Aspirin
  - Ibuprofen
  - Codeine/acetaminophen or codeine/aspirin
  - Caffeine/butabutal/ASA or acetaminophen
  - Ergotamine/caffeine
  - Dihydroergotamine nasal spray or IM, SC or IV w/ metoclopramide
  - 5-HT agonists: sumatriptan, rizatriptan, zolmitriptan, naratriptan, frovatriptan, eletriptan, almotriptan
    Narcotic analgesics in rare instances: meperidine intramuscularly or butorphanol tartrate by nasal spray

- Abortive agents for nausea
  - ➤ Promethazine
  - ➤ Prochlorperazine
  - ➤ Metaclopramide
- Prophylactic agents for head pain & nausea
  - ➤ Anti-inflammatory agents (above)
  - ➤ Tricyclic antidepressants
    - Amitriptyline
    - Nortriptyline
    - Doxepin
  - ➤ B-receptor antagonists
    - Propranolol
    - Nadolol
    - Atenolol
  - ➤ Calcium channel blockers
    - Verapamil
    - Amlodipine
  - ➤ Ergot preparations
    - Methysergide
  - ➤ Anticonvulsant: valproic acid
    Botulinum toxin type A

FOLLOW-UP
- Every 3–12 months depending on level of control

COMPLICATIONS AND PROGNOSIS
- Drug dependence to opiates & sedative meds
- Prognosis: good

MILIARIA

JEFFREY P. CALLEN, MD

HISTORY & PHYSICAL
- Pruritic rash on occluded areas or areas exposed to heat
- Caused by occlusion of the eccrine sweat ducts and pores, which leads to retention of sweat
- Back-up pressure causes rupture of sweat gland into adjacent tissue.
- Eruption is more common in hot, humid climates and hot summer months.
- May occur in hospitalized patients with a high fever

Different Forms of Miliaria

- Crystallina:
    - small, clear superficial vesicles without inflammation
    - appears often in bedridden patients or patients wearing tightly bound clothes
    - asymptomatic and self-limited
- Rubra:
    - discrete, extremely pruritic erythematous papulovesicles
    - sensation of prickling, burning or tingling
    - predilection for antecubital fossa, popliteal fossa, trunk, intertriginous areas, and waistline
- Pustulosa:
    - always preceded by a dermatitis that produces injury, destruction or blocking of the sweat duct
    - pustules are distinct and independent of hair follicles
    - intertriginous areas, flexural surface, scrotum, and back
- Profunda:
    - nonpruritic, flesh-colored, deep-seated white papules
    - asymptomatic
    - last about 1 hour after overheating has ended
    - concentrated on trunk and extremities
    - all sweat glands are nonfunctional except on face, axillae, hands and feet
    - observed usually in tropics and usually follows bout of miliaria rubra

TESTS

n/a

DIFFERENTIAL DIAGNOSIS

- Transient Acantholytic Dermatosis
- Pustular psoriasis
- Acute generalized exanthematous pustulosis
- Candidiasis
- Folliculitis

MANAGEMENT

- Place patient in cool environment.
- Circulating fans

SPECIFIC THERAPY

- Anhydrous lanolin helps to resolve occlusion of pores.

- Hydrophilic ointment helps to dissolve keratin plugs.
- Lotion with 1% menthol and glycerin and 4% Sal Ac in 95% alcohol dabbed on until desquamation starts

FOLLOW-UP

n/a

COMPLICATIONS AND PROGNOSIS

- Usually self-limited with cooling and treatment
- Postmiliarial hypohidrosis may result in sweating decreased up to half of normal for as long as 3 weeks.

MINERALOCORTICOID DISORDERS

RICHARD I. DORIN, MD

HISTORY & PHYSICAL

History

- Salt, potassium intake
- Review of prior BP determinations, electrolyte studies
- Vomiting, diarrhea
- Renal insufficiency
- Edema, cirrhosis, CHF, nephrotic syndrome
- Nocturia, polyuria, muscle weakness, cramps
- Purging, anorexia, surreptitious diuretic or laxative use or abuse
- Cushing's syndrome, adrenal insufficiency
- Diabetes mellitus
- Medications: diuretics, antibiotics, glucocorticoids, heparin, ACE inhibitors, spironolactone, amiloride, triamterene
- Family history of hypertension/hypokalemia
- Malignancy: history of malignancy, cigarette smoking, weight loss, bone pain, abdominal pain, flushing

Signs & Symptoms

- Mineralocorticoid excess: polyuria, nocturia, hypertension, edema (rarely)
- Mineralocorticoid deficiency: generally nonspecific, rarely hypotension or orthostatic hypotension

TESTS

Laboratory

- Basic blood studies:

- ➤ Mineralocorticoid excess: spontaneous or easily provoked hypokalemia, metabolic alkalosis, hypernatremia (mild), dilutional anemia, hypomagnasemia, kaliuresis
- ➤ Mineralocorticoid deficiency: hyperkalemia, hyperchloremic nonanion gap acidosis (type IV RTA)
- ▪ Basic urine studies:
    - ➤ 24-h urine potassium
- ▪ Specific Diagnostic Tests
    - ➤ Mineralocorticoid excess:
        - • Supine plasma renin activity (PRA), aldosterone level: ratio of aldosterone/PRA >30 with elevated plasma aldosterone concentration suggestive of primary hyperaldosteronism
        - • 24-h urine for aldosterone, creatinine
        - • Normal saline infusion 2.0 L over 4 h with serum aldosterone pre/post: aldosterone >10 ng/dL consistent with primary hyperaldosteronism
        - • 24-h urine for aldosterone, creatinine while off ACE inhibitors, beta-blockers for 1–2 wk, on high salt intake: aldosterone excretion >15 mcg/d consistent with primary hyperaldosteronism
        - • 18-OH-corticosterone: usually increased in adenoma
    - ➤ Mineralocorticoid deficiency:
        - • Serum PRA, aldosterone levels pre/post furosemide or 3-h upright
        - • Serum aldosterone 60 min post-Cosyntropin

Imaging
- ▪ Mineralocorticoid excess: CT/MRI of adrenals, radionuclide scintigraphy (not usually needed)
- ▪ Mineralocorticoid deficiency: none

Other Tests
- ▪ Mineralocorticoid excess: adrenal vein sampling of aldosterone pre/post-Cosyntropin, serum aldosterone post-dexamethasone

DIFFERENTIAL DIAGNOSIS
- ▪ Mineralocorticoid excess:
    - ➤ Primary hyperaldosteronism: adenoma, hyperplasia; glucocorticoid-remediable hyperaldosteronism; licorice (glycyrrhetinic acid) ingestion
    - ➤ Secondary hyperaldosteronism
    - ➤ Low renin hypertension
    - ➤ Liddle syndrome

- Cushing's syndrome (esp. associated with ectopic ACTH)
- Congenital adrenal hyperplasia
- Barter's syndrome
- Gittelman's syndrome
- Renovascular or malignant hypertension
- Diuretics, diarrhea, vomiting
- CHF, nephrotic syndrome, cirrhosis
- Inhibitors of 11-beta-hydroxysteroid dehydrogenase II (e.g., carbenoxone, licorice)
- Mineralocorticoid deficiency:
  - Primary hypoaldosteronism; heparin-induced
  - Congenital adrenal hyperplasia
  - Primary adrenal insufficiency
  - Chronic interstitial nephritis with mild renal insufficiency
  - Renal failure
  - Medications: NSAIDs, ACE inhibitors, cyclosporine, amiloride, spironolactone, triamterene, trimethoprim, pentamidine
  - Pseudohypoaldosteronism

MANAGEMENT

What to Do First
- Normalize serum potassium
- Discontinue confounding medications

General Measures
- Exclude common causes
- Evaluate laboratory data in context of dietary salt intake
- Use PRA to distinguish primary vs secondary disorders
- Confirm, establish cause
- Treat hypertension
- Restrict salt in mineralocorticoid excess
- Liberalize salt in mineralocorticoid deficiency

SPECIFIC THERAPY
- Mineralocorticoid excess: amiloride, spironolactone, triamterene; dexamethasone for glucocorticoid-remediable hyperaldosteronism (rare); surgery indicated for unilateral adenoma
- Mineralocorticoid deficiency: thiazide or furosemide for mild secondary causes; fludrocortisone
- Side Effects & Contraindications
  - Mineralocorticoid excess: hyperkalemia, gynecomastia, impotence, rash, liver function abnormalities

➤ Mineralocorticoid deficiency: hypertension, edema, hypokalemia

FOLLOW-UP
- Monitor serum potassium, renal function
- Monior BP, treat hypertension

COMPLICATIONS AND PROGNOSIS
- Hypertension persists after surgical resection of aldosterone-secreting adenoma in about 35% of patients.

MISCELLANEOUS INTESTINAL PROTOZOA

J. GORDON FRIERSON, MD

HISTORY & PHYSICAL

History
- Exposure: Ingestion of fecally contaminated food and water containing cysts of Entamoeba hartmanni, Entamoeba coli, Endolimax nana, Iodamoeba butschlii, or Chilomastix mesnili

Signs & Symptoms
- None. These are all non-pathogens.

TESTS
- Basic tests: blood: normal
- Basic tests: urine: normal
- Specific tests: Stool O&P exam finds organisms.
- Other tests: none

DIFFERENTIAL DIAGNOSIS
- None; no symptoms

MANAGEMENT

What to Do First
- If GI symptoms are present and no pathogenic organisms are seen, check more stools (up to 4–6), as presence of these non-pathogens is a marker for contamination.

General Measures
- Same

SPECIFIC THERAPY

Indications
- None

Treatment Options
- None

Contraindications
- Absolute: All patients

FOLLOW-UP

During Treatment
- None

Routine
- None

COMPLICATIONS AND PROGNOSIS
- N/A

MITRAL INSUFFICIENCY (MR)

JUDITH A. WISNESKI, MD

HISTORY & PHYSICAL

Etiology
- Abnormality in valve or subvalvular apparatus
  - Myxomatous degeneration (most common)
  - Coronary artery disease (papillary muscle ischemia or infarct)
  - Chordae tendineae rupture
  - Endocarditis
  - Marfan syndrome
  - Collagen vascular disease
- MR secondary to LV deformity
  - Inferior wall dyskinesis
  - Left ventricular (LV) dilation due to cardiomyopathy

History
- Symptoms of pulmonary congestion: DOE, orthopnea, or PND
- Hemoptysis (more common with mitral stenosis)
- Systemic emboli (rare)

Signs & Symptoms

- Holosytolic or crescendo systolic murmur, which radiates to axilla or back
- PMI – hyperdynamic and displaced to left and downward
- Soft S1
- S3 present
- Increased P2 and parasternal lift (pulmonary artery hypertension present)
- Elevated JVP and ascites (pulmonary artery hypertension and right heart failure present)

TESTS

- ECG
  - Left atrial abnormality
  - Atrial fibrillation
  - Left ventricular hypertrophy
  - ST and T wave changes, Q waves (papillary muscle dysfunction)
- Chest X-Ray
  - Cardiomegaly (chronic MR)
  - Enlarged and giant left atrium (chronic MR)
  - Normal heart and left atrial size (acute MR)
  - Pulmonary venous congestion may be present
- Echo/Doppler (very important)
  - Detect and quantitate MR
  - LV systolic function
  - LV diastolic and systolic dimensions
  - Enlarged left atrium with moderate/severe MR
- Cardiac Catheterization
  - Pulmonary capillary wedge elevated
    - Elevated and prominent V wave in acute MR
    - V wave may be normal in chronic MR
  - Pulmonary artery hypertension
  - Cardiac output and index low and not increase with exercise
  - Assess severity of MR, LV systolic function, and LV diastolic and systolic volumes
  - Coronary angiography required prior to valve repair/replacement in older patients

DIFFERENTIAL DIAGNOSIS

- Idiopathic hypertrophic subaortic stenosis
- Ventricular septal defect

MANAGEMENT
- Medical
  - ➤ Antibiotic prophylaxis in all patients
  - ➤ Vasodilator therapy
  - ➤ Atrial fibrillation
    - Rate control with digoxin, beta-blockers or calcium blockers
    - Anticoagulation with warfarin

SPECIFIC THERAPY
- Surgical repair or replacement of mitral valve
- Complications of mitral valve replacement
  - ➤ Acute
    - Complications of cardiopulmonary bypass
    - Increased acute mortality if LV systolic function depressed
  - ➤ Long-term
    - Thromboembolism
    - Valve failure
    - Bleeding from anticoagulation therap
    - Endocarditis

Mitral valve repair preferred over replacement
- Long-term complications significantly less with repair versus replacement: anticoagulation may not be required with repair and risk of valve failure not present (*TEE helps predict repair vs. replacement*)

Indications for mitral valve surgery for patients with moderate/severe MR:
- Moderate/severe symptoms due to MR
- Asymptomatic with LV dysfunction (LVEF < 60% or end-systolic dimension > 45 mm)
- Asymptomatic with normal LV function
  - ➤ If TEE indicates repair possible – perform surgery
  - ➤ If TEE indicates replacement – delay surgery until symptoms or LV dysfunction occur

FOLLOW-UP
n/a

COMPLICATIONS AND PROGNOSIS

Prognosis
- Post mitral valve surgery
  - ➤ Survival very good if LVEF >60% and end-systolic dimension < 45 mm prior to surgery

MITRAL STENOSIS (MS)

JUDITH A. WISNESKI, MD

HISTORY & PHYSICAL
- Most common – rheumatic heart disease (women 3–4 × more common than men)
- Congenital
- Malignant carcinoid (rare)

History
- Symptoms of pulmonary congestion: DOE, orthopnea, PND
- Symptoms of right heart failure: peripheral edema, elevated JVP, ascites (more severe)
- Hemoptysis – due to pulmonary hypertension (more severe)
- Hoarseness or dysphasia – due to enlarged left atrium (rare)
- Systemic emboli (common, especially with atrial fibrillation)
- Rapid atrial fibrillation poorly tolerated

Signs & Symptoms
- Diastolic rumble and possible diastolic thrill (best appreciated in left lateral decubitus position)
- Opening Snap (OS)
- Normal PMI
- S1 intensity increased (mild MS)
- Soft S1 (more severe MS)
- P2 increased with right ventricular lift (more severe MS)
- S2-OS interval shorter with more severe MS (<0.10 sec − severe MS)
- S3 and S4 absent with significant MS

TESTS
- ECG
  - Left atrial enlargement
  - Right axis deviation
  - Right ventricular hypertrophy
  - Atrial fibrillation
- Chest X-Ray
  - Normal left ventricular size
  - Left atrial enlargement
  - Pulmonary arteries enlarged (pulmonary artery hypertension)

> Kerley B lines
> Calcium in mitral valve (MV) (best seen in lateral view)
- Echo/Doppler (most important test)
  > Motion of mitral valve leaflets reduced
  > Abnormality of subvalvular apparatus
  > Left atrial enlargement
  > Pressure gradient between left atrium and left ventricle
  > Quantitation of mitral valve area (MVA)
    - (*NOTE: if TTE not adequate for above, TEE recommended*)
- Cardiac Catheterization (Right and Left heart catheterization)
  > Mitral valve gradient – simultaneous pulmonary wedge (or left atrium) and left ventricular pressures
  > MVA – Gorlin formula using MV gradient and cardiac output
  > Pulmonary wedge and pulmonary artery pressures during exercise

DIFFERENTIAL DIAGNOSIS
- Left atrial myxoma
- Severe MR (diastolic murmur present without OS)
- Austin-Flint murmur of aortic insufficiency
- Cor triatriatum (congential fibromuscular diaphragm dividing left atrium)
- Carey-coombs murmur of acute rheumatic fever

MANAGEMENT
- Medical treatment
  > Antibiotic prophylaxis for all patients
  > Mild symptoms-diuretics
  > Atrial fibrillation
    - Warfarin to prevent systemic emboli
    - Rate control with digoxin, beta-blockers or calcium blockers (**very important to prolong diastolic intervals with MS**)
  > Moderate/severe symptoms (see specific therapy below)

SPECIFIC THERAPY
- For moderate/severe symptoms (NYHA Class III or IV) and MVA = or < 1.0 cm2, two options:
  > **Percutaneous balloon valvotomy, or**
  > **Surgical repair/replacement of MV**
  > Candidates for percutaneous balloon valvotomy must meet the following TEE criteria:

- No significant MR
- No significant calcifications in MV leaflets
- Only mild leaflet thickening
- Miminal subvalvular apparatus involvement
- No thrombus in left atrium
- ➤ **(Surgical MV replacement indicated, if any one of above not met)**

FOLLOW-UP
n/a

COMPLICATIONS AND PROGNOSIS

Complications
- Percutaneous balloon valvotomy
  - ➤ Acute
    - Systemic emboli 4–8% (thrombus or calcified debris)
    - Severe MR requiring immediate MV replacement 2–3% (Careful selection using TEE data is essential to avoid this complication)
    - Left to right atrial shunt (usually small, non-significant)
    - I.V perforation resulting in cardiac tamponade 2–4%
  - ➤ Long-term
    - Excellent long-term results in younger patients, without atrial fibrillation, and careful selection by TEE (see above criteria)-5% restenosis at 32 months follow-up
- Surgical replacement of mitral valve
  - ➤ Acute
    - Complications associated with cardiopulmonary bypass surgery
  - ➤ Long-term
    - Bleeding due to warfarin therapy
    - Endocarditis
    - Malfunction of mechanical or bioprosthetic mitral valve
    - Thromboembolism

Prognosis
- Slow progression from Class II to Class III/IV over 5–10 years
- Class III and IV medical treatment survival worse versus interventional or surgical groups
- Overall prognosis good in surgical and interventional groups unless severe right heart failure present

MITRAL VALVE PROLAPSE

JUDITH A. WISNESKI, MD

HISTORY & PHYSICAL
- Most common – no other associated illness
- Mitral valve prolapse associated with:
  - Marfan's syndrome
  - Ehlers-Danlos syndrome
  - Osteogenesis imperfecta
  - Pseudoxanthoma elastican
  - Periarteritis nodosa
  - Hyperthyroidism
  - Ebstein's anomaly of tricuspid valve
  - Straight-back syndrome

History
- Asymptomatic (most common)
- Palpitations
- Chest pain
- Syncope

Signs & Symptoms
- Midsystolic click +/– late systolic murmur
  - Valsalva maneuver – click occurs earlier in systole, murmur louder and longer

TESTS
- ECG
  - Most common – normal
  - If significant mitral insufficiency (MR) – see section on MR
- Chest X-Ray
  - Most common – normal
  - If significant MR – see section on MR
- Echo/Doppler (most important in diagnosis)
  - Prolapse of mitral valve leaflets
  - Detect presence and severity of MR – see section on MR

DIFFERENTIAL DIAGNOSIS
- Other causes of mitral insufficiency

MANAGEMENT
- Medical

- ➤ Antibiotic prophylaxis
  - MR present on exam or echo
  - No antibiotic prophylaxis for click and prolapse only
- ➤ Palpitations and chest pain syndrome (r/o CAD)
  - Beta-blocker therapy – variable results

SPECIFIC THERAPY

n/a

FOLLOW-UP

n/a

COMPLICATIONS AND PROGNOSIS

Complications
- Endocarditis
- Stroke
- Progressive MR

Prognosis
- Systolic click only – excellent prognosis
- 10% progress to significant MR (usually men and older patients)
  - ➤ Obtain echo/Doppler every 1–2 years to assess severity of MR and left ventricular function
  - ➤ Consider mitral valve surgery if MR moderate/severe – see section on MR

MOLLUSCUM CONTAGIOSUM

JEFFREY P. CALLEN, MD

HISTORY & PHYSICAL

History
- Asymptomatic
- Facial and truncal lesions are common in children.
- Genital lesions are common in adults and are transmitted by direct contact with an infected individual.
- Facial lesions in adults are associated with immunosuppressed state.

Signs & Symptoms
- Flesh-colored or slight pink globose papules with a central dell
- Lesions may be single or may coalesce.

TESTS
- Biopsy is confirmatory.
- Potassium hydroxide preparation often reveal molluscum bodies.

DIFFERENTIAL DIAGNOSIS
- Clinically characteristic
- In immunosuppressed patients, cryptococcal infection may masquerade as molluscum.

MANAGEMENT
What to Do First
- Establish diagnosis.
- Examine contacts.

General Measures
- Assess for other sexually transmitted diseases in adults.

SPECIFIC THERAPY
- Removal or destruction – liquid nitrogen, sharp curettage or laser ablation

FOLLOW-UP
- Reassess for recurrences at 2–3 months following the last observed lesion.

COMPLICATIONS AND PROGNOSIS
- Self-limited disease except in immunocompromised patients

MOTOR NEURON DISEASES

MICHAEL J. AMINOFF, MD, DSc

HISTORY & PHYSICAL
- Diffuse weakness, w/o sensory or sphincter disturbance
  - Spinal muscular atrophy: lower motor neuron deficit mainly in limbs
  - Primary lateral sclerosis: upper motor neuron deficit in limbs
  - Progressive bulbar palsy: lower motor neuron deficit in bulbar muscles

> Pseudobulbar palsy: upper motor neuron deficit in bulbar muscles
> Amyotrophic lateral sclerosis: mixed upper & lower motor neuron deficit in limbs

TESTS
- EMG: chronic partial degeneration & reinnervation
- NCS: normal motor & sensory conduction studies
  > No evidence of motor conduction block
- CSF: normal
- Serum & WBC hexosaminidase A: normal
- Serum protein electrophoresis & immunoelectrophoresis: normal

DIFFERENTIAL DIAGNOSIS
- Hexosaminidase deficiency or monoclonal gammopathy may be associated w/ similar clinical picture
- Multifocal motor neuropathy excluded by NCS
- Compressive lesion excluded by imaging studies
- Familial forms excluded by genetic studies

MANAGEMENT
- Ensure ventilation & nutrition
- Anticholinergics for drooling
- Baclofen or diazepam for spasticity
- Palliative care in terminal stages

SPECIFIC THERAPY
- Riluzole may slow progression of ALS (monitor liver enzymes, blood count & electrolytes)

FOLLOW-UP
- Regularly assess ventilatory function & nutritional status
  > May require semiliquid diet, nasogastric feeding, gastrotomy or cricopharyngomyotomy
  > May require ventilator support

COMPLICATIONS AND PROGNOSIS
- Dysphagia is common
- Dysarthia or dysphonia
- Aspiration pneumonia
- Respiratory insufficiency

MUCOPOLYSACCHARIDOSES

GREGORY M. ENNS, MD

HISTORY & PHYSICAL

History

- history of consanguinity or family history of disease
- autosomal recessive or X-linked inheritance (Type II)

Signs & Symptoms

- most appear normal at birth with first signs in infancy
- wide spectrum of clinical severity – CNS symptoms appear later in MPS III, normal IQ in MPS IS, IV, VI, prominent skeletal dysplasia in MPS IV
- Common abnormalities: progressive mental deterioration, coarse features, macrocephaly, cloudy corneas, hearing loss, otitis media with effusion, chronic rhinitis, deafness, gum hypertrophy, obstructive airway disease, kyphoscoliosis, gibbus, claw hand, joint contractures, carpal tunnel syndrome, hepatosplenomegaly, umbilical and inguinal hernias
- silent cardiac abnormalities common late features (esp. mitral & aortic valve disease, valve thickening, coronary artery narrowing, endocardial fibroelastosis)
- Occasional abnormalities: hyperactivity, aggressive behavior, seizures, hydrocephalus, nystagmus, glaucoma, spinal cord compression, hydrops fetalis (MPS I, IVA, VII), neonatal/infantile cardiomegaly (MPS I, VI), diarrhea

Classification

- MPS Type: IH
  - ➤ Syndrome: Hurler
  - ➤ Enzyme deficiency: alpha-L-iduronidase
  - ➤ MPS excretion: DS, HS
- MPS Type: IS
  - ➤ Syndrome: Scheie
  - ➤ Enzyme deficiency: alpha-L-iduronidase
  - ➤ MPS excretion: DS, HS
- MPS Type: IHS
  - ➤ Syndrome: Hurler/Scheie
  - ➤ Enzyme deficiency: alpha-L-iduronidase
  - ➤ MPS excretion: DS, HS

- MPS Type: II
  - ➤ Syndrome: Hunter
  - ➤ Enzyme deficiency: iduronate sulfatase
  - ➤ MPS excretion: DS, HS
- MPS Type: IIIA
  - ➤ Syndrome: Sanfilippo type A
  - ➤ Enzyme deficiency: heparan N-sulfatase
  - ➤ MPS excretion: HS
- MPS Type: IIIB
  - ➤ Syndrome: Sanfilippo type B
  - ➤ Enzyme deficiency: alpha-N-acetylglucosaminidase
  - ➤ MPS excretion: HS
- MPS Type: IIIC
  - ➤ Syndrome: Sanfilippo type C
  - ➤ Enzyme deficiency: acetyl CoA: alpha-D-glucosaminidine-N-acetyl transferase
  - ➤ MPS excretion: HS
- MPS Type: IIID
  - ➤ Syndrome: Sanfilippo type D
  - ➤ Enzyme deficiency: N-acetyl-alpha-D-glucosaminidine-6-sulfatase
  - ➤ MPS excretion: HS
- MPS Type: IVA
  - ➤ Syndrome: Morquio type A
  - ➤ Enzyme deficiency: N-acetylgalactosamine-6-sulfatase
  - ➤ MPS excretion: KS, C6S
- MPS Type: IVB
  - ➤ Syndrome: Morquio type B
  - ➤ Enzyme deficiency: beta-galactosidase
  - ➤ MPS excretion: KS
- MPS Type: VI
  - ➤ Syndrome: Maroteaux-Lamy
  - ➤ Enzyme deficiency: N-acetylgalactosamine-4-sulfatase
  - ➤ MPS excretion: DS, C4S
- MPS Type: VII
  - ➤ Syndrome: Sly
  - ➤ Enzyme deficiency: beta-glucuronidase
  - ➤ MPS excretion: DS, HS, CS
- MPS Type: IX
  - ➤ Syndrome: Natowicz
  - ➤ Enzyme deficiency: hyaluronidase

➤ MPS excretion: CS

DS = dermatan sulfate; HS = heparan sulfate; KS = keratan sulfate; CS = chondroitin sulfate; C4S = chondroitin 4-sulfate; C6S = chondroitin 6-sulfate

TESTS

Laboratory
- basic blood studies:
  - ➤ normal routine studies
- basic urine studies:
  - ➤ normal routine studies

Screening
- urine mucopolysaccharides
  - ➤ thin-layer chromatography
- one-dimensional electrophoresis
  - ➤ high false +/− with spot or turbidity tests

Confirmatory Tests
- enzyme assay (lymphocytes, fibroblasts)
- prenatal diagnosis (enzyme activity in amniocytes, chorionic villi)

Imaging
- skeletal X-ray: dysostosis multiplex
- echocardiography: valve disease, endocardial fibroelastosis

DIFFERENTIAL DIAGNOSIS
- anticonvulsant therapy
- congenital hypothyroidism
- oligosaccharidoses/other lysosomal disorders:
  - ➤ mannosidosis
  - ➤ fucosidosis
  - ➤ sialidosis
  - ➤ galactosialidosis
  - ➤ aspartylglycosaminuria
- GM1 gangliosidosis
  - ➤ multiple sulfatase deficiency
    - I-cell disease (normal urine mucopolysaccharides, increased serum lysosomal enzyme activities diagnostic)
- genetic syndromes:
  - ➤ Coffin-Lowry syndrome
    - Coffin-Siris syndrome

- Costello syndrome
- Schinzel-Giedeon syndrome

■ other causes of increased urine mucopolysaccharides: Kniest dysplasia, Lowe syndrome, Grave's disease, scleroderma, rheumatoid arthritis, psoriasis, diabetes mellitus, cystic fibrosis

MANAGEMENT

What to Do First

■ assess severity of neurologic, eye, cardiac, bone disease

General Measures

■ developmental assessment
■ physical therapy for contractures

SPECIFIC THERAPY

■ referral to biochemical genetics center
■ supportive measures only
  ➤ corneal transplant
  ➤ VP shunt for hydrocephalus
  ➤ hearing aids, PE tubes
  ➤ aortic/mitral valve replacement
  ➤ bacterial endocarditis prophylaxis for patients with cardiac abnormalities
  ➤ decompression for carpal tunnel syndrome
  ➤ cervical spine fusion (MPS IV)
  ➤ total knee arthroplasty (MPS IV)
■ bone marrow or umbilical cord blood transplantation may arrest or reverse systemic manifestations (except bone disease), esp. for MPS I, but is not standard therapy for all disorders
■ enzyme replacement therapy is available for MPS I and in clinical trials for MPS II, MPS VI (improves systemic manifestations, but does not cross blood-brain barrier)
■ gene therapy experimental

FOLLOW-UP

■ regular monitoring for complications of disease
■ spinal fusion may be needed to prevent paralysis
■ genetic counseling

COMPLICATIONS AND PROGNOSIS

Complications

■ spinal cord compression (esp. in anesthesia)

- atlanto-axial subluxation
- aspiration pneumonia
- heart failure
- obstructive apnea
- graft-versus-host disease and autoimmune hemolytic anemia after BM transplant
- difficulty with surgery (25% difficult intubation, 8% fail intubation in general; 54% difficult intubation, 23% fail intubation in MPS IH)

Prognosis
- progressive impairment
- slowly progressive forms (MPS III) may survive into adulthood, but most have early demise (<10 years)
- peak of intellectual function 2–4 years in most patients, after which there is regression
- death secondary to pneumonia, cardiac dysfunction

MUCORMYCOSIS

RICHARD A. JACOBS, MD, PhD

HISTORY & PHYSICAL

History
- Name given to several opportunistic infections caused by fungi of the Mucorales order (Rhizopus, Mucor, *Absidia* and *Cunninghamella*)
- Think of the risk factors to assess susceptibility: diabetes mellitus
  - ➤ particularly diabetic ketoacidosis, chronic renal failure, steroids, other immunosuppressive therapy
- Ubiquitous fungi; exposure is common

Signs & Symptoms
- Can be classified into several different presentations based on anatomy: rhinocerebral, pulmonary, cutaneous, GI, CNS, other sites
  - ➤ Disseminated disease is also possible
  - ➤ Black eschars and discharge are clues to diagnosis
- Rhinocerebral:
  - ➤ Usually found in diabetic patients, neutropenic cancer patients
  - ➤ Pts complain of headache, facial pain, fever.
  - ➤ If eye involved, may see proptosis, orbital cellulitis, conjunctival swelling

- ➤ Vision loss may be due to retinal artery thrombosis.
- ➤ Ptosis and dilation of pupils seen if cranial nerve involvement
- ■ Pulmonary:
  - ➤ Usually found in neutropenic cancer patients, usually have received broad-spectrum antibiotics in the hospital
  - ➤ May present with fever and dyspnea; hemoptysis if vessel invasion
- ■ Cutaneous:
  - ➤ Primary: results from direct inoculation of the organism into the skin
  - ➤ Necrosis may develop if there is vessel invasion
  - ➤ Secondary: develops as a result of fungemia
- ■ GI:
  - ➤ Found in patients with severe malnutrition
- ■ May be introduced with contaminated food
  - ➤ Abdominal pain, nausea, vomiting, fever and hematochezia possible
- ■ CNS:
  - ➤ Usually via extension from sinuses or nose into brain
  - ➤ Altered mental status, cranial nerve findings
  - ➤ If via direct inoculation via trauma into brain, may present as black discharge from wound

TESTS

Laboratory
- ■ Basic studies: blood culture rarely positive
- ■ Basic studies: serology not used
- ■ Basic studies: tissue biopsy
  - ➤ Fungal hyphae can be seen in tissue that has been hematoxylin and eosin, methenamine silver or periodic acid-Schiff stained
- ■ The fungi appear as broad, nonseptate hyphae with right angle branching.

Imaging
- ■ Rhinocerebral mucormycosis:
- ■ Sinus films: mucosal thickening, air-fluid levels possible
- ■ CT may better define eroded bone in more advanced disease.
- ■ MRI also used, with similar findings
- ■ Pulmonary mucormycosis:
- ■ Chest X-ray: consolidation (66%), cavitation (40%)

DIFFERENTIAL DIAGNOSIS

- Aspergillus, neoplasm, cavernous sinus thrombosis (rhinocerebral mucormycosis), pulmonary embolism (pulmonary mucormycosis)

MANAGEMENT

What to Do First

- Correct the underlying problem!
  - ➤ Reverse acidosis in diabetic ketoacidosis (fluids, insulin, electrolyte abnormalities); strive for good glycemic control; discontinue immunosuppressive drugs if possible; await reversal of neutropenia.
- Start Amphotericin B immediately (see below).
- Call the surgeon to advise on aggressive debridement.

SPECIFIC THERAPY

Indications

- Every one, once mucormycosis is suspected; this is a rapidly progressive disease with fatal consequences.

Treatment Options

- Usually mucormycosis is refractory to medical treatment, necessitating larger doses of Amphotericin B.
- Aggressive surgical debridement is essential; may be cosmetically disfiguring.
- Repeated surgical intervention is usually needed to resect necrotic tissue.
- Can reduce to qod dosing if improvement
  - ➤ Lipid formulations of Amphotericin may have utility because of the ability to use higher doses over shorter periods of time

Side Effects & Contraindications

- Amphotericin B
  - ➤ Side effects: fevers, chills, nausea, vomiting and headaches; rigors may be prevented by the addition of hydrocortisone 25 mg to bag, meperidine 25–50 mg may treat rigors; nephrotoxicity; electrolyte disturbance (renal tubular acidosis, hypokalemia, hypomagnesemia)
- Contraindications: if Cr 2.5–3.0, may consider giving lipid-based Amphotericin products

Voriconazole, echinocandins not effective

FOLLOW-UP
- Assess response to therapy
- May need prolonged treatment with antifungal agents

COMPLICATIONS AND PROGNOSIS

Complications
- May be cosmetically disfiguring, and major reconstructive surgery is usually needed

Prognosis
- Depends to a large part on the prognosis of the underlying disease (neoplasm, etc.)
- Overall mortality rate 50%
- Pulmonary disease may have worse outcome because of later diagnosis.

Prevention
- No cost-effective method known
  - Use of rooms with high-efficiency particulate air filters (HEPA) in severely neutropenic patients (such as bone marrow transplant) may have efficacy.

MULTIFOCAL ATRIAL TACHYCARDIA (MAT)

EDMUND C. KEUNG, MD

HISTORY & PHYSICAL

History
- Most common in elderly patients with significant COPD.

Signs & Symptoms
- Palpitation with irregular rapid pulses. Predominant symptom: exacerbation of COPD with hypoxia

TESTS
- Basic Tests
  - 12-lead ECG:
  - Narrow QRS tachycardia unless pre-existing conduction defect or rate-related aberrant ventricular conduction. At least 3 different P wave morphologies. P-P and P-R intervals highly variable. Atrial rate 100–130 bpm. AV nodal block usually not present.
- Specific Diagnostic Test
  - none

DIFFERENTIAL DIAGNOSIS
- Atrial fibrillation: irregularly irregular QRS but no recognizable P waves.

MANAGEMENT

What to Do First
- Treatment of underlying pulmonary process. Administration of oxygen to correct hypoxia.

General Measures
- As above

SPECIFIC THERAPY
- Antiarrhythmic drugs ineffective. Amiodarone and calcium channel blockers may be tried. Potassium and magnesium replacement.

Side Effects & Contraindications
- Excessive suppression of AVN by calcium channel blockers or amiodarone. Exacerbation of existing lung disease from amiodarone lung toxicity. beta blockers usually contraindicated because of underlying COPD.

FOLLOW-UP
- Optimize chronic treatment for underlying lung disease.

COMPLICATIONS AND PROGNOSIS
- Deterioration of exiting lung disease.

MULTIPLE ENDOCRINE NEOPLASIA 1

COLEMAN GROSS, MD
REVISED BY ANDREW R. HOFFMAN, MD

HISTORY & PHYSICAL

History
- Hypercalcemia (hyperparathyroidism) presenting abnormality in 85%; eventually almost all develop hyperparathyroidism
- Pancreatic islet cell tumors second commonest; as many as 80%; many malignant or multifocal; gastrinoma with peptic ulcer disease most common
- Other islet tumors: insulinoma, glucagonoma, VIPoma, somatostatinoma, pancreatic polypeptide, GHRH-producing

- Pituitary adenoma, prolactinoma most common
- Other tumors: carcinoid, adrenocortical, lipoma
- Autosomal dominant inheritance; high penetrance but with different constellation of tumors among family members; mutation in *MEN1* gene

Signs & Symptoms

- Mostly due to hormone hypersecretion
- Hyperparathyroidism: usually no signs
- Islet cell tumor:
  - Gastrinoma: peptic ulcer symptoms, diarrhea
  - nsulinoma: hypoglycemic symptoms
  - Glucagonoma: hyperglycemia, necrolytic migratory erythema
  - VIPoma: watery diarrhea syndrome
- Pituitary: hypogonadism, amenorrhea, galactorrhea (prolactinoma), acromegaly, Cushing syndrome; visual field cut

TESTS

Laboratory

- Blood tests: random and dynamic: directed by symptom complex
  - Elevated calcium and PTH levels
  - Elevated gastrin (>300 pg/mL): may require secretin/calcium test
  - Hyperinsulinemic hypoglycemia (may require 72-h fast)
- Anterior pituitary axis testing: random prolactin, dexamethasone suppression (Cushing disease), growth hormone (after glucose load), IGF-1

Imaging

- Parathyoid: sestimibi radionuclide scan useful; US, MRI, CT adjunctive
- Pancreas: MRI or CT may be useful; ^{111}In-octreotide scan may detect lesions with (−) MRI or CT findings; intraoperative US increases detection
- Pituitary: MRI

Screening

- Family members: if mutation is known, screen all at-risk family members
- Complete physical and biochemical testing (calcium, gastrin, prolactin) q 3–5 y
- Pituitary and abdominal imaging at baseline and q 5–10 y if hyperparathryoid, depending on symptoms and biochemistry; if no hyperparathyroidism by age 40 y, no need to do routine screening

DIFFERENTIAL DIAGNOSIS

- Straightforward if hyperparathyroidism and family history of MEN1
- Can see familial hyperparathyroidism and overlap syndromes
- Hypercalcemia from isolated hyperparathyroidism may elevate serum gastrin levels

MANAGEMENT

What to Do First

- Detailed medical and family history (identify index case: important for screening)

General Measures

- History and physical exam dictate biochemical testing
- Measure calcium, gastrin, prolactin
- Significant morbidity/mortality from malignant islet cell tumors: maintain high index of suspicion

SPECIFIC THERAPY

- Hyperparathyroidism: for calcium >11 mg/dL, or end-organ damage (kidney stones, osteitis, osteoporosis, renal failure, hypercalciuria), surgical removal of 3 1/2 glands with tagging or transplant of remaining tissue; hyperplasia of all glands, can have more than 4 glands
- Islet cell tumor: proton pump inhibitors for gastrinoma, surgical excision, including partial pancreatectomy (multifocal tumors), chemotherapy if malignant (streptozotocin, somatostatin, others)
- Pituitary tumors: bromocriptine, cabergoline (prolactinoma), transphenoidal resection, somatostatin (acromegaly)

Side Effects

- Parathyroidectomy: hypoparathyroidism, recurrent laryngeal nerve injury
- Proton pump inhibitors: no increased risk of carcinoid
- Pancreatectomy: high morbidity, diabetes, pancreatic insufficiency
- Streptozotocin: diabetes
- Somatostatin: hyperglycemia, gallstones
- Bromocriptine, cabergoline: nausea, orthostatic hypotension.
- Transphenoidal resection: hypopituitarism, diabetes insipidus, CSF leak, infection

FOLLOW-UP

During Treatment

- Assess response to interventions:

➤ Parathyroidectomy: 75–90% of subjects with initial response many recur; follow calcium for hypoparathyroidism shortly after surgery, hungry bone syndrome (hypocalcemia) immediately postop; recurrent hypercalcemia

➤ Islet cell tumor: symptoms and hormone levels for response to intervention (surgery, medical)

➤ Pituitary tumor:
  • Prolactinoma: monitor prolactin and tumor size
  • Acromegaly: monitor GH and IGF-1 levels; GH target <1.0 mcg/L after oral glucose challenge (surgery or somatostatin); IGF-1 levels should be in normal age-and sex-adjusted range
  • Surgery: short-term monitor for posterior and anterior pituitary hypofunction (esp pituitary/adrenal and pituitary/thyroid axis)

Routine
▪ Monitor recurrence by symptomatology, lab screening, and imaging
▪ Screen for development of other tumors yearly:
  ➤ Pancreatic tumors in 30–80% (gastrin or other hormone, depending on symptoms and signs)
  ➤ Pituitary tumors in 15–90% (prolactin or other)

COMPLICATIONS AND PROGNOSIS
▪ Most serious: malignant islet cell tumor; most gastrinomas malignant; 10% of insulinomas malignant
▪ Due to hormone overproduction syndromes and therapies:
  ➤ Hyperparathyroidism: kidney stones, renal failure, osteitis, osteoporosis
  ➤ Pancreatic tumor:
    • Gastrinoma: luminal perforation, hemorrhage
    • Insulinoma: hypoglycemia with neuoglycopenic symptoms including seizures
  ➤ Pituitary tumor: mass effect, optic chiasm compression, hypopituitarism
    • Prolactinoma: hypogonadism, galactorrhea
    • Acromegaly: osteoarthritis, sleep apnea, cardiomyopathy, glucose intolerance, colonic polyps and cancer, increased mortality
    • Cushing disease: increased risk of infection, osteoporosis, hypogonadism, hypertension, diabetes mellitus

Prognosis
- Lifespan normal
- Prognosis excellent with regular screening
- Genetic testing reduces need for frequent biochemical screening, increases early diagnosis and intervention, improves quality of life

---

MULTIPLE ENDOCRINE NEOPLASIA 2

COLEMAN GROSS, MD
REVISED BY ANDREW R. HOFFMAN, MD

HISTORY & PHYSICAL

History
- Family history of MEN2: autosomal dominant, may occur sporadically
- MEN 2A: medullary thyroid carcinoma (MTC), pheochromocytoma, hyperparathyroidism.
- MEN2B: MTC, pheochromocytoma, mucosal neuromas.
- Familial isolated MTC is a third MEN2 syndrome
- MTC usually first tumor, defines MEN2 if family history of MTC and other tumors; thyroid nodule; may be multifocal; MTC may present with paraneoplastic syndrome due to production of variety of peptide hormones
- Pheochromocytomas may be bilateral or rarely malignant; present in 50% or more of MEN2A and 2B; associated symptoms: paroxysmal headache, palpitations, etc
- Hyperparathyroidism occurs in up to 1/3 of MEN 2A cases; often asymptomatic
- Mucosal neuromas in MEN2B; GI tract involvement can cause colic in children

Signs & Symptoms
- MEN2A and 2B:
  - ➢ Hypertension variable, may be sustained
  - ➢ Thyroid mass
- MEN2A:
  - ➢ Occasional papular skin changes: cutaneous lichen amyloidosis often involving upper back

- MEN2B:
  - Mucosal neuromas on lips and tongue
  - Marfanoid habitus

MTC more often metastatic

TESTS

Laboratory

- Basic blood studies:
  - MTC: pentagastrin-stimulated calcitonin
  - Hyperparathryoidism: elevated calcium and intact PTH
- Basic urine studies:
  - Pheochromocytoma: 24-h urine for catecholamines and meta-nephrines; plasma metanephrines and catecholamines; helpful at time of symptoms
- Specific Diagnostic Tests
  - Index case diagnosis and screening done by genetic analysis
  - MEN2A and 2B due to mutations in RET tyrosine kinase proto-oncogene; most common MEN2A mutations in exons 10 and 11; MEN2B mutations at codon 918
  - Familial MTC (no other MEN2A tumors) mutations in exon 10 and 11

Imaging

- MTC: radioiodine not useful; sestimibi and 111 I-octreotide scanning useful as adjunct to CT or MRI
- Pheochromocytoma: MRI useful; 131 I-MIBG nuclear scan less sensitive but more specific than CT or MRI
- Hyperparathyoidism: sestimibi scan preoperatively and in recurrent disease; US, MRI, CT adjunctive
- Thyroid Biopsy
  - FNA biopsy of thyroid nodule

DIFFERENTIAL DIAGNOSIS

- MTC with family history of MTC and MEN2 tumor points to diagnosis
- Sporadic, new mutations occur, so family history not obvious
- Familial MTC occurs without other MEN2 findings; 20% of all MTC

MANAGEMENT

What to Do First

- Detailed medical and family history (identify index case; important for screening)

General Measures
■ Established cases:
  ➤ Thyroidectomy for MTC
  ➤ Screen for pheochromocytoma prior to thyroidectomy
  ➤ Evaluate for hypercalcemia

Screening
■ RET gene analysis in index case and family members
■ Petagastrin-stimulated calcitonin annually in RET mutation (−) family
■ Urine catecholamines and metanephrines yearly
■ Calcium (MEN2A) yearly

SPECIFIC THERAPY
■ MTC: total thyroidectomy; thyroidectomy as early as age 4–7 y for RET (+) cases or abnormal calcitonin results; in MEN2B, screening and surgery before age 1 year often recommended continue calcitonin screening after surgery; screen for pheochromocytoma prior to surgery; chemotherapy for metastatic disease
■ Pheochromocytoma: adrenalectomy after alpha/beta-blockade (beta only after alpha) and hydration; bilateral adrenalectomy possible given high risk of developing contralateral pheochromocytoma
■ Hyperparathyroidism: indicated for calcium >11 mg/dL, or end-organ damage (kidney stones, osteitis, osteoporosis, renal failure, hypercalciuria); surgical removal of 3 1/2 glands with tagging or transplant of remaining tissue, hyperplasia of all glands and can have more than 4 glands

Side Effects
■ MTC and thyroidectomy: hypoparathyroidism, recurrent laryngeal nerve injury, metastatic disease
■ Pheochromocytoma and adrenalectomy: hypertensive crisis, recurrent tumor, adrenal insufficiency (bilateral adrenalectomy)
■ Hyperparathyroidism and parathyroidectomy: hypoparathyroidism, hypocalcemia (hungry bone syndrome), recurrent laryngeal nerve injury

Contraindications
■ Thyroidectomy only after pheochromocytoma ruled out

■ Adrenalectomy prior to thyroidectomy if pheochromocytoma present; alpha-blockade prior to beta-blockade to mitigate unopposed alpha vasoconstriction

FOLLOW-UP

■ Regularly assess for recurrent disease, esp MTC, because of high metastatic potential
■ Calcitonin (stimulated) annually for first 5 y after thyroidectomy, then periodically
■ 24-h urine catecholamines and metanephrines 1 wk after adrenalectomy
■ Calcium after parathroidectomy
■ 24-hr urine catecholamines and metanephrines yearly
■ Calcium yearly

COMPLICATIONS AND PROGNOSIS

Complications

■ MTC:
  ➤ Incidence of metastatic disease decreased with improved screening
  ➤ Up to 95% cure rate with thyrroidectomy, many have local spread
  ➤ Hypertensive crisis possible if not screened for pheochromocytoma
■ Pheochromocytoma:
  ➤ Surgical risk: 2–3% mortality, requires adequate adrenergic blockade and fluid resuscitation with expert anesthetic care
  ➤ Laparoscopic procedure reduces risk
  ➤ Risk of contralateral pheochromocytoma 50% at 10 y
  ➤ Adrenal insufficiency from bilateral adrenalectomy
■ Parathyroidectomy:
  ➤ Recurrent hyperparathyroidism common
  ➤ Subsequent surgery guided with imaging and venous sampling for PTH

Prognosis

■ Greatly improved with availability of genetic screening
■ 5-y survival for TNM I or II MTC 95%; delayed diagnosis dramatically reduces survival
■ Prognosis good after unilateral adrenalectomy; hypertension cured in 75%
■ Recurrent hyperparathyroidism less common than in MEN1

MULTIPLE SCLEROSIS

MICHAEL J. AMINOFF, MD, DSc

HISTORY & PHYSICAL

- Onset typically btwn 15 & 55 years
- Weakness, sensory disturbances, ataxia, dysarthria, vertigo, sphincter disturbances, retrobulbar optic neuritis, diplopia occur alone or in any combination
- Symptoms develop episodically, followed often by partial remission, leading to progressive disability; sometimes progressive from onset or after initial relapsing-remitting course
- Variable interval (sometimes of years) btwn episodes; in a few pts, disorder is progressive from onset
- Relapses may be triggered by infection or in postpartum period
- Findings vary in different pts & at different times in the same pt
- Cognitive deficits, emotional lability, dysarthria are common
- Cranial nerve deficits include optic atrophy, nystagmus, internuclear ophthalmoplegia, facial sensory loss
- Deficits in limbs include spasticity, pyramidal weakness, ataxia, intention tremor, sensory loss, hyperreflexia, extensor plantar responses

TESTS

- Cranial & spinal MRI reveals multiple white-matter lesions
- Cerebral evoked potentials may reveal subclinical involvement of afferent pathways
- CSF may show mild pleocytosis, elevated IgG, oligoclonal bands

DIFFERENTIAL DIAGNOSIS

- Depends on symptoms & signs; should be evidence of multiple lesions affecting CNS white matter & developing at different times
- If deficit can be attributed by lesion at a single site, a structural lesion must be excluded by imaging

MANAGEMENT

- Acute optic neuritis treated w/ IV methylprednisolone
- Acute relapses require steroids (eg, prednisone daily for 1 week, followed by taper)

SPECIFIC THERAPY

- Beta-interferon or copolymer reduces relapse frequency in relapsing-remitting disease
- Cyclophosphamide, azathioprine, methotrexate, cladribine, mitoxantrone are sometimes used in secondary progressive disease
- IV immunoglobulins may be used to reduce the attack rate in relapsing-remitting disease
- Spasticity is treated w/ gradually increasing doses of baclofen, diazepam or tizanidine

FOLLOW-UP

- Depends on disease stage & course
- Urinary or other infections & decubitus ulcers should be treated vigorously

COMPLICATIONS AND PROGNOSIS

- Increasing disability is likely
- Prognosis worse w/ progressive than relapsing remitting course
- Prognosis worse w/ brain stem/cerebellar deficit

MUMPS

CAROL A. GLASER, MD

HISTORY & PHYSICAL

History

- Paramyxovirus
- Humans only known natural host
- Airborne transmission, droplet spread or direct contact (from saliva of infected person)
- Incubation period: usually 16–18 days (12–25 days)
- Most common in 5–14 years
- Reportable
- Infection adulthood, more likely to be severe
- Late winter/early spring more common
- Marked decreased incidence since introduction of vaccine in 1967

Signs & Symptoms

- Many times – asymptomatic/ "subclinical" (25–30% of cases)
    - ➤ Classic symptoms: parotid salivary glands swelling

➤ Swelling salivary gland; can be uni-or bilateral, sometimes sublingual or submandibular swelling
➤ Fever – if present only moderately elevated for 3–4 days
➤ Variably present: respiratory symptoms, especially <5 years
➤ Headache, photophobia, anorexia, abdominal pain (due to pancreatic involvement)

TESTS

Nonspecific:
- Amylase often elevated
- CSF pleocytosis – ~50% of cases will have CSF pleocytosis

Specific:
Serology is diagnostic test of choice
- enzyme immunoassay (EIA or ELISA) methods widely available
- Complement fixation (CF), neutralization or hemagglutination (HAI) can also be used
- 4 fold change indicative of acute infection
- mumps-specific IgM is available and can be used to detect acute infection (note false positive can occur due to interference with rheumatoid factors/false negative can occur in mumps-infected individuals previously immunized but not fully protected)
- IgG antibody is an indication of previous infection/immunization and is predictive of immunity
- Skin test – not reliable
- Isolation saliva/urine; acute stages illness,
  ➤ virus can be isolated from respiratory specimens (48 hrs. before and up to 7 days following onset parotid swelling) urine (up to 14 days after onset) and CSF (up to 9 days after onset)
  ➤ these methods are expensive, slow and not uniformly available and should be used only in special circumstances

DIFFERENTIAL DIAGNOSIS
- Parotid swelling – other viruses such as influenza, parainfluenza types 1and 2/CMV-viral isolation/detection can help distinguish
- Bacterial infection parotid gland – exquisite tenderness/leukocytosis and pus from Wharton duct
- Stone/parotid gland

MANAGEMENT
- No specific antiviral
- Hydration/Analgesics

➤ Reportable in certain areas
➤ Immunize susceptible pts
➤ Respiratory isolation for 9 days after onset parotid swelling

SPECIFIC THERAPY
n/a

FOLLOW-UP
n/a

COMPLICATIONS AND PROGNOSIS

Complications
■ Orchitis: around 30–40% postpubertal males
  ➤ Usually unilateral
  ➤ Sterility not common
■ Oophoritis (inflammation of ovaries); ~7% of postpubertal females
  ➤ Usually unilateral
  ➤ Pelvic pain, lower abdominal tenderness
  ➤ Risk of sterility very low
■ Mastitis: 30% postpubertal females
■ Senso-neural hearing loss; 5/100,000 cases
  ➤ Central Nervous System
    • up to 15% of cases have signs of meningeal inflammation
    • Encephalitis; more common in patients >15 years
    • 2.6 encephalitis/1000 cases mumps
  ➤ Pancreatitis: often mild, ~4% of cases
    • 1st trimester; spontaneous abortions, no congenital malformations
    • other complications: arthritis, renal involvement, thyroiditis
    • Diabetes mellitus: association has been suggested, unproven

Prevention
■ For active cases;
  ➤ Exclude child from school/day care center
  ➤ Droplet precautions until 9 days after parotid swelling
    • Mumps vaccine does not prevent infection when given to individuals incubating mumps.
■ General:
  ➤ vaccine is live-virus vaccine
  ➤ Vaccine – lasting immunity
  ➤ Vaccine recommended to all children during 2nd year of life and booster at 4–6 years

MUSCULAR DYSTROPHIES

MICHAEL J. AMINOFF, MD, DSc

HISTORY & PHYSICAL

- Progressive muscle wasting & weakness occurring in a particular pattern depending on individual disorder
- Characteristic age of onset & pattern of inheritance for different dystrophies
- Weak, wasted muscles in characteristic distribution
- May be pseudohypertrophy of muscles, muscle contractures, intellectual changes, skeletal deformities or cardiac involvement w/ certain dystrophies
- Myotonia is present in myotonic dystrophy

TESTS

- Genetic testing permits a specific diagnosis in many dystrophies
- Serum CK is elevated, but level varies w/ the type of dystrophy
- EMG typically shows myopathic features; myotonia is also present in myotonic dystrophy
- ECG may reveal conduction defects
- Muscle biopsy confirms clinical diagnosis

DIFFERENTIAL DIAGNOSIS

- Various dystrophies are distinguished from each other by genetic studies & by pattern of inheritance & muscle involvement; Duchenne & Becker dystrophies are X-linked dystrophinopathies

MANAGEMENT

- Supportive care includes passive stretching of joints, bracing and assistive devices
- Tenotomies & surgical stabilization procedures, depending of type of dystrophy
- Cardiac pacemaker & treatment for CHF, especially in emerin deficiency (Emery-Dreifuss dystrophy)
- Steroids may slow progression of Duchenne dystrophy

SPECIFIC THERAPY

- None, except as above
- Genetic counseling is important

FOLLOW-UP

- Close follow-up by experienced medical team is important to prevent complications & optimize mobility

COMPLICATIONS AND PROGNOSIS

■ Depends on type of dystrophy; Duchenne dystrophy characterized by rapid progression leading to disability & death; progression is slow in Becker, FSH & distal dystrophies; prognosis more variable or unclear in other varieties

MUSCULOSKELETAL PROBLEMS

CHRIS WISE, MD

HISTORY & PHYSICAL

History

■ Cervical spine (whiplash, strain): history of neck injury, pain on motion
■ Mechanical back pain: onset often after activity, heavy labor
  ➤ Worse w/ activity
  ➤ Radicular symptoms: herniated disc
■ Shoulder (rotator cuff) pain: middle-aged, overhead arm activities
  ➤ Pain worse w/ reaching, lying on it in bed
■ Chest wall pain: arm or extremity activities
  ➤ Pain reproduced by pressure
■ Elbow pain: lateral epicondylitis: lateral arm pain, worse w/ forearm activities
  ➤ Olecranon bursitis: local trauma, swelling
■ Hand & wrist pain
  ➤ Flexor tenosynovitis: palmar hand pain, fingers catching/ triggering
  ➤ Carpal tunnel syndrome: repetitive use, diabetes, pregnancy, RA, diffuse pain, tingling, median nerve distribution
  ➤ DeQuervain's tenosynovitis: repetitive use, radial wrist pain,
■ Hip girdle pain
  ➤ Trochanteric bursitis: lateral hip pain, worse lying on affected side
  ➤ Meralgia paresthetica: anterior upper thigh numbness, tight garment
■ Knee & lower leg pain
  ➤ Anserine bursitis: medial knee pain, worse in bed, associated OA
  ➤ Popliteal cyst: posterior knee pain, swelling, known joint disease

- Ankle & foot pain
  - Plantar fasciitis: plantar pain, worse w/ weight bearing
  - Achilles' tendinitis: posterior heel pain, overactivity
  - Morton's neuroma: interdigital pain, paresthesias
  - Tarsal tunnel syndrome: plantar pain, paresthesias

Signs & Symptoms
- Cervical sprain, whiplash: localized tenderness, spasm
- Mechanical back pain: localized tenderness, spasm
  - Negative straight-leg raising
- Shoulder (rotator cuff) pain: pain and/or weakness on resisted abduction, rotation
  - Limited abduction, rotation, lateral tenderness
- Chest wall pain: pain reproduced by pressure
- Elbow pain
  - Lateral epicondylitis: localized tenderness, worse w/ wrist extension
  - Olecranon bursitis: localized swelling over olecranon process
- Hand & wrist pain
  - Flexor tenosynovitis: localized tenderness, thickening over tendon
  - Carpal tunnel syndrome: reproduce paresthesias w/ percussion or wrist flexion
  - Thenar weakness or atrophy
  - DeQuervain's tenosynovitis: localized tenderness, reproduce pain w/ ulnar wrist distraction
- Hip girdle pain
  - Trochanteric bursitis: localized tenderness, lateral hip, normal range of motion in hip joint
  - Meralgia paresthetica: localized area of decreased sensation, anterior thigh
- Knee & lower leg pain
  - Anserine bursitis: medial knee tenderness, below joint line
  - Popliteal cyst: posterior knee swelling, small knee effusion
- Ankle & foot pain
  - Plantar fasciitis: localized tenderness, plantar surface of heel
  - Achilles' tendinitis: localized tenderness, posterior heel & tendon
  - Morton's neuroma: interdigital tenderness, paresthesia
  - Tarsal tunnel syndrome: plantar pain w/ percussion behind medial malleolus

TESTS

Lab Tests

- Blood studies only to detect underlying cause (eg, thyroid tests for carpal tunnel syndrome)
- Synovial fluid analysis for infection (WBC >1,000/mm3, culture positive), crystals; may be important in olecranon bursitis in particular
- Nerve conduction studies for carpal or tarsal tunnel syndrome
  Imaging
- Radiographs useful only to rule out underlying joint & bony pathology in selective situations (persistent back, shoulder, foot, knee pain)
- MRI or ultrasound in refractory shoulder rotator cuff symptoms
- MRI or CT for persistent back pain w/ sciatica for herniated disc

DIFFERENTIAL DIAGNOSIS

- For local syndromes
  - Arthritis, fracture or other bony lesion
- For low back pain
  - Ankylosing spondylitis (young male, chronic symptoms, morning stiffness)
  - Fracture (trauma history, known or risk for osteoporosis)
  - Septic disc or bone lesion (fever, immunocompromised)
  - Malignancy (older, rest pain, weight loss)

MANAGEMENT

What to Do First

- Search for generalized medical illness, history of injury, underlying articular process

General Measures

- Local ice for acute symptoms, heat for more chronic symptoms
- Range-of-motion exercises, local support (splint, elastic)
- Strengthening exercises during recovery
- Analgesics, NSAIDs

SPECIFIC THERAPY

Indications

- Pain interfering w/ function, sleep

Treatment Options
- Mechanical back pain: limited bed rest (2–4 days) w/ gradual resumption of activities
  - Cyclobenzaprine for rest in acute phase
  - Physical therapy, exercises during recovery
- Shoulder (rotator cuff) pain: ROM exercises, rotator cuff strengthening
  - Steroid injection
  - Surgery for recurrent or refractory symptoms
- Chest wall pain: local heat, analgesics, chest wall stretching exercises
- Elbow pain
  - Lateral epicondylitis: local heat, elastic support, steroid injections
  - Olecranon bursitis: aspiration of fluid
  - Antibiotics for infected bursa
  - Steroid injection for noninfected bursa
- Hand & wrist pain
  - Flexor tenosynovitis: steroid injection
  - Carpal tunnel syndrome: night splint, steroid injections, surgical release for persistent symptoms, motor weakness
  - DeQuervain's tenosynovitis: thumb splint, steroid injections
- Hip girdle pain
  - Trochanteric bursitis: steroid injection
  - Meralgia paresthetica: looser garments, time
- Knee & lower leg pain
  - Anserine bursitis: steroid injection
  - Popliteal cyst: knee joint aspiration, steroid injection
- Ankle & foot pain
  - Plantar fasciitis: local heat, heel cord & plantar stretching
  - Steroid injection for most, rarely surgery
  - Achilles' tendinitis: heel lift, heat, stretching, do *not* inject steroids
  - Morton's neuroma: wider shoes, steroid injection, occasional surgery
  - Tarsal tunnel syndrome: ankle support, steroid injection

Side Effects & Contraindications
- NSAIDs
  - Renal impairment, salt & fluid retention
    - Caution: hypertension, heart failure, edematous states
  - GI hemorrhage

> Risk factors
  - Previous peptic ulcer disease
  - Age >65
  - Concomitant use of oral steroids, anticoagulants
> Protective measures
  - Misoprostol
  - Proton pump inhibitor
  - COX-2 selective NSAID (celecoxib)
- Steroid injections
  > Local soft tissue atrophy, skin pigment changes
  > Rarely local inflammatory reaction
  > Very rarely infection

FOLLOW-UP
- Most localized syndromes respond eventually over weeks to months

COMPLICATIONS & PROGNOSIS
- Most conditions respond w/out long-term sequelae
- Mechanical low back pain: for symptoms >6 months continued disability likely
- Shoulder pain: "frozen shoulder" (adhesive capsulitis) or reflex sympathetic dystrophy (shoulder-hand syndrome)
- Carpal tunnel syndrome: permanent thenar weakness & atrophy

MYASTHENIA GRAVIS

MICHAEL J. AMINOFF, MD, DSc

HISTORY & PHYSICAL
- Variable weakness, leading to ptosis, dysphagia, diplopia, respiratory difficulty or limb weakness depending on pattern of muscle involvement
- Weakness aggravated by activity
- No sensory complaints
- Exam reveals weakness & fatigability of affected muscles, ptosis or extraocular palsies, aggravated by activity & relieved by rest
- Pattern of involvement varies w/ the pt

TESTS
- Clinical response to short-acting anticholinesterase (IV edrophonium)
- CT scan of chest for thymoma

- Electrophysiologic studies to detect impaired neuromuscular transmission
- Assay of serum acetylcholine receptor antibody & muscle-specific tyrosine kinase (MuSK) antibody levels

DIFFERENTIAL DIAGNOSIS
- Drug-induced myasthenia is distinguished by history of use of causal agent
- Pattern & variability of weakness distinguishes myopathies, motor neuropathies, motor neuronopathies

MANAGEMENT
- Assess severity of disease & adequacy of ventilation; provide ventilatory support as needed
- Avoid or replace meds interfering w/ neuromuscular transmission (eg, aminoglycoside antibiotics, beta blockers, calcium channel blockers, magnesium salts)

SPECIFIC THERAPY
- Anticholinesterases (eg, pyridostigmine) may relieve or reduce symptoms; dose has to be individualized; overmedication enhances weakness
- Steroids often helpful when response to anticholinesterases is poor, but may lead to initial worsening of symptoms; dose is individualized, but initial high dose is tapered to lower maintenance dose
- Azathioprine or mycophenolate mofetil may be helpful if above measures are inadequate
- Thymectomy may lead to remission
- Plasmapheresis or IV immunoglobulins often helpful for major or acute disability, or prior to thymectomy

FOLLOW-UP
- Regular follow-up needed to avoid complications & ensure optimal therapy

COMPLICATIONS AND PROGNOSIS
- Involvement remains purely ocular in 20% of cases
- Disorder may worsen during systemic infections, thyroid disease, pregnancy or w/ drugs affecting neuromuscular transmission
- Thymoma is present in 10–20% of pts & is assoc w/ more severe disease
- Avoid inhalational anesthesia if possible; avoid or use neuromuscular blockers w/ great care

MYASTHENIC (LAMBERT-EATON) SYNDROME

MICHAEL J. AMINOFF, MD, DSc

HISTORY & PHYSICAL
- Variable weakness, esp. proximally in limbs, typically improving w/ activity
- Diplopia or dysphagia may occur
- Xerostoma, postural dizziness, constipation, impotence common
- May be history of malignancy
- Exam reveals weakness in variable distribution; improves after exercise
- Depressed tendon reflexes, augmented after exercise

TESTS
- May be mild response to IV edrophonium
- Electrodiagnostic findings are characteristic
- Chest x-ray may reveal underlying lung cancer

DIFFERENTIAL DIAGNOSIS
- Dysautonomic symptoms, response to activity & association with malignancy distinguish it from myasthenia gravis
- Pattern & variability of weakness distinguishes myopathies, motor neuropathies, motor neuronopathies

MANAGEMENT
- Underlying malignancy (usually small cell lung cancer) should be sought & treated
- Ensure ventilation is adequate & prevent aspiration

SPECIFIC THERAPY
- Cholinesterase inhibitors (pyridostigmine) may have mild benefit
- Guanidine sometimes helpful in escalating dose
- Diaminopyridine (not available in U.S.)
- Occasional pts require steroids, azathioprine, plasmapheresis or IV immunoglobulins, as for myasthenia gravis

FOLLOW-UP
- Close follow-up required to monitor neurologic disorder & underlying malignancy

COMPLICATIONS AND PROGNOSIS
- 50% of pts have underlying malignancy
- Aspiration pneumonia & ventilatory inadequacy may have fatal outcome

MYELODYSPLASTIC SYNDROME

D. GARY GILLILAND, MD, PhD

HISTORY & PHYSICAL

History
- Majority of cases are sporadic
- Risks: exposure to chemical solvents (e.g., benzene) or pesticides; significant exposure to ionizing radiation or chemotherapy (alkylating agents, topoisomerase inhibitors). Risk increases with age (median age at diagnosis approximately 65).
- Incidence approximately 1/100,000 per year all ages; 50/100,00 per year over 65
- High risk of progression to acute myelogenous leukemia (AML)

Signs & Symptoms
- Related to cytopenia of one or more hematopoietic lineages
- Neutropenia: bacterial infections (presentation with opportunistic infections rare)
- Anemia: fatigue, dyspnea on exertion, or angina in older patients
- Thrombocytopenia: easy bruisability, epistaxis, petechiae

TESTS

Basic Blood Tests
- CBC: neutropenia, anemia or thrombocytopenia. Absolute lymphocyte count usually normal
- Blood smear:
  - Granulocytes: poorly granulated, hyposegmented, Pelger-Huet anomaly
  - Red cells: hypochromic, polychromasia, teardrops, nucleated RBC
- Mild macrocytosis (MCV 100–105)
- Platelets: large, megakaryocyte fragments may be present
- Specific Diagnostic Tests:
- Bone marrow aspiration and biopsy:
  - BONE MARROW DYSPLASIA IS DIAGNOSTIC HALLMARK OF MDS
- Dysmyelopoiesis: large primary granules, decreased granules numbers, bizarre nuclear forms, Pelger-Huet cells.

- Dyserythropoiesis: multinuclear forms, nuclear fragments, megaloblastic changes, nuclear:cytoplasmic dyssynchrony, ringed sideroblasts on iron stain
- Dysthrombopoiesis: bizarre nuclear forms, decreased ploidy, "pawn ball" nuclei, micromegakaryocytes
- Increased myeloblasts

Other Tests:
- Cytogenetics on bone marrow; characteristic abnormalities = deletions (e.g., 5q-, 7q-, 20q); numerical abnormalities (monosomy 7, trisomy 8); translocations (e.g., t(3;21), t(5;12), t(1 1;16))
- Classification: undergoing revision. Current FAB nomenclature (French-American-British) categories: refractory anemia (RA, <5% marrow blasts); refractory anemia with ringed sideroblasts (RARS, <5% marrow blasts, >15% ringed sideroblasts); refractory anemia with excess blasts (RAEB, 5–20% marrow blasts); refractory anemia with excess blasts in transformation (RAEB-T, 20–30% marrow blasts). AML ≥30% marrow blasts.
- Chronic myelomonocytic leukemia (CMML) requires >1,000 moncytes/ml. Newer classification schemes: >20% marrow blasts = AML.

DIFFERENTIAL DIAGNOSIS
- Congenital Disorders
- Hereditary sideroblastic anemia (usually microcytic rather than macrocytic)
  - Fanconi's anemia (short stature, radial abnormalities)
  - Diamond-Blackfan syndrome
  - Kostmann's syndrome
  - Shwachman's syndrome
  - Down syndrome
- Vitamin Deficiency
  - B12, folate or iron deficiency
- Drug toxicity
- Marrow suppression from oral or parenteral medications
  - Toxins
  - Chemotherapy and/or radiation therapy
  - Alcohol
- Anemia of Chronic Disease
- Renal failure
  - Chronic infection, including tuberculosis
  - Rheumatologic and autoimmune disorders

- Viral marrow suppression
  - ➤ Epstein-Barr, hepatitis, parvovirus B19, HIV and others
- Marrow infiltration
  - ➤ Acute and chronic leukemias
  - ➤ Metastatic solid tumor infiltration
- Paroxysmal Nocturnal Hemoglobinuria
- Hypersplenism

MANAGEMENT

What to Do First

- Assess severity of pancytopenia; treat with supportive care
- Evaluate candidacy for allogeneic stem cell transplantation, especially in high-risk patients (see Prognosis)

General Measures

- Immediate attention to signs or symptoms of infection. Consider prophylactic antibiotics for repeat infections.
- Transfuse PRBC for symptomatic anemia
  - ➤ Treat iron overload with chelation therapy
- Minimize platelet transfusion to avoid alloimmunization. Transfusion guidelines: platelets <10,000/mcl, clinically significant bleeding, surgical procedure.

SPECIFIC THERAPY

Indications

- Symptomatic cytopenias are a general indication for treatment of MDS. Treatment options have improved recently, with FDA approval of methyltransferase inhibitors (5-Azadytidine, and anti-angiogenic agents (lenalidomide, Revlimid, Celgene).
  - ➤ Acute infection with neutropenia: Consider granulocyte colony-stimulating factor (G-CSF,Neupogen)
  - ➤ Symptomatic anemia: 15–30% of MDS patients with erythropoietin (Epo) level <2,500 mU/mL will respond to erythropoietin (Procrit) therapy. For patients refractory to monotherapy, dose escalation and/or c-administration of G-CSF may further increase response rate. Most recently, darbepoietin-alpha (DA, Aransep), a hypersialylated erythropoietic stimulating protein with a prolonged half-life, has shown erythroid responses comparable to rhuEP, with less frequent dosing, although optimal dosing and schedule of DA for MDS have not yet been established.

Treatment Options

- *5-Azacytidine* (Vidaza, Pharmion, Inc.) interferes with DNA methylation and prolongs median time of progression to AML, and median survival. 5-Azacytidine is now FDA approved for treatment of MDS and is indicated for MDS patients with symptomatic cytopenias. Another methyltransferase inhibitor, decitabine (Dacogen, MGI-Pharma), also has activity and is currently under review at the FDA.

- *Lenalidomide:* Agents with putative anti-angiogenic activity have been at the forefront of one of the most promising developments in treatment of MDS, although their precise mechanism of action in MDS is not fully understood. Lenaliodmide (CC-5013, Revlimid, Celgene) is a 4-amino-glutaramide analog of thalidomide and has remarkable activity in treatment of MDS. A landmark safety and efficacy study with oral lenalidomide in erythropoietin-unresponsive MDS patients resulted in a remarkable 58% overall response rate; the majority of pts achieved transfusion independence. Response rate was karyotype-dependent and highest in patients with chromosomal deletions of 5q31.1 (83%) compared with 56% of MDS patients with normal karyotype, and only 12% of patients with other karyotypic abnormalities. Based on these findings and results of additional phase II studies, lenalidomide has recently been approved by the FDA for treatment of transfusion-dependent patients with del5q.

- *G-CSF* (Neupogen) for treatment of selected cases of MDS with neutropenia, in particular in setting of acute infection

- *Erythropoietin* as above for treatment of symptomatic anemia

- *Allogeneic or Unrelated Donor Stem Cell Transplantation (SCT)*
  - ➤ Only curative therapy. Disease-free survival (DFS) variable, depends on age of recipient, stage of MDS, performance status, donor match. 70–80% DFS in best prognostic groups (age <40, good performance status, low risk MDS, HLA identical donor).

OR

- Enrollment in Clinical Trial

Side Effects and Complications of SCT

- May be severe and life-threatening; morbidity and/or mortality from infection, failure of engraftment, pulmonary hemorrhage, acute and/or graft vs. host disease, veno-occlusive disease, among others.

Contraindications to SCT for MDS

■ Age >65, poor performance status, lack of suitable donor, significant pulmonary, renal, cardiac or hepatic dysfunction. Patients with suitable donors who are not candidates for conventional SCT may be considered for non-myeloablative transplantation protocols.

FOLLOW-UP

During Treatment

■ Monitor patients treated with 5-azacytidine, lenalidomide, erythropoietin or G-CSF for evidence of hematologic response.

Routine

■ Off-protocol patients: monitor CBC to determine transfusion requirement for PRBC and/or platelets. Attentive monitoring and patient education for signs and symptoms of infection, especially in neutropenic patients.

■ For frequent PRBC, monitor for iron overload (Fe, TIBC, ferritin; consider MRI liver; definitive test = liver biopsy); treat overload with desferroxamine chelation.

COMPLICATIONS AND PROGNOSIS

■ Pancytopenia: morbidity and/or mortality from infection, bleeding
■ Progression to AML: morbidity and/or mortality from refractory AML, complications of chemotherapy.
■ International Prognostic Scoring System (IPSS). 4 risk categories that correlate with survival: Low, Intermediate-1, Intermediate-2, High

Score Value

■ Points:
  ➤ 0 for marrow blasts <5%, good karotype*, 0 or 1 cytopenias
  ➤ 0.5 for marrow blast 5–10%, intermediate karotype*, 2 or 3 cytopenias
  ➤ 1.0 for poor karyotype*
  ➤ 1.5 for marrow blasts 11–20%
  ➤ 2.0 for marrow blasts 21–30%
■ *Good: normal, -Y, del(5q), del(20q); Poor: complex (>3), any chromosome 7 abnormality; Intermediate: any other abnormality
■ #Hemoglobin <10 g/dl; Absolute neutrophil count <1,500/mi; Platelets <100,000/ml
■ SCORE: Low = 0; Intermediate-1 = 0.5–1.0; Intermediate-2 = 1.5–2.0; High ≥2.5

MYELOMA AND GAMMOPATHIES

KENNETH C. ANDERSON, MD

HISTORY & PHYSICAL

■ Less than two fold increased risk in farmers, paper producers, furniture manufacturers, and wood workers

■ Bone pain or pathologic fracture; recurrent infections; symptomatic anemia, renal insufficiency, hypercalcemia, or hyperviscosity; nerve root or spinal cord compression

TESTS

Basic Blood Studies:

■ anemia, leukopenia, thrombocytopenia, renal insufficiency, hypercalcemia, quantitative monoclonal protein with associated hypogammaglobulinemia

Basic Urine Studies:

■ Quantitative monoclonal protein and albumin

Basic Bone Studies:

■ Lytic lesions and/or osteoporosis on bone survey

Specific Diagnostic Tests

■ Excess plasma cells on bone marrow biopsy

■ Excess plasma cells on tissue biopsy of plasmacytoma

Other Tests as Appropriate

■ serum ß2 microglobulin

■ C reactive protein

■ Lactic dehydrogenase

■ Serum viscosity

■ Nuclear magnetic resonance imaging of spine (suspected cord compression or solitary plasmacytoma of bone)

■ Computerized tomographic scan (plasmacytoma)

■ Cytogenetics

■ Plasma cell labelling index

■ Bone marrow flow cytometry

DIFFERENTIAL DIAGNOSIS

■ Monoclonal gammopathy of unknown significance: low level monoclonal protein in blood and/or urine without other symptoms or signs of myeloma

- Primary amyloidosis (AL): fibrils consisting of variable region of immunoglobulin light chain in heart, tongue, gastrointestinal tract, and skin; in 20% cases associated with myeloma
- Waldenstrom's macroglobulinemia: elevated serum IgM, excess bone marrow lymphoplasmacytoid cells, visceral but rare bone involvement
- Non-Hodgkin's lymphoma: lymph node, visceral, and/or bone marrow infiltration with monoclonal B cells, occasionally associated with serum monoclonal protein
- Other lymphoproliferative syndromes: distinct histopathology

MANAGEMENT

What to Do First
- Assess severity and pace of disease, complications, and candidacy for treatment

General Measures
- Vigorous hydration
- Avoid nephrotoxic medications

SPECIFIC THERAPY

Observation
- Systemic, indolent or smoldering myeloma, Stage I myeloma (low level monoclonal protein and bone marrow plasmacytosis, no bone disease, asymptomatic)

Conventional Chemotherapy and Supportive Care
- All other stages of myeloma

Conventional Therapy
- Melphalan/prednisone; dexamethasone; vincristine/doxorubicin/dexamethasone; thalidomide/dexamethasone; other combination chemotherapy
- All cytotoxic; equivalent response rates but responses more rapid to combination chemotherapy
- Limit exposure to myelotoxic agents (including alkylating agents and nitrosoureas) to avoid compromising stem cell reserve prior to stem cell harvest in candidates for transplant

High-Dose Therapy
- Autologous stem cell transplant for patients with adequate cardiac, pulmonary, renal, and hepatic function; modest prolongation of survival, but no cures to date.
- Allogeneic transplantation in clinical trial

Radiotherapy

■ Involved field: (45–50 Gy) for solitary plasmacytoma; 30 Gy for palliation

■ Total body irradiation: component of preparative regimen for transplant

FOLLOW-UP

■ Quantitative immunoglobulins and quantitation of M protein (with alternate cycles of therapy and every 3 months thereafter)

■ Complete blood count, differential, platelets

■ BUN, creatinine, calcium

■ Bone survey annually or for symptoms

■ Bone marrow biopsy as clinically indicated

Maintenance Therapy

■ Steroids: every other day prednisone modestly prolongs progression free survival after conventional therapy

■ Interferon: slight prolongation of progression-free, but not overall, survival; multiple adverse sequelae

COMPLICATIONS AND PROGNOSIS

Response

■ Complete response: Disappearance of monoclonal protein and plasmacytomas, <5% bone marrow plasma cells, and no increase in size and number of bone lesions for at least 6 weeks

■ Partial response: ≥50% reduction in serum monoclonal protein, reduction in 24 hour urinary light chain excretion by either >90% or to <200 mg/24 h, >50% reduction in size of plasmacytomas, and no increase in size or number of lytic lesions for at least 6 weeks

■ Minimal response: ≥25% to ≤49% reduction in serum monoclonal protein, 50 to 89% reduction in 24 h light chain excretion (which still exceeds 200 mg/d), 25 to 49% reduction in size of plasmacytomas, and no increase in size or number of lytic lesions for at least 6 weeks

■ No change: not meeting criteria for minimal or partial response

■ Disease progression: reappearance of monoclonal protein; a sustained > 25% rise in monoclonal protein in serum or urine; development of new sites of lytic disease or hypercalcemia

Salvage Therapy for Progressive Disease

■ Repeat primary conventional dose therapy (if relapse at >6 months)

- Cyclophosphamide-VAD (hyperCVAD), etoposide/dexamethasone/ara-C/cisplatin (EDAP), high dose cyclophosphamide: responses but myelosuppressive
- Dexamethasone, thalidomide, Bortezomib as single agents or in combination: responses without significant myelosuppression
- Autologous stem cell tranplant: can prolong survival, but no cures
- Allogeneic transplant: responses from graft-versus myeloma effect, but high related morbidity and mortality

Supportive Care
- *Bone disease*
  - Bisphosphonates in all patients with documented bone disease including osteopenia
  - Bisphosphonates in smoldering or stage I disease in clinical trial
  - Bone survey yearly; bone densitometry or metabolic studies reserved for clinical trial
- Radiation therapy
  - Low dose (20–30Gy) radiation therapy for palliation of uncontrolled pain, for impending pathologic fracture, or impending cord compression
  - Consider impact on stem cell harvest
  - Orthopedic consultation for long bone fractures, bony compression of spinal cord or vertebral column instability
- *Hypercalcemia*
  - Hydration and steroids supplemented with furosemide, bisphosphonates, and/or calcitonin
- *Hyperviscosity*
  - Plasmapheresis as adjunctive therapy for symptomatic hyperviscosity
- *Anemia*
  - Consider erythropoietin for anemic patients
- *Infection*
  - Prophylactic antibiotics as adjunct to specific myeloma therapy, i.e. dexamethasone
  - Intravenous immunoglobulin therapy only in the setting of recurrent life-threatening infection
- *Renal dysfunction*
  - Vigorous hydration
  - Avoid non-steroidal anti-inflammatory drugs and intravenous contrast
  - Plasmapheresis and combination chemotherapy

Prognosis

- Dependent upon stage of disease; overall median survival is 3–4 years for conventional therapy and 4–5 years posttransplant.

MYELOPROLIFERATIVE DISORDERS

ALISON R. MOLITERNO, MD

HISTORY & PHYSICAL

- MPDs are acquired bone marrow stem cell disorders that share varying degrees of elevated peripheral cell counts, marrow fibrosis and splenomegaly
- Many patients are identified by routine blood work and are otherwise asymptomatic
- Symptoms and signs related to polycythemia include headaches, itching especially after bathing, plethora, hypertension, gastrointestinal ulcers and venous or arterial thrombosis
- Symptoms related to splenomegaly include early satiety, left upper quadrant fullness or pain
- Symptoms associated with high platelet counts include migraine headaches, visual disturbances, erythromelalgia, easy bruising or bleeding, transient ischemic attacks and venous or arterial thrombosis

TESTS

Molecular basis of these disorders is heterogeneous; diagnosis rests on assembling clinical findings and laboratory tests

Basic Tests

- complete blood count with differential
- peripheral blood smear
- bone marrow exam to assess cellularity, fibrosis, karyotype
- peripheral blood assessment for JAK2 V617F mutation

Specific Tests

- Polycythemia vera
  - ➤ elevated red cell mass by isotope dilution
  - ➤ normal oxygen saturation > 92%
  - ➤ erythropoietin level – low or normal in PV

JAK2 V617F positive in 90% of PV

- Idiopathic myelofibrosis

> teardrop poikilocytosis with early myeloid forms, nucleated red cells on the peripheral blood smear

> bone marrow fibrosis in absence of a secondary cause

JAK2 V617F positive in 50% of IMF

■ Essential thrombocythemia

> exclusion of the above two diseases, exclusion of secondary causes of high platelets

JAK2 V617F positive in 40% of ET

DIFFERENTIAL DIAGNOSIS

■ Polycythemia vera

> secondary causes of erythrocytosis:

- hypoxemia, carbon monoxide, high affinity hemoglobin, lung disease, pulmonary shunts, sleep apnea, testosterone excess, polycystic kidney disease, renal cell carcinoma, liver cysts/tumors, plasma volume contraction

■ IMF

> other causes of myelofibrosis: metastatic carcinoma, infection (HIV, TB), other hematologic disorders (acute leukemia, CML, myelodysplasia, hairy cell leukemia), SLE, renal osteodystrophy

- Essential thrombocytosis
  - other causes of thrombocytosis: PV, IMF, iron deficiency, CML, malignancy, inflammation, post-splenectomy state, chronic inflammatory conditions

MANAGEMENT

What to Do First:

■ lower hemoglobin – target males to 14 gm/dl, females to 12 gm/dl by weekly phlebotomy if necessary

■ exclude Philadelphia chromosome by karyotype or PCR in cases of idiopathic myelofibrosis or essential thrombocythemia

SPECIFIC THERAPY

Indications for treatment

■ PV

> control red cell mass via phlebotomy, hydroxyurea, or interferon

> pruritys may respond to antihistamines, interferon or hydrea

> low-dose aspirin for thromboprophylaxis

■ IMF

> supportive care

> consider hydrea, splenectomy or splenic irradiation for symptomatic splenomegaly

> thalidomide and prednisone, or erythropoietin trials for anemia

➤ consider allogeneic bone marrow transplant for younger patients
with progressive IMF
- Symptomatic thrombocytosis
  ➤ bleeding or thrombosis may respond to platelet lowering agents,
  such as anagrelide, hydroxyurea
  ➤ low dose aspirin for erythromelalgia

FOLLOW-UP
- PV – hemoglobin should be monitored monthly then q 3 months
once a stable regimen is achieved
- IMF – q 3 month CBC and physical
- ET – q 6 month CBC and physical

COMPLICATIONS AND PROGNOSIS
- Poor prognostic indicators for any of the MPDs include the development of anemia in the setting of marrow fibrosis
- Thrombotic complications
  ➤ Intra-abdominal thromboses (portal vein, hepatic vein) and
  stroke are very high in patients with an uncontrolled red cell
  mass
  ➤ Thrombotic risk due to high platelet count alone is controversial
  ➤ consider anti-platelet agent or lowering platelet count if history
  of or strong risk factors for thrombosis are present
- Massive splenomegaly may result in splenic infarctions, portal
hypertension, varices, and worsening anemia
- Many patients with ET will progress to PV or IMF over years to
decades
- Poor prognostic indicators for IMF include hemoglobin <10 gm/dl,
age, percentage of blasts in periphery, presence of night sweats,
weight loss, fevers. Approximately 20% patients with IMF will progress to leukemia.

MYOCLONUS

CHAD CHRISTINE, MD

HISTORY & PHYSICAL
- Episodic uncontrolled focal or generalized jerks
- Occasionally assoc w/ seizure disorder
- May be spontaneous or stimulus dependent (action myoclonus)
- Sudden, rapid, twitch-like muscle contractions
- Distribution may be focal segmental or generalized
- May be assoc w/ infectious, degenerative or metabolic disease

TESTS
- Diagnosis made clinically
- Blood & urine: normal in essential myoclonus
- Brain & spinal cord imaging: normal in essential myoclonus
- EEG: may show abnormalities in myoclonic epilepsies

DIFFERENTIAL DIAGNOSIS
- Epilepsy: excluded by history & EEG
- Degenerative disorders: Alzheimer's disease, Huntington's disease, Wilson's disease, Lafora body disease excluded clinically
- Infectious disorders: AIDS dementia, prion disorders; viral encephalitis, subacute sclerosing panencephalitis excluded by history & serologic studies
- Metabolic: drug intoxications or withdrawal; hypo- or hyperglycemia; uremia, hepatic encephalopathy excluded by history, blood & urine studies
- CNS injury: head injury, stroke or tumor excluded by neuroimaging

MANAGEMENT
- Depends on cause

SPECIFIC THERAPY
- Epileptic myoclonus may respond to valproic acid or benzodiazepines
- Postanoxic myoclonus may respond to 5-hydroxytryptophan or levetiracetam

FOLLOW-UP
- Depends on cause & severity

COMPLICATIONS AND PROGNOSIS
- Depend on cause

NARCOLEPSY

CHAD CHRISTINE, MD

HISTORY & PHYSICAL
- Excessive daytime sleepiness requiring daytime naps in setting of adequate sleep
- Onset in 2–4th decade
- Cataplexy may also occur & is often triggered by emotional events.
- Sleep paralysis & hypnagogic hallucinations may occur.

TESTS

- Diagnosis made clinically
- Routine blood studies are normal.
- Brain imaging is normal.
- Histocompatability antigens (HLA-DR2, HLA-DQw1) are present in all Japanese & most white pts.
- Sleep studies are abnormal (overnight polysomnogram & multiple sleep latency tests).

DIFFERENTIAL DIAGNOSIS

- Sleep apnea, restless legs syndrome & psychiatric disorder excluded by history & by sleep studies (overnight polysomnogram & multiple sleep latency tests)
- Structural lesions (pituitary adenoma, midbrain glioma, etc) excluded by brain imaging

MANAGEMENT

What to Do First

- Educate pt about the disorder

General measures

- Determine severity
- Determine driving safety: many attacks are predictable & can be prevented by short daytime naps (15–20 minutes in duration)
- Exercise & caffeinated beverages may prevent attacks
- Avoid heavy meals before period when alertness is required

SPECIFIC THERAPY

Indications

- Excessive daytime sleepiness that does not respond to general measures
  - ➤ Modafinil
  - ➤ Pemoline
  - ➤ Methylphenidate
  - ➤ Dextroamphetamine
- Sleep paralysis & cataplexy
  - ➤ Tricyclic antidepressants
    - Protriptyline
    - Imipramine
    - Nortriptyline

FOLLOW-UP
- Depends on severity & response to treatment

COMPLICATIONS AND PROGNOSIS

Prognosis
- Cataplexy, hypnagogic hallucinations & sleep paralysis may improve
- Chronic disorder

NEPHROGENIC DIABETES INSIPIDUS

MICHEL BAUM, MD

HISTORY & PHYSICAL
- Congenital nephrogenic DI – neonate with irritability, vomiting, constipation, fever, failure to thrive
- Adults – polydipsia and polyuria

TESTS
- Neonates with hypernatremic dehydration with low Uosm – no response to vasopressin
- Adults and children – Water deprivation test – inappropriately low Uosm – no response to vasopressin

DIFFERENTIAL DIAGNOSIS
- X-linked – defect in vasopressin 2 receptor
- Autosomal dominant and recessive forms – defect in aquaporin 2 water channel
- Acquired – Li, demeclocycline, hypokalemia, hypercalcemia, sickle cell disease, obstructive uropathy, medullary cystic disease, amyloidosis, polycystic kidney disease, amphotericin
- Distinguish from other causes if polyuria/polydipsia: central diabetes insipidus, psychogenic polydipsia, and osmotic diuresis

MANAGEMENT
- Allow free access to water.
- Inherited – thiazide diuretics to decrease GFR and filtered load of water
- Acquired – treat primary cause

SPECIFIC THERAPY
N/A

FOLLOW-UP
- To monitor electrolytes and response to therapy
- Close observation during episodes of fluid loss such as vomiting or diarrhea

COMPLICATIONS AND PROGNOSIS
- Infants with repeated episodes of hypernatremia may have developmental delay.

NEUROFIBROMATOSIS

TOR SHWAYDER, MD

HISTORY & PHYSICAL

Basic Criteria
- NF-1 diagnosed by 2 or more of the following 7 criteria:
  - Six or more café-au-lait macules (CALM) (>5 mm in children, >15 mm in adults)
    - Occur at birth and later on (80% will have 5 CALMs by age 1 yr)
    - Increase in number through adulthood
    - Randomly distributed over body
    - Most are 2–15 mm
  - Two or more neurofibromas (usually by early teens) or one plexiform neurofibroma (seen in childhood, 25%)
  - Axillary or inguinal freckling (Crowe's sign) (75% of pts w/ NF-1 have this)
  - Optic glioma (present in childhood)
  - Two or more Lisch nodules (Iris hamartomas)
    - Infrequent <6 years old
    - 50% by age 30, 100% by age 60
    - Need slit-lamp exam to tell for sure
  - Bone lesions (seen in childhood)
    - Scoliosis 10–30%
    - Pseudoarthrosis – bowing of long bones (tibia most common, also seen in ulna, radius, clavicle, femur. Represents failure of union after fracture.)
    - Long bone problems
      - Scalloping of cortex
      - Lytic areas resembling fibrous cortical defects

- Calcifying subperiosteal hematomas (s/p trauma) can mimic neoplasia.
- Cranial
    - Hypoplasia of wing of sphenoid bone (5–10%)
➤ First-degree relative with NF-1

NB: Diagnostic criteria do not provide insight into severity or prognosis. Diagnosis can be made in 95% of cases by age 11 years.

Other Problems in NF-1
- Brain Problems
    ➤ Astrocytomas most common tumors
    ➤ Meningiomas
    ➤ Head circumference often large compared with height and weight
    ➤ MRI – Unidentified bright objects
        Unrelated to learning disabilities
        Frank mental retardation (IQ < 70) in 4–8%
- Other eye problems
    ➤ Enlarged corneal nerves
    ➤ Congenital glaucoma
    ➤ Optic nerve gliomas
        - About 15% of NF-1
        - Develop by age 10
        - Associated with precocious puberty
- Hypertension (2–5%)
    ➤ Look for pheochromocytoma, renal artery stenosis, NFs around the kidneys, Wilms' tumor, coarctation of aorta.
- GI problems
    ➤ Constipation frequent complaint
    ➤ Abdominal dyspepsia and angina
    ➤ Carcinoid tumors
    ➤ Obstruction, ischemia, perforation
- Arterial Lesions
    ➤ Intramural Schwann cell proliferation in large arteries leads to aneurysms

NF-2
- Central NF
- Bilateral VIII n. masses (acoustic neuromas)
- Meningiomas, gliomas, schwannomas
- Juvenile posterior subcapsular lenticular opacities

■ CALMs tend to be large, pale, few in number.

NF-1 NEVER progresses to NF-2; they are separate diseases.

Other types of NF (3–8) now thought to be mosaics of NF-1

TESTS

■ NF is a clinical diagnosis.

Skin biopsy of CALM is nonspecific.

■ Skin biopsy for neurofibroma

■ Slit-lamp exam for Lisch nodules

■ Other tests depending on organ affected

■ Genetic counseling strongly suggested

■ Causative Gene:

■ NF-1
> 17q11.2
> ras-GAP protein
A tumor suppressor gene
Gene product: neurofibromin

■ NF-2
> 22q11

■ Prenatal Testing
> Only if DNA data from family members known

■ Genetics
> Autosomal Dominant
> 30–50% cases are spontaneous mutations
> Postzygotic mutation is the probable cause of segmental NF

■ Statistics
> NF-1 occurs in 1 in 3,500
> NF-1 represents 96–97% of all NF cases
> NF-2 occurs in 3%

NB: No consistent prenatal complications

Check parents of NF-1 child; they may be mosaics.

If parent is a mosaic, chance of second child with full NF-1 <3%.

DIFFERENTIAL DIAGNOSIS

■ CALM
> Single CALMs do occur frequently in Caucasians, more occur in dark-skinned races.
> Multiple CALMs are strongly suggestive of NF-1, but not a sine qua non.
> Solitary large segmental CALMs exist frequently unrelated to any syndromes.

➤ Do occur in other genetic diseases
- Other Conditions with CALMs
  - McCune-Albright's syndrome
  - Polyostotic fibrous dysplasia
    - Russell-Silver
    - Bloom
    - Noonan
    - Watson
    - LEOPARD/multiple lentigines
    - Sotos
    - Proteus

MANAGEMENT
N/A

SPECIFIC THERAPY
n/a

FOLLOW-UP
- Check child's blood pressure regularly.
- Evaluate neurodevelopmental progress – e.g., learning disabilities.
- Growth velocity increase or decrease may indicate intracranial process.
- Evaluate for optic pathway tumors, esp. if precocious puberty and tall stature.
- Evaluate for skeletal changes (scoliosis).
- Support group (National NF Foundation)

COMPLICATIONS AND PROGNOSIS

Complications
- Response to nondepolarizing anesthetics
  - ➤ Old data that are incorrect
  - ➤ Recent data show no problem
- Psychological
  - ➤ Stigma of the "Elephant Man"
  - ➤ Proteus syndrome, not NF-1
- Malignancy
  - ➤ Neurofibrosarcomas
    - 5–10% degeneration rate
  - ➤ Focal neurologic signs
  - ➤ Rapid growth of plexiform NF
  - ➤ Persistent pain
  - ➤ Host of other neuroid malignancies reported

Prognosis

- Majority (>60%) of NF-1 patients have mild forms of disease, lead healthy and productive lives
- 20% have problems that need correction
- 20% have severe problems
- A progressive disorder; time, pregnancy, adolescence make it worse
- 25–40% have learning disabilities
- 5–10% have mental retardation
- LISTEN TO SPEECH, an early clue.
- Behavior problems
- Mean age of death is about 60
  - ➤ Due to malignancies and complications of neurofibromas

Manifestations	Age of clinical expression
Café-au-lait macules	Infancy to early childhood
Crowe's sign	Childhood
Neurofibromas	Late childhood – adolescence – adulthood
Plexiform NF	Infancy to adulthood
Lisch nodules	Late childhood to adulthood
Optic path tumors	Early childhood
Sphenoid wing dysplasia	Infancy
Long-bone bowing	Infancy
Scoliosis	Childhood
Hypertension	Childhood to adulthood
Learning disabilities	early childhood to adolescence
Nerve sheath tumors	Adolescence to adulthood

(adapted from Viskochil D. Management of Genetic Syndromes. 2nd Ed. 2005. Wiley-Liss, Inc.)

NEVI AND PIGMENTED LESIONS

JEFFREY P. CALLEN, MD

HISTORY & PHYSICAL

History

- Personal or family hx of melanoma, atypical moles or non-melanoma skin cancer?
- A change in the mole
- "Newly" recognized mole

- Nevi have a lifespan – may disappear as pt ages
- Nevi are common.

Signs and Symptoms
- Junctional nevus = flat lesion, characterized by pigmentation w/ sharp margin; usually symmetrical & small
- Intradermal nevus = elevated, sharply demarcated lesion, usually nonpigmented
- Compound nevus = combination of features of junctional & intradermal nevi; elevated, sharply marginated pigmented mole
- Atypical mole = has one or more characteristics of melanoma (see below)
  - ➤ Clinically suspicious lesions, suggestive of melanoma:
    - Morphology (A, B, C, Ds):
      - Asymmetry
      - Border irregularity
      - Color – variation w/in lesion
      - Diameter >6 mm
    - Pruritus or other sx
    - Recent accelerated growth pattern
    - Changes in "mole" such as growth, bleeding, irritation

TESTS

Laboratory
- Excisional biopsy of suspicious lesions for dermatopathology examination
- Histologic evaluation of margins

Clinical
- Dermoscopy (epiluminesence microscopy): reserved for experts in this technique
- Photography of all areas w/ nevi can be used to evaluate presence of new lesions or changes to existing lesions.

DIFFERENTIAL DIAGNOSIS
- Melanoma
- Atypical nevus
- Seborrheic keratosis – sharply marginated
- Lentigo (freckle)
- Dermatofibroma (biopsy)
- Thrombosed hemangioma (biopsy)
- Pigmented basal cell carcinoma (biopsy)

MANAGEMENT

Benign
- Lesions may be observed or removed for cosmesis.
- Atypical (dysplastic) nevi are removed if they have changed or there is high degree of suspicion for melanoma; they should be excised completely w/ small margin of clinically normal skin; often saucerized excision is acceptable.
- Narrow excision (2-mm margins) of lesions suspected to be melanoma

Malignant
- See "Melanoma."

SPECIFIC THERAPY
N/A

FOLLOW-UP

Benign
- Observation
- Cosmetic considerations
- Patients w/ multiple atypical moles or positive family hx of malignant melanoma:
  - At increased risk for developing melanoma
  - Regular follow-up at q 6–12 month intervals
  - Use of baseline photographs for evaluation of new &/or changing lesions

Counseling
- Sun protection measures
- Behavioral alteration
- Protective clothing: hats, tightly woven clothing
- Avoid midday sun.
- Regular use of broad-spectrum sunscreens SPF 15 or higher
- Avoid tanning salons.

COMPLICATIONS AND PROGNOSIS

Complications
- Surgical complications (bleeding, infection, scarring)

Prognosis Dysplastic nevi
- Lifetime risk of developing subsequent melanoma:
  - 7% if no family hx of melanoma
  - 50–100% w/ personal &/or family hx of melanoma

NIACIN DEFICIENCY

ELISABETH RYZEN, MD

HISTORY & PHYSICAL

History
- high corn protein diets, diarrhea, cirrhosis, alcoholism, prolonged infusions without vitamins, prolonged isoniazide treatment, malignant carcinoid

Signs & Symptoms
- dermatitis, diarrhea, dementia = symptoms of pellagra; cutaneous erythema, intertrigo, cutaneous hypertrophy, mucous membrane inflammation, tongue edema, abdominal distention, psychosis, encephalopathy, stomatitis

TESTS

Laboratory
- Basic urine studies:
  - N-methylnicotinamide excretion <0.8 mg/day

DIFFERENTIAL DIAGNOSIS
n/a

MANAGEMENT
n/a

SPECIFIC THERAPY
- balanced diet, niacinamide orally in divided doses

Side Effects & Contraindications
- None

FOLLOW-UP
n/a

COMPLICATIONS AND PROGNOSIS
- Reversible with replacement

NOCARDIOSIS

RICHARD A. JACOBS, MD, PhD

HISTORY & PHYSICAL

History

- *Nocardia* are aerobic, Gram-positive, branching filamentous organisms that appear beaded on Gram stain and are acid-fast.
- They are ubiquitous in nature, found in soil and organic matter.
- *N. asteroides* is most common species causing human infection; other human pathogens include *N. brasiliensis, N. farcinica, N. nova, N. transvalensis, N. otitidiscaviarum.*
- Transmission to humans is by inhalation or direct inoculation into skin; human-to-human transmission does not occur.
- Risk factors include immunosuppression (organ transplantation), corticosteroids, chronic lung disease (especially alveolar proteinosis) and diabetes; one third have no predisposing conditions.

Signs & Symptoms

- Pulmonary infection presents as cough, fever, weight loss, malaise and can be insidious or acute.
- Cutaneous disease results from direct inoculation and presents as mycetoma (usually tropical areas), chronic nodular lymphangitis with nodular lesions following the distribution of lymphatics (usually *N. brasilinsis*) or as cellulitis indistinguishable from other bacterial causes of cellulitis; cutaneous involvement resulting from hematogenous dissemination manifests as multiple, diffuse subcutaneous nodules that may be tender
- CNS disease presents insidiously with headache, nausea, vomiting, visual changes or focal neurologic findings resulting from abscess formation; meningitis occurs less frequently and usually presents subacutely with headache

TESTS

- Routine laboratory tests rarely helpful in making diagnosis; blood cultures almost always negative; in meningitis, CSF may be culture positive with hypoglycorrhachia and a neutrophilic pleocytosis
- Chest x-ray nonspecific-consolidation, nodules with or without cavitation, reticulonodular pattern and effusion all described
- CT or MRI of brain may reveal abscess

- Definitive diagnosis made by culturing organism from sputum, aspirate of lung nodule, lung abscess, brain abscess or cutaneous lesion
- Although Nocardia spp grow on most routine media, the laboratory should be notified to look for the organism since it can take 3–5 days to grow and colonies may be difficult to detect if mixed with other respiratory flora.

PCR not yet widely clinically available

DIFFERENTIAL DIAGNOSIS
- Other causes of pneumonia – in the immunocompromised patient Cryptococcus neoformans, Aspergillus spp, other fungi, *M. tuberculosis*, atypical mycobacteria, aspiration, other bacteria; other causes of brain abscess – bacterial and fungal; cutaneous lesions – fungal and mycobacterial

MANAGEMENT
- Nocardiosis should be considered in any immunocompromised patient with pulmonary, cutaneous and/or CNS disease.

SPECIFIC THERAPY
- Sensitivities of various species of Nocardia vary (*N. farcinica* is most resistant) and sensitivity testing should be performed on all clinical isolates.
- Trimethoprim-sulfamethoxazole (TMP-SMX) at a dose of TMP 5–10 mg/kg per day, in 2 or 3 divided doses, is the drug of choice with the most clinical experience; alternatives include imipenem, third-generation cephalosporins (cefotaxime and ceftriaxone), amikacin, amoxicillin-clavulanate, minocycline and fluoroquinolones (ciprofloxacin and levofloxacin)
- Combination therapy with TMP-SMX and amikacin or imipenem or a third-generation cephalosporin has been advocated as initial therapy for patients who are immunocompromised with systemic disease
- Duration of therapy depends on site of infection and the immune status of the host; cutaneous disease treated for 1–3 months; in the non-immunosuppressed patient, pulmonary and non-CNS disseminated disease treated for at least 6 months and CNS disease treated at least 12 months; immunocompromised patients treated at least 12 months
- Immunosuppressive medications should be decreased or discontinued, if possible

■ Surgical intervention is indicated to drain or excise large abscesses and in those who do not clinically respond after several weeks of therapy; in patients with brain abscesses, surgery indicated if abscess does not decrease in size after 1 month of therapy or increases in size after 2 weeks of therapy

FOLLOW-UP
■ Careful early follow-up to ensure clinical response; usually see improvement in 1–2 weeks; repeat radiographic studies of chest and/or brain in 2–4 weeks
■ When improved and clinically stable (usually after 1–2 months), parenteral regimen can be changed to oral therapy and the dose of TMP-SMX can be reduced to 5–10 mg/kg/day of TMP; serum concentration of sulfamethoxazole should be measured 2 hours after an oral dose to ensure adequate absorption (level should be 100–150 micrograms/mL) and dose should be adjusted as needed
■ Relapse after therapy, particularly in the immunocompromised patient, warrants careful follow-up for 6 months after completion of therapy.

COMPLICATIONS AND PROGNOSIS
■ Prognosis depends on site of infection and immune status of host; cutaneous disease is 100% curable; pulmonary disease associated with 10–20% mortality and brain abscess 20–30% mortality; mortality higher in all groups if underlying immunosuppression present

NONALCOHOLIC FATTY LIVER DISEASE

EMMET B. KEEFFE, MD

HISTORY & PHYSICAL

History
■ spectrum of NAFLD ranges from simple nonalcoholic fatty liver (NAFL) to nonalcoholic steatohepatitis (NASH) with cirrhosis.
■ NAFL found in 12–15% of general population, NASH found in 3–4%
■ common risk factors: metabolic syndrome (insulin resistance with obesity, type II diabetes mellitus, lipid abnormalities, hypertension)
■ less common associated conditions: TPN, rapid weight loss, abetalipoproteinemia, JI bypass, and drugs

- simple fatty liver: found in 70% of patients >10% over ideal body weight
- steatosis present in 1/3 of type II diabetics

Signs and Symptoms
- usually asymptomatic
- if symptoms present: constitutional and nonspecific, such as fatigue, weakness and malaise; hepatomegaly common on physical examination.

TESTS

Basic Studies: Blood
- increased AST and ALT and occasionally alkaline phosphatase

Other Tests
- exclusion of viral, autoimmune and genetic liver diseases

Imaging
- fatty liver by ultrasound, CT or MRI
- liver biopsy
  - ➤ diagnosis of NASH requires liver biopsy, showing characteristic findings of fatty change, lobular inflammation, hepatocellular injury and Mallory's hyaline, with or without fibrosis
  - ➤ histologic features of NASH and alcoholic hepatitis overlap
  - ➤ simple fatty liver characterized by hepatic steatosis without inflammation, necrosis or fibrosis
  - ➤ role of liver biopsy in diagnosis of NASH in routine clinical practice debated, with most clinicians not recommending biopsy, unless needed to exclude suspected alternative liver diseases

DIFFERENTIAL DIAGNOSIS
- Alcoholic hepatitis
- Hemochromatosis
- Chronic hepatitis C

MANAGEMENT

What to Do First
- Exclude alcohol abuse by collateral history if required
- Exclude viral, autoimmune, and genetic liver diseases by specific laboratory tests

General Measures

- No therapy has been proven beneficial, although metformin and thiazolidinediones show promise.
- Standard treatment includes gradual and sustained weight loss, exercise, control of diabetes and use of lipid-lowering agents, as necessary to control hypertriglyceridemia

SPECIFIC THERAPY

Treatment Options: Routine

- Gradual and sustained weight loss
- Exercise
- Control of diabetes mellitus
- Use of lipid-lowering agents, as needed

Treatment Options: Experimental

- Metformin: early results promising; long-term studies underway
- Rosiglitazone and pioglitazone: early results promising; large, multicenter studies underway
- Ursodeoxycholic acid: large randomized trial showed no benefit
- Vitamin E: small pilot studies suggest benefit
- Other hepatoprotective agents
- Phlebotomy, if associated iron overload
- Betaine: benefit demonstrated in one pilot study
- Liver transplantation for end-stage liver disease

FOLLOW-UP

During Treatment

- regularly assess diet compliance, body weight, blood sugar and lipids

Routine

- Hepatic panel every 3 months

COMPLICATIONS AND PROGNOSIS

- Advanced fibrosis or cirrhosis in 10–50%
- Treat end-stage liver disease when occurs in standard fashion
- Refer for liver transplantation if end-stage liver disease

Prognosis

- Prognosis of simple fatty liver: benign
- Prognosis of NASH: risk of advanced fibrosis or cirrhosis, including liver failure
- NASH: may recur after liver transplantation

NONGRANULOMATOUS SYSTEMIC VASCULITIS

ERIC L. MATTESON, MD

HISTORY & PHYSICAL

- Polyarteritis nodosa (PAN)
  - ➤ Pts of any age; no gender difference
  - ➤ Fever, weight loss, hypertension, abdominal pain, peripheral neuropathy, vasculitic skin rash, abnormal kidney function or urine sediment due to renal ischemia or infarction, microaneurysms in visceral arteries
- Microscopic polyangiitis (MPA)
  - ➤ Like classic PAN but w/ renal disease w/ active sediment due to necrotizing glomerulonephritis
  - ➤ Cough (w/ hemoptysis)
- Essential cryoglobulinemic vasculitis (ECV)
  - ➤ Similar to MPA; often w/ Raynaud's phenomenon, livido reticularis
- Cutaneous leukocytoclastic angiitis (LCA)
  - ➤ New-onset purpuric rash confined to skin, often w/ other rheumatic disease or drug exposure
  - ➤ No systemic involvement
- Behçet's disease (BD)
  - ➤ Male:female 2:1; mean age about 30 yrs
  - ➤ More common in pts of Asian or Mediterranean descent
  - ➤ Aphthous oral (100%) and/or genital (70%) ulcers, uveitis (75%), meningoencephalitis 20%, arthritis (usually oligoarticular occasionally sacroiliitis) (40%), cutaneous vasculitis (50%)
- Cogan's syndrome (CS)
  - ➤ Interstitial keratitis (scleritis, uveitis, other forms of ocular inflammation); visual disturbance, hearing loss arteritis, aortitis, renal disease, abdominal pain
- Henoch-Schönlein purpura (HSP)
  - ➤ Children of any age; adults less often
  - ➤ Peak incidence in spring & fall
  - ➤ Upper respiratory infection in preceding 1–3 weeks
  - ➤ Palpable purpura, especially lower extremities (100%)
  - ➤ Abdominal pain (70%), mild renal abnormalities (40%)
- Kawasaki's disease (KD)
  - ➤ Children generally <8 yrs (usually <4 yrs) of age

➤ Bilateral conjunctival injection, fever >5 days, rash, mucus membrane changes ("strawberry tongue," etc), cervical lymphadenopathy

TESTS

Lab Tests
- CBC (anemia, thrombocytosis)
- ESR and/or C-reactive protein elevated
- Urinalysis for glomerulonephritis, esp. in MPA, ECV

Other Tests
- Skin biopsy: necrotizing vasculitis w/ leukocytoclasis in most forms; few or no immune deposits in MPA; IgA immune deposits in HSP; cryoglobulin immune deposits in ECV
- Sural nerve biopsy (esp. in PAN, MPA): necrotizing inflammation of small arteries
- ANCA: p-ANCA (anti-MPO) positive in MPA (40–80%)
- Cryoglobulins, rheumatoid factor in ECV
- Complement, ANA in some pts w/ LCV
- Hepatitis B, C, esp. in PAN, ECV
  ➤ Blood cultures to exclude endocarditis
  ➤ Antiphospholipid antibodies
- Other: In MPA, renal biopsy: necrotizing glomerulonephritis; pulmonary capillaritis

Imaging
- Angiogram often shows aneurysms & vessel narrowing in PAN; coronary aneurysms in 60% of pts who die of KD
- Echocardiography in CS: aortic root aneurysm
- Endoscopy in BD: mucosal ulcers, most often in right colon
- Chest X-ray: pulmonary infiltrates, hemorrhage; evaluate for emboli in BD; infiltrates in MPA
- Audiogram (CS)
- Ophthalmologic exam (CS)

DIFFERENTIAL DIAGNOSIS
- Bacterial sepsis, especially endocarditis, also disseminated Neisseria, rickettsiae
- Viral diseases, esp. hepatitis B, C
- Paraneoplastic syndromes assoc w/ cancers, esp. hematopoietic malignancies & adenocarcinomas

➤ Assoc w/ rheumatic disease (eg, SLE, rheumatoid arthritis, Sjogren syndrome)
- Cholesterol, mycotic emboli
- Drug reactions
- Atrial myxoma
- Serum sickness
- Systemic amyloidosis
- Familial Mediterranean fever

MANAGEMENT

What to Do First
- Assess extent & severity of vascular disease
- Control blood pressure; assessment of end-organ vascular integrity
- In cases of threatened organs (eg, abdominal angina w/ PAN, rapidly progressive glomerulonephritis, CNS disease or rapidly progressive mononeuritis multiplex, pulmonary disease; meningoencephalitis, eye disease in BD; rapidly progressive hearing loss in CS), begin "pulse" corticosteroids (eg, methylprednisolone, 1 g/d for 3 days)
- In MPA, ECV w/ severe progressive neuropathy, renal or severe pulmonary disease, add cyclophosphamide, adjusting dose for WBC; plasmapheresis sometimes also employed.
- In KD, aspirin or IV IgG, not corticosteroids

SPECIFIC THERAPY
- Microscopic polyangiitis
  ➤ Prednisone given initially & over the first 2–4 weeks then tapering; cyclophosphamide may be necessary
- Polyarteritis nodosa, essential cryoglobulinemic vasculitis
  ➤ As for MPA
  ➤ Antiviral agents in hepatitis B, C-associated disease
- Cogan's syndrome
  ➤ Prednisone, w/ methotrexate added
- Limited cutaneous angiitis
  ➤ Prednisone, w/ dapsone or cytotoxic agents
- Kawasaki's disease
  ➤ As outlined above under initial management
- Henoch-Schönlein purpura
  ➤ Most pts will do well w/ supportive care & NSAIDs
  ➤ Corticosteroids may be required for nonsurgical GI problems & cytotoxic agents for progressive renal disease
- Behçet's disease

➤ Oral, genital ulcers: azathioprine, thalidomide, corticosteroids (low dose), many other meds used

➤ Eye, CNS disease: azathioprine, cyclosporine, chlorambucil, cyclophosphamide

■ Other options for treatment of systemic vasculitis include TNF-alpha antagonists, azathioprine, mycophenolate mofetil

Side Effects & Contraindications

■ Side effects

➤ Corticosteroids: diabetes, weight gain, osteoporosis, cataracts, hypertension, increased susceptibility to infection

➤ Cytotoxic agents: cytopenias, cancers, alopecia, hepatotoxicity, infections; use prophylaxis against P. jiroveci pneumonia w/ cytotoxics & high-dose corticosteroids

■ Contraindications

➤ Corticosteroid therapy: none absolute

➤ Cytotoxics & thalidomide: pregnancy, cytopenias, active serious infection

FOLLOW-UP

■ Every 2–4 weeks, assess disease activity by history & physical exam

■ ESR or C-reactive protein every 1–2 months (may not normalize even w/ good disease control)

■ After 2–4 weeks, taper steroid dose by ~5 mg every 2 weeks to 10–15 mg/day, then more slowly

■ Continue cytotoxic agents, slowly adjusting downward

■ Watch for relapses, esp. in BD, MPA, CS, ECV, LCA

COMPLICATIONS & PROGNOSIS

■ BD

➤ Visual loss, blindness, aneurysm rupture, arterial or venous clotting disorders

■ MPA, ECV

➤ Progressive renal failure, central & peripheral neuropathy w/ stroke & paralysis, pulmonary hemorrhage, infarction of other arteries

■ PAN

➤ Renal failure, infarction of GI & other arteries; peripheral, central neuropathies

■ KD

➤ Acute thrombosis of coronary artery, coronary or other aneurysms

- HSP
  - GI complications, including intussusception, obstruction, bleeding, infarction, perforation
  - Progressive renal failure (rare)
- CS
  - Deafness, visual loss, heart failure

NONMELANOMA SKIN CANCERS: BASAL CELL CARCINOMA

ROGER I. CEILLEY, MD

HISTORY & PHYSICAL

- 80% of non-melanoma skin cancers
- Increasing incidence with age; most >40 years of age
- Usually begins as a small, slow-growing, waxy, semi-translucent nodule with central depression and telangiectasia
- May appear as reddish eczematous patch (superficial type) an irregular pigmented nodule (pigmented type) or as a waxy white sclerotic plaque (morphea or sclerotic type)
- Most often on head, neck and other sun-exposed areas of fair-skinned individuals with light-colored hair and eyes
- Ulceration, crusting and bleeding on slight injury common
- Usually history of extensive sun exposure, also seen in old burn scars, vaccination sites, previous x-ray treatment areas, immunosuppression and chronic arsenic exposure
- Genetic and congenital factors: basal cell nevus syndrome (Gorlin syndrome), Bazex syndrome, albinism, epidermolysis bullosa dystrophica, nevus sebaceus of Jadassohn and xeroderma pigmentosum

TESTS

Biospy:
- Tangential (shave) if lesion is elevated
- Saucerization if lesion is flat
- Excision or punch biopsy if sclerotic or recurrent

Full body examination to detect other cancerous or precancerous lesions

Palpate regional nodes

DIFFERENTIAL DIAGNOSIS
SCC

- Often indistinguishable from small BCC. Usually faster-growing, more common on dorsum of hands, involve vermillion surface of lower lip. Horny keratotic material not seen with BCC.

Nevus:

- Softer, non-ulcerated, no bleeding or telangiectasia and longer duration

Sebaceous hyperplasia

- Yellowish nodules with depressed center. No bleeding or crusting.
  Scar or morpheaform:
- Usually no bleeding, crusting or progression of size

Seborrheic keratosis

- Waxy, brown with "stuck-on" appearance

Malignant melanoma

- May be indistinguishable from pigmented variety. No translucent appearance or telangiectasia.

Psoriasis/chronic dermatitis:

- Easily mistaken for superficial BCC (do not clear with topical treatment)

MANAGEMENT

- Treatment depends on age, size, type of lesion, previous treatment, cosmetic concerns, medical status.
- Prophylaxis (sun safety recommendations):
  - ➤ Seek shade between 10 AM & 4 PM.
  - ➤ Wear light-colored, tightly woven, protective clothing.
  - ➤ Apply sunscreens with a SPF of at least 15 and reapply frequently, esp. with prolonged sun exposure, sweating, or swimming.

SPECIFIC THERAPY

Excision:

- Ideal for lesions 5–7 mm or less with discrete clinical borders

Curettage/C&D:

- Small nodular lesions not in central facial areas
- Superficial lesions, esp. on trunk
- Poor for large, recurrent or sclerotic types

Mohs micrographic surgery (MMS):

- Highest cure rate, esp. for recurrent tumors and poorly defined margins, tissue sparing, allows for immediate repair with clear margins
- Tumors in the "H zone" of the face (nose, nasolabial folds, periorbital, periauricular areas)

- Aggressive histologic types: morphea-like, micronodular sclerosing, recurrent, baso-squamous type
- Size: >2 cm
- Immunosuppressed patients

Cryosurgery:

- Best for smaller lesions not in the "H zone", <2 cm in size
- Not for recurrent lesions or tumors involving bone or cartilage

Radiation therapy:

- Best for older patients with small lesions or patients unable or unwilling to have surgery
- Not for previously x-rayed lesions
- Not for scalp or forehead, where permanent alopecia or bone necrosis may develop

Topical 5-FU:

- Only approved for superficial BCC
- Disadvantages: prolonged treatment time, discomfort, and risk of eliminating the superficial component with persistence of deeper subclinical foci

Laser surgery:

- Blind treatment similar to C&D, cryosurgery or radiation
 Investigational:
- Intralesional 5-FU
- Systemic retinoids: patients with BCC nevus syndrome, xeroderma pigmentosum and for chemoprevention
- Other: Imiquimod
  - ➤ Immunotherapy (IL-1, IL-2, interferon, Alfa-2A, interferon g)
  - ➤ Photodynamic therapy

FOLLOW-UP

- Self-examination and regular follow-up by a physician with expertise in skin cancer to detect new primary skin cancers and precancerous lesions
- Life-long follow-up, since recurrences have been reported after 10 years (80% will occur in 2–5 years)
- Most patients q 6–12 months, but higher-risk patients (multiple BCC, XP, BC nevus syndrome, chronic radiation dermatitis and immunosuppression) need to be seen more frequently
- Periodic general medical evaluation – some reports indicate an increased incidence of internal malignancy (salivary glands, larynx, lung, breast, kidney and non-Hodgkin's lymphoma)

- Patients with BCC prior to age 60 may have a higher rate of breast cancer, testicular cancer and non-Hodgkin's lymphoma.

COMPLICATIONS AND PROGNOSIS

- Deep invasion and local destruction (eye, ear, nose, even into the brain are the greatest risk)
- Recurrence varies with treatment; lowest with MMS
- Metastasis is extremely rare (0.0028%) since there is a need for supporting stromal tissue for cell survival. Usually in the head or neck with extremely large or multiply recurrent lesions.
- Very likely to develop other primary skin cancers, especially if positive family history, extensive sun exposure, history with multiple AKs, or immunosuppressed.

NONMELANOMA SKIN CANCERS: SQUAMOUS CELL CARCINOMA

ROGER I. CEILLEY, MD

HISTORY & PHYSICAL

- Often begins as a reddish, indurated nodule with a hard keratotic or ulcerated surface on ears, face, lips, dorsum of hands and arms
- May begin as small keratotic papule or scaly plaque
- Usually in individuals with fair skin, eyes and hair, and individuals (>60%) with actinic damage and actinic keratoses. Head and neck most common, 90% on sun-exposed areas.
- Incidence increases with age; most are >40 years old
- May develop in old scars, x-ray-damaged skin, chronic ulcers and chronic HPV infections (esp. in types 16, 18, 31 and 33)
- May grow in a few months, become large, ulcerated and deeply invasive
- Metastasis may be early if lesion large and ulcerated, patient is immunosuppressed or with tumors arising in chronic ulcers
- Lower lip lesions often develop in actinic cheilitis.
- Palpate regional nodules.

TESTS

- Biopsy
- Chest x-ray, CT scan, needle aspirate or node biopsy if metastasis suspected

DIFFERENTIAL DIAGNOSIS
- Basal cell carcinoma
- Warts
- Chronic ulcer
- Discoid lupus erythematosus
- Psoriasis or nummular eczema
- Seborrheic keratosis
- Other non-melanoma skin cancers
- Hypertrophic actinic keratosis

MANAGEMENT
- Examination to determine invasion or metastasis

SPECIFIC THERAPY
- Based on location, etiology, size, histologic type and immune status
- Smaller lesions: excisional biopsy with 2-mm margin with an ellipse or tangential (saucer) excision
- Large flat lesion: incisional or punch biopsy
- Large bulky lesion: incisional biopsy
- Biopsy technique: injection of local anesthetic around and not into the lesion

TREATMENT
- CURETTAGE & ELECTRODESICCATION (C&D)
  - ➤ Best for superficial or small, nodular non-recurrent lesions
  - ➤ May lead to hypertrophic or hypopigmented scars and notching of eyelids or lips
  - ➤ Residual tumor may be buried under scar, making detection of recurrence difficult.
- MOHS MICROGRAPHIC SURGERY
  - ➤ Best for large, invasive, recurrent or in dangerous areas such as the "H" area of the face (nose, nasolabial folds, periorbital or periauricular area). Excellent histologic control of margins.
  - ➤ Immunosuppressed patients
  - ➤ Aggressive histologic pattern with poor differentiation, perineural or lymphatic invasion
- CRYOSURGERY
  - ➤ Smaller (<2 cm), well differentiated, superficially invasive, and not in areas with high risk of recurrence
  - ➤ Disadvantages includes prolonged healing and hypopigmented scars.

- RADIATION THERAPY
  - ➤ Best for patients >55 with smaller lesions or those unwilling or unable to have surgery
  - ➤ Mainly if perineural invasion
  - ➤ May be an adjunct to excision of large and/or aggressive histologic types
  - ➤ May be used as palliation of nonresectable tumors
  - ➤ Disadvantages: scars worsen with time, risk of secondary cancer after many years, may lead to permanent alopecia and bone necrosis on scalp or forehead. Not for previously x-rayed tumors or most recurrent lesions.
- TOPICAL 5 Fluorouracil (5-FU)
  - ➤ For very superficial, noninvasive, and Bowen's disease
  - ➤ Disadvantage: may eliminate the superficial component with persistence of deeper subclinical foci
- LASER
  - ➤ Blind destructive procedure. Similar results with Cryo, C&D and x-ray.
  - ➤ May be more costly
- Photodynamic Therapy
  - ➤ Application of photosensitizing agent followed by light exposure
  - ➤ Another form of destruction
  - ➤ Requires at least 2 visits per treatment
- INVESTIGATIONAL
  - ➤ Intralesional 5-FU
  - ➤ Systemic retinoids
  - ➤ Interferon

FOLLOW-UP
- Self-examination with regular follow-up by a physician with expertise in skin cancer
- Life-long follow-up to detect new primary skin cancers and recurrence of previously treated lesions. Examination to include regional lymph nodes.
- Most follow up q6–12 months unless "high-risk patient" w/ multiple CAs, severe photodamage, immunosuppression, presence of multiple precancerous lesions such as HPV or AKs.
- Periodic general medical evaluation to detect other cancers such as cancer of the respiratory organs, oral cavity, small intestine, non-Hodgkin's lymphoma and leukemia
- PREVENTION

➤ Sun safety behavior life-long:
- Seek shade between 10 AM & 4 PM.
- Wear light-colored, tightly woven, protective clothing
- Apply sunscreens with a broad-spectrum SPF 15 or greater and reapply every 2 hours when outdoors for long periods.

➤ Treat precancerous lesions or in situ lesions such as AKs and HPV infections.

COMPLICATIONS AND PROGNOSIS

■ Recurrence rates vary with tumor type and treatment.

■ Lowest recurrence rate 10% for small well-differentiated lesions by MME, 40%+ if perineural spread

■ Metastasis with mortality of 18% if lesions arise on sun-damaged skin; 20–30% or more if they develop in a scarring process such as an ulcer

■ Very likely to develop other skin cancers, esp. if positive family history, extreme photodamage, actinic keratoses present, HPV infections or immunosuppression.

NON-STEROIDAL ANTI-INFLAMMATORY DRUGS

MICHAEL B. KIMMEY, MD

HISTORY & PHYSICAL

History

■ Dyspepsia most common side effect of NSAIDs
➤ occurs in 15% of chronic users on a daily basis
➤ less common with cyclo-oxygenase (COX) – 2 specific NSAIDs
➤ does not correlate with endoscopic findings of ulcers

■ Gastric and duodenal ulcers are usually asymptomatic until they bleed or perforate

■ Small intestinal ulcers and strictures are uncommon but can cause symptoms of intestinal obstruction or chronic GI bleeding and anemia

■ Type of NSAID important when considering the risk of GI side effects
➤ NSAIDs can inhibit COX-1 and/or COX-2 isoenzymes. COX-1 inhibition is responsible for GI ulceration and antiplatelet effects, while COX-2 inhibition reduces pain and inflammation
➤ most NSAIDs inhibit both COX-1 and COX-2 isoenzymes and are considered "non-selective" NSAIDs; these NSAIDs linked to

➤ gastroduodenal ulcers and their complications, including bleeding and perforation

➤ some NSAIDs have relatively less COX-1 inhibition and may have lower risks of GI complications (etodolac, nabumetone, and meloxicam)

➤ COX-2 specific NSAIDs (celecoxib and rofecoxib) do not cause gastroduodenal ulcers and have been shown in prospective randomized studies to cause 60% fewer GI bleeds and perforations than nonselective NSAIDs; these drugs do not have effects on platelet function and are therefore not effective for cardiovascular prophylaxis

➤ aspirin is a nonselective NSAID and is associated with GI bleeds and perforations even when used in low doses for cardiovascular prophylaxis; enteric-coating and buffering with antacids do not protect against the GI complications

Signs & Symptoms
■ dyspepsia
■ upper GI bleeding
■ chronic iron deficiency anemia

TESTS

Laboratory Tests
■ laboratory tests in dyspeptic patients are usually normal
■ patients with GI bleeding may have anemia and/or iron deficiency
■ patients with ulcers should be tested by serology for H pylori infection, although this infection neither enhances or reduces the risk of NSAID associated ulcers

Imaging Tests
■ Endoscopy
➤ upper GI endoscopy is the most sensitive and specific test for the diagnosis of NSAID related ulcers and associated mucosal damage
➤ gastric ulcers are found in 15% and duodenal ulcers in 5% of chronic NSAID users
➤ erosions are more common, but are superficial and rarely cause clinical problems
➤ endoscopic treatment of bleeding ulcers is effective in over 90% of patients and reduces mortality and the need for surgery

- **Upper GI X-rays**
  - ➤ less sensitive than endoscopy for detecting ulcers and should NEVER be obtained in patients with GI bleeding

DIFFERENTIAL DIAGNOSIS

- Dyspepsia: gastroesophageal reflux disease, peptic ulcer disease, gallstones, chronic pancreatitis, other drugs
- Upper GI bleeding: erosive esophagitis, esophageal varices, other causes of ulcers, Mallory-Weiss tears, vascular lesions
- Chronic anemia: colorectal cancer or polyps, small intestinal ulcers

MANAGEMENT

Dyspepsia:

- stop or change to another NSAID (e.g. a COX-2 inhibitor)
- trial of H2 receptor antagonist or proton pump inhibitor
- if symptoms persist despite above, upper GI endoscopy

GI bleeding

- hospitalize if hemodynamically significant or transfusion needed
- upper endoscopy to determine cause and treat

Severe abdominal pain

- plain and upright abdominal x-rays to diagnose GI perforation
- hospitalization and surgery usually required for GI perforation

SPECIFIC THERAPY

- H2 receptor antagonists
  - ➤ for persistent dyspepsia despite changing NSAID
  - ➤ ranitidine or nizatidine
  - ➤ famotidine
  - ➤ cimetidine
  - ➤ side effects: (rare) bone marrow suppression, gynecomastia (with cimetidine)
  - ➤ contraindications: gastric atrophy and achlorhydria
- Proton pump inhibitors
  - ➤ for persistent dyspepsia despite changing NSAID
  - ➤ for ulcer healing when NSAID must be continued
  - ➤ omeprazole, esoeprazole or rabeprazole
  - ➤ lansoprazole
  - ➤ pantoprazole
  - ➤ side effects: headache, diarrhea
  - ➤ contraindications: gastric atrophy and achlorhydria

FOLLOW-UP

- patients with dyspepsia whose symptoms do not respond to H2 receptor antagonists or proton pump inhibitors within 1 week should be endoscoped to look for ulcer or other cause of symptoms
- patients with gastric ulcers should have repeat upper endoscopy after 8 weeks of treatment to confirm healing (to exclude gastric cancer)

COMPLICATIONS AND PROGNOSIS

- dyspepsia is not life threatening and is usually responsive to stopping medications or use of acid reducing drugs as noted above
- ulcers almost always heal with acid reducing drugs but can recur
- ulcer complications (bleeding and perforation) occur in 2% of users of nonselective NSAIDs per year but can be avoided by using COX-2 specific inhibitors. The risk of dying from a major GI hemorrhage is 5–10%

NONTUBERCULOUS MYCOBACTERIAL INFECTIONS

RICHARD A. JACOBS, MD, PhD

HISTORY & PHYSICAL

History

- Nontuberculous or atypical mycobacteria are a heterogeneous group of acid-fast bacilli that are ubiquitous in nature.
- Cause disease in normal hosts, immunocompromised pts (especially HIV) and those with underlying pulmonary disease (bronchiectasis)
- Not transmissible from person to person
- Most species NOT sensitive to usual antituberculous drugs
- Most common pathogens are Mycobacterium avium complex (MAC), M. kansasii, M. fortuitum, M. chelonae, M. abscessus, M. marinum, M. scrofulaceum

Signs & Symptoms

- Pulmonary – MAC and M. kansasii most common causes; M. fortuitum and M. abscessus less common; presentation insidious with chronic cough, fatigue, weight loss over months
- Lymphadenitis – in children MAC and M. scrofulaceum most common causes, with M. tuberculosis less common; in adults M.

tuberculosis most common etiology; presents as painless enlargement of cervical nodes that may form sinus tract with chronic drainage

- Skin and Soft Tissue – M. fortuitum, M. chelonae, M. abscessus and M. marinum (fish tank granuloma) cause localized skin nodules following traumatic inoculation; lesions may ulcerate and M. marinum may cause sporotrichoid lesions (nodular lymphangitis)
- Disseminated disease – seen in advanced HIV disease; caused by MAC; present with persistent fevers and weight loss

TESTS

- Atypical mycobacteria can colonize respiratory tract; diagnosis requires two positive sputum cultures if one is smear positive, or three positive sputum cultures if none are smear positive, or pathologic confirmation of invasive disease on biopsy in symptomatic patients with CXR or chest CT showing cavitary upper lobe disease, diffuse nodular infiltrates or bronchiectasis
- Other forms of disease require positive cultures
- In disseminated disease in HIV, blood cultures positive in ≥95%

DIFFERENTIAL DIAGNOSIS

- Other causes of chronic cough and pulmonary infiltrate, especially M. tuberculosis, fungal infection, neoplasia, sarcoidosis
- Other causes of cervical adenopathy (see lymphadenopathy and lymphangitis)

MANAGEMENT

- Consider diagnosis in patients with chronic cough and infiltrates
- Obtain specimens for culture
- If AFB smear positive, empirical therapy for M. tuberculosis started while awaiting results of culture and speciation

SPECIFIC THERAPY

- Pulmonary – MAC treated with clarithromycin 500 mg bid (or azithromycin), plus ethambutol 15 mg/kg daily, plus rifampin 600 mg daily (or rifabutin) until cultures negative for 1 year; M. kansasii treated with INH 300 mg daily, plus ethambutol, plus rifampin for 18 months (M. kansasii resistant to pyrazinamide); M. abscessus treated with IV amikacin 15 mg/kg daily plus IV cefoxitin 12 g daily in divided doses for several weeks followed by 6 months of clarithromycin
- Lymphadenitis – treated by surgical excision; antituberculous therapy not required

- Skin and Soft Tissue – M. marinum sensitive to clarithromycin, ethambutol, doxycycline, minocycline, rifampin and trimethoprim-sulfamethoxazole; two drugs used for at least 3 months; M. fortuitum sensitive to amikacin, cefoxitin, trimethoprim-sulfamethoxazole, erythromycin and ciprofloxacin; therapy based on sensitivity testing; initial IV therapy for several weeks with two drugs intravenously, followed by oral therapy with two drugs for 3 months after resolution of lesions; surgical debridement may be needed

FOLLOW-UP
- Pulmonary symptoms take months to improve, even with appropriate therapy.
- Monthly sputum cultures until negative
- Periodic radiographic studies to ensure resolution
- Skin infections followed clinically

COMPLICATIONS AND PROGNOSIS
- Cure rate for pulmonary MAC 70–80%; progressive pulmonary insufficiency and death in those who fail to respond
- Cure of M. abscessus and M. chelonae pulmonary disease rare; intermittent therapy for symptomatic recurrences long-term strategy

OBESITY

PATSY OBAYASHI, MS, RD, CNSD, CDE

HISTORY & PHYSICAL

History
- Chronic excessive accumulation of body fat
- Calorie intake exceeds energy expenditure

Physical Signs
- Body mass index (BMI = weight in kg/height in m2)
    - BMI = 25–30 = overweight
    - BMI = ≥30 = obesity
    - BMI = ≥40 = extreme obesity
- Waist circumference >35 inches = risk for women
- Waist circumference >40 inches = risk for men
- Percent ideal body weight >120%

TESTS

Basic Tests: Blood
- Glucose, fasting
- Cholesterol: HDL, LDL, total
- Uric acid
- T3, T4

Basic Tests: Other
- Weight
- Height
- Blood pressure

DIFFERENTIAL DIAGNOSIS
- Chronic liver disease
- Renal failure
- Chronic steroid use
- Thyroid dysfunction
- Pregnancy

MANAGEMENT

What to Do First
- Create energy deficit
- Assess attitudes, motivation, present behaviors

General Measures
- 1 lb. Body fat = 3500 kilocalories
  - ➤ 500 kcal energy change/day = 1 lb weight change/week
- Physical activity, gradual increase to ≥30 minutes daily
- Specific, realistic, individualized short and long-term goals
- If <1200 kcal for women/1500 kcal for men, multivitamins needed

SPECIFIC THERAPY

Indications for Treatment
- BMI >30 (obese)
- BMI = 25–29.9 (overweight) with ≥2 comorbidities or increased waist circumference

Treatment Options
- Revised dietary guidelines for Americans (USDA)
- Physical activity each day
- Decreased:
  - ➤ saturated fats, cholesterol, total fats
  - ➤ sugars

> salt
> alcohol
- 50–60% carbohydrate calories, ≤30% fat calories (≤10% saturated fat), 10–20% protein calories
- Size acceptance approach (maintain healthy behavior, body size de-emphasized)
- Calorie-reduced diets (500–1000 kcal/day deficit for 1–2 lb. weight loss/week)
- VLCD (Very low calorie diets)
  > 400–800 kcal/day usually liquid form
- BMI ≥30
  > Generally 12–16 weeks with 3–6 weeks for carbohydrate reintroduction
- Pre-packaged Meal Programs
- Fad diets (promise miracle cures, minimal effort)
- Physical activity/exercise (goal: ≥30 minutes physical activity daily)
- Behavior modification
- Pharmacotherapy
  > Combined with low-calorie, low-fat diet, increased physical activity, behavioral therapy
- Prescriptions only for BMI ≥30 kg/m2 or ≥27 kg/m2 with comorbidities

Surgery
- Only if BMI ≥40 kg/m2 or 35–40 kg/m2 with high risk comorbidities
- Include structured behavioral modification, extensive follow-up

Alternative Weight Loss Products (ie, ephedra, caffeine, chitosan, pyruvate)
- Side Effects and Complications

Revised Dietary Guidelines for Americans (USDA)
- No gimmicks, not "glamorous"
- Slow/no results if volume eaten not reduced

Size Acceptance Approach
- Increased yo-yo dieting (slower basal metabolic rate, loss of lean body mass, increased body fat)
- Sense of failure, low self-esteem
- Eating and exercise disorders

Calorie-Reduced Diets
- Poor long-term weight loss maintenance
- Total calorie reduction causes weight loss

- Severe restriction (<1000 kcal/day) not recommended
- Difficult compliance
- May reduce resting metabolic rate, promoting weight gain when restriction stopped

VLCD
- Poor long-term weight loss maintenance

Pre-Packaged Meal Programs
- Must learn food preparation, sensible dining out, self-controlled social eating for long-term maintenance

Fad Diets
- Weight loss from lower total calorie levels or diuresis, not diet composition
- No documentation of safety or long-term weight loss effectiveness

Physical Activity/Exercise
- Musculoskeletal complaints
- Requires individualized guidance

Behavior Modification
- No known side effects or complications

Pharmacotherapy
- Addiction/severe dehydration possible
- Long-term consequences unknown, i.e., fenfluramine and dexfenfluramine (primary pulmonary hypertension)
- Sibutramine (hypertension, bradycardia)
- Xenical (oily diarrhea, potential malabsorption of fat-soluable vitamins, carotenoids)
- Surgery
- Risk of death
- Potential vitamin B12, calcium, iron malabsorption, anemia
- Weight loss may not meet expectations, especially if high calorie foods eaten
- Alternate weight loss products
- Ephedra (17 deaths)
- Caffeine (dehydration, irregular heart beat, no weight loss shown)
- Chitosan (vitamin E malabsorption, increased calcium excretion, decreased bone density, no significant weight loss)
- Pyruvate (no physiologically relevant weight loss)

FOLLOW-UP

During Treatment
- Weekly weight documentation
- Regular reinforcement/supportive encouragement to maintain calorie and
- activity changes

Long-Term Maintenance
- Regular physical activity crucial
- Individualized lifestyle changes
- Maintain energy equilibrium (calorie intake ≤ energy output)

COMPLICATIONS AND PROGNOSIS
- Diabetes Mellitus: two-fold in mild obesity
  - ➤ five-fold in moderate obesity
  - ➤ ten-fold in morbid besity
- Hypertension: two-fold
  - ➤ 10% weight gain = 6.5 mm Hg increased blood pressure
- Coronary artery disease: 1.8–3.9 times relative risk
  - ➤ 10% weight loss can = 20% reduction CAD risk
- Osteoarthritis: 0.4–1.45% risk
- Gallstones: 18–35% risk
- Hyperlipidemia: 22 mg increase cholesterol synthesis/day with excess weight
- Sleep apnea: increased risk closely associated, no specific data
- Long-term weight loss maintenance extremely difficult
  - ➤ Inactive lifestyles
  - ➤ Overabundant foods
- Require lifelong commitment

OBSTRUCTIVE SLEEP APNEA

DAVID CLAMAN, MD

HISTORY & PHYSICAL

History
- Focused history key to diagnosis
- Pts often don't recognize symptoms
- Men affected more than women (4% vs 2% prevalence)
- Associated w/ obesity (esp BMI >27–30) & hypertension

Signs & Symptoms
- Snoring (often disturbs housemates)
- Excessive sleepiness or fatigue during daytime
- May manifest as frequent napping or dozing accidentally
- Morning headache
- Witnessed apnea
- Obesity
- Large neck size
- Overbite (retrognathia)
- Enlarged tonsils
- Narrowed airway noted in posterior pharynx
- Nasal obstruction

TESTS

Basic Blood Studies
- TSH (estimated prevalence of hypothyroidism 1–3% in apnea pts)

Screening Studies
- Oximetry during sleep often less helpful, because airflow not measured
- Home respiratory studies in selected pts

Specific Diagnostic Tests
- Formal polysomnography:
  - Gold standard
  - Measures airflow, chest movement, exhaled gases
  - Includes EEG staging of REM & non-REM sleep
  - Quantifies frequency of apneas & hypopneas
  - Index is # of events/h: usually referred to as
    - apnea-hypopnea index (AHI) or
    - respiratory disturbance index (RDI)

DIFFERENTIAL DIAGNOSIS
- Associated w/ abnormal breathing patterns:
  - Central sleep apnea
  - Upper airway resistance syndrome
  - Cheyne-Stokes respiration
  - Obesity hypoventilation (pickwickian syndrome)
- Other sleep disorders:
  - Narcolepsy
  - Idiopathic CNS hypersomnia
  - Periodic limb movements of sleep

- Diseases that may interefere w/ sleep & cause sleep-related symptoms:
  - COPD/emphysema/asthma
  - Sinusitis & postnasal drip
  - GERD
  - CHF
  - Anxiety & panic attacks

MANAGEMENT

What to Do First

- Weight loss (only 10–20% of obese pts can maintain significant weight loss)
- Avoid alcohol & sedatives for 4 h before bedtime
- Sleep in the lateral position (sew 1–2 tennis balls in back of T-shirt to prevent lying on back)
- Treat nasal allergies or obstruction

SPECIFIC THERAPY

Treatment Options

- After confirmatory sleep study:
  - CPAP:
    - Most consistently effective medical therapy if pt adherent
    - BiPAP (BiLevel) may be superior to CPAP in 10–20% of pts
    - Proper fit & settings can improve adherence
  - Oral appliances can be used during sleep to pull jaw forward (fit by dentist)
  - Surgery:
    - Surgical treatment not always curative; need good follow-up
    - Tracheotomy most effective, but a morbid procedure
  - Antidepressants: protriptyline or SSRIs options if other therapies ineffective
  - Oxygen: may be used if other therapies not tolerated, but does not open obstructed airway

FOLLOW-UP

- Clinical follow-up to see if symptoms improve
- For CPAP, follow-up in first 2–4 wk improves adherence
- For surgery or oral appliances, follow-up sleep study to document effectiveness
- If pt has significant change in weight or symptoms, repeat sleep study often recommended

COMPLICATIONS AND PROGNOSIS

Complications

- Sleepiness may lead to decreased job performance or reduced quality of life
- If sleepiness while driving or sleep-related auto accidents present, check local DMV reporting requirements
- Cardiovascular risk subject of ongoing study
- W/o treatment, excess risk of MI or CVA may approach 5–10% over 6–8 y

Prognosis

- Prognosis excellent, particularly for pts compliant on CPAP, & those w/ curative surgery

OCCUPATIONAL PULMONARY DISEASE

STEPHEN F. WINTERMEYER, MD, MPH

HISTORY & PHYSICAL

- Focused history critical
- Ask what patients do at work and what materials they handle

History

- Occupational asthma (OA):
  - \>250 known causative agents
  - common: isocyanates, latex, western red cedar
  - low chronic exposure leads to gradual (latent) sensitization
  - heavy acute exposure leads to immediate symptoms (reactive airways dysfunction syndrome/RADS)
- Pneumoconioses ("dusty lungs"):
  - Asbestosis:
    - pipe fitters, plumbers, ship builders
    - latency: >15 y
  - Silicosis:
    - sand blasters, highway workers
    - latency: variable, typically >10 y
  - Coal workers pneumoconiosis (CWP, black lung):
    - coal workers, graphite workers
    - latency: variable

➤ Hypersensitivity pneumonitis (HP):
  • fungi, thermophilic actinomycetes, animal products, certain chemicals
  • acute or chronic

Signs & Symptoms
■ Occupational asthma:
  ➤ chest tightness, dyspnea, cough, wheezing, prolonged expiration
  ➤ often worse during, after work day; better after days away
■ Pneumoconioses:
  ➤ dyspnea, crackles (esp basilar in asbestosis)
■ Hypersensitivity pneumonitis:
  ➤ fever, productive cough, dyspnea, rales

TESTS
Laboratory

Basic Blood Studies
■ occupational asthma, pneumocomioses: normal
■ hypersensitivity pneumonitis: elevated WBC, ESR, HP antibody panel (low sensitivity)

Specific Diagnostic Tests
■ Occupational asthma:
  ➤ Peak flow (to document temporal relationship to work): cheap, done by patient
    • ideally 4 times per day (after waking, noontime, after work, before bedtime)
    • do ≥2 weeks when working and ≥1 week when not working
  ➤ Spirometry
    • reproducible
    • gold standard in diagnosing obstruction
  ➤ Challenge testing (aerosol bronchoprovocation)
    • nonspecific (methacholine or histamine)
    • safe, done commonly
    • documents nonspecific bronchial hyperresponsiveness
    • confirms diagnosis of asthma
    • following hyperresponsiveness over time can be helpful
    • specific (the suspected agent)
    • some regard as gold standard in diagnosing OA
    • more common in Europe, Canada than in U.S.
    • more risks than nonspecific bronchoprovocation

- Pneumoconioses
  - Bronchoscopy, BAL/Bx usually not necessary
  - Asbestosis:
    - CXR: increased basilar interstitial markings
    - International Labor Office (ILO) classification used to grade
    - pleural plaques are marker of exposure
    - chest CT: similar findings with increased sensitivity
- PFTs: decreased FVC, TLC, DLCO (comorbid conditions may complicate interpretation)
  - Silicosis:
    - CXR: upper lung nodules, egg shell calcification of hilar nodes (ILO classification)
    - chest CT: similar findings with increased sensitivity
    - PFTs: decreased FEV_1, FEV_1/FVC; possibly reduced FVC, TLC, DLCO
  - Coal workers pneumoconiosis:
    - CXR: increased interstitial markings (ILO classification)
    - PFTs: decreased DLCO, FVC
  - Hypersensitivity pneumonitis:
    - CXR:
      - acute HP-infiltrate
      - chronic HP-increased interstitial markings, fibrosis
    - PFTs: chronic HP-decreased DLCO
    - Bronchoscopy/BAL/biopsy: increased CD8+ lymphocytes, granulomas

DIFFERENTIAL DIAGNOSIS
- Occupational Asthma
  - nonoccupational asthma
  - work-aggravated asthma (asthma exacerbated by exposures at work but not caused by exposures at work)
  - bronchitis
  - emphysema
  - vocal cord dysfunction
  - cardiac disease
- Pneumoconioses
  - other pneumoconioses
  - hypersensitivity pneumonitis
  - other interstitial lung diseases
- Hypersensitivity pneumonitis

> acute HP
  - pneumonia, bronchitis
> chronic HP
  - pneumoconioses
  - other interstitial lung diseases

MANAGEMENT

Occupational Asthma

- Environmental
  > avoidance of exposure single most critical element
  > avoidance can have significant financial impact (job change) so accurate diagnosis is important
- Clinical management
  > supplemental to exposure management
  > treat as for nonoccupational asthma
  > follow with spirometry

Pneumoconioses

- No effective treatment for any pneumoconiosis
- Asbestosis:
  > Environmental
    - minimize future exposure
  > Clinical
    - smoking cessation
    - cardiopulmonary rehabilitation
    - screen for mesothelioma
    - follow periodically
- Silicosis:
  > Environmental
    - minimize future exposure
  > Clinical
    - cardiopulmonary rehabilitation
    - screen for TB
    - follow periodically
- Coal workers pneumoconiosis:
  > Environmental
    - minimize future exposure (change jobs)
  > Clinical
    - cardiopulmonary rehabilitation
    - follow periodically

■ Hypersensitivity pneumonitis:
  ➤ goal: prevent chronic fibrotic changes
  ➤ avoidance of further exposure is critical
  ➤ steroids can be helpful
  ➤ cardiopulmonary rehabilitation
  ➤ follow periodically

SPECIFIC THERAPY

n/a

FOLLOW-UP

■ Occupational asthma
  ➤ depends on severity
  ➤ typically q 3–6 mo for 2 y after removal from exposure
  ➤ can do impairment rating 2 y after removal from exposure
■ Pneumoconioses (asbestosis, silicosis, coal workers):
  ➤ Exam, CXR/CT, PFTs q 6–12 mo
■ Hypersensitivity pneumonitis:
  ➤ acute:
    • follow frequently until symptoms have resolved
  ➤ chronic:
    • history, physical, PFTs q 3–6 mo
    • if stable, annually

COMPLICATIONS AND PROGNOSIS

Complications

■ Continued exposure leads to progressive impairment
■ Pneumoconioses, HP may cause chronic respiratory insufficiency
■ Asbestosis associated with mesothelioma and cancer
■ Increased risk of tuberculosis with silicosis > CWP

Prognosis

■ Occupational asthma
  ➤ variable
  ➤ best prognosis if diagnosis is made early and patient is removed from exposure
  ➤ poor prognostic factors
    • long duration of exposure, symptoms
    • poor FEV_1
    • development of non-specific bronchial hyperreactivity
■ Pneumoconioses (asbestosis, silicosis, coal workers)
  ➤ variable

- ➤ generally progressive
- ➤ poor prognostic factors
  - long duration of exposure/symptoms
  - high severity of exposure
  - short latency to symptoms
  - high degree of impairment
  - greater severity of radiographic findings
- ➤ cigarette smoking + asbestos exposure increases risk of bronchogenic carcinoma multiplicatively
- ➤ TB more common with silicosis and worsens prognosis
- ■ Hypersensitivity pneumonitis:
  - ➤ variable; can resolve
  - ➤ poor prognostic factors
    - long duration of exposure/symptoms
    - high severity of exposure
    - high degree of impairment (low FVC, TLC, DLCO)
    - fibrotic changes on imaging

ONYCHOMYCOSIS – TINEA UNGUIUM

BONI E. ELEWSKI, MD and JEFFREY P. CALLEN, MD

HISTORY & PHYSICAL

History
- ■ Toenail – Tinea pedis, athletic activities
- ■ Fingernail – Tinea manuum

Signs & Symptoms
- ■ Thick, dystrophic toenail or fingernail
- ■ Toenails more common than fingernails
- ■ May be painful in 40–50% of patients

TESTS

Laboratory
- ■ KOH tests – hyphae in subungual debris
- ■ Fungal culture – growth of dermatophyte – about 60% are culture positive
- ■ *Trichophyton rubrum* most common pathogen
- ■ Nail biopsy/clippings
- ■ PAS stain may reveal fungal hyphae
- ■ No Blood tests

DIFFERENTIAL DIAGNOSIS
- Psoriasis
  - ➤ Family history of psoriasis, presence of silvery red plaques on scalp, elbows, knees, gluteal area and nail pits
- Nail trauma
  - ➤ One nail
    - History of trauma, hematoma
    - No tinea pedis
- Lichen planus
  - ➤ Nail biopsy will confirm diagnosis.

MANAGEMENT
What to Do First
- Make correct diagnosis.

General Measures
- Oral antifungal agents required
- Debridement of dystrophic nail
- Topical agents are available and might be used as adjunctive therapy.

SPECIFIC THERAPY
- Terbinafine 12 weeks for toenail disease and 6 weeks for fingernail disease (pulse therapy appears to be less effective than continuous therapy) (NOTE – terbinafine has been demonstrated to be more effective than either of the other oral agents)
- Itraconazole – pulse therapy daily for 7 days, 1 week per month for 3–4 consecutive months for toenail disease and 2 consecutive months for fingernail disease
- Fluconazole – once weekly for 6–9 months

FOLLOW-UP
During Treatment
- Liver profile – baseline and periodic monitoring may be helpful

After Treatment
- Regularly assess response – evidence of continuous healthy nail growth
- Additional oral antifungal drug may be required in some patients.

COMPLICATIONS AND PROGNOSIS
- Not all patients respond to therapy.
- Mycologic cure rates vary from 40–90%.
- Some nails may be incapable of growth.
- Prevent reinfection – regular use of topical antifungal product on feet

ORAL CANCER

SOL SILVERMAN Jr, DDS

HISTORY & PHYSICAL
- squamous cell carcinoma accounts for >90% of oral cancers
- 95% occur beyond age of 40; men 2:1 over women
- increased risk with tobacco and alcohol usage
- can occur on any mucosal site; tongue most common
- may appear as white, red, red-white, ulcer and lump
- often firm to indurated
- pain varies from minimal to severe, depending upon stage
- palpable lymph nodes in neck or size >3 cm indicates advanced disease
- overall 5-year survival rate approximates 50%

TESTS
- incisional biopsy to confirm diagnosis
- MRI and PET scan for staging
- fine needle aspiration biopsy for suspected nodes

DIFFERENTIAL DIAGNOSIS
- leukoplakia, lichen planus, inflammatory disease, acute/chronic trauma, infection
- disappearance rules out cancer

MANAGEMENT
- refer to oncologist for staging and treatment options
- analgesics if necessary

SPECIFIC THERAPY
- surgery and/or radiation depends upon tumor type, location, stage
- surgery can cause functional defects
- radiation can cause changes in salivary flow, taste, blood supply (necrosis), mucositis
- chemotherapy is adjunctive (can cause severe mucositis)
- pretreatment dental care including hygiene and topical fluoride use

FOLLOW-UP
- high recurrence rate; routine visits
- about 20% will develop second head and neck primary cancers
- treatment for complications

COMPLICATIONS AND PROGNOSIS

- prognosis good for early-stage lesions; less than 50% for advanced lesions
- xerostomia requires frequent water sips/rinses, sugarless gum, topical lubricants (e.g., Oral Balance), and sialogogues (pilocarpine, cevimeline)
- candidiasis requires antifungal medications (systemic or topical)
- necrosis requires analgesics, antibiotics, possible surgery and hyperbaric oxygen
- dental decay requires restorative dentistry
- extractions require antibiotic coverage and may cause an osteoradionecrosis
- optimal oral hygiene is essential; fluoride dentifrices helpful
- dietary consult to maintain weight
- maxillofacial prosthetic consultation to ensure optimal function
- patients on bisphosphonates are at risk for osteonecrosis following an invasive dental procedure (i.e., extraction)

ORAL LICHEN PLANUS

SOL SILVERMAN Jr, DDS

HISTORY & PHYSICAL

- reticular form: lace-like white changes
- atrophic form: reticular changes with erythema
- erosive form: reticular + atrophic forms + ulcerations
- immunologic (autoimmune) etiology; sudden and spontaneous onset
- usually no family history
- primarily adult onset
- can be mucocutaneous
- small risk for malignant transformation; not contagious

TESTS

- clinical recognition
- biopsy

DIFFERENTIAL DIAGNOSIS

- epithelial dysplasia, carcinoma, candidiasis, hypersensitivity, erythema multiforme

MANAGEMENT
- no curative treatment
- establish diagnosis
- control pain

SPECIFIC THERAPY
- topical or systemic corticosteroids to control offending lymphocytes
- prednisone
- fluocinonide 0.05% ointment mixed with equal parts Orabase B paste; use 3–5 × daily
- clobetasol 0.05% gel; use 3–5 × daily

FOLLOW-UP
- periodic and as necessry for flares

COMPLICATIONS AND PROGNOSIS
- no cure; control symptoms
- small risk for malignant transformation to squamous cell carcinoma

---

ORBITAL CELLULITIS

RICHARD A. JACOBS, MD, PhD

HISTORY & PHYSICAL

History
- Predisposing factors include sinusitis, dental infection, trauma and spread of contiguous infections (conjunctivitis, dacrocystitis).
- Two distinct clinical syndromes: preseptal cellulitis (anterior to the orbital septum) and postseptal or orbital cellulitis involving the orbital contents
- Preseptal cellulitis caused by *Staphylococcus aureus* and streptococci
- Orbital cellulitis caused by organisms that cause acute and chronic sinusitis – *S. pneumoniae* and other streptococci, Haemophilus influenzae, Moraxella catarrhalis, S. aureus and anaerobes

Signs & Symptoms
- Preseptal cellulitis – chemosis, conjunctival injection; pain, swelling and erythema of eyelid
- Orbital cellulitis – signs and symptoms as above plus proptosis, impaired ocular mobility and decreased vision (late manifestation); fever and headache common

TESTS
- Gram stain and culture of any purulent drainage
- Blood cultures, if febrile
- Thin-section CT and/or MRI to document orbital and sinus involvement

DIFFERENTIAL DIAGNOSIS
- Pseudotumor and orbital tumors – fever and inflammation NOT present in these entities

MANAGEMENT
- Distinguish preseptal from orbital cellulitis.
- Orbital cellulitis always hospitalized; consult ENT and ophthalmology to assess need to drain sinuses and orbit
- Preseptal cellulitis can be treated as outpatient, if disease mild.

SPECIFIC THERAPY
- Preseptal cellulitis – dicloxacillin, cephalexin or clindamycin (severe penicillin allergy) as outpatient; naficillin, cefazolin or vancomycin for hospitalized patient
- Orbital cellulitis – Unasyn, Zosyn or ceftriaxone plus metronidazole; clindamycin plus a fluoroquinolone, if penicillin allergic

FOLLOW-UP
- Preseptal cellulitis responds in several days.
- Orbital cellulitis slower response to therapy; evaluate vision once or twice daily – if not improved or worsens in 48 hours, repeat CT or MRI

COMPLICATIONS AND PROGNOSIS
- Preseptal cellulitis – eyelid abscess (S. aureus) requiring drainage, but recovery complete
- Orbital cellulitis – vision loss, cavernous sinus thrombosis, enucleation

ORBITAL TUMORS

DEVRON H. CHAR, MD

HISTORY & PHYSICAL
- Proptosis, diplopia, decreased vision, or eyelid abnormalities.

TESTS
- Ophthalmic oncologic evaluation.

- Non-invasive imaging studies (CT, MRI, rarely ultrasound)
- CT direct fine needle biopsy has >98% accuracy.

DIFFERENTIAL DIAGNOSIS
- Most common cause of unilateral/ bilateral adult proptosis is thyroid orbitopathy:
- In younger adults, orbital proptosis is usually due to a benign process
- Differential diagnosis includes a gamut of benign and malignant processes: inflammatory, vascular lesions (cavernous hemangiomas) benign mesenchymal tumors, idiopathic lymphoid/ inflammatory process, and malignancies.
- Orbital lymphoma may be the first sign of systemic lymphoma.
- 5–10% of orbital turnefactions in older age groups are orbital metastases that may be the initial presentation of a lung, renal or gastrointestinal malignancy.

MANAGEMENT
- Surgery, radiation, less commonly chemotherapy, depending on histology.
- Specific therapy depends on the histology and known therapy response.

SPECIFIC THERAPY
n/a

FOLLOW-UP
- Follow-up is predicated in the histology of the lesion.

COMPLICATIONS AND PROGNOSIS
n/a

ORCHITIS AND EPIDIDYMITIS

JAMES W. SMITH, MD and DANIEL BRAILITA, MD

HISTORY & PHYSICAL

History
- Patients with epididymitis and orchitis present with recent onset of painful swelling of the scrotum.
- Infection can follow sexually transmitted diseases such as urethritis in patients <35 years of age.
- In patients >35 years of age, bacterial infection of urinary tract with enteric pathogens is most frequent.

- Patients may have history of urinary tract infection as dysuria or frequency.
- Infection could follow urinary tract instrumentation or surgery.
- <5 years of age, it is often associated with anatomic defects.

Signs & Symptoms

- Tender swelling of the posterior aspect of the scrotum with erythema is found early.
- Later, involvement of the entire scrotum and the testes may be present.
- Temperature elevation is present in about one third of pts.
- A urethral discharge could be apparent in patients with sexually transmitted infections.
- A hydrocele can be present.
- Findings consistent with viral infections are present with mumps (rare with vaccine) or other viral infections.

TESTS

Laboratory

- Urinalysis with culture is indicated in those >35 years of age.
- Do Gram stain of urethral exudate or first void urine (5 ml) for polymorphonuclear leukocytes, if <35.
- Do nucleic acid amplification test (Gen-probe on intraurethral swab or LCR or PCR on first void urine for Neisseria gonorrhoeae and Chlamydia trachomatis).

Other Screening Tests

- If sexually transmitted, do syphilis serology and HIV counseling and testing.
- If urinary tract infection with fever, do blood cultures two times.

Imaging

- If symptoms do not improve within 3 days of antibiotic therapy or if complications occur during the course of epididymitis, do ultrasound.

Biopsy

- Biopsy may be indicated in patients with chronic epididymitis.

DIFFERENTIAL DIAGNOSIS

- Testicular torsion is a surgical emergency to be considered in adolescent boys with onset of sudden pain: do high-resolution ultrasound.

- Testicular infarction or tumors such as lymphoma can cause swelling.
- Abscess can develop from a perforated viscus.
- External infection of scrotum with Candida can occur in immuno-compromised or diabetic patients.

MANAGEMENT

What to Do First
- Examine the urethral secretions or first void urine.
- If <5 years of age, initiate urologic evaluation.
- If <15 years of age with no evidence of urinary tract infection, observe without specific treatment.

General Measures
- Bed rest, scrotal elevations, analgesic, and local ice packs are helpful.
- Discontinue amiodarone, as may be a side effect of drug.

SPECIFIC THERAPY
- If sexually transmitted, administer ceftriaxone 250 mg IM in single dose PLUS Doxycycline 100 mg p.o. bid for 21 days for Chlamydial and gonococcal infections.
- If urinary tract infection is present in patient >35 years of age, administer levofloxacin 500 mg q day or gatifloxacin 400 mg QD for 21 days.
- If systemic symptoms with evidence of sepsis, hospitalize and administer parenteral therapy as levofloxacin 500 mg IV q day or combination of extended-spectrum cephalosporin as Cefepime 1–2 g q12h with an aminoglycoside as gentamicin 5–7 mg/kg q24h.
- If evidence of chronic granulomatous infection, do biopsy of epididymal tissue and administer appropriate antituberculous or antifungal therapy.

Side Effects & Contraindications
- Ceftriaxone
  - ➤ Side effects: rare allergic reactions
  - ➤ Contraindications:
    - absolute: penicillin hypersensitivity. Give alternative therapy with spectinomycin or quinolone.
- Doxycycline
  - ➤ Side effects: nausea, vomiting, diarrhea, photosensitivity and rarely liver function abnormalities
  - ➤ Contraindications:
    - absolute: hypersensivity to tetracycline
    - relative: patient unlikely to be compliant

- Levofloxacin
  - ➤ Side effects: gastrointestinal upset, diarrhea, rare skin rash and mental status changes in the elderly
  - ➤ Contraindications:
    - absolute: If patient has sexual contact with persons from Southeast Asia or sexual contact in Hawaii, California, or New England or is a male who has sex with males (resistant gonococci)

FOLLOW-UP
- During treatment, patient should be examined at 3 days and re-evaluated if failure to improve.
- If symptoms worsen, consider ultrasonography.
- If abscess formation or pyocele of the scrotum develops, do surgery.
- Persistent swelling after antimicrobial therapy could be evidence of chronic epididymitis due to Mycobacteria or fungal infections.
- Patients with epididymitis due to sexually transmitted organisms should refer all sex partners within the last 60 days for examination and treatment and avoid sexual intercourse until therapy is completed.
- If patient has viral orchitis, semen analysis is indicated.

COMPLICATIONS AND PROGNOSIS
- Most patients recover. Sterility is a rare feature of epididymitis; it does occur in viral orchitis.
- Rarely, abscess formation, pyocele, testicular infarction, chronic epididymitis occur.

OSTEOARTHRITIS

CHRIS WISE, MD

HISTORY & PHYSICAL
History
- Pain in affected joint
- Symptoms worse w/ activity or weight bearing
- Most common in knees, hips, lumbar or cervical spine, specific hand joints (carpal-metacarpal of thumb, proximal & distal interphalangeals)
- Morning stiffness usually <1 h

- Swelling usually bony (from bony spurs), knee effusions in some
- Risk factors for primary osteoarthritis
  - Age
  - Obesity (for weight-bearing joints)
  - Trauma or major joint injuries
  - Occupational factors for knees, shoulders, hips
  - Hereditary factors (eg, finger involvement in women)
- Causes of secondary osteoarthritis
  - Previous inflammatory arthritis
  - Joint dysplasias
  - Underlying bone disorders (osteonecrosis, Paget's disease)
  - Metabolic diseases (hemochromatosis, acromegaly, bleeding disorders)

Signs & Symptoms
- Pain on motion
- Tenderness
- Limited motion
- Crepitus (palpable grating sensation on motion)
- Prominent bony enlargement, soft tissue swelling or effusion
- In finger joints, bony enlargement of proximal interphalangeal (Bouchard's nodes) & distal interphalangeal (Heberden's nodes)

TESTS

Lab Tests
- All blood & serum lab studies are normal
- Synovial fluid has good viscosity, clear appearance, WBC <2,000, no crystals

Imaging
- Plain radiographs are diagnostic
- Weight-bearing films are useful for knees
- Radiographic features
  - Joint space narrowing
  - Subchondral bony sclerosis
  - Osteophytes (spurs)
  - Subchondral bone cysts
  - Bone density is normal or increased

DIFFERENTIAL DIAGNOSIS
- Rheumatoid arthritis: more soft tissue swelling, morning stiffness, systemic symptoms, different joint distribution (wrists, MCPs,

elbows, shoulders, ankles), elevated ESR, positive rheumatoid factor, erosive changes on radiograph
- Crystal-induced arthritis (gout, pseudogout): acute attacks w/ swelling, inflammatory synovial fluid, crystals in fluid
- Polymyalgia rheumatica: elderly patients, recent onset, predominant shoulder & hip girdle symptoms, prolonged morning stiffness, elevated ESR
- Localized bone disorders near joint (eg, fracture, osteonecrosis, Paget's disease)
- Psoriatic arthritis: involvement of IP finger joints resembles OA, younger age
  - ➤ Psoriatic skin or nail changes
- Localized musculoskeletal problems: localized to specific periarticular structures (tendons, bursae), pain w/ specific maneuvers, radiographs normal or only incidental age-related degenerative changes

MANAGEMENT

What to Do First
- Confirm diagnosis
- Assess degree of joint limitation, functional impairment

General Measures
- Modify activities to protect involved joint, but not total rest
- Local heat, other local pain relief measures
- Exercise to increase mobility, strength of periarticular muscles
- Walking program for knee involvement
- Weight loss w/ knee, hip & probably lumbar spine disease
- No known current therapy affects long-term outcome
Braces, canes or crutches as needed

SPECIFIC THERAPY

Indications
- Pain & limitation of activity
- Asymptomatic or minimally symptomatic OA need not be treated w/ specific measures

Treatment Options
- Analgesics: acetaminophen, tramadol, narcotics w/ caution in some
- Topical capsaicin
  - ➤ NSAIDs in low to moderate doses
  - ➤ Goal of therapy is pain relief

- Local corticosteroid injections
  - Useful in less severe disease
  - Limit to 4x/yr
- Local hyaluronic acid injections: series of 3–5 weekly injections
  - Approved only for knees
  - Benefit may last 6–12 months

Surgical Options
- Arthroscopic surgery: often useful in knees, shoulders
- Total joint arthroplasty for hips, knees, shoulders
- Fusion, osteotomy, for selected joints

Side Effects & Contraindications
- Analgesics: acetaminophen used w/ caution w/ liver disease, alcohol use
- NSAIDs: renal impairment, salt & fluid retention
  - Caution: hypertension, heart failure, edematous states
  - GI hemorrhage
    - Risk factors
      - Previous peptic ulcer disease
      - Age >65
      - Concomitant use of oral steroids, anticoagulants
    - Protective measures
      - Misoprostol
      - Proton pump inhibitor
      - COX-2 selective NSAID (celecoxib)
- Steroid injections: transient local pain, infection (rare)
- Surgery: general surgical risks (cardiac, pulmonary, thrombosis)
  - Infection
  - Long-term loosening

FOLLOW-UP
- Initial assessment of response to therapies (every 2–4 months)
- Long-term assessment for loss of response (every 6–12 months)
- Watch for complications of NSAIDs

COMPLICATIONS & PROGNOSIS
- Progression to end-stage joint disease, but is usually slow (over 5–20 years)
- End-stage joint disease leading to severe disability most common in knees, hips

OSTEOGENESIS IMPERFECTA

JAY R. SHAPIRO, MD

HISTORY & PHYSICAL

History

- heritable disorder of connective tissue with mutations in type I collagen in 90%: in 10% protein defect not identified
  - Usually dominant mutations, rare recessive or "mosaic" pattern of inheritance
- multiple fractures: vertebral bodies, extremities
- first fractures at birth, may be delayed until first decade or later
- fracture incidence falls at puberty, increases in 50s
- positive family history in 65% of cases: new mutation in 35%

Signs & Symptoms

- Patient appearance (phenotype) highly variable
- No defined relation of severity or phenotype to genotype
- Clinical classification: 4 major types have collagen mutations
  - Type I: Mild, little deformity, blue sclerae, dominant inheritance
  - Type II: Perinatal lethal shortly after birth, pulmonary insufficiency, severe skeletal deformities, "beaded" ribs from fractures, "broad bone" extremities
  - Type III: Severe, progressive, fractures at birth, marked skeletal fragility with deformities upper and lower extremities, scoliosis, height 3 feet, wheelchair-bound, frequently white sclerae, scoliosis, "helmet" skull, blue or white sclerae, dentigenesis imperfecta
  - Type IV: Moderately severe skeletal fragility with long-bone deformities, prominent scoliosis. Blue sclerae in childhood, lighter scleral hue in adults. Usually use aids to ambulate because of deformities.
  - Type V: Moderate to severe bone fragility, white sclerae, calcification of forearm interosseous membrane, history of hyperplastic callus after fractures, no collagen mutation
  - Type VI and VII (presumed) reported in single publications only, no collagen mutation
- Diagnosis may be apparent at birth, especially if type II, III or IV: multiple fractures, short limbs, pulmonary insufficiency, x-rays show healing (prenatal) fractures of ribs and extremities
- Short stature, especially with more severe disease

- Dentinogenesis imperfecta (DI) in 15% regardless of phenotype
  > "A" designation denotes DI absent, "B" indicates DI present
- Teeth fragile especially in children, brownish translucent quality
- Mixed sensory or conductive hearing loss appears 2nd-3rd decade
- Basilar invagination of the skull in severe cases: neurologic symptoms include headache, nerve compression, brain stem compression

Hydrocephalus in infants, etiology uncertain
- Scoliosis: more severe in types III and IV
- Joint hyperextensibility of digits, elbows and knees is mild
- Easy skin bruising, mild. Specific coagulation defect not defined.

Aortic and mitral insufficiency very infrequent

TESTS

Imaging
- Wormian bone (unmineralized cranial occipito-pareital islands) in 60% of infants or young children.
- Bone mineral density decreased by DXA. Accurate standards for children being developed.
- Mild cases: normal overall bone architecture even after fractures, but decreased cortical width and osteoporosis
- Severe cases: irregular fracture healing and skeletal deformities: Narrow or broad diaphyses in long bones
- Marked remodeling defect in II, III, IV: broad or narrow remodeling defect
- Epiphyseal dysplasia with persistent whorls of calcified fibrous tissue ("popcorn epiphysis") in III, IV
- epiphyseal plate may be absent, accounting for growth defect Vertebral fractures may occur in children
- dentinogenesis imperfecta: coronal constriction, absent pulp space
- Test hearing in children and young adults

Biochemical Testing
- Standard blood tests including alkaline phosphatase normal except after fracture
- Urine bone biomarker excretion (collagen crosslink, N-telopeptide, pyridinoline crosslink) elevated in 20%: increased bone turnover in children, low bone turnover in adults
- Hypercalciuria in approximately 15%: no clinical sequelae
- Renal calculi in a small percentage, independent of urine calcium

Pulmonary function studies

Sleep apnea in some type III/IV/V OI

Genetic Testing
- Gene sequencing to determine type I collagen alpha 1 or alpha 2 mutations:
- Large genes, 50 exons
- Collagen protein analysis: obtain skin biopsy: culture fibroblasts
- Prenatal diagnosis: Ultrasound at 16–18 weeks; chorionic villus sampling, amniocentesis with DNA testing

DIFFERENTIAL DIAGNOSIS
- Infants and Children:
  - Thanatophoric dwarfism
  - Achondroplasia
  - Hypophosphatasia: severe perinatal and infantile
- Teenagers
  - Idiopathic juvenile osteoporosis
  - Occult endocrinopathy
  - Leukemia, lymphoma
  - Malabsorption syndromes
- Adults
  - Hypophosphatasia: adult, recessive
  - Osteomalacia
  - Idiopathic osteoporosis
  - Endocrinopathy
  - Malignancy: multiple myeloma, leukemia, lymphoma

MANAGEMENT
- Team Concept
  - Orthopedic
  - Medicine
  - Physical therapy
  - Social support

SPECIFIC THERAPY

Fracture Treatment
- Scoliosis surgery advised to limit deterioration of pulmonary function
- Fixed and extensible rods to correct deformities, improve function and assist ambulation: advise rodding when function requires intervention

Medical
- Maintain calcium and vitamin D intake appropriate for age and weight.

■ Bisphosphonate therapy, oral (alendronate, residronate) or intravenous (pamidronate; zoledronic acid not reported): decreases fracture rate, increases bone density in children. In adults may increase bone density transiently, but effect on fracture rate not defined.

Physical Therapy
■ Rehabilitation after fractures: Limit immobilization, counteract joint hyperextensibility, maintain gait
■ Pool therapy
■ Maintain strength and function in upper and lower extremities

FOLLOW-UP
■ Pulmonary function studies
■ DXA bone density
■ Maintain adequate calcium and vitamin D intake

COMPLICATIONS AND PROGNOSIS
■ Type II OI dies shortly after birth
■ Pulmonary insufficiency in type III
■ Neurologic complications due to posterior fossa and spinal cord compression in basilar invagination
■ Hearing loss in 2nd-3rd decade
■ Significant aortic or mitral insufficiency rarely occurs
■ Renal calculi
■ Traumatic injury is main risk: patients may live to 70s

OSTEOMALACIA AND RICKETS

DAVID FELDMAN, MD

HISTORY & PHYSICAL

History
■ Decreased dietary intake of vitamin D
■ Deficient sun exposure
■ Growth retardation
■ Fractures
■ Family history
■ Kidney disease
■ Chronic diarrhea

Signs & Symptoms
- Children: rickets, bowing of long bones, muscle weakness, joint pains, rachitic rosary
- Adults: osteomalacia, increased susceptibility to bone fracture

TESTS

Laboratory
- Basic blood tests:
  - Calcium, phosphate, alkaline phosphatase, 25-hydroxy vitamin D, creatinine clearance
- Specific Diagnostic Tests
  - 1,25-dihydroxyvitamin D, parathyroid hormone (PTH), 24-h urine for phosphate and calcium

Imaging
- Metabolic bone survey: bowing of long bones, widening, cupping, fraying of metaphyses; subperiosteal erosions; pseudofractures (Looser zones)
- Adults: bone mineral density of hip and spine; bone x-rays for fracture

DIFFERENTIAL DIAGNOSIS
- Nutritional: vitamin D deficiency:
  - Decreased 25-hydroxyvitamin D
  - Hypocalcemia
  - Hypophosphatemia
  - Secondary hyperparathyroidism
- GI disorders/malabsorption syndrome: as nutritional +
  - Signs of malabsorption of other nutrients
  - Diarrhea
- Renal insufficiency:
  - With hypocalcemia and secondary hyperparathyroidism
  - Deficiency of 1-alpha-hydroxylase activity
  - Normal 25-hydroxy vitamin D
  - Deficient 1,25-dihydroxy vitamin D
- Oncogenic osteomalacia:
  - Tumor-induced osteomalacia
  - Usually difficult to find benign mesenchymal tumor
  - Tumor product with renal phosphate wasting and elevated urine phosphate

- ➤ Hypophosphatemia and osteomalacia in adults: fractures and muscle weakness; may resemble late onset X-linked hypophosphatemia
- ■ Hereditary causes:
  - ➤ X-linked hypophosphatemic rickets:
  - ➤ Mutation of Phex gene
  - ➤ Phosphaturia due to renal phosphate wasting
  - ➤ Hypophosphatemia
  - ➤ Relatively deficient in 1,25-dihydroxy vitamin D
  - ➤ X-linked or sporadic
  - ➤ Can have late onset
- ■ 1-alpha-hydroxylase deficiency (vitamin D-dependent rickets, type I):
  - ➤ Mutations in 1-alpha-hydroxylase gene
  - ➤ Inadequate conversion of 25- to 1,25-dihydroxy vitamin D
  - ➤ Hypocalcemia
  - ➤ Hypophosphatemia
  - ➤ Secondary hyperparathyroidism
  - ➤ Normal 25-hydroxy vitamin D
  - ➤ Deficient 1,25-dihydroxy vitamin D
- ■ Hereditary vitamin D-resistant rickets (HVDRR, vitamin D-dependent rickets, type II):
  - ➤ Mutations in the vitamin D receptor
  - ➤ Elevated 1,25-dihydroxy vitamin D
  - ➤ Hypocalcemia
  - ➤ Hypophosphatemia
  - ➤ Secondary hyperparathyroidism
  - ➤ May have alopecia

MANAGEMENT

What to Do First

- ■ Assess severity of rickets and hypocalcemia
- ■ Obtain family history
- ■ Assess growth of children
- ■ Perform routine lab tests and imaging
- ■ Assess kidney function

General Measures

- ■ Infants and children susceptible to pneumonia because of poor chest wall movement; consider chest-x-ray and treatment of pneumonia if present

SPECIFIC THERAPY

Indications
- Rickets, hypocalcemia, hypophosphatemia, fractures, growth retardation, muscle weakness or pain

Treatment Options
- Nutritional rickets: vitamin D and calcium
- Hypocalcemic rickets: calcium and vitamin D
- Hypophosphatemic rickets: phosphate and vitamin D
- Renal failure and 1-alpha-hydroxylase deficiency: calcitriol, phosphate binders to reduce hyperphosphatemia
- HVDRR: high-dose calcium and calcitriol; may require IV infusions of calcium
- Oncogenic osteomalacia: removal of offending tumor

Side Effects
- Excessive replacement of calcium and vitamin D: hypercalcemia, hypercalciuria, renal stones
- Excessive vitamin D or calcitriol: hypervitaminosis D
- Excessive oral phosphate: diarrhea

FOLLOW-UP

During Treatment
- Monitor calcium and phosphate, observe vitamin D and PTH levels
- Assess symptom reduction
- Assess fracture healing
- Adults: monitor bone mineral density
- Intermittently check bone x-rays for evidence of healing of rickets

Routine
- Monitor growth
- Observe family members for hereditary syndromes

COMPLICATIONS AND PROGNOSIS
- Nutritional rickets responds well to vitamin D and calcium
- Renal osteodystrophy dramatically improved by preventing hyperphosphatemia and secondary hyperparathyroidism with calcitriol
- Oncogenic osteomalacia responds dramatically to tumor removal; patients should be observed for recurrence of syndrome, implying tumor recurrence
- Hereditary syndromes show improvement in rickets if calcium, phosphate and vitamin D can be normalized; healing of rickets can

be achieved; normal growth and full predicted height difficult to attain

- HVDRR most difficult syndrome to treat; may require months of IV calcium infusions; rickets can be improved after calcium and phosphate return to normal
- Alopecia does not respond to normalization of calcium
- All patients must be observed for hypercalcemia
- High urinary calcium x phosphate product indicates increased risk of renal stones

---

OSTEOMYELITIS

RICHARD A. JACOBS, MD, PhD

HISTORY & PHYSICAL

History

- Acute osteomyelitis results from hematogenous dissemination; most common organism *Staphylococcus aureus*; long bones and vertebrae most common sites; in IV drug users unusual organisms (*Serratia*, *Pseudomonas*, and *Candida albicans*) infect unusual sites (clavicles and symphysis pubis); sickle cell disease predisposes to *Salmonella osteomyelitis*
- Spread of infection to bone from contiguous site seen in open fractures, post-operatively in joint replacement surgery or from an adjacent chronic skin infection; S. aureus most common organism, but *S. epidermidis* (with prosthetic devices), Gram-negative bacilli and anaerobes also involved
- Osteomyelitis in association with diabetes and vascular insufficiency polymicrobial and includes *S. aureus*, enterococci, anaerobes and Gram-negative bacilli
- Inability to control initial infection may lead to chronic osteomyelitis; often polymicrobial
- Other organisms less commonly involved include *M. tuberculosis*, atypical mycobacteria, Coccidioides immitis, Histoplasma capsulatum and Blastomyces dermatitidis

Signs & Symptoms

- Hematogenous osteomyelitis presents either acutely with fever, chills and localized pain, or more chronically over a period of months with fatigue, malaise and poorly localized pain.

- Cellulitis, pain, drainage and an open wound seen in osteomyelitis associated with vascular insufficiency or a contiguous infection
- Chronic osteomyelitis associated with chronic draining sinus tract

TESTS

- In febrile patient, blood cultures may reveal etiologic agent.
- Cultures of sinus tracts, open wounds or ulcers unreliable in predicting pathogen and are not recommended
- WBC and sedimentation rate may be elevated; will decrease with successful therapy and can be used to monitor therapy
- Periosteal reaction and destructive lesions on bone films accurate in making diagnosis, but may take 2 weeks or longer to appear
- Technetium radionuclide scan positive as early as 2–3 days after onset of infection, but false-positive scans can occur if adjacent soft tissue infection present; negative scan helpful in excluding diagnosis
- CT and MRI may be useful in making diagnosis and defining extent of disease; correlation of abnormalities with pathologic confirmation of osteomyelitis has not been done and overinterpretation of scans is a concern
- Definitive diagnosis made by biopsy and culture

DIFFERENTIAL DIAGNOSIS

- Acute hematogenous osteomyelitis must be differentiated from tumor; osteomyelitis associated with diabetes or vascular insufficiency confused with Charcot joint, osteoarthritis, disuse osteopenia

MANAGEMENT

- Since therapy prolonged, attempt to define bacteriology
- Blood cultures in febrile patient
- Bone biopsy or surgical debridement encouraged to isolate causative organism(s) and aid in choosing best antibiotic regimen

SPECIFIC THERAPY

- IV antibiotic therapy for 4–6 weeks; use of oral antibiotics not well studied for acute osteomyelitis in adults
- Debride necrotic tissue
- Obliteration of dead space and revascularization of bone often accomplished with myocutaneous flaps
- Role of hyperbaric oxygen therapy for chronic osteomyelitis or osteomyelitis associated with vascular insufficiency unclear; dramatic successes anecdotally reported

FOLLOW-UP
- In acute hematogenous osteomyelitis clinical response seen in 48–72 hours; response slower in other forms
- X-rays every 1–2 months may be helpful, but radiographic improvement lags behind clinical response
- Sedimentation rate falls with therapy, but may take months to normalize
- Most important follow-up is careful clinical assessment after antibiotics completed

COMPLICATIONS AND PROGNOSIS
- Soft tissue abscesses, extension of infection into adjacent joints, epidural or psoas abscesses (in vertebral osteomyelitis) require surgical intervention.
- Osteomyelitis associated with vascular insufficiency and diabetes requires some form of amputation in up to 50% over long term.
- Hematogenous osteomyelitis has excellent prognosis, but inadequate or delayed therapy can result in chronic disease.

OSTEONECROSIS

MICHAEL WARD, MD

HISTORY & PHYSICAL

History
- Alcohol use
- Corticosteroid use
- Trauma or femoral neck fracture
- Sickle cell disease, thalassemia
- Gaucher, Cushing's, Caisson (diver's) disease
- Radiation therapy
- SLE
- Chronic renal failure
- Pancreatitis
- Pregnancy
- Gout
- Coagulopathy
- Hyperlipidemia
- Diabetes mellitus
- Marrow infiltrating tumors (leukemia, lymphoma)
- Congenital hip dislocation, slipped capital femoral epiphysis

Signs and Symptoms
- Most commonly involves femoral head, but can involve femoral condyles, humeral head, tibial plateau, small bones of hands/feet
- Gradual onset mild vague pain in groin or buttock
- Pain worse with activity
- Reduced exercise or activity
- Can progress to pain at rest or night
- Can develop limp, reduced ROM late in course
- Can be asymptomatic and discovered incidentally on radiographs
- Exam unremarkable early
- Late in course may have painful restricted joint motion

TESTS
- Basic Tests
  - None, except to evaluate risk factors
- Specific Diagnostic Tests
  - Biopsy and histology of bone, measurement of bone marrow pressure, venography (invasive and rarely performed)

Imaging
- Plain x-rays:
  - Stage 0 and 1: normal
  - Stage 2: focal osteopenia, sclerosis, and cysts
  - Stage 3: radiolucent line under subchondral end plate (crescent sign)
  - Stage 4: flattening of femoral head and collapse
  - Stage 5: joint space narrowing with secondary osteoarthritis
  - Stage 6: joint destruction
  - May not progress sequentially through all stages
- Radionuclide bone scans: may be positive in stages 1–6; useful in stage 1 (cold spot) when radiographs are normal
- MRI:
  - Positive in stages 1–6
  - Useful in stage 1 when radiographs are normal
  - Sensitivity almost 100%
- CT:
  - Normal in stages 0 and 1
  - Used to define extent of bone changes in stages 2 and 4
- Symptoms may precede radiographic changes by months or years
- Radiographic abnormalities present in asymptomatic contralateral hip in 30–70%

DIFFERENTIAL DIAGNOSIS

■ Osteoarthritis of hip involves both femoral head and acetabulum early in course; late-stage osteonecrosis indistinguishable from late-stage osteoarthritis

■ Inflammatory arthritis of hip: no characteristic radiographic changes of osteonecrosis

■ Synovial osteochondromatosis, synovial tumors, labrum tears: detected by specific imaging findings

■ Transient osteoporosis of hip: similar on radiographic and radionuclide scan; differs on MRI

MANAGEMENT

What to Do First

■ Plain x-rays will detect bone changes; if normal, MRI

General Measures

■ Minimize alcohol intake and corticosteroid use

■ Control hyperlipidemia, diabetes, sickle cell disease, renal failure

■ Education for divers on slow decompression

■ Analgesics, NSAIDs, canes

■ Limited weightbearing; weight loss if obese

SPECIFIC THERAPY

■ No specific medical treatments other than analgesics

■ Surgical Treatment
  ➤ Core decompression of femoral head:
    • Decreases intraosseous pressure
    • Prevents progression
    • Useful in stages 0 to 2
  ➤ Core decompression with bone grafting or free vascularized fibular graft:
    • Decreases intraosseous pressure
    • Promotes growth of viable bone
    • Useful in stages 0 to 2
    • Outcomes may be better than decompression alone

■ Osteotomy:
  ➤ Prevents collapse of femoral head by redirecting mechanical load
  ➤ Can preserve femoral head in young patients
  ➤ Useful in stage 3

■ Femoral head replacement useful in stage 4

■ Total hip replacement useful in stages 4 to 6

FOLLOW-UP
- Minimize risk factors
- Monitor for signs and symptoms of osteonecrosis at other sites

COMPLICATIONS AND PROGNOSIS
- Secondary osteoarthritis in joints next to affected bone
- Progression to joint destruction inevitable without surgery
- Progression to total hip replacement may occur in many with core decompression +/− grafting, but progression may be delayed by years

OSTEOPOROSIS

ROBERT MARCUS, MD

HISTORY & PHYSICAL

History
- Family history of osteoporosis
- Caucasian
- Amenorrhea
- Hypogonadism
- Avoidance of dietary calcium
- Lack of habitual weight-bearing exercise
- Bone toxic exposures: glucocorticosteroids, antiseizure medication, systemic illness
- Smoking
- Alcoholism
- Thyrotoxicosis
- Celiac disease and other forms of intestinal malabsorption

Signs & Symptoms
- Asymptomatic until fractures
- Only 1/3 of vertebral fractures symptomatic
- Height loss can be early clue
- Deformity (kyphosis)
- Low-trauma fractures of spine and throughout the skeleton are the essential clinical consequences of osteoporosis.

TESTS

Laboratory
- Basic blood studies:

➤ Calcium, phosphorus, alkaline phosphatase: usually normal
➤ PTH if calcium elevated
➤ 25-hydroxy vitamin D. Vitamin D inadequacy very common, must be corrected before any treatment for osteoporosis can be effective.
➤ Free T4, TSH
➤ Serum testosterone in men
➤ Serum protein electrophoresis if suspicion for myeloma

■ Basic urine studies:
➤ 24-h urine calcium
➤ 24-h urine free cortisol if suspicion for Cushing syndrome
➤ Urine protein electrophoresis if suspicion for myeloma

■ Specific Diagnostic Tests
➤ Bone mineral density (BMD) evaluation: dual-energy x-ray absorptiometry (DXA), quantitative CT (QCT)

■ World Health Organization BMD Categories:
➤ Osteoporosis: >2.5 SD below standard (T >< −2.5)
➤ Osteopenia: −1 to −2.5 SD below standard (T < −1)
➤ Normal: <1 SD below standard (T = +2 to −1)

Imaging

■ PA and lateral films of thoracic and lumbar spine to identify vertebral compression fractures. Presence of a single compression fracture increases subsequent fracture risk 5-fold.
■ Metabolic bone series if lab abnormalities; not routinely indicated

DIFFERENTIAL DIAGNOSIS

■ Common medical conditions associated with osteoporosis:
➤ Alcoholism
➤ Rheumatic diseases
➤ Intestinal malabsorption syndromes
➤ Adrenal cortical excess
➤ Osteomalacia
➤ Various malignancies
➤ Thyrotoxicosis
   Primary hyperparathyroidism

MANAGEMENT

What to Do first

■ Establish whether secondary causes
■ Consider specific pharmacologic therapy

General Measures

- Hygienic program of adequate calcium intake unless patient hyper-calciuric (24-h urine calcium >300 mg/d)
- Vitamin D maintenance: At least 800 IU/day. Can use 50,000 IU vitamin D capsule once each week. For vitamin D-deficient patients, 3 months repletion with 50,000 IU/week should precede maintenance. Vitamin D3 superior to Vitamin D2.
- Program of daily weight-bearing exercise adjusted by individual tolerability
- Attention to risk of fall

Indications

Criteria for treatment

- History of low-trauma fracture
- BMD T-score of −2.5 or lower
- BMD T-score of −2 or lower in presence of additional risk factors (family history, menopausal status)
- For higher BMD values, and no low-trauma fractures, pharmacologic treatment not recommended

SPECIFIC THERAPY

- Established osteoporosis:
- Antiresorptive medications: act to reduce osteoclastic bone resorption
  - ➤ Bisphosphonates:
    - Alendronate, risedronate taken fasting with 6 oz water only
    - Wait 30 min in upright position before taking other medications or food
    - Decrease risk of subsequent vertebral and non-vertebral fractures, including hip fracture, by 40–50% when given for 3 y
    - Reduced vertebral fracture incidence within 1 y of treatment
    - Ibandronate, vertebral fracture reduction, no reduction in non-vertebral fracture
  - ➤ Selective estradiol receptor modulator (SERM):
- Raloxifene
  - ➤ Decrease vertebral fracture incidence by ~40% in women with osteoporosis; fracture efficacy at other sites less certain
- Calcitonin:
  - ➤ Decreases vertebral compression fracture incidence by ~40%, but no effect on non-vertebral fractures
  - ➤ Prevention of osteoporosis:

- Estrogen/HRT:
  - ➤ Conjugated equine estrogens
  - ➤ Conserves BMD at menopause
  - ➤ Long-term (>5 y) estrogen reduces risk of all fractures
  - ➤ Decision to prescribe requires individualized assessment of multiple health risks
  - ➤ Selective estradiol receptor modulator (SERM): raloxifene
- Bisphosphonates: alendronate, risedronate
- Side Effects & Contraindications
- Bisphosphonates:
  - ➤ Side effects: esophageal irritation, ~10% of patients; if intolerant to one, try another bisphosphonate
  - ➤ Contraindications: previous severe intolerance, intestinal malabsorption due to disease or surgery
- Raloxifene:
  - ➤ Side effects: occasional increase in frequency and severity of hot flashes; rarely, deep venous thrombosis
  - ➤ Contraindications: premenopausal, pregnancy, history of venous thrombosis, pulmonary emboli
- Calcitonin:
  - ➤ Side effects: rhinorrhea, nasal irritation
  - ➤ Contraindications: none
- Estrogen/HRT:
  - ➤ Side effects: vaginal bleeding, venous thrombosis, pulmonary embolus, breast cancer, endometrial cancer
  - ➤ Contraindications: women with recent (<3 y) MI, recent (<5 y) breast cancer, recurrent DVT or pulmonary embolus

BONE ANABOLIC THERAPY:

- Teriparatide (recombinant human PTH1–34): directly stimulates new bone formation, increases trabecular and cortical bone throughout skeleton. 65% reduction in all vertebral fractures, 80% reduction in moderate/severe vertebral fractures within 18 months. 53% reduction in non-vertebral fractures. Given by single daily injection of 20 mcg for up to 2 years. Preclinical finding of osteosarcoma in rats, but no evidence of human equivalent.

FOLLOW-UP

- Assess annually for fractures, functional status, height loss
- Reevaluate BMD not less than 2 y after initiating treatment

COMPLICATIONS AND PROGNOSIS

- Multiple compression fractures severely restrict functional activity, promote loss of esteem, depression, increased hospitalization, increased mortality rate
- Treatment of fractures considerably less satisfactory than prevention

---

OTHER CARDIOMYOPATHIES

JOHN R. TEERLINK, MD

HISTORY & PHYSICAL

Also see congestive heart failure, acute heart failure, and myocarditides

- Three main types of cardiomyopathies: Dilated, Hypertrophic, Restrictive.

History

- Family history of cardiomyopathy and/or sudden death
- Dilated cardiomyopathy may result form alcohol or other toxic exposure

Signs & Symptoms

- Dilated: usually present with gradual onset of CHF symptoms, occasionally symptomatic ventricular arrhythmias
- Hypertrophic: most frequently present with chest pain and dyspnea, although postexertional syncope is more suggestive
- Restrictive: usually present with gradual onset of CHF symptoms, occasionally symptomatic ventricular arrhythmias, or conduction disturbances, depending on etiology
  - ➤ Dilated: consistent with CHF
  - ➤ Hypertrophic: bisferiens carotid upstroke, loud S4, triple apical impulse, systolic murmur that augments with Valsalva or upright posture and decreases with squatting
  - ➤ Restrictive: elevated JVP, Kussmaul's sign, edema, consistent with CHF with diastolic dysfunction

TESTS

- Basic Tests
  - ➤ As per CHF
- Specific Diagnostic Tests
  - ➤ Electrocardiogram: ST-T wave changes, conduction abnormalities (all); septal Q waves, LVH (hypertrophic); low voltage (restrictive)

- ➤ Chest X-ray: enlarged heart, pulmonary congestion (dilated); mild cardiomegaly (hypertrophic); normal to mild cardiomegaly (restrictive)
- ➤ Echocardiogram: LV dilation and reduced function (dilated); LVH, asymmetric septal hypertrophy, apical hypertrophy, systolic anterior motion of mitral valve leaflet, diastolic dysfunction, possible dynamic outflow tract obstruction (hypertrophic); small or normal LV size, in amyloid- scintillating appearance of myocardium (restrictive)
- ➤ Cardiac Catheterization: LV dilation and dysfunction, high filling pressures, low cardiac output (dilated); hypercontractile LV, dynamic outflow tract obstruction (hypertrophic); normal or mildly reduced LV function, high diastolic pressures, square root sign (restrictive)
- ■ Other Tests as Appropriate
  - ➤ Biopsy (fat pad, rectal. gingival, etc) with immunohistochemical staining for amyloidosis
  - ➤ Myocardial biopsy
  - ➤ Other tests for specific underlying etiologies (i.e. serum iron and ferritin for hemochromatosis)

DIFFERENTIAL DIAGNOSIS

- ■ Dilated cardiomyopathy: idiopathic, alcoholic, myocarditides, familial, post-partum, cobalt; also arrhythmogenic right ventricular hypertrophy
- ■ Hypertrophic: Hereditary (some forms autosomal dominant with incomplete penetrance)
- ■ Restrictive: Amyloidosis, endomyocardial fibrosis, inherited disorders (Fabry disease, Gaucher disease, hemochromatosis, glycogen storage diseases), sarcoidosis

MANAGEMENT

What to Do First

- ■ Assess underlying etiology and distinguish type of cardiomyopathy

General Measures

- ■ Remove possible toxins and toxic exposures (i.e. cease cocaine, alcohol)

SPECIFIC THERAPY

- ■ Dilated cardiomyopathy: as per CHF

- Hypertrophic cardiomyopathy: invasive interventions only required by 5–10% of patients
  - Beta blockers: improve symptoms, probably reduce risk of sudden death
  - Calcium channel blockers: alternative to beta blockers, usually verapamil
  - Dual chamber DDD pacemaker: assist with reduction of outflow tract gradient; improve symptoms
  - AICD: use in patients with sustained VT or aborted sudden death
  - Septal ablation: percutaneous infarction of septum to reduce outflow tract obstruction; heart block major complication
  - Surgical myectomy: large center surgical mortality about 3%
- Restrictive: As per underlying etiology (i.e. primary amyloidosis: consider alkylating agents; some centers use autologous stem cell transplantation)

FOLLOW-UP

During Treatment & Routine
- Repeat assessment of LV function 6 months after treatment or with deterioration of clinical course

COMPLICATIONS AND PROGNOSIS
- Highly variable and dependent on underlying etiology

OTHER CLOTTING FACTOR DEFICIENCIES

MARGARET V. RAGNI, MD, MPH

HISTORY & PHYSICAL

History
- easy bruising, epistaxis postoperative or traumatic bleeding
- GI, GU, or soft tissue bleeding
- menorrhagia in women
- family history of bleeding, consanguinity
- intracranial bleeding at birth (F VII, XIII deficiency)
- splenic rupture (F I deficiency)
- umbilical bleeding, spontaneous abortion (F I, XIII deficiency)
- poor wound healing (F I, XIII deficiency)

Signs & Symptoms

- excessive postoperative bleeding
- previous transfusions of red cells; anemia or iron therapy; excess bleeding with NSAIDs, aspirin

TESTS

Screening

- prolonged PT, APTT, TT (thrombin time), RT (reptilase time), shortened euglobulin clot lysis

Confirmatory

- decreased factor I, II, V, VII, X, XI, XIII activity

DIFFERENTIAL DIAGNOSIS

- lupus anticoagulant, acquired anti-VIII – APTT mix
- hemophilia A or B – factor VIII or IX levels
- von Willebrand disease – ristocetin cofactor, vW antigen
- vitamin K deficiency – factor II, VII, IX, X deficiency
- thrombocytopenia, platelet dysfunction – platelet count, closure time
- liver disease – may mimic factor deficiency

MANAGEMENT

What to Do First

- use history, exam to assess severity, location of hemorrhage assess pain, loss of motion, degree of blood loss, organ system damage
- initiate factor replacement 100% level immediately
- provide adequate pain relief and assess ongoing need
- monitor vital signs, blood pressure, heart rate, temperature
- obtain hemoglobin, platelet count, monitor factor level, PT, APTT
- keep patient at bed rest until assessment complete, improvement occurs

General Measures

- estimate ongoing blood loss by vital signs, frequent CBC, APTT, PT, and non-invasive tests, e.g. ultrasound
- maintain hemostasis with factor replacement on the half-life to start
- taper factor once bleeding slows
- avoid NSAIDs, ASA, platelet inhibitory drugs, heparin, or heparin flush

- if surgery required, use estimated blood loss to estimate factor replacement
- discuss safest, least invasive approach for procedures with surgeons

SPECIFIC THERAPY

Indications

- emergency replacement for trauma or spontaneous bleeding
- perioperative replacement for elective or emergency procedures
- prophylactic replacement to prevent bleeding

Treatment Options

- cryoprecipitate – replacement for factor I, XIII deficiency 6 bags 1200 mg fibrinogen for 80–100 mg level
- fresh frozen plasma – replacement for factor II, V, VII, X, XI, XIII deficiency 5 units = 5–15% factor level increment
- recombinant factor VIIa – replacement for factor VII deficiency or acquired anti-VIII inhibitor 90 mcg/kg q 2–3 hr = 100% factor level, then taper to q 4 hr; for anti-VIII inhibitor, once bleeding slows, may switch to FEIBA, Autoplex
- FEIBA, Autoplex, Konyne (factor IX complex): factor II, V, X, XI 75–100 U/kg = 100% level; then 50 U/kg q 8–24 hours

Side Effects & Contraindications

- FFP, cryoprecipitate – hepatitis, HIV, parvovirus, CJD, hives, hypotension contraindicated if uncontrolled allergic reactions
- rFVIIa – thrombosis, phlebitis
- FEIBA, Autoplex, Konyne – thrombosis, hepatitis, inhibitor contraindicated if allergic reactions, thrombosis present

FOLLOW-UP

During Treatment

- close monitoring for efficacy by blood loss, vital signs, and hematocrit; potential neurologic, orthopedic, musculoskeletal complications of continued bleeding: hypotension, neurologic sequelae
- assessment for complications of treatment:
  - ➤ FFP/cryoprecipitate – potential hepatitis A, B, C, HIV, parvovirus
  - ➤ FEIBA, Autoplex, Konyne – thrombosis, inhibitor, hepatitis
  - ➤ rFVIIa – thrombosis

Routine

- CBC, LFTs, inhibitor, HIV and hepatitis serologies q 6–12 months
- orthopedic, dental evaluation, review all bleeds & Rx q 6–12 month

- HCV RNA PCR at baseline, evaluate for biopsy, hepatitis Rx
- CD4, HIV RNA PCR q 3–6 months, evaluate for antiretroviral Rx

COMPLICATIONS AND PROGNOSIS

Complications

- at birth, CNS bleeding, intracranial bleeding, cephalhematoma, especially with forceps, vacuum extraction
- at diagnosis, bleeding with procedures, surgery, when no family history taken or no factor replacement given
- bleeding associated with drugs – e.g., NSAIDs, aspirin, or analgesics, platelet inhibitory drugs, Coumadin, antibiotics
- bleeding associated with other disorders that cause platelet dysfunction – e.g., uremia, ITP, liver disease, portal hypertension
- bacterial infection of body cavity hematomas
- compartment syndrome due to severe, large hemorrhage – e.g., of the extremities
- entrapment neuropathies associated with large hematomas (retoperitoneal)
- thrombosis, hepatitis complications from blood products, transfusions orthopedic, soft tissue, neurologic complications of hemorrhages: headaches, mental status change, or peripheral neuropathies associated with hematomas
- traumatic bleeds which block airway, causing mental status change, CNS bleed, cord compression
- anemia, iron deficiency, transfusion requirement, when preoperative treatment is inadequate by product, dose, or duration
- AIDS among those with chronic HIV infection
- end-stage liver disease, drug interactions, or hepatocellular carcinoma among those with chronic HCV infection

Prognosis

- homozygotes may die at birth or shortly thereafter
- heterozygotes may be symptomatic with trauma, procedures; most live normal life with adequate treatment, followup
- women with menorrhagia may develop iron deficiency anemia, undergo unnecessary gynecologic procedures, and more bleeding
- recurrent bleeding into joints in those with severe factor deficiency may lead to chronic arthritis and disability
- shortened lifespan, morbidity in areas without expertise in coagulation

OTITIS EXTERNA

STEVEN W. CHEUNG, MD

HISTORY & PHYSICAL

Classification
- Bacterial otitis externa (BOE): swimmer's ear
- Fungal otitis externa (FOE)
- Chronic otitis externa (COE)
- Malignant otitis externa (MOE): skull base osteomyelitis

History
- Otalgia
- Irritability (in infants)
- Trauma or instrumentation
- Water contamination
- Hearing loss
- Otorrhea
- Vertigo
- Bilateral disease not uncommon
- Diplopia
- Cranial neuropathies (CN 7, 9–12)

Signs & Symptoms
- Tender, painful auricle; worse w/ pinna movements
- Swollen, narrowed external auditory canal (EAC) associated w/ purulent otorrhea & debris
- Periauricular cellulitis in advanced OE
- Otoscopy: hyperemic, macerated skin of EAC w/ overlying skin debris; TM usually thickened, pts can have concomitant COM
- Cranial neuropathies (CN 7, 9–12) in MOE

TESTS
- Culture otorrhea in recalcitrant infections
- Temporal bone CT in suspected MOE to determine bony erosion
- Gallium/technetium bone scan in suspected MOE to evaluate for marrow infection

DIFFERENTIAL DIAGNOSIS
- Perichondritis, furunculosis, carbunculosis, psoriasis & seborrheic dermatitis of external ear

- Squamous cell carcinoma, adenoid cystic carcinoma, basal cell carcinoma, melanoma or metastatic carcinoma can present as infections of EAC

MANAGEMENT

- Aural toilet under microscope control
- Antibiotic otic drops to cover Pseudomonas & S aureus in BOE; oral antibiotics (eg, ciprofloxacin) may be necessary
- Antifungal otic preparations for FOE
- Otic wicks are used to deliver otic antibiotic drops when EAC is swollen shut.
- Dry ear precautions
- Directed IV antibiotic therapy required to treat MOE
- Otitis externa often requires multiple cleaning sessions; Dx of FOE vs BOE difficult; MOE often referred to specialist for management

Side Effects

- Neomycin otic drops can cause contact allergy in 6–8% of pts

SPECIFIC THERAPY

n/a

FOLLOW-UP

- Close follow-up critical: untreated OE can progress to MOE (particularly in diabetics)
- IV antibiotic therapy for MOE
- Follow-up until external canal infection-free
- Return to swimming when EAC makes normal wax

COMPLICATIONS AND PROGNOSIS

Complications

- MOE & skull base osteomyelitis with cranial neuropathies
- Stenosis of EAC
- Cellulitis of face & neck

Prognosis

- Most cases of BOE & FOE are treated effectively w/ meticulous aural hygiene & antibiotics
- MOE associated w/ worse prognosis & can result in death if not identified early & treated aggressively

OTITIS MEDIA

STEVEN W. CHEUNG, MD

HISTORY & PHYSICAL

Classification
- Acute otitis media (AOM)
- Chronic otitis media (COM)
- Otitis media w/ effusion (OME)

Epidemiology
- 2nd most common childhood disease after URI
- 13% of children have at least 1 episode of AOM before 3 mo old
- 65% of children have at least 1 episode of AOM before 1 y old
- Increased incidence of AOM in winter; decreased in summer
- Increased incidence of AOM in children whose caretaker smokes cigarettes
- Decreased incidence of AOM in children who are breast-fed
- Presence of effusion after AOM: 70% at 2 wk, 40% at 4 wk, 10% at 12 wk

History
- Otalgia
- Irritability (in infants)
- Fever
- Hearing loss
- Otorrhea
- Vertigo
- Facial nerve paralysis

Signs & Symptoms
- Tympanic membrane (TM) may be erythematous, bulging, or retracted
- Pneumatic otoscopy shows decreased mobility, consistent w/ effusion
- In AOM, TM erythematous, inflamed, & hypervascular
- In COM, TM may be perforated & draining fluid
- In otitis externa, movement of pinna elicits discomfort

TESTS
- Audiogram w/ tympanometry; impedance audiometry for infants

- Behavioral audiometry for younger children; acoustic audiometry for older children/adults
- CT scan with contrast if complications of OM (cranial neuropathy, brain abscess, etc.) are suspected
- Tympanocentesis to determine microbiology in refractory cases of COM

DIFFERENTIAL DIAGNOSIS
n/a

MANAGEMENT
n/a

SPECIFIC THERAPY

Treatment Options
- Antibiotics:
  - Amoxicillin, cefaclor, amoxicillin-clavulanate, trimethoprim-sulfamethoxazole, erythromycin-sulfisoxazole, cefixime, cefuroxime axetil
- Prophylaxis:
  - S pneumoniae vaccination, chronic prophylactic antibiotics
  - Tympanostomy tubes for recurrent otitis media (5 episodes/y) or 3+ mo of OME
  - Adenoidectomy +/− tonsillectomy with tubes

Side Effects
- Drug allergies
- Tympanostomy tubes: otorrhea & recurrent infection due to retrograde flow of water into middle ear; pt must keep ears dry
- Adenoidectomy/tonsillectomy: acute bleeding, velopharyngeal insufficiency (VPI)

FOLLOW-UP
- 7–10 d of antibiotics for AOM; follow-up in 1–2 wk
- Surveillance to 3 mo if effusion persists; then tympanostomy tubes indicated; refer to otolaryngologist.
- If any complications from OM such as vertigo, facial nerve weakness, sensorineural hearing loss, cholesteatoma, TM perforation, retraction pocket, or other abnormality, refer to specialist.
- If >3 episodes of AOM in 6 mo or >4 episodes/y, refer to specialist.

COMPLICATIONS AND PROGNOSIS

Complications

- Perforated TM & purulent otorrhea, speech delay, cholesteatoma, tympanosclerosis, ossicular discontinuity/fixation, sensorineural hearing loss, coalescent mastoiditis, petrositis, labyrinthitis, facial nerve paralysis, meningitis, extradural abscess, subdural empyema, brain abscess, sigmoid sinus thrombosis, otic hydrocephalus, & death
- Complications of OM should be referred to a specialist.

Prognosis

- 10% of children w/ OME will continue to have effusion at 3 mo after episode of AOM & will require tympanostomy tubes.
- Children not treated for OM have been found to have significantly greater incidence of speech delay & hearing loss in addition to other complications.

PAGET DISEASE

ROBERT A. MARCUS, MD

HISTORY & PHYSICAL

History

- Family history of Paget disease, rarely

Signs & Symptoms

- Bone aches, involving skull, spine, pelvis, femur, tibia
- Hearing loss
- May be asymptomatic
- Incidental radiographic finding
- Local increase in skin temperature at involved sites
- Gross deformity of affected bones after long-term untreated disease
- Swelling, deformity of skull

TESTS

Laboratory

- Basic blood studies:
  - ➤ Serum alkaline phosphatase elevated in most patients
  - ➤ Serum calcium normal unless patient immobilized, then elevated

- Specific Diagnostic Tests
  - Bone biopsy usually not indicated
  - Audiogram if skull involvement

Imaging
- Plain films of affected bone: osteolysis early, then thickened sclerotic bone
- Radionuclide bone scan highly sensitive for active disease

DIFFERENTIAL DIAGNOSIS
- Osteoblastic metastases
  - Sclerotic bone disorders (generally rare)

MANAGEMENT
What to Do First
- Establish diagnosis

General Measures
- NSAIDs for managing secondary degenerative arthritis

SPECIFIC THERAPY
- Bisphosphonates:
  - Treatment of choice
  - Alendronate, risedronate, tiludronate taken fasting with 6 oz water only
  - Wait 30 min in upright position before taking other medications or food
  - When oral therapy contraindicated or not tolerated: intravenous pamidronate
- Calcitonin:
  - SC injection or nasal spray
  - Rapidly diminishes disease activity
  - Less effective than bisphosphonates
- Side Effects & Contraindications
- Bisphosphonates:
  - Side effects: oral-esophageal irritation, ~10% of patients; IV: fever, arthralgias; if intolerant to one, try another bisphosphonate
    - Rare occurrence of osteonecrosis of jaw, particularly with IV bisphosphonates
  - Contraindications: previous severe intolerance, intestinal malabsorption due to disease or surgery

- Calcitonin:
  - Side effects: occasional abdominal cramps (SQ), rhinorrhea, nasal irritation
  - Contraindications: none

FOLLOW-UP
- Alkaline phosphatase q 4–6 wks
- Monitor pain
- Bone scan at end of treatment or when disease activity in doubt
- Audiogram repeated periodically if skull involved

COMPLICATIONS AND PROGNOSIS
- Degenerative joint disease adjacent to involved bone
- Deafness from temporal bone impinging on 8th cranial nerve or direct involvement of middle ear ossicles
- Spinal stenosis
- Other foraminal occlusion less common
- Fracture at involved weight-bearing sites
- Osteogenic sarcoma rare but lethal
- High-output cardiac failure uncommon; improves with successful therapy of Paget disease

---

PAIN SYNDROMES

MICHAEL J. AMINOFF, MD, DSc

HISTORY & PHYSICAL
- Acute or chronic pain: document onset, character, distribution, progression, duration, severity
- Sharp, short-duration, stabbing pain, sometimes on background of constant burning pain, suggests neuropathic pain that may radiate in nerve or root territory
- Associated symptoms
  - Local or systemic disease may suggest pain felt at one site is referred from another (eg, chest/arm pain from cardiac ischemia)
  - Limb pain may be accompanied by swelling, discoloration, temperature change, disuse (reflex sympathetic dystrophy or complex regional pain syndrome type 1 after seemingly minor injury or CRPS 2 after severe nerve injury)
  - Preceding rash suggests shingles or postherpetic neuralgia
- Past medical history may suggest cause of pain

- Psychogenic factors may perpetuate, exacerbate or result from the pain syndrome
- Exam findings depend on cause of pain
- See separate entries for findings w/ back or neck pain, peripheral neuropathy or visceral disease

TESTS
- Lab & imaging studies depend on likely cause

DIFFERENTIAL DIAGNOSIS
- Nature of pain & associated symptoms & signs suggest likely cause

MANAGEMENT
- Depends on cause of pain & clinical context
- For neuropathic pain, use tricyclic agents, topiramate or gabapentin
- For chronic pain & in terminally ill, pain should be controlled rapidly & as completely as possible, w/ adequate doses of opiates if needed; give medication on regular schedule; titrate dose upward rapidly; give opiates if NSAIDs are insufficient
- Surgical procedures (eg, nerve blocks, dorsal rhizotomy or central ablations) or
- Modulatory procedures (eg, transcutaneous electrical nerve stimulation) may be helpful; consider referral to multidisciplinary pain clinic

SPECIFIC THERAPY
- Treat underlying cause

FOLLOW-UP
- Depends on cause

COMPLICATIONS AND PROGNOSIS
- Depend on cause

PANCREATIC CANCER

ANSON W. LOWE, MD

HISTORY & PHYSICAL

Risk Factors
- Environmental
- An increased risk is associated with cigarette smoking

- Genetic
- familial hereditary pancreatic cancer
- hereditary pancreatitis
- familial adenomatous polyposis syndrome
- familial atypical multiple mole melanoma
- HNPCC1 – hereditary nonpolyposis colon cancer syndrome
- Associated diseases with an increased risk of pancreatic cancer
- recent onset of diabetes present in >50% of patients afflicted with pancreatic cancer
- chronic pancreatitis
- intraductal papillary mucinous tumor

Symptoms and Signs
- Abdominal or back pain
- Jaundice (often painless)
- Weight loss
- unexplained pancreatitis in an elderly patient > 50 yrs

TESTS
- endoscopic ultrasound (EUS) – may be the most sensitive (~99%) and can be used to obtain tissue at the time of examination
- high resolution spiral abdominal CT scan (sensitivity ~90%)
  - ➤ patients at high risk secondary to genetic causes should be entered into a screening program using high resolution CT or EUS.
- conventional CT scan (sensitivity ~75%)
- ERCP is also useful in detecting pancreatic cancer in specific cases

Blood Tests
- CA19-9 assays are often used but its sensitivity is poor and inadequate for screening purposes.
- serum amylase levels are not useful
- Abnormal liver function tests (bilirubin, alkaline phosphatase, aminotransminases) are often seen with cancers in the pancreatic head.

DIFFERENTIAL DIAGNOSIS
- Biliary tract disease must be considered in patients who are jaundiced or have liver function test abnormalities. Diseases should include:
- choledocholithiasis
- cholangiocarcinoma

- bile duct strictures
- sclerosing cholangitis

MANAGEMENT

What to Do First

- Initial assessment is directed toward whether the lesion is resectable. Staging and resectability are performed using high-resolution spiral CT scans and/or EUS.

SPECIFIC THERAPY

- If resection is considered, the surgery should be performed at experienced institutions.
- Palliation
  - biliary obstruction
    - surgery
    - endoscopic stent placement
  - duodenal obstruction
    - surgery (e.g., gastrojejunostomy with biliary bypass)
    - endoscopic stent (expandable metal stents)
  - pain
    - opiate analgesics
    - intraoperative splanchnicetomy or celiac block
    - percutaneous celiac block
- Chemotherapy
  - long-term survival benefit is rare.
  - only 5-FU and gemcitabine have demonstrated a survival benefit of >5 months.
  - gemcitabine may be useful for the palliation of pain.
  - adjuvant chemoradiotherapy should be considered for patients undergoing surgery.
  - patients should be entered in investigational trials when considering chemo- or radiotherapy.

FOLLOW-UP

n/a

COMPLICATIONS AND PROGNOSIS

- Prognosis remains very poor, even in many cases that initially appear surgically resectable.
- Average 5-year survival is <5% for all patients and 17% with localized resectable disease.
- Survival is better in carefully selected patients for surgical resection.

PANCREATIC CYSTS

ANSON W. LOWE, MD

HISTORY & PHYSICAL
- Pancreatitis vs. non-pancreatitis associated cysts
- Pancreatitis associated cysts are treated as pseudocysts. (see section on acute an chronic pancreatitis for further details)
- pseudocysts usually develop in the setting of chronic pancreatitis or acute necrotizing pancreatitis
- Non-pancreatitis associated cysts may represent neoplastic lesions.

Symptoms and Signs
- Because of improved imaging techniques, pancreatic cysts are often incidentally found.
- Abdominal or back pain
- Weight loss
- Early satiety
- Nausea and vomiting

TESTS
- no standard approach to pancreatic cysts has been established. There is currently no definitive approach aside from surgical resection to determine whether a cyst represents a neoplastic lesion. Commonly used diagnostic approaches include:
  - endoscopic ultrasound (EUS) – may be the most sensitive and can be used to obtain cyst fluid at the time of examination
- cytology of the cyst fluid is often of insufficient sensitivity
- analysis of the cyst fluid should be considered investigational and may include:
  - viscosity
  - amylase
  - CEA
  - CA 19-9
  - CA 72-4
- high resolution spiral abdominal CT scan
- cystic features such as the thickness of the wall and septae may help differentiate benign from neoplastic lesions.
- ERCP may reveal a communication of the cysts with the pancreatic duct which occurs in 65% of pseudocysts and almost never with neoplastic cysts.

Blood Tests

■ elevated serum amylase suggests a pseudocyst secondary to pancreatitis
■ CA19-9 and CEA may be elevated. Sensitivity is insufficient to be used for screening purposes.

DIFFERENTIAL DIAGNOSIS

■ Truly benign pancreatic cysts are rare. Most often, the goal is to differentiate mucinous cystic tumors from serous cystadenomas. Differentiation between different cyst types is often difficult to distinguish from each other prior to resection.
■ The most common lesions are mucinous cystic tumors and serous cystadenomas
  ➤ mucinous cystadenoma
  ➤ mucinous cystadenocarcinoma
  ➤ serous cystadenoma – malignant transformation is rare and thus can be treated as a benign lesion
■ Less common cystic lesions include
  ➤ papillary cystic tumor
  ➤ cystic neuroendocrine tumor
  ➤ adenocarcinoma of the pancreas with cystic degeneration
  ➤ acinar cystadenocarcinoma
  ➤ cystic teratoma
  ➤ lymphangioma
  ➤ hemangioma

MANAGEMENT

■ Because current diagnostic modalities are often quite poor in determining whether a cystic lesion is malignant, evaluation and surgery should be carried out in a facility experienced in the medical and surgical management of pancreatic disease
■ The only definitive approach in determining the identity of a cystic lesion is surgical resection. Surgical outcomes of pancreatic resections are much better in institutions where the volume is high and the necessary expertise is present.

SPECIFIC THERAPY

n/a

FOLLOW-UP

■ dictated by the approach chosen

■ observation is sometimes chosen over surgical resection. These patients are followed with serial CT scans to monitor any change in the cysts.

COMPLICATIONS AND PROGNOSIS
■ Prognosis is excellent for serous cystadenomas
■ Resected mucinous cystadenocarcinomas possess better 5-year survival rates than the more common adenocarcinomas.
■ unresectable mucinous tumors carry a poor prognosis

PAPILLARY MUSCLE DYSFUNCTION AND RUPTURE

JUDITH A. WISNESKI, MD

HISTORY & PHYSICAL

History
■ Myocardial ischemia and infarction (most common)
  ➤ Rupture of posterior papillary muscle with infarction of right coronary artery (most common); rupture of anterolateral papillary muscle with infarction of diagonal or obtuse marginal branches off left coronary artery (less frequent)
■ Severe anemia
■ Shock
■ Trauma

Signs & Symptoms
■ Transient mid or late systolic or holosystolic heart murmur and pulmonary congestion during angina (papillary muscle dysfunction during ischemia)
■ Pulmonary congestion or acute pulmonary edema with new heart murmur (holosystolic or mid systolic) following an acute MI (papillary muscle rupture)
■ Hypotension may be present; cardiogenic shock can occur

TESTS
■ ECG
  ➤ ST and T wave changes of ischemia or infarction
  ➤ New Q waves may be present (usually present prior to rupture)
■ Blood
  ➤ Elevation of troponin I and other cardiac enzymes prior to rupture of papillary muscle (enzyme elevation may be small)

➤ Enzymes normal with ischemia and transient papillary muscle dysfunction
- Chest X Ray
  ➤ Heart size may be normal
  ➤ Normal size left atrium
  ➤ Pulmonary venous congestion present
- Echo/Doppler
  ➤ Detect and quantitate MR
  ➤ Flail mitral valve leaflet may be visualized after rupture
  ➤ Detect left ventricular (LV) wall motion abnormality
  ➤ Assess LV dimensions (usually normal for acute MR)
  ➤ Assess LV function (may be normal pending othe conditions)
- Cardiac Catheterization
  ➤ Prominent V wave in pulmonary capillary wedge pressure
  ➤ Low cardiac output and index
  ➤ Detect and quantitate mitral regurgitation during left ventriculography
  ➤ Wall motion abnormality present on left ventriculogram
  ➤ Detect high grade/total occlusion of vessel (usually the right coronary artery) and presence of other coronary stenoses by coronary angiography

DIFFERENTIAL DIAGNOSIS
- Ventricular septal defect

MANAGEMENT
Medical
- Afterload reduction therapy with vasodilators
- Intra-aortic balloon pump for hypotension

SPECIFIC THERAPY
- Surgical repair/replacement of mitral valve with coronary revascularization (usually surgical emergency) See discussion under Mitral Insufficiency

FOLLOW-UP
n/a

COMPLICATIONS AND PROGNOSIS
Complications – see section Mitral Insufficiency

Prognosis
- Depends on co-existing CAD and LV function
- See section Mitral Insufficiency

PARACOCCIDIOIDOMYCOSIS

RICHARD A. JACOBS, MD, PhD

HISTORY & PHYSICAL

History

- Caused by *Paracoccidioides brasiliensis*, a dimorphic fungus
  - ➤ Very narrow geographic zone of infection; from Mexico to Argentina with Brazil at the center of the endemic area
  - ➤ Cases reported in the US, Canada, Asia and Europe, but patients were previous residents of endemic country
  - ➤ The route of transmission is still debated; generally most agree that the respiratory route is most likely
- No person-to-person transmission has been established
- Significant for long periods of latency (as long as 30 years)

Signs & Symptoms

- Primary infection is usually asymptomatic
- Two main forms: pulmonary and mucocutaneous
  - ➤ Pulmonary disease:
  - ➤ Dyspnea is common, cough may not be productive of sputum
  - ➤ Patients may also present with weight loss, fever and malaise mimicking tuberculosis
  - ➤ Mucocutaneous disease:
  - ➤ Ulceration in the nasopharynx or oropharynx may be the first symptom
  - ➤ Facial or nasal mucosal ulcers may coalesce with destruction of uvula and vocal cords
  - ➤ May present with odynophagia or dysphonia, lymphadenopathy (especially cervical) may ulcerate and form draining sinuses
  - ➤ Pediatric disease:
  - ➤ more subacute symptoms; fewer respiratory complaints, can be more severe
- HIV patients:
  - ➤ presentation similar to pediatric disease

TESTS

Laboratory

- Other studies: sputum or exudates may by diagnostic in over 90% patients
  - ➤ At 37 degrees, seen as ovoid yeast cell with numerous cells around the mother cell in a "pilot wheel" or "ship wheel" formation

■ Other studies: serology can be helpful
> agar gel immunodiffusion (ID) test can be 98% sensitive
> does not give an indication about burden of disease
> the complement fixation test can be followed for response to therapy
> can cross-react with Histoplasma antigens
■ Other studies: skin testing is not useful

Imaging
■ Chest X-ray: patchy and bilateral nodular infiltrates, usually symmetrical, spares the apices

Pathology
■ If direct examination does not provide a diagnosis, may get biopsy with Gomori staining

DIFFERENTIAL DIAGNOSIS
■ Tuberculosis, histoplasmosis, leprosy, syphilis, mucocutaneous leishmaniasis

MANAGEMENT

General Measures
■ General supportive care

SPECIFIC THERAPY

Treatment Options
■ Itraconazole for 6 months
> Itraconazole cyclodextrin solution has increased bioavailability
■ Alternatives:
■ For severe disease: Amphotericin B IV
■ Others: sulfonamides (e.g., sulfadiazine)
■ Others: ketoconazole for 6–12 months

Side Effects & Contraindications
■ Itraconazole
> Side effects: nausea, vomiting, anorexia, abdominal pain, rash; rarely hypokalemia and hepatitis
> Contraindications: end stage renal disease for cyclodextran solution; lower cyclosporin dose when concomitantly given; may dangerously increase serum levels of digoxin, astemizole and loratidine, causing fatal arrhythmias

- Amphotericin B
  - Side effects: fevers, chills, nausea, vomiting and headaches; rigors may be prevented by the addition of hydrocortisone to bag, meperidine may treat rigors; nephrotoxicity; electrolyte disturbance (renal tubular acidosis, hypokalemia, hypomagnesemia)
- Contraindications: if Cr 2.5–3.0, may consider giving lipid-based Amphotericin products

FOLLOW-UP
- Follow-up chest radiographs as necessary
- May also follow complement fixation titers for response to therapy

COMPLICATIONS AND PROGNOSIS
Complications
- Pulmonary disease may progress to right ventricular hypertrophy and right heart failure

Prognosis
- Good with treatment; may need prolonged course of therapy

PARAINFLUENZA

CAROL A. GLASER, MD

HISTORY & PHYSICAL
History
- RNA virus – paramyxoviruses; 4 distinct types – 1, 2, 3, and 4
- Several animal species hosts to parainfluenza but human infection from humans only
- Transmission person to person – direct contact, contaminated secretions and fomites
- incubation period: 2–6 days
- type 1: outbreaks (usually croup) in fall (2–6 yr old)
- type 2: sometimes cause outbreaks but less severe/irregular > type 1 (2–6 yr old)
- type 3: must prominent spring/summer
- type 4: can cause disease young chickens but is rarely isolated
- Reinfections can occur at any age milder > initial.
- Nosocomial infections are common.

- Major cause of laryngotracheitis bronchitis
- At least 50% croup due to parainfluenza
- Major problem infancy

Signs & Symptoms

- Croup: hoarseness, cough, inspiratory stridor with laryngeal obstruction and fever, peak incidence 1–2 yrs
- Upper respiratory infection
- Pneumonia
- Bronchiolitis
- Expiratory wheezing with tachypnea, air trapping and retractions
- Mostly in first year of life
- Tracheobronchitis
- Cough, fever, large airway auscultation
- Occurs throughout childhood and adolescence
- Otitis media
- Pharyngitis
- Conjunctivitis
- Coryza

TESTS

Specific

- Antigen detection (DFA or ELISA) in respiratory secretions available most settings
  - Isolation of virus in respiratory secretions
  - Serology of limited value

DIFFERENTIAL DIAGNOSIS

n/a

MANAGEMENT

- For hospitalized patients – contact precautions

SPECIFIC THERAPY

- No specific antiviral
- Supportive management
- Racemic epinephrine is sometimes given to reduce airway obstruction.
- Steroids sometimes used

FOLLOW-UP

n/a

COMPLICATIONS AND PROGNOSIS

- Neurologic disease/case reports of:

> associated with Guillain-Barre syndrome
> demyelinating syndrome
> meningitis children/adults
- Immunocompromised host
  > can cause serious and sometimes fatal lower respiratory tract infections in immunocompromised children + adults
  > Giant – cell pneumonia – SCIDS, AML and s/p BMT
  > Persistent respiratory tract infection has been described in immunocompromised (e.g., DiGeorge rejection episodes in renal + liver transplant [type 3])
  > Fever and neutropenia in children

PARALYTIC POLIOMYELITIS

MICHAEL J. AMINOFF, MD, DSc

HISTORY & PHYSICAL
- Weakness of muscles in one or more limbs or the trunk, or supplied by the lower cranial nerves; may progress for 3–5 days
- Minor GI disturbance, fever, malaise, headache or neck stiffness in preceding 10 days
- May have been recent recipient or contact of recipient of oral polio vaccine
- Neck stiffness or other evidence of aseptic meningitis
- Flaccid weakness or paralysis of affected muscles
- No sensory deficit
- Tendon reflexes normal or reduced

TESTS
- CSF shows pleocytosis & increased protein level
- Poliovirus may be isolated from stool, throat swabs, CSF
- Acute & convalescent serum to detect increase in polio antibody titers
- EMG evidence of denervation in affected muscles

DIFFERENTIAL DIAGNOSIS
- Infections w/other enteroviruses are distinguished serologically & by virus isolation studies
- Acute weakness of LMN type due to cord or peripheral nerve disease is distinguished by the associated clinical deficits; organophosphate

toxicity is suggested by history of exposure; multifocal motor neuropathy has a more prolonged course

MANAGEMENT
- Assess adequacy of ventilation; provide support if needed
- Supportive care
- Notify local public health/communicable disease control unit

SPECIFIC THERAPY
- None available

FOLLOW-UP
- Depends on severity of disease

COMPLICATIONS AND PROGNOSIS
- Mortality <10% except in bulbar cases, when it approaches 50%
- Survivors may develop increasing weakness after some years in affected limb ("postpolio syndrome")

PARKINSON'S DISEASE AND PARKINSONISM

CHAD CHRISTINE, MD

HISTORY & PHYSICAL
- Tremor at rest
- Slowness of voluntary movement (bradykinesia)
- Stooped posture, short steps
- Reduced facial expression
- Hypophonia
- Increased muscle tone; cogwheel rigidity
- Reduced postural stability
- Dementia may occur

TESTS
- Diagnosis made clinically
- Lab: blood tests unremarkable
- Imaging: CT or MRI of brain is typically unremarkable
- Specific tests: genetic tests available for rare familial forms (research)

DIFFERENTIAL DIAGNOSIS
- Degenerative diseases such as progressive supranuclear palsy, multisystem atrophy, corticobasal ganglionic degeneration, dementia w/ Lewy bodies excluded clinically

- Drug-induced parkinsonism (esp dopamine receptor antagonists) excluded by history
- Infectious & postinfectious causes excluded by history
- Toxic exposures (MPTP, pesticides) excluded by history

MANAGEMENT
- Depends on cause & type of symptoms
  - For PD, treatment is symptomatic

SPECIFIC THERAPY
- Tremor
  - Amantadine
  - Benztropine or trihexyphenidyl
- Bradykinesia
  - Dopamine agonists
    - Bromocriptine
    - Pergolide
    - Pramipexole
    - Ropinirole
    - Apomorphine (IM) for rescue of disabling akinesia
  - L-dopa/carbidopa may also be used
  - COMT inhibitors
    - Extend half-life of L-dopa in moderate/advanced PD
    - Entacapone: w/ each dose of L-dopa
    - Tolcapone (monitor liver enzymes)
  - L-dopa/carbidopa/entacapone combination
- Drug-induced confusion, paranoia, hallucinations
  - Quetiapine
  - Clozapine (requires routine complete blood counts)

FOLLOW-UP
- Depends on cause & severity of symptoms

COMPLICATIONS AND PROGNOSIS
- PD is a chronic progressive disorder
- Clinical course is variable
- 40% develop depression that responds to treatment (TCAs, SSRIs, etc.)
- 30% develop dementia
- Most die of aspiration pneumonia

PARONYCHIA

JEFFREY P. CALLEN, MD

HISTORY & PHYSICAL

History

- Inflammation around the periungual structures (nail fold)
- May be due to bacteria (acute) or candida (chronic) or a combination of bacteria and yeast
- Excessive moisture may predispose – e.g., bartenders, healthcare workers, children who suck their fingers
- Trauma may be involved

Signs & Symptoms

- Inflammation characterized by erythema, tenderness, swelling and occasional discharge of pus in a periungual location
- May result in disturbance of the nail growth with eventual ridging

TESTS

- Basic tests: none needed
- Basic Tests: none needed
- Specific Diagnostic Tests
    - ➤ culture for bacteria
    - ➤ fungal culture
    - ➤ Tzanck smear or viral culture if herpes simplex is considered
- Imaging studies
    - ➤ Radiographs for recurrent or non-responsive disease to rule out osteomyelitis

DIFFERENTIAL DIAGNOSIS

- The process is clinically characteristic; the main differential diagnosis is among the infecting organism.
- Herpetic whitlow may be considered a viral form of paronychia.
- Eczema

MANAGEMENT

What to Do First

- Assess the risk factors such as trauma, exposure to excess moisture.

General Measures

- Keep area dry.
- Avoid manipulation of the cuticle.

- Consider the need for incision and drainage of the area.
- Assess the need for systemic therapy vs. local therapy.

SPECIFIC THERAPY
- Acute Paronychia
  - ➤ consider incision and drainage
  - ➤ Antibiotics – cephalexin, erythromycin or dicloxacillin
- Chronic paronychia
  - ➤ Drying maneuvers
  - ➤ Avoidance of trauma
  - ➤ Topical antifungal cream (e.g., clotrimazole) may be combined with a mild corticosteroid (e.g., triamcinolone) cream.

FOLLOW-UP

During Treatment
- Re-evaluate patient 1–2 weeks after initiating therapy

COMPLICATIONS AND PROGNOSIS
- Nail dystrophy may occur.

PARVOVIRUS B19

CAROL A. GLASER, MD

HISTORY & PHYSICAL

History
- Parvovirus B19 is a small single-stranded DNA virus.
- Humans only known hosts, not related to canine or feline parvovirus
- Mode of spread: respiratory secretions, blood transfusions
- Incubation period: usually 4–24 days (may be up to 21 days)
- Focal outbreaks elementary, community epidemics
- Winter/Spring
- 50% of adults are immune.
- Erythema Infectiosum (EI) aka "fifth disease"

Signs & Symptoms
- Classic; Erythema infection (EI) – mild systemic symptoms
  - ➤ fever: 15–30%
    - "distinct rash" (described below)
    - not infectious at time of rash

- Prior onset EI nonspecific symptoms fever, malaise, myalgias, headache that lasts 2–3 days, followed 7–10 days later with characteristic exanthem
- Exanthem: 3 stages;
  - facial rash; fiery red rash and cheeks (slapped cheek)
  - symmetric maculopapular rash on arms, move caudally to trunk, buttocks, thighs
  - central clearing of rash leads to a lacy or reticular pattern
  - rash can recur, fluctuating in intensity, weeks or months
  - rash is often pruritic, and take any form such as morbilliform, hemorrhagic/urticarial/vesicular/erythema-multiforme like
- arthralgia/arthritis – peripheral joints, symmetric, common in adults, especially adult female patient
- Sometimes asymptomatic
  - Sometimes mild respiratory illness without rash

TESTS

Nonspecific
- WBC is usually normal/mild eosinophilia occasionally noted

Specific
- Serum B19- IgM antibody best test for acute infection in normal hosts-single serum usually sufficient to establish diagnosis, IgM is almost always present at time of rash, these tests may not be widely available
- B19-IgG antibody-useful for demonstrating past infection and immunity
- IgM and IgG antibody tests are immunoblot assays or EIA
- PCR tests on clinical specimens available in some settings and may be particularly useful in immunocompromised host
- Antigen detection methods available in some settings, especially for tissue specimens
- Electron microscopy can be used for tissues

DIFFERENTIAL DIAGNOSIS
- Rubella – rash may be similar, serology can distinguish
- Scarlet fever – lack of pharyngitis in EI, positive Strep culture in Scarlet fever
- Collagen vascular disease
- Drug reactions

- Aplastic crisis – Parvo B19 is most common cause of aplastic crisis but may need to distinguish from systemic bacterial infections (Salmonella, Streptococcus pneumoniae)

MANAGEMENT
- Supportive
- Transient aplastic crisis – may require transfusion
- Chronic anemia immunodeficient patient – IVIG
- Pregnancy – monitor closely, B19 immune hydrops may require intrauterine blood transfusion

SPECIFIC THERAPY
- No specific antiviral indicated

FOLLOW-UP
n/a

COMPLICATIONS AND PROGNOSIS
- Chronic infection with anemia: immunodeficient (especially congenital immunodeficiency syndromes, leukemia, cancer, HIV, tissue transplant patients) patients
- Aplastic crisis: in chronic hemolytic anemia* (often present with pallor, weakness, lethargy, anemia. Rash usually absent)
  - ➤ (*includes sickle cell anemia/hereditary spherocytosis/thalassemia/G6PD deficiency, PK deficiency)
- congenital infection – fetal hydrops or death – risk of fetal death is 0.6–1.25% based on rate of fetal death after maternal infection (2.5–5%), rate of susceptibility (50% in women of childbearing age) and rate of infection after given exposure (50%)
- case reports described: transient hemolytic anemia, meningitis/encephalitis, HSP, myocarditis and pseudo-appendicitis

PATENT DUCTUS ARTERIOSUS

MARIA ANSARI, MD

HISTORY & PHYSICAL

History
- Females: Males 2:1
- Associated with maternal rubella
- Usually an isolated defect, but may coexist with coarctation, VSD, pulmonic stenosis, aortic stenosis
- Represents 5–10% of adult congenital heart disease

Signs & Symptoms

- Rare for adult PDA to have associated symptoms, but if it occasionally patient will develop CHF, DOE, CP, and palpitations
- Continuous "machinery" murmur, peaks in late systole, best heard in left infraclavicular area, 2nd ICS
- Widened pulse pressure if significant left-to-right shunt is present
- Differential cyanosis with sparing of upper extremities in presence of severe pulmonary hypertension

TESTS

Screening

- Physical examination with classic murmur

Imaging

- CXR may show calcification of the ductus, left atrial enlargement or pulmonary artery enlargement
- ECHO: Color flow Doppler shows continuous high velocity flow within the main pulmonary artery near the left branch; estimate gradient across the PDA from velocity across ductus
- Right heart catheterization: gold standard; if PVR < 10 U/m^2, surgery for ligation and division of the PDA is low risk

DIFFERENTIAL DIAGNOSIS

DDx of continuous murmur

- Pulmonary A-V fistula
- Coronary-cameral fistula (coronary to cardiac chamber)
- Anomalous origin of left coronary artery from pulmonary artery
- VSD with aortic regurgitation
- Venous hum (external jugular compression obliterates murmur)
- Aortopulmonary window
- Coarctation of aorta (rarely causes a continuous murmur)

MANAGEMENT

- Assess for evidence of shunt reversal and pulmonary hypertension (physical exam/echo)
- Endocarditis prophylaxis indicated

SPECIFIC THERAPY

- Surgical ligation is curative, can be done thorascopically or by catheter based approach
- Contraindication: high PVR >10 U/m^2 or predominantly right-to-left shunting

FOLLOW-UP

■ No endocarditis prophylaxis required after curative surgery

COMPLICATIONS AND PROGNOSIS

Complications

■ Potential for infective endarteritis before surgical correction
■ CHF may develop due to long term left-to-right shunting
■ Eisenmenger's physiology: occurs with large PDA due to progressive right-sided pressure and volume overload from long term left-to-right shunting. Results in pulmonary hypertension and reversal of shunt.

Prognosis

■ Near normal long-term survival for PDA corrected in childhood
■ Survival in later repair depends on presence of pulmonary vascular disease and LV dilation

PEDICULOSIS

MICHAEL DACEY, MD and JEFFREY P. CALLEN, MD
REVISED BY JEFFREY P. CALLEN, MD

HISTORY & PHYSICAL

■ Can occur at any age, independent of hygiene
■ Three types: corporis (body), capitis (scalp), pubis (groin)
■ Transmitted person to person, or via fomites (blankets, combs, towels); overcrowded conditions are a risk factor
■ Pruritus becomes extreme, often accompanied by excoriations and secondary infection (especially impetigo), local adenopathy
■ Egg sacs, or nits, found on proximal hair shaft on scalp, groin
■ Organisms seen in pubic hair of adults; eyelashes of children

TESTS

■ No systemic work up required

DIFFERENTIAL DIAGNOSIS

■ Scalp: seborrheic dermatitis, psoriasis, atopic eczema, delusions of parasitosis
■ Body: acne, xerosis, dermatitis herpetiformis, delusions of parasitosis, scabies
■ Groin: tinea cruris, candidiasis, intertrigo, folliculitis

MANAGEMENT

- Eradication of all live lice, destroying incubating larvae, nit removal, treatment of secondary infection
- Treat all family members, regardless of symptoms
- Instruct family that personal use items and bedding must be deloused

SPECIFIC THERAPY

- Pyrethrins (RID): OTC, not ovicidal so require repeat application 1 week later
- Pyrethroids (Permethrin = Nix): single, 10-minute treatment application
- Lindane (Kwell): removes adults but not nits; requires second application
- Ivermectin might be used in extremely severe or recalcitrant cases

FOLLOW-UP

- One month to assess treatment response

COMPLICATIONS AND PROGNOSIS

- Commonly secondarily infected, particularly impetigo, requiring further therapy
- No long-term sequelae if properly treated

PELVIC INFLAMMATORY DISEASE

SARAH STAEDKE, MD

HISTORY & PHYSICAL

History

- Pelvic inflammatory disease (PID) encompasses a spectrum of female genital tract disorders including endometritis, salpingitis, tubo-ovarian abscess, and peritonitis.
- PID is typically an ascending, polymicrobial infection caused by N. gonorrhoeae, C. trachomatis, vaginal flora (anaerobes and facultative organisms), and possibly M. hominis and U. urealyticum.
- Risk factors: young age; contraception (decreased risk with barrier methods and OCPs, increased with IUDs); habits (douching, smoking); invasive procedures (IUD insertion, dilatation and curettage, induced abortion, hysterosalpingography), menses
- HIV infection may increase risk and influence clinical course of PID

- Epidemiology of PID complicated by imprecise terminology, lack of well-defined diagnostic criteria, inconsistent disease reporting requirements, frequency of asymptomatic infection, reliance on cervical rather than upper genital tract cultures, and polymicrobial nature of PID

Signs & Symptoms

- 10–20% of women with gonorrhea (GC) or chlamydia (CT) infections of the lower genital tract progress to PID
- Subclinical PID occurs in 60% (commonly caused by CT); mild to moderate in 30–40%; severe in <5%
- Symptoms: lower abdominal pain, vaginal discharge, vaginal bleeding, dysuria, dyspareunia, nausea or vomiting, anorectal symptoms
- Signs: fever, mucopurulent cervical discharge, cervical motion tenderness, uterine and adenexal tenderness, adenexal fullness or mass, abdominal guarding or rebound tenderness; elevated WBC count, ESR, C-reactive protein (CRP)

TESTS

Basic Tests: Blood

- WBC count: elevation particularly associated with GC PID
- ESR ≥15 mm/hr; elevated C-reactive protein (CRP)

Basic Tests: Other

- Urinalysis: pyuria, hematuria with urethral GC or CT infection
- Vaginal wet mount: ≥3 WBC/hpf, sensitive but not specific

Specific Diagnostic Tests

- Gram's stained endocervical specimen: Positive for GC = intracellular gram negative diplococci within leukocytes, ≥10 WBC/hpf
- Non-culture assays for GC and CT: EIA, DFA, DNA probe, nucleic acid amplification (LCR, PCR)
- Cervical culture for GC or CT; GC/CT co-infection in 20–30%
- Upper genital tract culture: may be positive for GC, CT, and vaginal flora including anaerobes
- Endometrial biopsy: histologic evidence of endometritis = intraepithelial polymorphonuclear leukocytes (PMNs) and plasma cells; sensitivity 92% and specificity 87% but may be lower depending on sampling
- Laparoscopy: "gold standard" but impractical for routine diagnosis; abnormalities include tubal erythema, swelling, exudate

Other Tests

- Peritoneal fluid analysis: increased WBC, bacteria
- Imaging: ultrasound, CT, MRI – enlarged, fluid-filled fallopian tubes, tubo-ovarian abscess

DIFFERENTIAL DIAGNOSIS

- Gynecological: ectopic pregnancy, ovarian cyst torsion/rupture, endometriosis
- GI: acute appendicitis, mesenteric lymphadenitis, IBD
- Urinary: UTI, pyelonephritis, nephrolithiasis and renal colic

MANAGEMENT

What to Do First

- Check pregnancy test to rule out ectopic
- Indications for hospitalization: unable to rule out surgical emergencies, pregnancy, immunodeficiency (including HIV), severe illness, tubo-ovarian abscess, patient unable to tolerate oral regimen, unsuccessful outpatient treatment
- Consider hospitalization for adolescents and patients likely to be non-compliant

General Measures

- Maintain high index of suspicion for PID and low threshold for treatment
- If present, remove IUD after starting antibiotics
- Report cases to local public health authorities and **refer** sexual contacts for evaluation and treatment
- Advise patient to abstain from sexual activity during therapy

SPECIFIC THERAPY

Indications

- Diagnosis of PID is based on clinical findings
- Treat all sexually active young women that meet minimum criteria:
  - Lower abdominal pain
  - Cervical motion tenderness
  - Adnexal tenderness
- Additional diagnostic criteria:
  - Temperature >38.3°C (>101°F)
  - Abnormal cervical or vaginal discharge
  - Presence of mucopus or vaginal WBCs
  - Elevated ESR

➤ Elevated CRP
➤ Positive GC or CT test
■ Definitive criteria:
  ➤ Histopathologic evidence of endometritis
  ➤ Abnormal imaging study (US, CT, or MRI)
  ➤ Laparoscopic abnormalities

Treatment Options

Now often treated as outpatient, but low threshold to admit if adolescent, appears acutely ill, or does not tolerate or respond to oral treatment. Should return for evaluation in 24–72 h.

Parenteral Regimens:

A. Cefotetan OR Cefoxitin; PLUS Doxycycline
B. Clindamycin PLUS Gentamicin

■ Continue parenteral regimen for 24 h after clinical improvement, then change to Doxycycline to complete 14 days of therapy; add Clindamycin or Metronidazole if tubo-ovarian abscess present
■ Alternative parenterals: Ofloxacin PLUS Metronidazole; Ampicillin/Sulbactam PLUS Doxycycline; Ciprofloxacin PLUS Doxycycline PLUS Metronidazole Oral Regimens: A. Ofloxacin PLUS Metronidazole B. Ceftriaxone OR Cefoxitin PLUS Probenecid OR other third-generation cephalosporin; PLUS Doxycycline
■ Consider adding Metronidazole if bacterial vaginosis present
■ Alternative oral regimens: Amoxicillin/clavulanate PLUS Doxycycline; insufficient data to recommend Azithromycin

Side Effects & Contraindications

■ Cefotetan: side effects: disulfiram-like reaction with alcohol, diarrhea; contraindicated in penicillin allergy; pregnancy = B
■ Ceftriaxone: side effects: pain with IM injection, phlebitis, diarrhea, cholestasis; contraindicated with penicillin allergy; pregnancy = B
■ Clindamycin: side effects: diarrhea, *C. difficile colitis*, rash, GI intolerance; caution in pregnancy but no risk with extensive experience
■ Doxycycline: side effects: GI distress, photosensitivity, erosive esophagitis; contraindicated in pregnancy (D) and growing children
■ Gentamicin: side effects: nephrotoxicity, ototoxicity, vestibular toxicity; contraindicated in pregnancy (C); avoid in renal or hepatic insufficiency
■ Metronidazole: side effects: disulfiram-like reaction with alcohol, GI distress, headache, metallic taste; pregnancy = B; avoid in first trimester

- Ofloxacin: side effects: GI intolerance, CNS stimulation, dizziness; contraindicated in pregnancy (C) and patients < 18 years

FOLLOW-UP

- Must re-examine patients receiving outpatient care in 24–72 h; if no clinical improvement pursue additional diagnostic tests, hospitalization, surgical intervention; if improving, continue follow-up at 7 and 21 days
- Consider re-screening for GC and CT 4–6 weeks after completion of therapy with cervical cultures and/or non-culture assays

COMPLICATIONS AND PROGNOSIS

- Perihepatitis: inflammation of liver capsule and adjacent peritoneum; presents with RUQ pain, LFTs usually normal; occurs in 5–15% of patients with acute salpingitis
- 25% of cases experience long-term sequelae (tubal infertility, ectopic pregnancy, chronic pelvic pain); increased risk with severe disease and repeated infections; decreased risk if antibiotics are started within 3 days of symptom onset
- Mortality is rare, usually occurs with ruptured tubo-ovarian abscess (mortality 3–8%)

PEMPHIGUS VULGARIS AND PEMPHIGUS FOLIACEUS

DANIEL J. SHEEHAN, MD; ROBERT SWERLICK, MD; and
JEFFREY P. CALLEN, MD

HISTORY & PHYSICAL

- Mucosal erosions and ulcerations are the most common initial manifestation in pemphigus vulgaris.
- Flaccid bullae or erosions or crusted skin lesions may occur initially in pemphigus foliaceus and following oral lesions in pemphigus vulgaris.
- Pemphigus foliaceus does not involve the mucous membranes and often follows a seborrheic distribution.

TESTS

Basic Blood Tests

- Electrolytes

Specific Diagnostic Tests

- Skin biopsy from small bulla or margin of larger bulla shows intra-epidermal blistering

- Biopsy of the oral mucosa demonstrates similar findings.
- DIF – intercellular IgG and C3
- IIF – circulating IgG that binds to cell surface of keratinocytes
- ELISA for antibodies to desmoglein 1 and or 3 may be predictive of clinical activity (desmoglein 3 is associated with pemphigus vulgaris and desmoglein 1 with pemphigus foliaceus).

DIFFERENTIAL DIAGNOSIS
- Impetigo: Does not cause mucosal erosions
- Bullous pemphigoid: BP has tense as opposed to flaccid bullae
- Erythema multiforme: Negative immunofluorescence studies

MANAGEMENT
What to Do First
- Correct fluid and electrolyte imbalances.

General Measures
- Antibiotics for bacterial infection, cleansing baths, wet dressings, pain management

SPECIFIC THERAPY
- Mild/localized disease can be treated with topical and intralesional corticosteroids along with dapsone or a tetracycline.
- Generalized PV – use systemic corticosteroids along with a steroid-sparing agent
- Prednisone as a single daily dose, 50% respond. May require divided-dose corticosteroids.
- Steroid-sparing agents:
  - dapsone
  - minocycline
  - azathioprine
  - mycophenolate mofetil
  - cyclophosphamide
  - methotrexate
  - Intravenous immune globulin
  - Rituximab
- Side Effects & Contraindications
  - Prednisone, azathioprine, mycophenolate mofetil, cyclophosphamide, methotrexate, dapsone, rituximab, tetracyclines – see Specific Therapy for Bullous Pemphigoid

FOLLOW-UP

During Treatment

- Azathioprine, cyclophosphamide, methotrexate – see Follow-Up During Treatment for Bullous Pemphigoid

Routine

- Clinical for improvement of skin lesions and development of drug-related side effects
- Rough correlation of IgG autoantibody titers with disease activity; the use of desmoglein antibodies by ELISA may be better correlated with disease activity

COMPLICATIONS AND PROGNOSIS

- Prior to corticosteroids, disease mortality was 100% at 5 years.
- Current mortality <5%, usually due to sepsis associated with immunosuppression
- Chronic course, but spontaneous resolution can occur after 3–5 years

---

PEPTIC ULCER DISEASE

M. BRIAN FENNERTY, MD

HISTORY & PHYSICAL

History

Risk Factors for Ulcers

- *Helicobacter pylori* (see section on *H. pylori*) 50–70%
- NSAIDs 30–40%
- Idiopathic 10–20%
- Smoking increases risk of recurrence of ulcer

Symptoms

- Epigastric pain
- Food may alleviate or worsen symptoms
- Pain usually relieved with acid reduction
- Nausea/vomiting unusual
- Weight loss is unusual unless malignant
- Hematemesis and/or melena if ulcer bleeds

Physical Findings

- Epigastric tenderness
- Melena in bleeding patients

- Physical findings of malignant ulcer:
  - ➤ anemia
  - ➤ weight loss
  - ➤ abdominal mass

TESTS

Specific Diagnostic Tests
- Upper GI barium study
- Endoscopy

Indirect Tests
- *H. pylori* antibody, urea breath tests, fecal antigen tests

DIFFERENTIAL DIAGNOSIS
- Nonulcer dyspepsia (diagnosis made by negative imaging study)
- Gastroesophageal reflux (diagnosis made by endoscopy, pH study, response to empirical trial of therapy, etc.)
- Cholelithiasis (diagnosis made by ultrasound or CT imaging)
- Gastroparesis (diagnosis made by nuclear medicine gastric emptying study)

* Gastric neoplasia (diagnosis made by endoscopy or barium radiography)

MANAGEMENT

What To Do First
- Should I empirically treat for an ulcer or make a definitive diagnosis by specific testing?
  - ➤ This is a philosophical issue and should be decided in conjunction with the patient's needs.
- If I decide to empirically treat, do I use an anti-secretory agent or anti-*Helicobacter pylori* therapy?
  - ➤ Both are acceptable approaches, but a response to either therapy does not exclude nonulcer dyspepsia, GERD or malignancy.
- If I decide to do a diagnostic test, should it be *H. pylori* testing or evaluating for an ulcer with endoscopy or a barium UGI study?
- Endoscopy vs. barium UGI
  - ➤ Endoscopy is:
    - more accurate than an UGI
    - allows for biopsy to exclude malignancy or diagnose *Helicobacter pylori*
    - can diagnose esophagitis

- more expensive than an UGI
- more invasive than an UGI

General Measures
- Stop smoking
- Stop and/or avoid NSAIDs
- Use anti-secretory agents or antacids for breakthrough symptoms

SPECIFIC THERAPY

Indications
- A confirmed or suspected diagnosis of an ulcer

Treatment Options
- *Helicobacter pylori* therapy if positive (see section on *H. pylori*)
- Anti-secretory therapy with a H2-receptor antagonist or proton pump inhibitor for 4–6 weeks

Side Effects
- Dyspepsia, nausea, vomiting, metallic taste with some *Helicobacter pylori* treatments (usually mild)
- Side effects rare with H2RAs or PPIs

Contraindications
- Absolute: allergy to drug

FOLLOW-UP

Routine
- Complicated peptic ulcer
- Suspected malignant ulcer
- Worried patient

COMPLICATIONS AND PROGNOSIS

Complications

Peptic Ulcer
- Bleeding
- Perforation
- Obstruction
- Symptomatic ulcer

Prognosis
- 80% of individuals with *H. pylori*-related peptic ulcer will relapse within one year once anti-secretory therapy is discontinued if H. pylori is not eradicated

- Maintenance therapy with an H2RA or PPI decreases relapse rate to 10–15%
- Of those infected with and cured of their *H. pylori* only 20% will still have an ulcer relapse
- Patients developing an ulcer while on NSAIDs
  - NSAIDs are relatively contraindicated in future
  - If NSAID is absolutely needed (which should be a rare event) use
    - Co-therapy with PPI or misoprostol
    - A COX-2 sparing agent

PERICARDIAL TAMPONADE

ANDREW D. MICHAELS, MD

HISTORY & PHYSICAL

Signs & Symptoms
- lightheadedness
- dyspnea
- tachycardia, hypotension
- elevated neck veins
- pulsus paradoxus
- clear lung fields

TESTS
ECG
- low QRS voltage

Chest x-ray
- enlarged cardiac silhouette

Echo
- diastolic collapse of right atrium/ventricle
- respiratory variation in tricuspid/mitral inflow velocities
- dilated inferior vena cava

DIFFERENTIAL DIAGNOSIS
- consider other causes of hypotension (hypovolemia, sepsis, MI, tension pneumothorax, aortic dissection, CHF)

MANAGEMENT
- emergent pericardiocentesis is treatment of choice

SPECIFIC THERAPY
- consider balloon pericardiotomy or surgical drainage for recurrent effusions

FOLLOW-UP
- repeat echo after drainage
- during hospitalization, regularly assess for reaccumulation of effusion

COMPLICATIONS AND PROGNOSIS

Complications
- death from untreated tamponade is most immediate complication
- complications of pericardiocentesis include pneumothorax, bleeding, cardiac perforation

Prognosis
- largely depends on underlying etiology of pericardial effusion

---

PERIPHERAL NEUROPATHIES

MICHAEL J. AMINOFF, MD, DSc

HISTORY & PHYSICAL
- Numbness, paresthesias, dysesthesias or hyperpathia
- Weakness, fasciculations or cramps of affected muscles
- Pain, often deep & burning, commonly present during rest
- Symptoms may be in distribution of single nerves (mononeuropathy), multiple individual nerves (mononeuropathy multiplex) or diffusely (polyneuropathy)
- May be family history of neuropathy
- May be history of systemic illness (eg, diabetes, uremia, AIDS, vasculitis, connective tissue disease, malignancy, infections), toxin exposure or use of medication assoc w/ neuropathy
- May be history of repetitive strain injury or recurrent trauma
- Distribution of deficit depends on nerves affected; depending on type of neuropathy, may be motor, sensory or mixed deficit
- Motor: weakness, wasting or both in muscles supplied by affected nerves
- Sensory: loss or impairment depending on nerve fibers affected, in stocking-and-glove distribution (polyneuropathy) or territory of individual nerves

> Small fibers: pain & temperature appreciation
> Large fibers: vibration & joint position sense
- Tendon reflexes depressed or absent
- Ataxia if marked sensory loss
- Localized dysautonomia (eg, cold or discoloration, impaired sweating) when small fibers affected

TESTS
- EMG & NCS confirm presence of neuropathy, suggest type of involvement (axonal or demyelination) & identify site of focal involvement or entrapment
- For polyneuropathy or mononeuropathy multiplex, some or all of the following tests may be required: CBC, differential count, ESR, FBS, liver & kidney function tests, TFTs, serum proteins, protein electrophoresis & immunoelectrophoresis, serum autoantibody studies (eg, anti-Hu, anti-MAG, anti-GM1), serum vitamin B12 & folate, RPR, HIV serology, CSF cell count & protein level, ANA, genetic studies, nerve biopsy

DIFFERENTIAL DIAGNOSIS
- Clinical exam distinguishes myelopathies or radiculopathies from neuropathies
- Clinical onset & course, nature of deficit & results of investigations distinguish different causes of neuropathy

MANAGEMENT
- For acute neuropathy, ensure adequacy of ventilation & cardiovascular function
- Protect airway, maintain blood pressure & assist ventilation as needed
- Simple analgesics, tricyclic antidepressants, gabapentin or carbamazepine may be helpful for neuropathic pain; dose is individualized depending on response & tolerance
- For acute weakness or paralysis, ensure joint mobility by passive range-of-motion exercises twice daily

SPECIFIC THERAPY
- Treat underlying cause of neuropathy when possible
- Guillain-Barre syndrome: plasmapheresis or IVIg, except in mild cases
- Chronic inflammatory demyelinating neuropathy: steroids, plasmapheresis or IVIg

■ Local treatment to minimize pressure damage for entrapment neuropathy; surgical decompression sometimes needed

FOLLOW-UP
■ Depends on individual disorder

COMPLICATIONS AND PROGNOSIS
■ Depend on individual disorder

PERIRECTAL ABSCESSES AND FISTULAS

MARK A. VIERRA, MD

HISTORY & PHYSICAL

Abscess
■ Rectal pain most common presenting symptom.
■ Pain tends to be of relatively short duration (hours or days), progressive, and present continuously, rather than pain only with bowel movements, as occurs with a fissure
■ Tenderness, swelling, induration, fluctulence usually, but not always present
■ Complicated abscesses may require examination under anesthesia for diagnosis
■ Fever and leukocytosis unreliably present

Fistula
■ Following drainage 25%–50% of abscesses will go on to persist as a fistula
■ Not usually painful, though may develop recurrent abscesses at the site
■ Small external opening with mucoid or prurulent drainage is usually easily visible

TESTS

Laboratory Tests
■ Anorectal abscesses or fistulas complicated by abscess may be accompanied by leukocytosis, though this is variable
■ CT scan or endorectal ultrasound may very rarely be necessary to delineate abscess or fistula
■ Barium enema or fistulogram may be necessary to delineate complex fistulas

- Barium enema and/or endoscopy may be necessary to look for Crohn's disease
- Exam under anesthesia occasionally necessary to identify a deep or complex abscess in a patient with pain but no clear external signs of infection

DIFFERENTIAL DIAGNOSIS
- Fissure in ano will severe pain with defecation
- Anodynia causes chronic pain without signs or symptoms of inflammation
- Consider Crohn's disease with unusual or multiple fistulae
- Rarely, tumors such as Kaposi's sarcoma may be mistaken for an abscess
- Hemorrhoids should not cause pain

MANAGEMENT
- Perirectal abscesses should be drained surgically, often but not necessarily always in the operating room
- Antibiotics should be given for complex abscesses and may be given by some, but not all surgeons at the time of drainage of an abscess
- Fistulae are best treated electively after the inflammation of an abscess has subsided

SPECIFIC THERAPY
- Superficial abscesses may be opened under local anesthesia in the office.
- More complex abscesses should be treated in the operating room.
- Occasionally, debridement of devitalized tissue may be necessary associated with drainage of the abscess
- Rarely, a fistula may be treated definitively at the same time as drainage of a perirectal abscess
- Fistulae typically require surgery to open the tract. Complex fistulae may require staged repairs, sometimes including the use of a seton, (a tie that will cut through the sphincter muscles slowly in order to prevent incontinence), and occasionally may even require a colostomy
- Some fistulae may respond to injection of the tract with fibrin glue
- Fistulae associated with Crohn's disease may respond to anti-TNF antibodies (infliximab)

FOLLOW-UP
- An abscess that resolves completely with drainage requires no further followup

- Recurrent abscesses at the same site suggest a fistula
- Consider inflammatory bowel disease or malignancy in patients with unusual or recurrent abscesses or fistulae
- Don't forget colon cancer screening!

COMPLICATIONS AND PROGNOSIS
- Neglected abscesses may result in extensive necrosis and can result in incontinence, considerable tissue loss, even death
- 25–50% of abscesses will go on to produce a fistula in spite of (not because of) appropriate drainage of the fistula
- Fecal incontinence is a risk of fistulae treatment by any technique; the risk is greater the more of the sphincter that is involved and more likely in women than in men, especially women with prior vaginal deliveries
- Most fistulae respond well to surgical treatment
- Fistula recurrence much greater in Crohn's patients
- Anti-TNF antibodies may allow Crohn's fistulae to close

PERITONEAL TUMORS

MINDIE H. NGUYEN, MD

HISTORY & PHYSICAL

History
- primary peritoneal tumors in general rare
  - mesotheliomas: most are malignant; found 35–40 years after exposure to asbestos
  - pelvic lipomatosis: nonmalignant growth of adipose tissue with or without fibrosis in the perirectal and perivesical spaces; predominantly in black males (male:female ratio 18:1) between 20–60 yr of age; may cause proliferative cystitis, urinary tract obstruction, hypertension, and occasionally gastrointestinal symptoms
- benign peritoneal cysts: rare condition
  - benign cystic mesothelioma: usually in adult women who present with pain; usually recurs after resection
  - benign cystic lymphangioma: usually in young men who present with abdominal mass; seldom recurs after resection
- metastatic peritoneal tumors (peritoneal carcinomatosis): by far the most common peritoneal tumors
  - tissues of origin:

- adenocarcinoma
- ovarian, breast, colon, stomach, pancreas, lung
- ➤ lymphoma and sarcoma
- ➤ ovary and appendix in the case of pseudotumor peritonei

Signs & Symptoms
- ■ ascites (abdominal distention less well tolerated by these patients than in cirrhotics)
- ■ bowel obstruction as ascites is replaced by solid tumor as the malignancy progresses

TESTS
- ■ ascitic fluid analysis:
- ■ cytology: positive in 60% of all malignant ascites and >90% peritoneal carcinomatosis with malignant cells lining the peritoneum
- ■ imaging tests: identify mass lesions, including primary tumor and peritoneal seeding

Diagnosis
- ■ ascitic fluid cytology
- ■ image-guide biopsy of mass
- ■ diagnostic laparoscopy or laparotomy usually required for mesothelioma

DIFFERENTIAL DIAGNOSIS
n/a

MANAGEMENT
What To Do First
- ■ confirm diagnosis with ascitic fluid for cytology, imaging study, or biopsy

General Measures
- ■ therapeutic paracentesis for comfort
- ■ determine options for palliative therapy

SPECIFIC THERAPY
- ■ diuretics not effective in most cases
- ■ therapeutic paracentesis usually required for symptomatic relief
- ■ mesothelioma: best results with radiation in combination with intravenous and intraperitoneal chemotherapy
- ■ pelvic lipomatosis: diversion indicated if significant urinary obstruction

- peritoneal carcinomatosis: intraperitoneal chemotherapy advocated by some
- ovarian cancer: surgical debulking and chemotherapy most promising

FOLLOW-UP

n/a

COMPLICATIONS AND PROGNOSIS

- overall very poor: survival 70% at 1 month, 25% at 3 months, 12% at 6 months, and 4% at 12 months after diagnosis of peritoneal carcinomatosis

PERITONITIS

MINDIE H. NGUYEN, MD

HISTORY & PHYSICAL

History

- bacterial peritonitis common in ambulatory peritoneal dialysis (1.4 events per patient-year)
- tuberculous peritonitis: in the US, 50% of the cases are associated with cirrhosis, usually alcoholic; in third-world countries, most cases occur without underlying cirrhosis
- Fitz-Hugh-Curtis syndrome = Chlamydia (less commonly gonococcus) peritonitis; actually a perihepatitis; very rare in men
- fungal peritonitis: usually due to Candida albicans and associated with perforated viscus or ambulatory peritoneal dialysis
- peritoneal histoplasmosis, coccidioidomycosis, and cryptococcal infection: rare in the US; usually seen in the setting of AIDS
- parasitic peritonitis: schistosomiasis, pinworms, ascariasis, strongyloidiasis, amebiasis; rare
- rare causes of peritonitis: connective-tissue diseases (lupus, polyarteritis, and scleroderma); familial Mediterranean fever (very rare in the US, common in Europe and in the Far East)

Signs and Symptoms

- peritoneal dialysis: abdominal pain and tenderness in 75% but fever only in 33%
- Fitz-Hugh-Curtis syndrome: RUQ pain, fever, hepatic friction rub; ascites may not be detectable clinically

TESTS

Basic Tests: Blood
- increased WBC, with or without left shift in bacterial peritonitis; lymphocytosis in tuberculous peritonitis

Special Tests

Peritoneal Fluid (Bacterial Peritonitis):
- >100 WBC/mm3 with >50% PMNs, or >100 PMNs/mm3
- organisms on Gram's stain: 70% of isolates are gram-positive, usually from the skin flora
- Fitz-Hugh-Curtis: usually neutrocytic; highest reported total protein of any cause of ascites

Laparoscopy:
- 100% sensitive for diagnosis of tuberculous peritonitis
- laparoscopy shows characteristic "violin-string" or "bridal veil" adhesions from abdominal to liver in Fitz-Hugh-Curtis syndrome

DIFFERENTIAL DIAGNOSIS
- peritonitis associated with AIDS: patients are predisposed to opportunistic infections that may involve the peritoneum:
  - viruses [i.e., CMV]
  - parasites [i.e., Pneumocystis carinii]
  - fungus [i.e., Histoplasma, Cryptococcus, and Coccidioides]
  - mycobacteria [i.e., Mycobacterium tuberculosis and Mycobacterium avium-intracellulare]
  - Non-Hodgkin's lymphoma and Karposi sarcoma

MANAGEMENT

What To Do First
- assess stability of patient and nature of underlying diseases
- perform diagnostic paracentesis

General Measures
- assess likelihood of bacterial peritonitis and need for empiric antibiotic therapy pending cultures

SPECIFIC THERAPY
- presumed bacterial peritonitis: empiric IV or intraperitoneal (in dialysis-related peritonitis) second- or third-generation cephalosporin while awaiting culture result. Coverage for gram positive cocci and anarobes should be considered in cases of

suspected dialysis-related cases and intestinal ischemia/perforation, respectively
- tuberculous peritonitis: 8 weeks of isoniazid, rifampin, and pyrazinamide, followed by 4 more months of isoniazid and rifampin
- Fitz-Hugh-Curtis: doxycycline usually curative
- fungal peritonitits: amphotericin B (intraperitoneal and intravenous combination therapy) may be curative

FOLLOW-UP
- repeat paracentesis to access improvement in peritonitis with decreasing WBC

COMPLICATIONS AND PROGNOSIS
- recurrent infection is common and may require replacement or removal of peritoneal catheter in dialysis patients
- fungal peritonitis more difficult to cure
- worse in AIDS patients

PERSISTENT VEGETATIVE STATE

MICHAEL J. AMINOFF, MD, DSc

HISTORY & PHYSICAL
- Pt previously in coma from bihemispheric disease appears awake, but w/o evidence of mental awareness or responsiveness
- Is totally dependent
- No evidence of mental activity
- Periods w/ opened eyes but no environmental contact
- May be decerebrate or decorticate posturing, recovery of brain stem reflexes, but no purposive responses
- Pt has sleep-wake cycles

TESTS
- EEG abnormal but shows evidence of sleep-wake cycles in previously comatose pt

DIFFERENTIAL DIAGNOSIS
- History of preceding coma distinguishes this disorder from de-efferented state ("locked-in syndrome") in which pt is conscious but mute & quadriplegic

MANAGEMENT
- Supportive care
- Discuss poor prognosis w/ family & consider withdrawal of support

SPECIFIC THERAPY
- None

FOLLOW-UP
n/a

COMPLICATIONS AND PROGNOSIS
- Most pts will die in weeks/months
- Recovery is rare & typically insufficient to permit independent living

---

PHARYNGITIS

RICHARD A. JACOBS, MD, PhD

HISTORY & PHYSICAL

History
- Viral (rhinovirus, coronavirus, adenovirus, herpes simplex, influenza, Epstein-Barr virus) etiology in 40%
- Bacteria cause 15–30%; most common etiology is group A streptococcus, but group C streptococcus, *Chlamydia pneumoniae*, and *Neisseria gonorrhoeae* also causes
- In 30% no known etiology
- Young age, crowding, temperate climate, contact with infected individual, sexual practices (gonorrhea and acute HIV) predispose to illness
- Major clinical distinction is between group A streptococcus and all the others

Signs & Symptoms
- Acute onset of sore throat, painful swallowing and fever; erythema of posterior pharynx and tonsils, with or without exudate, with tender enlarged anterior cervical nodes
- Signs and symptoms NOT specific for group A streptococcus-seen with viruses and other bacteria
- Absence of fever and presence of conjunctivitis, viral exanthem, diarrhea or pharyngeal vesicles suggests viral etiology

TESTS
- Leukocytosis may be present
- Pharyngeal swab for rapid antigen test 80–90% sensitive for diagnosis of group A streptococcus and >95% specific
- If rapid antigen test negative, culture should be obtained

■ Culture for gonorrhea and test for acute HIV if epidemiologic suspicion

DIFFERENTIAL DIAGNOSIS
■ Diphtheria (membrane present), parapharyngeal and retropharyngeal abscesses (bulging of posterior or lateral pharyngeal wall), epiglottitis (severe sore throat, hoarseness, stridor, drooling with minimal findings on exam-exclude by direct visualization of epiglottis) and foreign body (especially infants and children)

MANAGEMENT
■ Supportive care – rest, analgesics (ibuprofen, acetaminophen), fluids

SPECIFIC THERAPY
■ For group A streptococcus, penicillin or amoxicillin for 10 days (erythromycin for the penicillin allergic patient) or benzathine penicillin (single dose)
■ See gonorrhea for therapy of GC pharyngitis

FOLLOW-UP
■ Symptoms resolve in 2–3 days
■ Follow-up cultures NOT recommended for test of cure

COMPLICATIONS AND PROGNOSIS
■ Pyogenic complications include peritonsillar, retropharyngeal and parapharyngeal abscesses
■ Nonpyogenic complications include rheumatic fever (preventable if infection treated within 10 days of onset) and glomerulonephritis (not prevented with therapy)
■ Penicillin prophylaxis indicated for patients with rheumatic fever

---

PHEOCHROMOCYTOMA

RICHARD I. DORIN, MD

HISTORY & PHYSICAL

History
■ Headaches, paroxysms
■ Adrenergic excess: tachycardia, excessive sweating
■ Hypermetabolism: fever, weight loss
■ Hypertension, stable or paroxysmal
■ Chest or abdominal pain

- Unusual BP response to surgery, anesthesia, or trauma
- Family history of pheochromocytoma, adrenal tumor, medullary carcinoma of the thyroid, hypercalcemia/hyperparathyroidism
- Genetic associations: neurofibromatosis, Von-Hippel Landau disease, multiple endocrine neoplasia (MEN) II
- Medications: antihypertensives, decongestants, stimulants, adrenergic bronchodilators, MAO inhibitors, labetolol and buspirone (interfere with catecholamine tests), clonidine or beta-blocker withdrawal
- Diabetes, constipation
- Psychiatric disorders, alcohol or illicit drug use, spinal cord injury
- History of angina, MI, CVA

Signs & Symptoms
- Episodic headache, sweating, and palpitations
- Orthostatic hypotension, chest pain, abdominal pain
- Blurred vision, weight loss, polyuria, polydipsia
- Constipation, anxiety, "spells" or panic attacks
- Labile or difficult to control hypertension
- Orthostatic hypotension (due to volume contraction)
- Lid lag, papilledema
- Neurocutaneous disease
- Pallor (due to vasoconstriction)
- Abdominal mass, dilated cardiomyopathy
- Cutaneous flushing
- Thyroid nodule or mucosal/eyelid neuromas (in association in MEN IIA or IIB)

TESTS
- Basic Tests
  - ➤ 24-h urine collection for fractionated urinary metanephrines (metanephrine and normetanephrine), free catecholamines (norepinephrine and epinephrine); creatinine (to ensure complete collection of urine)
- Confirmatory Tests
  - ➤ Plasma catecholamines; perform in resting conditions with indwelling catheter after 30 min of rest, avoid setting of acute illness
  - ➤ Clonidine suppression test: plasma catecholamines before and 3 h after oral clonidine.
  - ➤ Plasma chromogranin
  - ➤ Plasma calcitonin: for MEN-2

Imaging

- CT or MRI only after biochemical diagnosis confirmed
- CT and MRI have limited specificity due to high prevalence of incidental adrenal mass
- CT of abdomen: pretreat with alpha-blockers to avoid aggravation of hypertension that may occur during administration of IV CT contrast dye; 90% of pheochromocytoma localize to adrenals; 95% of pheochromocytomas are intraabdominal
- MRI: On T2-weighted imaging, pheochromocytomas often appear hyperintense
- Nuclear Medicine Studies
- For extraadrenal, extraabdominal, or metastatic pheochromocytomas where CT or MRI nondiagnostic
- 131-I-metalobenzylguanidine (MIBG) (a catechol precursor)
- 111-Indium pentetreotide (labels neuroendocrine tissues expressing somatostatin receptor)

DIFFERENTIAL DIAGNOSIS

- Catecholamine excess from nonpheochromocytoma source (drugs, panic attacks, medical/surgical illness, spinal cord injury)
- Bilateral pheochromocytoma in 10% of cases, esp in setting of genetic predisposition
- Extraadrenal pheochromocytoma (paraganglionoma): paraaortic, bladder, thorax, head and neck, pelvis

MANAGEMENT

What to Do First

- Initiate medical therapy prior to surgery

General Measures

- Avoid extremes of hypo/hypertension
- Avoid catecholamine-releasing agents
- Volume replacement
- Management of cardiovascular risk

SPECIFIC THERAPY

- Alpha-adrenergic blockade:
    - Phenoxybenzamine until symptoms and BP controlled or titrated to clinical parameters (nasal stuffiness, orthostatic hypotension)
    - Calcium channel blockers as alternatives to pheonoxybenzamine

➤ Phentolamine: IV alpha-adrenergic blocker for acute management of hypertension or adrenergic crisis
■ Beta-adrenergic blockade:
  ➤ After alpha-blockade established, initiate beta-blockade for heart-rate control (Note: beta blockers alone lead to unopposed alpha-blockade and exacerbated hypertension)
■ Inhibition of catecholamine synthesis:
  ➤ Metyrosine (alpha-methyl-tyrosine) inhibits catecholamine synthesis

Surgery:
■ Usually abdominal approach, occasionally flank or laparoscopic approach
■ Intraoperative hypotension best avoided by preoperative alpha-blockade and vigorous IV fluid replacement
■ Medical and surgical coordination with anesthesia team

FOLLOW-UP

During Medical Treatment:
■ Evaluate q 3–4 d to monitor heart rate, BP, orthostatic BP and pulse, and side effects (eg, nasal stuffiness) to gradually increase dose of alpha-blockers

Postoperative:
■ Intraoperative fluids and volume replacement for hypotension
■ During 1st wk postop, monitor blood glucose or CBG q 4–6 h for hypoglycemia
■ 1–2 wks: repeat catecholamine tests to assess biochemical cure of catecholamine excess

Long-Term:
■ Difficult to distinguish benign vs malignant pheochromocytoma at pathology, so review for pheochromocytoma recurrence or metastases
■ Annual evaluation to assess and manage hypertension, screen for recurrence of symptoms, and measure urinary catecholamines and metabolites

COMPLICATIONS AND PROGNOSIS
■ Acute: hypertensive encephalopathy, hypotension, cardiovascular collapse
■ Chronic: dilated cardiomyopathy, angina and MI, CVA

Prognosis
- Benign pheochromocytoma:
  - Complete resection cures hypertension in 75%
  - Patients may remain hypertensive despite normal catecholamine levels
- Malignant pheochromocytoma:
  - 50% 5-y mortality

PHIMOSIS AND PARAPHIMOSIS

KEY H. STAGE, MD, FACS

HISTORY & PHYSICAL

Signs & Symptoms of Phimosis
- May be congenital or acquired, incidence 1% males >16 yrs
  - Foreskin cannot be retracted behind the glans penis
  - Normal in boys under age 4, even into early teens
  - Usually not painful, but may result in difficulty voiding, balloon appearance of distal foreskin with voiding due to obstruction

Signs & Symptoms of Paraphimosis
- Foreskin has been retracted behind the glans penis/coronal sulcus
- If not reduced, vascular engorgement with swelling and pain

TESTS
- Physical examination alone is sufficient for diagnosing phimosis and paraphimosis.

DIFFERENTIAL DIAGNOSIS
- Phimosis may be congenital or a result of trauma, forceful retraction of congenital phimosis, inflammation, poor hygiene.
- Paraphimosis is often iatrogenic, due to health care personnel carelessly leaving foreskin retracted, i.e., in a patient with a Foley catheter, chronic balanoposthitis, vigorous prolonged intercourse, popularity of body piercing.

MANAGEMENT

Phimosis
- Initially consists of topical cream and warm soaks for patient comfort
- If difficulty voiding, a dorsal slit may be performed in an emergency situation – dorsal aspect of foreskin incised using local anesthesia,

exposing glans and urethral meatus. Elective circumcision accomplished at a later date.

Paraphimosis

- Management must be immediate.
- Using analgesics and gentle, firm traction, foreskin may be drawn distally over the edematous coronal sulcus with immediate relief.
- Edema takes several hours to resolve. Manual compression using the hand or a pediatric blood pressure cuff around the penile shaft to squeeze out edema also a useful technique. Manual traction may result in successful replacement of the foreskin to normal position.
- If these measures fail, emergency dorsal slit may be necessary.

SPECIFIC THERAPY

Phimosis

- If foreskin cannot be retracted for hygienic and inspection purposes, circumcision recommended

Paraphimosis

- Management must be immediate.
- Manual compression technique described above.
- If previously mentioned measures fail, emergency dorsal slit may be necessary.

FOLLOW-UP

Phimosis and Paraphimosis

- Ensure that foreskin can be retracted.
- If not possible, circumcision recommended
- If circumcision is done and no neoplasia, no long-term follow-up necessary post-operatively

COMPLICATIONS AND PROGNOSIS

Phimosis

- Left untreated, long-term complications may include higher incidence of squamous cell carcinoma

Paraphimosis

- Left untreated, long-term complications include continued vascular congestion with edema, possible partial necrosis of penile skin

PHOSPHATE DEFICIENCY

ELISABETH RYZEN, MD

HISTORY AND PHYSICAL

History:

alcoholism, diabetic ketoacidosis, severe burns, TPN, malnutrition, hyperparathyroidism, Vitamin D deficiency, malabsorption syndrome, hypomagnesemia, chronic ingestion of phosphate-binding antacids, refeeding (transcellular shifts)

Physical:

muscle weakness (including respiratory muscles), anorexia, rhabdomyolysis, impaired cardiac output, osteomalacia (chronic), hemolytic anemia, impaired leukocyte and platelet function

TESTS

Laboratory

- Basic studies: blood (serum phosphate <2.5 mg/dL)
- Severe symptoms (e.g., hemolytic anemia, impaired cardiac output) only develop with phosphate <1 mg/dL)
- DDx N/A

MANAGEMENT

What to Do First

- Assess severity of symptoms (respiratory, cardiac)

General Measures

- Treat underlying cause, feed patient phosphate-rich foods if possible (e.g., skim milk)

SPECIFIC THERAPY

- oral replacement with sodium or potassium phosphate (e.g., Neutra-Phos 500 mg p.o. qid) – may cause diarrhea
- IV for severe hypophosphatemia and symptoms (assess renal function first):
  - ➤ e.g., 2–5 mg/kg IV phosphate as K-phosphate slowly over 6–8 h

Contraindications to Treatment

- Absolute
  - ➤ Elevated serum phosphate level; inability to accurately control amount of phosphate given
- Relative
  - ➤ Renal failure – use with extreme caution even if mild creatinine elevations, lower doses

FOLLOW-UP

■ Monitor serum phosphate, creatinine, calcium to avoid hypocalcemia, hyperphosphatemia, hypotension

COMPLICATIONS AND PROGNOSIS
n/a

PHOTOSENSITIVITY

JEFFREY P. CALLEN, MD

HISTORY & PHYSICAL

History

■ Eruption on exposed surfaces, patient may note the relationship to the exposure.
■ Classification:
  ➤ Phototoxicity – increased reaction to sun or UVB light commonly caused by drugs, particularly sulfonamides, thiazide diuretics, and tetracyclines
  ➤ Photoallergy – cell-mediated response that requires both a drug/antigen and light, most often UVA light. Most common: fragrances and sunscreens containing PABA or PABA esters
  ➤ Endogenous diseases – polymorphous light eruption (PMLE) and lupus erythematosus (LE) are the most common, porphyria cutanea tarda (PCT) and pseudoporphyria are less common
    • PMLE – often occurs with intense exposure or early in the spring/summer and lessens in its severity toward fall even with continued exposure (hardening). It is often extremely pruritic.
    • LE – patients may have accompanying systemic complaints (see chapter on Cutaneous LE)
    • PCT/Pseudoporphyria may complain of fragility of the skin
      • PCT often associated with Hepatitis C infection
      • Pseudoporphyria is caused by drugs (particularly the NSAIDs naproxen, nabumetone and oxaprozin), tanning beds, and is associated with hemodialysis
  ➤ Photoaggravated Diseases
    • Acne vulgaris
    • Darier's disease (keratosis follicularis)
    • Dermatomyositis
    • Grover's disease (transient acantholytic dermatosis)
    • Herpes simplex

Signs & Symptoms

- Phototoxicity is manifest by erythema in a photodistribution
- Photoallergy is manifest by an eczematous eruption in a photodistribution
- Polymorphous light eruption – most often erythematous papules or plaques without epidermal change
- Lupus erythematosus may be manifest as discoid lesions, or non-scarring lesions (see Cutaneous LE chapter)
- PCT and pseudoporphyria are manifest as blisters, erosions, scars and milia most commonly on the dorsal hands. Patients with PCT may have hyperpigmentation and/or hypertrichosis

TESTS

- Basic blood tests:
    - ANA, Anti Ro (SS-A), anti-nDNA in patients with PMLE or possible LE
    - None in patients with phototoxicity and photoallergy
- Basic urine tests:
    - Urinary porphyrins in patients with fragility or blisters of the dorsal hands
- Specific diagnostic tests –
    - Hepatitis C antibody in patients diagnosed with PCT
    - Skin biopsy is helpful for diagnosis of LE

DIFFERENTIAL DIAGNOSIS

- PMLE and LE may be at times difficult to distinguish. LE often has antibodies and the skin biopsy may help.
- PCT and pseudoporphyria can be differentiated by hypertrichosis that occurs with PCT, both must be differentiated from epidermolysis bullosa acquisita – immunofluorescence microscopy is useful

MANAGEMENT

What to Do First

- Establish the possibility that sunlight is involved with the condition
- Determine the pattern of the disease – phototoxicity vs. allergy vs. endogenous disease vs. photoaggravated disease
- Determine the action spectrum – the wavelength of light that causes or aggravates the disease. Phototesting may be helpful in reproducing the disease.
- Consider skin biopsy and other diagnostic tests

General Measures
- Remove the patient from exposure – light and drug/antigen where appropriate

SPECIFIC THERAPY
- PMLE – Avoidance of light, topical or systemic corticosteroids, oral antimalarials
- LE – broad spectrum sunscreens, photoprotective clothing, topical corticosteroids, oral antimalarials
- PCT – treat concomitant Hepatitis C, phlebotomy or antimalarials
  - ➤ Antimalarial therapy may result in a toxic reaction, so the dose must start very low.
- Pseudoporphyria – discontinue the causative agent

FOLLOW-UP
- PMLE – follow to be certain that LE is not the correct diagnosis
- LE – see cutaneous LE chapter
- Pseudoporphyria – some of the NSAIDs cross-react. It may take weeks to months for the eruption to clear.

COMPLICATIONS AND PROGNOSIS
- Dependent upon the diagnosis

PITUITARY TUMORS

ANDREW R. HOFFMAN, MD

HISTORY & PHYSICAL

History
- Weakness, fatigue
- Infertility
- Amenorrhea/oligoamenorrhea
- Weight loss
- Absent or delayed puberty
- Cushing syndrome
- Acromegaly, galactorrhea

Signs & Symptoms
- General: headache, visual field cut, decreased libido, impotence
- Hypopituitarism: fatigue, cachexia, cold intolerance, constipation, diminished pubic/axillary hair, inability to lactate, orthostatic hypotension, hypoglycemia, dry, pale, wrinkled skin

- Cushing's disease: central obesity, emotional lability, hypertension, diabetes mellitus; weakness, striae
- Acromegaly: enlarged hands and feet, sleep apnea, loose teeth, prognathic jaw, frontal bossing, diabetes, carpal tunnel syndrome
- TSH-secreting tumor (rare): thyrotoxicosis
- LH/FSH-secreting tumor: asymptomatic; hypopituitarism
- Prolactinoma: galactorrhea, amenorrhea, impotence
- Diabetes insipidus: polydipsia, polyuria, nocturia

TESTS

Laboratory
- Basic blood studies:
    - LH, FSH, prolactin, free T4, TSH, testosterone, ACTH
    - Cortisol after Cosyntropin or insulin tolerance test
      24-hour urine free cortisol
        8:00 AM cortisol after 1 mg (low dose) or 8 mg (high dose) dexamethasone at midnight
    - Insulin-like growth factor-I (IGF-I)
    - Growth hormone (GH)
    - Electrolytes, glucose
    - Urinalysis
- Ancillary blood tests:
    - Estradiol
    - ACE

Imaging
- MRI of pituitary and brain.
Pituitary tumors classified as macroadenomas (≥ 1 cm) or microadenomas (<1 cm); microadenomas rarely grow on follow-up exams

DIFFERENTIAL DIAGNOSIS
- Pituitary tumor:
    - Nonsecretory, prolactinoma, acromegaly, Cushing syndrome
    - Usually causes partial or complete anterior pituitary insufficiency
    - Most common deficiencies: GH > LH, FSH > TSH, ACTH
- Enlarged pituitary without mass: lymphocytic hypophysitis, severe primary hypothyroidism
- Aneurysm, meningioma
- Pituitary apoplexy
- Rathke pouch cyst

- Hypothalamic mass: craniopharyngioma, dysgerminoma
- Metastatic tumor: breast and lung most common
- Granulomatous disease and histiocytosis: may cause anterior and posterior pituitary deficiency 10% of people have small microadenomas that are nonsecretory. Clinically silent tumors may be found when patient has MRI for other causes ("incidentaloma").

MANAGEMENT

What to Do First
- Determine hormone deficiencies (partial or panhypopituitarism) and excesses
- Assess size and resectability of tumor
- Rule out apoplexy
- Obtain tissue for diagnosis if possible

Treatment Goals
- Treat hormone deficiencies and excesses
- Resect or diminish size of pituitary or CNS mass

SPECIFIC THERAPY
- Hormone replacement therapy:
  - Cortisol
  - Thyroid hormone
  - Testosterone
  - Estrogen/progestin
  - DDAVP
  - Growth hormone
  - Gonadotropins for fertility only
- Normalize prolactin, ACTH, or GH hypersecretion
- Surgical resection of tumor
- Medical therapy for prolactinoma and acromegaly
- Radiation therapy
- Treat granulomatous diseases
- Observation with repeated pituitary MRI to determine if tumor growing
- Side Effects & Contraindications
  - Surgery and radiation: panhypopituitarism, CNS injury

FOLLOW-UP
- Assess adequacy of hormone replacement therapy annually
- Repeat pituitary MRI in 3–6 mo to assess tumor growth

COMPLICATIONS AND PROGNOSIS
- Pituitary apoplexy
- Visual field changes
- Patients require lifelong observation

PITYRIASIS ROSEA

DENISE W. METRY, MD

HISTORY & PHYSICAL
- Most common in adolescents and young adults in spring and autumn months
- Most patients are asymptomatic prior to onset; viral prodrome (mild malaise and/or sore throat) is uncommon
- Usually begins with a single, large, oval "herald" patch, followed 1–2 weeks later by oval or annular patches or plaques with thin "collarette" of scale near inner side of lesion
  - Symmetrical distribution with long axis of lesions parallel to lines of the ribs on trunk and proximal extremities ("Christmas tree" pattern); face, palms and soles usually spared
  - Pruritus common with onset of generalized eruption
- Atypical variants (more common in children): pustular, purpuric, erythema-multiforme-like, "inverse" (axillae and groin)
- Oral lesions consisting of petechiae, ulcers, erythematous macules or vesicles/bullae may occur and seem to be more common in children, black patients and more severely affected individuals
- Viral etiology is highly suspected because of the seasonal occurrence and finding of human herpes virus 6 & 7 in some patients

TESTS
- No specific laboratory abnormalities
- Histopathology may be helpful in atypical cases and demonstrates perivascular lymphohistiocytic infiltrate in the dermis with extravasated red blood cells.

DIFFERENTIAL DIAGNOSIS
- Herald patch: tinea corporis (fungal hyphae apparent on KOH/ microscopic exam)
- Generalized symmetrical eruption: secondary syphilis (involvement of palms, soles and mucous membranes, shotty adenopathy, positive

serology); guttate psoriasis (no collarette of scale, herald patch or "Christmas tree" pattern)

■ Pityriasis rosea-like drug eruptions may occur with gold, captopril, D-penicillamine, metronidazole, isotretinoin, barbiturates, pyribenzamine, ketotifen, combined use of anti-inflammatory and antipyretic drugs, mustard oil, ergotamine, linsinopril

MANAGEMENT

■ Exclusion of syphilis with VDRL or FTA-ABS if clinical suspicion warrants

SPECIFIC THERAPY

■ Due to the self-limiting nature, therapy needed only for significant pruritus or cosmetic concerns

■ Treatment options include oral erythromycin (for 2 weeks), ultraviolet B phototherapy or modest amounts of natural sunlight, low- to mid-potency topical corticosteroids, oral corticosteroids (short course), and/or antihistamines.

■ Recently high-dose oral acyclovir has been advocated as a potential treatment.

FOLLOW-UP

■ Generally unnecessary

COMPLICATIONS AND PROGNOSIS

■ Usual course: 6 to 8 weeks with spontaneous resolution; rarely lasts longer than 3 months and rarely recurs

PLEURAL DISEASES: EFFUSION/EMPYEMA

GEORGE SU, MD

HISTORY & PHYSICAL

Signs & Symptoms

■ Often asymptomatic

■ Pleuritic chest pain

■ Dyspnea (large effusion)

■ Fevers

■ Tracheal deviation

■ Absent fremitus

■ Percussion dullness

■ Decreased breath sounds

- Pleural rub
- Cardiomegaly, JVD, edema, S3 (CHF)
- Arthropathy, subcutaneous nodules (rheumatoid, lupus)
- Nodular liver, osteoarthropathy, breast masses (metastases)
- Abdominal tenderness (subdiaphragmatic process)
- Ascites (hepatic hydrothorax)
- Lymphadenopathy (lymphoma, metastases, sarcoidosis)

TESTS

CXR
- Costophrenic blunting, subpulmonic, "pseudotumor"
- Sensitivity: lateral decubitus (10 cc) > lateral (75 cc) > PA
- CBC/diff, LDH, total protein, glucose

Thoracentesis
- Contraindications: bleeding diathesis, anticoagulation, uncooperative patient, obliterated pleural space, co-morbidity making pneumothorax hazardous
- Avoid removing >1000 ml at one time (re-expansion pulmonary edema)

Pleural Fluid Analysis
- Color, turbidity, RBC, WBC/diff, protein, LDH, pH, glucose, gram stain, culture
- Other: hematocrit, amylase, cytology, ANA, lupus erythematosus (LE) cells, Rh factor, triglycerides, chylomicrons, cholesterol, KOH, fungal culture, creatinine

Transudate vs. Exudate
- Exudate = at least one:
    - Pleural fluid/serum protein >0.5
    - Pleural fluid/serum LDH >0.6
    - Pleural fluid LDH >2/3 upper limit of serum normal
- Suggestive of exudate:
    - Pleural fluid protein >2.9 g/dL
    - Pleural fluid cholesterol >45 mg/dL

Ultrasound
- Simple: hypoechoic
- Hemorrhage/empyema: echogenic

CT with Contrast

- Loculations, airway or parenchymal lesions, abscesses, bronchopleural fistula, pleural plaques

Percutaneous Pleural Biopsy

- Lymphocytic effusion (TB). Rarely for sarcoidosis or rheumatoid (necrobiotic nodule) Malignancy (low yield)

Thoracoscopy

- Malignancy, TB

Bronchoscopy

- Hemoptysis, parenchymal or endobronchial lesion

DIFFERENTIAL DIAGNOSIS

Transudate

- CHF, hepatic hydrothorax, nephrotic syndrome, peritoneal dialysis (protein <1 g/dL; glucose 300–400 mg/dL), hypoalbuminemia, urinothorax (pleural fluid/serum creatinine >1.0), atelectasis, constrictive pericarditis, trapped lung, SVC obstruction
- "Classically exudative" that can be transudative: malignancy, PE, sarcoidosis, hypothyroid

Exudate:

Infectious

- *Iatrogenic*: drugs; esophageal perforation, sclerotherapy; misplaced central venous catheter or feeding tube
- *Malignancy*: +cytology (60–90%), pleural biopsy (17%), thoracoscopy (>90%);
- associated chylothorax (triglycerides >110 mg/dL)
- *Inflammatory*: pancreatitis, asbestos, pulmonary embolism, radiation, uremia, sarcoidosis, post-cardiac injury, hemothorax (pleural fluid/blood *hematocrit >0.5*)
- *Negative intrapleural pressu*re: atelectasis, trapped lung
- *Connective tissue*: lupus (+LE cells, pleural fluid/serum ANA >1.0), rheumatoid, MCTD, Churg-Strauss, Wegener's
- *Endocrine*: hypothyroidism, ovarian hyperstimulation
- *Lymphatic*: yellow-nail syndrome, lymphangiomyomatosis
- *Abdominal Translocation*: pancreatitis, pseudocyst, Meigs', chylous ascites, urinothorax

Exudate: Lab-Based Differential

- Protein
  - \>4.0 g/dL: TB
  - 7.0–8.0 g/dL: Waldenstrom's, myeloma
- LDH >1000 IU/L: complicated parapneumonic/empyema, rheumatoid, malignancy, paragonimiasis
- Pleural fluid/serum LDH >1.0 and pleural fluid/serum protein < 0.5: PCP
- Glucose <60 mg/dL, or pleural fluid/serum glucose < 0.5: rheumatoid, complicated parapneumonic/empyema, malignancy, TB, esophageal rupture
- pH <7.30: rheumatoid, complicated parapneumonic/empyema, malignancy, TB, lupus, esophageal rupture (as low as 6.00)
- Pleural fluid/serum amylase >1.0: pancreatitis, esophageal rupture, malignancy, pneumonia, ectopic pregnancy, hydronephrosis, cirrhosis
- Total nucleated cells:
  - <5000/mcl: TB, malignancy
  - \>10,000/mcl: parapneumonic effusion, pancreatitis, lupus
  - \>50,000/mcl: complicated parapneumonic effusion/empyema
- Differential cell count:
  - 50–70% lymphocytes: malignancy
  - 85 to 95% lymphocytes: TB, lymphoma, sarcoidosis, rheumatoid, yellow-nail syndrome, chylothorax
  - \>10% eosinophils: pneumothorax, hemothorax, pulmonary infarction, asbestos, parasitic, fungal, drugs, malignancy
  - \>5% mesothelial cells: TB unlikely

MANAGEMENT

Parapneumonic Effusions/Empyema

- Antibiotics, consider drainage, oxygen, analgesia

Staging

- I. Uncomplicated parapneumonic: exudative, neutrophilic
- II. Complicated parapneumonic: neutrophilic, pH <7.30, glucose <60 mg/dL, LDH >1000 IU/L. Often sterile
- III. Empyema: +gram stain or pus (+culture not required)
- Anaerobes, strep pneumonia, staph aureus (post-surgery/trauma), GNRs (nosocomial, diabetes, EtOH)

SPECIFIC THERAPY

I. Uncomplicated parapneumonic: antibiotics; serial CXR/exams

II. Complicated parapneumonic: as for empyema
III. Empyema:

Nonsurgical:
- Sterilization: ≥4–6 weeks antibiotics
- Early drainage (loculations form quickly)
- Large thoracostomy tubes or smaller radiologically guided catheters
- Multiple tubes if multiloculated
- Chest tube until <50 mL/day and closure of cavity
- No role for serial thoracenteses

Intrapleural fibrinolytics:
- Multiloculated stage II/III
- Streptokinase or urokinase (in 100 mL NS) into largest loculation; clamp 2–4 hours

Surgical:
- Inadequate drainage or incomplete obliteration of cavity
- Thoracoscopy, open thoracostomy, open-flap drainage, thoracoscopic or open decortication

Special
- ***Empyema with bronchopleural fistula:* requires immediate drainage (risk of pneumonia)**
- ***Empyema distal to obstructed bronchus:* must relieve obstruction (radiotherapy or laser) to allow re-expansion**
- ***Recurrent effusion (e.g., malignant):* consider talc, bleomycin pleurodesis**
- ***Hemothorax:* insert tube early to monitor bleeding and prevent fibrothorax**

FOLLOW-UP
- Uniloculated stage II/III: CT 24 hours after chest tube
- Multiloculated stage II/III: Marginal/poor surgical candidates; tube drainage with
- Fibrinolysis: CT in 72 hours

COMPLICATIONS AND PROGNOSIS
- Average 1.8 procedures/patient for empyema
- Success rates:
  - ➤ chest tube alone: 11% (better for aerobic infection)
  - ➤ image-directed catheter: 57%
  - ➤ decortication: 95%
- Follow for recurrent infections, persistent intrapleural space

PLEURAL TUMORS

STEPHEN C. LAZARUS, MD

HISTORY & PHYSICAL

History
- Depends on diagnosis
  - *Malignant Mesothelioma*
    - 2/3 of patients – known asbestos exposure
    - latent period 30–45 years; most patients 50–75 years old
    - high prevalence in Cappadocian region of Turkey
  - *Benign Fibrous Mesothelioma*
    - Not associated with asbestos
    - Often an "incidental" finding on routine chest Xray
  - *Primary Effusion Lymphoma*
    - homosexual men with AIDS + KS-associated HHV-8
  - *Metastatic Pleural Disease*
    - 75% due to lung (30%), breast (25%), and lymphoma (20%) primary
    - 6% ovarian, 3% sarcomas, 6% no primary found

Signs & Symptoms
- *Malignant Mesothelioma*
  - chest pain most common presenting symptom
  - dyspnea in 40%; also chills, fever, sweats, weakness
  - large effusion in 50%; progressive encasement of lung
- *Benign Fibrous Mesothelioma*
  - 50% asymptomatic
  - Cough, chest pain, dyspnea and fever may occur
  - Hypertrophic pulmonary osteoarthropathy (20%) – may resolve after resection
  - Symptomatic hypoglycemia (4%; due to insulin-like GFII)
- *Primary Effusion Lymphoma*
  - malignant lymphomatous effusion without mass
- *Metastatic Pleural Disease*
  - Dyspnea (>50%); chest pain (25%), anorexia, weight loss, malaise
  - 20% asymptomatic

TESTS

Imaging
- *Chest X-ray*: may demonstrate effusion, pleural plaques, pleural-based mass, underlying lung mass
- *CT Scan*: better visualization of pleural surface, mediastinum

Thoracentesis:
- diagnosis often made by pleural fluid analysis – combination of cytology and immunohistochemistry

Pleural Biopsy: low yield ($\leq$15–20% positive)

Thoracoscopic or Open Biopsy: often required, especially for mesothelioma

Specific Diagnostic Tests:
- Immunohistochemical markers
- Electron Microscopy

DIFFERENTIAL DIAGNOSIS

Malignant Mesothelioma
- effusion in 75%:
  - ➤ exudate; 50% serosanguinous
  - ➤ cytol positive in 25% (hard to distinguish from adenocarcinoma)
  - ➤ Immunohistochemistry: CEA, B72.3, Leu M1, Ber(EP4)
    - $\geq$2 positive = adenocarcinoma
    - 0 positive = mesothelioma
- pleural plaques in 30%
- EM of tissue can be diagnostic

Benign Fibrous Mesothelioma
- solitary, well-defined, often lobulated mass; 70% visceral, 30% parietal
- 10% with associated effusion
- highly vascular, often enhances with contrast on CT

Primary Effusion Lymphoma
- Distinctive cytologic morphology

Metastatic Pleural Disease
- exudative effusion; >50% are bloody
- cytology positive in 60–90%, especially adenocarcinoma
- thoracoscopy positive in 90%

MANAGEMENT

What to Do First
- Thoracentesis, for diagnosis, and symptom relief
  - ➤ May reveal underlying pathology

General Measures
- *Imaging*: Chest X-ray, CT for staging

- *Pleurodesis*
  - Indication: recurrent effusion with symptoms
  - Contraindication: mediastinal shift toward effusion usually means lung can't expand and pleurodesis will fail
  - Complications: pain; loculations; ARDS with talc
  - Efficacy: 70–90% in selected patients; talc > doxycycline > bleomycin
  - Most common cause of failure is incomplete drainage of effusion
- Technique
  - tube thoracostomy
  - wait for apposition of pleural surfaces (if not apposed, can't adhere)
  - volume of drainage not important
  - sedation/analgesia with opiates
  - inject sclerosing agent + saline
  - clamp tube x 2 hours
  - positional rotation may be important for talc
- *Other measures*
  - pleuroperitoneal shunt
  - serial therapeutic thoracenteses
  - pleurectomy

SPECIFIC THERAPY

Malignant Mesothelioma
- Surgery + Chemotherapy + Radiotherapy
- Immunotherapy
- Palliation: pleurodesis, pleurectomy, pain control

Benign Fibrous Mesothelioma
- Resection

Primary Effusion Lymphoma
- Chemotherapy for lymphoma

Metastatic Pleural Disease
- Chemotherapy for primary
- If positive cytology without obvious primary – get CT scan of chest, abdomen, pelvis, and mammogram, since 75% originate from lung, breast, lymphoma
- Pleurodesis

FOLLOW-UP

- Most follow-up is directed at the specific disease
- Benign fibrous mesothelioma, because of late recurrences, should have annual Chest X-ray

COMPLICATIONS AND PROGNOSIS

- *Malignant mesothelioma*:
  - ➤ Median Survival:
    - Stage I (resectable without LN involvement): 22 months
    - Stage II (resectable with LN involvement): 17 months
    - Stage III (unresectable): 11 months
- *Benign Fibrous Mesothelioma*:
  - ➤ 90% cure; 10% recurrence (may occur late)
- *Primary Effusion Lymphoma*:
  - ➤ Survival: 4–6 months
- *Metastatic Pleural Disease*
  - ➤ Mean survival with positive cytology = 3 months
  - ➤ Effusion decreases with chemotherapy in 40% of breast and 35% of small cell cancers

---

PNEUMOTHORAX

MESHELL D. JOHNSON, MD

HISTORY & PHYSICAL

History

- Spontaneous pneumothorax (ptx)
- Primary – no underlying lung disease
  - ➤ Incidence 18 /100,000 in men, 6/100,000 in women
  - ➤ Usually tall, thin males 10–30 years old; uncommon over 40;
    - 4:1 male predominance; cigarette smoking increases rate
- Secondary – history of underlying COPD, emphysema, cystic fibrosis, status asthmaticus, PCP, necrotizing pneumonias, sarcoidosis, IPF, EG, LAM, tuberous sclerosis, connective tissue disease, Marfan's, Ehlers-Danlos, cancer, thoracic endometriosis
  - ➤ Incidence 6/100,000 in men, 2/100,000 in women; in COPD, incidence is 26/100,000
  - ➤ Peak incidence 60–65 years of age
- Traumatic ptx – penetrating or blunt chest injury (rib fracture, bronchial rupture, esophageal injury)
- Iatrogenic ptx – transthoracic needle aspiration, central line, thoracentesis, pleural biopsy, positive pressure ventilation

Signs & Symptoms

- Ipsilateral pleuritic chest pain, acute dyspnea, tachycardia, cough
- Primary spontaneous ptx usually occurs at rest; strenuous activity associated with ~20% of cases
- Small ptx (<15% hemithorax) may yield normal exam
- Larger ptx (>15% hemithorax): tachypnea, splinting, decreased chest wall movement, hyperresonance, decreased fremitus, decreased or absent breath sounds on affected side

TESTS

Imaging

- upright PA CXR: thin visceral pleural line
- expiratory film can uncover small apical ptx
- Chest CT: to distinguish large bullae from ptx; shows subpleural blebs and underlying lung disease
- ECG: decreased QRS in limb leads, decreased precordial R wave; inverted T waves with L sided ptx
- ABG: increased A-a gradient, acute respiratory alkalosis; hypoxemia and hypercapnia in patients with underlying lung disease.

DIFFERENTIAL DIAGNOSIS

- PA CXR often confirms diagnosis. Giant bullae may mimic ptx on CXR; obtain chest CT for confirmation

MANAGEMENT

What to Do First

- R/o tension ptx
- treat hypoxemia and continue Rx of any underlying lung disease

General Measures

- history and physical to r/o underlying lung disease
- Encourage smoking cessation

SPECIFIC THERAPY

- Observation – for young healthy patients with small primary spontaneous ptx, no SOB, and no hemodynamic instability; hospitalization not required.
- Oxygen – accclerates rate of reabsorption 4-fold; administer to all hospitalized patients.
- Needle aspiration – recommended for first large (>15% hemithorax) primary spontaneous ptx; success rate ~ 70%; not for recurrent primary or secondary ptx (success rate only ~30%)

- Chest tube-for primary spontaneous ptx that failed aspiration, recurrent primary spontaneous ptx, or secondary spontaneous ptx.
  - Insert into 2nd intercostal space anteriorly or directly into loculated air under CT or fluoroscopic guidance
  - Place initially to waterseal
  - If air leak >24 hours, connect to 20 cm H_2O wall suction
  - 24 hours after resolution (no air leak, nl CXR), place tube to waterseal; repeat expiratory CXR in 3–6 hours
  - If no recurrence, clamp tube for 12–24 hours under close observation to look for slow air leaks
  - If ptx recurs, return to suction; if no recurrence, remove tube.
  - Side effects-pain, pleural infections, reexpansion pulmonary edema
  - Contraindications – unclear anatomy (ptx vs bulla); obtain chest CT
- Pleurodesis – recurrent primary spontaneous or secondary spontaneous ptx associated with respiratory compromise.
  - Sclerosing agents: talc, tetracycline, minocycline, bleomycin, doxycycline
    - Side effects – pain, fever, ARDS
    - Contraindications –
      - absolute: allergy to chemical sclerosing agent, trapped or unexpanded lung
      - relative: likelihood of future lung transplant; young patient with emphysema – treat these patients with VATS with stapling of blebs and abrasion of apical pleura
  - Multiple sclerosing strategies:
    - Instillation via chest tube
    - Surgical thoracoscopy, thoracotomy -for air leaks >7 days, failed chemical pleurodesis, recurrent ptx; blebs/bullae are resected; pleurodesis via partial pleurectomy, physical abrasion of pleural surfaces or installation of sclerosing agents
    - Side effects- fevers, wound infection, air leaks, pneumonia, risks of general anesthesia. Thoracoscopic procedures require longer OR time, greater treatment failures, but require less anesthesia, lesser post-op lung function abnormalities, and less wound pain
    - Contraindications for thoracoscopic surgery:
      - inability to tolerate one lung ventilation, extensive
        - adhesion in thoracic cavity, complex anatomical
        - variation, small thoracic cavity

Special Situations

■ HIV infection and ptx: most often secondary to PCP; contralateral recurrences common; high rate of recurrence with tube drainage alone; pleurodesis recommended even without air leak (therapy depends on underlying prognosis – outpatient care with small-bore chest catheter and Heimlich valve is an alternative)

FOLLOW-UP

■ As needed for recurring symptoms; no routine follow up if CXR is normal after removal of chest tube

COMPLICATIONS AND PROGNOSIS

Complications

■ *Acute complications*
> ➤ Tension ptx: progressive dyspnea and tachycardia, tracheal shift away from and increasing tympany of affected side, HR>140, hypotension, increased JVP, cyanosis.
> ➤ Management: decompress immediately with transthoracic needle into affected side (waiting for CXR can be lethal)
> ➤ Acute respiratory failure: assisted ventilation as needed

■ *Long-term complications*
> ➤ Failure to reexpand
> ➤ Recurrence rates: healthy patients with primary spontaneous ptx treated with observation, needle aspiration or chest tube drainage ~ 30%; secondary spontaneous ptx recurrence rate 39–47%; most occur within 6–24 months; asthenic habitus, smoking history, younger age are independent risk factors for recurrence; bullae not predictive of recurrence.

Prognosis

■ Good in healthy patients with primary spontaneous ptx
■ Poor in patients with AIDS (most die of AIDS-related complications within 3–6 months of initial ptx), and COPD

POLYMYOSITIS AND RELATED DISORDERS

ROBERT WORTMANN, MD

HISTORY & PHYSICAL

■ Polymyositis (PM)
> ➤ Insidious onset
> ➤ Proximal (shoulder & pelvic girdle) muscle weakness

➤ Other possible complaints
  • Fatigue, morning stiffness, anorexia, fever (rare)
  • Dysphagia
  • Cough or dyspnea
  • Arthralgia more common than true arthritis
  • Raynaud's phenomenon
➤ Physical examination shows proximal muscle weakness
➤ Remainder of neurologic exam normal

■ Dermatomyositis (DM)
  ➤ Like PM plus rash
    • Gottron's sign: pink raised plaques over knuckles, elbows, knees
  ➤ Heliotrope rash on eyelids
  ➤ Rash in sun-exposed areas
  ➤ Malar
    • Anterior chest (V sign)
    • Upper back (shawl sign)
  ➤ Nail fold capillary changes

■ Variations
  ➤ Juvenile dermatomyositis
    • Like DM plus vasculitis (mainly GI)
    • Subcutaneous calcifications, lipodystrophy
  ➤ DM or PM w/ another collagen vascular disease
    • SLE, scleroderma, mixed connective tissue disease
  ➤ DM or PM w/ malignancy (any cancer but especially ovarian)
  ➤ Inclusion body myositis (IBM)
    • More common in older people
    • Like polymyositis but may have distal or asymmetric weakness & rarely responds to therapy

TESTS

Lab Tests

■ Blood (essential)
  ➤ Elevated CK, aldolase, AST, ALT, LDH
■ Electromyography (usually required)
  ➤ Myopathic changes (IBM may also show neuropathic changes)

Imaging (Discretionary)

■ MRI w/T2-weighted imaging or STIR shows inflammation in involved muscles
■ Muscle biopsy (essential to distinguish IBM)
■ PM: muscle fiber degeneration & regeneration w/ CD8+ lymphocyte endomyseal infiltrate

- DM: CD4+ lymphocytes in perimyseal & perivascular distribution, perifascicular atrophy
- IBM-like PM w/ rimmed vacuoles in fibers & inclusions on electron microscopy
- Autoantibodies (useful for prognosis)
  - Nonspecific ANA in 15–30%
  - Myositis specific autoantibodies
    - Anti-synthetase (eg, anti-Jo-1)
      - More common in PM than DM
      - Interstitial lung disease
      - Arthritis
      - Raynaud's
      - Fever
      - Mechanic's hands
      - Fair treatment response
    - Anti-Signal Recognition Peptide (SRP)
      - PM
      - Sudden onset
      - Cardiomyopathy
      - Poor prognosis
    - Anti-Mi-2
      - DM
      - Very good prognosis

DIFFERENTIAL DIAGNOSIS

- Myasthenia gravis, muscular dystrophies
- Thyroid disease (hyper, hypo), adrenal disease (hyper, hypo), hyperparathyroism, aldosteronism, carcinoid
- Abnormal Na, K, Ca, P, Mg
- Trichinosis, viruses (influenza, Coxsackie, HIV)
- Eaton-Lambert, paraneoplastic neuromyopathy
- Alcohol, beta-blockers, cholesterol-lowering agents
  - Clozapine, cocaine, colchicine, cylcosporine, hydroxycholoquine, glucocorticosteroids, penicillamine
- Glycogen storage disease, carnitine deficiency, mitochondrial myopathy
- Sarcoid, amyloidosis, sarcopenia of aging, hysteria

MANAGEMENT

What to Do First

- Assess baseline strength objectively: grade specific muscle groups on 1 to 5 scale
- Check baseline CK & other muscle enzymes

General Measures

- Check baseline labs used to screen side effects of meds
- CXR & pulmonary function tests if concerned for interstitial lung disease
- Swallowing study if there is dysphagia or hoarseness
- Physical therapy to prevent contracture & maintain strength of unaffected muscles
- Screen for malignancy as appropriate for pt's age & gender

SPECIFIC THERAPY

Treatment Options

- High-dose oral prednisone
- In severe disease, add methotrexate or azathioprine
- In DM, topical steroids or hydroxychloroquine may help rash but not muscle weakness
- In refractory cases, IVIg may lead to improvement
- Cylcosporine, tacrolimus & alkylating agents such as cyclophosphamide & chlorambucil have also been reported as effective
- Case reports also describe the efficacy of tumor necrosis factor inhibitors such as infliximab

Side Effects & Contraindications

- Prednisone: hypertension, glucose intolerance, sodium retention, hypokalemia, rash, cushingoid appearance, osteoporosis, aseptic necrosis, cataracts, infection
- Methotrexate: mucositis, GI distress, cirrhosis, bone marrow depression, pneumonitis, pseudolymphoma, infection. Avoid use w/alcohol use or liver or renal dysfunction.
- Azathioprine: GI distress, bone marrow depression, serious infection. Increased risk of neoplasia if previously used alkylating agent. Avoid concomitant use of allopurinol.

FOLLOW-UP

- See every 4 to 6 weeks, checking muscle strength & CPK & for potential drug toxicities. Frequency can be decreased if remission is seen.
- Meds are gradually tapered over a 6-month period once remission has been achieved for 6 to 12 weeks.

COMPLICATIONS & PROGNOSIS

- Refractory disease may result in severe muscle weakness w/ atrophy, joint contractures, aspiration pneumonia

- Respiratory failure & congestive heart failure are rare. 50–75% of pts will go into complete remission.
- If pt fails to respond to treatment:
  - Add another drug
  - Consider steroid myopathy
  - Question the accuracy of the diagnosis
  - Question if dealing w/ known unresponsive disease-types-associated-malignancy IBM-anti-SRP or anti-synthetase syndrome
  - Consider using cyclosporine, cyclophosphamide, chlorambucil or IVIg

PORPHYRIA, ACUTE

D. MONTGOMERY BISSELL, MD

HISTORY & PHYSICAL

History

- Young adult, female more often than male, Caucasian more than African, Indian or Asian; very rare before puberty; declining incidence after age 50.
- Recent caloric restriction, due to illness or strict diet regimen.
- Use of porphyria-inducing medication, e.g. barbiturates, phenytoin, valproate, sulfa drugs, estrogens.
- Constipation: common, often chronic
- History of recurrent pain attacks; negative exploratory surgery; premenstrual pain attacks
- Steadily increasing nausea and pain (abdomen, back or extremities) over days (not hours).
- Dark urine, depending on the type of porphyria; in acute intermittent porphyria (AIP) urine color may be normal.
- Mental status change: often subtle (e.g., hysterical affect); seizures can occur; florid psychosis is unusual.
- Family history: often negative. Relatives with similar attacks of pain or a devastating, undiagnosed neurological condition.

Signs & Symptoms

- Tachycardia common; fever usually absent
- On abdominal exam, reduced bowel sounds (suggestive of ileus); diffuse or focal tenderness but less than degree of pain would suggest. No rebound tenderness.

- Early neurological findings (if present): extremity weakness, proximal muscles > distal.
- Late neurological presentation: flaccid paralysis and respiratory failure.

TESTS

- Urine porphobilinogen (PBG) and delta-aminolevulinic acid (ALA). NOTE: this is not a "porphyrin screen". For rapid PBG: Watson-Schwartz test. In patients with acute symptoms, urine PBG is > 20 mg/24 h (normal < 2 mg) and often 60–200 mg/24 h. Normal PBG in symptomatic patient excludes acute porphyria. Values in 2–20 mg/24 h range may identify a "silent" genetic carrier of the disease.
- CBC: mild leukocytosis; no left shift
- Serum electrolytes: hyponatriemia
- RBC uroporphyrinogen-1-synthetase (PBG deaminase): deficiency is constant in genetic carriers of AIP. Not useful for diagnosing acutely ill patients.
- Urine and fecal porphyrins: for identifying type of acute porphyria, for genetic screening of family members

DIFFERENTIAL DIAGNOSIS

- If localized pain, fever and leukocytosis or rebound tenderness are present, intra-abdominal inflammation (appendicitis, cholecystitis, pancreatitis, vasculitis, volvulus, etc) must be excluded. Markedly increased PBG otherwise is diagnostic.
- If urine shows predominant elevation of ALA with slightly elevated or normal PBG, consider heavy metal intoxication, especially lead. Check smear for basophilic stippling, and obtain blood lead level.
- Motor weakness can suggest Guillain-Barre syndrome. However, in G-B, CSF has lymphocytes and elevated protein, which are not present in porphyria.
- Elevation of urine coproporphyrin only (normal PBG) is non-specific, occurring in diseases of the liver, bone marrow, nervous system and others.
- Substantial elevation of uroporphyrin with normal PBG suggests porphyria cutanea tarda (PCT), which is a cutaneous disease. Acute pain attacks are not part of PCT.

MANAGEMENT

- Eliminate possible porphyria-inducing drugs; discontinue all but essential medications.
- Serial 24-hour urine collections for PBG

- Reverse fasting state by giving carbohydrate, by mouth if possible, otherwise as D10W by vein; monitor for hyponatremia.
- Give analgesia; generally parenteral opiates (meperidine, fentanyl).

SPECIFIC THERAPY

- If seizures present, control with short-acting benzodiazepine (e.g., i.v. diazepam) or magnesium.
- If neurological signs present or pain persists over 24–48 hours, start Panhematin (Ovation Pharmaceuticals; 800-455-1141) by slow i.v. push. Use a large peripheral vein or central line. Panhematin is supplied as powder, which is reconstituted immediately prior to infusion.

FOLLOW-UP

- Adequate hematin will produce a sharp drop in urinary PBG after 2–3 days, and resolution of pain after 3–5 days. Discontinue infusions when a clinical response is evident or after 8 days.
- Educate patient as to porphyria-inducing medications.
- Determine the type of acute porphyria (urine and stool porphyrins; RBC uroporphyrinogen-1 synthetase), and offer genetic screening to first-degree relatives.

COMPLICATIONS AND PROGNOSIS

- Outlook for acute abdominal attacks is good, particularly if an inciting agent is identified. Most genetic carriers have no symptoms provided they avoid inducing drugs. Spontaneous attacks can recur. Psychosis, if present, resolves completely; chronic mental illness not seen. Recovery from motor neuropathy is slow (many months) but in many cases is complete.

PORTAL HYPERTENSIVE BLEEDING

EMMET B. KEEFFE, MD

HISTORY & PHYSICAL

History

- Likelihood of developing varices in patients with cirrhosis: 35–80%
- 25–35% of cirrhotic patients with large varices will bleed
- risk of recurrent variceal bleeding: ~70% within 2 years of index bleed
- for each bleeding episode, mortality ranges 35–50%

Signs and Symptoms

- Compensated or decompensated liver disease prior to index bleed
- Manifestations include hematemesis and/or melena
- Bleeding brisk and may be exsanguinating from esophageal or gastric varices; bleeding from portal hypertensive gastropathy tends to be chronic

TESTS

Basic Studies

- blood: abnormal LFTs, including decreased albumin, increased bilirubin and increased INR, indicating various degrees of hepatic synthetic dysfunction
- Hemoccult positive stool

Other Tests

- imaging:
  - ultrasound or CT scan showing presence of cirrhosis, including evidence of portal hypertension
- endoscopy:
  - showing esophageal and/or gastric varices, with either blood in the lumen or evidence of active bleeding from the varix; exclusion of ulcer or other disease also important

DIFFERENTIAL DIAGNOSIS

- esophageal varices
- gastric varices
- portal hypertensive gastropathy
- peptic ulcer
- Dieulofoy's lesion

MANAGEMENT

What to Do First

- patients suspected of bleeding from varices require hospitalization and immediate endoscopy
- adequate venous access established
- resuscitation with restoration of blood volume with blood and fresh frozen plasma guided by CVP and urine output

General Measures

- care taken not to overexpand the plasma volume, which may increase portal pressure and exacerbate bleeding

- endotracheal intubation performed in patients with a major bleed or significant hepatic encephalopathy to protect the airway
- antibiotics such as norfloxacin administered to prevent spontaneous bacterial peritonitis

SPECIFIC THERAPY

Treatment Options: Routine

- vasoactive drugs: octreotide, or vasopressin and nitroglycerin, initiated to decrease portal flow
- endoscopic therapy: either variceal band ligation or sclerotherapy effective in control of acute hemorrhage
- band ligation is preferable to sclerotherapy because of less complications, lower rate of rebleeding, and decrease in the number of sessions required to obliterate varices
- gastric varices are more difficult to control, and typically require TIPS
- in rare circumstances, balloon tamponade, emergency portosystemic shunt or transection of the esophagus required for exsanguinating hemorrhage

Side Effects and Contraindications

- Vasopressin
  - ➤ side effects: bradycardia, angina, myocardial infarction, hypertension, abdominal pain
  - ➤ contraindications: caution in patients with coronary artery disease, congestive heart failure or elderly patients
- Octreotide (or somatostatin)
  - ➤ side effects: nausea, abdominal pain, flushing
  - ➤ contraindications: use with caution in diabetics or patients with renal dysfunction

Treatment Options: Alternative

- TIPS for patients with continued bleeding in spite of endoscopic variceal banding or sclerotherapy, or recurrent bleeding in spite of banding therapy
- technical success of TIPS in control of bleeding: 90–95% of cases
- side effects: early morbidity occurs in 20% of patients, including arrhythmias or intraperitoneal bleeding, early precipitation of liver failure, and exacerbation or precipitation of hepatic encephalopathy; early mortality is 5%; other problems include TIPS stenosis or occlusion that may require TIPS revision; late chronic encephalopathy uncommon, but may be severe in 5% of patients.

FOLLOW-UP

- patients at risk for recurrent bleeding and should be treated with endoscopic therapy to obliteration of varices and chronic beta blocker with or without nitroglycerin therapy
- endoscopy typically performed every 2–4 weeks until varices are obliterated, and beta blockers +/− nitroglycerin continued long-term
- routine monitoring of hepatic function with CBC, INR and LFTs every 2–4 months

COMPLICATIONS AND PROGNOSIS

- uncontrollable or recurrent variceal bleeding, which may be treatable in selected patients with reasonable hepatic function by TIPS, portosystemic shunt or esophageal transaction

Prognosis

- portal hypertensive bleeding indicates decompensation of chronic liver disease and reduced short-term and long-term survival mandating consideration of liver transplantation

---

POSTCONCUSSION SYNDROME OR POSTCONCUSSIVE SYNDROME

CHAD CHRISTINE, MD

HISTORY & PHYSICAL

- Impairment of neurologic function persisting days to weeks after mild to severe traumatic brain injury
- Headache, fatigue, dizziness most common symptoms
- Symptoms worsened by mental & physical effort
- Cognitive symptoms
- Neurologic signs typically unremarkable

TESTS

- Serum tests are unremarkable
- Brain CT or MRI usually normal; may show small subcortical hemorrhages
- Neuropsychological testing usually abnormal in severe cases

DIFFERENTIAL DIAGNOSIS

- Intracranial hemorrhage, epidural or subdural hematoma excluded by brain imaging

■ Drug intoxication or withdrawal excluded by history & toxicology tests

MANAGEMENT
■ Reassure pt that symptoms resolve over weeks to months
■ Many require no medical therapy

SPECIFIC THERAPY

Indications
■ Headache

Treatment Options
■ Abortive agents
  ➤ Acetaminophen
  ➤ Aspirin
  ➤ Ibuprofen
■ Prophylactic agents
  ➤ Anti-inflammatory agents (above)
  ➤ Tricyclic antidepressants
    • Amitriptyline
    • Nortriptyline
    • Doxepin

FOLLOW-UP
■ Depends on severity of symptoms

COMPLICATIONS AND PROGNOSIS
■ Most improve over weeks to months

PREECLAMPTIC LIVER DISEASE/HELLP

CAROLINE A. RIELY, MD

HISTORY & PHYSICAL

History
■ Third trimester, often primipara, or immediately post-partem
■ Signs and symptoms of preeclampsia (hypertension, proteinuria, headache, or none)
■ Abdominal/right lower chest pain
■ Common – 30% of severe preeclampsia

Signs and Symptoms
- Often none, other than hypertension. Rare jaundice

TESTS

Laboratory
- Hemolysis, mild (spur cells on smear)
- Elevated liver tests (AST <ALT)
- Low platelets (<100,000)
- Normal PT/INR, fibrinogen, unless very severe
- Elevated or normal uric acid (usually low in pregnancy)

Liver Biopsy
- Periportal hemorrhage and fibrin deposits, may have small amounts of fat. Usually not needed, base diagnosis on clinical grounds

DIFFERENTIAL DIAGNOSIS
- R/O acute fatty liver of pregnancy (prolonged PT, low fibrinogen)
- Consider viral hepatitis (+ serologies, risk factors)
- R/O cholestasis of pregnancy (+ hx of itching)

MANAGEMENT

What to Do First
- Consult with obstetrician, consider terminating pregnancy

General Measures
- Fetal monitoring, follow PT

SPECIFIC THERAPY
- Delivery; temporizing, corticosteriods only with extreme caution

FOLLOW-UP
- Monitor AST, ALT, PT
- Imaging with CT or MRI to r/o hepatic hematoma with rupture or infarct
- Expect full recovery

COMPLICATIONS AND PROGNOSIS
- Consider progression to hepatic rupture (shock, hemoperitoneum), infarct (marked ALT elevations > 4,000, geographic infarcts on CT or MRI)
- No sequellae, perhaps increased risk for repeat with subsequent pregnancies

PREGNANCY COMPLICATIONS FOR THE INTERNIST

MAXINE H. DORIN, MD
REVISED BY ANDREW R. HOFFMAN, MD;
FREDRIC B. KRAEMER, MD, and THOMAS F. McELRATH, MD, PhD

HISTORY & PHYSICAL

History
- Age, last normal menstrual period, menstrual pattern, birth control method (past/present), number of pregnancies and outcome; history of STD, PID, IUD use, infertility
    Has prenatal care been initiated?
    Has intrauterine pregnancy been documented?
    Prior pregnancy history
    Prior seizure disorder
- Hypertension, thromboembolic events, liver disease, renal disease, surgical history (esp. abdominal pelvic surgery)
- History of smoking
- Sexual activity

Signs & Symptoms
- Vaginal spotting/bleeding, abdominal/pelvic pain, breast tenderness, dizziness, gush of fluid
- Orthostatic changes, tachycardia, abdominal pain, peritoneal signs, blood in vagina, bluish cervix
- Cervical os may be open with or without tissues present
- Soft, enlarged uterus or firm, normal-sized uterus, adnexal tenderness/fullness

TESTS

Laboratory
- Beta-HCG: qualitative
- CBC, Rh factor
- Consider beta-HCG quantitative, serum progesterone, AST, creatinine, BUN
- Urinary protein excretion (dip, spot protein/creatinine ratio, 24-hour protein collection)
- Type/cross for blood

Screening
- Cervical cultures for GC/Chlamydia

Imaging

- Transvaginal US: more helpful than transabdominal US to assess intrauterine content and pelvis, adnexal mass or fetal cardiac activity, fluid or clots in pelvis, placenta previa

DIFFERENTIAL DIAGNOSIS

- Normal intrauterine pregnancy (IUP)
- Abortion: threatened, missed, inevitable (complete/incomplete), septic
- Gestational trophoblastic neoplasia (GTN): confirmed on US with characteristic "snowstorm" pattern
- Ectopic pregnancy: potentially life- and fertility-threatening
- Preeclampsia/eclampsia
- Placental abruption
- Membrane rupture

MANAGEMENT

What to Do First

- Beta-HCG (+)
- Order US
- Assess stability of patient: if unstable go straight to OR
- Assess risk factors for ectopic pregnancy: higher with history of prior ectopic, PID, STD, abdominal/pelvic surgery, infertility, poststerilization
- Assess likelihood of IUP vs ectopic pregnancy

General Measures

- Threatened & missed abortion: IUP, cervical os closed and minimal bleeding
- Inevitable abortion: os open, usually bleeding, assess likelihood of complete vs incomplete
- Septic abortion: start antibiotics before D&C
- GTN:
  - ➤ CXR
  - ➤ Assess high or low risk for persistent GTN post D&C: high risk factors include eclampsia, acute pulmonary insufficiency, theca-lutein cysts >5 cm, uterus >20 wks, coexistent fetus, uterus large for dates, beta-HCG >100,000 IU/mL, maternal age >40 y
  - ➤ Suspected ectopic pregnancy:
  - ➤ If stable with positive beta-HCG and no IUP seen on US, obtain quantitative beta-HCG and rapid serum progesterone

➤ If pregnancy not desired or progesterone below threshold for viability or beta-HCG >2000 mIU/mL or beta-HCG increases >66% in 48 h, D&C indicated

➤ No chorionic villi in D&C: treat for presumed ectopic pregnancy

➤ Serum progesterone above threshold of viability and beta-HCG increases >66% in 48 h: repeat beta-HCG q 48 h until it reaches 2000 mIU/mL; no intrauterine gestational sac seen on US, treat for ectopic pregnancy

■ Specific Treatment

➤ Threatened abortion: reassurance and bed rest, but 50% abort

➤ Missed abortion: D&C vs expectant management (may spontaneously abort)

➤ Inevitable abortion: D&C if incomplete; otherwise, expectant management

➤ Septic abortion: broad-spectrum antibiotics, D&

➤ GTN: D&C followed by weekly beta-HC

• When beta-HCG (–) for 2 consecutive wks, monitor beta-HCG monthly for 1 y

• Treat with contraception for 1 y

• 80% cured with D&C

➤ Ectopic pregnancy: Surgical vs. medical management

• Surgical management by laparoscopy or laparotomy, salpingectomy or linear salpingostomy

• Medical management appropriate if ALL the following present:

• Beta-HCG <5–10,000 mIU/mL, hemodynamically stable, no significant pain, adnexal mass <3.5 cm, no cardiac activity in the adnexal mass, no significant fluid in pelvis per US and AST, creatinine and BUN normal

• Treat with IM methotrexate

• Check beta-HCG days 4 and 7; if <15% beta-HCG decline, repeat dose if patient stable

■ Side Effects

➤ Methotrexate: nausea, vomiting, rash, pruritus, dizziness, fatigue, headache, neurotoxicity, leukoencephalopathy, renal failure, photosensitivity, seizure, thrombocytopenia, hepatoxicity

■ Contraindications

➤ Methotrexate: lactation, alcohol abuse, liver dysfunction, infection, renal impairment

■ Special Situations

➤ Cornual ectopic: cornual resection vs hysterectomy +/– methotrexate prior

➤ Ovarian ectopic: partial vs complete oophorectomy

➤ Cervical ectopic: cone of cervix vs hysterectomy; uterine artery embolization or methotrexate prior to surgery possible

➤ Abdominal pregnancy: 10% fetal salvage rate, placenta can be removed later, after cessation of function by beta-HCG

➤ Preeclampsia, preterm labor or preterm membrane rupture – Seek specialized obstetrical consultation

SPECIFIC THERAPY

n/a

FOLLOW-UP

■ Rh (–) with (–) antibody screen:
  ➤ 50 mcg RhoGAM IM for ectopic and <12 wks gestation
  ➤ 300 mcg RhoGAM IM I >12 wks

COMPLICATIONS AND PROGNOSIS

■ Persistent GTN requires chemotherapy
■ Infertility in ectopic pregnancies, infectious complications

---

PRESSURE ULCERS

JEFFREY P. CALLEN, MD

HISTORY & PHYSICAL

History

■ Also known as decubitus ulcer
■ Due to pressure often associated with bedridden or wheelchair-bound patient
■ Friction, moisture may contribute.

Signs & Symptoms

■ Ulceration over the sacrum, coccygeal, ischial tuberosities or greater trochanter
■ Begins as an erythematous, induration
■ Ulcer may be very deep.

TESTS

■ Basic tests: none needed
■ Imaging studies – Radiographs to rule out osteomyelitis

DIFFERENTIAL DIAGNOSIS
■ The process is clinically characteristic.

MANAGEMENT

What to Do First
■ Assess the risk factors such as trauma, exposure to excess moisture.
■ Relieve pressure.

General Measures
■ Keep area dry.
■ Surgical beds to redistribute weight

SPECIFIC THERAPY
n/a

FOLLOW-UP

During Treatment
■ Re-evaluate patient 1–2 weeks after initiating therapy
■ Culture if drainage is purulent

COMPLICATIONS AND PROGNOSIS
■ Osteomyelitis is possible.

PRIAPISM

SHAHRAM S. GHOLAMI, MD; WILLIAM O. BRANT, MD; ANTHONY J. BELLA, MD; and TOM F. LUE, MD

HISTORY & PHYSICAL
Priapism is a persistent penile erection that continues hours beyond, or is unrelated to, sexual stimulation (4 hours is considered the usual time frame). Typically, only the corpora cavernosa are affected.

History
■ Regarding trauma, medication/drug use, medical conditions, or enlarged lymph nodes
■ Time of onset of erection
■ Association with sexual activity, sleep
■ Associated with pain

Signs & Symptoms
■ Evaluation of rigidity of erection (glans, shaft), penile pain
■ Perineal/scrotal/penile trauma or bruising

- Signs of fever
- Abdominal or pelvic lymph nodes or masses

TESTS
- CBC, electrolytes and sickle cell prep or electrophoresis
- Aspiration of penile blood (from corpus cavernosum) for blood gas determination
- Blood gas values of PO2 <40, PCO2 >60 and pH <7.25 suggest an ischemic state.
- Blood gas values P02 >65, PC02 <40 and pH >7.3 suggest arterial priapism.
- Color Doppler ultrasound of penis showing localized pooling of arterial flow
  - Study of choice for arterial priapism
  - If positive, requires angiography to locate and embolize the ruptured artery

DIFFERENTIAL DIAGNOSIS
Priapism should be distinguished from
- Penile carcinoma
- Penile induration
- Severe infection of penis
- Cavernositis
- Penile prosthesis

Causes of priapism
Idiopathic (50%)
- Medications
  - Penile injection with papaverine, phentolamine, alprostadil or any combination
  - Phosphodiesterase-5 inhibitors (very rare) or intraurethral alprostadil
  - Antidepressants (trazodone)
  - Antipsychotics (chlorpromazine, phenothiazine, clozapine)
  - Antihypertensives (hydralazine, prazosin, guanethidine)
  - Total parenteral nutrition (high fat content)
  - Drugs of abuse (alcohol, cocaine)
  - Anticoagulants (heparin, coumadin)
- Thrombotic/hyper-viscosity syndromes
- Hematologic conditions
  - Sickle cell disease or trait (up to 35% incidence)
  - Lymphoma
  - Leukemia (esp. CGL)
- Pelvic infections

- Oncologic lesions
  - Compression or obstruction of venous drainage of the penis
- Neurologic disease
  - Spinal trauma and stenosis
  - General anesthesia
- Trauma

MANAGEMENT

Classification:
- Non-ischemic (arterial or high-flow) priapism
  - Rare
  - Associated with injury to a branch of the cavernosal artery
  - Usually after perineal or direct penile trauma
  - Results in uncontrolled high arterial inflow within the corpora cavernosa
  - Painless
  - Not emergent – may be followed for many months safely
  - May require eventual angiographic embolization of rupture cavernosal artery
  - Assess function of contralateral artery prior to embolization of ruptured vessel.
- Ischemic priapism
  - More common
  - Inadequate venous outflow creates an acidotic and hypoxic environment.
  - Painful prolonged erection
  - Most common identified causes: intracavernous agents for erections or sickle cell disease
  - Emergency
  - Goal of therapy to evacuate the old blood and re-establish circulation
- Untreated penile ischemia leads to edema, endothelial, nerve terminal and smooth muscle destruction and necrosis.
- If untreated within 24 hours, penile fibrosis and erectile dysfunction can occur.
- Initial therapy consists of corporeal aspiration of blood and intracavernous therapy with sympathomimetic drugs (phenylephrine, drug of choice).

SPECIFIC THERAPY
- Sickle cell disease
  - Treated with intracavernosal sympathomimetic drug as soon as possible

- ➤ Supplement with hydration, alkalinization, and hypertransfusion
- ➤ Recurrent cases treated with gonadotropin-releasing hormone agonist or antiandrogen
- Lymphoma and Leukemia
  - ➤ Treatment of primary disease with chemotherapy or radiotherapy
- Pelvic malignancy/metastatic lesions
  - ➤ Indicative of advanced and incurable disease
  - ➤ Secondary to compression or obstruction of venous drainage of the penis
  - ➤ Treated symptomatically
- Intermittent or stuttering ischemic priapism
  - ➤ Associated with spinal trauma or stenosis and sickle cell disease
  - ➤ Treated with LHRH agonist or antiandrogen
- Severe recalcitrant ischemic priapism requires surgical shunt procedures:
  - ➤ Initial therapy: distal (glans-cavernosum) shunt
    - Surgical blade to create communication between the glans and corpus cavernosum
    - Decompress corpora cavernosa
  - ➤ If distal shunt fails, proceed with proximal shunt procedures:
    - Cavernosal-spongiosal shunt
    - Cavernosal-penile dorsal vein shunt
    - Cavernosal-saphenous vein shunt

FOLLOW-UP

- Each 3–6 months to assess erectile function
- Patients with mild erectile dysfunction treated medically
  - ➤ Phosphodiesterase-5 inhibitor (sildenafil, vardenafil, tadalafil)
  - ➤ Vacuum constriction device
  - ➤ Intracavernous injection therapy
- Patients with severe erectile dysfunction given penile prosthesis

COMPLICATIONS AND PROGNOSIS

- Permanent erectile dysfunction is most severe complication
  - ➤ Associated with ischemic priapism lasting >24 hours
  - ➤ Penile fibrosis and damage increase as duration of ischemic priapism increases.
- Severe fibrosis of penile corporal tissue
  - ➤ Unresponsive to medications for erectile function
  - ➤ Difficulty with placement of penile prosthesis
  - ➤ Decrease in penile size

PRIMARY BILIARY CIRRHOSIS

ANDY S. YU, MD and JOANNE C. IMPERIAL, MD

HISTORY & PHYSICAL

History

- primarily affects middle-aged women (median age 50 at diagnosis)
- most cases are diagnosed while asymptomatic with incidental serum alkaline phosphatase elevation
- fatigue: most common symptom
- pruritus: most specific symptom
- association with extrahepatic diseases: arthritis (20%), sicca syndrome (70%), scleroderma/CREST (15%), thyroiditis (10–15%), type I & II renal tubular acidosis (50–60%), celiac disease (6%)

Physical Signs

- early disease: hyperpigmentation, hepatomegaly, splenomegaly, jaundice, xanthelasma
- advanced disease: liver failure

TESTS
Laboratory

Basic Studies: Blood

- early disease
  - ➤ alkaline phosphatase at least 3–4 x normal, increased GGT, increased IgM (95% of cases), increased serum cholesterol level, increased AST and ALT
- advanced disease
  - ➤ increased serum bilirubin and INR, decreased serum albumin
- serology
  - ➤ positive AMA ≥1:40; M2 antibody (highly sensitive and specific)
  - ➤ positive SMA, antithyroid antibody, antimicrosomal and antithyroglobulin antibodies, ANA, rheumatoid factor are nonspecific

Liver Biopsy

- may not be necessary if clinical, biochemical, and serological features are all typical of PBC; useful to exclude other causes of liver disease
- early disease: inflammatory destruction of intrahepatic bile ducts granulomatous destruction of bile ducts (florid duct lesion), proliferation of bile ductules
- advanced disease: scarring with regenerative nodules

Imaging

- abdominal ultrasound or CT is not diagnostic
- early disease: usually normal; excludes biliary obstruction
- MRCP utilized when the diagnosis of PBC is uncertain to visualize biliary tree (diagnostic ERCP if MRI contraindicated)
- advanced disease: hepatomegaly, nodular liver; venous collaterals suggestive of portal hypertension

DIFFERENTIAL DIAGNOSIS

- autoimmune hepatitis
- autoimmune cholangitis
- other causes of obstructive jaundice (stones, benign/malignant strictures)
- drug-induced cholestasis (estrogen, androgenic steroids)
- granulomatous hepatitis (including sarcoidosis)
- idiopathic adult ductopenia

MANAGEMENT

What to Do First

- attempt to establish a firm diagnosis of PBC before treatment

General Measures

- use liver biopsy, imaging studies to assess disease severity and rule out biliary obstruction, exclude other hepatic diagnoses
- identify and manage the specific complications of end-stage liver disease as they arise and complications of chronic cholestasis
- adjust or avoid potentially hepatotoxic medications

SPECIFIC THERAPY

- indicated for any patient diagnosed with PBC and abnormal liver enzymes:
  - ➤ ursodeoxycholic acid 13–15 mg/kg daily
- side effects and complications
  - ➤ ursodeoxycholic acid: diarrhea, rash, nausea, arthralgias

Specific Therapy for Complications Associated with PBC

- indications for treatment
  - ➤ cirrhosis/end stage liver disease: consider liver transplantation for patients with CTP score = 7; PBC may recur in transplanted liver
  - ➤ pruritus: cholestyramine, 4 grams QID, spaced 4 hours apart from other oral medications

- rifampin 150 mg BID-TID, as second-line therapy
- naltrexone 50 mg daily, for resistant cases
- liver transplantation for uncontrollable pruritus
➤ sicca syndrome: xerophthalmia: artificial tears without preservatives
➤ xerostomia: regular dental checkup for caries; oral moisturizers
➤ osteoporosis: bone mineral density with dual X-ray absorptiometry when the diagnosis of PBC is first established and yearly thereafter; regular and adequate exercise
  - calcium 1,500 grams daily
  - vitamin D 1,000 iu daily
  - hormonal replacement therapy for perimenopausal women
  - cyclical etidronate 400 mg daily (for documented osteoporosis)
  - liver transplantation for severe osteoporosis

FOLLOW-UP

During Treatment
- monitor biochemistry, including alkaline phosphatase and bilirubin every 3–6 months
- regularly assess potential complications of PBC, including osteoporosis, pruritus, portal hypertension, and other extrahepatic diseases

COMPLICATIONS AND PROGNOSIS
- serum bilirubin and Mayo risk score are both important indices that predict survival
- liver transplantation is cure, although recurrence post-OLT does occur
- post-OLT 1-year survival >90% and 5-year survival >60%

PRIMARY HYPERPARATHYROIDISM

DOLORES SHOBACK, MD

HISTORY & PHYSICAL

History
- Most common in women over age 60
- Symptomatic or asymptomatic presentation
- Renal stones (10–15%)

- Osteoporosis, fractures
- Psychological complaints – depression, fatigue
- May occur in MEN 1 (common, penetrance >90%), MEN 2A (up to 50%), MEN 2B (<10%)

Signs & Symptoms
- Height loss due to osteoporosis
- Band keratopathy
- Flank pain secondary to renal colic
- 50–70% patients asymptomatic
- Wide spectrum of symptoms
- CNS: decreased memory and concentration, lethargy, depression, somnolence
- Cardiovascular: hypertension
- Neuromuscular: myopathy
- Musculoskeletal: aches and pains, arthralgias, fractures, osteitis fibrosa cystica (rare)
- Gastrointestinal: anorexia, constipation, pancreatitis, peptic ulcer
- Renal: dehydration, thirst, polyuria, renal stones

TESTS
Laboratory
- Blood:
  - ➤ elevated total Ca (occasionally ionized Ca needed)
  - ➤ elevated or high normal intact PTH (90% of patients above normal)
  - ➤ low or normal serum P
  - ➤ elevated alk phos, if advanced skeletal disease
  - ➤ high or normal 1,25-OH-vitamin D
- Urine:
  - ➤ 24 h Ca (>100 mg)
  - ➤ Ca/creatinine clearance (>0.01): U-Ca X S-creat/S-Ca X U-creat

Screening
- Asymptomatic elevated Ca on routine chemistry

Confirmatory Tests
- Elevated Ca
- Inappropriately normal or frankly elevated PTH
- Elevated Ca/creat clearance

Imaging
- Sestamibi scanning sensitive and specific in localizing abnormal parathyroid gland(s)
- Bone densitometry to assess effects on bone mineral (spine, hip, radius)
- Nephrocalcinosis on abdominal X-ray

DIFFERENTIAL DIAGNOSIS
- Hypercalcemia of malignancy
- Familial benign hypercalcemia (FBH)
- Granulomatous disease
- Thyrotoxicosis
- Vitamin A or D toxicity
- Lithium or thiazide therapy

MANAGEMENT

What to Do First
- Determine if symptomatic or asymptomatic
- If asymptomatic, rule out FBH

General Measures
- Assess symptoms and end-organ complications (renal, bone, psychological, gastrointestinal)
- If complications present, consider surgery
- If symptomatic, refer to endocrine surgeon
- If hypercalcemic crisis present (rare, <10% of patients):
  - Urgent volume expansion
  - Loop diuretics
  - IV bisphosphonates
  - Refer for surgery

SPECIFIC THERAPY
- May be followed, if asymptomatic
- If symptomatic, end-organ complications or young (<age 50), refer to endocrine surgeon

Guidelines from NIH Consensus on Management of Primary HPTH (2002)
- If symptoms present, operate
- Consider surgery if:
  - Age < 50
  - U-Ca > 400 mg/24 h
  - Serum Ca 1 mg/dl above upper limit of normal

➤ Reduced creat clearance (<70% of normal)
➤ Renal stones
➤ Reduced bone mass (>–2.5 SD below sex-, and race-matched normals)

■ Small clinical trials show skeletal benefit with po alendronate

FOLLOW-UP

■ Twice-yearly or annual monitoring of symptoms, Ca, PTH, renal function, annual bone mineral density

COMPLICATIONS AND PROGNOSIS

■ Renal stones, deterioration of renal function, fractures, changes in mental status, depression, neurologic and myopathic changes

■ Prognosis: recent 10 year prospective study – no skeletal or functional deterioration in majority of patients with mild, asymptomatic disease

■ Symptomatic and severe disease – excellent response to parathyroidectomy (>95% curative) and gains in bone mass

---

PRIMARY SCLEROSING CHOLANGITIS

JOANNE C. IMPERIAL, MD

HISTORY & PHYSICAL

History

■ frequently a disease of men; onset usually below age 45

■ approximately 70% have IBD (usually ulcerative colitis), although only 4–5% of ulcerative colitis patients have PSC

■ often associated with other autoimmune diseases (Sjogren's, thyroiditis) and certain HLA haplotypes (HLA-B8)

■ must exclude other causes of chronic cholestasis in order to confirm the diagnosis

Signs and Symptoms

■ two potential patterns of disease progression have been described:

■ insidious development of abdominal discomfort, pruritus, diarrhea, malnutrition, osteoporosis

■ fluctuating course of fever, RUQ pain and jaundice associated with development of large dominant ductal strictures (possible increased association with cholangiocarcinoma)

➤ early disease: often asymptomatic and associated with few physical signs; often detected after routine chemistry panel shows increased LFTs

➤ advanced disease: liver failure

TESTS

Laboratory

Basic Studies: Blood

■ early disease: cholestatic pattern
  ➤ increased alkaline phosphatase and GGT, mild increased AST/ALT, normal or transiently increased bilirubin
  ➤ serology: autoantibodies nonspecific, nondiagnostic; ANA, SMA positive in 50%; p-ANCA positive in majority
■ advanced disease: increased bilirubin and INR; hypoalbuminemia, malnutrition

Imaging

■ ultrasound or CT scan: nonspecific/nondiagnostic
  ➤ early disease: normal or hepatomegaly; dilated ducts may be suggestive of malignancy
  ➤ advanced disease: hepatomegaly, venous collaterals, signs of portal hypertension
■ ERCP
  ➤ traditional "gold standard" for diagnosis of PSC: stricturing and dilation of the biliary ducts; ductal pseudodiverticula considered pathognomic
■ MRCP
  ➤ replacing ERCP for diagnosis of PSC (less invasive, fewer complications, excellent images; intrahepatic ducts less well visualized)

Liver Biopsy

■ helpful, but not necessary for diagnosis of PSC; excludes other or concurrent diagnoses; stages the disease
  ➤ early disease: bile duct epithelium infiltrated with inflammatory cells arranged in a concentric manner, previously named pericholangitis
  ➤ advanced disease: portal-to-portal bridging fibrosis; biliary ductular proliferation, periductular sclerosis and stenosis

DIFFERENTIAL DIAGNOSIS

■ secondary causes of sclerosing cholangitis: choledocholithiasis, chronic infections due to parasites or opportunistic organisms,

ischemic bile duct injury, drug-induced sclerosing cholangitis (floxuridine)
- sclerosing variant of cholangiocarcinoma
- idiopathic adulthood ductopenia
- autoimmune cholangitis
- drug-induced cholestasis

MANAGEMENT

What to Do First
- establish diagnosis by MRCP or ERCP; exclude secondary causes of sclerosing cholangitis, cholangiocarcinoma; look for evidence of inflammatory bowel disease (if patient has no colonic symptoms or has not been previously evaluated do flexible sigmoidoscopy, biopsies)

General Measures
- use liver biopsy, imaging studies to assess disease severity and rule out biliary obstruction or cirrhosis, exclude other diagnoses
- therapeutic ERCP if evidence of biliary ductular dilatation on ultrasound, CT or sudden change in liver function tests; do biliary brushings/biopsies to rule out cholangiocarcinoma
- identify and manage the silent complications of chronic cholestasis
- adjust or avoid potentially hepatotoxic medications
- optimize therapy of underlying inflammatory bowel disease

SPECIFIC THERAPY
- no proven medical therapy; UDCA commonly used in high doses (25–30 mg/kg/day)
- therapy directed at treating complications of the disease

FOLLOW-UP

Routine
- early disease: patients should be seen semi-annually and screened for possible silent complications of PSC (i.e. assess bone mineral density); manage biliary complications with therapeutic ERCP
- advanced disease: patients should be seen every 3–6 months and
- refer for liver transplantation (OLT) when minimal listing criteria are met (CPT score ≥7)

COMPLICATIONS AND PROGNOSIS

Complications
- cirrhosis/end-stage liver disease: refer for OLT, sooner rather than later, to avoid complication of cholangiocarcinoma

- cholangiocarcinoma: in approximately 30% of patients; more prevalent with long-standing PSC; no proven therapy although OLT increases survival in specific cases
- biliary obstruction: antibiotics either for acute episodes of cholangitis secondary to sludge/stones or strictures, or prior to endoscopic intervention; chronic antibiotic therapy may be indicated in certain patients with intrahepatic disease
- therapeutic ERCP and dilatation with/without temporary stenting of dominant bile duct strictures
- rule out cholangiocarcinoma with biliary brushings and biopsies as indicated (yield is <50%); CA 19–9 not validated as a screening marker for cholangiocarcinoma
- pruritus: cholestyramine, 4 grams QID spaced 4 hours apart from other oral medications
- rifampin 150 mg BID/TID
- naltrexone 50 mg daily, for resistant cases
- liver transplantation for uncontrollable pruritus
- osteoporosis: calcium 1500 mg daily supplementation, vitamin D 1000 IU daily; bone mineral density annually; regular exercise
- calcium and or vitamin D: side effects encountered when hypercalcemia occurs
- absolute contraindications: hypercalcemia, hypervitaminosis D

Prognosis
- 8-year survival of asymptomatic patients 80%
- 8-yr survival symptomatic patient 50%
- cirrhosis diagnosed at initial presentation has associated poor survival
- survival after OLT excellent ($\geq$90% at one year without cholangiocarcinoma), although disease recurrence has been reported to occur in up to 25% of patients

PRION DISORDERS (CREUTZFELDT-JAKOB DISEASE)

CHAD CHRISTINE, MD

HISTORY & PHYSICAL

Sporadic Form: May Present W/Diffuse or Localized Neurologic Dysfunction
- Onset at any age
- Dementia develops in all cases

- Progression to akinetic mutism or coma typically over months
- Accounts for 85% of all cases of CJD

Transmissible Form: Rare
- Human-to-human transmission
  - Cannibalism
  - Corneal transplantation
  - Improperly sterilized surgical instruments
  - Human growth hormone
- Animal to human transmission
  - New variant CJD (or bovine spongiform encephalopathy)
  - Characterized by early onset (mean age 30 yr)
  - More prolonged course than sporadic CJD
  - Prominent psychiatric abnormalities

Familial Forms
- Fatal familial insomnia (dementia & ataxia)
- Gerstmann-Straussler-Scheinker syndrome (disturbance of sleep, autonomic & endocrine function)
- Signs & symptoms include memory loss, behavioral abnormalities, myoclonus (often induced by startle), extrapyramidal signs (rigidity, bradykinesia, tremor, dystonia, chorea or athetosis), pyramidal signs, cerebellar signs

TESTS
- Diagnosis made clinically
- Lab tests: blood & urine unremarkable
- EEG may show a typical but nonspecific pattern of periodic sharp waves or spikes
- CSF protein may be mildly elevated
- Brain MRI may show mildly increased signal in the basal ganglia on T2 images
- Biopsy: detection of PrPsc protein in brain or tonsillar tissue is diagnostic
- Genetic testing (research): available in familial forms

DIFFERENTIAL DIAGNOSIS
- Alzheimer's disease, Parkinson's disease, progressive supranuclear palsy excluded by history
- Hashimoto's encephalopathy, drug intoxication (lithium), toxic exposure (bismuth) and sedative drug withdrawal may be differentiated by lab evaluation
- Intracerebral mass lesion excluded by brain imaging

MANAGEMENT
- Supportive

SPECIFIC THERAPY
- None available

FOLLOW-UP
n/a

COMPLICATIONS AND PROGNOSIS
- Relentlessly progressive, although transient improvement may occur
- In most sporadic cases, death occurs within 1 year
- In familial forms, disease duration depends on specific mutation

PROLACTINOMA AND GALACTORRHEA

ANDREW R. HOFFMAN, MD

HISTORY & PHYSICAL

History
- Infertility, amenorrhea or oligoamenorrhea, pregnancy, breast feeding
- Impotence
- Psychotropic drug use
- Hypothyroidism
- Renal failure
- Family history of pituitary tumor
- Persistence of galactorrhea after cessation of breast feeding

Signs & Symptoms
- Galactorrhea (rare in men)
- Headache
- Decreased libido
- Visual field defect
- Osteoporosis
- Hypopituitarism
- Occasionally occurs in acromegaly

TESTS

Laboratory
- Basic blood studies:
  - Prolactin, free T4, TSH, IGF I, GH
  - Serum pregnancy test (beta-hCG)

- Ancillary blood tests:
  - ➤ LH, FSH
  - ➤ Testosterone
  - ➤ Estradiol
  - ➤ DHEA-S

Imaging
- MRI of pituitary to determine if microadenoma (<1 cm), macroadenoma (>1 cm), or hypothalamic mass present

DIFFERENTIAL DIAGNOSIS
- Hyperprolactinemia without pituitary mass
- Primary hypothyroidism
- Pregnancy and breastfeeding cause physiologic hyperprolactinemia
- Nonsecretory pituitary macroadenoma; stalk compression leads to decreased dopamine transmission to pituitary and hyperprolactinemia
- Acromegaly; tumor may secrete both GH and Prolactin
- May be associated with polycystic ovarian disease
- Idiopathic galactorrhea with normal prolactin levels
Nipple stimulation may raise prolactin level (rare)

MANAGEMENT

What to Do First
- Rule out pregnancy and primary hypothyroidism
- Determine presence or absence of pituitary mass by MRI:
  - ➤ Macroadenoma, prolactin <100–150 ng/dL: nonsecretory pituitary mass
  - ➤ Macroadenoma, prolactin >150 ng/dL: macroprolactinoma
  - ➤ Microadenoma: microprolactinoma (may be incidental pituitary adenoma, esp if <4 mm); most commonly seen in women
  - ➤ No mass: idiopathic hyperprolactinemia

SPECIFIC THERAPY
- Nonsecretory macroadenoma:
  - ➤ Surgery to debulk tumor if visual field cut or headache
  - ➤ Observation with repeated pituitary MRI to determine if tumor growing
  - ➤ Radiation therapy (eg, gamma knife) if tumor grows
  - ➤ Dopaminergic agents (bromocriptine or cabergoline) to decrease prolactin levels and decrease galactorrhea

- Macroprolactinoma:
  - Dopaminergic agents (bromocriptine or cabergoline) as first-line therapy to decrease serum prolactin (successful >90% of cases) and shrink tumor (successful >70% of patients).
  - Transsphenoidal or transfrontal surgery to debulk tumor if dopaminergic agents are unsuccessful or if patient desires pregnancy and tumor is near optic chiasm
- Microprolactinoma:
  - Dopaminergic agents as first-line therapy to restore fertility in women
  - Transsphenoidal surgical removal of tumor if medications not tolerated; recurrence rate >30%
  - If fertility is not desired and menses occur at least every 2–3 mo, no therapy; repeat MRI in 3 mo, and then q 6–12 mo to determine if tumor growing; microadenomas rarely grow
  - If fertility not desired and no menses, may use oral contraceptive to provide estrogen and prevent osteoporosis
  - Idiopathic hyperprolactinemia:
    - Rule out use of medications that increase prolactin (eg, phenothiazines)
    - Treat like microprolactinoma

Treatment Goals
- Decrease or normalize serum prolactin
- Shrink pituitary tumor
- Maintain normal pituitary function
- Fertility
  - Cessation of galactorrhea
  - Restoration of libido/potency

Side Effects & Contraindications
- Bromocriptine and cabergoline:
  - Side effects (more prominent with bromocriptine): gastric upset, nasal stuffiness, orthostatic hypotension with initial doses; always take medications with food
  - Contraindications: not recommended to stop postpartum galactorrhea or normoprolactinemic galactorrhea

FOLLOW-UP
- Start bromocriptine with small doses and work up to full therapeutic dose (2–3 times daily) over at least 1–2 wks
- Cabergoline given once or twice weekly

- Measure serum prolactin after 4–6 wks of therapy
- Repeat pituitary MRI in 3–6 mo to assess pituitary growth/shrinkage

COMPLICATIONS AND PROGNOSIS
- Pituitary apoplexy (in patients with macroadenomas):
  - ➤ Very severe headache, altered consciousness, coma
  - ➤ Requires emergent surgical intervention and resection of tumor
- Visual field changes:
  - ➤ Signifies tumor growth
  - ➤ May occur in pregnancy with macroprolactinomas
  - ➤ Requires institution of dopaminergic agents or surgery
- Pregnancy
- Macroadenoma: requires lifelong therapy
- Microadenoma: may stop therapy at menopause

PROSTATE CANCER

JOHN D. McCONNELL, MD
REVISED BY BIFF F. PALMER MD

HISTORY & PHYSICAL

History
- Aging: Overall lifetime risk approximately 1 in 12; occult, clinically insignificant prostate cancer present in half of men over age 70
- Race: risk two-fold higher in African American, with a tendency to occur in younger men
- Family history: a brother or father with prostate cancer increases an individual's risk by two-fold

Signs & Symptoms
- Local, organ-confined cancer is usually asymptomatic.
- Locally and locally advanced disease:
  - ➤ Lower urinary tract symptoms (frequency, urgency, decreased force of stream, incomplete bladder emptying, nocturia)
  - ➤ Hematuria (especially with invasion of the bladder)
  - ➤ Hematospermia (blood in the semen, usually a benign symptom)
  - ➤ Rarely symptoms of renal failure from ureteral obstruction (nausea, vomiting, lethargy)
- Advanced, metastatic disease:
  - ➤ Bone pain (lumbar vertebrae, pelvis, femur, most common)
  - ➤ Weight loss, anorexia

> Lymphedema (from pelvic and retroperitoneal lymph node involvement)
> Severe anemia secondary to bone marrow replacement
> Symptoms of renal failure from ureteral obstruction
> Disseminated intravascular coagulation
■ Majority of men with cancer diagnosed on the basis of an elevated serum prostate specific antigen (PSA) have a normal rectal exam.
■ Nodularity, induration, asymmetry of the prostate on digital rectal examination (DRE)
■ Lymphedema and spinal cord compression (paraparesis, paraplegia)

TESTS
Laboratory
Serum PSA:
■ Prostate-specific antigen: a serine protease made by the normal prostate (not specific for prostate cancer)
■ Serum PSA is dependent on age and prostate size.
■ 25% of men with localized prostate cancer will have a normal PSA.
■ Only 25% of men with a serum PSA 4–10 ng/ml have prostate cancer; most have only benign prostatic hyperplasia (BPH).
■ Men with known prostate cancer and a PSA <10 ng/ml rarely have metastatic disease.

Urine:
■ Early disease: normal
■ Advanced disease: hematuria, especially if bladder involved

Other Tests:
■ Free (unbound) and complexed serum PSA may help distinguish cancer from BPH.
■ Acid phosphatase and prostatic acid phosphastase may be elevated in advanced disease.
■ CBC, serum creatinine and alkaline phosphatase

Screening
■ Annual digital rectal examination and serum PSA beginning at age 50
■ Begin testing at age 40 or 45 in African Americans and men with a family history.
■ Stop annual detection when expected life expectancy <10 years.

Prostate Biopsy
- 6–12 core needle biopsies of the prostate usually necessary

Other Imaging Studies
- Radionuclide bone scan if PSA >10 or poorly differentiated cancer
- Transrectal MRI may confirm extension beyond the prostate

DIFFERENTIAL DIAGNOSIS
- Elevated serum PSA may be due to BPH, prostate infection, or recent urinary tract procedures such as catheterization, endoscopy, or biopsy.
- Lower urinary tract symptoms may be due to BPH, UTI, neurogenic bladder disease, bladder cancer or urolithiasis.

MANAGEMENT
What to Do First
- Treat spinal cord compression and obstructive uropathy if present.

General Measures
- Estimate extent of disease by digital rectal examination, tumor grade (Gleason score), and serum PSA.
- Consider other staging studies (bone scan, CT scan).

SPECIFIC THERAPY
Indications
- Localized (organ-confined) disease in a patient with at least a 10-year life expectancy
- Metastatic bone disease
- Symptomatic, locally advanced

Treatment Options for Organ-Confined Cancer
- Radical prostatectomy, external beam radiotherapy, interstitial radiotherapy (brachytherapy or "seeds"), watchful waiting
- Surgery offers the highest probability of cancer-free survival, but radiotherapy results are comparable for small, well to moderately differentiated tumors.
- Major risks of surgery: significant incontinence 2–10%; erectile dysfunction 10–50% (age and tumor dependent, usually treatable)
- Major risks of radiation: rectal and bladder irritation, uncertain incidence of erectile dysfunction, urinary retention

Treatment Options for Locally Advanced Cancer
- Watchful waiting (followed by delayed hormonal therapy), hormonal therapy, hormonal therapy plus external beam radiotherapy
- Surgery not indicated

Treatment Options for Metastatic Cancer
- Hormonal Therapy:
  - Androgen deprivation: bilateral orchiectomy or injection of GnRH (LHRH) agonists (leads to depressed levels of LH and FSH)
  - Oral androgen receptor (AR) antagonists indicated during initial therapy of symptomatic bone disease with GnRH agonists
  - The average patient has evidence of disease progression after 3–5 years of androgen deprivation.
  - Side effects: loss of sexual function, osteoporosis, loss of muscle mass, hot flashes, hepatic dysfunction (AR antagonists)
- Emergency Treatment of Spinal Cord Compression:
  - Rapid lowering of serum testosterone if not already achieved: ketaconazole or orchiectomy
  - Decadron plus spot radiation or (rarely) surgical laminectomy
- Therapy for Androgen-Independent Cancer:
  - Chemotherapy: Taxol and taxane-based therapies, in combination with estramustine or alkalating agents
  - Spot radiation therapy to painful bone lesions

FOLLOW-UP
- Serum PSA and digital rectal examination q 3 6 months in patients following potentially curative therapy for localized disease
- Patients with advanced disease should have a periodic bone scan, hemoglobin and assessment of renal function.

COMPLICATIONS AND PROGNOSIS
n/a

PROSTATITIS

GARY SINCLAIR, MD

HISTORY & PHYSICAL

Acute Prostatitis
- Chills, back and perineal pain, urinary frequency, malaise, myalgias, lightheadedness

- Rectal exam reveals tender, swollen, and indurated prostate.
- Urinary retention revealed by bladder percussion

Chronic Prostatitis
- History and physical much more subtle
- May present as vague perineal or back pain with low-grade fever
- Digital exam reveals boggy enlarged prostate, without extraordinary tenderness.

TESTS
- Urine and blood cultures – suspect *Escherichia coli*, *Enterococcus sp.*, *Klebsiella sp.*, *Enterobacter sp.*, *Serratia sp.*, *Proteus sp.*, *Morganella sp.*, and *Providencia sp.*, in outpatient setting; *Pseudomonas sp.* in hospitalized patient
- In patients <35, consider *N. gonorrhea* and *C. trachomatis* (rare).
- Pre- and post-prostatic massage cultures of urine are only necessary/helpful for chronic prostatitis.
- Prostatic-specific antigen will be nonspecifically elevated.
- Transrectal ultrasound necessary to rule out prostatic abscess in cases refractory to treatment

DIFFERENTIAL DIAGNOSIS
- Prostatic hypertrophy, prostadynia, prostate cancer, prostatic abscess, proctitis, cystitis, pyelonephritis

MANAGEMENT
- Hydration
- Relief of urinary obstruction (catheter)

SPECIFIC THERAPY
- Treat empirically with quinolone or trimethoprim-sulfamethoxazole for at least 14 days for acute prostatitis.
- Some would argue for 28 days of treatment to prevent chronic prostatitis, prostatic abscess.
- Chronic prostatitis can require treatment courses of 6 weeks to 6 months.
- Due to increasing resistance in both inpatient and outpatient settings, treatment must be modified based on culture and sensitivity results. Do not assume that empiric choice is correct.

FOLLOW-UP
- Expect rapid (within 24 h) improvement for treatment of acute prostatitis.
- If improvement not rapid, consider complications (see below).

COMPLICATIONS AND PROGNOSIS

- Prostatic abscess (requires drainage – can be source of fever of unknown origin), pyelonephritis, bacteremia, chronic pain, urinary obstruction

---

PROTEIN-LOSING ENTEROPATHY

GARY M. GRAY, MD

HISTORY & PHYSICAL

History

- Fatigue, pedal edema, ascites
- Associated history of intra-abdominal disease of stomach, intestine, colon, lymph channels (especially lymphangiectasia) or functional blockage of major abdominal or thoracic veins.
- Underlying heart disease (chronic heart failure, pericarditis, tricuspid valve regurgitation) or after transplantation of heart or liver

Physical

- Pitting edema of lower extremities; ascites and pleural effusions

TESTS

Basic Blood

- hypoalbuminemia (albumin usually <2.5 g/dl); lymphopenia, hypogammaglobulinemia

Basic Urine

- none usually helpful; no proteinuria

Specific Diagnostic

- Increased fecal loss of macromolecules (alpha-1-antitrypsin) or enhanced loss into hollow gut by scintigraphy (technetium-99m-labeled) [Tc-99m]albumin; [Tc-99m]dextran

DIFFERENTIAL DIAGNOSIS

- Hypoabuminemia due to renal loss (proteinuria)
- Inadequate liver synthesis of albumin (especially in cirrhosis)
- Generalized protein calorie malnutrition due to an intestinal disease

MANAGEMENT

What to Do First

- Initial trial of fluid restriction and diuretics (often not successful)
- High protein diet

General Measures
- Identify and treat the primary disease by appropriate study of intestine, colon, heart, and large abdominal or thoracic veins

SPECIFIC THERAPY
- If PLE persists, prednisone 10–20 mg/day (30 days, gradual taper) may reverse the protein loss, regardless of cause
- Repeat courses of prednisone may be necessary

FOLLOW-UP
- Weekly body weights, monthly examinations, including estimation of pleural fluid (chest X-rays), ascites (measure abdominal girth, abdominal ultrasound), extent of residual pedal edema
- Monthly measurement of serum albumin

COMPLICATIONS AND PROGNOSIS
- Varies with underlying disease; mechanical correction, when possible, may be curative.
- Intermittent prednisone therapy may be required over the long-term

---

PRURITUS

JEFFREY P. CALLEN, MD

HISTORY & PHYSICAL

Signs & Symptoms
- Pruritus is the symptom of itching
- Scratching may result in excoriations, rubbing may result in lichenification
- Pruritus may be a symptom that accompanies a primary skin disorder, or may reflect an underlying systemic disease
- Pruritus may be localized or generalized

TESTS

Laboratory
- Basic blood studies:
  - ➤ CBC, comprehensive metabolic panel, hepatic enzymes (particularly alkaline phosphatase), thyroid panel, hepatitis C antibody, HIV test
  - ➤ Skin biopsy may be helpful in diagnosis of dermatitis herpetiformis, mycosis fungoides

Imaging

- Chest x-ray, particularly in the absence of a primary cutaneous disorder

DIFFERENTIAL DIAGNOSIS

- Primary dermatologic diseases:
  - Eczema – including atopic and contact
  - Psoriasis
  - Scabies
  - Mycosis fungoides
  - Dermatitis herpetiformis
  - Lichen planus
  - Insect bites
  - Xerosis
  - Drug reactions
- Systemic diseases:
  - Renal disease – hemodialysis associated, uremic pruritus
  - Hepatic dysfunction – biliary obstruction, primary biliary cirrhosis, hepatitis C
  - Hyper- or hypothyroidism
  - Iron deficiency anemia
  - Diabetes mellitus
  - Polycythemia vera
  - Lymphoma – particularly Hodgkin's disease
  - Parasitosis – intestinal
  - HIV infection
  - Pregnancy – might be due to cholestasis
- Localized pruritus:
  - Notalgia paresthetica – localized pruritus usually on the back of middle-aged to elderly women – may reflect an underlying spinal nerve impingement
  - Brachioradial pruritus – localized itching on the arm and forearm. This condition might also reflect underlying nerve impingement.
  - Lichen amyloidosis
  - Lichen simplex chronicus
  - Pruritus ani or pruritus vulvae

MANAGEMENT

What to Do First

- Assess severity of pruritus and possible causes

General Measures
- Emollients
- Topical antipruritic agents – menthol, pramoxine
  - Systemic antipruritic agents – soporific antihistamines such as hydroxyzine, doxepin, cyproheptadine

SPECIFIC THERAPY
- For localized pruritus – intralesional injection of triamcinolone
- For pruritus of hemodialysis, HIV, hepatic dysfunction – Ultraviolet B phototherapy
- Treat underlying cause of the pruritus.

FOLLOW-UP

During Rx
- Regularly assess potential complications of therapy; – irritation of the skin or drowsiness from antihistamines

COMPLICATIONS AND PROGNOSIS
- Dependent upon the cause of the pruritus

PSEUDOHYPOALDOSTERONISM

MICHEL BAUM, MD

HISTORY & PHYSICAL
- Pseudohypoaldosteronism type 1 (PHA) presents in the first week of life with volume depletion, hyponatremia and hyperkalemia.
- Autosomal recessive PHA also has recurrent episodes of chest congestion, coughing, and wheezing, not due to airway infections but due to pulmonary fluid accumulation.

TESTS
- Both forms have hyponatremia due to renal salt wasting and hyperkalemia and elevated aldosterone levels; have type 4 renal tubular acidosis.

DIFFERENTIAL DIAGNOSIS
- Autosomal recessive PHA is due to an inactivating mutation in the epithelial sodium channel. It is typically much more severe and presents earlier in life than the dominant form.
- Autosomal dominant PHA is due to inactivating mutations in the aldosterone receptor.

MANAGEMENT
■ Sodium supplements
■ Kayexalate and low-potassium diet

SPECIFIC THERAPY
■ N/A

FOLLOW-UP
■ Frequent follow-up to follow electrolytes, whether pt is thriving

COMPLICATIONS AND PROGNOSIS
■ Patients do not tolerate volume depletion from GI losses.
■ Hyperkalemia can be life-threatening.
■ Patients may have failure to thrive.

PSEUDOMONAS INFECTIONS

RICHARD A. JACOBS, MD, PhD

HISTORY & PHYSICAL

History
■ *Pseudomonas aeruginosa* is an oxidase-positive, aerobic Gram-negative bacillus that is ubiquitous in nature.
■ Predilection for moist environments; colonizes skin, ear canal, upper respiratory tract and gastrointestinal tract, particularly in hospitalized, burn, immunocompromised and intensive care unit patients and those receiving broad-spectrum antimicrobial therapy; colonization of the hospital environment and equipment common
■ Most infections nosocomial, but community-acquired infection seen in those with comorbid diseases

Signs & Symptoms
■ Urinary Tract Infections – usually associated with instrumentation or catheterization; outpatient infection associated with obstruction, stones or superinfection after antibiotic therapy; clinical manifestations same as infection with other bacteria
■ Pneumonia – usually nosocomial; seen in ventilator-dependant, neutropenic or immunosuppressed patients; outpatient pneumonia associated with chronic lung disease, cystic fibrosis, HIV infection and chronic care facilities; symptoms indistinguishable from other serious bacterial pneumonias

- Bacteremia – can be primary without source (neutropenic patients with presumed source the gastrointestinal tract) or secondary to pneumonia, genitourinary infection, intravascular devices or rarely endocarditis; manifestations similar to other causes of bacteremia; characteristic skin lesion, ecthyma gangrenosum, may be early clue to diagnosis – vesicular lesion that ulcerates, becomes necrotic and is surrounded by erythema; Gram stain of lesion reveals Gram-negative rods

- Bone and Joint Infections – secondary to hematogenous seeding or direct contiguous spread; predilection for fibrocartilaginous joints including the vertebrae, and in IV drug users the sternoclavicular joint and the symphysis pubis; osteochondritis of the foot following nail puncture wound common in children

- Ear Infections – otitis externa presents with pain, swelling, and marked tenderness with a waxy exudate in the ear canal; invasive disease (malignant otitis externa or basilar skull osteomyelitis) with involvement of bone seen almost exclusively in diabetics with microvascular disease

- Eye Disease – keratitis and ulcer from trauma or extended-wear contact lenses; ulcer that expands to include the sclera, associated with pain, decreased vision and purulent discharge; can be rapidly progressive and sight-threatening; Gram stain reveals characteristic organisms; endophthalmitis involving the anterior and/or posterior chamber with pain and decreased vision results from trauma or hematogenous seeding and is uncommon

- Skin Infections – ecthyma gangrenosum (see above), postoperative wound infection and infection of burns most common; burn wound infection presents with separation of eschar, black discoloration of wound, spread of cellulitis to adjacent normal skin with necrosis and bleeding; frequently associated with bacteremia and sepsis; hot tub dermatitis is a maculopapular or vesicular, erythematous rash involving swimming suit-covered areas (can be more diffuse) resulting from exposure to hot tubs, spas or swimming pools improperly maintained

- Meningitis, Endocarditis and Neutropenic Enterocolitis (typhlitis) – unusual manifestations of Pseudomonas infection

TESTS

- Culture of blood or specimen from suspected site of infection (sputum, urine, joint fluid, etc) confirms diagnosis in most cases.

- CXR with bilateral, diffuse bronchopneumonia; presence of nodular densities suggestive but not diagnostic of Pseudomonas
- Bone films, CT or MRI may be helpful in septic arthritis/osteomyelitis.
- MRI, bone scan and indium WBC scan helpful in diagnosing and following course of basilar skull osteomyelitis

DIFFERENTIAL DIAGNOSIS
- Includes other pyogenic bacteria that cause similar syndromes

MANAGEMENT
- Assess severity of illness; acute, rapidly progressive disease (meningitis, sepsis, necrotizing pneumonia, corneal ulcer, burn wound infection) or infection in an immunocompromised patient requires use of empiric antibiotics before culture results known.
- General supportive care

SPECIFIC THERAPY
- A number of antibiotics active against *Pseudomonas* including aminoglycosides (tobramycin, amikacin), cephalosporins (ceftazidime, cefipime), anti-pseudomonal penicillins (piperacillin, mezlocillin, ticarcillin), fluoroquinolones (ciprofloxcin the most active), monobactams (aztreonam), and carbapenems (imipenem, meropenem)
- No definitive evidence that use of two drugs improves outcome compared to single-drug therapy; however, in severe infections or infections in immunocompromised patients, two drugs are used initially (until clinical improvement), with completion of therapy with a single agent; common combinations include an anti-pseudomonal penicillin or cephalosporin plus an aminoglycoside or a fluoroquinolone; two beta-lactam drugs should be avoided (possible antagonism)
- Urinary Tract Infections – uncomplicated cystitis treated 3 days, pyelonephritis 2 weeks
- Pneumonia – 2–3 weeks; in cystic fibrosis higher doses of antibiotics required because of increased clearance and volume of distribution); nebulized tobramycin improves pulmonary function in colonized, clinically stable patients with cystic fibrosis, but inhaled antibiotics, though often used, are not of proven benefit in treating acute exacerbations
- Bacteremia – 2–3 weeks

- Bone and Joint Infections – osteomyelitis 6–8 weeks; septic arthritis 3–4 weeks with joint drainage; osteochondritis 2 weeks with debridement
- Ear Infections – otitis externa treated with antibiotic drops; basilar skull osteomyelitis 6–8 weeks with limited surgery to debride necrotic tissue and drain abscesses
- Eye Infections – topical aminoglycosides, subconjunctival or sub-Tenon antibiotic injections and intravenous antibiotics depending upon severity of disease
- Skin Infections – hot tub dermatitis resolves without therapy; other skin infections 10–14 days
- Meningitis – 2–3 weeks
- Endocarditis – 6–8 weeks plus surgery, as indicated

FOLLOW-UP
- Resolution of infection may be slow, especially in the immunocompromised patient.
- Routine follow-up required

COMPLICATIONS AND PROGNOSIS
- Variable; depends on organ system involved and immune status of host; acute, fulminant infections associated with high mortality

PSITTACOSIS

RICHARD A. JACOBS, MD, PhD

HISTORY & PHYSICAL

History
- Causative agent *Chlamydia psittaci*, an obligate intracellular bacteria
- Major reservoir is birds (any species can be infected, not just psitticines); rarely other animals (cattle, sheep, goats) can transmit disease; infected birds may be asymptomatic or ill, with ill birds excreting more organisms in their feces, urine and beaks than well birds
- Anyone with exposure to birds is at increased risk of infection, including bird owners, importers of birds, chicken and turkey farmers, veterinarians, abattoir and processing plant workers.
- Humans infected by inhalation of aerosolized organisms; person-to-person transmission rare

Signs & Symptoms

■ Pneumonia most common presentation, with fevers, chills, severe headache, myalgias and a nonproductive cough; the typhoidal presentation includes systemic symptoms listed above and relative bradycardia, hepatosplenomegaly, Horder's spots (erythematous, blanching, maculopapular rash) without respiratory symptoms.

TESTS

■ Routine laboratory tests often abnormal, but non-diagnostic; WBC may be low, normal or high; liver function tests mildly abnormal in 50%; lobar consolidation most commonly seen on CXR (75%), although other patterns described (may have extensive infiltrates with only minimal findings on exam); sputum shows numerous polymorphonuclear leukocytes and no organisms

■ Definitive diagnosis made serologically (fourfold or greater rise in titer confirms diagnosis; a single titer of 1:32 or higher in a patient with a compatible disease is a probable case)

DIFFERENTIAL DIAGNOSIS

■ Symptoms nonspecific and thus differential extensive; atypical pneumonia due to mycoplasma, *C. pneumoniae*, legionella, viruses; typhoidal presentation suggests typhoid fever, bacteremia, endocarditis, viral illness, mononucleosis; hepatitis suggests viral causes, brucella, Q fever, toxoplasmosis

MANAGEMENT

■ Careful epidemiologic history critical in making diagnosis
■ Routine supportive care

SPECIFIC THERAPY

■ Doxycycline or tetracycline for 2–3 weeks: drugs of choice
■ Erythromycin an alternative, but may be less effective

FOLLOW-UP

■ Clinical response very rapid with improvement in 1–2 days
■ CXR abnormalities slow to resolve (6–20 weeks)

COMPLICATIONS AND PROGNOSIS

■ Rare complications include cardiac involvement (myocarditis, pericarditis, culture-negative endocarditis) and neurologic disease (meningitis, encephalitis)
■ With therapy the mortality rate is 1%.

PSORIASIS

JEFFREY P. CALLEN, MD

HISTORY & PHYSICAL

History

- Psoriasis is a genetically determined disorder that affects the skin and nails
    - Plaque type psoriasis
    - Guttate psoriasis – small, drop-like scaly plaques, often in children or adolescents and triggered by streptococcal infection
    - Pustular psoriasis – localized v. generalized
    - Erythrodermic
- Environmental triggers
    - Heat and sunlight improve many patients
    - Trauma to the skin leads to development of lesions (Koebner phenomenon)
- Infections may exacerbate the disease – e.g., Group A beta-hemolytic streptococcal infection or HIV
- Stress may worsen the condition
- Flares with drugs – e.g. lithium, withdrawal of topical or systemic corticosteroids, occasionally beta blockers or angiotensin-converting enzyme inhibitors and possibly antimalarial agents

Signs & Symptoms

- Chronic Plaque Psoriasis
    - Well-demarcated erythematous plaques with micaceous scale
    - Most common on the elbows, knees, scalp, lower back, and nails
    - Inverse Psoriasis – occurs in the folds
- Guttate Psoriasis
    - Small scaly erythematous plaques primarily on the trunk
- Pustular psoriasis
    - Generalized – erythematous skin studded with small pustules
    - Localized – most often the palms or soles, a pustular eruption
- Erythrodermic psoriasis
    - Exfoliative erythroderma
    - Signs of high output cardiac failure, or hypovolemia may accompany the eruption
- Nail Changes
    - Common

➤ May present as pits, onycholysis, or hyperkeratotic debris under the nail

➤ May correlate with arthritis in nearby joints

■ Arthritis

➤ May occur as the major manifestation of psoriasis, or as a second major illness with major or minor skin involvement. Roughly 30% of patients with psoriasis have or will develop psoriatic arthritis. Most often the skin disease is present prior to the onset and diagnosis of psoriatic arthritis.

TESTS

■ Basic Blood Tests: N/A

■ Specific Diagnostic Tests

➤ Histopathology is helpful in differentiating other disorders, but when the disease is clinically atypical the histology is often atypical

■ Other Tests as Appropriate

➤ Joint x-rays for those with arthralgias or arthritis

DIFFERENTIAL DIAGNOSIS

■ Chronic Plaque Psoriasis

➤ Lichen planus

➤ Eczema

➤ Mycosis fungoides

➤ Tinea corporis

■ Inverse Psoriasis

➤ Candida Intertrigo

➤ Tinea cruris/corporis

➤ Benign familial pemphigus

➤ Contact dermatitis

■ Guttate psoriasis

➤ Pityriasis rosea

➤ Pityriasis lichenoides et varioliformis acuta

➤ Syphilis

➤ Tinea corporis

■ Pustular psoriasis

➤ Infection

■ Erythrodermic psoriasis

➤ Dermatitis

➤ Cutaneous T-cell lymphoma (Sezary syndrome)

➤ Drug eruption

> Lichen planus
> Pityriasis rubra pilaris – often islands of normal skin, palmoplantar hyperkeratosis

MANAGEMENT

What to Do First

- Assess the extent of the disease
- Assess the affect of the disease on the patient's life circumstances

General Measures

- Topical therapy for limited disease
- Phototherapy
- Systemic therapy for extensive disease or disease that interferes with daily activities or employment

SPECIFIC THERAPY

Topical Therapy

- Corticosteroids
  > Wide range of potencies and vehicles
  > Select a potency and vehicle for the specific site
- Tars – adjunctive therapy, messy
- Anthralin – difficult to use, should be handled by a dermatologist
- Calcipotriene (Dovonex)
  > Available as an ointment, cream or scalp solution
  > May use in combination with a superpotent corticosteroid – use the calcipotriene bid on Monday through Friday and the superpotent corticosteroid on Saturday and Sunday
- Retinoids (Tazarotene)
  > Available as a gel or cream

Phototherapy

- UVB phototherapy – heliotherapy or home or office UVB
  > May be delivered daily at home or 3–5 times per week in an office
  > Enhanced by tar application (Goeckerman therapy)
  > Side effects
  - Short term – burns, time away from work
  - Long-term – skin cancer risk
  > Contraindications
  - Inability to stand
  - Presence of skin cancers or a genetic predisposition – e.g., xeroderma pigmentosa

- ■ PUVA (photochemotherapy)
  - ➤ Office based procedure given 2 or 3 times per week
  - ➤ Psoralen (Oxsoralen ultra) is given based on body weight 1 hour prior to therapy
  - ➤ Contraindications
    - • History of photosensitivity diseases
    - • History or presence of skin cancer
    - • Inability to come to an office with appropriate equipment
- ■ PUVA should not be administered in an uncontrolled setting – e.g. a tanning salon
- ■ PUVA may be combined with systemic retinoids to enhance the effect and to limit the development of squamous cell carcinoma

Systemic Therapies
- ■ Methotrexate
  - ➤ Indication – disabling psoriasis, not responsive to less toxic therapy, generally >20% surface involvement, or disease of the hands
  - ➤ Begin at low dose (5 mg/week) and escalate gradually to 20–30 mg/wk
- ■ Acitretin
  - ➤ Indications for treatment
    - • Pustular psoriasis, erythrodermic psoriasis, PUVA or UVB failure
- ■ Cyclosporine
  - ➤ Indications for treatment – Patients with extensive psoriasis who have failed less toxic therapies
- ■ Biologic agents
  - ➤ Anti-TNF agents – etanercept, infliximab and adalimumab are approved for psoriasis (E) and psoriatic arthritis (E, I, A).
    - • Contraindicated in patients with active infection, history of tuberculosis, neurologic disease (particularly multiple sclerosis), unstable cardiac disease. May predispose to a greater risk of lymphoma.
  - ➤ Efalizumab – affects T cells and their ability to migrate into the skin
  - ➤ Alefacept – causes T-cell apoptosis; 20% of patients might have long-lasting remissions

FOLLOW-UP
- ■ Assess response to therapy monthly, monitor blood tests in patients on methotrexate, acitretin or cyclosporine every 2–4 weeks initially, then every 2–3 months once on stable dosage

COMPLICATIONS AND PROGNOSIS

- Arthritis may accompany psoriasis; treatment for the skin disease may be effective, methotrexate or anti-TNF agents are commonly used
- Psoriasis is a chronic disorder.

PULMONARY EMBOLISM

LESLIE H. ZIMMERMAN, MD

HISTORY & PHYSICAL

History

- 65–90% from leg DVTs
- Risk factors:
  - lower extremity or abdominal surgery
  - trauma
  - malignancy
  - MI
  - prior DVT
  - CHF
  - immobilization
  - hormone therapy
  - pregnancy
  - advanced age
  - thrombophilia

Signs & Symptoms

- >90% – dyspnea or tachypnea
- also: pleuritic pain, cough, leg pain or swelling (30%),
- hemoptysis, palpitations, wheezing, fever, syncope
- tachypnea, rales, tachycardia (30%), S4, increased P2 (25%), fever (rarely > 38.5o C), DVT

TESTS

ABG:

- usually low PaCO2
- hypoxemia, increased A-a gradient (correlates with size)
- normal ABG does not rule out PE

Other labs:

- D-dimers:

➤ <500 ng/ml may exclude; usefulness unclear, especially if malignancy or recent surgery

ECG:
- anterior T wave inversions, tachycardia
- less common: new RBBB, afib
- massive PE: 30% with RBBB, P-pulmonale, RAD, or S1 Q3 T3

CXR:
- atelectasis or non-specific
- also: effusion, elevated hemidiaphragm, prominent PA, cardiomegaly, focal oligemia (Westermark's sign)

Imaging:
- V/Q scans
  - ➤ Normal essentially rules out PE
  - ➤ PE present in:
    - 96% with high suspicion & high prob V/Q
    - 87% with high probability V/Q
    - 33% with intermediate probability V/Q
    - 12% with low probability V/Q
    - 4% with low suspicion & low prob V/Q
- Spiral CT (CT Angiogram)
  - ➤ Sensitivity 53 to 98%; greatest for main, lobar, & segmental arteries
  - ➤ If neg & high suspicion, consider conventional angiogram
  - ➤ Risk of nephrotoxicity
- Doppler-Ultrasound
  - ➤ High yield for symptomatic DVT
  - ➤ Consider with non-diagnostic V/Q
  - ➤ Clot in "superficial femoral vein" is a DVT
- Angiogram
  - ➤ Diagnostic in 96%
  - ➤ Complication rate (death & major): 1.2%
  - ➤ Risk of nephrotoxicity

DIFFERENTIAL DIAGNOSIS
- Pneumonia, COPD, asthma, CHF, MI, pneumothorax, rib fracture, pleurodynia

MANAGEMENT
- Assess oxygenation, vital signs, risk factors
- If high suspicion, start heparin

➤ Normal V/Q essentially rules out PE

➤ High prob V/Q: highly likely PE (unless prior PE or low suspicion)

➤ Low prob V/Q & low suspicion: consider other diagnosis (negative leg US adds confidence to "no PE" diagnosis)

■ Low prob V/Q & suspicion not low, or intermediate prob V/Q:

➤ consider spiral CT, treat if +

➤ consider leg US, treat if +

• if negative, consider angiogram or

• if patient stable, suspicion not high, & adequate cardiopulmonary reserve, consider serial leg studies over following week. If leg studies remain neg, low risk of subsequent PE

■ Evaluate for thrombophilia if age <50, family history, or recurrent thrombosis

SPECIFIC THERAPY

Treatment Options:

■ Weight-based unfractionated (Usual type) heparin

➤ check for contraindications

➤ baseline PT/INR, PTT, CBC

➤ daily platelet count

➤ PTT 4–6 hours after starting heparin & q6 hours 24 hours, then

• qAM unless out of therapeutic range

➤ Minimum 5 days, overlap with warfarin until INR 2.0–3.0 × 2 days

➤ Complications:

• Bleeding

• Thrombocytopenia

• Hypersensitivity reactions

• Osteoporosis with use >6 months

➤ Contraindications:

• Absolute: Hypersensitivity; thrombocytopenia; history of heparin induced thrombocytopenia; uncontrolled bleeding; intracranial hemorrhage

• Relative: bleeding disorders; GI bleeding or ulcer; severe liver disease; uncontrolled hypertension; recent surgery; need for invasive procedures

■ Low molecular weight heparin (LMWH)

➤ check for contraindications to heparin

➤ baseline PT/INR, PTT, CBC

➤ platelet count q2 days

➤ Minimum of 5 days, overlap with warfarin until INR 2.0–3.0 × 2 days

➤ Complications:
- See unfractionated heparin; also
- Follow anti-Xa activity levels if:
  - serum creatinine >2 mg/dl or calculated CrCl <30 ml/min)
  - Weight >100 or <45 kg
  - Pregnancy

➤ Contraindications
- See unfractionated heparin

■ Thrombolytics
➤ Indications: Documented PE with hemodynamic compromise
➤ Complications:
- Bleeding
- Intracranial hemorrhage, 2%
- Streptokinase: allergic reaction 1–4%, anaphylaxis 0.1%

➤ Contraindications:
- Absolute: Hemorrhagic stroke, intracranial tumor, AVM, aneurysm, intracranial or intraspinal surgery or trauma, uncontrolled hypertension, internal bleeding, bleeding diathesis
- Relative: Surgery, prolonged CPR, puncture of non-compressible vessel, hemorrhagic diabetic retinopathy, severe liver or renal disease, endocarditis, pericarditis, pregnancy, menstruation

■ IVC filters
➤ Indications:
- lower extremity DVT +/or PE AND
  - Contraindication to anticoagulation, or
  - Recurrent PE despite anticoagulation, or
  - Compromised pulmonary vascular bed and residual DVT

➤ Complications:
- Thrombosis at insertion or filter site, IVC obstruction, erosion through IVC
- Short term decreased risk of recurrent PE partially offset by higher long term risk of DVTs
- Consider continuation of anti-coagulation

➤ Contraindications
- Will not prevent PE from RV or upper extremity

■ Long-term therapy:
➤ Warfarin
- All should receive warfarin unless contraindication
- Adjust dose to INR of 2.0–3.0

- Drug interactions require more frequent testing
- Anti-phospholid antibody may require more intensive therapy
➤ Duration:
  - First DVT/PE, reversible risk factors: 3–6 months
  - Idiopathic DVT/PE: = six months.
  - Recurrent thromboembolism or continuing risk factors: optimum duration unclear, suggest 1 year then reassess
  - Consider indefinite if >2 episodes or irreversible risk factor
➤ Complications:
  - Bleeding
  - Skin necrosis: highest risk in first weeks & in Protein C or S deficiency
  - May increase complications from cholesterol emboli
  - Spontaneous abortions
  - Embryopathies
➤ Contraindications:
  - Absolute: Pregnancy; hypersensitivity to warfarin; blood dyscrasias; active bleeding; intracranial hemorrhage, inability to obtain/follow INRs
  - Relative: bleeding disorders; GI bleeding or active ulcer; severe liver disease; protein C or S deficiency; uncontrolled hypertension; recent surgery; need for invasive procedures; risk of falling

FOLLOW-UP
■ Monitor anti-coagulation
■ DVT prophylaxis with future hospitalizations/bed rest

COMPLICATIONS AND PROGNOSIS
■ PE mortality 2.5% at 1 year
■ Overall mortality 24% at 1 year (from underlying diseases)
■ 20–25% with idiopathic DVT/PE have recurrence in 5 years
■ Risk of major bleeding: 3–7% per year

PULMONARY HYPERTENSION

MARIA ANSARI, MD

HISTORY & PHYSICAL
History
■ **Primary Pulmonary HTN (PPH)**

➢ Idiopathic- seen in women> men (up to 3:1), mean age of onset $= 35$ years

➢ Familial- rare (6% of cases)

■ **Secondary Pulmonary HTN**

➢ Pre-capillary (pulmonary arteriolar vasoconstriction)

- Hypoxia due to chronic lung disease from COPD, restriction, insterstial lung dz, connective tissue disorders, granulomatous disease, sleep apnea
- Chronic pulmonary emboli (risk factors include trauma, HTN, malignancy, recent surgery/immobilization, oral contraceptives, smoking, obesity, and hypercoagulable states)
- High pulmonary blood flow from left to right intra-cardiac shunts
- Anorectic agents
- Cirrhosis with portal hypertension and subsequent porto-pulmonary HTN
- HIV infection

➢ Post-capillary (pulmonary venous hypertension)

- Left ventricular dysfunction
- Valvular heart disease (classically mitral stenosis)

Signs & Symptoms

■ Earliest symptoms (fatigue) are nonspecific leading to a delay in diagnosis

■ Dyspnea- most common

■ Chest pain from right ventricular ischemia

■ Syncope or near syncope

■ Lower extremity edema

■ Raynaud's phenomenon (10% of cases)

■ Ortner's syndrome (hoarseness due to laryngeal nerve compression by dilated pulmonary artery)

■ Exam may show

➢ prominent "a" waves in jugular venous contour

➢ prominent P2

➢ right-sided S4 or S3 gallop

➢ palpable pulm artery in 2nd left ICS

➢ right ventricular heave

■ If advanced, the Graham-Steel murmur of pulmonary insufficiency may be audible.

■ With tricuspid insufficiency, prominent CV wave and systolic murmur that increases with inspiration at lower left sternal border are common.

TESTS

Laboratory
- Basic blood tests
- Rule out secondary causes of PH (CBC, LFT's, HIV, serologic tests for connective tissue diseases and hypercoagulable states).

Imaging
- Basic imaging tests:
- CXR- rule out significant lung or cardiac disease
- Echocardiogram- noninvasively measures pulmonary pressure and evaluates for secondary causes of PH
- EKG-typically shows RA and RV enlargement, may show rsR' or RBBB, RAD

Specific Diagnostic Tests
- Pulmonary function tests
- Ventilation/perfusion lung scan to rule out occult pulmonary emboli
- Hi resolution chest CT if lung disease identified by CXR/PFT's or history of connective tissue disease
- Right heart catheterization: gold standard for diagnosis of pulmonary hypertension and for determining if there is a post-capillary component (elevated wedge pressure) or shunt
  - ➤ Diagnosis made by pulmonary artery systolic pressure >25 mm Hg at rest or >30 mm Hg with during exercise

DIFFERENTIAL DIAGNOSIS
- Diagnosis can be confirmed by right heart catheterization
- Symptoms of dyspnea may be related to other underlying lung or cardiac disease
- Secondary causes of pulmonary hypertension most commonly include: COPD with accompanying right heart failure (cor pulmonale), post capillary pulmonary hypertension to LV dysfunction, connective tissue diseases (scleroderma, lupus, rheumatoid arthritis), and chronic occult pulmonary emboli

MANAGEMENT
- Assess severity of pulmonary hypertension and severity of complications.
- Treat underlying causes for secondary PH.
- For primary PH, assess candidacy for transplant while initiating specific therapy.

- Patients should avoid significant physical exertion or high altitudes
- Discontinue potential offending medications (appetite suppressants) and other meds which may lead to pulmonary artery vasoconstriciton (decongestants)

SPECIFIC THERAPY

- Vasodilators
  - Some benefit in select patients
  - May improve symptoms and pulmonary artery pressures
  - No change in survival
  - Initiate slowly in CCU with cardiology consultation and with right heart catheter in place to monitor pressures
  - Only continue as outpatient if drug has a hemodynamic benefit
  - Calcium channel blockers traditionally used (diltiazem, nifedipine)
  - Inhaled nitric oxide used in acute situations especially in pediatric cases
- Epoprostenol (Prostacyclin)
  - Vasodilator and inhibitor of platelet aggregation
  - May improve symptoms, hemodynamics and survival in select patients
  - Must be initiated in CCU with cardiology consultation through IV
  - Continuous infusion requires indwelling central line
- Anticoagulation
  - Warfarin may have some benefit on survival based on uncontrolled trials
  - May prevent DVT's from venous stasis or in-situ thrombosis from PH
- Oxygen
  - For use in patients with demonstrated hypoxemia
- Diuretics and digoxin
  - May help with right heart failure and lower extremity edema
- Surgery
  - For patients with secondary PH from large pulmonary emboli, pulmonary thromboendarterectomy is indicated
  - For chronic small pulmonary emboli, patients should have a vena caval filter placed
  - In PPH, single or double lung transplantation is reserved for advanced cases in ideal candidates
  - Heart-lung transplantation is done for patients with a cardiac

contribution such as an intracardiac shunt, congenital heart disease, or an impaired RV
- Experimental treatments
  - Newer agents being tested include subcutaneous esoprostenol and oral endothelin receptor antagonists

Side Effects & Contraindications
- Vasodilators (oral)
  - Side effects: systemic hypotension, oxygen desaturation, or
  - increased cardiac output which may lead to increased right heart failure
  - Contraindications (relative): SBP <90 mm Hg,
- Esoprostenol
  - Side effects: nausea, headache, flushing, diarrhea, jaw claudication, joint pain, catheter related infection
  - Contraindications (absolute): pulmonary veno-occlusive disease
  - Contraindications (relative): thrombocytopenia

FOLLOW-UP

During Therapy
- With vasodilators and esoprostenol
  - Monitor for changes in pulmonary artery pressure, cardiac output, systemic BP, and oxygen saturation and symptoms.
  - Drugs need gradual up titration to achieve hemodynamic effect

Routine
- Esoprostenol dose must be gradually titrated upwards every 4–6 weeks as patients develop tolerance for the drug

COMPLICATIONS AND PROGNOSIS

Complications
- Right heart failure (63%)
- Hypoxemia and pneumonia
- Sudden death- usually due to arrhythmias

Prognosis
- Severe progressive symptoms in most patients
- 1 year survival 64%
- 3 year survival 48%

PULMONARY STENOSIS (PS)

JUDITH A. WISNESKI, MD

HISTORY & PHYSICAL

Etiology
- Congenital
- Carcinoid syndrome

History
- Fatigue
- Syncope – usually with exertion
- Chest pain – similar to angina

Signs & Symptoms
- Harsh systolic ejection murmur in pulmonic area
- Systolic click varies with respiration
- P2 increased (mild/moderate)
- P2 absent (severe or calcified valve)
- Right ventricular lift
- Signs of right ventricular failure
  - Elevated JVP
  - Hepatomegaly, ascites
  - Peripheral edema

TESTS
- ECG
  - Right ventricular hypertrophy
- Chest X-Ray
  - Post-stenotic dilation of pulmonary arteries
  - Calcifications in pulmonic valve (adults)
  - Enlarged right ventricule
  - Enlarged right atrium (severe)
- Echo/Doppler
  - Doming of pulmonic valve
  - Quantitate gradient across pulmonic valve
- Cardiac Catheterization
  - Measure gradient across pulmonic valve
  - Right ventricular and right atrial pressures elevated
  - Low cardiac output (severe)

DIFFERENTIAL DIAGNOSIS

- Aortic stenosis
- Pulmonary artery stenosis

MANAGEMENT

Medical Treatment

- Antiboitic prophylaxis

SPECIFIC THERAPY

- Balloon valvulotomy
  - ➤ Asymptomatic patients with gradient >75 mm Hg
  - ➤ Symptomatic patients with gradient >50 mm Hg

FOLLOW-UP

n/a

COMPLICATIONS AND PROGNOSIS

Complications

- Right ventricular failure with tricuspid valve insufficiency
- Right to left atrial shunt through patent foramen ovale

Prognosis

- Overall prognosis good, unless severe right ventricular failure

---

PULMONARY VALVE INSUFFICIENCY (PI)

JUDITH A. WISNESKI, MD

HISTORY & PHYSICAL

Etiology

- Pulmonary artery hypertension (most common)
- Idiopathic dilation of pulmonary artery
- Connective tissue disorders
- Congenital

History

- Symptoms of right ventricular failure and low cardiac output

Signs & Symptoms

- High pitched decrescendo or low pitched diastolic murmur left sternal border
- Right ventricular lift

- P2 increased (pulmonary artery hypertension present)
- P2 absent (congenital)
- S2 wide split
- Right ventricular S3
- Signs of right ventricular failure
  - ➤ Elevated JVP
  - ➤ Hepatomegaly, ascites
  - ➤ Edema

TESTS

ECG
- Incomplete or complete RBBB
- Right ventricular hypertrophy (pulmonary artery hypertension present)
- Right atrial abnormality

Chest X-Ray
- Pulmonary artery enlarged
- Right ventricle enlarged
- Right atrium enlarged
- Dilated superior vena cava and azygos veins (severe)

Echo/Doppler (most important)
- Detect pulmonary valve insufficiency
- Function and size of right ventricule
- Right atrial size
- Detect tricuspid insufficiency (TR) and assess pulmonary artery pressure (TR secondary to dilation of right ventricular)
- **If pulmonary artery hypertension present, assess other conditions which may be responsible: left ventricular dysfunction, mitral stenosis**

DIFFERENTIAL DIAGNOSIS
- Aortic insufficiency

MANAGEMENT
n/a

SPECIFIC THERAPY
- Primary pulmonary valve insufficiency
  - ➤ Medical
    - Diuretics and digoxin
  - ➤ Surgery

- Primary pulmonary insufficiency – rarely requires surgical valve replacement
■ Secondary to pulmonary artery hypertension
  ➤ Medical or surgical therapy for primary condition

FOLLOW-UP
n/a

COMPLICATIONS AND PROGNOSIS
■ Primary pulmonary valve insufficiency – usually good prognosis
■ Secondary to pulmonary artery hypertension or other conditions – progress depends on the associated pathology

PURINE AND PYRIMIDINE METABOLIC DISORDERS

GREGORY M. ENNS, MD

HISTORY & PHYSICAL

History:
■ most disorders are autosomal recessive
■ (history of parental consanguinity or affected siblings)
■ Lesch-Nyhan disease (HPRT deficiency) and PRPS superactivity are X-linked

Signs & Symptoms
■ Purine Disorders
  ➤ Lesch-Nyhan disease (hypoxanthine-guanine phosphoribosyl transferase [HPRT] deficiency): motor delays, cerebral palsy, self-injurious behavior, choreoathetosis, opisthotonic spasms, increased deep tendon reflexes, nephropathy, gout, urinary tract calculi, urinary tract infections
  ➤ Adenine phosphoribosyl transferase (APRT) deficiency: asymptomatic to renal failure, renal calculi, brownish diaper spots, crystalluria
  ➤ Phosphoribosyl pyrophosphate synthetase (PRPS) superactivity: developmental delay, ataxia, gout, renal disease, sensorineural deafness
  ➤ Adenylosuccinate lyase (ASL) deficiency: autism, developmental delay, seizures, hypotonia
  ➤ Xanthine dehydrogenase (XDH) deficiency: renal failure (urolithiasis), muscle pain (uncommon)

- ➤ Adenosine deaminase (ADA) deficiency: severe combined immunodeficiency (SCID), persistent diarrhea, pulmonary disease, moniliasis, absent lymph nodes, hepatic dysfunction
- ➤ Purine nucleoside phosphorylase (PNP) deficiency: recurrent infections (T-cell immunodeficiency), SCID (accounts for ~4% of SCID patients), 2/3 have neurologic dysfunction (hypotonia, cerebral palsy), 1/3 have autoimmune disease (hemolytic anemia, idiopathic thrombocytopenic purpura, systemic lupus erythematosus)
- ■ Pyrimidine disorders
  - ➤ Hereditary orotic aciduria (uridine monophosphate synthetase [UMPS] deficiency): crystalluria, pallor (megaloblastic anemia), failure to thrive
  - ➤ Uridine monophosphate hydrolase (UMPH1) deficiency (pyrimidine-5'-nucleotidase deficiency): splenomegaly, pallor (hemolytic anemia)
  - ➤ Dihydropyrimidine dehydrogenase (DHPD) deficiency: asymptomatic, seizures, developmental delay, severe toxicity to 5-fluorouracil
  - ➤ Dihydropyrimidinase (DHPA) deficiency: asymptomatic, seizures, developmental delay
  - ➤ Ureidopropionase deficiency: hypotonia, developmental delay, dystonia, optic atrophy, scoliosis

TESTS

Laboratory
- ■ basic blood studies:
  - ➤ anemia (UMPS, UMPH1 deficiencies)
  - ➤ increased BUN, creatinine (HPRT, APRT, XDH deficiencies, PRPS superactivity)
  - ➤ increased uric acid (HPRT deficiency, PRPS superactivity)
  - ➤ decreased uric acid (XDH, PNP deficiencies)
  - ➤ decreased immunoglobulins (ADA deficiency)
- ■ basic urine studies:
  - ➤ crystalluria (HPRT, APRT, UMPS defs.)
  - ➤ increased uric acid (HPRT deficiency, PRPS superactivity)

Screening
- ■ increased urine orotic acid (UMPS def.)
- ■ decreased CD4+ cells (ADA def., + PNP def.)
- ■ decreased CD8+ cells (ADA def.)

Confirmatory Tests
- increased urine hypoxanthine (HPRT def., PRPS superactivity)
- increased urine adenine 2,8-dihydroxy-adenosine (APRT def.)
- increased urine, plasma, CSF succinyl-aminoimidazole carboxamide riboside (ASL def.)
- increased blood and urine hypoxanthine, xanthine (XDH def.)
- increased erythrocyte dATP (ADA def.)
- increased urine 2'-deoxyadeosine (ADA def.)
- increased plasma inosine, guanosine, deoxyinosine, deoxyguanosine (PNP def.)
- increased urine uracil, thymine (DHPD, DHPA defs.)
- increased urine dihydrothymine, dihydrouracil (DHPA def.)
- increased urine beta-ureidoisobutyrate (Ureidopropionase def.)

Other Tests
- erythrocyte enzymology (HPRT, APRT, ADA, PNP, UMPS, UMPH1 defs., PRPS superactivity)
- liver biopsy enzymology (XDH def.)
- DNA analysis may be available in some centers
- prenatal diagnosis using enzymology or DNA analysis may be available in some centers

Imaging
- abdominal ultrasound: not diagnostic, may detect lithiasis (HPRT, APRT, XDH defs., PRPS superactivity), obstructive uropathy (UMPS def.), or splenomegaly (UMPH1 def.)

DIFFERENTIAL DIAGNOSIS
- gout
- other causes of renal failure/lithiasis
- other causes of immunodeficiency (AIDS, inherited disorders of T-/B-cell dysfunction)
- increased orotic acid is also seen in urea cycle defects (esp. ornithine transcarbamylase def.)
- self-injurious behavior may be seen in familial dysautonomia, Smith-Magenis syndrome, de Lange syndrome
- XDH deficiency may be part of molybdenum cofactor deficiency (combined XDH/sulfite oxidase deficiencies)

MANAGEMENT

What to Do First
- assess severity of immunologic, neurologic, renal and joint disease
- treat anemia

General Measures
■ referral to biochemical genetics center
■ adjust or avoid nephrotoxic medications (HPRT, APRT, XDH defs., PRPS superactivity)
■ high fluid intake (HPRT, APRT, XDH, UMPS defs., PRPS superactivity)
■ treat intercurrent infection (ADA, PNP defs.)
■ irradiated blood products (ADA, PNP defs.)
■ hearing testing (PRPS superactivity)

SPECIFIC THERAPY
■ indicated for all symptomatic patients

Treatment Options
■ HPRT deficiency: allopurinol, physical restraint, teeth removal, mouth guard, behavioral therapy for self-injurious behavior, pharmacotherapy (e.g., risperidone, gabapentin)
■ APRT deficiency: allopurinol, low purine diet, avoid alkali, renal transplantation
■ PRPS superactivity: allopurinol
■ XDH deficiency: low purine diet
■ ADA deficiency: bone marrow transplantation, polyethylene glycol (PEG) ADA, gene therapy in clinical trials
■ UMPS deficiency: uridine supplementation

Side Effects & Contraindications
■ allopurinol may cause xanthine stone formation in HPRT deficiency
■ decrease dose of allopurinol in renal failure
■ severe graft-versus-host disease may occur in ADA, PNP deficiencies if non-irradiated blood products used
■ patients with DHPD and DHPA deficiencies should not be given 5-fluorouracil (extremely toxic)

FOLLOW-UP

Routine
■ close monitoring of renal function (HPRT, APRT, XDH defs., PRPS superactivity)
■ periodic hearing testing (PRPS superactivity)
■ genetic counseling

COMPLICATIONS AND PROGNOSIS
■ HPRT deficiency: death secondary to renal failure, aspiration pneumonia in adolescence

- APRT deficiency: good prognosis if detected early and treatment started
- ASL deficiency: may be mild or have more severe neurologic disease, prognosis generally poor
- XDH deficiency: renal failure may occur
- ADA/PNP deficiencies: death in childhood from infection if not treated, bone marrow transplant may be curative, but some series report high mortality (grave prognosis in general for PNP def. – no patient survived to 3rd decade). ADA deficiency was the first inherited condition to be treated with gene therapy (long-term prognosis under study).
- UMPS, UMPH1 deficiencies: good prognosis in treated patients
- DHPD, DHPA deficiencies: variable prognosis ranging from asymptomatic individuals to severe neurologic illness

---

PYOGENIC GRANULOMA

JASON HUBERT, MD
REVISED BY JEFFREY P. CALLEN, MD

HISTORY & PHYSICAL
- May be related to minor trauma
- Present as red or pink pedunculated papules or nodules
- Common sites are the lips, periungual skin, and face
- Frequently arise on the gums and lips in pregnant women
- May have a history of profuse bleeding from the lesion

TESTS
- Skin biopsy usually diagnostic

DIFFERENTIAL DIAGNOSIS
- Includes Kaposi's sarcoma, bacillary angiomatosis, and nodular amelanotic melanoma

MANAGEMENT
- Dependent on size and location of the lesion
- Curettage and electrodesiccation often sufficient

SPECIFIC THERAPY
- Other options include carbon dioxide laser, cryotherapy, and surgical excision.

FOLLOW-UP
■ After removal, no follow-up is usually needed.

COMPLICATIONS AND PROGNOSIS
■ Recurrences and development of satellite lesions after therapy are relatively frequent.

PYOGENIC LIVER ABSCESS

AIJAZ AHMED, MD

HISTORY & PHYSICAL

History
■ Predisposing conditions: intraabdominal infection (diverticulitis, peritonitis); Crohn disease; cholangitis, stones, or endoscopic biliary intervention; previous abdominal surgery or liver biopsy, after trauma; diabetes; malignancy

Signs & Symptoms
■ Fever, chills, abdominal pain, nausea/vomiting, weight loss, pleuritic chest pain, cough/dyspnea, diarrhea, jaundice, tender hepatomegaly

TESTS

Laboratory
■ ESR, leukocytosis, anemia; other common findings: bilirubin, AST, ALT, alkaline phosphatase, & PT
■ Microbiology: positive blood cultures (50–100%); aspiration increases yield (in polymicrobial abscesses, all organisms may not be detected in blood)
■ E coli most common causative organism

Imaging
■ US: multiple (occasionally single) round/oval hypoechoeic lesions w/ irregular margins
■ CT: detects up to 95% lesions (reduced attenuation/enhance w/ contrast)

DIFFERENTIAL DIAGNOSIS
■ Amebic abscess, hydatid cyst

MANAGEMENT

What to Do First
- History (incl medical/surgical), physical exam, imaging

General Measures
- Admit to hospital (ICU if unstable)

SPECIFIC THERAPY

Treatment Options
- Percutaneous drainage/aspiration w/ antibiotics
- IV antibiotics: should cover gram-negatives, microaerophilics, & anaerobes; change to oral based on clinical response; total duration 2–3 wk
- Surgical intervention: unresponsive pts

FOLLOW-UP
n/a

COMPLICATIONS AND PROGNOSIS

Complications
- Septicemia, shock, metastatic abscesses, rupture, ARDS, renal failure

Prognosis
- W/ prompt diagnosis & therapy, mortality rate 10–30%, depending on underlying cause & comorbid conditions

---

PYRIDOXINE DEFICIENCY

ELISABETH RYZEN, MD

HISTORY & PHYSICAL

History
- malabsorption, alcoholism, oral contraceptives, inactivation by penicillamine, hydralazine, isoniazide

Signs & Symptoms
- glossitis, dermatitis, peripheral neuropathy, microcytic anemia

TESTS

Laboratory
- Basic studies: none

DIFFERENTIAL DIAGNOSIS
n/a

MANAGEMENT
n/a

SPECIFIC THERAPY
■ correct underlying causes; pyridoxine

Side Effects & Contraindications
■ None

FOLLOW-UP
n/a

COMPLICATIONS AND PROGNOSIS
■ Reversible with replacement

RABIES

CAROL A. GLASER, MD

HISTORY & PHYSICAL

History
■ RNA virus/Rhabdovirus family
■ Large animal reservoir of sylvatic rabies exists in U.S. (includes skunks, bats, raccoons, foxes)
■ Domestic animals occasionally infected by wild animals
■ Rodents, rabbits – RARE
■ Usually transmitted by bites (less commonly licking of mucosa or open wounds)
■ Transmission has occurred by transplantation of organs
■ A small number of "nonbite humans rabies" reported where exposure were in environments containing rabies virus in extremely high concentration
  ➤ e.g. caves/aerosolized rabies virus from bats
  ➤ e.g. laboratories working with infected tissues
■ incubation period dependent upon site of wound (in relation to richness nerve supply) and distance from brain as well as amount of virus present

- Incubation period: variable, has been reported, however most occur within 2 months after exposure
- Shorter incubation when bite on head vs. extremity
- Common in Asia/Africa/Latin America

Signs & Symptoms
Acute illness with rapidly progressive CNS systems; almost always progresses to coma and then death
- Initial neurologic signs may include hyperactivity, disorientation, hallucinations, seizures, bizarre behavior, nuchal stiffness or paralysis
- May have paresthesia/neuritic pain at site injury
- Other symptoms may include: fever, muscle fasciculations, hyperventilation, hypersalivation, focal or generalized convulsions, and priapism
- Some patients will complain of difficulty swallowing food and water (hydrophobia)
- Waxing and waning neurologic status the first week of illness
- In 20% of cases: paralysis dominates clinical course (may look like Guillain-Barre)
- Other organ failure commonly seen; renal and respiratory failure
- Coma usually occurs within 1 week onset neurologic symptoms

TESTS
Nonspecific:
- LP may be normal or show pleocytosis
- CSF pressure may be normal or elevated

Specific Tests:
Note: specimens should be from multiple sites. Consult with state health department or CDC prior to obtaining specimens.

Ante-mortem Tests:
- Serology: IFA tests are available and should be performed, but note that antibody does not appear until late in course, check serial samples in highly suspect cases
- Nuchal skin biopsy/saliva/CSF/cornea/skin; Rabies DFA is gold standard and is usually available at State Health Departments (PCR on these same specimens is sometimes used)
- Postmortem tests: Rabies DFA of brain stem, cerebellum and hippocampus (PCR on these same specimens is sometimes used)

DIFFERENTIAL DIAGNOSIS

In absence of exposure history; little to differentiate rabies from other viral encephalitides

- Tetanus: Muscle rigidity may resemble rabies/ CSF normal in tetanus/usually lucid in tetanus
- Rabies hysteria: a psychological reaction seen in persons exposed to an animal they believe has rabies
  - ➤ Paralytic rabies may resemble other paralytic neurologic disease; includes poliomyelitis, Guillain-Barre syndrome and transverse myelitis

MANAGEMENT

- Contact isolation is recommended.
- Personnel should avoid contact with patient's saliva, tears, urine or other body fluids (virus has not been found in blood).
- Although transmission from patient to hospital staff not documented, transmission is theoretically possible.
- Reportable

SPECIFIC THERAPY

- Once symptoms start, no drug or vaccine improves outcomes.
- Treatment consists of intensive supportive care.

FOLLOW-UP

n/a

COMPLICATIONS AND PROGNOSIS

Complications

- Almost invariably fatal
- Complications mostly occur during coma phase
  - ➤ SIADH
  - ➤ Autonomic dysfunction – hypertension, hypotension, cardiac arrhythmias, hypothermia
  - ➤ Seizures: generalized or focal
  - ➤ Acute renal failure
  - ➤ Secondary bacterial infection of lungs or urinary tract

Prevention

- Prevention is extremely important – if individual is exposed to potentially rabid animal, consult with local health department, consider post-exposure prophylaxis (PEP)
- Individuals in high-risk occupations (e.g., veterinarians) need pre-exposure vaccine.

RADIATION ENTERITIS AND COLITIS

ALVARO D. DAVILA, MD

HISTORY & PHYSICAL

History of Exposure

- Radiation injury depends on type and quantity of radiation energy delivered
- SI unit for measuring a dose of radiation: gray (Gy); one gray (Gy) equals 1 joule of energy deposited in 1 kg of tissue; 1 Gy = 100 rads
- Small intestine most vulnerable to radiation injury
  - Risk factors for radiation enteritis:
  - lack of mobility of the distal ileum and cecum, previous abdominal surgery, atherosclerotic vascular disease, lean body habitus, chemotherapy and other drugs
  - Minimal tolerance dose is 45 Gy
- Colon relatively radioresistant but incidence of colonic radiation injury greatest
  - Risk factors for radiation colitis:
  - high radiation doses for pelvic tumors, relative immobility of rectum and sigmoid colon; Minimal tolerance dose is 45 Gy for colon and 55 Gy for rectum

Signs and Symptoms

- Acute injury to the small intestine and colon frequent, dose dependent and usually transient
- Chronic radiation enteritis appears far less frequently (average incidence of 6%)
  - Onset of symptoms variable and latent (usually 1–2 yr, up to 20 yr after treatment)
  - Chronic bowel injury from ischemia and progressive fibrosis/atrophy, leading to stricture, obstruction, bacterial overgrowth, ulceration, fistulization, recurrent infection, and perforation
  - Chronic radiation colitis/proctitis from 5–15% of patients after pelvic irradiation for prostate, cervical, uterine, bladder, and testicular cancer
- Early symptoms and signs (acute injury, reversible)
  - Small intestinal injury: nausea, vomiting, abdominal cramping, and watery diarrhea
  - Colonic and/or rectal injury: tenesmus, diarrhea, mucorrhea, and rarely hematochezia

■ Late symptoms and signs (chronic injury, irreversible)
➤ Chronic radiation enteritis
➤ Small bowel obstruction
➤ Malabsorption
➤ Fistula (fecaluria, pneumaturia, feculent vaginal discharge)
➤ Abscess (with sepsis or peritonitis)
➤ Perforation with acute peritonitis
➤ Massive intestinal bleeding (rare)
➤ Chronic radiation colitis or proctitis
➤ Mild to chronic severe rectal bleeding
➤ Obstruction secondary to rectal or sigmoid strictures
➤ Fistula formation (rectovaginal, rectovesical, cystitis)
➤ Necrosis and gangrene with perforation (rare)

TESTS

Laboratory

Basic Studies: Blood
■ Mild to severe anemia, decreased albumin, vitamins B_{12}, D, A, and E deficiencies, abnormal D-xylose test, positive blood cultures

Basic Studies: Urine
■ Pyuria, fecaluria, abnormal D-xylose test

Basic Studies: Stool
■ Mild to severe steatorrhea, positive FOBT

Imaging
■ Plain abdominal films: ileus early and small or large bowel obstruction late
■ Barium contrast studies: small intestinal mucosal edema, separation of loops, excessive secretions, stricture, tubular appearance, and absent mucosal markings
■ CT: recurrent cancer, nonspecific bowel wall thickening, widened presacral space, fistulous disease
■ Endoscopy/colonoscopy: test of choice for colitis or proctitis; may reveal mucosal pallor, friability, edema, and telangiectasias

DIFFERENTIAL DIAGNOSIS
■ Crohn's disease, ulcerative colitis, colorectal cancer, small bowel tumors, celiac disease, intestinal tuberculosis, amyloidosis, scleroderma, immunodeficiency states, chronic intestinal ischemia, vasculitis, collagen vascular disorders

MANAGEMENT

What to Do First

■ Preventive measures and careful planning taken before radiation therapy is delivered

General Measures

■ Radiation therapy techniques to avoid tissue injury
■ Prophylactic dietary changes including elemental diets or low-fat, low-residue, lactose-free diets
■ Prophylactic use of antioxidants such as vitamin E or radioprotectors such as WR-2721 (amifostine)

SPECIFIC THERAPY

■ Control or ameliorate symptoms of acute or chronic radiation bowel injury

Treatment Options

■ Acute radiation enteritis and colitis
　➤ Symptoms usually reversible; supportive care only
　➤ Small radiation dose reduction (10%) may be sufficient
　➤ Mild diarrhea, abdominal cramping, and tenesmus managed with antispasmodics, bulk-forming agents, sitz baths, and anti-diarrheal agents (loperamide)
　➤ Sucralfate (4 g daily) for treatment of diarrhea
　➤ Cholestyramine a bile acid sequestrant for watery diarrhea due to bile salt malabsorption (4–12 g/day)
　➤ Ondansetron and other anti-emetics can be used to treat nausea
　➤ 5-ASA drugs (oral or enema form) such as mesalamine are ineffective at controlling tenesmus, diarrhea or hematochezia
■ Chronic radiation enteritis
　➤ Acute small bowel obstruction (SBO) managed conservatively
　➤ Surgery used as a last resort for SBO (high complication rate)
　➤ Surgery for persistent SBO from adhesions or strictures
　➤ Complete, wide resection of the involved segment indicated, with end-end anastomosis
　➤ Resection preferred over intestinal bypass procedures Surgery also indicated for management of fistulas, hemorrhage, and perforation with peritonitis or intra-abdominal abscess Malabsorption from bacterial overgrowth treated with antibiotics
　➤ Bacterial overgrowth caused by severe obstruction or fistula usually requires surgery (resection or bypass)

- ➤ Cholestyramine reduces bile salt malabsorption and diarrhea
- ➤ Trial of TPN for failed medical therapies or poor surgical candidates
- ■ Chronic radiation colitis or proctitis
  - ➤ Patients with anemia or persistent bleeding treated with endoscopic laser or electrocoagulation of bleeding ectasias
  - ➤ Formalin irrigation of the rectum and hyperbaric oxygen therapy also effective for control of bleeding
  - ➤ Mild obstruction from rectal or sigmoid strictures treated with stool softeners or mineral oil enemas
  - ➤ More severe strictures treated with endoscopic balloon dilation or Savary-Gilliard dilators
  - ➤ Long or tortuous strictures best managed with surgical resection and immediate reanastomosis
  - ➤ Abdominoperineal resection reserved for severe cases
  - ➤ Rectovaginal, rectovesical, enterocolic fistulas treated surgically
  - ➤ Presacral sympathectomy for severe uncontrolled pelvic pain

FOLLOW-UP
- ■ After diagnosis and treatment established, at least a half of patients continue to have symptoms, develop new complications, or both
- ■ Close monitoring indicated for the potential risk of secondary malignancy development

COMPLICATIONS AND PROGNOSIS
- ■ Complications — see above; manage on an individual basis
- ■ Mortality of surgery for complications of radiation enteritis up to 17%
- ■ About 50% of patients will continue to experience symptoms and/or develop complications (1/3 of these require further surgery)
- ■ 5-yr survival rates 40%, increasing to 70% for those surviving surgery

---

RAYNAUD'S SYNDROME

RAJABRATA SARKAR, MD

HISTORY & PHYSICAL
HISTORY
- ■ No associated connective tissue diseases = Primary Raynaud's
- ■ Collagen Vascular Disease (mainly scleroderma) = Secondary Raynaud's

- Episodic:
  - Coldness
  - Numbness
  - Pain
  - Cyanosis
  - Paresthesia
  - Almost always cold-induced

Signs & Symptoms
- Examination usually normal
- Fingertip ulceration seen in secondary Raynaud's
- Decreased pulses at wrist suggestive of vasculitis, atherosclerosis or other diagnosis
- Symptoms usually cannot be reproduced by immersion in cold water
- Capillary refill delayed after Allen's test

TESTS

Blood
- Sedimentation rate and antinuclear antibody to determine collagen vascular disease

Specific Diagnostic Tests
- Noninvasive vascular tests
  - Doppler ultrasound to exclude large vessel disease
  - Digital artery pressures
  - Decreased pressures at rest
    - proximal obstruction
    - secondary Raynaud's or other cause
  - Decreased pressures with cold
  - Consistent with either primary or secondary Raynaud's
- Arteriography
  - Used to determine etiology if noninvasive studies suggest proximal obstruction
  - Differentiates atherosclerosis from vasculitis
  - Intra-arterial vasodilators illustrate vasospastic component of obstruction

DIFFERENTIAL DIAGNOSIS
- Livido reticularis
  - Asymptomatic irregular patchy purple discoloration of skin in fishnet pattern
  - May be superimposed on Raynaud's

- ➤ Benign condition; presence of ulcers suggest vasculitis
- ➤ Cosmetic problem that requires no treatment
- ■ Acrocyanosis
  - ➤ Painless blue discoloration of fingertips, hands and feet
  - ➤ Associated with increased sweating
  - ➤ Cosmetic problem that requires no treatment
- ■ Upper extremity atherosclerosis
  - ➤ Usually in large vessels of the arm – decreased pulses at wrist
  - ➤ Older patients with risk factors for atherosclerosis
  - ➤ Emboli are common with painful ulceration and gangrene of fingertips
  - ➤ Digit pressures are decreased
  - ➤ Angiogram shows proximal lesion (usually subclavian) and embolic obstructions of hand
  - ➤ Emboli can be from non-palpable subclavian aneurysm

MANAGEMENT

General Measures
- ■ Conservative therapy
- ■ Avoidance of cold (whole body)
- ■ Mittens and hand warmers (chemical and electrical)
- ■ Discontinuation of smoking
- ■ Severe disease (ulceration, gangrene)
- ■ Define and aggressively treat associated large vessel disease and collagen vascular disease

SPECIFIC THERAPY

Indications
- ■ Raynaud's that interferes with daily activity

Treatment Options
- ■ Calcium channel blockers (Nifedipine)
- ■ Treatment of choice for most patients
- ■ Proven in placebo controlled studies
  - ➤ Side Effects
    - • Headache
    - • Ankle edema
    - • Light-headedness
    - • Flushing
    - • Dyspepsia
    - • Palpitation
    - • Gingival hyperplasia

- Alpha blocking agents (Prazosin)
  - 2/3 of patients have favorable response
  - Less well-tolerated than calcium channel blockers
  - Side effects
    - Palpitations
    - Orthostatic hypotension
    - Dizzyness
    - Headache
    - Fatigue
    - Edema
    - Diarrhea
- Nitroglycerin
  - May be used on hands or elsewhere
  - Response less common than calcium channel blockers
  - Side effects
  - Headache
- Cervical sympathectomy
  - Not of value in Raynaud's
  - Treatment of underlying collagen vascular disease generally does not reduce symptoms of Raynaud's

FOLLOW-UP

During Treatment
- Individual pt's response to a particular agent is variable
- Check for efficacy and side-effects
- Switch to other agents as needed

Routine
- Mild disease – no specific follow-up needed

COMPLICATIONS AND PROGNOSIS

Complications
- Ulceration, necrosis and finger gangrene
  - Due to associated collagen vascular disease or proximal occlusion or emboli
  - Define and treat specific occlusive lesions – surgical bypass
  - Aggressive treatment of collagen vascular disease

Prognosis
- Primary Raynaud's (10 year follow-up)
  - 1/6 symptoms disappear
  - 1/3 stable

➤ 1/3 improve
➤ 1/6 worse
■ Secondary Raynaud's
  ➤ Prognosis highly dependent on course of underlying collagen vascular disease

---

RECURRENT APHTHOUS STOMATITIS

SOL SILVERMAN Jr, DDS

HISTORY & PHYSICAL
■ usually a history of recurrent oral sores/ulcers
■ immunopathic; cause unknown; genetic influence (predisposition)
■ aggravated by various irritants, e.g. citrus, nuts, chocolate
■ single or multiple shallow ulcers; vary in size up to 6 mm
■ last up to 2 weeks; frequency of attacks variable
■ covered by pseudomembrane (fibrin) surrounded by red halo (inflammation)
■ occur on unkeratinized mucosa (cheeks, ventral-lateral tongue, floor of mouth,
■ soft palate, oropharynx)

TESTS
■ no tests are indicated; history and clinical appearance usually sufficient

DIFFERENTIAL DIAGNOSIS
■ Herpes simplex virus (occur on keratinized mucosa: hard palate, gingiva, lips)
■ erythema multiforme
■ Behcet's
■ trauma/injury

MANAGEMENT
■ self healing
■ topical or systemic analgesics

SPECIFIC THERAPY
■ systemic corticosteroids for severe signs/symptoms
  ➤ high dose, short course
■ topical corticosteroids; no contraindications; compliance problem;
  ➤ not reproducibly effective

- insomnia most common side-effect
- caution in diabetes, GI ulcers, fragile hypertension

FOLLOW-UP
- recurrence time (frequency of attacks) varies

COMPLICATIONS AND PROGNOSIS
- no association with other conditions
- no cure; treat symptoms; not contagious
- avoid events, agents that are associated with outbreaks

RED CELL ENZYMES

XYLINA GREGG, MD and JOSEF PRCHAL, MD

HISTORY & PHYSICAL

History
- Variety of phenotypes
  - Red cell phenotypes
    - Hemolysis – acute intermittent – G6PD, GC and GSH synthase deficiencies
    - Chronic – pyruvate kinase (PK), glucose-1-phosphate isomerase, 5′nucleotidase, hexokinase and rarely G6PD, GC and GSH synthase deficiencies
    - Polycythemia – biphosphoglyceratemutase deficiency – decreased 2,3 BPG levels result in increased hemoglobin oxygen affinity
    - Methemoglobinemia – cytochrome b5 deficiency
  - Other Phenotypes
    - Cataracts – galactokinase deficiency
    - Cataracts, deafness, developmental delay – galactose uridyl transferase deficiency
    - Glycogen storage disorders – aldolase deficiency, PGK deficiency
    - Metabolic acidosis and failure to thrive – cytochrome b5 deficiency (type 2 methemoglobinemia)
    - Myoglobinuria – PGK deficiency
    - Immune deficiency from B lymphocyte dysfunction – adenosine deaminase
- Inheritance Patterns
  - X-linked – PGK and G6PD
  - Autosomal recessive – all others; check for history of consanguinity or inbreeding

- Ethnic Groups – G6PD Deficiency
  - African descent (less severe defect; not subject to hemolysis induced by Fava beans),
  - Mediterranean (more severe defect; subject to more severe hemolysis that may be also induced by Fava beans)
  - Asian (Indian & Southeast Asian): several endemic variants

Signs & Symptoms
- Nonspecific
- Jaundice, leg ulcers, splenomegaly, gallstones, may be present in chronic hemolytic states

TESTS
- Basic blood tests
  - RBC morphology – mostly nonspecific
    - Heinz bodies – acute hemolytic episodes of G6PD, GC and GSH synthase and rare congenital glutathione reductase deficiencies
    - Only specific finding is basophilic stippling in 5′nucleotidase deficiency
  - Biochemical tests of hemolysis (hyperbilirubinemia, reticulocytosis etc), but none specific for hemolysis from erythrocyte enzyme defects
- Screening tests
  - Misses up to third of PK deficient mutants
  - G6PD screening tests not useful for heterozygous females (they have proportion of deficient erythrocytes that are subject to hemo-lysis) and may be falsely negative after acute hemolytic episodes in males as older G6PD deficient cells have been destroyed
- Specific quantitative assays and DNA-based assays
  - Only available in few reference laboratories (and decreasing in number)
- Polycythemia – low P50 by hemoglobin oxygen dissociation study or estimated from venous blood gasses is the best initial screening. Confirm by measuring 2,3 BPG level and differentiate from high-oxygen-affinity hemoglobin mutants.

DIFFERENTIAL DIAGNOSIS
- Other hemolytic states – autoimmune causes (positive Coombs test), PNH (CD55 and CD 59 deficient cells), fragmentation syndromes (schistocytes), and red cell membrane defects (characteristic erythrocyte abnormalities [i.e., spherocytes, elliptocytes, pyropoikilocytes])

MANAGEMENT
n/a

SPECIFIC THERAPY
- No specific therapy is available.
- Avoidance of hemolysis-inducing drugs (and in some instances Fava beans) in G6PD, GC and GSH synthase, and congenital glutathione reductase deficiencies
- Splenectomy – not curative, but may ameliorate hemolysis in PK and GPI deficiencies; may be necessary in infancy in transfusion-dependent patients

FOLLOW-UP
- Identify and counsel relatives at risk for defect.
- Prevent folate deficiency.
- Provide list of hemolysis-inducing agents to the patient to avoid recurrence.
- In life-threatening cases, consider prenatal diagnosis after identifying a specific mutation.

COMPLICATIONS AND PROGNOSIS
- Nonspecific complications of any chronic hemolytic state: jaundice, leg ulcers, splenomegaly, gallstones, aplastic crises from Parvovirus infection

---

REFRACTIVE DISORDERS (AMETROPIAS)

DAVID G. HWANG, MD, FACS

HISTORY & PHYSICAL
- Emmetropia (normal vision)
  - ➤ Refractive disorders: images are not formed in precise focus on the retina
  - ➤ Regular ametropias can be fully optically corrected using sphero-cylindrical lenses. Includes hyperopia (farsightedness), myopia (nearsightedness), regular astigmatism, and presbyopia (age-related loss of accommodation).
  - ➤ Irregular ametropias cannot be fully corrected using lenses, most commonly due to inhomogeneity in the corneal power (irregular corneal astigmatism), less commonly due to irregularities in

the lens power or the contour of the retina at its optical center (fovea).

■ Myopia

➤ Prevalence – most common, 10–60% of the population; in USA at 30%

➤ Definition – Myopia is characterized by a corneal power that is of excessive convex power (i.e., too steep), lens power with excessive convex power and/or an axial length that is too long.

➤ Myopic astigmatism – Myopia may be compounded by astigmatism, a condition known as myopic astigmatism.

➤ Onset in childhood and progression during puberty and early adult years. Pathologic myopia is uncommon, characterized by progressive myopia with scleral and retinal thinning that can cause permanent visual loss.

➤ Optical correction – Myopia can be corrected using minus or concave lenses, either in glasses or contact lenses.

➤ > Surgical correction – See below.

■ Hyperopia

➤ Prevalence – in USA, at 10%

➤ Definition – Hyperopia is characterized by inadequate corneal power (i.e., too flat), a lens power that is of inadequate convex power, and/or an axial length that is too short

➤ Hyperopic astigmatism – Hyperopia compounded by astigmatism

➤ Causes – most cases are naturally occurring, but can also be postsurgical, as from extraction of the crystalline lens without replacement (aphakia) or overcorrection following refractive surgery for myopia

➤ optical correction – Hyperopia can be corrected with plus or convex lenses, either in glasses or contact lenses

➤ Surgical correction – See below

Astigmatism

■ Prevalence – Most cases of myopia and hyperopia are compounded by the concurrent presence of astigmatism.

■ Definition – Astigmatism is a nonspherical refractive error. Commonly, astigmatism is corneal in origin; the cornea is toric (i.e., football-shaped) rather than spherical (i.e., basketball-shaped). In the case of irregular astigmatism, the curvature is irregularly distributed.

- Causes – whereas regular astigmatism is generally a naturally occurring condition, irregular astigmatism is generally caused by disorders that may cause irregularity of the corneal surface or tear film (e.g., dry eye; corneal scarring or irregularity due to infection, trauma, or surgery; or ectatic conditions such as keratoconus).
- Correction – regular astigmatism can be corrected with spectacles or toric soft contact lenses. Rigid gas-permeable contact lenses can be used to correct both regular astigmatism and irregular corneal astigmatism.

Presbyopia
- Prevalence – Presbyopia is a universal, progressive, age-related loss of accommodative power, with symptomatic onset typically between ages 42–46. Onset occurs earlier in hyperopes since a portion of the accommodative reserve must be used to correct the hyperopia.
- Definition – In accommodation, the ring-like ciliary muscle contracts, relaxing the zonules attached to the lens, thereby increasing convexity and refractive power, allowing focus on near images.
  - Causes – Presbyopia is caused by age-related oxidative and other changes to the lens proteins (crystallins), resulting in reduced deformability in response to ciliary muscle contraction.
  - Correction – presbyopia is commonly treated with bifocal spectacles, reading glasses, or bifocal contact lenses.

TESTS
Ametropias (refractive errors) can be diagnosed using subjective or objective means.

Subjective refraction is the process of determining the underlying refractive error by presenting lenses of varying powers until the patient reports that a small target image is in sharpest focus.

Objective refraction is the process of measuring the underlying refractive error using retinoscopy (manual or automated) or aberrometry.

Objective refraction is invaluable in measuring ametropias in children and in uncooperative patients.

DIFFERENTIAL DIAGNOSIS
n/a

MANAGEMENT
n/a

SPECIFIC THERAPY

■ Myopia

> ➤ Optical correction – Myopia can be corrected with a minus power, or concave spectacle or contact lens. Degree of myopia measured by the power of the concave lens to correct it, as expressed in units of diopters (D).

> ➤ Surgical correction – Myopia and myopic astigmatism can be corrected by a variety of methods:

> ➤ Keratorefractive procedures that flatten the central cornea or otherwise reduce the effective convex power of the cornea, or lens implant-based procedures that either replace the crystalline lens or add a lens implant that has reduced convex power.

Keratorefractive methods of myopia correction include:

■ LASIK (laser in situ keratomileusis) – a microkeratome or a femtosecond laser creates a thin flap of corneal tissue that is then lifted, and the underlying corneal stromal bed is precisely photoablated by an ArF 193 nm excimer laser.

■ PRK (photorefractive keratectomy) – the corneal tissue is ablated directly, without first creating and lifting a corneal flap

■ LASEK (laser subepithelial keratectomy) – in this variant of PRK, the epithelium is elevated manually or with a modified microkeratome, and excimer ablation is performed on the underlying stroma

■ RK (radial keratotomy) – deep incisions in the midperipheral and peripheral cornea made in radial fashion cause central flattening. Radial keratotomy, while common in the past, is uncommonly performed today.

■ ICRS (intrastromal corneal ring segment implantation) – arc-like segments of clear polymethylmethacrylate (Intacs) are inserted into the peripheral corneal mid-stroma, inducing central corneal flattening

Lens-based methods of myopia correction include:

■ Phakic intraocular lens implantation – an artificial lens is placed in the anterior or posterior chamber, but the natural crystalline lens is left intact

■ Lens extraction with intraocular lens implantation – in patients with cataract, a spherical or toric intraocular lens can be implanted after the cataract has been removed, thereby correcting any co-existing ametropia. Clear lens extraction in the absence of cataract is generally avoided as a means of correcting high myopia because of the elevated risk of postoperative retinal detachment in these patients.

■ Hyperopia

> ➤ Keratorefractive procedures that steepen the central cornea or otherwise increase the effective convex power of the cornea, or

lens implant-based procedures that either replace the crystalline
lens or add a lens implant that has added convex power

Keratorefractive methods of correcting hyperopia include:

- LASIK (laser in situ keratomileusis) – After creating and lifting a thin
  corneal flap, laser ablation is performed in the peripheral cornea,
  causing effective steepening of the central cornea. Regression over
  time may occur.
- PRK (photorefractive keratectomy) and LASEK (laser subepithelial
  keratectomy) – Peripheral corneal photoablation causes relative
  steepening centrally. As with LASIK, regression over time may occur.
- Thermokeratoplasty – using laser or non-laser approaches, thermal
  treatment is applied to the peripheral cornea, causing collagen contraction and central steepening. Regression of effect is a frequent
  occurrence with this method, particularly with correction of higher
  degrees of hyperopia.

Lens procedures that increase the net effective convex power of the
crystalline lens:

- Phakic intraocular lens implantation – an artificial lens is placed in
  the anterior or posterior chambers, but the natural crystalline lens
  is left intact
- Clear lens extraction with intraocular lens implantation – the
  undoubted effectiveness of this method of correcting higher degrees
  of hyperopia must be balanced against the uncommon but potentially serious complications of an intraocular surgical procedure.
  However, the risk of postoperative retinal detachments is lower in
  lens extraction performed in hyperopes than in myopes.
- Astigmatism
  ➤ Optical correction – Regular astigmatism corrected with lenses.
    Irregular astigmatism requires correction with a rigid contact
    lens that can "float" over the tear film, thus neutralizing the
    underlying irregular cornea.
  ➤ Surgical correction – Regular astigmatism can be corrected using
    the same metbods used to correct myopia and astigmatism, with
    modification. Irregular astigmatism is more difficult to correct
    and may require special techniques such as "custom corneal
    ablation," in which a small- or variable-diameter beam excimer
    laser is directed in a topographically or wavefront-guided fashion
    to "smooth" the irregular corneal surface.
- Presbyopia
  ➤ Optical correction – Convex ("plus") lenses can assist with view-
    ing near objects. Early presbyopes (e.g., those in their early 40s)

generally require a lens of modest power (e.g., +1.00 D), whereas a fully presbyopic individual generally requires a more powerful convex lens (e.g., +2.50 D). This convex power is "added" to any underlying lens power used to correct a co-existing ametropia, either in the form of bifocals or reading spectacles. Specially designed bifocal contact lenses can also be used to correct presbyopia. Monovision is a method of correcting one eye for distance and the other eye for reading, thereby sacrificing depth perception and stereopsis.

➤ Surgical correction – Multifocal and accommodating intraocular lens implants can correct presbyopia but require surgical removal of the crystalline lens as part of cataract surgery or clear lens extraction. Alternatively, a keratorefractive or lens-based procedure may be used to create a monovision correction. Other approaches, such as corneal inlay procedures, remain investigational.

FOLLOW-UP
n/a

COMPLICATIONS AND PROGNOSIS
n/a

RENAL ARTERY STENOSIS

STEPHEN C. TEXTOR, MD

HISTORY & PHYSICAL
- Fibromuscular disease: Early onset of hypertension: Women more likely than men
- Atherosclerosis: Risk Profile:
  ➤ Vascular/Coronary disease history, esp. claudication/aortic aneurysm
  ➤ Smoking history
  ➤ Hyperlipidemia
  ➤ Diabetes
- Clinical Syndromes
  ➤ May be asymptomatic, incidental finding during "screening"
  ➤ Progressive hypertension, when stenosis exceeds 70%
  ➤ Unexplained deterioration of renal function
  ➤ Acute change in renal function with ACE inhibitors or other BP meds

➤ Episodes of pulmonary congestion: "Flash" pulmonary edema
➤ Unexplained end-stage renal failure
➤ Accelerated hypertension

Signs & Symptoms
■ Hypertension (>140/90 mm Hg) at early or advanced age
■ Abdominal bruits
■ Lower extremity vascular insufficiency
■ Hypertensive retinopathy
■ Left ventricular hypertrophy

TESTS
■ Serum creatinine often normal in FMD/usually elevated with atherosclerosis
■ Plasma renin activity: depends on medications/conditions
■ Urinalysis: minimal to mild proteinuria is common; rarely, nephrotic range proteinuria that regresses with revascularization
■ Imaging:
■ Captopril-enhanced renogram (scintigraphy): Excludes high-grade functional stenosis when creatinine is normal. False positives from other conditions, particularly when creatinine >2.0 mg/dL.
■ Doppler ultrasound: Operator-dependent, but highly reliable when imaging satisfactory. 20% of subjects not able to obtain satisfactory studies. Inexpensive means of following lesions over time.
■ Magnetic resonance angiography (MRA): expensive, but most reliable non-nephrotoxic study in patients with renal dysfunction and atherosclerotic disease
■ CT angiography: good anatomic resolution but high contrast load
■ Digital arterial angiography: gold standard for diagnosis, often combined with endovascular intervention
■ Functional tests: Captopril renogram has been advocated to predict response to revascularization. Provides functional estimate before considering nephrectomy.
■ Lateralization of renal vein renins: strong positive predictive value (>90%) when ratio exceeds 1.5–2.0 for benefit regarding blood pressure response. However, >50% benefit even when no lateralization present.

DIFFERENTIAL DIAGNOSIS
■ Essential hypertension
■ Nephrosclerosis and other causes of parenchymal renal disease
■ Primary glomerular diseases as cause of proteinuria

MANAGEMENT

- Goals of therapy are reduction of morbidity/mortality of hypertension and preservation of renal function.
- Initial therapy is reduction of blood pressure using medical means consistent with recommendations of JNC VI.

SPECIFIC THERAPY

- Medical Therapy: This is often undertaken before the diagnosis of renal artery stenosis is considered or established. Unilateral renal artery disease often responds to blockade of renin angiotensin system (e.g., ACE inhibitors and angiotensin receptor blockers) in combination with other agents.
- CAUTION: these agents have potential to reduce glomerular filtration in post-stenotic kidneys due to loss of efferent arteriolar tone.
- Renal Revascularization: Percutaneous angioplasty (PTRA) with or without stenting. FMD often responds to PTRA alone if location is favorable.
- Atherosclerotic disease is more commonly located at ostium; primary patency is better with stents (>75%) as compared to PTRA alone (29%) after 6 months.
- Side effects include atheroemboli, vessel dissection, hematoma and small vessel occlusion (incidence of major events: 4–9%).
- Contraindications (relative): active atheroemboli, diffuse aortic disease, pre-existing vessel occlusion
- Surgical reconstruction usually part of aortic surgery: endarterectomy or renal artery bypass grafting: Morbidity dependent upon surgical expertise and support, co-existing cardiac and carotid disease. Proven long-term durability and patency in most cases, but higher early morbidity and surgical risk than endovascular techniques.

FOLLOW-UP

- Recheck blood pressure, medications and renal function at regular intervals – e.g., 1 month and 3 months thereafter. Blood pressure response to revascularization may develop over several months. Usually recheck vessel patency between 3–6 months (Doppler ultrasound).
- Goal is reduction in medication requirement and improved blood pressure control after successful renal revascularization. Renal function may improve in patients with pre-existing renal dysfunction (25–30%), remain unchanged 45–50%) and deteriorate in 20%.

COMPLICATIONS AND PROGNOSIS

- Progressive atherosclerotic disease: worsening vascular stenosis develops in 30–50% of lesions over 5 years. Total occlusion is relatively infrequent (3%) but does occur.
- Vascular restenosis after stenting (15–30% in 1 year): May appear as recurrent or refractory hypertension and declining renal function. May require re-imaging and repeat endovascular intervention.
- Atheroemboli may appear as progressive decline in renal function, occasionally with lower extremity focal tissue necrosis.

RENAL CALCULI

MARGARET S. PEARLE, MD

HISTORY & PHYSICAL

History

- personal or family history
- history of gout, chronic diarrhea secondary to to gastrointestinal disorders (intestinal resection, Crohn's disease, ulcerative colitis, celiac sprue, pancreatic insufficiency), chronic urinary tract infection, hyperthyroidism, primary hyperparathyroidism
- use of calcium supplements, vitamin C or D, acetazolamide

Signs & Symptoms

- abrupt onset sharp, paroxysmal pain lasting a few minutes or more at a time
- pain originates in flank, radiates to lower abdomen, groin or testicle (labia)
- nausea and vomiting
- gross hematuria
- irritative bladder symptoms (frequency, urgency) with distal ureteral stones
- elevated pulse and blood pressure secondary to pain
- low-grade temperature ($\leq 100°$F) not uncommon, but high fever should alert to possibility of pyelonephritis
- tenderness over flank or anterior abdomen but no peritoneal signs

TESTS

Basic Blood Tests

- CBC: mild leukocytosis common

- creatinine: assess before contrast imaging study
- Ca

Basic Urine Tests
- urinalysis: pH, microhematuria, pyuria, crystals; red blood cells absent in 10–25% of patients with a stone
- urine culture

Imaging
- non-enhanced, thin-cut (3 mm) helical CT of kidneys and ureters: study of choice for acute flank pain
- plain abdominal radiograph (KUB): to determine if stone seen on CT is radiopaque
- intravenous urogram or CT urogram: to assess degree of obstruction and define anatomy for consideration of treatment
- renal sonogram: may detect hydronephrosis, renal calculi, and some distal ureteral calculi, but less sensitive than CT

DIFFERENTIAL DIAGNOSIS
- appendicitis, perforated ulcer, colitis, diverticulitis, pelvic inflammatory disease, ectopic pregnancy, urinary tract infection
- no peritoneal signs or high fever with stone as is typical with acute abdomen
- non-enhanced CT scan highly sensitive for diagnosing stone; may also demonstrate appendicitis, free air, secondary signs of diverticulitis

MANAGEMENT
What to Do First
- relieve pain with narcotic analgesics: morphine sulfate or meperidine
- hydration; may use ketorolac with caution, but avoid in patients with renal insufficiency
- if obstruction with clinical signs of infection, immediately decompress collecting system with percutaneous nephrostomy or ureteral stent

Indications for Hospital Admission
- obstruction with signs of infection
- persistent vomiting and inability to retain fluids
- pain not relieved by oral narcotics
- solitary kidney

SPECIFIC THERAPY

- likelihood of spontaneous passage depends on stone size, stone location, and anatomy of urinary tract
- most small (<5 mm) ureteral stones will pass spontaneously
  - ➤ tamsulosin with or without short course of corticosteroids to facilitate spontaneous stone passage

Indications for Surgical Management

- high grade or complete obstruction for >1 week
- persistent or recurrent renal colic
- occupational requirements (i.e., airline pilot)
- failure of partially obstructing stone to pass within 4–6 weeks

Options for Surgical Management

- optimal treatment depends on stone size, location, composition

Shock Wave Lithotripsy (SWL)

- historically treatment of choice for most (>85%) renal and ureteral calculi, not cystine stones
- usually limited to stones <20 mm in kidney and <10 mm in proximal ureter
- complications: related to bleeding and obstruction from stone fragments
  - ➤ steinstrasse (column of stone fragments in ureter)
  - ➤ bleeding
  - ➤ infection
  - ➤ damage to surrounding organs
- absolute contraindications
  - ➤ pregnancy
  - ➤ middle and distal ureteral stones in women of child-bearing age

Ureteroscopy

- primarily, but not exclusively, used for ureteral stones
  - ➤ increasing use for renal calculi
- treatment of choice for cystine stones and salvage therapy for SWL failures
- controversy regarding optimal treatment for lower ureteral stones (stones below the pelvic bone): ureteroscopy versus SWL
- absolute contraindications
  - ➤ active urinary tract infection

Percutaneous Nephrostolithotomy (PCNL)
- endoscopic retrieval or fragmentation of stones via direct access to kidney through small flank incision
- reserved for large renal or proximal ureteral calculi
  - ➤ Treatment of choice for staghorn calculi
- salvage therapy for SWL and ureteroscopy failures

Open or Laparoscopic Ureterolithotomy or Pyelolithotomy
- rare salvage therapy for SWL or endoscopic failures

FOLLOW-UP

During Treatment
- Radiographic follow-up within approximately 1 month of surgical treatment to ensure stone-free state and absence of obstruction

Routine
- KUB every 6–12 months

Medical Evaluation
- for recurrent stone formers and high-risk (family history of stones, nephrocalcinosis, medical risk factors) first-time stone formers
- serum chemistries
  - ➤ creatinine, K, Ca, PO4, HCO3
  - ➤ uric acid
  - ➤ intact PTH
- urinalysis
- stone analysis
- 24-hour urine collection for total volume, pH, calcium, oxalate, sodium, citrate, uric acid, sulfate, phosphorus, magnesium

Medical Management – Conservative
- increased fluids
- sodium restriction
- limitation of animal protein
- mild calcium restriction if urinary calcium elevated
- limitation of oxalate-rich foods
- increased intake of citrus fruits and juices

Medical Management – Specific Drug Therapy
- hypercalciuria with normal serum calcium: thiazide diuretic and K citrate
- hypercalciuria with elevated serum calcium and PTH: parathyroidectomy

- hyperuricosuria: allopurinol, limited intake of animal protein
- hypocitraturia: K citrate
- hyperoxaluria: vitamin B6, low-oxalate diet
- low urine pH: K citrate
- cystinuria: K citrate and chelating agents
- infection stones: stone removal, suppressive antibiotics, rarely urease inhibitor

COMPLICATIONS AND PROGNOSIS
- recurrent stones: without medical prophylaxis, risk of recurrence at least 50% within 5 years
- renal failure from untreated, obstructing stones or staghorn calculi
- infection: due to obstruction or presence of infection stones

RENAL GLUCOSURIA

MICHEL BAUM, MD

HISTORY & PHYSICAL
- Glucosuria found in asymptomatic patient on routine urinalysis
- No history of polydipsia, polyuria, or polyphagia

TESTS
- Urinalysis positive for glucose
- Normal blood glucose and hemoglobin A1c
- Normal electrolytes and serum phosphorus

DIFFERENTIAL DIAGNOSIS
- Autosomal recessive disorder due to inactivating mutation of Na-glucose cotransporter (SGLT2) in proximal tubule

MANAGEMENT
n/a

SPECIFIC THERAPY
- No therapy indicated

FOLLOW-UP
n/a

COMPLICATIONS AND PROGNOSIS
Prognosis excellent

RENAL MASSES AND TUMORS

BENJAMIN N. HENDIN, MD

HISTORY & PHYSICAL
- Classic triad in Renal Cell Carcinoma (RCC)
- Gross hematuria, flank pain, and palpable mass
- Triad was previously found in 10–15% of patients
- Now less common due to earlier detection with increasing incidence of "incidentally detected" tumors

Paraneoplastic Syndromes
- Erythrocytosis
  - up to 3–10% of patients
  - consequence of increased erythropoietin production
- Stauffer's syndrome:
  - reversible hepatic dysfunction associated with non-metastatic RCC
  - Abnormalities include elevated Alk Phos and Bili, hypoalbuminemia, prolonged PTT, hypergammaglobulinemia. Fever, fatigue, weight loss occur in association
  - Resolves following nephrectomy
- Hypertension
- Hypercalcemia

TESTS

Blood Tests
- CBC to detect anemia, in late-stage RCC
- Serum Creatinine to assess global renal function
- Hepatocellular enzymes – elevated levels with either Stauffer's syndrome or hepatic metastases.
- Alkaline Phosphatase – to detect bone metastases

Radiographic
- Ultrasound
- CT Scan with and without IV contrast, renal imaging protocol
- MRI with Gadolinium
- CXR to evaluate for metastases.

DIFFERENTIAL DIAGNOSIS

Key is to Differentiate Cystic vs. Solid
- CT or MRI essential to evaluate indeterminate lesions
- Ultrasound may aid in diagnosis

■ Presence of fat within a solid lesion is virtually diagnostic of angiomyolipoma

Cystic Renal Masses

■ Vast majority of renal masses are simple cysts
■ Incidence of simple renal cysts: 25–33% among patients >50 years of age
■ Renal ultrasound can definitively diagnose a simple cyst:
■ Criteria: anechoic, through transmission, smooth-walled, without solid components or calcifications.
➤ Percutaneous cyst puncture generally not helpful in differentiating "benign" from malignant cysts
➤ Bloody fluid or high protein content is not diagnostic

Cyst Classification (Bosniak System)

■ Based on CT Criteria
■ Accurate delineation requires:
■ Pre- and post- contrast CT images with 5-mm cuts

Type I Cyst

■ Simple cyst
■ Smooth uncalcified walls, sonographic through-transmission,
■ Uncomplicated simple cysts are definitively diagnosed by sonography and/or CT, and are uniformly benign

Type II Cyst

■ Minimally complicated cysts – are benign but have some radiographic features of concern, including:
■ Septated cysts, minimally calcified cysts, infected cysts, and high-density cysts
■ < 20% incidence of malignancy

Type II Hyperdense Cyst

■ Smooth, round, sharply marginated, homogenous lesion
■ Does not enhance, configuration remains unchanged after IV contrast
■ 3 cm or less

Type III Cyst

■ More complicated cystic lesions that cannot be confidently be distinguished from malignancy on radiographic imaging
■ Should be surgically explored unless clinically contraindicated
■ Incidence of malignancy: 30–60%

Type IV Cyst
- Solid enhancing elements associated with cystic elements
- Incidence of malignancy 70–100%

Solid Renal Masses
- Solid renal tumors should be presumed malignant until surgical pathology demonstrates otherwise
- Percutaneous biopsy of solid renal neoplasms is rarely appropriate, and should be limited to cases in which the renal lesion is suspected to be a metastasis from another site. Consider formal urologic consultation prior to such biopsy.

Solid Renal Tumors
Renal Pseudotumors
- Hypertrophied Column of Bertin
  - ➤ Functional renal parenchyma
  - ➤ Distinguished from renal neoplasm by functional radioisotope study demonstrating normal uptake/excretion of tracer

Benign Neoplasm
- Oncocytoma (3–7% of solid renal tumors)
  - ➤ Note: 15–30% of oncocytomas may occur in conjunction with Renal Cell CA
- Angiomyolipoma
- Fibroma
- Leiomyoma
- Juxtaglomerular tumors
- Hemangioma
- Lipoma

Primary Malignant Neoplasm
- Renal Cell Carcinoma (85% of solid renal neoplasms)
- Transitional Cell Carcinoma/Urothelial Carcinoma (8% of renal malignancies)
- Sarcoma

Secondary Malignant Neoplasm
- Retroperitoneal sarcoma
- Pancreatic carcinoma, colon carcinoma (direct extension)
- Lung, breast, GI (hematogenous spread)
- Lymphoma, leukemia

MANAGEMENT
- RCC is primarily a surgical disease
- Non-surgical treatments are of limited efficacy at present

■ Surgery + Adjuvant/Neoadjuvant Therapy (Biologic Response Modifiers; i.e. cytokine-based therapy) for advanced disease

SPECIFIC THERAPY

Treatment Options

■ Partial Nephrectomy
➤ Indications (relative)
  • Tumor <4 cm
  • Bilateral renal neoplasms
  • Hypertension
  • Urolithiasis
  • Renal insufficiency
  • Solitary kidney
■ Radical Nephrectomy
➤ Open vs. Laparoscopic
  • Approach depends on:
  • Experience/expertise of surgeon
  • Anatomical considerations
    • Tumor size, location, extent
    • Prior abdominal/retroperitoneal surgery

FOLLOW-UP

■ Post-surgical follow-up at 2–4 weeks postop
■ CT Abdomen and Pelvis, CXR, and Alkaline Phosphatase as clinically indicated, based on stage/grade of disease

COMPLICATIONS AND PROGNOSIS

Stage/Treatment: 5-Year Survival

■ Nephron-sparing surgery: ~87%
■ Radical Nephrectomy, Stage I: ~75%
■ Radical Nephrectomy, Stage II: ~66%
■ Radical Nephrectomy, Stage III (venous extension): ~55%
■ Metastatic to Regional Nodes: ~25%
■ Distant Metastases: ~4.5%
■ Radical Nephrectomy w/ simultaneous excision of a solitary metastasis: ~22%
■ Excision of solitary metastasis following radical nephrectomy: ~40%

Cell Type

■ Clear Cell Alone: ~64%
■ Any Granular Cell: ~53%
■ Spindle, Sarcomatoid, Anaplastic: ~24%

Tumor Grade

- Grade I: ~69%
- Grade II: ~42%
- Grade III: ~27%

RENAL OSTEODYSTROPHY

KENNETH CHEN, MD; TIMOTHY MEYER, MD; and YIMING LIT, MD

HISTORY & PHYSICAL

History

- Chronic renal failure
- Bone pain, fractures
- Muscle weakness
- Dialysis
- Kidney transplant

Signs & Symptoms

- Asymptomatic until irreparable damage
- Musculoskeletal:
- Fractures: mineralization defects, impaired new bone formation, excess bone resorption
  - Bone pain in lower back, hips, legs
  - Proximal muscle aching, weakness (with high PTH)
- Ectopic calcification in arteries, cardiac conduction system, cornea with high values for Ca × PO4 product (>65):
  - Arrhythmia
  - Accelerated atherosclerosis
  - Calciphylaxis: ischemic necrosis of the skin, muscles, digits

TESTS

Laboratory

- Early disease:
  - Elevated PO4, low Ca (correct for albumin)
  - Elevated PTH, alkaline phosphatase
- Advanced disease:
  - Hypercalcemia from tertiary hyperparathyroidism
  - Alternatively low PTH from oversuppression by vitamin D and Ca

Imaging

- X-rays for symptomatic bone disease or elevated PTH:
- Early disease: radiologic findings usually absent
- Advanced disease: high PTH causes subperiosteal bone resorption (hands)

Bone Biopsy

- Performed infrequently; management guided by serum tests

DIFFERENTIAL DIAGNOSIS

- Muscle weakness: electrolyte disturbances, peripheral neuropathy, steroid-induced myopathy
- Bone pain: osteomyelitis, osteoporosis, fractures, bone tumors

MANAGEMENT

What to Do First

- Check serum PO4, Ca, albumin (to correct Ca level):
   - stage 3 (GFR 30–59 ml/min/1.73 m2) every 12 months
   - stage 4 (GFR 15–29 ml/min/1.73 m2) every 3 months
   - stage 5 (GFR <15 ml/min/1.73 m2) every month
- Check serum PTH:
   - stage 3 every 12 months
   - stage 4 every 3 months
   - stage 5 every 3 months
- Check 25(OH) vitamin D3 level if PTH is elevated

General Measures

- Normalize PO4 and Ca
- Monitor PTH
- Add vitamin D analogs when necessary
- Treatment for age-related and postmenopausal osteoporosis in renal insufficiency not established:
   - ➤ Bisphosphonates not approved for use
   - ➤ Standards for estrogen replacement not described

SPECIFIC THERAPY

- Indicated whenever PO4 and/or Ca values are chronically abnormal
- First lower PO4: target normal range:
   - ➤ Restrict dietary PO4: major sources: dairy products, meat
   - ➤ Phosphate binders to reduce gut PO4 absorption
   - ➤ Calcium carbonate or calcium acetate with each meal
   - ➤ If hypercalcemic, use sevelamer HCl or lanthanium carbonate with each meal

- Next correct Ca: target normal range: 8.4 to 9.5 mg/dl
- Calcitriol to increase gut Ca absorption and suppress PTH secretion:
  - Predialysis: oral
  - Dialysis: IV
- If corrected Ca or PO4 levels high, can try paricalcitol or doxercalciferol
- PTH target for stage 5: 150–300 pg/ml (intact PTH)
  - If PTH higher despite calcitrol or other vitamin D analogs, try calcimimetic agents that suppress PTH without increasing serum Ca: Cinacalcet
  - If PTH is low, discontinue vitamin D

Side Effects & Contraindications
- Calcium acetate and calcium carbonate:
  - Side effects: nausea, hypercalcemia, hypophosphatemia
  - Contraindications:
    - Absolute: hypercalcemia
    - Relative: GI motility disorders
- Sevelamer HCl:
  - Side effects: nausea, other GI symptoms
  - Relative contraindication: GI motility disorders
- Lanthanium carbonate: nausea, vomiting, diarrhea, abdominal pain, headache
- Calcitriol and other vitamin D analogs:
  - Side effects: hypercalcemia, hyperphosphatemia
  - Contraindications:
    - Absolute: hypercalcemia
    - Relative: hyperphosphatemia
    - Cinacalcet: hypocalamia, nausea, vomiting, diarrhea, myalgia

FOLLOW-UP
- Serum PO4, Ca, albumin monthly for dialysis patients
- Serum PTH q 3 mo in dialysis patients
- Test less frequently in predialysis patients

COMPLICATIONS AND PROGNOSIS

Complications
- Tertiary hyperparathyroidism: parathyroid hyperplasia not suppressed by high serum Ca; causes bone injury and hypercalcemia; may require parathyroidectomy
- Hypocalcemia postparathyroidectomy: may require IV Ca postop (hungry bone syndrome)

- Anemia unresponsive to erythropoietin due to marrow fibrosis
- Acceleration of atherosclerosis by calcification of arteries
- Arrhythmias from calcification of conduction system

Prognosis
- Good if PO4 and Ca kept near normal
- Increased mortality when P >6.5 mg/dL or Ca × PO4 product >72
- Prognosis with calciphylaxis is extremely poor; sepsis leading cause of death

---

RENAL VEIN THROMBOSIS

STEPHEN C. TEXTOR, MD

HISTORY & PHYSICAL
- Acute thrombosis produces pain:flank/loin pain
  - ➤ hematuria
  - ➤ Fever
  - ➤ Worsening proteinuria
  - ➤ Testicular pain and swelling (left renal vein)
- Chronic thrombosis – often asymptomatic
  - ➤ worsening proteinuria
  - ➤ loss of renal function in solitary kidney or if bilateral
  - ➤ First manifestation may be pulmonary embolus
- Acute thrombosis may be associated with clotting disorders elsewhere, e.g. antiphospholipid syndrome, venous trauma (e.g. surgery/venography/manipulation); renal allograft rejection, vena cava occlusion
- Chronic thrombosis often associated with nephrotic syndrome, particularly membranous nephropathy, renal cell carcinoma, or retroperitoneal fibrosis or other veno-occlusive diseases. Incidence estimated between 10–40% of overtly nephrotic patients.

TESTS
- Basic tests: creatinine elevation
- Urinalysis: hematuria/nephrotic sediment with heavy proteinuria
- Screening for hypercoagulable states: Protein S deficiency screen, protein C and antithrombin III are common inherited disorders with 8–10 fold relative increase in thrombotic events. Absolute risk not certain.
- Imaging:

> Routine imaging of nephrotic subjects is not usually performed. Often first consideration when abnormal pulmonary ventilation/perfusion scan noted.

■ Vena Cavagram and renal venogram are "gold standards". MRA angiography or CT scans can delineate extent and location of thrombus within the main renal vein and vena cava. Doppler ultrasound may identify lack of flow within renal vein but is operator dependent.

DIFFERENTIAL DIAGNOSIS

■ Loss of renal function and/or pain related to other disorders, including primary glomerular diseases.

■ Must exclude renal arterial occlusion and/or nephrolithiasis, extrinsic renal vein compression (e.g. retroperitoneal fibrosis).

MANAGEMENT

■ Exclude other causes of reversible acute renal failure

■ Hydration, volume expansion

■ anticoagulation: Risks/benefits of anticoagulation in asymptomatic RVT are uncertain and depend upon probability of embolic events. Avoidance of high risk venous stasis and edema (e.g. use of support hose) are preferred.

■ Anticoagulation for established disease.

■ role for thrombolytic therapy uncertain

SPECIFIC THERAPY

■ For established RVT and embolic events
> Heparin followed by oral warfarin
> Anticoagulation-oral coumadin until prothrombin INR 2.0–3.0
> anticoagulation should be continued as long as nephrotic state persists
> Inferior Vena Cava Filter (Greenfield Filter) may be considered if anticoagulation contraindicated or failure

FOLLOW-UP
n/a

COMPLICATIONS AND PROGNOSIS

■ Often asymptomatic with little or no clinical effect on proteinuria or renal function.

■ Occasional embolic events with pulmonary emboli and/or systemic emboli when intracardiac defect, e.g. atrial septal defect

- may slowly extend into right atrium, particularly when associated with renal cell carcinoma. Tumor resection in this case requires attention to avoid thrombus fracture and embolic phenomena.
- Surgical thrombectomy rarely warranted.

REPAIRED CONGENITAL HEART DISEASE

MARIA ANSARI, MD

HISTORY & PHYSICAL

History
- Prior surgical repair of teratology of Fallot, transposition of great arteries, coarctation of aorta

Signs & Symptoms
- Atrial and ventricular arrhythmias
- Eisenmenger's syndrome
- Hypertension recurrence after coarctation repair
- Heart failure symptoms (chest pain, dyspnea)

TESTS

Screening
- Accurate medical and surgical history

Imaging
- Transthoracic echocardiogram usually diagnostic

DIFFERENTIAL DIAGNOSIS
n/a

MANAGEMENT
- Endocarditis prophylaxis indicated
- Assess for development of heart failure, pulmonary hypertension, systemic hypertension

SPECIFIC THERAPY
n/a

FOLLOW-UP
- Patients should have regular follow-up with a cardiologist annually

COMPLICATIONS AND PROGNOSIS

Complications
- Endocarditis
- *Transposition and tetralogy repairs*
  - Right heart failure due to volume overload or pulmonary hypertension
  - Stenosis/thrombosis of palliative shunts or conduits
  - Atrial and ventricular arrhythmias
  - Sudden cardiac death
  - Residual VSD
  - Systemic (tricuspid valve) regurgitation (transposition repairs)
- *Coarctation repairs*
  - Recurrence of HTN
  - Aortic dissection
  - Premature CAD

Prognosis
- Tetralogy of Fallot (94% 25-year survival if repaired early)
- Transposition of great arteries (90% 20-year survival)
- Coarctation (91% 20-year survival if repaired before age 14)

RESTLESS LEGS SYNDROME

CHAD CHRISTINE, MD

HISTORY & PHYSICAL
- Tightness, tingling or burning discomfort in legs
- Exacerbated by rest; relief w/ activity
- Symptoms involve rhythmic movement of feet during sleep that disturbs sleep
- Hereditary
- Signs: unremarkable

TESTS
- Lab tests & neuroimaging are unremarkable
- Sleep study may demonstrate periodic limb movements & frequent arousals

DIFFERENTIAL DIAGNOSIS
- Polyneuropathy, radiculopathy, myelopathy excluded by exam & EMG/NCS
- Uremia & iron deficiency excluded by history & serum studies

MANAGEMENT
- General measures: increase exercise

SPECIFIC THERAPY
- Indications: symptoms that interfere significantly w/ lifestyle
  - ➤ L-dopa/carbidopa
  - ➤ Dopamine agonists (pramipexole, ropinirole)
  - ➤ Opiods: propoxyphene or oxycodone in combination w/ L-dopa or dopamine agonists

FOLLOW-UP
- Periodically depending on response to treatment

COMPLICATIONS AND PROGNOSIS
- Chronic disorder often responsive to treatment

RHEGMATOGENOUS RETINAL DETACHMENT

PATRICK M. MONAHAN, MD

HISTORY & PHYSICAL

History
- High myopia.
- Cataract surgery.
- Trauma – blunt or perforating.
- Inflammation.

Signs & Symptoms
- New floaters.
- Flashing lights – Small arcs lasting only seconds.
- Visual field deficit in one eye – possibly progressive.
- Vision decreased – very mild to severe.
- Usually painless.
- Visual acuity – normal to severe decrease,
- Afferent papillary defect – none to very positive.
- Slit Lamp Exam – Pigmented debris in anterior vitreous behind lens.
- Intraocular pressure – usually normal, but can be decreased or elevated in longstanding detachments.
- Posterior exam – new detachments appear as white elevated mobile retina. Old detachments may be clear or taut. Optic nerve looks pink to white. Retinal vessels usually normal or tortuous. Vitreous may contain blood or debris.

TESTS

- B scan ultrasound – performed when poor view of retina – shows elevated retina.

DIFFERENTIAL DIAGNOSIS

- Posterior vitreous detachment – floaters and flashing lights, vitreous debris. May precede retinal tears or detachments.
  - ➤ Differentiate on – clinical exam with scleral depression.
- Central or branch retinal artery occlusion – Portion or all of retina appears white.
  - ➤ Differentiate on – Clinical exam & Fluorescence angiogram.
- Vitreous hemorrhage – decreased vision, vitreous blood, possible retinal tear.
  - ➤ Differentiate on – clinical exam & B scan ultrasound.
- Retinoschisis (a splitting of retinal layers) – thin elevated peripheral retina.
  - ➤ Differentiate on – clinical exam with scleral depression.
- Choroidal detachment – usually after trauma or surgery.
  - ➤ Differentiate on – B scan ultra sound.

MANAGEMENT

- Referral to Ophthalmologist within 24 hours if possible.
- Patching eyes not necessary.
- Have patient position head back and keep still until evaluated.
- Stop ASA like products and coumadin if safe to do so.
- Keep NPO if surgery likely within 8 hours.

SPECIFIC THERAPY

- All therapy for rhegamatogenous retinal detachments involve surgery designed to oppose the retina to the underlying retinal pigmented epithelium and seal around the retinal tear.
- Laser photocoagulation –
  - ➤ Internally burns are placed around tear to create a scar to weld the retina to underlying tissue.
  - ➤ For retinal tears with or without small subclinical retinal detachments.
  - ➤ Requires clear view through media.
- Cryoretinopexy –
  - ➤ Externally freeze burns are placed through the wall of the eye to scar the retina to the underlying tissue.
  - ➤ For retinal tears with or without small subclinical retinal detachments.
  - ➤ Better for poor view, but requires local anesthesia.

- Pneumatoretinopexy –
  - A small expansile gas bubble is injected into the vitreous cavity after cryoretinopexy around breaks.
  - For partial or complete retinal detachments with retinal breaks in the superior portion of the retina.
  - Requires patient to position head so that bubble covers break for 5–7 days.
- Scleral Buckle –
  - A silicon rubber explant is sutured on to the external scleral wall in a way that causes the wall to buckle inward, thus forcing the internal eye wall up against the detached retina.
  - Performed in conjunction with cryoretinopexy with or without subretinal fluid drainage.
  - For partial or complete retinal detachment. Works well for inferior or multiple retinal breaks.
- Vitrectomy –
  - Internal surgery whereby vitreous is removed and the retina repositioned. Vitreous is replaced by gas that dissipates on its own. Performed in conjunction with laser or cryoretinopexy and scleral buckling.
  - For retinal detachments with multiple or giant tears, vitreous hemorrhage, cataract, inflammation, Proliferative vitreoretinopathy, or other complicating factors.
  - Requires head positioning 7–10 days.

FOLLOW-UP

- Initially daily, then weekly, and then monthly in postop period.
- Yearly once stable.

COMPLICATIONS AND PROGNOSIS

Complications

- Astigmatism or myopic shift – expected,
  - Get new glasses (6 mo postop).
- Cataract progression – expected with Vitrectomy.
  - Cataract surgery.
- Glaucoma (transient) – common.
  - Eye drops or oral meds (i.e., Diamox).
- Recurrent detachment – common till 2 mos., extremely rare after 6 mos.
  - Surgery.

- Proliferative Vitreoretinopathy (PVR) – uncommon, causes redetachment.
  - ➤ Surgery.
- Vitreous hemorrhage – uncommon.
  - ➤ May reabsorb, if not surgery.
- Epiretinal Membrane – rare, late complication.
  - ➤ Surgery to remove.
- Choroidal detachment- rare
  - ➤ Oral predmisone, rarely surgery.
- Glaucoma permanent – rare
  - ➤ Eye drops, meds or surgery.
- Infection – rare
  - ➤ Immediate attention with antibiotics and possible surgery
- Note: Patients with infection or severe post op glaucoma are most likely to present emergently with severe headache and nausea.

Prognosis
- Approximately 98% of new detachments are repairable with one or two
- operations.
- Good vision is obtainable if repair is performed within one week of central
- vision loss.
- Most complications are treatable.
- If PVR develops the risk of regrowth and redetachment may be as high as
- 50% even with successful initial surgical detachment repair.

RHEUMATOID ARTHRITIS

W. NEAL ROBERTS, MD

HISTORY & PHYSICAL

History
- Sine qua non: pain in the characteristic pattern, usually small joints of hands & feet
- 1% prevalence in population, 2–5% in first-degree relatives of pts w/ RA
- ~ 80% female

- 50% are women w/ onset 5 years before or after menopause
- Additional 25% are women in their late 20s
- Remainder spread evenly across age & gender

Signs & Symptoms
- Morning stiffness
- Symmetric joint pain, especially 2nd & 3rd MCPs, wrists
- Joint swelling & tenderness
- Palpable synovium
- Decreased range of motion
- Subcutaneous nodules on extensor surfaces
- Must last 6 weeks to exclude self-limited postviral synovitis

TESTS

Laboratory
General
- Urinalysis
- CBC
- Comprehensive metabolic panel as baseline for potentially toxic drug treatment & to exclude end-organ damage due to other diseases (eg, SLE)
- ESR or C-reactive protein usually elevated, not specific

Specific
- Rheumatoid factor
  - 60–80% sensitive
  - Takes up to 10 months to turn positive
  - Not very specific: occurs in other diseases w/ polyclonal B cell activation: hepatitis C w/ cryoglobulinemia, endocarditis, Sjögren's syndrome, other rheumatic diseases (eg, SLE)
- ANA to rule out lupus, especially in African Americans. Antibodies to cyclic citrullinated peptide (CCP) more specific (80–90%) but less sensitive (~55%) than rheumatoid factor

Imaging
- Chest radiograph for sarcoidosis
- Joint radiographs
  - Early: juxtarticular osteopenia
  - Erosions defined by cortical discontinuity on hand & foot are the most specific, take 6 months to develop
  - Joint space narrowing, indicating cartilage loss, comes later
  - Ultrasound or MRI of joint may be more sensitive, not widely available

DIFFERENTIAL DIAGNOSIS

- Hand & foot joint disease: SLE, viral diseases (eg, hepatitis C, parvovirus B19)
- Spine & few joints: psoriatic arthritis, Reiter's disease, other spondyloarthropathies
- Fibromyalgia not in differential. It has central pain & no swelling.

MANAGEMENT

What to Do First

- Begin pt education w/ Arthritis Foundation (or similar) pamphlets
- Communicate emotion-laden label in increments: "arthritis," "a type of inflammatory arthritis," "likely rheumatoid arthritis"
- Stratify risk by the following prognostic criteria:
  - ➤ Work loss in first 6 weeks
  - ➤ Joint count >20
  - ➤ Early radiographic changes
  - ➤ Positive rheumatoid factor
  - ➤ Elevated ESR
  - ➤ Family history
- Consultation to confirm diagnosis & begin disease-modifying antirheumatic drug (DMARD) in first 3 months

General Measures

- Team approach: primary care, subspecialist, orthopedist, therapists, family
- Physical therapy & occupational (hand) therapy as tolerated
- Surgery for destroyed joints or contractures

SPECIFIC THERAPY

Indications

- Symptoms & joint damage (erosions & joint space narrowing) drive treatment. Suppress both.

Treatment Options

- NSAID &/or acetaminophen for pain
- Low-dose prednisone to control disease temporarily
- DMARDs
  - ➤ Need a consult to choose appropriate agent
  - ➤ Begin DMARD w/in 3 months of onset for best results (most joint damage occurs in the first 2 years)
  - ➤ Good prognosis: sulfasalazine (SSZ), hydroxychloroquine (HCQ), minocycline

➤ Bad prognosis: methotrexate (MTX)
  - Best combination of efficacy, safety & cost: 70% of pts continue it for 5 years or more
  - If response inadequate, add SSZ, HCQ, leflunomide (2/3 of MTX responders require this "step up")
  - MTX + SSZ + HCQ substantially better than MTX or MTX + HCQ in randomized trial
  - If response still inadequate, add or switch to anti-TNF agent, including etanercept, infliximab, adalimumab (>70% response rate, serious infections as complications) or anti IL-1 agent, anakinra (30% response rate).

▦ Azathioprine, gold salts, cylcosporine are also options

Side Effects & Complications
▦ NSAIDs: decreased renal function, GI toxicity (selective COX-2 inhibitors [celecoxib] avoid GI but not renal problems)
▦ HCQ: retinal damage
▦ SSZ: leukopenia, rash
▦ MTX: cirrhosis, pneumonitis
▦ Minocycline: skin pigmentation
▦ Leflunomide: diarrhea & liver disease
▦ Anti-TNF or anti-IL-1 biologics: infections up to 5 per 100 pnt-years
▦ Azathioprine: liver disease, leukopenia
▦ Gold salts: rash, membranous glomerulopathy, cytopenia
▦ Cylcosporine: increased creatinine

Contraindications
▦ NSAIDS: renal failure, peptic ulcer disease
▦ All DMARDs: potential for pregnancy (prednisone safest)
▦ MTX: alcohol intake, liver disease, lung disease
▦ HCQ: retinal disease
▦ SSZ: allergy to sulfa drugs
▦ Leflunomide: liver disease
▦ Biologics: underlying infection, cost (>$10,000/yr)

FOLLOW-UP
▦ Initial treatment: 4–6 weeks while adjusting doses & choice of drugs
▦ Routine: 3-month intervals at a minimum while stable
▦ Monitor toxicities (eg, liver function on MTX) every 6–8 weeks

COMPLICATIONS & PROGNOSIS
▦ Extra-articular involvement

➤ Rheumatoid nodules in viscera (eg, lungs, heart)
➤ Eyes: sicca syndrome, part of Sjogren's syndrome, episcleritis
➤ Lungs: nodules, pleurisy w/ effusion, interstitial fibrosis
➤ Heart: pericarditis, nodules, valvulitis
➤ Vasculitis
■ Disability
➤ 30% of work capacity lost. Only about half still working at old job w/out adaptation at 5 yrs.
■ Death
➤ Excess mortality from 20–40%
➤ GI bleeding from NSAIDs is by far the most common drug side effect
➤ Infection in pts immunocompromised by DMARDs
➤ Lung or liver damage from MTX
➤ Increased cardiovascular disease
■ Prognosis (see risk factors in Management section above)
➤ Only 4% will achieve a complete remission
➤ W/ appropriate therapy, most pts will have some joint problems but maintain satisfactory overall function

RHINITIS

ANDREW N. GOLDBERG, MD

HISTORY & PHYSICAL

■ Nasal congestion
■ Nasal obstruction
■ Clear or white nasal discharge
➤ Sinusitis
➤ Pregnancy or high progesterone (e.g., BCPs)
➤ Underlying illness such as hypothyroidism, sarcoid, Wegener granulomatosis, sarcoid, lymphoma in a rare situation
➤ Topical nasal decongestant abuse (rhinitis medicamentosa)
➤ Systemic medications (e.g., beta blockers, reserpine)
➤ Atrophic rhinitis or ozena in the elderly where mucosa has thinned
➤ Two predominant types occur which may have similar symptoms and appearance
  • *Allergic Rhinitis*
    • Sneezing / itchy eyes / watery eyes / allergy symptoms

- Triggered by exposure to allergen (dust, animal dander, molds, grasses, trees, etc.)
- Seasonal component, but perennial symptoms can occur as well
- Pale white or bluish discoloration of nasal and specifically turbinate mucosa Mucosa typically boggy or edematous
- Erythematous mucosa can also be seen
- *Nonallergic (vasomotor) Rhinitis*
  - Nasal congestion that may occur suddenly with changes in temperature, humidity, or with smoke or chemical exposure (e.g. perfume).
  - Associated with pregnancy or pre-menstrual time frame
  - May be postural with nasal congestion on dependent side or both sides
  - Nasal congestion and clear rhinorrhea with food ingestion (gustatory rhinitis)
  - Boggy edematous mucosa
  - May appear similar to allergic rhinitis with pale or bluish discoloration of turbinate mucosa
  - Erythematous mucosa can also be seen

TESTS
- Allergic testing (skin or RAST) can reveal allergens to be avoided and desensitization therapy can proceed in selected cases
- CT scan of the sinuses (coronal CT with bone window 3 mm cuts) to rule out concomitant sinusitis
- Rarely, biopsy is rare needed for diagnosis of an underlying illness (e.g. Wegener's, sarcoid, lymphoma)
- Blood testing for systemic causes such as hypothyroidism, Wegener, sarcoid
- Some use smear of nasal secretions to look for eosinophils (NARES syndrome)

DIFFERENTIAL DIAGNOSIS
- Sinusitis/nasal polyposis with associated rhinitis
- Acute viral upper respiratory infection for acute rhinitis
- Normal nasal cycle where some patients notice congestion which alternates sides
- Deviated septum causing nasal obstruction
- Systemic processes such as Wegener granulomatosis, sarcoidosis
- Tumor or mass causing nasal obstruction
- Adenoid hypertrophy causing nasal obstruction and nasal drainage
- Foreign body

MANAGEMENT

- Nonallergic and allergic rhinitis are treated similarly
  - ➤ Avoidance of trigger in allergic or nonallergic rhinitis is suggested
  - ➤ Control or recognition of an identified underlying mechanism such as sinusitis, systemic disorders such as hypothyroidism, or conditions such as pregnancy)
- Topical and systemic medications are chosen by history (ie antihistimines for allergy) or are given empirically for a 2–4 week period and continued as indicated. Use of any medication or treatment in pregnancy should be carefully considered in consultation with the patient and obstetrician

SPECIFIC THERAPY

Treatment Options

- *Medications*
  - ➤ Use of topical nasal steroid sprays are often first measure used
  - ➤ Systemic antihistamines (Non-sedating are commonly used first)
  - ➤ Systemic decongestants such as pseudoephedrine
  - ➤ Systemic steroids are rarely, but sometimes used
  - ➤ Topical nasal cromolyn for allergic rhinitis
  - ➤ Topical ipratropium bromide 0.03% 30 minutes prior to meals for gustatory rhinitis
  - ➤ Topical nasal saline spray can be effective for symptom relief
  - ➤ Treatments are typically empiric and proceed with alternatives after a 2–4 week trial
- *Surgery*
  - ➤ Surgical treatment of the inferior turbinates is often used. Choices for treatment are multiple and may involve partial or submucosal resection of the turbinates or size reduction by mucosal cartery or radiofrequency ablation. Correction of a deviated septum may offer relief as well and is often done in conjunction with treatment of the turbinates.

Side Effects

- Topical nasal steroid sprays
  - ➤ Nasal bleeding, ulceration or rarely perforation of the nasal septum
- Systemic effects such as glaucoma, cataracts and adrenal suppression should be considered, but do not appear to be as significant as in pulmonary use
- The risks and benefits of the specific surgical procedures should be carefully reviewed with the patient and may be specific to the

procedure and anesthesia used Atrophic rhinitis can occur in certain patients and in patients in whom over resection of the turbinates has occurred

FOLLOW-UP
- Follow up can be performed as needed for progression or lack of resolution of symptoms
- Underlying conditions should be followed as appropriate

COMPLICATIONS AND PROGNOSIS
- In general, rhinitis is not a life threatening condition and there is no known impact on survival

RHINOVIRUS

CAROL A. GLASER, MD

HISTORY & PHYSICAL

History
- Rhinovirus principal cause of the "common cold"
- Rhinovirus; at least 100 antigenic serotypes (infection with one type confers type-specific immunity, but little or no protection against other types)
- Coronaviruses can also cause common cold (see Coronavirus)
- Humans only known host
- Transmission: direct contact or inhalation airborne droplets
- Household spread common
- Incubation period: 12–72 h
- Period of communicability around 24 h before onset and 5 days after onset
- Many persons have 1–6 colds/year
- Incidence highest in children <5 yr

Signs & Symptoms
- Coryza
- Sneezing
- Fever – occurs in 10–20% of cases, low-grade
- Variable symptoms; malaise, headache, cough (unremarkable chest exam)
- Last 2–7 days

TESTS
- Nonspecific:
  - ➤ WBC usually normal
- Specific:
  - ➤ Viral isolation-respiratory specimens
  - ➤ Serology-not practicable, not available

DIFFERENTIAL DIAGNOSIS
- Allergies
  - ➤ Other viruses; coronaviruses, RSV. Influenza, parainfluenza, adenoviruses, some enteroviruses (pts with influenza/adenovirus often have higher fever, more severe illness)

MANAGEMENT
n/a

SPECIFIC THERAPY
- For rhinovirus – no specific therapy usually indicated

FOLLOW-UP
n/a

COMPLICATIONS AND PROGNOSIS

Complications
- Predispose to bacterial sinusitis
- Predispose to otitis media
- May precipitate asthma attacks
- Exacerbation of bronchitis in COPD
- Possibly – predispose to bacterial pneumonia, unproven

Prevention
- Good handwashing
- No vaccine available

RIBOFLAVIN DEFICIENCY

ELISABETH RYZEN, MD

HISTORY & PHYSICAL

History
- Inadequate animal products, milk consumption, liver disease, alcoholism, chronic diarrhea, prolonged IV hydration without vitamins

Signs & Symptoms
- pallor, angular stomatitis, cheilosis, red tongue, shark skin, photophobia

TESTS

Laboratory
- Basic urine studies:
  - ➤ <30 mcg riboflavin/gram creatinine excretion

DIFFERENTIAL DIAGNOSIS
n/a

MANAGEMENT
n/a

SPECIFIC THERAPY
- Riboflavin 10–30 mg/day PO; treat associated vitamin deficiencies

Side Effects & Contraindications
- None

FOLLOW-UP
n/a

COMPLICATIONS AND PROGNOSIS
- Reversible with replacement

ROCKY MOUNTAIN SPOTTED FEVER

RICHARD A. JACOBS, MD, PhD

HISTORY & PHYSICAL

History
- Tick bite 3–12 days before onset of symptoms.
- Outdoor activity during spring or summer
- Disease reported in 48 states.
- Contact with dogs or rabbits
- Travel in highly endemic areas (N. Carolina, Missouri, Oklahoma, Georgia, Montana, S. Dakota)

Signs & Symptoms
- Fever >40°C and chills (100%), nausea and vomiting (50%), abdominal pain (<50%), diarrhea (<50%), cough (<25%), confusion and stupor (25%)

- Physical Signs: Nonpruritic rash (macular, maculopapular or petechial) beginning 3–5 days after onset of fever, usually around wrists and ankles or trunk. Rash present in 49% at day 3 and 80% day 6. Palm and sole distribution late and uncommon.
- Generalized lymphadenopathy, hepatosplenomegaly
- Neurologic defects (ataxia, seizures, coma, focal defects)
- Arrhythmias, peripheral edema
- Conjunctivitis
- May have evidence of tick bites

TESTS

Laboratory
- Basic Blood Tests
  - Hyponatremia more pronounced than with Colorado tick fever, ehrlichiosis, typhus, tularemia or dengue fever
  - Elevated BUN and Cr
  - Mildly elevated LFTs, especially ALT, alkaline phosphatase
  - Anemia and low platelets
  - Normal WBC with left shift
  - Prolonged PT, PTT

Specific Diagnostic Tests
- Blood cultures to rule out other bacterial etiologies
- Serology: Indirect immunofluorescence is usually negative at presentation, >1:64 by 7–10 days after onset. 94–100% sensitive; 100% specificity.
- Skin biopsy of rash with direct immunofluorescence and immunoperoxidase test: 70% sensitive, 100% specific.

DIFFERENTIAL DIAGNOSIS
- Measles, rubella, typhoid fever, murine typhus, upper respiratory infection, gastroenteritis, enteroviral infection, disseminated gonorrhea, secondary syphilis, rickettsial pox, ehrlichiosis, Lyme disease, leptospirosis, meningococcemia, boutonneuse fever, dengue fever, Colorado tick fever, tularemia, infectious mononucleosis, acute HIV infection, immune complex vasculitis, idiopathic thrombocytopenic purpura, thrombotic, thrombocytopenic purpura, drug reaction

MANAGEMENT

What to Do First
- Must maintain high diagnostic suspicion and treat based on clinical diagnosis

■ Patients with mild disease can be followed as outpatients.
■ Hospitalize moderately ill patients and those with multiple organ involvement.

General Measures
■ Hospitalized patients may require IV hydration and nutrition
   ➤ May need pulmonary-arterial line for hemodynamic monitoring
   ➤ Watch for increased vascular permeability leading to noncardiogenic pulmonary edema.
   ➤ Heparin not recommended
   ➤ Steroids used by some; not proven to be useful

SPECIFIC THERAPY
Indications
■ All patients in whom the disease is suspected should be treated while awaiting serologic confirmation – delay increases mortality.

Treatment Options
■ Doxycycline or Tetracycline 7–10 days
■ Contraindicated in children <9 or in pregnancy
■ Severe disease is treated with same drugs given IV.
■ Alternates: chloramphenicol in 4 divided doses for pregnant women and children <9 yr Ciprofloxacin 7–10 days

FOLLOW-UP
During Treatment
■ Mild disease followed outpatient.
■ Office visits every 2–3 days to follow symptoms
■ Monitor electrolytes, renal function and CBC

COMPLICATIONS AND PROGNOSIS
Complications
■ Managed with standard medical therapy. Thrombosis/vasculitis in multiple organs leads to complications.
■ Heparin not recommended.
   ➤ Azotemia and renal failure
   ➤ Encephalopathy
   ➤ Seizure activity
   ➤ Hepatitis and liver failure
   ➤ Heart failure
   ➤ Respiratory failure

Prognosis
- Mortality ≥25% untreated.
- 5% mortality with treatment, due to delays in diagnosis and treatment.

ROSACEA

JEFFREY P. CALLEN, MD

HISTORY & PHYSICAL

History
- Common condition in adults
- Facial erythema, papules and pustules
- Potentially exacerbated by hot foods, spicy foods, alcohol, and sunlight
- Patients most often with Celtic or Northern European background
- Ocular disease (ocular rosacea) has symptoms of burning or redness of the eyes

Signs & Symptoms
- Erythema and telangiectasia
- Papules and pustules on the central face
- Rare patients develop more fixed swellings known as "phymas," of which the most common is rhinophyma.

TESTS
- Clinical diagnosis
- Biopsy rarely needed

DIFFERENTIAL DIAGNOSIS
- Seborrheic dermatitis
- Acne vulgaris
- Lupus erythematosus
- Contact dermatitis

MANAGEMENT

What to Do First
- Establish a diagnosis

General Measures
- Gentle facial cleansers
- Consider dietary alterations
- Ophthalmologic referral for ocular symptoms

SPECIFIC THERAPY
- Oral antibiotic therapy – tetracycline 500 mg bid, doxycycline 100 mg bid or minocycline 100 mg bid
- Topical metronidazole, azeleic acid, sulfacetamide
- Mild topical corticosteroid combined with precipitated sulfur
- Rhinophyma may be treated surgically.

FOLLOW-UP
- Regular reassessment and alteration of therapy will generally lead to a control of the process.

COMPLICATIONS AND PROGNOSIS
- Phymas are not likely, even in untreated patients.
- Telangiectasia may be treated with lasers.

ROTOR SYNDROME

WILLIAM E. BERQUIST, MD

HISTORY & PHYSICAL
- incidence rare
- inheritance: autosomal recessive
- incidental finding of jaundice

TESTS

Basic Tests
- plasma bilirubin 1–20 mg/dL; usually <7 mg/dL with 60% conjugated
- normal liver enzymes

Specific Diagnostic Tests
- BSP retention abnormal (30–45%) at 45 min
- total urinary coproporphyrin elevated with relative coproporphyrin I increase

DIFFERENTIAL DIAGNOSIS
n/a

MANAGEMENT
- none

SPECIFIC THERAPY
n/a

FOLLOW-UP
n/a

COMPLICATIONS AND PROGNOSIS
- none; excellent prognosis

RSV/RESPIRATORY SYNCYTIAL VIRUS

CAROL A. GLASER, MD

HISTORY & PHYSICAL

History
- 2 major strains of RSV; A + B belong to family Paramyxovirus (large, enveloped RNA virus)
- Humans only source
- Transmission by direct or close contact with contaminated secretions (droplets or fomites)
- Incubation period: 2–8 days
- Viral shedding: 3–8 days, infants may have prolonged shedding
- Virus can persist on environment surface – many hours
- Hospital-acquired infections common
- Re-infection is common
- Winter and early spring

Signs & Symptoms
Severity highest extremes of ages
- preterm infants and/or infants <1 month old:
  - ➤ respiratory signs may be minimal + other symptoms such as lethargy, poor feeding + irritability may be more common
- Older children/ adults – URI

TESTS

Specific:
- DFA tests on respiratory specimens quick, sensitive method
- Viral isolation from nasopharyngeal secretions
- Serology of limited utility

DIFFERENTIAL DIAGNOSIS
n/a

MANAGEMENT
- For hospitalized patients – contact precautions are recommended for duration of illness
- Good hand washing should be emphasized.

SPECIFIC THERAPY
- In uncomplicated case – no treatment needed
- Ribavarin aerosol therapy may be considered for CHD, BPD, cystic fibrosis, and underlying immunodeficiency. Controversial in children; data to suggest that it reduces mortality in adults post BMT.
- RSV-IVIG may also be effective in certain high-risk patients.

FOLLOW-UP
n/a

COMPLICATIONS AND PROGNOSIS
- infants/young children –
  - ➤ important cause bronchiolitis and pneumonia
  - ➤ apnea can occur in preterm and <1-month-old infants
- High severity in infants with CHD, immunodeficiency, underlying pulmonary disease
- Exacerbation of asthma any age group

RUBELLA

CAROL A. GLASER, MD

HISTORY & PHYSICAL

History
- aka "German measles" or 3-day measles
- Togaviridae, RNA virus
- Transmission usually respiratory route, direct contact or droplet (congenital infection also possible)
- Incubation 16–18 days (14–23 days)
- Humans only host
- Maximal communicability: few days BEFORE and 5–7 days after ONSET rash
- Late winter/spring – peak incidence

Signs & Symptoms
- 25–50% infections asymptomatic

- generally mild disease with minimal morbidity and mortality (EXCEPT congenital infections; see complications below)
- lymphadenopathy common – suboccipital/posterior auricular nodes or generalized, precedes rash by 5–10 days
- exanthem appears on face first and spreads centrifugal pattern
- rash is usually erythematous, maculopapular, discrete
- adolescent – facial rash may be confused with acne
- in adult – exanthem frequently pruritic
- rash may NOT be present (up to half may not have rash)
- joint involvement: women more than men (usually athralgic, sometimes arthritis)
- fever variable, mild if present
- occasional features; palatal petechiae, mild pharyngitis, conjunctivitis,
- in utero infection may result in abortion, stillbirth and congenital anomalies

TESTS

Nonspecific:
- Low WBC, thrombocytopenia can occur

Specific:
For postnatal: best method is serology
- Single serum IgM (however note false positive can occur)
- 4-fold or greater change titer IgG
- EIA most available (IFA, CF, III or neutralizing antibody) for acute and/or convalescent titers.
- Viral isolation is possible but not practical – nasal/throat specimens (notify lab that rubella is suspected)
For congenital;
- best method – viral isolation urine and respiratory secretions (feces and CSF may also be suitable specimens)

DIFFERENTIAL DIAGNOSIS
- For postnatal infection;
  - Measles; rash generally more erythematous in measles than rubella
  - Scarlet fever; rash in Scarlet fever often spares the face
  - Infectious mononucleosis (especially when ampicillin is given)
  - Enterovirus; seasonality may be helpful
- For congenital:
  - Other TORCH agents-serology/viral isolation to distinguish

MANAGEMENT
- if pregnant woman exposed – need to check for immune status of rubella immediately and appropriate counseling offered
- Children with postnatal rubella should be excluded from school/DCC for 7 days after onset of rash.
- In hospital settings, patients should be managed under contact isolation precautions.
- Note: infants with congenital rubella syndrome (CRS) shed virus for prolonged period.
- Children are now routinely immunized at 15 months, 4–6 years.
- Presence of rubella virus antibody implies protection against subsequent infection.
- Reportable disease

SPECIFIC THERAPY
- Supportive

FOLLOW-UP
n/a

COMPLICATIONS AND PROGNOSIS

Complications
- Neurologic: encephalitis: 1/5000 cases
- SSPE – similar to measles, occurs years after primary infection
- Myocarditis/pericarditis
- Thrombocytopenia
- Congenital rubella syndrome (CRS) occurs in up to 90% infants born to women who are infected 1st trimester, risks fall 2nd/3rd trimesters
- CRS abnormalities include cataracts, neurosensory deafness, congenital heart disease, thrombocytopenia, hepatitis, encephalitis

---

SALMONELLA INFECTIONS OTHER THAN GASTROENTERITIS

RICHARD A. JACOBS, MD, PhD

HISTORY & PHYSICAL

History
- Salmonellae are a complex group of facultatively anaerobic Gram-negative bacilli that consist of over 2000 serotypes.

- Ubiquitous in nature, found primarily in the gastrointestinal tracts of wild and domestic animals; exceptions are *S. typhi* and *S. paratyphi*, which only colonize humans
- Humans become infected by eating contaminated food (poultry, eggs, ice cream, other dairy products, meat) or by direct contact with infected animals (particularly reptiles).
- Serotypes commonly causing human disease are *S. typhi, S. paratyphi, S. enteritidis, S. typhimurium, S. heidelberg*, and *S. choleraesuis*.

Signs & Symptoms
- Gastroenteritis – see GI section
- Enteric Fever – an illness characterized by systemic and gastrointestinal symptoms that can be caused by any serotype; when caused by S. typhi it is called typhoid fever; when caused by S. paratyphi it is called paratyphoid fever. Incubation period 5–20 days; early in course, there may be a brief period of diarrhea (invasion of mucosa by bacteria) followed by increasing fever, malaise, headache, cough, abdominal pain, constipation and confusion; symptoms peak in 10–14 days. Even without therapy there is slow improvement over the next 2 weeks. Anorexia, weight loss and lassitude can persist for several months and in 10% relapses occur. Physical findings may be minimal, even in the acutely ill patient. Findings include bradycardia (<50%), abdominal tenderness and distention, cervical adenopathy, hepatosplenomegaly (50%) and in 50%,an evanescent, pink, macular rash primarily on the trunk that lasts 3–4 days (rose spots).
- Bacteremia – can be due to any serotype, but S. choleraesuis and S. dublin are the most common; <5% of patients with gastroenteritis develop bacteremia; increased risk in immunocompromised (HIV) and the elderly; presents with prolonged or recurrent fevers
- Localized infections – seeding of any organ system can occur as a result of bacteremia; bone and joint (especially in patients with sickle cell disease), genitourinary, central nervous system and atherosclerotic abdominal aneurysms are the most common sites
- Asymptomatic chronic carrier – defined as presence of salmonella in the stool for >1 year; associated with biliary stones

TESTS
- Enteric fever diagnosed by obtaining positive blood culture; highest yield in first week (70–80%) and by third week only 20% positive; bone marrow aspirate sometimes positive when blood culture negative; stool culture, urine culture and duodenal aspirates also may be

positive; localized infection diagnosed by culturing abscess or tissue of involved organ system

DIFFERENTIAL DIAGNOSIS

- In patients with history of foreign travel, enteric fever may be confused with malaria, yellow fever, dengue and amebiasis; other systemic illnesses such as endocarditis, hepatitis, viral infections may be confused with enteric fever and bacteremia.

MANAGEMENT

- Assess possibility of food-borne outbreak and notify public health officials as indicated.
- Hospitalized patients should be placed on routine barrier precautions if stools positive.

SPECIFIC THERAPY

- Gastroenteritis not treated unless associated with bacteremia
- Increasing resistance of *Salmonella* to ampicillin and trimethoprim-sulfamethoxazole limits the use of these drugs until sensitivities known; empirical therapy with a fluoroquinolone (ciprofloxacin) or a third-generation cephalosporin (ceftriaxone) indicated
- Enteric fever and bacteremia secondary to gastroenteritis treated for 14 days; endovascular infections (endocarditis, infected aneurysm) and osteomyelitis treated for 6 weeks; amoxicillin, trimethoprim-sulfamethoxazole or ciprofloxacin for 4–6 weeks is 80% effective in eradicating the carrier state; in the presence of biliary stones, cholecystectomy in addition to antibiotics often needed to eradicate carrier state

FOLLOW-UP

- Clinical improvement seen within several days of antibiotic therapy

COMPLICATIONS AND PROGNOSIS

- Gastrointestinal hemorrhage most common complication of untreated enteric fever; relapses occur in 10–15%
- Mortality rate <5% in treated cases; higher in elderly and immunocompromised
- Vaccination with an inactivated preparation given parenterally or a live attenuated preparation given orally is available for travelers to high risk areas; efficacy 50–75%; booster doses needed every 2–5 years depending on the preparation used; live attenuated vaccine should not be used in the immunosuppressed
- Chronic carriers should not be employed as food handlers.

SARCOIDOSIS

LAURA L. KOTH, MD

HISTORY & PHYSICAL

History
- Elicit occupational or environmental exposures
- Symptoms vary depending on organs involved
- Hallmark of disease: clinically silent organ involvement with almost 50% of patients asymptomatic
- Fever, fatigue, weight loss (30%)
- Lungs involved (90%); dyspnea, dry cough, chest pain (50%)
- Hemoptysis rare
- Airway hyperreactivity (<20%)

Signs & Symptoms
- Eyes: uveitis, conjunctivitis
- Eye pain, rashes, or joint pain
- Skin: erythema nodosum, lupus pernio
- Lungs: crackles <20% of patients
- Abdomen: 15–20% with splenomegaly, hepatomegaly
- Extremities: clubbing rare; palpable peripheral lymph nodes in 30%
- Neurologic: facial palsies

Common Presentations:
- Acute:
  - Lofgren's syndrome (erythema nodosum, uveitis, hilar adenopathy, +/− migratory arthritis)
  - Heerfordt's syndrome (fever, parotid enlargement, anterior uveitis, facial nerve palsy)
- Subacute:
  - <2 y duration; often spontaneous remission
- Chronic:
  - >2 y duration; often leads to fibrosis in affected organs

TESTS

Laboratory
- Basic Blood Tests
  - Peripheral blood counts: WBC, RBC, platelets
  - Serum chemistries: calcium, liver enzymes (AST, ALT, AP) creatinine, BUN

■ Basic Urine Tests
> 24-h urine calcium indicated when hypercalcemia present

Specific Diagnostic Tests
■ ACE level, pulmonary function tests, spirometry & DLCO, ECG, routine ophthalmologic exam, tuberculin skin test
■ Kveim test used rarely and only in selected centers

Imaging
■ PA CXR useful for prognostic staging:
> Stage 0: normal CXR
> Stage I: bilateral hilar lymphadenopathy (BHL)
> Stage II: BHL plus pulmonary infiltrates
> Stage III: pulmonary infiltrates (without BHL)
> Stage IV: pulmonary fibrosis
■ High-resolution chest CT: helpful when parenchyma appears normal on CXR

Biopsy
■ A biopsy is required for definitive Dx in most cases
■ Choose proper site (lung, lymph node, skin, lip, granulomatous scar; E nodosum biopsy does not show granulomas)
■ If no easily accessible biopsy site, transbronchial biopsy procedure of choice (overall diagnostic yield 85%); other options: mediastinoscopy, VATS, open-lung biopsy

DIFFERENTIAL DIAGNOSIS
■ Conditions to exclude:
> Infections: TB, mycobacteriosis, cryptococcosis, histoplasmosis, coccidiodomycosis, blastomycosis, aspergillosis, P. carinii, mycoplasma
> Occupational & environmental: hypersensitivity pneumonitis, pneumoconiosis (beryllium, titanium, aluminum), drug reactions, aspiration of foreign materials
> Noninfectious: Wegener's granulomatosis, chronic interstitial pneumonia (LIP), necrotizing sarcoid granulomatosis, sarcoid reaction in lymph node to carcinoma

MANAGEMENT
What to Do First
■ Establish baseline studies

General Measures

- Assess extent & severity of organ involvement, whether disease stable or likely to progress & need for treatment

SPECIFIC THERAPY

Indications

- Controversial: many patients undergo remission without specific therapy
- Mild & focal disease (eg, skin lesions, anterior uveitis, cough) may respond to topical steroid therapy
- Systemic disease:
  - ➤ Absolute indications: cardiac or neurosarcoid, eye disease not responding to topical therapy, hypercalcemia
  - ➤ No treatment necessary: asymptomatic stage 0, I or II disease with no objective signs of pulmonary impairment
  - ➤ Less well-defined indications: severe symptoms in any organ, progression of symptoms or worsening pulmonary function

Treatment Options for Systemic Disease

- Treatment of choice: oral prednisone
  - ➤ Most pts require minimal effective dose steroid therapy for several mo, then slow taper to maintenance dose over 6 mo
  - ➤ After clinical response, alternate-day therapy is an option to decrease side effects
  - ➤ Total length of therapy approx 12 mo
  - ➤ Some pts require long-term therapy or increased doses due to relapse
- Second-line therapy: methotrexate, azathioprine, cyclophosphamide, cyclosporine & chloroquine (specialty referral recommended)
  - ➤ Used when oral steroid Rx contraindicated ineffective or as a steroid-sparing measure

Side Effects

- Prednisone: weight gain, osteoporosis, hyperglycemia, cushingoid syndrome, cataracts, avascular necrosis of the hip, peptic ulcer disease, skin fragility, myopathy
- Cyclophosphamide (bladder toxicity) & azathioprine; hematologic, carcinogenic, teratogenic
- Methotrexate: liver & lung toxicity, mucositis, teratogenic
- Chloroquine: retinal toxicity

FOLLOW-UP

During Treatment

- Assess clinical, biochemical and radiologic activity of disease (common markers: hypercalcemia, worsening lung function, liver function tests, ACE, progressive changes on CXR or CT)

COMPLICATIONS AND PROGNOSIS

Complications

- Blindness, pulmonary fibrosis, upper lung cavitations with mycetoma, cardiac involvement leading to arrhythmias, sudden death, CHF

Prognosis

- CXR stage as prognostic guide:
  - ➤ Stage I: remission of 55–90% of patients
  - ➤ Stage II: remission 40–70%
  - ➤ Stage III: remission 10–20%
  - ➤ Stage IV: remission 0%
  - ➤ Lofgren's syndrome: 90% remission
- >85% of spontaneous remissions occur within 2 y of presentation
- 10-fold increase in mortality with cardiac or neurosarcoid

SCABIES

KAREN GOULD, MD

HISTORY & PHYSICAL

History

- close household contacts or sexual partners
- clinical manifestations delayed 3–4 weeks after first exposure
  - ➤ symptoms appear earlier with subsequent infestations
- epidemics seen in nursing homes, hospitals

Signs & Symptoms

- pruritic eruption with excoriations
- pruritus worse at night
- lesions often bilateral, usually involving finger web spaces, wrists, penis
- linear burrows and small erythematous papules seen

- children with involvement of head, face, and scalp
  - ➤ crusted (Norwegian) scabies in immunocompromised, debilitated patients, or patients with neurologic disease
    - increased number of mites

TESTS

Basic Microscopic Tests
- skin scrapings or curettage of burrows or papules
- glass slide with drop of mineral oil and cover slip
- specimen examined under low power
- identification of mites, eggs, or fecal pellet

Biopsy
- identification of mites, eggs, or feces

DIFFERENTIAL DIAGNOSIS
- any pruritic dermatosis – atopic dermatitis, papular urticaria, insect bites, dermatitis herpetiformis

MANAGEMENT

General Measures
- treat all close symptomatic contacts
- launder all linens in hot water
- treat pruritus symptomatically with antihistamines
- symptoms may take 4–5 weeks to resolve after appropriate treatment

SPECIFIC THERAPY

Treatment Options
- permethrin 5% cream
  - ➤ entire cutaneous surface neck down (immunocompetent)
  - ➤ entire surface of body with scalp and face (immunosuppressed)
  - ➤ apply evening, wash off in AM
  - ➤ repeat 1 week
  - ➤ most effective topical treatment
- lindane 1% cream, lotion, or shampoo (Kwell)
  - ➤ apply for 8 hours, then wash off
  - ➤ entire cutaneous surface with scalp and face for immunosuppressed, without scalp and face for immunocompetent patients
  - ➤ repeat in 1 week
  - ➤ CNS side effects
- sulfur ointment 6–10%

➤ apply nightly for 3 consecutive nights
➤ wash off 24 hours after last application
➤ messy, odor, not as effective
- crotamiton cream and lotion
  ➤ two daily applications
  ➤ not very effective
- ivermectin tablets
  ➤ repeat 1 week

FOLLOW-UP

Routine
- if symptomatic, microscopic re-examination
- re-assess symptoms in 6 weeks

COMPLICATIONS AND PROGNOSIS
- secondary bacterial infection
- eczematous symptoms even after scabies eradicated
- prognosis is excellent

SCHISTOSOMIASIS

J. GORDON FRIERSON, MD

HISTORY & PHYSICAL

History
- Causative agents are Schistosoma mansoni, Schistosoma hematobium, Schistosoma japonicum.
  ➤ Life cycle: *S hematobium* adults live in venules around the bladder, *S mansoni* in venules around lower colon and rectum (inferior mesenteric plexus), and *S japonicum* in venules around the superior and inferior mesenteric plexus. Eggs pass out in either the urine or stool, depending on worm location, and hatch in fresh water into miracidia, which penetrate snails. Multiplication occurs and cercariae emerge as infective larval form. These penetrate skin and go via the circulation to the lungs, then to the portal circulation. After mating, the females move to the vesical, superior or inferior mesenteric plexus (dependant on species), where they lay eggs and start a new cycle. *S hematobium* found in tropical Africa and Egypt, S mansoni in tropical Africa, Egypt and parts of middle East, and South America, and *S japonicum* in

China, Philippines, Indonesia. *S mekongi* is variant of *S japonicum* found in Mekong Delta.

➤ Exposure: skin exposure to fresh water contaminated with cercariae through swimming, wading, rafting. Drinking water not established as mode of infection.

Signs & Symptoms

■ Dermal phase: penetration of cercariae causes an allergic dermatitis, called "swimmer's itch", at areas of exposed skin. Also seen with exposure to non-human (usually bird) schistosomes. Reaction to first exposure is mild, more severe to second.

■ Katayama fever: seen in heavy infections 5–7 weeks after exposure, after pulmonary phase but before eggs seen. Fever, chills, nausea, vomiting, diarrhea, abdominal pain, urticaria, cough, headache may be present in varying degrees. Signs include fever, tachycardia, urticaria, hepatosplenomegaly, lymphadenopathy, eosinophilia, elevated IgE.

■ Chronic phase: In *S hematobium* there is microscopic or gross hematuria, sometimes urgency, and in later stages symptoms due to ureteral obstruction or secondary urinary tract infection, often with salmonella. In *S mansoni* there is chronic abdominal discomfort or pain, low-grade diarrhea, sometimes passage of blood. In *S japonicum* symptoms are similar but may be more severe. All forms can develop portal hypertension, resulting in hematemesis, hepatosplenomegaly, dilated abdominal veins.

TESTS

■ Basic tests: blood: CBC shows eosinophilia, marked in Katayama syndrome, moderate in chronic phase. Also mild anemia. LFTs frequently mildly abnormal in both stages.

■ Basic tests: urine: hematuria in *S hematobium*. Sometimes proteinuria.

■ Specific tests: centrifuged urine collected between 10 AM and 3 PM (when egg emergence is at maximum) shows *S hematobium*. Stool O&P shows S mansoni and japonicum.

■ Serology becomes positive at 2–3 months, done at CDC by FAST-ELISA and immunoblot techniques – very sensitive and species specific.

■ Other tests: *S hematobium*: X-rays can show urinary tract deformity or obstruction. *S mansoni and japonicum*: barium enema can show polypoid changes in colon, irritability, and biopsy through sigmoidoscope can show eggs. Chest X-ray in Katayama syndrome may show scattered infiltrates, and in late stage of all 3 types may show fibrosis and pulmonary hypertension.

➤ Ultrasound shows signs of portal hypertension and periportal fibrosis. Liver biopsy can show eggs in all 3 types.

➤ Blood assay for schistosoma antigen available as research tool.

DIFFERENTIAL DIAGNOSIS

■ Cercarial dermatitis resembles other irritative and allergic dermatoses. Sharp delimitation at borders of water exposure characterize it.

■ Katayama syndrome confused with invasive stage of roundworms (hookworm, ascaris, strongyloides) and serum sickness.

■ Chronic stage: *S hematobium* confused with other bladder pathologies, including cancer. *S mansoni* and *japonicum* confused with other helminthic infections, amebiasis, ulcerative colitis, carcinoma of colon. Hepatosplenic stage confused with other causes of portal hypertension: chronic hepatitis B or C, cirrhosis of any type. These conditions can co-exist.

MANAGEMENT

What to Do First

■ Cercarial dermatitis: assess severity.

■ Katayama syndrome: assess need for hospitalization, fluids.

■ Chronic stage: assess for signs of portal hypertension and possible hemorrhage. In *S hematobium* assess for secondary urine infection.

General Measures

■ Fluids, transfusions as needed

SPECIFIC THERAPY

Indications

■ Probably all patients should be treated.

Treatment Options

■ Praziquantel for 1 day. This is drug of choice.

■ Oxamniquine once; give after a meal (less efficacious treatment, difficult to obtain)

Side Effects & Complications

■ Praziquantel: nausea, vomiting, abdominal pain, diarrhea may occur, usually in heavily infected patients, seldom in lightly infected. Headache, dizziness of mild degree, sometimes.

- Oxamniquine: drowsiness and dizziness (in up to 15%), and mild fever on day 3–4 after administration (probably due to worm death)
- Contraindications to treatment: absolute: first-trimester pregnancy, patients clinically unstable (such as hemorrhage, sepsis, etc.)
- Contraindications to treatment: relative: lesser degrees of instability (such as recent surgery, etc.)

FOLLOW-UP

During Treatment
- Katayama syndrome: Observation, stabilization
  - ➢ Chronic phase: little needed

Routine
- Chronic phase: Check urine or stool for O&P 3 months or more after treatment, and request assessment for viability of eggs found. In later stages, reassessment of portal fibrosis with ultrasound.

COMPLICATIONS AND PROGNOSIS

- Portal hypertension: low degree of reversibility with chemotherapy. May require shunting procedure to prevent recurrent bleeding.
- Genitourinary disease: Ureteral obstruction often reverses with chemotherapy, and bacteriuria responds better after worm therapy. Calcification and carcinoma of bladder occur in chronic hematobium. Granulomas, fibrotic lesions common in female genitalia, less in male, generally treated with excision.
- Pulmonary disease: presents as cor pulmonale, and some fibrosis, mainly around arterioles. Not usually reversible.
- CNS disease: *S japonicum* (2–4% of cases) or *hematobium* (infrequent) eggs may be in brain, causing seizures or mass effect. Diagnosed on CT or MRI in appropriate patient. Treated with praziquantel and often steroids.
- *S mansoni* eggs may occur in spinal cord, usually low, causing paraplegia, usually seen early in infection. Diagnosed by seeing swelling on MRI in patient with known disease, or at surgery. Treated with steroids and praziquantel.
- Salmonella-schistosome syndrome: chronic salmonella bacteremia can occur in all 3 schistosome infections, apparently due to salmonella attached to cuticle of adult worms. Presents as chronic fatigue, fever, weight loss, seldom acutely ill. Chronic salmonella urinary infection may co-exist in *S hematobium*. Responds to treatment of schistosomiasis and antibiotics.
- Ectopic eggs and worms can be found almost anywhere, responding to local excision or chemotherapy.

SCLERODERMA

GEORGE MOXLEY, MD

HISTORY & PHYSICAL

History

- Systemic sclerosis in two forms
  - ➤ Diffuse scleroderma
  - ➤ CREST syndrome (calcinosis, Raynaud's, esophageal dysmotility, sclerodactyly, telangiectasia)
- Possible association w/ exposure to silica dusts, organic solvents (vinyl chloride). Epidemiologic evidence shows no association w/ silicone breast implants.
- Localized scleroderma (morphea, linear scleroderma) – involves only skin, subcutaneous tissue & muscle. No Raynaud's or systemic disease.

Signs & Symptoms

- Raynaud's phenomenon (finger pain & numbness upon exposure to cold or stress, w/ two or three shades of discoloration [red, white, purplish]) is hallmark & usually first symptom. Raynaud's w/o underlying disease also extremely common. Associated w/ exposure to bleomycin, ergot alkaloids, beta blockers, methysergide, vinyl chloride, vibrating tools. Sometimes leads to digital ulcers or gangrene. 13% of pts w/ Raynaud's eventually develop an inflammatory rheumatic disease.
- Skin hypopigmentation over clavicular areas, hyperpigmentation over distal arms
- Subcutaneous hard nodules around joint capsules (calcinosis, subcutaneous calcific deposits)
- Reflux esophagitis (due to esophageal dilatation & hypomotility)
- Contracted tight thickened skin–sclerodactyly in fingers, also forearms, face, trunk. Pursed mouth, reduced oral aperture so gap between upper & lower teeth <2 cm.
- Telangiectasias on lips, face, hands
- Joint pain & stiffness (mild inflammatory arthropathy). Sometimes friction rubs of tendons within tendon sheaths.
- Resorption of terminal phalanges & overlying digital soft tissue
- Fatigue, simple myopathy or inflammatory myositis w/ weakness
- Dry mouth & dry eyes (Sjogren's syndrome)

- Bloating & emesis due to intestinal paresis, wide-mouthed colonic diverticula, malabsorption due to intestinal bacterial overgrowth
- Dyspnea from isolated pulmonary hypertension (CREST syndrome), interstitial pulmonary fibrosis, alveolitis, heart failure due to myocardial fibrosis
- Chest pain & angina (myocardial infarctions w/o coronary artery disease), pericarditis w/arrhythmias & effusions
- Hypertension, mild proteinuria, scleroderma renal crisis
- Numbness due to neuropathies, facial pain & numbness due to trigeminal neuralgia

TESTS

Basic Tests
- Assess end-organ involvement through CBC, serum creatinine, urinalysis

Specific Diagnostic Tests
- Antinuclear antibody (ANA) positive in >85%, typically nucleolar pattern. Specificities included antibodies against topoisomerase Scl-70, centromere, RNA polymerases I & III, fibrillarin, nucleolus organizer region protein. Sensitivity approx. 20–40%, specificity 95+%.
- Anticentromere ANAs w/CREST syndrome
- Anti-ribonucleoprotein w/diffuse & limited scleroderma

Other Tests as Appropriate
- Pulmonary function tests (PFTs) including lung volumes & diffusing capacity, possibly high-resolution CT scan to detect inflammatory alveolitis (ground-glass appearance)

DIFFERENTIAL DIAGNOSIS
- Raynaud's phenomenon alone, due to exposures listed above, or w/SLE or other inflammatory rheumatic disease
- Finger contractures w/longstanding poorly controlled diabetes (cheiropathy)

MANAGEMENT

What to Do First
- Check blood pressure & obtain blood tests for end-organ involvement
- Teach pt about potentially serious but treatable hypertension, lung & GI problems
- Consult rheumatologist

SPECIFIC THERAPY

- No specific treatment available. Treat the complications.
- Hypertension: invariably high renin; treat w/ACE inhibitors or angiotensin receptor blockers
- Pulmonary hypertension: oxygen therapy as indicated; endothelin receptor antagonist bosentan
- Alveolitis: life-threatening & potentially controllable w/oral cyclophosphamide & low-dose daily corticosteroids. Adverse reactions include serious bacterial, viral & opportunistic infections, hemorrhagic cystitis, transitional cell malignancies, lymphoproliferative disorders, suppression of gonadal function/infertility
- Esophageal dysfunction: proton pump inhibitor, elevate head of bed on masonry blocks, esophageal dilatation for strictures
- GI dysmotility: frequent small meals, metoclopramide, antibiotics for bacterial overgrowth
- Arthritis: analgesics & NSAIDs (selective COX-2 inhibitors for pts w/esophageal disease)
- Raynaud's: Avoid cold exposure. Stop smoking. Avoid vasoconstrictive agents (decongestants, caffeine, beta blockers, ergot alkaloids, amphetamines). Calcium channel blockers & sildenafil are both effective. For severe Raynaud's, sympathectomy.
- Digital ulcerations: topical or oral antibiotics as necessary for infections
- Sjogren's: methylcellulose eye drops, frequent dental prophylaxis, ophthalmic lubricants, lacrimal duct plugging–consult ophthalmologist

FOLLOW-UP

During Treatment

- Attain BP control <130/80, evaluate end-organ function through blood & urine tests
- PFTs w/lung volumes & diffusing capacity for carbon monoxide, resting & exercise ABGs
- Some recommend semiannual or annual 2-D echocardiogram to detect pulmonary hypertension

Routine

- Monitor BP daily if hypertensive, periodically if normal

COMPLICATIONS & PROGNOSIS

- Renal crisis, now uncommon, includes malignant hypertension, microangiopathic hemolytic anemia, oliguric renal failure. Consult nephrologist, control BP w/ACE inhibitors, dialyze if necessary. Pt may partially recover renal function after dialysis.

- Pulmonary: 10% of CREST pts develop severe pulmonary hypertension, 5-year survival <10%. Alveolitis & interstitial fibrosis in 45–75%, 5-year survival 45%. For cyclophosphamide therapy, consult rheumatologist for follow-up. Check blood counts frequently & adjust dose to achieve WBC 3.5–4.5, monitor urine for hematuria.
- Myocardial involvement 20–25%, pericardial 5–16%. Treat w/heart failure agents, anti-arrhythmic agents.
- Trigeminal neuralgia: analgesics, agents for neuropathic pain
- Barrett's esophagus, esophageal cancer, candidal esophagitis
- Pneumatosis intestinalis: gas dissection into abdominal wall, may burst into abdominal cavity, simulating perforated viscus
- Lung malignancy
- Mortality higher in diffuse disease, older onset age, pulmonary & renal involvement

SEBORRHEIC DERMATITIS

J. MARK JACKSON, MD

HISTORY & PHYSICAL
- History: scaly itchy patches, most often on scalp, central face, in and behind ears, may also be in central chest
- Physical-red, "greasy" scaly patches in scalp, mid face, nasal creases, in and behind ears, mid chest, and occasionally genital area (esp. glans penis)

TESTS
- Usually none
- Consider HIV testing in young adults with new onset or severe seborrhea.

DIFFERENTIAL DIAGNOSIS
- Psoriasis
- Lupus erythematosus
- Dermatomyositis
- Rosacea/perioral dermatitis
Contact dermatitis

MANAGEMENT
What to Do First
- Mild topical corticosteroids (Class 6 or 7) or the topical calcineurin inhibitors tacrolimus and pimecrolimus

➤ dandruff shampoos with ketoconazole, ciclopirox, or selenium sulfide

SPECIFIC THERAPY

- Mild topical corticosteroids (class 6 or 7) or the topical calcineurin inhibitors or antifungal creams
- Scalp involvement, use selenium sulfide, ketoconazole, cyclopirox or zinc shampoo; if severe in scalp, mid- to high-potency topical corticosteroid solution
- If severe facial involvement, use a mid-potency nonfluorinated topical steroid (Class 4 or 5) <7 days, then taper back to the milder forms
- Refractory cases may try oral azole antifungals

FOLLOW-UP

- Follow up for improvement and side effects

COMPLICATIONS AND PROGNOSIS

n/a

SEBORRHEIC KERATOSIS

JEFFREY P. CALLEN, MD

HISTORY & PHYSICAL

History

- Asymptomatic lesions
- Symptoms may occur from irritation from clothing or jewelry.
- Solitary lesions are less common than multiple lesions.

Signs & Symptoms

- Flat or elevated lesions
- Verrucous surface
- Sharply marginated
- "Stuck-on" appearance
- Small, multiple facial lesions in patients of color are known as dermatosis papulosa nigra.

TESTS

- None needed

DIFFERENTIAL DIAGNOSIS

- Warts

■ Melanoma
■ Squamous cell carcinoma

MANAGEMENT

What to Do First
■ Establish a diagnosis
■ Further treatment is needed only if the diagnosis is in question or if the lesion is symptomatic.

SPECIFIC THERAPY
■ Removal or destruction of symptomatic lesions

FOLLOW-UP
■ None

COMPLICATIONS AND PROGNOSIS
■ None

SELENIUM DEFCIENCY

ELISABETH RYZEN, MD

HISTORY AND PHYSICAL
Deficiency rare in humans; Keshan disease in China where selenium intake very low (cardiomyopathy symptoms), long-term TPN may cause, with muscle pain and tenderness

Tests/ DDx/Mgt/Specific Therapy/FU/Comps & Prognosis
N/A

SEVERE ACUTE RESPIRATORY SYNDROME

SUSAN PHILIP, MD, MPH

HISTORY & PHYSICAL

History
NOTE: NO reported cases since 2004. Please see CDC or WHO websites for most current epidemiology and advisories.

Epidemiology: Reported from Guangdong Province in China, Hong Kong, SE Asia and Canada. Major epidemic ended 2003, last lab related outbreaks in 2004.

- Exposure; Travel to affected area. Healthcare workers and those in contact with infected individuals. Adults infected more than children. Spread person to person via droplets.

Etiology: novel coronavirus (SARS CoV) isolated.

Incubation: 2–7 days before symptoms

Signs & Symptoms

Two stage: prodrome – fever, malaise, myalgias, can have diarrhea
Respiratory phase (begins in 3–7 days) – nonproductive cough, dyspnea and can have progressive respiratory distress.

- WHO case definition: Suspected case
  - ➤ Fever >38.0 AND
  - ➤ Cough or respiratory distress AND
  - ➤ Close contact with known patient with SARS or travel to area of known transmission in previous 10 days.
- Probable case:
  - ➤ CXR suggesting pneumonia or acute respiratory distress syndrome (ARDS) OR
  - ➤ Suspected case positive in one or more lab assays for SARS OR
  - ➤ Suspected case who dies of severe respiratory illness of unknown cause and pathology consistent with ARDS.

TESTS

- Basic tests: blood: lymphopenia may be present, LFTs and CK may be elevated.
- Radiology: CXR can range from normal to diffuse interstitial infiltrates of ARDS or focal consolidation. CT may reveal abnormalities with normal CXR.
- Pathology: diffuse alveolar damage
- Serology: ELISA may be available from CDC. IgG usually present, but may not be in early disease.
- Other tests: PCR in development, but not currently standardized.

DIFFERENTIAL DIAGNOSIS

Other treatable bacterial or viral causes of severe pneumonia must be considered.

MANAGEMENT

What to Do First

- Assess severity and whether suspected case

General measures
Admit to isolation in negative pressure room, contact precautions and N95 masks on entering. Prepare for full respiratory support, seek consultation with infectious diseases and CDC

SPECIFIC THERAPY
Treatment Options
- No specific treatment available. Ribavirin shown to be of no benefit.

FOLLOW-UP
- Supportive care as needed

COMPLICATIONS AND PROGNOSIS
- High morbidity and mortality. Worse prognosis with age, comorbid conditions, elevated LDH on admission, atypical symptoms.

SEX DIFFERENTIATION DISORDERS

KIRK NEELY, MD

HISTORY & PHYSICAL
History
- Exposure to androgens or teratogens
- Family history of genital ambiguity, hypospadias, delayed puberty
- Delayed puberty:
  - Females: no breast tissue by age 13 y
  - Males: no testicular enlargement by age 14 y
- Amenorrhea, virilization, infertility
  - Primary amenorrhea: no menarche by age 16 y
  - Secondary amenorrhea: fewer than 2 menstrual cycles/y after normal menses

Signs & Symptoms
- Ambiguity of external genitalia:
  - Incomplete or excessive midline fusion from fetal androgen exposure
  - Inappropriate phallic size
- Virilized female:
  - Complete labial fusion or posterior fusion
  - Single urogenital orifice
  - Clitoromegaly
  - Labioscrotal rugation, pigmentation

- Undervirilized male:
  - Bifid scrotum
  - Micropenis
  - Hypospadias
- Cryptorchidism:
  - Usually w/o genital ambiguity
  - Idiopathic, syndromal, or with hypopituitarism
  - Common at birth, resolving by 3 mo

TESTS

Laboratory
- Blood tests for partial virilization:
  - Karyotype for sex chromosomes
  - LH, FSH
  - Sex steroids: virilized female:
    - 17-hydroxyprogesterone
    - DHEA
    - Androstenedione
    - Testosterone
  - Sex steroids: undervirilized male:
    - Testosterone
    - Dihydrotestosterone
    - Testosterone precursors
    - Antimullerian hormone
- Delayed puberty:
  - T4, TSH
  - Prolactin
  - Estradiol or testosterone
LH, FSH; if elevated, karyotype

Imaging
- MRI of hypothalamus/pituitary
- Pelvic/abdominal US

DIFFERENTIAL DIAGNOSIS
- Undervirilized male:
  - Phenotype:
    - 46,XY with normal testes
    - External genitalia undervirilized
  - Internal genitalia normal
  - Dysmorphology syndromes

➤ Leydig cell agenesis
➤ Defects in testosterone biosynthesis:
  • External genitalia range from female to ambiguous
  • Some virilization at puberty from androgen precursors
  • Responds to testosterone
➤ 5-alpha-reductase deficiency:
  • Failed conversion of T to more potent DHT
  • Decreased body and facial hair, no balding, small prostate
  • Poor response to testosterone injections
  • Some masculinization at puberty with changes in gender identity

■ Androgen insensitivity:
  ➤ Complete form:
    • Breast development at puberty, amenorrhea
    • Pubic, axillary hair sparse
    • Testes in inguinal hernia
    • Gonadectomy indicated
    • Normal female external genitalia with blind vagina
    • Uterus, cervix, upper vagina, fallopian tubes absent
  ➤ Incomplete forms present with genital ambiguity, infertility
■ Virilized female:
  ➤ 46,XX with normal ovaries and mullerian structures
  ➤ Ambiguous external genitalia from androgen exposure in utero
  ➤ Placental aromatase deficiency
  ➤ Virilizing adrenal or ovarian tumor
  ➤ Congenital adrenal hyperplasia (CAH)
  ➤ 21-hydoxylase deficiency most common
  ➤ Classical CAH:
  ➤ Presents in neonate
    • Genital ambiguity in females
    • Decreased cortisol in all
    • In salt losers: Hyponatremia, hyperkalemia, hyperreninemia, hypoaldosteronism
      • Elevated serum 17-hydroxyprogesterone (17-OHP)
  ➤ Nonclassical CAH:
    • Presents later
    • Progressive virilization: acne, hirsutism, clitoromegaly
    • Menstrual disorder
■ Gonadal dysgenesis:
  ➤ True hermaphroditism:
    • Both ovary and testis

- Ambiguous external genitalia
- Internal genitalia may be asymmetric
- Most often 46,XX
- Further virilization at puberty
- Mixed gonadal dysgenesis: 45,X/46,XY
- Turner syndrome:
  - 45,X, but usually mosaicism
  - Fetal and neonatal lymphedema
  - Streak gonads, primary amenorrhea
  - Osteopenia from lack of estrogen
  - Short stature responds to growth hormone
  - Aortic coarctation and aortic valve defects
  - Renal anomalies
  - Hearing loss
- Klinefelter syndrome:
  - 47,XXY
  - Normal masculinization
  - Small testes, infertility
  - Testosterone slightly low
  - Mild developmental delay, learning disorders
  - Tall stature, gynecomastia

MANAGEMENT

- Surgical management of genital ambiguity controversial
  - Females:
    - Clitoral recession in infancy
    - Vaginoplasty at puberty
  - Males:
    - Early repair of incomplete midline and hypospadias
    - Testosterone therapy
    - Female sex of rearing in complete androgen insensitivity
  - Gonadectomy in gonadal dysgenesis due to tumor risk:
    - If Y chromosome or testis present in female
    - Monitor descended testes in male
  - Cryptorchidism:
    - Orchiopexy in early childhood to reduce risk of tumor, infertility
- Sex steroid replacement:
  - Males: testosterone (injection, patch, gel)
  - Females:
    - Estrogen alone initially; then cycle with progestin after 1–2 y
    - Alternative: oral contraceptives

- Maintenance medications in CAH:
  - Hydrocortisone: monitor 17-OHP, testosterone
  - Mineralocorticoids for salt losers: fludrocortisone; monitor plasma renin activity and BP

SPECIFIC THERAPY
n/a

FOLLOW-UP
n/a

COMPLICATIONS AND PROGNOSIS
n/a

SHOCK

THOMAS SHAUGHNESSY, MD

HISTORY & PHYSICAL

History
- Hypoperfusion resulting in inadequate oxygen delivery to vital organs
- Hypovolemia – dehydration, hemorrhage
- Cardiogenic – myocardial infarction, cardiomyopathy
- Septic – endotoxemia, abscess +/– drainage
- Neurogenic – cervical spinal cord lesion

Signs & Symptoms
- Oliguria, altered mental status, tachypnea, pallor, tachycardia
- Hypovolemic, Cardiogenic:
  - Cold, clammy, diaphoretic decreased pulse pressure (SBP-DBP) and capillary refill
- Septic, Neurogenic:
  - Bounding pulse, dry skin, increased pulse pressure

TESTS
- Shock is predominately diagnosed by clinical observations

Laboratory
- Basic Studies:
  - Anion Gap $(Na - [Cl + HCO_3])$
    - Normal: 13–15 mEq/L

> Lactate Level >2 mEq/L
  - Most accurate marker of shock; consider empiric therapy if laboratory turnaround >1 hr

- Advanced Studies:
  > A-VDO$_2$ >5 ml/dl
    - requires PA catheter; may be normal in sepsis
    - Mixed Venous O$_2$ <70%
  > requires PA catheter; may be normal in sepsis
- Urine:
  > Fractional Excretion Sodium <1%
  > (UNa × PCr)/(UCr × PNa) ×100
  > Urine Sodium <20 mEq/ml (hypovolemia)
- Other Tests:
  > ECG – signs of ischemia, MI
  > Cardiac Output – PA catheter, Echocardiography

DIFFERENTIAL DIAGNOSIS

Hypovolemic vs Cardiogenic

- Hypovolemia: Low PCWP, inadequate RA or LV filling on echocardiography
- Cardiogenic: ECG changes, hypodynamic LV on echo, increased troponin, CPK, adequate PCWP

Septic vs Neurogenic

- Septic: Fever, leukocytosis, bacteremia, normal mixed venous O$_2$, AVDO$_2$
- Neurogenic: Acute spinal trauma

MANAGEMENT

What to Do First:

- Secure airway: Endotracheal intubation if mentally altered
- Institute respiratory support: bag-valve or mechanical ventilation
  > Caution: Positive pressure will exacerbate hypotension
  > Continuous monitoring with arterial catheter is recommended
- Augment preload: Fluid Challenge: 20 cc/kg crystalloid, 10 cc/kg colloid
- Raise systemic perfusion pressure: Dopamine, phenylepherine, epinepherine, norepinepherine
- Caution: Dobutamine may exacerbate hypotension

General Measures

■ Prompt resuscitation to avoid end organ damage (renal failure, hypoxic encephalopathy, ARDS, MI, ischemic colitis)

■ Monitor in intensive care setting

■ If hypotension fails to improve after two acute fluid challenges, hypovolemia is unlikely; consider inotropes

■ Consider vasopressors when patient has a marked tachycardia

■ No vasoactive agent is superior in shock. Choice should be guided by side effect profile of agent

SPECIFIC THERAPY

Indications

■ Institute therapy upon diagnosis while etiology is sought

Treatment Options

■ Fluids

➤ *Crystalloids* (Lactated Ringers, 0.9% NaCl, 3% NaCl)

  • Most studies show no significant difference between colloid and crystalloid resuscitation

➤ *Colloid* (Albumin, Hetastarch, Fresh Frozen Plasma)

  • Certain outcome parameters support use of Hetastarch

  • FFP should only be used if coagulopathy is present

➤ *Packed RBC*

  • Outcome is unaffected if Hgb >7 gm/dl

■ Vasopressors: Phenylepherine, Vasopressin

➤ Emerging literature support use of Vasopressin in ACLS protocols

■ Inotropes: (ephedrine, dopamine, epinephrine, norepinephrine, dobutamine)

Other

■ *Cardiogenic:*

➤ Intraaortic Balloon Pump: Indicated for cardiogenic shock unresponsive to pharmacologic therapy

■ *Neurogenic:*

➤ Naloxone; Steroids for acute spinal cord trauma as neuroprotective agents

■ *Septic:*

➤ Panculture

➤ Cytokine inhibitors have not proven effective

➤ Initiate broad spectrum antibiotic therapy

- *Hypovolemic*:
  - ➤ Investigate and control all possible sources of hemorrhage Consider NG lavage

Side Effects & Complications
- Fluids
  - ➤ Crystalloids: NaCl associated with hyperchloremic metabolic acidosis and coagulopathy
  - ➤ Albumin: Expensive; beneficial for preexisting hypoalbuminemic states (ESLD, malnutrition)
  - ➤ PRBC, FFP: Blood-borne disease transmission; transfusion reaction
- Vasopressors: Splanchnic ischemia when hypovolemia uncorrected
- Inotropes: Increased myocardial oxygen consumption, similar risk profile to vasopressors
- Balloon Pump: gas embolization, limb ischemia

Contraindications
- Absolute:
  - ➤ Balloon Pump: Aortic regurgitation, femoral vascular disease, atrial fibrillation, aortic vascular disease
- Relative:
  - ➤ Fluids: Pulmonary edema, CHF
  - ➤ Vasopressors: Persistent hypovolemia
  - ➤ Inotropes: Tachycardia, ventricular arrhythmia.
    - Myocardial ischemia may resolve with enhanced inotropy and systemic perfusion. Consider therapeutic trial to treat myocardial ischemia

FOLLOW-UP

During Treatment
- Monitor serial lactate level and anion gap
- Monitor hypotension
- Administer fluids until CVP or PA pressures are adequate
- Increased A-aDO$_2$ (onset of pulmonary edema) may indicate optimization of ventricular filling. Consider inotropes to further enhance CO
- Monitor CO; titrate fluid and vasoactive agent to achieve Cardiac Index of 2.0 L/min/m^2

Routine
- Monitor Urine Output, serum creatinine
- Address etiology of hypoperfusion

COMPLICATIONS AND PROGNOSIS
- Renal failure: 2 days -2 weeks; may be permanent
- Hypoxic encephalopathy: may manifest as focal or global event
- Likelihood increased in the presence of CNS vascular disease
- ARDS: Typically 1 week -1 month; 50% mortality mostly secondary to Multiple Organ Failure Syndrome
- MI: Extent and prognosis depends on preexisting CAD.
- Ischemic colitis: Associated with prolonged hypotension
  - May result in acalculous cholecystitis, pancreatitis, or mesenteric infarction
  - Mortality from these events as a result of shock is >90%

SHORT BOWEL SYNDROME

GARY M. GRAY, MD

HISTORY & PHYSICAL

History
- Weight loss
- Watery, bulky stools containing undigested food
- Malnutrition
- Conditions that result in insufficient small intestinal mucosa for adequate nutrition:
  - neonatal congenital anomalies (intestinal atresia, gastroschisis)
  - necrotizing enterocolitis
  - volvulus
  - trauma
  - extensive enteropathy (especially Crohn's disease)
  - mesenteric vascular ischemia
  - collagen vascular disease (especially periarteritis nodosa)

Physical
- Smooth, red tongue
- Cracking at mouth corners
- Pitting edema of lower extremities
- Mental slowness

TESTS

Basic Blood
- Anemia (iron deficiency, folate/vitamin B_{12} deficiency)
- Hypoalbuminemia (albumin often <2.5 gm/dl)

Basic Urine
- Usually normal

Specific Diagnostic
- Small intestine by barium contrast X-ray usually less than 25% of the normal length; not infrequently 10% of the normal length
- Functional tests of malabsorption: quantitative fecal fat (72-hour) elevated; xylose absorption reduced (25 gm ingested; 5-hour urine excretion)

DIFFERENTIAL DIAGNOSIS
- Maldigestion due to primary enteric diseases (especially celiac sprue, hypogammaglobulinemia, tropical sprue, Whipple's disease); pancreatic insufficiency (chronic pancreatitis; fecal fat elevated but xylose absorption normal) or pancreatic duct obstruction (pancreatic carcinoma)

MANAGEMENT

What to Do First
- Confirm short bowel syndrome by history, barium studies and functional tests of malabsorption

General Measures
- Increased caloric intake to tolerance with high protein diet; 4000 cal/day may be required, if tolerated
- High protein diet, nutritional supplements
- Add vitamin supplements (multivitamins, folic acid, fat-soluble vitamins [A,D,E]) and mineral supplements (especially magnesium, calcium)

SPECIFIC THERAPY
- Total parenteral nutrition (TPN) if enteric nutrition is insufficient to maintain normal body weight and nutrition
- If TPN cannot be maintained (vascular access, liver dysfunction), consider small intestinal (or intestinal plus hepatic) transplantation
- Parenteral epidermal growth factor (EGF), growth hormone (GH), glucacon-like peptides, interleukin-11 (IR-11), and glutamine (oral or parenteral) have been proposed to enhance intestinal adaptation and consequent nutrient assimilation; more studies needed to establish their effectiveness

FOLLOW-UP

■ Weekly body weights, monthly examinations, nutritional assessment to include vitamin assays [(B12), folate, vitamins A, D, and prothrombin time (INR)], magnesium, calcium

COMPLICATIONS AND PROGNOSIS

■ Varies with underlying disease with potential of recurrence (Crohn's, intestinal ischemia, collagen vascular disease)

SICKLE CELL SYNDROMES

ORAH S. PLATT, MD

HISTORY & PHYSICAL

History

■ Family history of sickle syndrome (common syndromes include sickle trait, disease, SC disease, sickle cell anemia, S/thalassemia)
■ Most states in the US screen newborns for homozygous disease (SS = sickle cell anemia)
■ History of anemia – no anemia in sickle trait, no or mild anemia in SC disease and some patients with S/thalassemia
■ History of pain crises, acute chest syndrome, priapism, stroke – not found in sickle trait, less common in SC disease than SS

Signs & Symptoms

■ Pallor, icterus, mild tachycardia only in syndromes with anemia – ie NOT in sickle trait
■ Splenomegaly absent in sickle trait and most adults with SS (because of autoinfarction)
■ Splenomegaly common in children with SS, and adults and children with SC disease and S/thalassemia
■ Hepatomegaly common in SS (increased RE system)
■ Flow murmur found in essentially all anemic patients
■ Signs of hemiparesis found in the <20% of adults with SS who have had a stroke
■ Leg ulcers found in <5% of adults with SS, even rarer in childhood or in other sickle syndromes
■ Retinal lesions (proliferative and non-proliferative) most common in adults with SC disease

TESTS

Basic Blood Tests

- Sickle trait: normal CBC, normal LFTs
- SS: Hematocrit in 20's, reticulocytes in 20's, elevated MCV, elevated WBC, elevated platelets, many sickle forms, Howell-Jolly bodies, increased indirect bilirubin, low haptoglobin, mild increase in LFTs
- SC disease: Hematocrit in low 30's, reticulocytes in 5–10 range, rare sickle forms, slightly low MCV, rare mild increase in indirect bilirubin
- SS/thalassemia: Hematocrit in 20–30's, reticulocytes in 5–20's, decreased MCV, ± Howell-Jolly bodies, ± increased indirect bilirubin

Basic Urine Tests

- All sickle syndromes (including sickle trait) – isosthenuria
- In SS, proteinuria can be early sign of sickle glomerulopathy and should be monitored yearly
- Hematuria a fairly common problem in SC disease, can occur in sickle trait, but specific non-sickle related causes must be ruled out

Recommended Tests in SS :

- Extended panel RBC typing (to assure appropriate choice in case of transfusion)
- Yearly ophthalmologic exam to detect early retinopathy
- In children, transcranial Doppler to detect those at high risk for stroke
- Yearly baseline PFTs, ABGs, and ECG to compare with studies at time of acute event
  Periodic echocardiogram to identify adults with pulmonary hypertension

DIFFERENTIAL DIAGNOSIS

- Hemoglobin electrophoresis and CBC can distinguish sickle trait, SS, SC disease, and S/thalassemia.

MANAGEMENT

Routine Health Maintenance

- Anticipatory testing as above
- Pneumococcal and influenza vaccines
- Prophylactic folate

Specific Complications

- High incidence of pain crises and/or acute chest syndrome use hydroxyurea prophylaxis

- Elevated transcranial Doppler, use chronic transfusion program to prevent first stroke

  Stroke, use exchange transfusion followed by maintenance transfusions with iron chelation regimen
- Pain crisis use incentive spirometry, narcotic analgesics as appropriate
- Acute chest syndrome use empiric antibiotics to cover chlamydia, mycoplasma, pneumococcus, oxygen supplementation, bronchodilators, incentive spirometry simple or exchange transfusion, mechanical ventilation, inhaled NO as indicated
- Cholecystitis, perform elective cholecystectomy after resolution of acute episode
- Osteomyelitis use empiric antibiotics to cover salmonella and staph
- Priapism use exchange transfusion and operative shunting procedure if necessary

SPECIFIC THERAPY
- Hydroxyurea therapy follow CBC every 2 weeks, fetal hemoglobin level monthly, LFTs monthly, birth control for males and females
- Chronic transfusion therapy, monitor for alloantibodies, Fe, ferritin monthly. Start parenteral deferoxamine when iron overload present.
- Cholecystectomy can be done laparoscopically, most safely done with preoperative simple or exchange transfusion. Similar guidelines pertain to other operative procedures.

FOLLOW-UP
- Patients on hydroxyurea monitor for toxicity as above, visits every two weeks, tapering to every month once chronic stable dose is achieved
- Patients on chronic transfusion typically get 2–3 units of packed cells every 3–4 weeks.
- Relatively asymptomatic adults can be seen every 6 months

COMPLICATIONS AND PROGNOSIS
- Sickle trait is not a disease, and has no measurable morbidity or mortality associated with it.
- SS patients have average life expectancy in the 45–50 year range. Those with increased morbidity (higher rates of pain, acute chest syndrome, pulmonary hypertension, etc.) have a shorter life expectancy. This can be influenced by the use of prophylactic hydroxyurea.

- SC patients are generally less severe than those with SS, and have a life expectancy that is ~10 years longer. However, individual patients may be extremely symptomatic with high rates of pain crises, etc.
- S/thalassemia patients can be very symptomatic if they have a beta$_0$ genotype (i.e., no hemoglobin A) and should be treated the same as those with SS. Patients with a beta+ genotype (i.e., some hemoglobin A) are clinically more like those with SC disease.

SIGMOID VOLVULUS

BASSEM SAFADI, MD and ROY SOETIKNO, MD, MS

HISTORY & PHYSICAL

Risk Factors
- elongated or narrow-based mesentery
- distended colon with gas and feces
- adhesions
- elderly male in chronic care
- chronic constipation

Symptoms & Signs
- rapid onset of lower abdominal pain, distention and obstipation
- prior episodes may be less severe
- abdominal distention and tympany
- fever, tachycardia and peritoneal signs in ischemia or perforation

TESTS
- abdominal X-ray: diagnostic in 40–50% of cases
- markedly distended sigmoid colon loop in the right upper quadrant with both ends pointing to the left lower quadrant
- Gastrograffin or barium enema
- contrast in the rectum and distal sigmoid: tapers and ends at the torsion
- abdominal and pelvic CAT scan can de diagnostic

DIFFERENTIAL DIAGNOSIS
- Obstruction from intra and extra colorectal malignancies
- Strictures
- Pseudo-obstruction
- Severe constipation

MANAGEMENT

What to Do First
▪ Confirm diagnosis with abdominal X-ray, barium enema or CT scan

General Measures
▪ Assess for presence or absence of peritoneal signs

SPECIFIC THERAPY
▪ peritoneal signs absent
  ➤ endoscopic reduction, decompression, and placement of a rectal tube; mucosa assessed for viability
    • successful in 85%, recurs in 50%
    • bowel preparation and elective surgery should follow
    • reduction with Gastrograffin enema may be useful
▪ peritoneal signs present
  ➤ urgent laparotomy
    • sigmoid resection, colostomy and Hartmann's pouch in most cases
    • primary anastomosis in selected cases

FOLLOW-UP
▪ Return visits for recurrent symptoms if decompressed endoscopically
▪ Usual postoperative visits to ensure wound healing

COMPLICATIONS AND PROGNOSIS
▪ recurrence rate <1%
▪ mortality 10–30% with viable and 40–80% with non-viable bowel

---

SINOATRIAL BLOCK

EDMUND C. KEUNG, MD

HISTORY & PHYSICAL

History
▪ Infarction and fibrosis of the atrium, excessive vagal discharge, acute myocarditis, drugs such as beta blocker, calcium channel blocker, clonidine, procainamide, quinidine. Most common in elderly (beta blocker in ophthalmic solutions).

Signs & Symptoms

■ Generally asymptomatic. Fatigue, worsening of congestive heart failure, syncope or near-syncope may occur.

TESTS

■ Basic Tests
  ➤ 12-lead ECG:
  ➤ Pauses due to periodic absence of P waves.
  ➤ First Degree SA exit block: cannot be recognized on ECG (conduction defect occurs within the SA node)
  ➤ Second Degree SA exit block:
  ➤ Type I SA exit block (SA Wenckebach): P-P interval duration progressively shortens before pause. The longest P-P interval (pause) is shorter than 2 times the shortest P-P interval.
  ➤ Type II SA exit block (Mobitz II SA exit block): Duration of pause is a multiple of the regular P-P intervals.
  ➤ Third degree SA block: cannot be distinguished on ECG. Suggested by complete absence of P waves.
■ Specific Diagnostic Test
  ➤ Holter monitoring. In electrophysiology study, intracardiac recording records atrial depolarization but not sinus node activity.

DIFFERENTIAL DIAGNOSIS

■ Sinus pauses or arrest from absence of sinus node activity (in SA block, sinus node impulse is present but fails to depolarize the atrium).
■ AV nodal block: P-P interval is always regular.

MANAGEMENT

What to Do First

■ Usually requires no treatment. Adjustment of existing beta and calcium blockers, clonidine, and antiarrhythmic drug regimen.

General Measures

■ As above

SPECIFIC THERAPY

Permanent Pacemaker Implantation

■ If chronotropic incompetence from SA exit block causes fatigue, worsening of congestive heart failure, syncope or near-syncope (Type I indication).

- If heart rate < 40 bpm when a clear association between significant symptoms and actual presence of SA block has not been documented (Type IIa indication).
- Chronic HR < 30 bpm while awake in patients with minimal symptoms.

Side Effects & Contraindications
- none

FOLLOW-UP
- ECG and Holter monitoring if symptoms appear.

COMPLICATIONS AND PROGNOSIS
- In asymptomatic patients, no long term complication.
- Pacemaker: cardiac perforation, lead dislodgement, infected pacemaker pocket, lead fracture, failure to sense, failure to pace, pulse generator depletion. Requires specialized pacemaker followup.

SINUSITIS

ANDREW N. GOLDBERG, MD

HISTORY & PHYSICAL
- Diagnosis supported by 3 components:
- History, exam, imaging (CT)

History
- Frequency, duration, intensity of symptoms
- Adequacy and extent of previous treatment (antibiotics, systemic or topical steroids, decongestants, triggers of infection, seasonality)
- Predisposing conditions
  - Allergy
  - Immunocompromise
  - Smoking/irritants
  - Asthma and aspirin sensitivity
  - Other causes of nasal edema

Signs & Symptoms
- Purulent nasal discharge
- Facial fullness
- Facial pain or pressure
- Hyposmia or anosmia

- Nasal obstruction
- Fever (variable)
- Malaise or fatigue headache
- Dental pain
- Ear pressure or fullness
- Cough
- Halitosis
- Reduced resonance of voice, or "hyponasal voice" due to inflammation in sinuses

Physical Examination
- Nasal speculum: erythema, edema, purulent discharge, nasal polyps
- Nasal endoscopy with fiberoptic scope: offers more sensitive exam and better localization of site of involvement: erythema, edema, purulent discharge, nasal polyps
- Oral cavity: purulent discharge sometimes visible on posterior pharyngeal wall
- Facial: in acute cases, tenderness may be present over frontal or maxillary sinuses and edema or swelling around eyes (may indicate extension of infection and should be investigated)
- Be wary of orbital, intracranial complications (mental status change, periorbital swelling, proptosis, visual acuity change, severe headache, meningismus)
- Complications less common with chronic sinusitis
- Mucocele or mucopyocele can occur with chronic infection
- Rhinosinusitis Classification
  - Acute: <4 weeks often preceded by a viral URI
  - Recurrent acute 4 or more episodes/year resolution of symptoms between episodes
  - Subacute: 4–12 weeks intermediate classification
  - Chronic: >12 weeks may have acute exacerbations

TESTS

Laboratory
- CBC, immunologic evaluation, blood cultures as clinically indicated

Radiography
- Uncomplicated sinusitis: coronal CT of sinuses: 3 mm cuts, bone windows, no contrast
- If complications suspected:
  - Coronal and axial CT of sinuses and brain
  - 3 mm cuts, soft tissue and bone windows, with contrast

Culture
- Nasal swab inadequate; swab of purulent drainage taken on endoscopic exam or from maxillary sinus puncture needed
- Culture from maxillary sinus puncture

Other Tests
- Allergy testing may be needed as indicated by symptoms

DIFFERENTIAL DIAGNOSIS
- Rhinitis
- Allergy exacerbation
- Cystic fibrosis (should be tested in all children with nasal polyps)
- Sampter's triad (nasal polyps, athsma, asprin sensitivity)
- Kartagener's (immotile cilia) syndrome (chronic sinusitis, bronchiectasis, situs inversus)
- Facial pain syndrome (eg, tic doloureaux,)
- Headache syndrome (eg, cluster, migrane, tension headache, temporomandibular joint syndrome)
- Dental origin (periapical or other abscess, pain of other dental origin)
- Wegener's granulomatosis
- Sarcoid
- Facial cellulitis (rare)
- Nasal papilloma (eg, inverting papilloma)
- Neoplasm (nasopharyngeal cancer, maxillary sinus cancer, lymphoma, benign tumor)
- Foreign body

MANAGEMENT
n/a

SPECIFIC THERAPY
Treatment Options
- Acute Sinusitis
  - ➤ Adjunctive care only for viral causes mitigated by intensity or persistence for >5 days
  - ➤ If bacterial cause suspected, add antibiotic
  - ➤ Antibiotics for 10–14 days (strep, H. Flu, M. Cat, Staph)
  - ➤ Immunocompromised patients may have other infectious agents including fungus
  - ➤ First line: Amoxicillin, trimeth/sulfa, erythromycin, and others
  - ➤ Second line: Amoxicillin/clavulanate, cefaroxime, clarithromycin, azithromycin, clindamycin, levofloxacin, gatifloxacin, and others

- ➤ Adjunctive treatments
  - Topical steroids, decongestants, mucolytics as indicated
  - Warm compresses
  - Humidification
  - Nasal saline
  - Antipyretics
- ➤ Surgery
  - Maxillary sinus puncture for culture/treatment in selected cases
  - Recurrent acute sinusitis may be treated successfully with endoscopic or open techniques to reduce frequency, duration, intensity of infections
- ■ Side Effects
  - ➤ Medical
    - Allergy/reaction to antibiotic
    - Psuedomembranous colitis
    - Usual side effects of decongestants/steroids (see Rhinitis chapter)
  - ➤ Surgery
    - Rare complication from maxillary sinus puncture
    - Rare orbital/intracranial or other complications of sinus surgery
    - Recurrence or persistence of infection
    - Unusual surgical complications (eg, bleeding, anesthesia related)
    - Rarely may require hospitalization for persistent infection, complications
- ■ Chronic Sinusitis
- ■ Antibiotics for 3 weeks (same bacteria as acute sinusitis + anaerobes, higher incidence of Staph, Pseudomonas)
- ■ Immunocompromised patients may have other infectious agents including fungus
- ■ Treat with second line antibiotics as listed above
- ■ Consider oral prednisone
- ■ Topical nasal steroids
  - ➤ Adjunctive Treatments
  - ➤ Decongestants, mucolytics as indicated
  - ➤ Humidification
  - ➤ Nasal saline
  - ➤ Surgery

- Chronic sinusitis may be treated successfully with endoscopic or open techniques to reduce frequency, duration, intensity of infections
- Side Effects
- Medical
  - Allergy/reaction to antibiotic
  - Pseudomembranous colitis
  - Usual side effects of decongestants/steroids (see Rhinitis chapter)
- Surgery
  - Rare orbital/intracranial or other complications of sinus surgery
  - Usual surgical complications (eg, bleeding, anesthesia related)
  - Rarely require hospitalization

FOLLOW-UP

- Acute Sinusitis
  - 1 month as needed. Reassess in 2–4 days if no improvement
  - May require second course of antibiotics or rarely, addition of oral steroids
  - For recurrent infection, CT when patient at baseline (without symptoms)
  - If diagnosis uncertain, CT during exacerbation (with symptoms)
- Chronic Sinusitis
  - Reassess in 4–6 weeks
  - May require additional courses of antibiotics or, rarely, chronic oral steroids
  - CT approximately 1 month after therapy is completed (guided by history)

COMPLICATIONS AND PROGNOSIS

- Acute Sinusitis
  - Rarely life threatening
  - Excellent prognosis for virtually all infections
  - Intracranial and orbital complications rare, but need to be diagnosed early for optimal outcome
- Chronic Sinusitis
  - Rarely life threatening
  - Can have intracranial or orbital complications
  - Quality of life compromised by chronic infection
  - Difficult to eradicate completely
  - Chronic treatments commonly needed

SMALL BOWEL TUMORS

ALVARO D. DAVILA, MD

HISTORY & PHYSICAL

Risk Factors
- Small bowel tumors rare; account for 5–10% of GI tumors
- Risk from direct exposure to carcinogens:
  - Diet – high in animal fat, protein, red meat, smoked or cured foods
- Risk from predisposing conditions:
  - Peutz-Jeghers syndrome (malignant degeneration of hamartomatous polyps)
  - Gardner's syndrome (duodenal adenomas)
  - Crohn's disease (adenocarcinoma)
  - Familial adenomatous polyposis (adenoma)
  - Celiac disease (lymphoma, adenocarcinoma)
  - Immunodeficiency states (HIV – Kaposi's sarcoma, lymphoma)
  - Autoimmune disorders (lymphoma)

Signs and Symptoms
- Often asymptomatic until late in the course
- No group of signs or symptoms specific for benign or malignant tumors
- Most common presenting symptoms: intermittent obstructive GI symptoms, intussusception, chronic occult bleeding, weight loss, and abdominal pain
- Less common manifestations: perforation, acute hemorrhage, jaundice, pancreatitis
- Advanced disease: jaundice, ascites, cachexia, hepatomegaly, carcinoid syndrome (hepatic metastases)
- Physical exam usually benign; palpable abdominal mass (25%), signs of obstruction (25%), positive fecal occult blood test

Types of Tumors by Pathology
- Benign neoplasms:
  - Adenomas: tubular, villous, or Brunner's gland
  - Leiomyomas
  - Lipomas: mostly ileum/duodenum
  - Others: desmoid tumors, fibromas, lymphangiomas, hemangiomas, neurofibromas

- Malignant neoplasms:
  - Adenocarcinoma
    - accounts for 25–50% of small bowel malignancies
    - incidence decreases from duodenum to jejunum
    - 60% periampullary
    - Crohn's disease, predominantly involves ileum
    - tendency to metastasize early to regional lymph nodes
- Carcinoid tumors
  - see chapter on carcinoid tumor
- Lymphoma
  - small bowel often involved (most common extranodal site)
  - mostly non-Hodgkin's lymphomas
  - all types, including B-cell, large cell, immunoblastic, T-cell, intermediate or high grade
  - most common in the ileum
  - typical symptoms are fatigue, weight loss, pain
- Sarcomas
  - rare (1% of small bowel malignancies)
  - most common in jejunum, ileum, and Meckel's diverticula most common type is leiomyosarcoma
  - symptoms include obstruction, bleeding, or pain
  - criteria for malignancy: number of mitoses, nuclear atypia, presence of necrosis, cellularity
  - local or hematogenous spread
- Metastatic tumors
  - predominantly melanoma; also breast, lung, kidney, colon, cervical, ovarian
  - may cause symptoms of obstruction, bleeding and pain
- Neuroendocrine tumors
  - gastrinoma, somatostatinoma, schwannoma, paraganglionoma
  - present with hormone-specific symptoms or as a mass lesion

TESTS

Basic Studies: Blood
- Early disease: usually normal
- Advanced disease: variable by tumor; microcytic anemia with GI bleeding; elevated alkaline phosphatase and bilirubin with biliary obstruction; elevated CEA with metastatic adenocarcinoma; elevated beta-$_2$-microglobulin, LDH, or monoclonal gammopathy with lymphoma

Imaging

- Plain abdominal films: usually nondiagnostic; may demonstrate obstruction, free subdiaphragmatic air
- Barium contrast studies (UGI with small bowel follow-through or enteroclysis): best tests to locate and possibly define small bowel lesions; enteroclysis has a reported sensitivity of 90% versus 33% for conventional SBFT
- Computed tomography (CT): useful in identifying a tumor mass and may define extraluminal or metastatic disease
- Upper endoscopy: direct visualization limited to duodenum; may perform biopsy or polypectomy
- Push enteroscopy: extends endoscopic visualization to jejunum; biopsy capability

DIFFERENTIAL DIAGNOSIS

- Symptoms of obstruction, bleeding or pain lead to broad diagnostic categories: common causes include ulcer disease, vascular ectasias, bleeding vascular lesions, Meckel's diverticulum, portal hypertension, hemobilia, endometriosis, pneumatosis intestinalis, adhesions, enteric duplication cysts, strictures, pancreatic rest, inflammatory bowel disease, and other ulcerative diseases

MANAGEMENT

What to Do First

- Assess the type of neoplasm (benign versus malignant, histology) and evaluate extent of disease

General Measures

- History, physical, and appropriate tests to evaluate extent of disease
- Surgical consultation often necessary

SPECIFIC THERAPY

- Some form of therapy indicated for all patients regardless of histology or symptoms

Treatment Options

- Benign neoplasms: resection by endoscopy (biopsy or polypectomy) or laparotomy; choice of therapy depends on size of lesion, growth pattern, and location
- Malignant neoplasms:
- Adenocarcinoma – surgical treatment is indicated with wide segmental resection; pancreaticoduodenectomy may be required for tumors in the first or second portions of the duodenum; role of chemotherapy or radiation therapy uncertain

- Lymphomas – optimal treatments have not been defined due to large variety and rarity of these tumors; treatments include (alone or in combination): antibiotics, surgical resection, chemotherapy, radiation therapy, nutritional support, bone marrow transplantation
- Sarcomas – treatment of choice is surgical resection with wide excision; palliative resection or bypass for extensive disease; minimal or no benefit to adjuvant chemotherapy or radiotherapy
- Metastatic tumors – palliative treatment with surgical resection or intestinal bypass

FOLLOW-UP
- Continued clinical and/or endoscopic surveillance for indeterminate periods indicated due to aggressive or indolent nature of these tumors

COMPLICATIONS AND PROGNOSIS

Complications
- Endoscopic therapy
  - ➤ bleeding, perforation, cardiopulmonary
- Surgery
  - ➤ bleeding, infections, obstruction, death
- Chemotherapy
  - ➤ variable by chemotherapeutic agent
- Radiation therapy
  - ➤ fatigue, nausea, nephritis; bleeding and perforation rare

Prognosis
- Most favorable for surgically or endoscopically resected early carcinoids, sarcomas, lymphomas and benign neoplasms
- Prognosis of malignant bowel tumors is determined by resectability, status of surgical margins, histologic grade, lymph node involvement, and metastases
- Poor prognosis for late presentations of adenocarcinomas, high grade smooth muscle tumors and cancers metastatic to small bowel

---

SPERMATOCELE

ARTHUR I. SAGALOWSKY, MD

HISTORY & PHYSICAL
- painless cystic mass containing sperm
- usually in head of epididymis
- asymptomatic unless large

TESTS
- usually transilluminates
- ultrasound

DIFFERENTIAL DIAGNOSIS
- exclude tumor of testis or spermatic cord

MANAGEMENT
n/a

SPECIFIC THERAPY
- observation strongly advised unless large and painful
- surgical excision; risks testis infarction or epididymal obstruction

FOLLOW-UP
n/a

COMPLICATIONS AND PROGNOSIS
n/a

SPINE & SPINAL CORD INJURY

MICHAEL J. AMINOFF, MD, DSc

HISTORY & PHYSICAL
- History of injury to head, spine or both
- Pain over neck or back often present, may be worse w/movement
- Weakness, paralysis or sensory disturbance below level of injury; symptoms are transient w/mild injuries
- Sphincter disturbance may be present
- No deficit w/mild injuries
- Spinal tenderness or misalignment of spinal processes may be present
- Weakness or paralysis depending on level and severity of injury
  - Cervical injury: all limbs may be affected
  - Injury below T1: weakness confined to legs
  - Lateral cord injury: weakness ipsilateral to injury
  - Central cord injury: LMN weakness at level of lesion
- Sensory impairment below lesion level; perianal sensation may be impaired; w/lateral cord injury or hemisection, ipsilateral hyperesthesia & contralateral analgesia occur
- Tone may be reduced acutely below lesion level & then increased (spasticity)
- Tendon reflexes may be normal, absent or increased; Babinski responses indicate pyramidal deficit

- Sphincters may be impaired, typically w/urinary and fecal retention
- Complete cord injury: no motor or sensory function preserved below lesion level

TESTS
- Stabilize spine before any imaging studies
- Lateral film of neck on all pts w/head, cervical or multiple injuries
- MRI to visualize cord & soft tissues

DIFFERENTIAL DIAGNOSIS
- Imaging studies will suggest nature & extent of cord injury.

MANAGEMENT
- Maintain spinal stability
- Assess adequacy of ventilation; support may be required after cervical or upper thoracic injuries
- Analgesia as needed
- Assess for presence & severity of cord injury
- Methylprednisolone for 24–48 hr if cord injury has occurred
- Care of skin, bladder, bowels
- Physical therapy to maintain joint mobility & muscle function

SPECIFIC THERAPY
- Subdural or epidural hematomas may require evacuation
- No specific therapy otherwise except as indicated for mgt as above

FOLLOW-UP
- Depends on nature & severity of injury

COMPLICATIONS AND PROGNOSIS
- Prognosis for recovery is better w/incomplete than complete lesions

SPONDYLOARTHROPATHIES

DAVID TAK YAN YU, MD

HISTORY & PHYSICAL

Classification
- Ankylosing spondylitis (the prototype)
- Undifferentiated spondyloarthropathy
- Reactive arthritis: preceded within 1 month by urethritis, cervicitis or acute diarrhea caused by Chlamydia, Yersinia, Shigella, Salmonella & Campylobacter

- Reiter's syndrome: triad of arthritis, urethritis, conjunctivitis
- Assoc w/psoriasis or inflammatory bowel disease

History

- Firm diagnosis of spondyloarthropathy requires at least 1 of the following:
  - Spinal pain esp. in low back, inflammatory in type (insidious onset, <40 years of age at onset, persisting >3 months, improves w/exercise, assoc w/morning stiffness)
  - Joint swelling in 4 or fewer joints; asymmetrical or predominantly of the lower extremities
  - And one of the following additional features:
    - Positive family history of spondyloarthropathy, psoriasis, inflammatory bowel diseases or iritis
    - Psoriasis
    - Inflammatory bowel disease
    - Urethritis, cervicitis or acute diarrhea within 1 month before arthritis, alternating buttock pain
    - Enthesopathy (eg, Achilles tendinitis, plantar fasciitis or sausage digits)

Other Features

- Unilateral iritis (~30%)
- Mucocutaneous lesions: painless erythematous lesions of the glans penis or oral mucosa (infrequent)
- Keratoderma blennorrhagica: lesions resembling pustular psoriasis on the soles (infrequent)
- In advanced & severe disease:
  - Limitation of range of motion of lumbar and/or cervical spine
  - Decreased chest expansion
  - Flexion contracture of neck
  - Hip pain & limitation of motion
  - Aortic insufficiency (rare)
  - Cauda equina syndrome from arachnoiditis

TESTS

Blood Tests

- HLA-B27 is very helpful in 2 ways. If it is negative, the probability of ankylosing spondylitis is very low. If a pt has inflammatory low back pain & positive HLA-B27, there is a high probability of ankylosing spondylitis even though other features are negative.

Imaging

- Always do plain AP view of the pelvis to evaluate for sacroiliitis.
- The diagnosis of spondyloarthropathy is almost certain if there is significant sacroiliitis.
- If plain x-ray for sacroiliitis is ambiguous or negative but spondyloarthropathy is highly suspected on clinical grounds, proceed to MRI of the sacroiliac joint. Bone edema as visualized by STIR or T2 w/ fat absorption technique is characteristic of spondyloarthropathy.
- Plain x-ray of AP view of pelvis also allows assessment of hip joints.
- If assessment of spine is needed, a single lateral view of the lumbar & cervical spine will allow visualization of squaring of vertebrae, syndesmophytes or fusion as "bamboo spine."

DIFFERENTIAL DIAGNOSIS
N/A

MANAGEMENT

What to Do First

- Assess disease activity & functional status & impending disability (see "Assessment" in http://www.asas-group.org)
- Begin pt education

GENERAL MEASURES

- Posture training to prevent flexion contracture of cervical spine
- Stretching exercises to improve mobility
- Daily exercise (eg, swimming)

SPECIFIC THERAPY

- NSAIDs, selective COX-2 inhibitor, celecoxib, if indicated
- CT-guided steroid injection of sacroiliac joints may provide local relief of pain from sacroiliitis up to 10 months
- Sulfasalazine w/ gradual increase in dose for early or mild disease w/ peripheral joint involvement. Stop if not effective after a 4-month trial. Not useful for spinal pain.
- Methotrexate is of unproven efficacy. Discontinue if not effective after a 6-month trial.
- TNF antagonists (eg, etanercept, infliximab, adalumimab) may provide dramatic response within days of initiating therapy. Risk of infection & high cost mandate reserving for refractory disease (For guideline, see "Publications" in http://www.asas-group.org).
- Total hip replacement for unrelieved hip pain or disability

- Spine surgery for awkward flexion deformities
- Valve replacement for life-threatening aortic insufficiency

Side Effects & Complications
- As in rheumatoid arthritis

FOLLOW-UP
- Assess adequacy of control of disease activity
- Monitor functional status every 3–6 months, more often w/very active disease (see "Assessment" in http://www.asas-group.org)
- Reinforce education about daily exercise, stretching, activity

COMPLICATIONS AND PROGNOSIS

Complications
- Aortic incompetence in 3.5% after 15 years, 10% after 30 years
- Fibrosis of upper lungs after 20+ years (infrequent), cystic changes, Aspergillus infection
- Neurologic complications of spinal involvement
- Spinal fracture at C5, 6, 7 after minor trauma
- C1–C2 subluxation & cord compression
- Cauda equina syndrome
- IgA nephropathy (frequent, but functional significance unclear)
- Osteoporosis w/spinal compression fracture
- Secondary amyloidosis

Prognosis
- Vast majority of pts do well, w/o disabling disease
- Indicators of poor prognosis
  - Hip arthritis
  - ESR >30 mm/hr
  - Poor response to NSAIDs
  - Limitation of motion in lumbar spine
  - Sausage-like finger or toe
  - Onset at or before 16 years of age

SPONTANEOUS BACTERIAL PERITONITIS

ANDY S. YU, MD and EMMET B. KEEFFE, MD

HISTORY & PHYSICAL

History
- cirrhotic ascites or ascites due to subacute liver failure
- fever, chills, rigors, abdominal pain, encephalopathy

Physical Signs
- fever, hypotension, tachycardia, abdominal tenderness, asterixis
- one-third without the classical signs

TESTS
- laboratory features: azotemia, peripheral leukocytosis, acidosis
- diagnostic paracentesis
  - ➤ cell count
    - neutrophil (PMN) count $\geq$250/mm^3 presumed to be infection
  - ➤ culture
    - bedside inoculation of 10 mL of ascitic fluid into each of two culture bottles
    - most infections are caused by Escherichia coli, streptococci (mostly pneumococci), and Klebsiella, with only 1% contribution from anaerobes
  - ➤ gram stain
    - too insensitive for detecting spontaneous bacterial peritonitis
  - ➤ patients with neutrocytic ascites and meeting 2 of the following 3 criteria may have surgical peritonitis:
    - ascitic fluid total protein >1.0 gm/dL,
    - ascitic fluid glucose <50 mg/dL
    - ascitic fluid LDH level > upper limit of normal for serum

DIFFERENTIAL DIAGNOSIS
- spontaneous ascitic fluid infection is divided into subcategories:
  - ➤ spontaneous bacterial peritonitis (SBP)
    - elevated ascitic fluid PMN $\geq$250 cells/mm(3), monomicrobial ascitic fluid culture, and absence of surgical source of intra-abdominal infection
  - ➤ monomicrobial non-neutrocytic bacterascites (MNB)
    - non-elevated ascitic fluid PMN $\leq$250 cells per mm^3, monomicrobial ascitic fluid culture, and absence of surgical infection
    - early stage and common variant of SBP; progresses to SBP in 40% and resolve spontaneously in 60%
  - ➤ culture-negative neutrocytic ascites (CNNA)
    - elevated ascitic fluid PMN $\geq$250 cells/mm3, negative ascitic fluid culture, absence of surgical infection, absence of other causes for elevated ascitic fluid PMN, and absence of any antibiotics given within 30 days
- secondary bacterial peritonitis: ascitic fluid PMN $\geq$250 cells/mm3, positive ascitic fluid culture that is usually polymicrobial, and presence of intra-abdominal infection due to either free perforation of a viscus or loculated abscess

- polymicrobial bacterascites: gut perforation due to paracentesis needle, with diagnosis based on ascitic fluid PMN <250 cells/mm3 and polymicrobial Gram stain and/or culture

MANAGEMENT

What to Do First

- diagnostic paracentesis, including cell count and culture
- empirical broad-spectrum intravenous antibiotic without delay

General Measures

- err on the side of overtreatment if initial presentation is uncertain
- avoid nephrotoxic medications, including aminoglycosides

SPECIFIC THERAPY

Indications for Treatment

- ascitic fluid PMN > 250 cells/mm3
- convincing signs and symptoms of infection

Treatment Options for SBP

- cefotaxime or a similar third-generation cephalosporin antibiotic of choice for spontaneous ascitic fluid infection
- intravenous albumin can further reduce the morbidity and mortality oral
- ofloxacin effective in uncomplicated SBP

Treatment of Other Spontaneous Ascitic Fluid Infections

- treatment of MNB
  - ➤ symptomatic patients without neutrocytic ascites: empiric initiated on cefotaxime, with follow-up paracentesis performed at 48 hours; if culture results demonstrate no growth 2–3 days later, antibiotics can be discontinued
  - ➤ asymptomatic patients: do not need treatment immediately but require repeat paracentesis for cell count and culture; if ascitic fluid becomes neutrocytic or signs and symptoms of infection develop, antibiotics should be initiated
- treatment of CNNA
  - ➤ patient is already initiated empirically on antibiotics since the turn-around time for ascitic fluid culture takes a few days
  - ➤ repeat paracentesis; a decline in ascitic fluid PMN count confirms response and warrants a few more days of antibiotics; a stable ascitic fluid PMN count suggests a nonbacterial cause and warrants further investigation

Treatment of Secondary Ascitic Fluid Infections
- treatment of secondary bacterial peritonitis
  - intravenous cefotaxime and metronidazole initiated immediately for broad-spectrum coverage
  - studies to localize site of perforation
  - emergent surgical laparotomy

Treatment of Polymicrobial Bacterascites
- intravenous cefotaxime and metronidazole, with duration of therapy dictated by clinical response and serial ascitic fluid PMN levels and cultures

Side Effects and Contraindications
- antibiotics
  - side effects: hypersensitivity reactions, thrombophlebitis, and Clostridium difficile infection for cefotaxime

FOLLOW-UP

During Treatment
- spectrum of antibiotic coverage narrowed once culture and sensitivity become available
- may repeat diagnostic paracentesis 48 hours after initiation of therapy to monitor therapeutic response

Routine
- long term antibiotic prophylaxis after initial SBP episode
- antibiotic choices include oral norfloxacin 400 mg daily, ciprofloxacin 750 mg weekly, and trimethoprim-sulfamethoxazole double-strength 5 times per week
- short-term inpatient antibiotic prophylaxis for cirrhotic patients with ascitic fluid total protein <1 gm/dL or variceal hemorrhage

COMPLICATIONS AND PROGNOSIS

Complications
- renal impairment in 33% of patients with SBP treated with cefotaxime alone; intravenous albumin reduces renal impairment and mortality

Prognosis
- spontaneous ascitic fluid infection
  - one-year survival as low as 20% after treatment
  - established indication for OLT

SPOROTRICHOSIS

RICHARD A. JACOBS, MD, PhD

HISTORY & PHYSICAL

History

- Chronic infection caused by Sporothrix schenckii, a dimorphic fungus able to grow in yeast form in culture and tissue at 37 degrees Celsius or as a mold at 25 degrees
- Found in plants, soil, decaying wood, rose thorns; worldwide
  - The organism is usually inoculated into the skin, typically from a penetrating skin injury; rarely is it inhaled

Signs & Symptoms

- Two main forms: cutaneous and extracutaneous
- Cutaneous:
  - Usually begins as a firm, painless subcutaneous nodule at the site of inoculation
- This may later ulcerate
- Within several days to weeks, these nodules may extend along the path of the lymphatics
  - These lesions usually appear and disappear in waves over months to years; rarely do they regress spontaneously

Extracutaneous:

- Osteoarticular (extremity joint arthritis, carpal tunnel syndrome) may lead to severe bone and joint destruction if left untreated
- Pulmonary (older males, productive cough, fever and weight loss; CXR with cavitary lesions)
- Meningitis (usually indolent, CSF with lymphocytic predominance)
- HIV patients:
- Disseminated disease usually in advanced AIDS patients (CD4 <200)
- Skin lesions tend to ulcerate more, are more extensive, and are associated with arthritis
- Multiple organs have been described: brain, eye, intestines, liver, bone marrow

TESTS

Laboratory

- Basic studies: Blood cultures: positive blood cultures seen in disseminated disease
- Other studies: Tissue culture: diagnostic of infection

➤ Other studies: Serology may be useful for extracutaneous disease (particularly central nervous system disease) but is not standardized

Pathology
■ Granulomas with cigar-like yeast forms

DIFFERENTIAL DIAGNOSIS
■ Single lesions may suggest foreign body granuloma, dermatophytic infection, blastomycosis, bacterial pyoderma
■ Nodular lymphatic spread may suggest non-tuberculous mycobacteria, nocardia, leishmania.
■ Less commonly, blastomycosis, coccidioidomycosis, cryptococcosis, anthrax, tularemia, and streptococcal Group A and Staphylococcus aureus infections

MANAGEMENT
What to Do First
■ Assess whether or not patient is immunocompromised and is at risk for dissemination

General Measures
■ If fevers or ill-appearing, draw blood cultures; skin biopsy if cutaneous disease

SPECIFIC THERAPY
Treatment Options
■ For cutaneous/localized disease:
  ➤ Iodides such as potassium iodide (SSKI) can be cheap and effective: start with 5–10 drops po TID, advancing to 40–50 drops po TID for adults; can mix in juice or other beverage; take for several months until lesions have cleared
  ➤ OR Itraconazole for more than 2 months
  ➤ Itraconazole cyclodextrin solution has increased bioavailability
  ➤ If relapse, treat again for more prolonged course
■ For disseminated disease:
  ➤ Amphotericin B (preferred in meningitis and severe disseminated disease)
  ➤ OR Itraconazole for 6–18 months
  ➤ Surgery has an uncertain role in treatment; may be necessary in Pulmonary disease
  ➤ For HIV patients:
  ➤ Treat as above but may need to follow with lifetime suppressive doses of Itraconazole because of higher likelihood of relapse and dissemination

Side Effects & Complications
- Potassium Iodide (SSKI)
- Side effects: bitter taste, nausea, anorexia, diarrhea, rash, parotid gland enlargement
- Itraconazole
  - Side effects: nausea, vomiting, anorexia, abdominal pain, rash; rarely hypokalemia and hepatitis
  - Contraindications: end-stage renal disease for cyclodextran solution; lower cyclosporin dose when concomitantly given; may dangerously increase serum levels of digoxin, astemizole and loratadine, causing fatal arrhythmias
- Amphotericin B
  - Side effects: fevers, chills, nausea, vomiting and headaches; rigors may be prevented by the addition of hydrocortisone 25 mg to bag, meperidine 25–50 mg may treat rigors; nephrotoxicity; electrolyte disturbance (renal tubular acidosis, hypokalemia, hypomagnesemia)
- Contraindications: if Cr 2.5–3.0, may consider giving lipid-based Amphotericin products

FOLLOW-UP
- For cutaneous disease: assess resolution of nodules
- Treat for as long as needed, may require several months

COMPLICATIONS AND PROGNOSIS

Complications
- Functional impairment with bone and joint destruction in osteoarticular disease

Prognosis
- For cutaneous/localized disease: excellent prognosis
- For disseminated disease: poor prognosis, may be fatal

STAPHYLOCOCCAL INFECTIONS

RICHARD A. JACOBS, MD, PhD

HISTORY & PHYSICAL

History
- Clinically relevant species: *Staphylococcus aureus*, *Staphylococcus epidermidis* and other coagulase-negative staphylococci

- Most humans become intermittently colonized with *S. aureus* in (by order of frequency) the nasopharynx (most), skin, vagina (as in toxic shock syndrome) and rectum
- The skin is an effective barrier to infection and when integrity is disrupted as in surgery, intravenous lines or trauma, *S. aureus* may gain entry and create its trademark local abscess lesion, with subsequent dissemination
- *S. epidermidis* is a common colonizer of skin
- Infection related to intravenous catheters and insertion of other devices; wounds can also give rise to osteomyelitis

Increasing prevalence of methicillin-resistant S. aureus without recent hospitalization – community acquired or CA-MRSA. Strains are distinct from hospital strains. Has been reported as a cause most commonly of skin and soft tissue infection and has been associated with risk groups including MSM (men who have sex with men) athletes, military personnel.

S. aureus isolates intermediate or resistant to vancomycin have also been reported in hospitalized patients.

Signs & Symptoms
- Skin and soft tissue disease:
  - Primarily due to S. aureus
  - Folliculitis:
  - Local infection of hair follicle seen as raised, tender pustules at the base of a hair follicle
  - Furuncles (boils):
  - Begin as a tender, erythematous nodule that becomes more fluctuant
  - Sometimes creamy discharge; hairy areas of body; usually one hair follicle involve
  - Carbuncles:
  - Deeper seated infection; sinus tracts can develop; may be associated with more systemic symptoms with fevers and chills; multiple follicles involves
  - Impetigo:
  - Superficial infection; usually localized to exposed skin (face, extremities)
  - Multiple lesions of different ages; honey-colored crusting
  - Cellulitis:
  - May develop as an extension of the processes outlined above; indistinguishable from infections caused by Streptococcal spp

- Osteomyelitis:
  - *S. aureus* cause of 60% cases of osteomyelitis
  - Can be direct (e.g.: open fracture) or by hematogenous spread
  - Present acutely or insidiously with localized pain
  - Epidural abscesses may arise from vertebral osteomyelitis; suspect if fever, back pain and radiculopathy
- Bacteremia:
  - Usually a result of direct infection or inoculation (e.g.: intravenous devices, intravenous drug use) but no source identified in 30%
  - May present with fevers, chills or rigors, arthralgias, myalgias; patient looks acutely ill
  - Careful examination of the patient may reveal the source (e.g., infected intravenous catheter, petechiae or other stigmata of endocarditis)
- Device associated infections:
  - Primarily due to S. epidermidis
  - May present as bacteremia in a patient who does not look ill and whose intravenous catheter does not appear infected
  - In CSF shunt infections, the patient may present with a low-grade fever or local wound but without meningismus
  - Common cause of peritonitis in chronic ambulatory peritoneal dialysis patients
  - Prosthetic joint infection may be suggested by joint pain, swelling and fevers
- Endocarditis:
  - Presentation may be fever and malaise only; peripheral stigmata of endocarditis often absent
  - Compared to other etiologies, S aureus endocarditis is noted for its rapid onset, high fevers, involvement of previously normal valves and lack of physical findings supporting endocarditis on admission
  - *S. aureus* endocarditis usually related to intravenous drug use; often right sided disease
  - Prosthetic valve endocarditis is usually due to *S. epidermidis*
  - Suspect in any patient with a prosthetic heart valve with a fever and bacteremia
  - High rate of complications with sewing ring dehiscence and arrhythmias
- Metastatic infections:
  - Primarily *S. aureus*

➤ May present in bones, joints, lungs and kidneys as suppurative collections via hematogenous spread

➤ Suspect metastatic infections if persistent fevers despite treatment for bacteremia or endocarditis

■ Food poisoning:

➤ Toxin-mediated disease due to S. aureus

➤ Presents with nausea, vomiting followed by abdominal cramps and watery diarrhea 2–4 hours following ingestion of contaminated food

➤ Usually appears in outbreaks

➤ Patients not febrile and without rash

■ Toxic shock syndrome:

➤ Toxin-mediated disease due to S. aureus

➤ In 1980–81 became increasingly seen with the introduction of super absorbent tampons

➤ Appears abruptly with fever, vomiting, diarrhea and myalgias; hypotension follows and a "sunburn" rash later appears with desquamation of the palms and soles; multiorgan involvement is common

➤ Non-menstrual cases may be associated with surgery or localized infections and present in a similar way

TESTS

Laboratory

■ Blood culture or specimen gram stain and culture from suspected site of infection (sputum, urine, joint fluid, etc) confirms diagnosis in most cases

Imaging

■ CXR: can give clues as to etiology; think of right-sided endocarditis if nodular appearance of septic emboli; can become cavitary in a few days

■ Bone films, CT or MRI: can be helpful in diagnosis of septic arthritis/ osteomyelitis

■ Bone scan and indium WBC scan: can be used to diagnose osteomyelitis

➤ Transesophageal echocardiogram: preferred over transthoracic echocardiogram for diagnosis of endocarditis

DIFFERENTIAL DIAGNOSIS

■ Includes other pyogenic bacteria that cause similar syndromes

MANAGEMENT

What to Do First

- In serious infections (e.g.: sepsis, endocarditis, neurosurgical shunt infection), empiric antibiotics are important before definitive microbiological diagnosis
- Septic joints need immediate drainage
  - ➤ In suspected intravenous catheter infection, early removal of the line is important (particularly in S. aureus infections)

General Measures

- General supportive care

SPECIFIC THERAPY

Treatment Options

- The first-line drugs are the anti-staphylococcal penicillins (nafcillin IV, dicloxicillin po). The first-generation cephalosporins (cefazolin IV cephalexin po) also have excellent staphylococcal activity. Fluoroquinolones such as levofloxacin also have very good activity. The beta-lactam/beta-lactamase inhibitor combinations (ampicillin-sulbactam, piperacillin-tazobactam, ticarcillin-clavulanate) are outstanding. Vancomycin is an important agent for methicillin resistant *S. aureus*. Trimethoprim-sulfamethoxazole, clindamycin, or minocycline can be tried if the patient cannot tolerate Vancomycin. Quinupristin/dalfopristin (Synercid), linezolid, tigecycline, and daptomycin have activity against methicillin-resistant *S. aureus* but at present these agents should be reserved for vancomycin-resistant enterococcus (VRE). For vancomycin intermediate (VISA) and resistant S. aureus (VRSA), obtain infectious disease consultation, and isolates should be sent to CDC for susceptibility testing. Isolates reported to date have been susceptible to other drugs.
- For *S. aureus* bacteremia, would treat for 2 weeks if no evidence of endocarditis. If evidence of metastatic disease, may need longer therapy (4 weeks). For endocarditis and osteomyelitis, the duration of therapy is 4–6 weeks. For uncomplicated right-sided endocarditis, can treat for 2 weeks if synergistic doses of gentamicin or tobramycin are concomitantly administered with nafcillin. Rifampin is added to regimen for prosthetic valve endocarditis.
- For line-infections, use vancomycin empirically, if etiology is *S. aureus*, need to remove catheter, treat for at least 2 weeks. If etiology is *S. epidermidis*, can try to "save" catheter (>80% cure rate if infection limited to exit site).

FOLLOW-UP
- For cases of bacteremia, may follow-up with blood cultures to ensure that bacteremia is cleared off antibiotics
- Recurrence of bacteremia suggests wrong diagnosis (e.g., missed endocarditis) or may necessitate removal of medical device (intravenous catheter, prosthetic joint).

COMPLICATIONS AND PROGNOSIS

Prognosis
- Generally good if localized disease
  - ➤ *S. aureus* bacteremia has a mortality rate of 10–40%; higher if age >50 or more comorbidities; lower in catheter-related infections.
  - ➤ The mortality is lower for young intravenous drug users with uncomplicated right-sided endocarditis; higher (20–45%) in the other cases (older patients, left-sided disease, prosthetic valve infections).

Prevention
- Elimination of nasal carriage (using Mupirocin) may be helpful in preventing infection in high-risk populations (surgical or hemodialysis patients or those with recurrent disease).
- Using hospital infection control principles, nosocomial infection with Staphylococcus spp can be dramatically reduced.

STASIS DERMATITIS

J. MARK JACKSON, MD

HISTORY & PHYSICAL
- History – swelling of lower extremity, pruritus
- Physical – erythematous, scaly, patches and plaques over edematous skin, with or without hyper/hypopigmentation and lichenification. Ulceration may occur as a consequence.

TESTS
n/a

DIFFERENTIAL DIAGNOSIS
- Cellulitis usually warm and tender with fever, unilateral (not always)
- Contact/irritant dermatitis

MANAGEMENT

What to Do First

- Eliminate swelling/edema and irritants, treat involved skin

SPECIFIC THERAPY

- Support Hose 30–40 mmHg pressure, leg elevation
- Level 4 or 5 topical corticosteroids and moisturizers
- If severe short course corticosteroids, side effects and contraindications per atopic dermatitis
- Avoid development of contact allergy to topical antibiotics

FOLLOW-UP

n/a

COMPLICATIONS AND PROGNOSIS

Chronic course if swelling not eliminated. If swelling is eliminated, then resolution may occur. Residual hyperpigmentation may still be present after dermatitis has resolved.

STATUS EPILEPTICUS

MICHAEL J. AMINOFF, MD, DSc

HISTORY & PHYSICAL

- Recurrent convulsions w/o recovery of consciousness btwn attacks or a fixed epileptic state continuing for 20 minutes or more; non-convulsive status may present simply as a fluctuating alteration in mental status
- Continuing seizures: precise findings depend on seizure type
- May be findings of underlying neurologic deficit

TESTS

- Blood should be obtained at initiation of treatment, but mgt should start immediately; do not wait for test results
- Lab studies: CBC, differential, LFTs, BUN & electrolytes, FBS, ESR, blood levels of anticonvulsants (if being taken prior to status epilepticus), toxicology screen, CSF exam
- Cranial CT scan or MRI
- CXR

DIFFERENTIAL DIAGNOSIS

- Status epilepticus is a syndrome of many causes, not a specific diagnosis

MANAGEMENT
- Postpone diagnostic studies until seizures are controlled; follow protocol, providing assisted ventilation or pressor agents as needed
  - Ensure adequate airway & oxygenation; maintain vital functions
  - Administer thiamine followed by 50% dextrose IV (to counteract possible underlying hypoglycemia)
  - Administer diazepam or lorazepam IV; repeat after 5 min if necessary to control seizures in short term
  - Administer phenytoin IV or phosphenytoin to control seizures in longer term (regardless of response to diazepam or lorazepam); monitor ECG & blood pressure; avoid glucose-containing solutions w/ phenytoin
  - If status continues, give further phenytoin or phosphenytoin IV w/o delay
  - If status continues, give phenobarbital IV
  - If status continues, induce anesthesia w/ midazolam, propofol or pentobarbital IV; will require ventilatory assistance; EEG is needed to monitor depth of anesthesia & to determine whether seizures continue (if pt is pharmacologically paralyzed); lighten anesthesia level after 12 hr unless seizures recur

SPECIFIC THERAPY
- Seizures managed as above; specific therapy directed at underlying cause

FOLLOW-UP
- Depends on underlying cause

COMPLICATIONS AND PROGNOSIS
- Delay in initiating effective treatment may lead to fatal outcome or to residual neurologic deficits (eg, cognitive deficit)

STRABISMUS

WILLIAM V. GOOD, MD

HISTORY & PHYSICAL

History
- Congenital esotropia is usually noted in the first 4 months of life. Accommodative esotropia onset at 1 1/2 to 3 years. Intermittent exotropia usual onset after 3 years. Vertical strabismus usually acquired (e.g. Graves disease, blowout fracture).

■ Family history may be positive. Congenital esotropia more common in neurologically impaired children. Maternal smoking is a risk factor.

Signs & Symptoms
■ Esotropia is crossed eyes. Look for light reflex displaced temporally.
■ Accommodative esotropes may show variable strabismus, worse with near visual tasks.
■ Amblyopia (loss of vision due to non-usage of eye) most likely in accommodative esotropia.
■ Depth perception affected with misaligned eyes-may not recover with correction of strabismus.
■ Exotropes usually squint one eye in bright light. Eyes diverge. Look for light reflex displaced nasally.
■ Vertical strabismus patients take an anomalous head position to keep eyes aligned and avoid double vision.
■ Sixth nerve palsy causes esotropia. Involved eye won't abduct (turn out). Third nerve palsy usually shows involved eye "down and out." Fourth nerve palsy causes head tilt.

TESTS
■ Physical Exam
  ➤ Usually the only "test." Cover test – cover fixing eye and look to see whether uncovered eye shifts to look at the visual target. Forced duction (traction on eye to palpate resistance to movement of eye) for restrictive disease diagnosis (e.g., tight muscle in Graves disease). Myasthenia suspect – Tensilon test.
■ Imaging
  ➤ Brain for suspected space-occupying lesion: cases late in onset (esotropia after age 5); other neuro signs, esp. cranial nerve loss; papilledema; constant exotropia first year of life

DIFFERENTIAL DIAGNOSIS
■ Esotropia
  ➤ 1. Pseudoesotropia occurs when epicanthal folds cause illusion of esotropia. Look for light reflex off center of corneas and normal cover test.
  2. Sixth nerve palsy causes poor abduction movement of affected eye.
  3. Duane syndrome is anomalous innervation of extraocular muscles. Left eye usually affected and won't abduct or adduct.

- Exotropia
  - ➤ 1. pontine lesions may cause paralytic exotropia – look to see whether each eye fully adducts.
  - 2. craniofacial disorders may cause true exotropia.
  - 3. High myopia also may cause exotropia that can be corrected with glasses.
- Vertical strabismus (hypertropia)
- Myasthenia gravis may mimic any sort of strabismus. Skew deviation is coirritant hypertropia seen in patients with brainstem disease. Causes of true vertical strabismus are 4th nerve palsy, Graves disease, blowout fracture, double elevator palsy (congenital fibrosis of inferior rectus muscle), orbit tumor.
- Amblyopia
  - ➤ Diagnosed when decreased visual acuity occurs with normal eye. Differential includes strabismus, anisometropia (unequal refractive error), and occlusion (e.g., congenital cataracts).

MANAGEMENT

What to Do First
- Rule out neurologic cause-sixth nerve palsy, papilledema. Assess visual acuity and start treating amblyopia.

General Measures
- Measure severity of strabismus, measure refraction to see whether glasses are indicated.

SPECIFIC THERAPY
- For congenital esotropia, usually surgery. First treat amblyopia and refractive error.
- For accommodative esotropia, treat with glasses first for hyperopia. If still esotropia, surgery. Manage amblyopia as necessary.
- For exotropia, first try over-minus with glasses to induce accommodative convergence. May need surgery.
- For vertical strabismus, surgery when uncomfortable or double vision can't be managed with glasses and prism. For adults, adjustable suture technique may improve outcome.

Side Effects & Contraindications
- Rate of reoperation at least 1/3 for congenital esotropia. Surgery may overcorrect esotropia or exotropia. Surgical complications include conjunctival cyst, change in eyelid position (especially for vertical strabismus surgery), endophthalmitis (rare).

■ Compliance with patching and glasses may be difficult in young children.

FOLLOW-UP

■ After surgery, children still may develop amblyopia or need glasses. Follow at least to age 5, longer for some conditions. Routine follow-up 3–4 times per year.

COMPLICATIONS AND PROGNOSIS

■ Cycloplegic agents used to measure refraction have systemic absorption. Cyclopentolate most likely to cause problems, esp. in developmentally delayed children.

■ Patching for amblyopia may cause amblyopia of patched eye. Follow the rule of 1 week occlusion per year of life with careful follow-up.

■ Prognosis for alignment good. May take several operations plus glasses.

■ Prognosis for good depth perception (stereopsis) is mixed. Early surgery may improve depth perception prognosis.

STREPTOCOCCAL INFECTIONS

RICHARD A. JACOBS, MD, PhD

HISTORY & PHYSICAL

History

■ Clinically relevant species: Streptococcus pyogenes (group A streptococcus), Streptococcus pneumoniae, Streptococcus agalactiae (group B streptococcus), Streptococcus bovis, viridans streptococci and groups C and G streptococci

■ Streptococci not universally part of normal skin flora

■ Colonization by contact with infected persons, usually in extreme crowding

  ➤ Streptococcal pharyngitis transmitted by saliva droplet or nasal transmission; crowding facilitates infection

  ➤ Acute rheumatic fever can occur 2–4 weeks afterwards, usually in school-age children; uncommon in the US

  ➤ Group B streptococcus can be colonized in about 20% female genital and gastrointestinal tracts; vertical transmission responsible for neonatal sepsis, especially if early rupture of membranes, early gestational age

Signs & Symptoms
- Pharyngitis
  - Primarily seen in Group A streptococci
  - Incubation 2–4 days
  - Sudden onset of sore throat with pain on swallowing, fevers, headaches, malaise
  - Large, hyperemic tonsils with or without grayish-white exudates; cervical lymphadenopathy
- Scarlet fever
  - Any streptococcal infection that elaborates pyrogenic exotoxins; usually with pharyngitis
  - Diffusely erythematous; superimposed fine red papules; blanches on pressure; "strawberry tongue"; Can be followed by desquamation
- Skin and soft-tissue infections
  - Usually due to Group A streptococci; Groups B, C and G also possible
- Erysipelas:
  - Well demarcated raised inflammation that usually involves the face
  - Can spread rapidly with swelling
  - Fever and chills common
- Cellulitis:
  - Presents with pain, erythema and swelling; lesions are not raised or well-demarcated
- Necrotizing fasciitis:
  - Presents as severe cellulitis, but pain out of proportion to findings
  - Anesthesia of the skin as the infection rapidly extends along the deep muscle fascia
- Streptococcal toxic shock syndrome may develop with the sudden onset of shock and multiorgan failure
- Rheumatic fever
  - Follows group A streptococcal pharyngeal infections (not skin infections)
  - Inflammatory lesions involving the heart (carditis), joints (arthritis), subcutaneous tissue (subcutaneous nodules), skin (erythema marginatum begins as a macule that enlarges with a clear center) and central nervous system (Sydenham's chorea)
  - Non-specific manifestations: heart block, fever, arthralgias and acute-phase reactants (increased erythrocyte sedimentation rate, positive C reactive protein)

➤ Presents as acute onset polyarthritis (75%), insidiously as carditis or uncommonly with chorea

■ Pneumonia
➤ S. pneumoniae: most common cause of community acquired pyogenic pneumonia
➤ Presents with productive cough, high fevers, and pleuritic chest pain
➤ Malaise and shortness of breath common
➤ Ill-appearing

■ Meningitis
➤ S. pneumoniae: most common cause of bacterial meningitis in adults
➤ Present with rapid onset of fever, headaches, altered mental status
➤ Meningismus is common
➤ Focal neurologic findings and obtundation are more common than in meningococcal meningitis

■ Endocarditis
■ Viridans streptococci: most common cause of native valve endocarditis, particularly if underlying valvular disease
➤ Insidious onset with a subacute course over several weeks before diagnosis
➤ Present with fever and constitutional signs (weight loss, anorexia, fatigue) as well as the usual diagnostic hallmarks of endocarditis (murmurs, peripheral stigmata etc)
➤ Also seen in S. pneumoniae, S. bovis (50% also have bowel malignancy), Streptococci groups C and G

■ Neonatal sepsis
➤ Group B streptococci: cause of neonatal sepsis, bacteremia and meningitis
➤ Also thought to be the etiology for endometritis, peripartum infections or septic abortions

TESTS

Laboratory
■ Basic blood studies:
■ Normal or elevated WBC (compare to baseline especially in HIV patients) with neutrophil predominance; abnormal liver function tests in systemic disease and shock; elevated creatinine phosphokinase levels may be clue in necrotizing fasciitis; high C-reactive

protein and erythrocyte sedimentation rate: nonspecific but may be seen in acute rheumatic fever and endocarditis
- Basic urine studies:
- Hematuria may be seen in endocarditis and post-streptococcal glomerulonephritis
  - Basic studies: gram stain (slightly elongated gram-positive cocci in pairs and chains) or culture of blood or specimen from suspected site of infection (sputum, CSF, joint fluid etc.) can confirm the diagnosis in most cases
  - An adequate sputum expectorate (large number of PMNs, few epithelial cells) that is analyzed promptly can lead to early diagnosis of pneumococcal pneumonia
  - Other studies: rapid antigen-detection tests
  - Can detect presence of group A streptococcal (carbohydrate) antigen in minutes from throat swabs
  - Highly specific (>95%) but lower sensitivity: if clinical suspicion is high, need to confirm negative throat swabs with culture
- Other studies: serology
  - Can be helpful in diagnosis of rheumatic fever but not specific (three samples sent for ASO >95% sensitivity two months after onset); can also help in poststreptococcal glomerulonephritis

Imaging
- CXR: usually infiltrates in a single lobe seen in pneumococcal pneumonia; pleural effusion generally uncommon, but suspect empyema if seen in pneumonia due to S. pyogenes
- Plain films, CT and MRI rarely helpful in necrotizing fasciitis and often delay diagnosis

DIFFERENTIAL DIAGNOSIS
- Streptococcal pharyngitis can be identical to adenovirus and Epstein-Barr virus; always think of acute HIV in the right host. Also distinguish from diphtheria, epiglottitis, Neisseria spp and Mycoplasma
- Streptococcal skin infections may be difficult to those caused by S. aureus

MANAGEMENT
What to Do First
- Empiric antibiotics in serious disease is necessary (endocarditis, meningitis, pneumonia) before definitive diagnosis

■ Prompt evaluation for surgical exploration in cases of suspected necrotizing fasciitis can be life-saving

General Measures
■ General supportive care

SPECIFIC THERAPY

Treatment Options
■ The antibiotic of choice for serious streptococcal infections remains penicillin, with some exceptions.
■ For serious streptococcal skin infections, may need to treat as possible staphylococcal infection (Cefazolin 500 mg IV TID or with Nafcillin 1.5 g IV QID). Treat with parental antibiotics for facial erysipelas: Penicillin 2 million units IV q4h. For patients with serious penicillin allergy, Vancomycin 1 g IV q12h is used.
■ In necrotizing fasciitis and other conditions that lead to streptococcal toxic shock syndrome, some advocate the addition of clindamycin (may suppress exotoxin production by group A streptococcus).
■ For endocarditis caused by the viridans streptococci and S. bovis, gentamicin is added for the duration of therapy at synergistic doses (1 mg/kg IV q8h for 4–6 weeks)
■ For S. pneumoniae, increasing penicillin-resistance (MIC > 0.1) may necessitate high-dose penicillin therapy. High level resistance (MIC > 2.0) should be treated with Ceftriaxone or a fluoroquinolone such as levofloxacin.
■ In meningitis, Vancomycin is now indicated as empiric therapy with Ceftriaxone, given the increasing prevalence of penicillin-resistant pneumococcus.
■ In streptococcal pharyngitis, therapy has a minimal effect on resolution of symptoms but prevent complications; consider treatment if clinical suspicion high even before definitive diagnosis by culture; benzathine penicillin G 1.2 million units IM X1 is preferred or penicillin V potassium 500 mg po QID for 10 days
■ Control of rheumatic fever involves both treatment of primary streptococcal pharyngitis and secondary prevention of recurrent disease; patients who have had rheumatic fever need prophylaxis for at least 5 years (1.2 million unit q 4 weeks IM or 250 mg po BID)

FOLLOW-UP
■ Routine follow-up depending on the disease

COMPLICATIONS AND PROGNOSIS

Complications

- Sequelae of streptococcus group A pharyngitis: acute rheumatic fever and poststreptococcal glomerulonephritis (can also get from impetigo)

Prognosis

- Good for most soft-tissue infections except necrotizing fasciitis; 20–70% mortality despite antibiotics
- In general, highest mortality in the elderly, immunocompromised, presence of other co-morbidities; invasive pneumococcal disease have a case-fatality rate of 40% in the elderly
- The prevalence of later heart disease after acute rheumatic fever depends on the severity of heart disease during the initial attack

Prevention

- Pneumococcal vaccine:
- Contains capsular polysaccharides from 23 common infecting sero-types of S. pneumoniae
- Studies show an efficacy of 60–70%, particularly in reducing bacteremia
- The U.S. Preventive Services Task Force recommends vaccines for individuals >65, or institutionalized people >50, or if over 2 years with cardiac, pulmonary disease, diabetes or asplenia
- Revaccination is not routinely recommended.

STRONGYLOIDIASIS

J. GORDON FRIERSON, MD

HISTORY & PHYSICAL

History

- Infection due to infestation with strongyloides stercoralis
- Life cycle: pregnant females are embedded in wall of upper small intestine, eggs laid which hatch in small intestine, producing filariform (infective) and rhabditiform (non-infective) larvae, which pass in stool. Some filariform larvae re-invade through the small or large bowel or perianal skin. In soil, rhabditiform larvae may become infective filariform) and penetrate skin. Re-invading larvae pass in

circulation to lungs, go to alveolae, migrate up bronchial tree and are swallowed, and mate in small intestine.

■ Exposure: by contact of skin with feces, contaminated soil, or ingestion of food contaminated with larvae. Autoinfection occurs continuously through bowel wall and perianal skin. Massive autoinfection (hyperinfection syndrome) occurs in immunocompromised patients (steroids, hematologic malignancies, starvation, immunosuppressive drugs, transplant patients, etc.)

Signs & Symptoms

■ Penetration phase (skin): local itching, sometimes subcutaneous larval tracts visible, especially on buttocks or perianal area.

■ Migratory phase: In heavy infections may have cough, wheeze, eosinophilia, and transient pulmonary infiltrates (Loeffler's syndrome).

■ Intestinal Phase: may have no symptoms, or may have varying degrees of epigastric pain, dyspepsia, bloating, diarrhea, sometimes with passage of blood in heavy infections. Allergic symptoms or urticaria, asthma may occur at any time. AIDS patients usually have standard syndromes, but sometimes hyperinfection.

■ Hyperinfection syndrome: this may give exaggerated intestinal symptoms such as diarrhea, bloating, abdominal pain. If sufficient tissue invasion has occurred there may be fever, hypotension, inanition, pulmonary infiltrates, meningeal signs.

TESTS

■ Basic tests: blood: CBC almost always shows eosinophilia, sometimes anemia. In severe disease eosinophilia may be absent.

■ Basic tests: urine: normal

■ Specific tests: Stool O&P shows the larvae in 50–70% of cases. Organism more easily seen using concentration methods: (1) the Baermann method (putting stool in gauze in funnel over warm water, larvae migrate to water), or, (2) a similar method using filter paper (Harada-Mori technique), or, (3) culture on nutrient agar (probably most sensitive but not readily available).

■ Other tests: Larvae may be seen in duodenal juices using the Enterotest, or intubation. Serology is sensitive, positive in 95% of cases, done at CDC, may cross-react with filariasis and may be false-negative in immunocompromised host. Occasionally larvae are coughed up or seen at bronchoscopy. In hyperinfection syndrome larvae are plentiful in stool, blood cultures often positive for enteric organisms, and CSF may show PMNs and culture gram negative organisms.

DIFFERENTIAL DIAGNOSIS

■ Skin lesions mimic cutaneous larva migrans due to Ancylostoma of dogs and cats. Intestinal symptoms are confused with ulcers, other causes of diarrhea, enteritis, colitis. Eosinophilia and allergic symptoms may mimic noninfectious causes. In the hyperinfection state, gram negative sepsis, shock, meningitis, and pulmonary infiltrates direct attention away from a parasitic cause.

MANAGEMENT

What to Do First

■ Correct any fluid and electrolyte problems. If a hyperinfection state exists, sepsis and hypotension need treatment.

General Measures

■ Stabilization of patient. Identify source of infection.

SPECIFIC THERAPY

Indications

■ All patients should be treated since the infection does not heal spontaneously.

Treatment Options

■ Ivermectin for 1 or 2 days
■ Thiabendazole for 2–3 days
■ Albendazole for 5–7 days
■ It is probably best to repeat the treatment in a week, if tolerated. Ivermectin and thiabendazole are approximately equivalent in effectiveness, curing about 90% with one course. Albendazole is a little less effective.

Side Effects & Complications

■ Ivermectin: well tolerated, may be itching, light-headedness
■ Thiabendazole: side effects common, consisting of dizziness, nausea, vomiting, rash, occasionally Stevens-Johnson syndrome.
■ Albendazole: well tolerated, may get mild intestinal complaints, light-headedness, rash.
■ Contraindications to treatment: absolute: First trimester pregnancy in mild infection. Treat any stage in hyperinfection syndrome, where Ivermectin is drug of choice.
■ Contraindications to treatment:relative:none

FOLLOW-UP

During Treatment
- If thiabendazole given, patient should be watched if sick, or given early follow-up if out-patient. Hyperinfection patients need attention to fluids, diarrhea, electrolytes, and frequently need multiple courses of treatment or even maintenance therapy.

Routine
- Assess patient for cure. Criteria are: absence of larvae on stool exam by Baermann, Harada-Mori, or culture techniques, disappearance of eosinophilia, and disappearance of symptoms. Retreat if necessary.

COMPLICATIONS AND PROGNOSIS
- Prognosis of light infections is good, though retreatment may be necessary. In hyperinfection syndrome the prognosis is guarded. The infection is controllable if treated promptly, but may need either several courses or maintenance of periodic treatment. Reduction of immunocompromising factors (such as steroids) if possible, and treatment of complications such as gram negative sepsis/meningitis.

SUBARACHNOID HEMORRHAGE (SAH)

MICHAEL J. AMINOFF, MD, DSc

HISTORY & PHYSICAL
- Sudden severe headache ("worst headache in my life")
- Nausea, vomiting, obtundation common
- Obtunded or comatose pt
- Signs of meningeal irritation
- Often no focal neurologic deficits except bilateral Babinski signs
- Middle cerebral artery aneurysm may cause aphasia, weakness of arm & face
- Posterior communicating artery aneurysm may cause pupil-sparing 3rd nerve palsy
- Cerebral AVM usually causes deficit depending on lesion location

TESTS
- Lab studies: usually normal; peripheral leukocytosis or transient glycosuria may occur
- Cranial CT: subarachnoid & intraventricular blood
- CSF (if CT scan normal): blood-stained

- Four-vessel angiography: to identify source of bleeding & any coexisting vascular anomalies
- ECG may show arrhythmia or myocardial ischemia (as secondary phenomenon due to central sympathetic activation)

DIFFERENTIAL DIAGNOSIS

- Imaging studies will distinguish btwn aneurysm & AVM, and btwn subarachnoid & intracerebral hemorrhage; primary intracerebral hemorrhage leads to marked focal deficit
- Traumatic cause of SAH usually evident from history
- Acute bacterial meningitis is distinguished by CSF findings

MANAGEMENT

- Supportive care
- Strict bed rest
- Analgesics for headache (but avoid antiplatelet meds)
- Keep pt sedated & blood pressure at low-normal levels
- Anticonvulsant prophylaxis for seizures
- Nimodipine to reduce risk of vasospasm

SPECIFIC THERAPY

- Early surgery or endovascular treatment for accessible aneurysm or AVM, if feasible, unless pt deeply comatose

FOLLOW-UP

n/a

COMPLICATIONS AND PROGNOSIS

Complications

- Recurrence of hemorrhage common w/ aneurysmal source; prevented by early surgery
- Vasospasm: may lead to ischemic neurologic deficit in first 21 days after SAH despite prophylaxis w/ nimodipine; treat w/ volume expansion & induced hypertension only if underlying lesion has been surgically treated & no other lesions exist; angioplasty may be required
- Acute hydrocephalus (from impaired CSF absorption) suggested by somnolence, poor attention, confusion; treat by shunt
- Cardiac arrhythmias: treat as appropriate
- Cerebral salt-wasting may lead to hyponatremia

Prognosis

- After first aneurysmal SAH, approximately 50% of pts die, many before arriving in hospital; another 20% die from re-bleeding unless the aneurysm is corrected; approximately 90% of pts survive after bleeding from an AVM; focal deficit more likely among survivors of SAH from AVM than aneurysm

---

SUNBURN

JEFFREY P. CALLEN, MD

HISTORY & PHYSICAL

History
- Outdoor activities or tanning bed use
  - ➤ Photosensitizing medications – i.e., sulfonamides, thiazide diuretics, tetracyclines, psoralens, NSAIDs
  - ➤ Topical photosensitizers – e.g., coal tar extracts, lime juice
  - ➤ Ultraviolet light (UVL) radiation increases with altitude
  - ➤ Reflection from sand, snow, water of UVL

Signs & Symptoms
- Warmth, pain, itching on sun-exposed areas
- Blistering may occur with severe sunburns
- Sharply demarcated areas of involvement
- Inflammation
  - ➤ Appears within 2–4 hours
  - ➤ Peaks at 12–24 hours
  - ➤ Abates slowly over several days
- Daily sun exposure is additive and a "tan" does not protect well against sunburn
- UVA tanning (tanning beds/salons) is only mildly protective against UVB-induced erythema

TESTS
- None are needed

DIFFERENTIAL DIAGNOSIS
- Photosensitivity diseases – polymorphous light eruption, lupus erythematosus, dermatomyositis, photoallergic dermatitis

MANAGEMENT

What to Do First
- Assess the severity of the sunburn – is there vesiculation?
- Assess the role of medications as a factor in the photosensitivity.

■ Recommend complete avoidance of further exposure until resolution.

General Measures
■ Stress the need for future sun protection.
■ Substitute an alternative agent for a photosensitizing medication.

SPECIFIC THERAPY
■ Cool compresses
■ Aspirin or indomethacin, or other NSAID
■ Topical antibiotic for vesicular, bullous or erosive lesion

Specific Situations
■ UVL is an immunosuppressant
■ UVB phototherapy or Psoralen + UVA (PUVA) photochemotherapy is used to treat a variety of skin diseases, and may cause "sunburn" reactions

FOLLOW-UP
■ Yearly full body examination for patients who sustained a blistering sunburn
■ Teach self-examination to patients or family members.
■ Educate patients and family members about the hazards of acute or chronic sun exposure.

COMPLICATIONS AND PROGNOSIS
■ Freckles, lentigines, poikiloderma as signs of actinic damage (photo-aging)
■ Increased risk of development of melanoma and non-melanoma skin cancer

SUPERFICIAL THROMBOPHLEBITIS

RAJABRATA SARKAR, MD

HISTORY & PHYSICAL

History
■ Pain and swelling in the distribution of a superficial vein
■ Can occur spontaneously or after trauma, venipuncture or IV placement
■ No history of fevers in most cases
■ Septic thrombophlebitis

➤ Spiking fevers, leukocytosis
➤ Recent indwelling catheter (either peripheral IV or PICC or central line)

Signs & Symptoms

▪ Swelling, tenderness and erythema over a superficial vein
▪ Pus or induration at the venipuncture site is suspicious for septic thrombophlebitis
▪ Swelling of the whole extremity is unusual

TESTS

Blood

▪ Blood cultures and CBC for detection of septicemia in pts with fevers

DIFFERENTIAL DIAGNOSIS

n/a

MANAGEMENT

General Measures

▪ In non-septic thrombophlebitis, inflammation is sterile and due to thrombus in vein
   ➤ no need for antibiotics
   ➤ no need for anticoagulation
▪ Treat with
   ➤ elevation
   ➤ warm compresses
   ➤ nonsteroidal anti-inflammatory medications
▪ Septic thrombophlebitis
   ➤ prevent with aseptic technique during line placement
   ➤ vigilant surveillance of all IV sites to prevent infection
   ➤ surgical exploration of any suspicious prior venipuncture site
   ➤ if pus is found in vein, complete excision of vein
   ➤ high dose antibiotic therapy based on vein culture
   ➤ start presumptive antibiotics for S. aureus
   ➤ high morbidity and mortality if diagnosis is missed

SPECIFIC THERAPY

n/a

FOLLOW-UP

n/a

COMPLICATIONS AND PROGNOSIS

Complications (of Septic Thrombophlebitis)
- Bacterial endocarditis (often fatal)
- Abscess at site of venipuncture
- Septic emboli to lungs or other organs (splenic abscess, etc.)

Prognosis
- Superficial thrombophlebitis
  - ➤ prognosis is excellent
- Septic thrombophlebitis
  - ➤ prognosis is related to the timeliness of diagnosis
  - ➤ early excision of the septic vein – good prognosis
  - ➤ *S. aureus* endocarditis – poor prognosis

SYNCOPE

MICHAEL J. AMINOFF, MD, DSc

HISTORY & PHYSICAL
- Transient loss of consciousness
- Prodromal malaise, nausea, pallor, diaphoresis, weakness
- Loss of muscle tone is common
- Rapid recovery once pt is recumbent
- Urinary incontinence sometimes occurs during episode
- Episodes may be precipitated by acute or anticipated pain, emotional stress, fluid loss, obstructed venous return, intense activity in the heat, prolonged standing, postural hypotension, cardiac arrhythmia
- Examination usually normal in vasovagal syncope
- Cardiac arrhythmia or evidence of dysautonomia (eg, postural hypotension, impaired sweating, pupillary abnormalities) may be found when syncope is secondary
- With dysautonomias, associated abnormalities may be found in CNS or PNS

TESTS
- Normal in vasovagal syncope
- Abnormal autonomic function studies indicate dysautonomia
- Tilt-table testing may reproduce symptoms & indicate cardiac abnormality

- ECG & Holter monitoring may indicate disturbance of cardiac rhythm
- Lab studies may reveal systemic cause (eg, anemia or cardiac, metabolic, toxic or endocrine disorder; hypovolemia)
- In pts w/ neurologic abnormalities on examination, CT scan or MRI may reveal structural cause in CNS; NCS may reveal abnormalities in PNS

DIFFERENTIAL DIAGNOSIS
- Cause of syncope may be revealed by testing as above; in many cases, no specific cause found
- Prodromal symptoms, loss of muscle tone, precipitating circumstances, rapid recovery w/ recumbency distinguish syncope from seizures

MANAGEMENT
- During syncopal episode, ensure pt becomes recumbent
- Syncope may be averted by placing pt recumbent during precipitating circumstances or presyncopal events

SPECIFIC THERAPY
- Treat underlying cause

FOLLOW-UP
- As needed, depending on cause

COMPLICATIONS AND PROGNOSIS
- Depend on underlying cause
- Usually good prognosis in typical vasovagal syncope

SYPHILIS

SARAH STAEDKE, MD

HISTORY & PHYSICAL

History
- Syphilis is a complex systemic illness caused by the spirochete Treponema pallidum; natural course of disease is divided into three stages
- Modes of transmission: sexual contact, blood transfusion, direct inoculation, vertically to fetus

- Risk factors: young age, race/ethnicity (highest reported rates in African-Americans and Hispanics); lower socioeconomic status, urban residence, illicit drug use, prostitution
- 30–40% risk of transmission following sexual contact with infected case

Signs & Symptoms

- Primary syphilis
  - Incubation period averages 21 days, range 10–90 d
  - Chancre: painless, indurated, usually single, multiple in 25% cases
  - Lymphadenopathy: nontender, rubbery
  - Lesions heal spontaneously without treatment in 3–6 weeks
- Secondary syphilis
  - Incubation period 3–6 weeks after development of chancre
  - Constitutional symptoms (70%): fever, malaise, arthralgias
  - Skin rash (90%): diffuse, typically involving palms and soles
  - Condyloma lata: painless, moist mucosal lesions; highly infectious
  - Lymphadenopathy: generalized, painless
  - CNS: asymptomatic involvement in 8–40%, symptomatic 1–2%
  - Other: patchy alopecia (40%), mucous patches (35%), glomerulonephritis, hepatitis, arthritis, osteitis
  - Symptoms resolve spontaneously; recurrent episodes in 25% untreated patients usually within first year of infection
- Latent syphilis
  - Positive treponemal serologic tests with no clinical manifestations
  - Early = disease of <1 year duration
  - Late ≥1 year duration or disease of unknown duration
- Tertiary syphilis
  - Late complications occur in 30% of untreated patients
  - Gummas: rare, granulomatous lesions of skin, bone, brain, heart
  - Cardivascular: ascending aortic aneurysm, aortic insufficiency
  - Neurosyphilis – can occur at any stage of disease
    - Asymptomatic: CSF abnormalities only
    - Meningeal: acute meningitis
    - Meningovascular: stroke syndrome, seizures
    - Parenchymal: general paresis, tabes dorsalis

TESTS

Basic Tests

■ CSF examination: pleocytosis (>5 WBC/mm3), elevated protein, +VDRL

Specific Diagnostic Tests

■ Darkfield examination: examine fresh specimen of serous exudate from lesions; identify characteristic corkscrew motility of spirochete; test of choice (if available) for primary syphilis; not for oral or anal specimens due to presence of nonpathogenic treponemes.

■ Fluorescent antibody microscopy: use if darkfield not available and for oral and anal specimens

■ Non-treponemal serologic tests (RPR and VDRL): Inexpensive, rapid, quantitative, screening tests, titers correlate with disease activity and response to therapy:
  ➤ RPR + in 80% primary, 99% secondary, 56% tertiary
  ➤ VDRL + in 70% primary, 99% secondary, 56% tertiary
  ➤ False positive results: IV drug use, pregnancy, autoimmune disease, immunization, infections (EBV, TB, SBE, malaria)
  ➤ False negatives: early infection, prozone phenomenon (rare)

■ Treponemal serologic tests (FTA-ABS, MHA-TP, TPHA): More sensitive, expensive, confirmatory tests
  ➤ FTA-ABS + in 85% primary, 100% secondary, 98% tertiary
  ➤ MHA-TP + in 65% primary, 100% secondary, 95% tertiary

Other Tests

■ Chest Xray: linear calcifications in ascending aorta suggestive of cardiovascular syphilis 1/1/2001

DIFFERENTIAL DIAGNOSIS

■ Primary: HSV, chancroid, lymphogranulorna venereum, fixed drug eruption, traumatic ulcer, aphthous ulcer

■ Secondary: drug reaction, pityriasis rosea, viral exanthem, tinea versicolor, acute guttate psoriasis, condyloma acuminata

MANAGEMENT

What to Do First

■ Obtain specimens for darkfield microscopy, if available

General Measures

■ Test for HIV; consider testing for gonorrhea, chlamydia

- Clinical manifestations, serologic tests, and response to therapy may be atypical in HIV-infected patients
- Indications for CSF evaluation
  - Neurologic or ophthalmologic signs or symptoms
  - Evidence of tertiary disease (gummas, cardiovascular)
  - Early syphilis treatment failure
  - HIV infection with late latent (>1 yr) or disease of unknown duration
- Some experts recommend CSF examination in all HIV-infected patients
- Report case to local public health authorities and refer sexual partners for evaluation and treatment

SPECIFIC THERAPY

Indications
- Sexual partner of infected contact within past 3 months
- Positive darkfield examination or direct fluorescent antibody test
- Positive serologic tests:
  - Newly positive non-treponemal and/or treponemal test
  - Four-fold increase in non-treponemal serologic titer
- Neurosyphilis: no single test is diagnostic
  - Positive CSF VDRL
  - >5 WBCs/mm3 in CSF
  - Elevated protein

Treatment Options
Primary, Secondary, and Early Latent Syphilis and Epidemiologic treatment
- Benzathine penicillin (PCN) IM in single dose
- PCN allergic: Doxycycline orally OR Tetracycline orally
Late Latent Syphilis (>1 year duration) and Tertiary (gumma, cardiovascular)
- Benzathine PCN IM weekly ×3
- PCN allergic (consider CSF examination before using alternative drugs): Doxycycline orally OR Tetracycline

Neurosyphilis
- Aqueous crystalline PCN G
- OR (for compliant patients only) Procaine PCN IM daily, for 10–14 days PLUS Probenecid orally for 10–14 days
- PCN allergic: skin test and desensitize to PCN

Special Considerations

- Pregnancy: PCN is only recommended therapy; if PCN allergic, skin test and desensitize; consider 4.8 mil U of Benzathine PCN for treatment of patients with early (primary, secondary, early latent) disease or those with ultrasound findings consistent with fetal syphilis
- HIV: for primary, secondary, and early latent disease, consider additional doses of benzathine PCN (7.2 mil U total)

Side Effects & Contraindications

- Penicillin: side effects: hypersensitivity reaction, rash, diarrhea, GI distress; contraindicated in penicillin allergy; pregnancy = B
- Doxycycline/Tetracycline: side effects: GI distress, photosensitivity, erosive esophagitis; contraindicated in pregnancy (D) and growing children

FOLLOW-UP

Primary, Secondary, Early Latent

- Re-examine clinically and serologically at 6 and 12 mo (3, 6, 9, 12, and 24 in HIV+)
- Repeat serology in pregnant women in 3rd trimester and at delivery
- Recommend repeat HIV test and CSF evaluation if. –
  - ➤ Signs or symptoms persist
  - ➤ Non-treponemal titers fail to decrease four-fold in 6 mo
  - ➤ Non-treponemal titers increase four-fold
- Consider CSF evaluation at 6 mo in HIV+ patients

Late Latent

- Repeat non-treponemal serologic tests at 6, 12, and 24 mo (re-evaluate clinically and serologically at 6, 12, 18, and 24 in HIV+)
- Repeat HIV test and evaluate CSF if:
  - ➤ Signs or symptoms develop
  - ➤ Non-treponemal titers fail to decrease four-fold in 12–24 mo
  - ➤ Non-treponemal titers increase four-fold

Neurosyphilis

- If CSF abnormal initially, repeat CSF evaluations every 6 months
- Consider retreatment if:
  - ➤ Elevated CSF WBC persists after 6 months
  - ➤ CSF is remains abnormal after 2 years

COMPLICATIONS AND PROGNOSIS

- Jarisch-Herxheimer reaction: develops within 24 h of treatment; self-limited but potentially severe; 50% primary, 90% secondary, and 25%

early latent cases; may precipitate preterm delivery and fetal distress in pregnancy
- Prognosis: PCN remains highly effective against T. pallidum; failure to respond to therapy likely due to reinfection, undiagnosed neurosyphilis, or non-compliance with alternative treatment regimen

---

SYSTEMIC LUPUS ERYTHEMATOSUS

JOHN B. WINFIELD, MD

HISTORY & PHYSICAL

Risk Factors
- young women (M:F = 1:5), but may occur at any age
- associations: complement deficiencies, MHC class II genes, Fc receptor genes
- ~10% have affected relatives
- UV light exposure,
- Drugs: procainamide, isoniazid, hydantoins, minocycline, many others silica dust
- flare during pregnancy or postnatally (20–60%)

Signs & Symptoms
- at onset: constitutional, arthralgia/arthritis, malar rash, alopecia, Raynaud's disease, pleuritis, pericarditis, mesangial glomerulonephritis (GN)
- established SLE: above plus other rashes (discoid, generalized erythema ± photosensitivity) oral/nasal ulcerations, vasculitis, neurologic disease, hematological manifestations, glomerulonephritis (mesangial, membranous, focal proliferative or diffuse), peritonitis
- less common: bullous rash, myositis, pancreatitis, myocarditis, endocarditis, pulmonary disease (diffuse interstitial pneumonitis, hemorrhage, pulmonary hypertension)

TESTS

Laboratory
- Basic blood studies:
  - ➤ CBC: anemia (usually of chronic disease, occasionally hemolytic), lymphopenia, thrombocytopenia
  - ➤ ESR: increased
  - ➤ BUN/creatinine: increased in renal disease
  - ➤ Decreased complement (CH_{50} or C3 & C4)

- Basic urine studies:
  - Proteinuria
  - Hematuria (RBC casts suggest diffuse proliferative GN)
  - Pyuria in the absence of infection

Specific Tests
- Antinuclear antibody test (ANA) nearly always positive: low titers non-specific, occur in other autoimmune diseases; specificity for SLE increases with titer
- Anti-Ro/SSA & anti-La/SSB may be positive in rare "ANA-negative" lupus
- Highly specific for SLE:
  - antibodies to Sm antigen
  - antibodies to double-stranded DNA

Biopsy
- Renal:
  - mesangial widening, mild hypercellularity most common;
  - significant renal disease shows glomerular lesions (focal segmental or focal proliferative, diffuse proliferative, membranous, sclerosing, or combinations thereof)
  - granular glomerular Ig deposits by immunofluorescence
  - mesangial and subendothelial deposits by electron microscopy
  - mild renal disease may develop into more severe forms
- Other biopsies, e.g., skin, as indicated

DIFFERENTIAL DIAGNOSIS
- rheumatoid arthritis,
- fever of unknown origin
- infection, especially subacute bacterial endocarditis
- fibromyalgia
- systemic vasculitis

MANAGEMENT

What to Do First
- Assess disease activity, assess presence /severity of major organ system involvement
- Discontinue any drugs that might be responsible for SLE
- Assess for co-morbid fibromyalgia
- Patient education, psychosocial support
- Establish plan for follow-up clinical and laboratory monitoring

General Measures
- prophylaxis regarding sun exposure
- birth control or estrogen replacement
- treat hypertension aggressively
- control hyperlipidemia

SPECIFIC THERAPY
- Conservative Management
  - arthritis/arthralga and myalgia: acetaminophen, NSAIDs, hydroxychloroquine, low-dose corticosteroids if quality of life impaired
- cutaneous lupus:
  - sunscreens, topical corticosteroids, hydroxychloroquine,
  - dapsone, etretinate for resistant rashes
- fatigue:
  - often due to comorbid fibromyalgia
  - may requires oral corticosteroids
- serositis:
  - NSAIDs or low-moderate dose corticosteroids
  - alternative to low-dose corticosteroids: methotrexate
- Aggressive Management
  - initial therapy of severe organ system involvement:
    - prednisone for 6–8 wks with gradual tapering
    - for diffuse proliferative GN, or for other life-threatening disease, e.g. severe pneumonitis, vasculitis, and CNS lupus:
- IV cyclophosphamide repeated monthly for 6 months and then every 3 months for 18–24 months, with escalation unless WBC is <1500; optional initial pulse methylprednisolone
- monitor WBC at 10 and 14 d post cyclophosphamide treatment, adjusting dose to keep nadir WBC >1500
- alternative 1: mycophenolate mofetil (500 mg BID escalating to max. 3 gm/d) for minimum of two years, then taper; optional initial pulse methylprednisolone
- alternative 2: azathioprine (1–3 mg/kg/d); optional initial pulse methylprednisolone
- alternative 3: IV pulse methylprednisolone (7 mg/kg) daily ×3 d, then repeated monthly for 6 months

Special Situations
- Arterial or venous thrombosis (manifestation of antiphospholipid syndrome): warfarin to keep INR 3–3.5, low-dose aspirin, avoid estrogens

- Severe thrombocytopenia: high-dose prednisone and/or IV IgG; danazol, or splenectomy
- CNS lupus: with stroke, treat anti-phospholipid antibody mediated hypercoagulation; for seizures, diffuse cerebritis, cranial neuropathies, use moderate-high-dose corticosteroids plus psychoactive drugs for psychiatric manifestations
- Membranous glomerulonephritis: high-dose corticosteroids for 2–4 months or no treatment
- chronic stable glomerulonephritis: no treatment
- pregnancy:
  - ➤ with recurrent fetal loss (manifestation of antiphospholipid syndrome): low-dose aspirin, moderate-high-dose corticosteroids or heparin
  - ➤ screen for anti-Ro (SS-A)
- SLE in older persons: generally more benign with more musculoskeletal complaints, less renal disease; consider drug-induced lupus

Side Effects/Toxicities
- NSAIDs: see section in Osteoarthritis
- Corticosteroids: see section on Polymyositis
- Hydroxychloroquine: retinopathy, indigestion, rash
- Cyclophosphamide:
  - ➤ Hemorrhagic cystitis (leads to bladder carcinoma),
  - ➤ infection, suppression of gonadal function/infertility
- Azathioprine:
  - ➤ nausea, vomiting, diarrhea, bone marrow suppression, hepatitis, increased risk of lymphoproliferative malignancies
- Mycophenolate mofetil:
  - ➤ bone marrow suppression, hepatitis, nausea, vomiting diarrhea, long-term risk of malignancy

Contraindications
- Corticosteroids: relative: uncontrollable diabetes or hypertension, severe osteoporosis, steroid psychosis, life-threatening infection
- Hydroxychloroquine: absolute: retinopathy
- Cyclophosphamide:
  - ➤ absolute: cytopenia due to marrow suppression, life-threatening infection, irreversible renal disease, refusal to accept risk of infertility
  - ➤ relative: refractory hemorrhagic cystitis, severe nausea and vomiting, previous radiation therapy, history of malignancy

- Mycophenolate mofetil:
  - ➤ absolute: inability to comply with contraception; cytopenia due to marrow suppression, life-threatening infection, irreversible renal disease
  - ➤ relative: gastrointestinal side effects

FOLLOW-UP

Routine

- Every 3–6 months; CBC; BUN, creatinine, and electrolytes; urinalysis; anti-dsDNA; CH_{50} or C3 and C4
- Yearly: bone densitometry with corticosteroid therapy; eye checks with hydroxychloroquine flow chart for clinical and laboratory indices of disease activity
- During Treatment of severe organ system involvement: monitor organ function, drug complications

COMPLICATIONS AND PROGNOSIS

- Drug-induced SLE usually remits when the offending drug is discontinued
- overall survival ~95% at 1 year, ~75% at 10 years
- poorer prognosis in renal disease with elevated creatinine at time of biopsy, glomerular and tubulointerstitial scarring, initial Hct <26%, male sex, and black race
- renal allograft survival at 1 year ~70%, at 5 years, ~50%

TAKAYASU ARTERITIS

ERIC L. MATTESON, MD

HISTORY & PHYSICAL

History

- Female:Male 10:1; <40 years of age

Signs & Symptoms

- dizziness, syncope, upper or lower extremity
- claudication
- vascular bruits and pulse deficits
- hypertension more common than in GCA.

TESTS

n/a

DIFFERENTIAL DIAGNOSIS
n/a

MANAGEMENT
n/a

SPECIFIC THERAPY
n/a

FOLLOW-UP
n/a

COMPLICATIONS AND PROGNOSIS
n/a

TAPEWORM INFECTIONS

J. GORDON FRIERSON, MD

HISTORY & PHYSICAL

History
- Exposure: *Taenia saginata* (beef tapeworm): eating raw or undercooked beef containing encysted larvae.
  - *Taenia solium* (pork tapeworm): eating raw or undercooked pork containing encysted larvae (see cysticercosis).
  - *Diphyllobothrium* infections (fish tapeworm): eating raw or undercooked fresh or brackish water fish containing encysted larvae. Several species infest humans.
  - *Hymenolepis nana*: fecal-oral route: eating contaminated food or putting fecally contaminated fingers into mouth thus conveying eggs to mouth. Auto-infection occurs, can produce heavy infections.

Signs & Symptoms
- *T saginata*: passage of individual segments (proglottids) or parts of worm. Rarely any GI symptoms.
- *T solium*: passage of individual segments (proglottids) or parts of worm. Rarely any GI symptoms. Symptoms and signs of cysticercosis may be present.
- *Diphyllobothrium latum*: passage of individual segments (proglottids) or parts of worm. Rarely any GI symptoms. Occasionally fatigue and vitamin B12 deficiency.

- *Hymenolepis nana*: usually seen in children. Light infections: no symptoms. Heavy infections: diarrhea, abdominal pain, irritability. Passage of proglottids.

TESTS
- Basic tests: blood: normal
- Basic tests: urine: normal.
- Specific tests:
  - *T saginata* and *solium*: identification of submitted proglottid is diagnostic. O&P exam may be negative or if positive cannot distinguish between solium and saginata.
  - *Diphyllobothrium* species: Stool O&P usually finds eggs identifying genus but not species. Whole segments occasionally passed and are genus-specific. To speciate scolex is required (but not needed for treatment).
  - *Hymenolepis nana*: Stool O&P finds diagnostic ova. Proglottids not usually found.
- Other tests: B12 levels sometimes low in *Diphyllobothrium* infections.

DIFFERENTIAL DIAGNOSIS
- None

MANAGEMENT
What to Do First
- Ascertain source of infection if possible. In *T solium*, assess for presence of cysticercosis (serology, presence of SQ nodules, possibly brain imaging).

General Measures
- Education of patient on epidemiology, to avoid future infections. With *T solium*, other household members should be evaluated for cysticercosis.

SPECIFIC THERAPY
Indications
- All infected patients.

Treatment Options
- *T saginata* and *solium*, *Diphyllobothrium*:
  - Praziquantel single dose. With *T solium*, follow this with a saline purge 2 hours later, instructing patient to exercise care disposing of stool to avoid auto-infection.

- *Hymenolepis nana*:
  - ➤ Praziquantel single dose

Side Effects & Complications
- All infections: occasional mild nausea, pain, occasional dizziness. Theoretical risk of auto-infection with *T solium*, leading to cysticercosis.
- Contraindications to treatment: absolute: allergy to medication.
- Contraindications to treatment: relative: none.

FOLLOW-UP

During Treatment
- *T solium*: treat any nausea. Vomiting should be avoided.

Routine
- *T saginata*: If no segments or proglottids seen at 3 months, patient cured.
- *T solium*: check stools at 2–3 months. If no eggs and no segments or proglottids, patient cured.
- *Diphyllobothrium*: check stool O&P at 3 months.
- *Hymenolepis nana*: check stool O&P at one month.

COMPLICATIONS AND PROGNOSIS
- Prognosis is excellent regarding elimination of worms. Patients with *T solium* may have cysticercosis (see cysticercosis).

TARDIVE DYSKINESIA

CHAD CHRISTINE, MD

HISTORY & PHYSICAL
- Typically develops after long-term treatment w/ dopamine receptor antagonists (may occur w/ both typical & atypical neuroleptics)
- Occurs in 15–30% of pts on long-term neuroleptic treatment
- May develop during treatment or just after discontinuing treatment
- Higher risk in women, advanced age or prolonged exposure
- Higher risk in pts w/ diabetes, HIV or depression
- Movement can be suppressed voluntarily
- Choreoathetoid movement especially conspicuous about the lower face (eg, lip smacking, puckering, chewing movements, tongue twisting)
- Limb involvement usually symmetric

- Body rocking & swaying motions of the trunk
- Gait may be abnormal w/ leg jerking
- While standing in place, may shift weight
- Breathing may be irregular

TESTS
- Diagnosis made clinically
- Laby tests & brain imaging are normal

DIFFERENTIAL DIAGNOSIS
- Acute drug-induced movement disorders, stroke, neurodegenerative disorders (Huntington's disease, Wilson's disease, Tourette syndrome, edentulouness (or poorly fitting dentures), vasculitis, psychogenic causes excluded clinically
- Metabolic disorders (hyperparathyroidism, hyperthyroidism, hepatocerebral degeneration) & vasculitis (lupus erythematosus, periarteritis nodosa) excluded by lab tests & brain imaging

MANAGEMENT
- Preventive: avoid long-term, high-dose treatment w/ neuroleptics
  - ➤ Taper dopamine receptor antagonist slowly
  - ➤ Substitute atypical neuroleptics for high-potency D2 antagonists

SPECIFIC THERAPY
- No definitive treatment available
- If symptoms persist & are significantly disruptive, consider treatment w/:
  - ➤ Reserpine
  - ➤ Tetrabenazine (not available in U.S.)
  - ➤ L-dopa, dopamine agonists in low doses may help some pts
  - ➤ Amantadine, lithium, valproate, benzodiazepines, baclofen may also be tried
  - ➤ If these agents not helpful (or for those who suffer ongoing psychosis), atypical neuroleptics (eg, quetiapine, olanzapine, clozapine) helpful

FOLLOW-UP
- Depends on severity & whether treatment is indicated

COMPLICATIONS AND PROGNOSIS
- Symptoms regress spontaneously in 5–30% (but may take years)
- Better prognosis for younger pts

TENSION-TYPE HEADACHE

CHAD CHRISTINE, MD

HISTORY & PHYSICAL
- Recurrent headache disorder
- Pressing/tightening (nonpulsatile) holocephalic pain of mild to moderate severity
- Contraction of neck & scalp muscles common
- Develops over minutes to hours
- May occur daily
- Absence of nausea, vomiting, photophobia, phonophobia
- Normal exam

TESTS
- Diagnosis made clinically
- Lab tests & brain imaging are normal
- Lumbar puncture opening pressure & CSF studies are normal

DIFFERENTIAL DIAGNOSIS
- Brain mass lesion & subdural hematoma excluded by history & brain imaging
- Migraine headache distinguished by history
- Pseudotumor cerebri, postconcussion syndrome, metabolic disorders (eg, hypothyroidism) excluded by history & serum studies
- Dental pathology, sinus disease, poor posture or unphysiologic work conditions, inadequate sleep, sleep apnea, depression excluded clinically
- Brain imaging indicated for prominent change in headache quality or frequency

MANAGEMENT
- Depends on severity & prior treatment
- General measures
  - ➤ Headache diary may elucidate precipitants
  - ➤ Ensure adequate relaxation, exercise & sleep

SPECIFIC THERAPY

Indications
- Abortive meds indicated for rare headaches (2 or fewer a week); prophylactic meds are used for more frequent moderate to severe headaches

Treatment options
- Abortive agents
  - Acetaminophen
  - Aspirin
  - Ibuprofen
- Prophylactic agents
  - Tricyclic antidepressants
    - Amitriptyline
    - Nortriptyline
    - Doxepin
  - Botulinum toxin

FOLLOW-UP
- Every 3–12 months depending on level of control

COMPLICATIONS AND PROGNOSIS
- Good

TESTIS TUMORS

ARTHUR I. SAGALOWSKY, MD

HISTORY & PHYSICAL
- the most common male cancer ages 15–35 years
- cryptorchidism risk ratio for tumor 3–14× normal; contralateral testis also at increased risk
- Primary testis tumors: 5 most common histologies:
  - seminoma 40%
  - teratocarcinoma 25–30%
  - embryonal carcinoma 20-25%
  - teratoma 5–10%
  - choriocarcinoma 1%

Symptoms & Signs
- painless or painful testis mass
- testis may feel heavy
- often first noticed after minor trauma, so-called "trauma decoy"
- may have reactive epididymitis, orchitis, or hydrocele due to sudden tumor growth or blood
- any solid testis mass should be considered a germ cell tumor until proven otherwise

■ possible secondary signs: supraclavicular mass, abdominal epigastric mass, back pain, gynecomastia

TESTS

Diagnostic
■ Physical exam alone strongly suggests Dx in most cases
■ scrotal ultrasound a helpful adjunct if exam equivocal
■ initial biopsy not recommended routinely
■ Dx established by inguinal orchiectomy
■ positive urine pregnancy test (HCG) proves germ cell tumor in males (see below under tumor markers)

Staging
■ metastasis is common via predictable retroperitoneal lymph nodes draining testis in all cell types
■ hematogenous spread uncommon except in choriocarcinoma
■ involved sites in advanced disease (in descending order): lung >> liver, or bone >> brain
■ 3-pronged approach to staging:
   ➤ primary pathology predictors for spread
      • lymphovascular invasion in testis
      • embryonal carcinoma predominance
      • invasion into epididymis, rete testis, and/or spermatic cord
   ➤ serum tumor markers
      • alpha fetoprotein (AFP) in embryonal carcinoma
      • beta subunit human chorionic gonadotropin (HCG) in chorio-carcinoma, some seminoma
      • lactic dehydrogenase (LDH) in advanced embryonal carcinoma
   ➤ imaging
      • CXR in all cases
      • abdominal CT in all cases
      • chest CT if positive abdominal CT or positive tumor markers after orchiectomy

Definition of Clinical Stages
■ I: Abd CT, CXR, serum markers all neg
■ II: Abd CT pos; CXR and chest CT neg; serum markers pos or neg
   ➤ IIA: 2–5 cm mass
   ➤ IIB: 5 to 9 cm mass
   ➤ IIC: >10 cm mass

■ III: Chest CT pos; Abd CT pos or neg; markers pos or neg
■ Seropositive: only markers pos; all else neg

DIFFERENTIAL DIAGNOSIS
■ secondary testis tumors: lymphoma, leukemia
■ rare benign testis tumors: Leydig cell, gonadal stromal
■ benign or malignant paratesticular tumors: adenomatoid, rhabdomyosarcoma, leiomyosarcoma
■ other benign scrotal masses (see preceding section)

MANAGEMENT
n/a

SPECIFIC THERAPY
■ Refer to a urologist
■ inguinal orchiectomy is first step
■ initiation of chemotherapy in proven advanced disease (measurable
metastasis and positive markers) may precede orchiectomy as timing
critical due to rapid tumor growth
■ seminoma is radiosensitive
■ all cell types are chemosensitive: platinum, etoposide, bleomycin
(PEB) most common regimen
■ highly successful multimodal therapy allows a variety of Rx
approaches; nuances of specific choice are beyond the scope of this
article
■ acceptable treatment options for each clinical stage:
  ➤ Stage I: retroperitoneal lymph node dissection (RPLND): Open
  RPLND remains the standard, but experience with laparoscopic
  RPLND also is evolving; surveillance; primary chemotherapy
  (platinum, etoposide, bleomycin) 2 courses; retroperitoneal
  radiation therapy (pure seminoma only)
  ➤ Stage II, limited: RPLND; PEB chemotherapy 3–4 courses
  ➤ Stage II, advanced, and Stage III: PEB chemotherapy 3–4 courses;
  possible debulking RPLND after chemotherapy
  ➤ Seropositive: PEB chemotherapy 2–4 courses

FOLLOW-UP
■ 90% of relapse is within 12 months
■ 95% of relapse is within 24 months
■ general guideline: interval extent and duration of evaluation vary by
initial stage and extent of treatment
■ for good-risk patients (low stage, low tumor volume):

➤ PE, CXR, tumor markers q 1–3 months 1st year; q 3–6 months 2nd year; q 6 months year 3; then annually
➤ abd CT q 3–6 months 1st year; q 6–12 months 2nd year
■ for high-risk patients (advanced stage, high tumor volume):
➤ PE, CXR, tumor markers q month 1st year; q 2–3 months 2nd year; q 3–6 months 3rd year; q 6 months 4th and 5th years; then annually
➤ abd CT, ± chest CT q 3 months 1st year; q 6 months 2nd, 3rd, and 4th years; then annually

COMPLICATIONS AND PROGNOSIS
■ cure rate most dependent on tumor volume
■ 98% cure if no nodal involvement
■ >90% cure with minimal lymph node and lung involvement
■ 60–70% cure extensive lymph node and lung involvement
■ complications related to Rx (surgery, XRT, chemotherapy) currently low overall

TETANUS

RICHARD A. JACOBS, MD, PhD

HISTORY & PHYSICAL

History
■ In US, most cases are in adults with inadequate immunity to tetanus and follow puncture or laceration.
■ The wound may be trivial.
■ Can also follow burns, surgery, childbirth, abortion, injection drug use (skin-popping), and frostbite.
■ Symptoms: 3–10 days after injury, increase in muscle tone and rigidity, progressing to painful spasms. Classically short nerves (head) are affected more than long nerves (limbs). Dysphagia and trismus, pain and stiffness in shoulders, neck and back.
■ Hands and feet relatively spared.

Signs & Symptoms
■ Trismus, facial grimace (risus sardonicus), arched back (opisthotonos),
■ Painful Spasms (face > trunk > extremities) without loss of consciousness
■ Hyperactive deep tendon reflexes

- May have fever
- In severe cases, autonomic dysfunction may occur

TESTS

- Basic Tests: Blood. May have increased WBC, May have increased CPK, normal calcium
- Basic Tests, other: may have urine myoglobin
- Specific Diagnostic Tests: Diagnosis is clinical. Serum antitoxin level of 0.01 units/ml is usually protective, but doesn't rule out the diagnosis.
- Other Tests: Cerebrospinal fluid is normal
- Toxicology for strychnine is negative.

DIFFERENTIAL DIAGNOSIS

- Strychnine poisoning, hypocalcemia, rabies, dystonic reaction, meningitis/encephalitis. Trismus can also be caused by alveolar abscess.

MANAGEMENT

What to Do First

- Assess airway and ventilation-upper airway can be obstructed or diaphragm can be involved by spasms. May require intubation with early tracheostomy.
- Draw labs
- Given tetanus immune globulin and dT at separate sites.
- ICU monitoring and care
- Clean and debride wound.

General Measures

- Antispasmodics: Benzodiazepines do not oversedate or depress respiratory function.
- Minimize paralysis duration to avoid prolonged paralysis.
  - ➤ Use non-depolarizing paralytic: consider propofol, dantrolene, baclofen
  - ➤ Treat autonomic dysfunction, which usually occurs several days after onset of symptoms, with drips if labile (labetalol, esmolol).

SPECIFIC THERAPY

Indications

- Antibiotics of unproven efficacy but often used.
- Antitoxin neutralizes circulating toxin and unbound toxin in wound, lowering mortality.

Treatment Options
- Human tetanus immune globulin (TIG) IM.
- Low dose as effective as higher dose. Best given before manipulating wound. Consider infiltrating wound with TIG.
- Pooled IVIG is second line
- Equine tetanus immune toxin works, available, causes serum sickness.
- If using antibiotics, metronidazole associated with better survival rate than penicillin (a GABA antagonist).

FOLLOW-UP
- Immunize since immunity not induced by disease. 2nd dT at time of discharge, and 3rd 4 weeks later.
- During Treatment: Patients require rehabilitation and supportive psychotherapy as they recover.

COMPLICATIONS AND PROGNOSIS

Complications
- Airway compromise – Intubation and mechanical ventilation, may require early tracheostomy.
- Spasms (very common) – benzodiazepines
- Autonomic dysfunction from excessive catecholamine release- labetalol or esmolol.
- Hypotension (uncommon) – may require norepinephrine
- High caloric and protein needs (common) – may require enteral and parenteral nutrition begun early.

Prognosis
- Mortality for mild-moderate disease is 6%; 60% for severe disease
- Disease course may be 4–6 weeks
- Shorter incubation periods and more rapid progression from stiffness to spasms associated with worse prognosis.
- Survivors often have post traumatic stress disorder requiring psychotherapy.

THALASSEMIA

AKIKO SHIMAMURA, MD, PhD

HISTORY & PHYSICAL
- Family history of thalassemia syndrome
- History of anemia. No anemia with single alpha gene deletion (alpha thalassemia "silent carrier")

- Family history of splenomegaly, splenectomy, jaundice, gallstones
- Alpha and beta thalassemia common in Mediterranean basin, Southeast Asia, southern China, India, and Africa

Signs & Symptoms

- Heterogyzotes (beta thalassemia trait or deletion of one or two alpha globin genes) are asymptomatic.
- Clinical manifestations of beta thalassemia intermedia are variable (mild to severe)
- Beta thalassemia not expressed clinically during first months of life (due to presence of Hb F)
- Pallor
- Maxillary hyperplasia and frontal bossing secondary to extramedullary hematopoiesis
- Short stature
- Splenomegaly
- Hepatomegaly
- Jaundice
- Congestive heart failure
- Hydrops fetalis associated with alpha thalassemia major (absence of all four alpha globin genes). Found in Southeast Asian and Mediterranean population, rare in African population.

TESTS

Blood

- Alpha thalassemia silent carrier: normal
- microcytic, hypochromic anemia (normal to mild with alpha or beta thalassemia trait), target cells, variable basophilic stippling
- Hb H (beta$_4$) inclusion bodies can be stained with brilliant cresyl blue and may be seen with alpha thalassemia
- elevated red cell count
- increased indirect bilirubin
- hemoglobin electrophoresis:
  - beta thalassemia: elevated Hb A$_2$. Note: normal Hb A$_2$ does not rule out beta thalassemia (eg: delta beta thalassemia).
  - beta thalassemia major: predominance of Hb F, no Hb A
  - alpha thalassemia trait (2 alpha gene deletions): Hb Barts (gamma$_4$) in newborn period, no increase in Hb A$_2$ or Hb F
  - Hb H disease (3 alpha gene deletions): 20–40% Hb Barts at birth, 5–40% Hb H by few months of life, decreased Hb A$_2$
  - alpha thalassemia major: Hb Barts, Hb H, Hb Portland (zeta and epsilon chains), no HbF or Hb A.

Recommended Tests for Beta Thalassemia Major/Intermedia:
- Extended panel RBC typing to minimize alloantibodies following transfusion
- Echocardiogram and EKG

DIFFERENTIAL DIAGNOSIS
- Iron deficiency vs. alpha or beta thalassemia trait:
  - Distinguish with iron, total iron-binding capacity (TIBC) and ferritin (generally normal in thalassemia trait)
  - Mentzer index (MCV/RBC):
    - \>13 iron deficiency
    - <13 thalassemia trait
  - Hemoglobin electrophoresis (elevations in Hb A_2 and Hb F may be masked if iron deficiency occurs concurrently with beta thalassemia)
  - Parental CBC, MCV, and blood smears
- Hb E: common in Southeast Asian populations
- diagnosis by hemoglobin electrophoresis

MANAGEMENT
- Routine health maintenance
  - Anticipatory testing
  - Monitor growth, development
  - Hepatitis B vaccination
  - Alpha thalassemia trait (1 or 2 gene deletion) or beta thalassemia trait: no treatment. Genetic counseling. Avoid inappropriate iron supplementation (increased gastrointestinal iron absorption).
  - Hb H disease: avoidance of oxidant drugs, splenectomy for severe anemia, judicious use of transfusion therapy.

SPECIFIC THERAPY

Chronic Transfusion Therapy
- Goal:
  - promote normal growth and development
  - Promote normal activity
  - Suppress extramedullary hematopoiesis

Complications:
- Iron overload
  - Use minimum required red cell transfusions

➤ Diagnosis: serum ferritin, left ventricular ejection fraction (LVEF) and myocardial T2* magnetic resonance (MR) measurements, liver biopsy

➤ Toxicities: cardiac, liver, endocrine (hypogonadism, hypothyroidism, diabetes, hypoparathyroidism)

➤ Treatment: Desferrioxamine, given as continuous subcutaneous or intravenous infusion (monitor for local skin reaction)

- ICL670, given orally (monitor skin rash, renal effects)
- iron chelation may be associated with an increased risk of *Yersinia enterocolitica* infection, auditory and visual losses

■ Infection (particularly hepatitis B, C and HIV)

■ Allosensitization

■ Transfusion reaction (acute or delayed)

Splenectomy

■ Indications: increased or excessive transfusional requirements
➤ risk of splenic rupture hypersplenism

■ Complications: increased risk of infection with encapsulated bacteria (immunize patient against pneumococcus, *Haemophilus influenzae*, and meningococcus prior to splenectomy, prophylactic penicillin)

Bone Marrow Transplantation

■ Only curative therapy.

■ Guidelines regarding this treatment still under investigation.

FOLLOW-UP

■ Patients on chronic transfusions/iron chelation
➤ Monthly: CBC
➤ Every 3 months: serum ferritin, glucose, creatinine, iron, TIBC, alkaline phosphatase, AST, ALT, LDH
➤ Yearly: echocardiogram and EKG

- Viral serologies (hepatitis B and C, HIV)
- Endocrine evaluation
- Bone age (in children)
- Ophthalmology exam
- Audiology exam
- Cardiac T2* MR, LVEF measurements
- Liver biopsy if iron overload

■ Patients with mild-moderate beta thalassemia intermedia may develop complications with age (bone deformity, osteoporosis, leg ulcers, folate deficiency, hypersplenism, progressive anemia, iron overload secondary to increased iron absorption)

COMPLICATIONS AND PROGNOSIS

Complications
- Beta thalassemia major/intermedia:
  - osteoporosis
  - hypersplenism
  - cholecystitis
  - iron overload from increased intestinal absorption
  - if untreated severe anemia: heart failure, bone deformities, poor growth, fatigue, hypogonadism.
- Untransfused beta thalassemia intermedia may develop folate deficiency

Prognosis
- Alpha or beta thalassemia trait is not associated with morbidity or mortality.
- Beta thalassemia intermedia follows a variable course, and may develop increasing complications with age.
- Untransfused beta thalassemia major is fatal in childhood.
- Alpha thalassemia major is fatal in utero or in the neonatal period.
- In transfused patients, mortality is mainly related to complications of blood transfusions and iron overload.

THIAMINE DEFICIENCY

ELISABETH RYZEN, MD

HISTORY & PHYSICAL

History
- diet high in polished rice, alcoholism, lactation, pregnancy, malabsorption, liver disease, prolonged dextrose infusions

Signs & Symptoms
- irritability, sleep disturbances, abdominal complaints, peripheral neuropathy, cardiomyopathy (beriberi), Wernicke-Korsakoff syndrome with mental confusion, ophthalmoplegia, coma

TESTS

Laboratory
- Basic blood studies:
  - ➤ high blood pyruvate and lactate
- Basic urine studies:
  - ➤ diminished urinary thiamine excretion (<50 mcg/day)

DIFFERENTIAL DIAGNOSIS
n/a

MANAGEMENT
n/a

SPECIFIC THERAPY
- nutritious diet, thiamine

Side Effects & Contraindications
- None

FOLLOW-UP
n/a

COMPLICATIONS AND PROGNOSIS
- Reversible with replacement

THORACIC AORTIC ANEURYSM

KENDRICK A. SHUNK, MD, PhD

HISTORY & PHYSICAL

History
- Syphilis, Atherosclerosis, hypertension, inherited connective tissue disorders (Marfans, Ehlers-Danlos, others), rheumatic (ankylosing spondylitis), trauma, pregnancy, prior staph/strep/salmonella sepsis (mycotic aneurysm)

Signs & Symptoms
- Pain, cough, hoarseness, dysphagia, SVC syndrome
- Occasionally visible pulsatile masses on thorax
- Signs of sequelae, e.g. Aortic insufficiency (diastolic AI murmur, widened pulse pressure)
- Signs of other manifestations of underlying etiology (e.g. Marfanoid features, + Shober's test, etc)

TESTS
- Specific diagnostic tests: chest x-ray
  - ➤ Usually apparent on standard PA and lateral films, however small saccular aneurysms may not be seen and are still prone to rupture
- Other imaging tests
  - ➤ CT and TEE good, comparable for defining thoracic aneurysm
  - ➤ MRI/MRA usually offers even better anatomic definition, may replace angiography
  - ➤ Angiography remains gold standard for many or most surgeons

DIFFERENTIAL DIAGNOSIS
- Peri-aortic thoracic mass

MANAGEMENT
What to Do First
- Assess risk of rupture, treat hypertension if present

General Measures
- Determine size (>6 cm indicates surgery)

SPECIFIC THERAPY
Indication for surgical therapy: aneurysm >6 cm

Treatment Options
- Surgical repair, generally with Dacron prosthesis.

Side Effects & Contraindications
- Side effects: major hemorrhage, spinal cord injury (>−5%), death (~6–9%), CVA/MI/renal failure mainly related to patients with atherosclerotic etiology
- Contraindications: Absolute: severe pulmonary disease, contraindications to systemic anticoagulation

FOLLOW-UP
- If aneurysm <5 cm, follow with imaging every 6–12 months, treat hypertension if present

COMPLICATIONS AND PROGNOSIS
- Complications: see side effects
- Prognosis: 5 year survival ~66% with surgery; 27% if symptomatic or 58% if asymptomatic and medically managed

THROMBOPHILIA

MIGUEL A. ESCOBAR, MD; ALICE D. MA; MD and
HAROLD R. ROBERTS, MD

HISTORY & PHYSICAL

Thrombophilia is a multi-causal condition in which genetic and acquired risk factors interact increasing the risk of thrombosis.

Several features suggest the presence of a hypercoagulable state.

- Thromboembolism before age 45 y
- Family history of thrombosis
  - Idiopathic thromboembolism
- Recurrent thromboembolism
- Thrombosis in an unusual site
  - Warfarin-induced skin necrosis (protein C or S deficiency)
  - Neonatal purpura fulminans (homozygous protein C or protein S deficiency)

Conditions predisposing to arterial and venous thrombosis are not the same.

Congenital Conditions Predisposing only to Venous Thrombosis

- Factor V Leiden mutation
- Prothrombin gene mutation
- AT deficiency
- Protein C Deficiency
- Protein S Deficiency

Congenital Conditions Predisposing to Both Venous and Arterial Thrombosis

- Dysfibrinogenemia
- Elevated levels of lipoprotein (a)

Acquired Conditions Predisposing only to Venous Thrombosis

- Pregnancy and puerperium
- Estrogen use
  - Thalidomide
  - Tamoxifen/Raloxifene
- Malignancy
- Trauma, surgery, immobility
  - Previous venous thrombosis
  - Nephrotic syndrome
- Congestive heart failure
- Hyperviscosity syndromes
- High levels of fibrinogen

- High levels of FVIII, FIX, FXI (above the 90th percentile)
- Caval filter
- Post-thrombotic syndrome

Acquired Conditions Predisposing to Both Venous and Arterial Thrombosis

- Hyperhomocysteinemia
- Paroxysmal nocturnal hemoglobinuria
- Antiphospholipid antibodies (anticardiolipin antibodies, lupus anticoagulant)
- Myeloproliferative diseases
- Heparin-induced thrombocytopenia
- Tobacco use
- Vasculitis

Acquired Conditions Predisposing only to Arterial Thrombosis

- Hyperlipidemia

Factor V Leiden

- Caused by a point mutation in the factor V gene, leading to change at the major Protein C cleavage site (FV R506Q)
- Frequency varies from 1% to 8%. Found mainly in Caucasians.
- Found in 20–50% of patients with venous thrombosis
- Relative risk for thrombosis is 5-fold in heterozygous patients.
- Relative risk for thrombosis is 50-fold in homozygotes.
- Oral contraceptives increase risk in heterozygous patients by 48-fold.

Prothrombin Mutation

- Caused by a point mutation in the 3′ untranslated region of the prothrombin gene (G20210A)
- Leads to increased levels of prothrombin
- Frequency varies from 0.7–4.0%.
- Found in 6–20% of patients with venous thrombosis
- Relative risk for thrombosis is 2.5.

Protein C Deficiency

- Frequency estimated to be 0.2%
- Found in 3% of patients with venous thrombosis
- Homozygotes develop neonatal purpura fulminans, cerebral vein thrombosis.
- Heterozygotes have 10-fold increased relative risk for venous thrombosis and increased risk of developing warfarin skin necrosis.

Protein S Deficiency
- Unknown frequency in general population
- Found in 1–2% of patients with venous thrombosis
- Homozygotes develop neonatal purpura fulminans, cerebral vein thrombosis.
- Heterozygotes have 10-fold increased relative risk for venous thrombosis.

Antithrombin Deficiency
- Frequency: 0.02% of general population
- Found in 1% of patients with venous thrombosis
- Homozygous state is lethal in utero.
- Heterozygotes have 25-fold increased relative risk for venous thrombosis.
- Pregnancy leads to thrombosis in as many as 60% of patients.
- AT concentrates are available for patients with acquired or congenital AT deficiency.

Lupus Anticoagulant (LA)
- Criteria for diagnosis:
  - Prolonged aPTT that fails to correct after 1:1 plasma mix
  - Prolongation of at least 1 phospholipid-dependent clotting assay
  - Correction after addition of exogenous phospholipid
- Frequency is 0–2% of general population.
- Found in 5–15% of patients with venous thrombosis
- Estimated relative risk for thrombosis is about 10-fold.

Hyperhomocysteinemia
- Elevated levels of hymocysteine can arise from congenital mutations in either Cystathionine beta-syntethase or methyl tetrahydrofolate reductase, but are more commonly acquired.
- Secondary causes of elevated homocysteine levels:
  - renal insufficiency
  - hypothyroidism
  - smoking
  - deficiencies of either folate or B12
  - drugs (theophylline, methotrexate, phenytoin)
  - increase age
- Hyperhomocysteinemia can be found in ~10% of patients with venous thromboembolism.
- Elevated homocysteine levels increase risk of venous clots by 2- to 4-fold.

■ Elevated homocysteine levels increase risk of atherosclerotic disease – risk is multiplied in patients with hypertension and in smokers.

TESTS
Once thromboembolism has been diagnosed, the physician must decide whether to screen for thrombophilic risks. About one third of individuals with idiopathic thromboembolism will have a positive test for thrombophilia.

In general, the following guidelines apply:

■ Most patients should be screened for common disorders such as Factor V Leiden and the Prothrombin gene mutation, the lupus anticoagulant, anticardiolipin antibodies, and hyperhomocysteinemia.

■ Younger patients with unprovoked thromboses and/or a strong family history of clots or patients with clots in unusual sites should be screened for the more uncommon congenital and acquired disorders.

■ Hepatic vein thrombosis (Budd-Chiari syndrome) should also prompt a search for paroxysmal nocturnal hemoglobinuria and myeloproliferative syndromes.

Screening Laboratory Evaluation for Individuals with Venous Thromboembolism
■ Whole blood (heparin or ACD tube) for the following:
➤ Genetic test for Factor V Leiden mutation
➤ Genetic test for Prothrombin mutation
■ Plasma (citrate tube):
➤ Functional assay for AT (may be affected by heparin)
➤ Functional assay for protein C (affected by warfarin)
➤ Functional assay for protein S (affected by warfarin)
➤ Immunologic assays for total and free protein S (can be affected by estrogen use and pregnancy)
➤ Screen for dysfibrinogenemia (immunologic and functional assays for fibrinogen, thrombin time, reptilase time)
➤ Clotting assays for lupus anticoagulant
➤ Serologic tests for anticardiolipin antibodies
■ Serum or plasma for the following:
➤ Fasting homocysteine (Collect on ice and centrifuge within 1 hour)

DIFFERENTIAL DIAGNOSIS
n/a

MANAGEMENT

Initial therapy for venous thromboembolism is usually unfractionated heparin (UFH) or low-molecular-weight heparin (LMWH) followed by long-term treatment with warfarin. Target INR for oral anticoagulation is 2.0–3.0.

Duration of anticoagulation depends on the balance between recurrent thrombosis and risk of bleeding.

Guidelines for duration of anticoagulation:

- In the absence of contraindications, most patients with a first clot require 3–6 months of anticoagulation.
- Underlying malignancy, AT deficiency, protein S and C deficiency, homozygosity for factor V Leiden or the prothrombin gene mutation or double heterozygosity, or persistent antiphospholipid antibodies, may require longer, perhaps indefinite, duration of therapy.
- A second spontaneous thrombosis, or a first clot with two or more biochemical/genetic thrombophilic risk factors might also warrant indefinite anticoagulation.

Consider thrombolytic therapy, if no contraindications in the following circumstances:

- For local lytic therapy, a large thrombus in the following areas:
  - ➤ portal system
  - ➤ mesenteric system
  - ➤ vena cava
  - ➤ upper extremity
  - ➤ limb-threatening thrombosis
- For a hemodynamically-significant PE, consider systemic lytic therapy.

Once thrombophilia is diagnosed, need prophylaxis for high-risk situations – i.e., pregnancy, surgery, prolonged bed rest, prolonged car or plane trips

SPECIFIC THERAPY

Lupus Anticoagulant (LA)

- Women with the LA may have recurrent spontaneous miscarriages.
  - ➤ Heparin plus aspirin has been shown to improve outcomes.
  - ➤ No benefit with steroids
- Patients with the LA that have a baseline prolongation of the prothrombin time and INR may require monitoring of FXa by chromogenic method (keep levels between 10–30%).

Hyperhomocysteinemia – Vitamin therapy can decrease levels of homocysteine

- 1–5 mg folate PO daily will decrease homocysteine levels by 25% – even if levels are normal to start.
- 0.5 mg B12 PO daily will further decrease homocysteine levels by 7%.
- Start treatment with 2–5 mg folate daily, then recheck fasting homocysteine levels in 8 weeks. If no change, then add B12 +/– B6.

FOLLOW-UP
n/a

COMPLICATIONS AND PROGNOSIS
- Complications from anticoagulation include bleeding (1–7%), heparin-induced thrombocytopenia (UFH > LMWH) and osteoporosis (UFH > LMWH).
- Platelet counts should be checked every few days while patients are on UFH or LMWH to monitor for the development of heparin-induced thrombocytopenia.
- Patients with active cancer and venous thromboembolism have an increased risk of recurrence when treated with warfarin. LMWH should be considered the treatment of choice for these individuals.
- Inferior vena cava (IVC) filters are recommended in patients who have contraindication for anticoagulation or failed treatment with oral anticoagulants. The long-term use of these filters is associated with recurrent venous thrombosis for which anticoagulation should be started when safe. More recently, removable IVC filters are been used for short-term periods without the administration of anticoagulation.

THYROID NODULES AND CANCER

LAWRENCE CRAPO, MD, PhD

HISTORY & PHYSICAL

History
- Personal/family history of thyroid nodules or cancer
- Hypertension or pheochromocytoma
- Neck irradiation

Signs & Symptoms
- Thyroid mass: soft or firm, tender or not, mobile or fixed, large or small
- Fever, sweats, chills

- Sudden appearance
- Growth rate of nodule
- Hoarseness, dysphagia
- Cervical adenopathy: present or absent
- Elevated temperature or BP

TESTS

Laboratory
- Basic blood tests: free T4, TSH
- Specific Diagnostic Tests
  - FNA biopsy
  - Blood:
  - Calcitonin: if FNA shows medullary CA
  - Calcium: if nodule is parathyroid or if clinical suspicion of hyper-parathyroidism
  - Thyroglobulin: to follow treatment of papillary or follicular thyroid CA

Imaging
- I-123 uptake and scan (if TSH low)
- Thyroid US (if diagnostic uncertainty or to follow growth)

DIFFERENTIAL DIAGNOSIS
- Benign nodules:
  - Cysts: simple, infected, hemorrhagic, thyroglossal duct
  - Solid: follicular adenoma, thyroiditis, parathyroid adenoma
- Malignant nodules:
  - Well-differentiated: papillary CA, follicular CA,
  - Not well-differentiated: medullary, anaplastic, other (rare)

MANAGEMENT

What to Do First
- Assess for likelihood of malignancy, infection, hemorrhage
- Consider FNA or surgical resection

General Measures
- Assess for possibility of hyperparathyroidism or pheochromocytoma
- Assess for general risks of surgery

SPECIFIC THERAPY
- Drainage by FNA: benign, hemorrhagic, or infected cysts; antibiotics for suppurative infection

- Partial thyroidectomy: follicular adenoma, small intrathyroidal papillary CA, occasional anaplastic CA
- Total thyroidectomy: all other malignancies
- High-dose I-131 ablation: follicular/papillary CA 1 mo after total thyroidectomy when hypothyroid

FOLLOW-UP

During Treatment
- Assess for hypocalcemia and hoarseness after total thyroidectomy
- Suppressive levothyroxine therapy after total thyroidectomy or I-131 ablation

Routine
- Adjust levothyroxine q 6–8 wks so that TSH completely suppressed for follicular/papillary CA, or TSH normal for medullary/anaplastic CA
- 1 y after initial I-131 ablation: obtain serum thyroglobulin and whole body I-131 scan after T4 levothyroxine withdrawal; repeat high-dose I-131 ablation if thyroid CA still present
- Reiterate above process annually until thyroid CA no longer present; may use thyrogen (human TSH) injection for evaluation; best evidence for cure: undetectable serum thyroglobulin and negative I-131 whole body scan when serum TSH >30 mcU/mL or after thyrogen injection

COMPLICATIONS AND PROGNOSIS

Complications
- Total thyroidectomy: hypothyroidism, hypoparathyroidism, recurrent laryngeal nerve injury
- Repeated I-131 ablation: hypothyroidism; leukemia (rare); radiation fibrosis of lung for metastatic follicular/papillary CA
- Suppressive dose of levothyroxine T4: osteoporosis, cardiac toxicity

Prognosis
- Benign cysts/nodules: excellent
- Papillary/follicular CA: good
- Medullary CA: moderate
- Anaplastic CA: poor

TICS

CHAD CHRISTINE, MD

HISTORY & PHYSICAL
- Involuntary recurrent, jerk-like movements or vocalizations
- Uncomfortable sensation may precede & be relieved by movement or vocalization
- Typically begin in childhood
- May occur transiently in children
- Worse w/ stress; diminish w/ activity
- Absent during sleep
- Sudden, recurrent, coordinated abnormal movements or vocalizations
- Simple tics: eye blinking, facial grimacing, head jerking
- Complex tics: more complicated movements that may appear purposeful
- Simple vocal tic: throat clearing, grunting, sniffing
- Complex vocal tic: full or truncated words, may repeat words

TESTS
- Diagnosis made clinically
- Lab tests & brain imaging usually normal

DIFFERENTIAL DIAGNOSIS
- Degenerative diseases (Huntington's disease, Hallervoden-Spatz) & torsion dystonia excluded clinically
- Acquired injuries: head injury, stroke, encephalitis, developmental neuropsychiatric disorders, toxins (carbon monoxide) excluded by history & brain imaging
- Drugs: neuroleptics, stimulants, anticonvulsants excluded by history & toxicology screen
- Childhood onset, motor & vocal tics likely represent Tourette syndrome

MANAGEMENT
- What to do first: search for underlying cause
- Education about the disorder for family, friends & teachers

SPECIFIC THERAPY
- Many will not require treatment
- Fluphenazine or pimozide (if not effective, haloperidol)

- Nicotine gum or patch may provide days of relief
- Botulinum toxin may help simple tics

FOLLOW-UP
- Depends on cause & treatment

COMPLICATIONS AND PROGNOSIS
- Neuroleptic treatment can cause tardive dyskinesia
- Prognosis depends on cause

TINEA CAPITIS

BONI E. ELEWSKI, MD and JEFFREY P. CALLEN, MD

HISTORY & PHYSICAL

History
- Prepubertal children and those of African or Hispanic descent
- Rare in Adults – except in immunocompromised patients
- Adults exposed to young children – i.e. teachers
- Exposure to cats or dogs

Signs & Symptoms
- Hair loss, scale, crusting, pustules or abscesses in the scalp
- Black dots – broken hairs
- Posterior cervical and postauricular lymphadenopathy
- Scarring alopecia in end stage infections

TESTS

Laboratory
- KOH – spore within or without hair shaft
- Fungal culture of a dermatophyte
- *Trichophyton tonsurans* most common in U.S.
- Woods light – yellow fluorescent in Microsporum canis

DIFFERENTIAL DIAGNOSIS
- Alopecia areata
- Trichotillomania (hair pulling tics)
- Seborrheic dermatitis/psoriasis
- Folliculitis

MANAGEMENT

Oral Antifungal Drugs
- Oral antifungal drugs required

SPECIFIC THERAPY
- Griseofulvin 20 mg/kg/d for 8–12 weeks
- Terbinafine 250 mg/d for people >35 kg, 187 mg for children 25–25 kg and 125 mg/d for children <25 kg 4 weeks
- Itraconazole capsules
- Fluconazole solution or tablets

Topical Antifungal Drugs
- Adjunct usage to reduce fungal shedding/transmission in patients and family members
- 2% Ketoconazole shampoo
  - Ciclopirox shampoo
- 2.5% Selenium sulfide lotion/shampoo
  - Prednisone should only be used in rare patients with severe inflammation in conjunction with antifungal therapy.

FOLLOW-UP

During Treatment
- Regularly assess response to therapy – clinical evidence of reduced symptoms and new hair growth

Laboratory
- Not generally indicated

COMPLICATIONS AND PROGNOSIS
- Dermatophytid reaction – lichenoid pinpoint papules develop during treatment generally on head/neck and progress to trunk and extremities – up to 10%
  - Resolves without specific therapy
  - Not an allergic eruption
- Treat a secondary bacterial infection, if present.
- Scarring alopecia if left untreated

TINEA CRURIS/CORPORIS/PEDIS

BONI E. ELEWSKI, MD and JEFFREY P. CALLEN, MD

HISTORY & PHYSICAL

History
- Wrestlers, athletes, contact sports
- Exposure to animals – cats, dogs
- Onychomycosis/tinea capitis are risk factors

Signs & Symptoms
- Pruritic rash on feet, groin or body skin – exposed areas most affected, annular patches
- Feet – plantar surface, dry scale, macerated, fissured toe webs
- Onychomycosis

TESTS
- KOH – septate hyphae
- Fungal culture – growth of dermatophyte
- No blood work indicated

DIFFERENTIAL DIAGNOSIS
- *Tinea pedis*
  - Eczema, dyshidrosis
  - Psoriasis
  - Bacterial infection (toe web)
- *Tinea cruris*
  - Cutaneous candidiasis
  - Erythrasma
  - Inverse psoriasis
- *Tinea corporis*
  - Nummular eczema
  - Pityriasis rosea
  - Psoriasis (guttate type)
  - Granuloma annulare
  - Discoid lupus

MANAGEMENT

What to Do First
- Confirm diagnosis by KOH/fungal culture

General Measures
- Topical antifungal agent applied to affected site for 6 weeks depending on location of infection and product used

SPECIFIC THERAPY
- Topical antimycotics – clotrimazole, econazole, ketoconazole, and ciclopirox olamine
- 4–6 weeks – tinea pedis
- 2–4 weeks – tinea corporis/cruris

- terbinafine, naftifine, butenafine
- 2–4 weeks – tinea pedis
- 1–2 weeks – tinea corporis/cruris
- Prevent reinfection: disinfect/discard shoes
- Oral therapy may be used in patients with widespread disease or recurrent disease.
  - ➣ Options – griseofulvin, itraconazole, fluconazole, terbinafine

FOLLOW-UP
- Rash should clear during therapy.

COMPLICATIONS AND PROGNOSIS
- Total clearing expected
- Treat onychomycosis to prevent recurrent disease.
  - ➣ Recurrent or severe widespread disease may be indicative of an underlying immune disorder.

TORSION OF APPENDIX TESTIS

ARTHUR I. SAGALOWSKY, MD

HISTORY & PHYSICAL
- vestigial mullerian remnant at upper pole of testis
- most often in children
- acute pain
- palpable, tender "BB-like" dot
- diffuse scrotal swelling may mask signs

TESTS
- urinalysis usually normal
- elevated WBC, fever variable
- ultrasound highly effective

DIFFERENTIAL DIAGNOSIS
n/a

MANAGEMENT
n/a

SPECIFIC THERAPY
- observation if Dx confident; self-limited
- prompt exploration if cannot exclude torsion of spermatic cord

FOLLOW-UP
n/a

COMPLICATIONS AND PROGNOSIS
n/a

TORSION OF TESTIS AND SPERMATIC CORD

ARTHUR I. SAGALOWSKY, MD

HISTORY & PHYSICAL
- most common in adolescents
- due to a medial rotation of spermatic cord acutely occluding testis blood supply
- sudden, severe pain over testis
- scrotal pain may produce nausea, abdominal pain
- early, may detect testis high in scrotum, transverse lie, epididymis draped anteriorly
- later, diffuse swelling masks signs
- scrotal skin may be inflamed

TESTS
- urinalysis usually normal
- ultrasound and/or nuclear scan highly sensitive – shows hyperemic ring surrounding "cold testis," i.e., no uptake of tracer

DIFFERENTIAL DIAGNOSIS
- Torsion of appendix testis – vestigial mullerian remnant at upper pole of testis; most often in children; no treatment necessary

MANAGEMENT
n/a

SPECIFIC THERAPY
- emergency surgical repair within 3–4 hours of onset to prevent testis atrophy
  - ➤ detorsion of affected side
  - ➤ orchiopexy on both sides

FOLLOW-UP
- for resolution of acute event
- potential long term impact on fertility, testosterone secretion

COMPLICATIONS AND PROGNOSIS
n/a

TORTICOLLIS

CHAD CHRISTINE, MD

HISTORY & PHYSICAL
- Involuntary turning of head & neck
- Typical onset in 3rd or 4th decade; may occur at any age
- May be family history
- Sensory trick (touching chin, occiput, etc.) often temporarily relieves deviation
- Pain is common
- Involuntary contraction of selective neck muscles causing head deviation
- Simultaneous activation of agonist & antagonist muscles
- Shoulder may be elevated
- Movement may be slow or jerky
- Spasms worse w/ activity

TESTS
- Diagnosis made clinically
- Laboratory: genetic tests available for hereditary forms; rule out Wilson's disease
- Imaging: indicated if torticollis follows head or neck injury or if other neurologic features are present
- EMG may show sustained or intermittent activity of cervical muscles

DIFFERENTIAL DIAGNOSIS
- Structural lesion, Wilson's disease

MANAGEMENT
- General measures
  - ➤ Treat pain w/ NSAIDs
  - ➤ Physical therapy & prosthetic devices that take advantage of sensory trick may be helpful

SPECIFIC THERAPY
- Indications: symptoms that interfere w/ function
- Botulinum toxin local injection
  - ➤ Injected into abnormally contracting muscles
  - ➤ Must be repeated every 3–5 months in most pts
- Oral meds
  - ➤ Anticholinergics: benztropine or trihexyphenidyl
  - ➤ GABA agonists: baclofen, clonazepam, diazepam

■ Surgery: pallidotomy or deep brain stimulation to globus pallidus or thalamus may be helpful

FOLLOW-UP
■ Depends on cause & severity

COMPLICATIONS AND PROGNOSIS
■ May resolve w/o therapy in 10–15%
■ Symptoms may slowly progress in untreated pts

TOURETTE SYNDROME

CHAD CHRISTINE, MD

HISTORY & PHYSICAL
■ Syndrome of involuntary motor & vocal tics
■ First motor tic often involves face (sniffing, blinking, etc.)
■ Vocal tics usually follow (eg, grunts, barks, hisses, coughing, copro-lalia or echolalia)
■ Obsessive-compulsive disorder & attention deficit/hyperactivity disorder common
■ Onset between 2 & 21 yr
■ Hereditary
■ Males > females 3:1
■ Poor impulse control is common
■ Multiple motor & vocal tics

TESTS
■ Diagnosis made clinically
■ Lab tests & brain imaging normal

DIFFERENTIAL DIAGNOSIS
■ Wilson's disease, Sydenham's chorea, bobble-head syndrome excluded clinically

MANAGEMENT
■ What to do first: education of pt, family & teachers
■ General measures: extra break periods at school, extra time on tests
■ Counseling, behavior modification may be sufficient

SPECIFIC THERAPY
■ Many will not require treatment
Tics
■ Fluphenazine or pimozide increased every 5–7 d

- If not effective, haloperidol
- Nicotine gum or patch may provide days of relief
- Botulinum toxin: may help simple tics

Attention deficit w/ or w/o hyperactivity
- Clonidine patch: start TTS1 patch; may increase to TTS3 if necessary
- Guanfacine
- Pemoline
- Methylphenidate
- Dextroamphetamine

Obsessive-compulsive disorder
- Sertraline, fluoxetine, citalopram, fluvoxamine
- Clomipramine

FOLLOW-UP
- Depends on severity of symptoms & treatment

COMPLICATIONS AND PROGNOSIS
- Tardive dyskinesia may occur in 30% of those treated w/ neuroleptics
- TS is a lifelong illness but is not progressive
- Some symptoms may improve

TOXOPLASMOSIS

J. GORDON FRIERSON, MD

HISTORY & PHYSICAL

History
- Life cycle: Cats are principal host, pass oocysts in stool, ingested by human and pass through bowel wall to reach various tissues where they encyst. Humans and cats also infected by eating rare meat that contains cysts (includes lamb, beef, pork).
- Exposure: Ingesting oocysts through contaminated food, fingers, or eating rare or raw meat containing toxoplasma cysts.

Signs & Symptoms
- Acute infection: fever, headache, myalgias, lymphadenopathy, splenomegaly, rash. Incubation period is 10–12 days.
- Ocular toxoplasmosis: acutely presents as painless, focal, unilateral retinochoroiditis. Later there is retinal scar.
  In AIDS, usually presents at CD4 <100 (reactivation) as cerebral abscess or encephalitis.

- Neonatal toxoplasmosis: variable picture from few findings to severe illness. May see chorioretinitis, encephalitis, hepatosplenomegaly, rash, fever, hydrocephalus, lymphadenopathy.
- Acute infection in pregnancy: fetus infected in 10–25% of first trimester infections, rising to 65% for third trimester, but babies infected in third trimester usually clinically normal or near normal at term.

TESTS
- Basic tests: blood: Acute infection: CBC shows atypical lymphocytosis, increased monocytes. LFTs may be mildly abnormal.
- Basic tests: urine: not helpful
- Specific tests: Serology, using ELISA, useful. IGG rises early and usually positive at time of symptoms. Presence of IGM confirms acute infection. Biopsy of lymph node shows characteristic morphology (highly suggestive but not diagnostic), and sometimes parasite cysts seen.
- Other tests: Chest X-ray can show interstitial infiltrate. For cerebral toxoplasmosis in AIDS, MRI more sensitive than CT.

DIFFERENTIAL DIAGNOSIS
- Acute infection: infectious mononucleosis, CMV infection, lymphoma.
- Congenital infection: CMV disease, rubella, syphilis, tuberculosis.

MANAGEMENT
What to Do First
- Assess organs involved. Neonatal case may need IVs, nutritional help

General Measures
- Teach patient and family about epidemiology

SPECIFIC THERAPY
Indications
- Clinically ill acute case, neonatal disease, active chorioretinitis, any immunocompromised patient, and infection acquired during pregnancy (if abortion not requested).

Treatment Options
- Pyrimethamine plus:
- Sulfadiazine
- Folinic acid
- Another regimen: clindamycin plus pyrimethamine and folinic acid

Side Effects & Complications
- Pyrimethamine: bone marrow suppression, GI distress, bad taste in mouth.
- Sulfadiaziine: skin rashes, crystal-induced nephrotoxicity, encephalopathic symptoms.
- Clindamycin: rash, nausea, vomiting, pseudomembranous colitis.
- Contraindications to treatment: absolute: drug allergies, Pyrimethamine cannot be given in first trimester of pregnancy.
- Contraindications to treatment: relative: asymptomatic or lightly symptomatic acute cases. Treatment in pregnancy not always curative for fetus, though severity of neonatal disease decreased. Risks and benefits need discussion.

FOLLOW-UP

During Treatment
- Watch blood count for signs of marrow suppression, and urine and renal function for signs of nephritis. Administer liberal fluids to prevent nephritis.

Routine
- Clinical follow. In neonatal disease intellectual function needs follow. IGG remains up for years and not helpful. Chorioretinitis can be chronic and recurrent, may need retreatment.

AIDS – secondary prophylaxis required until CD4 >200.

COMPLICATIONS AND PROGNOSIS
- Acute infection: good prognosis.
- Neonatal infection: prognosis depends on extent of pathology at birth.
- Retinal disease: treatment arrests disease, but may reactivate.
- Immunocompromised patients have poorer prognosis, require larger doses of drugs and longer therapy.

TRANSFUSION REACTIONS

RICHARD KAUFMAN, MD; FRANK STROBL, MD;
JONATHAN KURTIS, MD; and LESLIE SILBERSTEIN, MD

HISTORY & PHYSICAL

History
- Acute transfusion reaction: transfusion w/ any blood product within several hr:

- Acute hemolytic transfusion reaction: most common w/ transfusion of ABO-incompatible RBCs
- Febrile nonhemolytic transfusion reaction: most common w/ platelet & RBC transfusions
- Allergic transfusion reaction: most common w/ platelet & FFP transfusions
- Acute transfusion-associated lung injury (TRALI): most common w/ FFP transfusions but can occur with any plasma-containing component
- Volume overload
- Bacterial contamination: most common w/ platelet blood products
■ Delayed transfusion reaction: transfusion w/ any blood product within past 4 wk:
  - Delayed hemolytic transfusion reaction: most common w/ RBC transfusions
  - Transfusion-associated GVHD
  - Post-transfusion purpura (PTP): almost always in multiparous women

Signs & Symptoms
■ Acute transfusion reactions:
  - Acute hemolytic transfusion reaction: fever, flank pain, chest pain, hypotension, respiratory distress, hemoglobinuria, DIC, renal failure, impending sense of doom
  - Febrile transfusion reaction: temperature increase of 1 degree C during or immediately after transfusion
  - Allergic transfusion reaction: urticaria, pruritus, wheezing, cough laryngeal edema, flushing, hypoxemia, nausea, vomiting, diarrhea, hypotension, shock
  - TRALI: respiratory distress w/ pulmonary edema in absence of heart failure within several hr of transfusion
  - Volume overload: respiratory distress w/ pulmonary edema within several hr of transfusion
■ Delayed transfusion reactions:
  - Delayed hemolytic transfusion reaction: fever, unexplained anemia, jaundice days to weeks after transfusion
  - Transfusion-associated GVHD: fever, rash, enterocolitis, hepatitis, pancytopenia
  - PTP: severe thrombocytopenia within several d after transfusion

TESTS
Stop transfusion; send transfusion reaction report form and samples to blood bank

Basic Blood & Urine Tests
- Repeat clerical check
- Visually inspect blood & urine samples for hemolysis
- Perform direct antiglobulin test; if positive, perform eluate
- Repeat ABO/Rh on pre- & post-transfusion samples & donor unit
- Repeat antibody screen on pre- & post-transfusion samples
- Repeat cross-match on pre- & post-transfusion samples
- Gram stain & culture component
- TRALI: look for antibodies against HLA, neutrophils
- Anaphylaxis: look for antibodies against IgA

DIFFERENTIAL DIAGNOSIS
- Presentation of transfusion reactions myriad; suspect transfusion reaction when pt's clinical status changes in temporal association w/ transfusion
- Must integrate pt's pretransfusion clinical status w/ intra- & post-transfusion signs & symptoms & results of transfusion reaction workup
- Signs & symptoms of transfusion reactions can mimic exacerbations of transfusion recipient's underlying disease processes
- Neither presence nor absence of any sign or symptom can exclude hemolytic transfusion reaction
- If transfusion reaction is in DDx for pt's signs & symptoms, stop transfusion, send transfusion reaction report & samples to the blood bank for workup

MANAGEMENT

What to Do First
- Stop transfusion: keep IV open
- Record vital signs (T, BP, P, R)
- Treat pt as needed (fluids, pressors, O2, antihistamines, meperidine, antimicrobials, etc)
- Perform clerical check of pt & component
- Obtain post-transfusion blood samples (red-top & purple-top tubes) & urine sample
- Complete transfusion reaction report form

■ Send component bag/IV tubing, blood samples & transfusion reaction report form to blood bank. Send fresh urine specimen to lab to check for hemoglobinuria.

SPECIFIC THERAPY

■ Dictated by type of transfusion reaction: informed by results of transfusion reaction workup

■ Acute hemolytic transfusion reaction: stop transfusion; IV fluids, promote diuresis (furosemide), coagulation factor & platelet replacement PRN

■ Febrile nonhemolytic transfusion reaction: leukoreduction, antipyretics, meperidine

■ Allergic transfusion reaction: pre- & post-medication w/ antihistamines; if anaphylactic reaction, aggressive hemodynamic & respiratory support incl O2, IV fluids, epinephrine, & steroids

■ TRALI: O2, ventilatory & circulatory support

■ Volume overload: diuresis, transfuse w/ smaller volumes over greater time

■ Bacterial contamination: IV fluids, broad-spectrum antibiotics, coagulation factor & platelet replacement

■ Delayed hemolytic transfusion reaction: transfuse w/ antigen-negative RBCs if necessary

■ Transfusion-associated GVHD: no effective therapy, although corticosteroid & immunosuppressive therapy employed w/ limited efficacy. Prevented by blood product irradiation.

■ PTP: IVIg, steroids, plasmapheresis, PLA-1-negative blood products

FOLLOW-UP

n/a

COMPLICATIONS AND PROGNOSIS

■ Acute hemolytic transfusion reaction: 1/30,000 transfusions w/ 5% mortality

■ Febrile nonhemolytic transfusion reaction: 1/200 transfusions w/ no impact on morbidity & mortality

■ Allergic transfusion reaction: mild urticaria in 1/100 transfusions w/ no impact on morbidity & mortality; anaphylaxis in 1/20,000 to 1/50,000 transfusions w/ appreciable morbidity & mortality

■ TRALI: 1/5,000 transfusions w/ up to 5–10% mortality

■ Bacterial contamination leading to sepsis: 1/20,000 apheresis platelet transfusions & 1/500,000 RBC transfusions w/ significant morbidity & mortality

- Delayed hemolytic transfusion reaction: 1/4,000 transfusions w/ little impact on morbidity & mortality
- Transfusion-associated GVHD: very rare, w/ mortality approaching 100%
- PTP: very rare, w/ appreciable morbidity & mortality secondary to prolonged thrombocytopenia

TRANSIENT ISCHEMIC ATTACKS

MICHAEL J. AMINOFF, MD, DSc

HISTORY & PHYSICAL

- Acute, focal ischemic neurologic deficit that clears completely within 24 hours, usually within a few minutes; nature & distribution of symptoms depend on site of lesion; may consist of weakness, heaviness, paresthesias, numbness, aphasia, amaurosis fugax, dysarthria, diplopia or vertigo
- No abnormality except during attack, when may be pyramidal deficit, sensory changes, speech disturbance, ataxia, reflex changes; may be carotid bruit or cardiac arrhythmia

TESTS

- Basic: CBC, differential count, ESR, PT, PTT, FBS, lipid profile, RP, electrolytes; consider also SPEP, fibrinogen, proteins C & S, ANA, antiphospholipid antibody, antithrombin III, factor V Leiden
- Chest x-ray
- Cranial CT scan to show absence of hemorrhage; cranial & cervical MRA – may show evidence of diffuse or localized vascular disease; carotid duplex ultrasonography may reveal localized disease
- Cardiac studies: ECG, Echo

DIFFERENTIAL DIAGNOSIS

- Other causes of episodic neurologic deficit; focal seizures consist of positive phenomena (clonic motor activity or paresthesias) rather than negative phenomena (weakness, paralysis, numbness) & may spread ("march"); pt's age & family and past history may help to distinguish migrainous phenomena
- Distinguish by above tests btwn intrinsic cerebrovascular disease, other vasculopathies (fibromuscular dysplasia, vasculitides, meningovascular syphilis), cardiac causes of cerebral emboli,

hematologic causes of TIAs (polycythemia, sickle cell disease, hyperviscosity syndromes)

MANAGEMENT
- Aspirin (optimal dose not established)
- Ticlopidine
- Initiate anticoagulant treatment w/ heparin & introduce warfarin (to INR 2–3) for cardiogenic embolism

SPECIFIC THERAPY
Carotid endarterectomy for ipsilateral localized stenotic lesion (70% or more)

Treat or control cardiac arrhythmia or continue warfarin

General measures: stop cigarette smoking, treat underlying medical disorders (polycythemia, hypertension, diabetes, hyperlipidemia)

FOLLOW-UP
- As necessary to control anticoagulants for disturbance of cardiac rhythm
- Every 3 months to ensure no further TIAs or episodes of amaurosis fugax

COMPLICATIONS AND PROGNOSIS
- 30% of pts w/ stroke have history of previous TIAs
- Pts w/ TIA overall have an average 4% per year risk of stroke
- Symptomatic carotid stenosis >70% has a 13% risk over 2 years of major or fatal stroke

---

TRICHINOSIS

J. GORDON FRIERSON, MD

HISTORY & PHYSICAL

History
- Exposure: Eating undercooked pork, bear, wild boar, walrus, meat of other carnivores, occasionally horsemeat. Larvae digested out of muscle, penetrate small intestine, go to skeletal and cardiac muscle via the circulation, encyst there.

Signs & Symptoms
- Intestinal phase: no symptoms, or mild diarrhea, bloating, abdominal pain 2–7 days after exposure.

- Muscle stage: starts second week after infection, fever, chills, tachycardia, myalgias, headache, periorbital edema, conjunctivitis, rashes (usually macular, brief duration), urticaria, pruritis, dry cough, swelling of masseter muscles, splinter subungual hemorrhages.

TESTS
- Basic tests: blood: eosinopohilia, often high, present. Sed rate normal or slightly elevated. CPK and aldolase elevated.
- Basic tests: urine: normal or proteinuria
- Specific tests: muscle biopsy on deltoid or gastrocnemius, larvae most numerous at 5–6 weeks after infection. Serologic tests become positive 3–4 weeks after infection. Most used are bentonite flocculation, IFA, and ELISA.
- Other tests: EKG may show tachycardia, ST-T changes, and arrythmias due to myocarditis.

DIFFERENTIAL DIAGNOSIS
- Myositis of various types, especially dermatomyositis – distinguished by normal sed rate, muscle biopsy. Other allergic diseases, serum sickness, Katayama syndrome.

MANAGEMENT
What to Do First
- Hospitalize if ill enough. Obtain history of other contacts, determine source.

General Measures
- Fluid and electrolyte support if needed. Watch for signs of myocarditis, use cardiac monitor if severe case.

SPECIFIC THERAPY
Indications
- Intestinal phase: anyone suspected to be infected. Treatment in this phase kills larvae before invasion.
- Muscle invasion phase: cases with moderate or severe symptoms. Treatment of mild cases is optional.

Treatment Options
- Intestinal phase: Mebendazole for 5 days
    ➤ Albendazole for 3 days.
- Muscle invasion phase, moderate to severe cases:

➤ Prednisone, depending on severity of symptoms, until fever and allergic signs regress. Start steroids before antihelminthic thrapy.
➤ Mebendazole (graduated dose because of occasional herxheimer reaction)
➤ Albendazole (dose not standardized)
■ Mild cases: steroids as needed.

Side Effects & Complications
■ Prednisone: usual side effects.
■ Mebendazole: mild intestinal complaints, rarely leukopenia. Herxheimer reaction at onset.
■ Albendazole: mild intestinal complaints, liver function abnormalities, leukopenia, alopecia (usually with longer treatment). Herxheimer reaction may occur early.
■ Contraindications to treatment: absolute: allergy to medication, pregnancy
■ Contraindications to treatment: relative: mild cases.

FOLLOW-UP
During Treatment
■ Watch for herxheimer reaction. Watch for myocarditis: prolonged tachycardia, any rhythm disturbance, hypotension, pericardial effusion. Have patient monitored in severe case or if significant myocarditis suspected.

Routine
■ Recovery is the rule, clinical follow-up is adequate

COMPLICATIONS AND PROGNOSIS
■ Myocarditis, retinal hemorrhage, CNS invasion with encephalopathic picture. Most cases have full recovery, sometimes prolonged muscle weakness in severe cases. Main cause of death is myocarditis.

TRICHURIASIS

J. GORDON FRIERSON, MD

HISTORY & PHYSICAL
History
■ Life cycle: eggs of *Trichuris trichura* passed in feces, must incubate in soil at least 10–14 days to be infective. Then ingested through

contaminated food, water, or soil, hatch and mature in intestine, and the head of the worm lodges in mucosa of cecum. Females pass fertilized eggs.

Signs & Symptoms
- Light infections: none
- Medium infections: mild diarrhea
- Heavy infections: more diarrhea, abdominal discomfort, blood in stool, and rectal prolapse (in children).

TESTS
- Basic tests: blood: sometimes eosinophilia is seen
- Basic tests: urine: normal
- Specific tests: Stool exam for O&P shows diagnostic eggs. Charcot-Leydon crystals may be seen.
- Other tests: Worms can be seen on sigmoidoscopy.

DIFFERENTIAL DIAGNOSIS
- Almost anything that causes diarrhea can suggest moderate to heavy trichuriasis. Stool exam is specific.

MANAGEMENT
What to Do First
- Assess severity of infection. In heavy infection fluid and electrolyte replacement may be needed. Anemia rarely needs transfusion.

General Measures
- Find source of infection.

SPECIFIC THERAPY
Indications
- Any patient with symptoms. Treatment of light infections is optional.

Treatment Options
- Mebendazole for 3 days
- Albendazole for 1–3 days depending on intensity of infection.

Side Effects & Complications
- Mebendazole – almost none, perhaps mild intestinal complaints
- Albendazole – rare in this dosage. Possibly mild intestinal complaints.

- Contraindications: absolute: Pregnancy if light infection. Hold treatment to second or third trimester if heavy infection (heavy infections rare in adults), and use mebendazole.
- Contraindications: relative: none

FOLLOW-UP

Routine

- Usually not needed, since a few remaining worms are not clinically significant. Repeat O&P can be done.

COMPLICATIONS AND PROGNOSIS

- Recovery is the rule. Untreated worms die off within 4–5 years. Severe cases in children can cause rectal prolapse.

TRICUSPID VALVE INSUFFICIENCY (TR)

JUDITH A. WISNESKI, MD

HISTORY & PHYSICAL

Etiology

- Secondary due to right ventricular dilatation due to pressure or volume overload (*most common*)
  - ➤ Left ventricular systolic or diastolic dysfunction
  - ➤ Mitral stenosis
  - ➤ Cor pulmonale
  - ➤ Primary pulmonary hypertension
  - ➤ Pulmonic stenosis
  - ➤ Left to right shunt
- Primary due to structural damage to tricuspid valve
  - ➤ Endocarditis (most common primary etiology)
  - ➤ Carcinoid syndrome
  - ➤ Rheumatic heart disease
  - ➤ Right ventricular infarct
  - ➤ Ebstein's anomaly
  - ➤ Trauma

History

- Symptoms
  - ➤ Right ventricular failure

Signs & Symptoms

- Right ventricular lift

- Holosystolic murmur right sternal border, which may increase with inspiration
- Right ventricular S3
- Elevated JVP with prominent V wave
- Enlarged pulsatile liver
- Ascites
- Edema

TESTS
- ECG
  - Right atrial abnormality
  - Right ventricular hypertrophy
  - Right axis deviation
  - Atrial fibrillation
- Chest X-Ray
  - Enlarged right ventricle
  - Enlarged right atrium
  - Dilated superior vena cava and azygos veins
- Echo/Doppler (*most important*)
  - Detect and quantitate TR
  - Assess pulmonary artery pressure and other conditions which may cause TR: left ventricular dysfunction, mitral stenosis
- Cardiac Catheterization
  - **Limited role in assessing primary TR**
    - Measure pulmonary artery pressure (< 40 mm Hg suggests primary TR)
    - Right atrial and right ventricular diastolic pressures elevated
  - **Major role in assessing conditions which may cause right ventricular dilation and TR**

DIFFERENTIAL DIAGNOSIS
- Pericardial effusion/tamponade
- Aortic stenosis

MANAGEMENT
- Secondary TR
  - Treatment of primary condition
- Primary TR
  - Medical – diuretics
  - Surgery – most cases with primary TR, valve surgery not necessary; severe/poorly tolerated TR with medical therapy, tricuspid valve repair with annuloplasty ring

SPECIFIC THERAPY
n/a

FOLLOW-UP
n/a

COMPLICATIONS AND PROGNOSIS
- Absence of pulmonary artery hypertension – prognosis good
- Presence of pulmonary artery hypertension – prognosis depends on primary condition

TRICUSPID VALVE STENOSIS (TS)

JUDITH A. WISNESKI, MD

HISTORY & PHYSICAL

Etiology
- Isolated TS not common
- Rheumatic heart disease (*almost never isolated TS, but associated with mitral*
  ➤ *and aortic valve disease*)
- Carcinoid syndrome (*usually tricuspid insufficiency, TS rare*)

History
- Symptoms of right heart failure: fatigue, elevated JVP, hepatomegaly, ascites, peripheral edema
- Symptoms associated with other valvular disease
- Flushing and diarrhea: carcinoid syndrome

Signs & Symptoms
- PMI – normal
- JVP – elevated
- Diastolic rumble right sternal border or lower left sternal border, increases
  ➤ with inspiration or leg raising
- Opening snap varies with respiration
- P2-normal
- Hepatic enlargement, ascites
- Peripheral edema

TESTS

Note: findings below for isolated tricuspid valve stenosis without pathology on other cardiac valves

ECG
- Right atrial enlargement
- Atrial fibrillation

Chest X-Ray
- Cardiomegaly with right atrial enlargement
- Dilated superior vena cava and azygos vein
- No pulmonary congestion

Echo/Doppler
- Thickening and immobility of tricuspid valve leaflets
- Diastolic gradient across tricuspid valve
- Enlarged right atrium
- Normal right ventricle (isolated TS)
  - ➤ (*Note, rheumatic in etiology – pathology usually present on other heart valves, such as mitral valve*)

Cardiac Catheterization
- Right ventricular/right atrial diastolic gradient; mean gradient of 5 mm Hg associated with signs of systemic venous congestion
- Cardiac output reduced at baseline or decreases with exercise

DIFFERENTIAL DIAGNOSIS
- Mitral stenosis
- Right atrial tumors
- Tricuspid atresia

MANAGEMENT

Medical
- Antibiotic prophylaxis
- Diuretics

SPECIFIC THERAPY
- Tricuspid commissurotomy during surgery for other heart valve
  - ➤ pathology
- Percutaneous balloon tricuspid valvotomy for isolated TS

FOLLOW-UP

n/a

COMPLICATIONS AND PROGNOSIS

■ Overall prognosis usually depends on other conditions (rheumatic involvement of other valves and left ventricular function, or carcinoid syndrome)

TROUSSEAU SYNDROME

WILLIAM BELL, PhD, MD

HISTORY & PHYSICAL

History

■ Characterized by recurrent migratory thrombophlebitis – thrombosis simultaneously in superficial and deep veins & arterial systems in any anatomic location

■ Associated with underlying neoplastic disease

■ Patient complains of:
  ➤ painful venous cords often associated with linear erythematous cutaneous streaks accompanied by cold distal extremities with absence of arterial pulse in involved area
  ➤ Rarely: fever, weight loss, headache, decline in appetite or any other systemic constitutional signs & symptoms

Signs & Symptoms

■ Usually no systemic complaints

■ Most commonly: normal, healthy-appearing pt; normal vital signs. Occasionally, minimal, questionable weight loss.

■ Most common: palpable venous cords; exquisitely tender to minimal manipulation
  ➤ Often venous or arterial cord can be picked up by examiner's fingers
  ➤ Heat immed above cut surface over involved vessel
  ➤ Cutaneous erythematous streaks
  ➤ Minimal to modest degree of edema (surrounding & distal to involved site)
  ➤ Flexion & distention of involved site – painful
  ➤ Body weight cannot be supported without discomfort
  ➤ Reasonably frequent: concomitant overlapping thrombophlebitis, arterial emboli, etc.

TESTS

Laboratory Studies
- Most studies non-specific & unrevealing
- Approx 40–60% pts may demonstrate features of DIC characterized by prolongation of prothrombin time, activated partial thromboplastin & thrombin time; hypofibrinogenemia & appreciable elevated quantities of fibrinogen-fibrin degradation products in the serum
- Histologic evidence of neoplastic tissue is essential to make Dx of Trousseau syndrome.

DIFFERENTIAL DIAGNOSIS
- Thrombophlebitis
- Acute arterial occlusion
- Pulmonary emboli
- All known neoplastic diseases
- CNS stroke
- Non-bacterial thrombotic endocarditis
- SBE
- Anti phospholipid syndrome
- Budd-Chiari syndrome

MANAGEMENT
- Venography promptly indicated: whenever indicated any place in body (usually initially lower extremities). PET imaging to locate primary and extent of metastases. Removal of primary may provide therapeutic benefit.
- Presence of distended venous network; in particular, if there are tender cutaneous erythematous streaks
- If prob involves both lower extremities simultaneously: prompt intense investigation for presence of a neoplasm must be initiated.
- The primary may be in any organ.
- In order of frequency, following must be exhaustively studied:
  - ➤ Lung; stomach; prostate; pancreas; blood (for acute leukemia); colon; ovary; gall bladder; liver; cholangiocarcinoma; reticulum cell carcinoma; melanoma; neuroblastoma; hepatoma; breast; tonsil; & site for unknown primary
- If any invasive studies needed: do immediately
- Tumor markers – employing noninvasive techniques such as CEA, PSA, chest radiography, upper GI endoscopy, abdominal ultrasound, and computed axial tomography scan may be very helpful in early detection of neoplasia

SPECIFIC THERAPY
- IV heparin loading dose followed by continuous IV infusion of heparin to prolong the APTT to twice normal baseline value:
- As soon as Dx of thrombosis (thrombophlebitis) is made; after a baseline PT, TT, APTT, FDP-fdp & fibrinogen have been obtained (as well as any other blood study needed [e.g., hem-8, M-12])
- IV heparin must be continued until underlying neoplasm is identified & completely removed
- If neoplasm can be completely removed: prompt return of all lab values to normal without any other treatment. As this takes place, IV heparin can be discontinued.
- If neoplasm cannot be found or found & cannot be removed: pt must remain on IV heparin for life
- Only way to successfully treat this disease: complete elimination of the neoplastic disease
- All other therapeutic maneuvers are palliative.
- If continuous IV heparin is being employed: may be possible to discharge pt home where pt receives continuous IV heparin via battery-driven pump attached to pt with waist belt. Pt & family must be thoroughly instructed in detail about all aspects of pump use, etc. before discharge home.
- Pt should be seen by the attending physician at least once/wk – if as outpt everything is in excellent functional order, pt can be managed without hospitalization. Close monitoring is needed to achieve this.

FOLLOW-UP
n/a

COMPLICATIONS AND PROGNOSIS
n/a

TRYPANOSOMIASIS, AFRICAN

J. GORDON FRIERSON, MD

HISTORY & PHYSICAL

History
- Exposure: bite of tsetse fly in tropical Africa. The fly transmits *Trypanosoma brucei rhodiense* in E. and S. Africa, and *Trypanosoma brucei gambiense* in Central and W. Africa.

Signs & Symptoms

- *T.b. rhodiense*: Chancre at site of Tsetse fly bite, 5–15 days after bite, which is red, indurated, raised, often with local adenopathy. Shortly thereafter, sudden onset of fever, chills, headache, lymphadenopathy, and often serpiginous erythematous skin lesions.
- *T.b. gambiense*: gradual onset weeks or months after bite of lethargy, headaches, fatigue, myalgias, malaise, followed by progressive deterioration of mental function. Lymphadenopathy, especially of posterior cervical nodes, is common. Gradual progress to death with psychosis, seizures, coma, etc. on the way.

TESTS

- Basic tests: blood: *T.b. rhodiense*: CBC may show anemia, thrombocytopenia. High sed rate. LFTs normal or mildly abnormal.
- T.b. gambiense: CBC shows anemia, maybe thrombocytopenia. High IGM (up to 4 times normal), mild LFT abnormalities.
- Basic tests: urine: not helpful
- Specific tests: *T.b. rhodiense*: thick blood smear stained with Giemsa for trypanosomes, or (more sensitive) examine buffy coat by Giemsa stain for trypanosomes.
  - ➤ *T.b. gambiense*: same smear techniques, but parasites are scarce, multiple smears may be needed. Lymph node (usually posterior cervical) aspirate usually positive for trypanosomes.
  - ➤ Other tests: CSF shows increased lymphocytes and protein, and centrifuged specimen often shows trypanosomes in gambiense, only later in rhodiense. High CSF IGM in *gambiense*. No serology available in U.S.

DIFFERENTIAL DIAGNOSIS

- *T.b. rhodiense*: any acute fever, such as malaria, African tick typhus, dengue fever, possibly typhoid fever.
- *T.b. gambiense*: chronic and subacute causes of fever, deterioration of mental function, such as syphilis, tuberculous meningitis, HIV-associated diseases.

MANAGEMENT

What to Do First

- Stabilize patient, may need IV fluids, fever control. Spinal tap.

General Measures

- Same.

SPECIFIC THERAPY

Indications
- All patients with both forms.

Treatment Options
- *T.b. rhodiense* without CNS involvement: Suramin (obtainable from CDC)
- *T.b. gambiense* without CNS involvement: pentamidine IV or IM
- *T.b. rhodiense* with CNS involvement (trypanosomes in CSF): melarsoprol, given in graduated dosage
- *T.b. gambiense* with CNS involvement: melarsoprol; Eflornithine is more effective, but not available in US.

Side Effects & Complications
- Suramin: fever, malaise, proteinuria, urticaria, paresthesias.
- Melarsoprol: reactive encephalopathy (considered autoimmune) in 4–8%, sometimes fatal, treated with steroids. Also peripheral neuropathy – can be severe
- Pentamidine: hypotension, hypoglycemia, renal failure, hypocalcemia, hyperkalemia, neutropenia.
- Contraindications to treatment: absolute: none, except allergy to intended agent.
- Contraindications to treatment: relative: same.

FOLLOW-UP

During Treatment
- In both forms, drugs are toxic, and close clinical follow needed, usually in a hospital. CSF examination to assess presence of parasites.

Routine
- Good nutrition, general care, treatment of coexisting illness.

COMPLICATIONS AND PROGNOSIS
- *T.b. rhodiensis*: in early stage, before CNS invasion and treated promptly, prognosis is good. If CNS invasion has occurred, prognosis is more guarded and melarsoprol can be very toxic and result in encephalopathy or death.
- *T.b. gambiense*: early stage: some hazard with pentamidine, otherwise good prognosis. In late stage, there is not complete reversal of brain damage, and without eflornithine treatment melarsoprol must be used which is very toxic (see T.b. rhodiesiense).

TRYPANOSOMIASIS, AMERICAN (CHAGAS' DISEASE)

J. GORDON FRIERSON, MD

HISTORY & PHYSICAL

History

■ Exposure: Disease most prevalent in South America, especially Brazil, Bolivia, now less common in Venezuela, Chile, Argentina, Paraguay, Uruguay, Colombia. Parasite exists in Central America and Mexico but clinical disease less common. Many mammals, including dogs serve as reservoir hosts. Transmitted by triatomine bugs, which live in ceilings and walls of mud and thatched huts. Bite is painless, trypanosomes defecated on skin during feeding, then rubbed or scratched into wound.

Signs & Symptoms

■ Acute phase: usually children, swelling develops at site of bite, sometimes indurated (chagoma). If conjunctiva infected, periorbital tissues swell (Romana's sign). Then ensues fever, adenopathy, hepatosplenomegaly, often meningeal signs. Resolves in 4–8 weeks.
■ Indeterminate phase: no symptoms. Parasites settled in myocardium, nerve plexus of esophagus and colon. Lasts 10 or more years.
■ Chronic phase: characterized by: a) myocardopathy, with enlarged heart, congestive heart failure, ventricular aneurysms, and arrhythmias; b) megasyndromes, such as megaesophagus and megacolon. Due to destruction of nerve plexus in bowel, these areas lose motility and dilate producing a baggy, flaccid esophagus or colon or both, and dysphagia and constipation.

TESTS

■ Basic tests: blood: CBC shows anemia and lymphocytosis in acute phase, normal later.
■ Basic tests: urine: no help
■ Specific tests: in acute phase, can see trypanosomes in spun specimen or buffy coat (most sensitive). In indeterminate and chronic phase, parasites seldom seen, may be detected by xenodiagnosis (feed triatomine bugs on patient) in about 50%.
■ Upper GI or barium enema results are very typical, almost diagnostic in endemic area.
■ Other tests: EKG usually shows RBBB, often other abnormalities, and rhythm disturbances. PCR useful in detecting parasites in

indeterminate and chronic phases, more sensitive than xenodiagnosis. Commercial ELISA kits available in US, or serology can be performed at CDC.

DIFFERENTIAL DIAGNOSIS
- Acute phase: Fever can resemble many other febrile diseases, including typhoid, leishmaniasis, malaria, mononucleosis. Presence of chagoma or Romana's sign helps distinguish. In chronic stage, other causes of myocardiopathy, rheumatic heart disease, endomyocardial fibrosis. Megasyndromes are quite distinct.

MANAGEMENT

What to Do First
- Acute phase: Treat fever; attention to fluids, nutrition.
- Chronic phase: evaluate heart and GI tract.

General Measures
- Same. Fumigate housing and vicinity.

SPECIFIC THERAPY

Indications
- Any acute case. Treatment in indeterminate and chronic phase is controversial. Recent papers suggest parasites can be eliminated in some, but pathology not reversed.

Treatment Options
- Acute stage: Nifurtimox for 30–120 days (available only through CDC)
- Benznidazole for 30–60 days, all ages (not available in US)

Side Effects & Complications
- Nifurtimox: peripheral neuropathy is most serious effect. Also tremor, excitation, anorexia, rashes, exfoliation.
- Benznidazole: rash, exfoliation, peripheral neuropathy, anorexia, hematologic abnormalities.
- Contraindications to treatment: absolute: allergy to drug, pregnancy (but treat newborn of infected), and indeterminate cases with no pathology.
- Contraindications to treatment: relative: chronic cases with advanced manifestations.

FOLLOW-UP

During Treatment
- Observe for side effects, which can be severe. Monitor CBC.

Routine

■ Prolonged follow-up for development of or persistence of myocardial or bowel pathology.

COMPLICATIONS AND PROGNOSIS

■ Treatment of acute phase prevents chronic parasitization in about 50% of cases. Immunosuppressed states can lead to renewal of acute disease with trypanosomes in blood, fever, and sometimes cerebral masses. Treatment can still be effective. Cardiac transplant done for advanced myocardial disease.

TUBERCULOSIS

RICHARD A. JACOBS, MD, PhD

HISTORY & PHYSICAL

History

■ Etiologic agent *Mycobacterium tuberculosis*, an aerobic, acid-fast bacillus

■ Humans only known reservoir; infection results from inhalation of aerosolized droplets containing viable organisms

■ Risk factors for infection include close contact with infected individuals, immunosuppression (15 mg prednisone daily for at least a month, HIV, organ transplantation), residence in or recent (within 5 years) immigration from high prevalence areas (Asia, Africa, Central America, Mexico), intravenous drug use, homelessness, incarceration in prison, residents and employees of nursing homes (including health care workers with exposure to TB) and the presence of certain underlying diseases (diabetes, chronic renal insufficiency, hematologic and solid malignancies, malnutrition, gastrectomy, ileojejunal bypass, silicosis)

Signs & Symptoms

■ Pulmonary – cough (initially dry, then becoming productive of purulent sputum that may be blood tinged) and constitutional symptoms (fever, chills, night sweats, anorexia, weight loss, fatigue) hallmarks of disease; rales or consolidation on exam

■ Extra-pulmonary – any organ can be involved; most common include: meningitis (presentation over several weeks with fever, headache, nausea, vomiting, seizures, confusion and cranial nerve palsies); skeletal – spine infection or Pott's disease (localized pain)

and arthritis (chronic, monoarticular, involving large, weight bearing joints); genitourinary – renal (back pain, fever, dysuria), prostate, epididymis, endometrium, ovaries; gastrointestinal – small bowel, particularly ileocecal area (fever, pain, diarrhea, obstruction), but colon, duodenum, stomach, liver and peritoneum (fever, weight loss, abdominal pain over several weeks) can also be involved; pericarditis (acute presentation with tamponade or chronic constrictive with shortness of breath, pleural effusions, ascites)

TESTS

- Definitive diagnosis made by culturing *M. tuberculosis* from involved tissue; growth on solid media in 6–8 weeks; radiometric media (Bactec) positive in 1–2 weeks depending on inoculum
- Pulmonary – 3 sputums on successive days; sputum induction or bronchoscopy may be needed if cough nonproductive; early morning gastric aspirate and blood cultures (up to15% positive) may be helpful; direct nucleic amplification test on sputum of smear negative cases, with high or intermediate likelihood of disease, has sensitivity of 40–70%
- Extra-pulmonary – must obtain tissue or fluid for culture; negative culture does not exclude disease; pleural, peritoneal, pericardial, joint and cerebrospinal fluids positive in only 25–50% of cases; presence of granulomas suggestive, but not diagnostic, of M. tuberculosis (non-tuberculous mycobacteria, fungi, other bacteria also cause granulomas)
- Chest x-ray in primary tuberculosis usually shows infiltrate in upper lobes, hilar and/or paratracheal adenopathy; pleural effusion less common; in reactivation tuberculosis nodular infiltrates or cavities in the posterior segment or the upper lobe or superior segment or lower lobe in 70%; infiltrates in other areas in 30%
- Infected tuberculous fluid classically exudative with lymphocytic predominance and low glucose, but great deal of variability exits
- Tuberculin skin test (PPD) positive in 75% with active infection; negative test does not exclude disease; positive test may reflect previous, inactive disease

Latent TB infection (LTBI) previously diagnosed by PPD. Now, whole blood interferon-gamma assays are available that require only one visit and are not subject to reader interpretation. Not yet validated in all groups.

DIFFERENTIAL DIAGNOSIS

- Pulmonary disease must be differentiated from other bacterial and fungal causes of pneumonia as well as neoplastic and non-infectious causes of pulmonary infiltrates
- Extra-pulmonary disease usually insidious and must be distinguished from neoplasm and fungal infection

MANAGEMENT

- Consider diagnosis in any high risk person with pulmonary infiltrates, especially in presence of hilar or paratracheal adenopathy
- Hospitalization required if patient unreliable or too ill for self-care; respiratory isolation in negative pressure private room until active disease excluded by 3 negative AFB smears of sputum
- All documented or highly probable cases should be reported to public health authorities

SPECIFIC THERAPY

- Therapy based on sensitivities of organism, but results take weeks
- Because of increasing resistance, empirical therapy includes four drugs: isoniazid (INH), rifampin (RIF), ethambutol (ETH), and pyrazinamide (PZA) 25 mg/kg daily; PZA discontinued after 8 weeks; ETH discontinued if organism sensitive to INH and RIF; total duration at least 6 months, or 3 months after cultures negative; fixed combinations of INH and RIF (Rifamate) and INH, RIF and PZA (Rifater) available to simplify regimen
- If drugs other than INH, RIF and PZA used because of adverse drug reactions or resistance, longer courses of therapy (9–24 months) required
- Directly observed therapy highly recommended to improve compliance and decrease development of drug resistance; employs less frequent administration of drugs (2 or 3 times weekly) at higher doses
- Duration of therapy for extra-pulmonary tuberculosis (especially osteomyelitis and meningitis) 9–12 months
- Adjunctive corticosteroids used in tuberculous meningitis and pericarditis
- Baseline liver function tests obtained before starting INH, RIF or PZA; visual acuity and test for red-green color discrimination before starting ETH; monitoring of adverse reactions can be done by monthly symptom checks

FOLLOW-UP

- Clinical improvement seen within weeks

- Monthly cultures of sputum indicated; if positive beyond 3 months, consider noncompliance (institute directly observed therapy) or drug resistance (check sensitivities)
  - Two weeks of therapy with active drugs considered to render patients no longer infectious

COMPLICATIONS AND PROGNOSIS
- With appropriate therapy, prognosis good and relapse rate <5%
- Chemoprophylaxis indicated for some with positive PPD or positive whole blood interferon-gamma assay.
- PPD positive if 48–72 hours after intradermal injection, induration >5 mm present in those with HIV, those receiving immunosuppressive medications, those with close contact with known case of TB and those with CXRs consistent with TB and not previously treated; ≥ 10 mm considered positive in other high risk groups (see risk factors above); for all others, ≥ 15 mm considered positive
- Those with positive PPD should receive prophylaxis, regardless of age, if they are HIV positive, are close contacts of known active cases, are recent converters (defined as increase of 10 mm or more within 2 years) or have predisposing medical conditions; others with positive PPD treated only if under age 35 years
- Several prophylactic regimens recommended: 9 months of INH, 2 months of RIF plus PZA, or 4 months of RIF
  - Exclude active disease with CXR and cultures (if indicated) before starting prophylaxis

---

TUBULOINTERSTITIAL RENAL DISEASE

CHARLES B. CANGRO, MD, PhD and WILLIAM L. HENRICH, MD

HISTORY & PHYSICAL
- There are two forms: acute and chronic
- Acute TIN may present with:
  - asymptomatic increase in BUN and creatinine
  - rapid onset acute renal failure
  - azotemia
  - oliguria (25%-40% of cases)
  - need for dialysis (30% of cases)
  - flank pain (up to 50% of patients) (distention of renal capsule)
  - hypersensitivity rash (maculopapular in 25%-50% of cases)

- fever (75% of cases)
- nonspecific arthralgias (10% of cases)

■ Chronic TIN may present with:
- insidious, symptomatic increase in BUN and creatinine
- hypertension
- inability to concentrate urine
- polyuria, nocturia
- azotemia, malaise, anemia
- renal tubular acidosis
- advanced renal insufficiency/need for dialysis

TESTS

Laboratory

■ Hematology – CBC (add differential with acute TIN)
- Acute TIN: eosinophilia – in 80% of cases caused by methicillin – 39% of cases caused by other drugs
- Chronic TIN: anemia (decreased EPO production)

■ Metabolic Profile
- Acute TIN:
  - frequently has increased BUN and creatinine
  - no specific pattern of RTA, electrolyte or acid-base disturbance
  - mimics ARF
- Chronic TIN:
  - elevated BUN and creatinine

■ Urinalysis
- Abnormalities reflect site and severity of tubular damage
- Acute TIN:
  - mild to moderate proteinuria, <2 g/24 hours (60%–80% of cases)
  - nephrotic range proteinuria rare except with minimal change disease associated with NSAID use
  - microscopic hematuria (50%–90% of cases), RBC casts rare
  - pyuria (50% 0f cases), WBC casts
  - eosinophiluria – >5% of urine WBC stain with Hansel's stain (low positive predictive value – also seen with ARF)
  - glucosuria (with normal serum glucoses)
  - bicarbonaturia (proximal RTA)
  - inability to acidify urine (urine pH > 5.5)
  - distal RTA
- Chronic TIN
  - inability to concentrate urine, low specific gravity

- non nephrotic proteinuria
- inactive urine sediment

Imaging
- Acute TIN:
  - ultrasound: kidneys may be swollen and enlarged
  - may have increased cortical echo density
- Chronic TIN:
  - ultrasound: kidneys may be small, echo dense
  - blunted calyx with reflux

Renal Biopsy
- definitive diagnostic test
- not always necessary
- perform when history and evidence are not strong
- consider in patients with ARF, who are not prerenal, and not obstructed by ultrasound
- perform biopsy when information obtained will alter therapy
  - Acute TIN:
    - increased interstitial volume and edema
    - focal infiltrates of mononuclear cells primarily peritubular location with sparing of glomeruli and vessels
    - immunoglobulin deposits rarely seen by immunofluorescence
    - amount of fibrosis may aid in determining aggressiveness of therapy
  - Chronic TIN:
    - increased interstitial volume-primary fibrosis and tubular atrophy
    - extent of fibrosis has prognostic value

DIFFERENTIAL DIAGNOSIS
- Clinical entities which must be distinguished from TIN
  - Acute TIN: any cause of pre-renal, post renal or renal ARF
  - Chronic TIN: any cause of chronic renal failure

Causes of ATIN
- Common causes:
  - Drug induced (immune mediated)
  - Systemic disease
  - Infection (frequently immune mediated)
  - Idiopathic

- Drug Induced
  - most common cause of acute TIN
  - occurs 2–60 days after beginning drug
  - not dose related
  - cannot be ruled out by prior exposure without adverse reaction
  - recurs with exposure to the same or similar drugs
  - may be accompanied by systemic manifestation of hypersensitivity, rash (50% of cases) fever (75% of cases), eosinophilia (40%-80% of cases)
- Drugs Implicated include:
  - Antibiotics:
    - ampicillin, penicillin, methicillin and congeners, cephalosporins, ciprofloxacin, rifampin, sulfonamides, ethambutol, polymixin, trimethoprim/sulfamethoxazole, and many others
  - Anticonvulsants:
    - phenytoin, carbamazepine, phenobarbital
  - Diuretics:
    - furosemide, metolazone, thiazides, triamterene
  - NSAIDs: see chapter on analgesic nephropathy
  - Miscellaneous:
    - Allopurinol, azathioprine, captopril, cimetadine, clofibrate, cyclosporine, gold, interferon, lithium, warfarin, herbal preparations
  - List of implicated drugs continues to expand; however biopsy confirmation often lacking
- Systemic Disease
  - Anti-tubular basement membrane mediated
  - Sjogren's syndrome
  - Sarcoidosis (hypercalcemia, hypercalciuria granulomatous disease)
  - Systemic lupus erythematosus
  - Cryoglobulinemia
- Infection
  - Direct Involvement of renal parenchyma
    - classic cause is bacterial pyelonephritis
    - may also be fungal, viral, parasitic
  - Systemic Infection
    - occurs with or without infectious agent identified in renal interstitium
    - Bacteria – beta streptococci, Legionella, Brucella, Mycoplasma, Treponema

- Viral – EBV, CMV, HIV, rubella, polyoma, Hanta, HSV, Hepatitis B
- Parasites – Leishmania, Toxoplasma
- Fungal – Histoplasmosis
- Rickettsia

➤ Idiopathic
  - TINU – anterior uveitis and acute TIN
  - diagnosed after exclusion of infection, drug or systemic disease

■ Chronic Tubulointerstitial Nephritis (CTIN)

➤ common causes:
  - immune disease
  - drugs
  - infection
  - obstruction and reflux
  - hematopoietic disease
  - heavy metals
  - metabolic disease
  - hereditary disease
  - granulomatous disease
  - others
  - idiopathic

➤ Immune disease
  - Lupus nephritis
  - Mixed cryoglobulinemia
  - Goodpasture's syndrome
  - Chronic rejection of renal transplant
  - Amyloidosis
  - Sjogren's disease

➤ Drugs
  - prolonged and excessive exposure
  - analgesics / NSAIDS
  - Lithium
  - Cis-platinum
  - Nitrosoureas
  - Cyclosporine / FK 506
  - Chinese herbs

➤ Infections
  - increased risk with concurrent UTI and obstruction or vesicoureteral reflux

➤ Obstruction and Reflux
  - obstruction and vesicoureteral reflux can result in tubulointerstitial damage even without infection

- magnitude and duration of back pressure determine severity of chronic TIN
- Hematopoietic disease
  - Sickle cell disease and trait – may cause papillary necrosis
  - Plasma Cell Dyscrasias
  - Lymphoproliferative disease (non-Hodgkin's lymphoma and lymphoblastic leukemia)
- Heavy Metals
  - Lead (hyperuricemia, hypertension)
  - Cadmium
  - Mercury
  - Uranium
  - Arsenic
- Metabolic Disease
  - Hypercalcemia
  - Hyperuricemia
  - Hyperoxaluria
  - Cystinosis
  - Chronic hypokalemia
- Hereditary Disease
  - Polycystic kidney disease
  - Alport's syndrome
  - Medullary sponge kidney
  - Hereditary nephritis
- Granulomatous Disease
  - Sarcoidosis
  - Tuberculosis
  - Wegener's
  - Heroin nephropathy
- Others
  - Radiation
  - Hypertensive nephrosclerosis
  - Balkan nephropathy
- Idiopathic
  - no definite etiology for 15–20% of cases of biopsy-proven chronic TIN

MANAGEMENT

What to Do First

- obtain detailed history and physical exam
- assess severity of renal dysfunction
- what is rate of rise of serum creatinine (days, weeks, months, years)

- Acute vs. Chronic TIN or other cause of ARF?
- Is patient non-oliguric, oliguric or anuric?
- assess volume status (pre-renal, euvolemic, volume overloaded)
- Is a life-threatening electrolyte, acid-base abnormality present?
- Call Nephrology Consult

General Measures
- avoid nephrotoxic drugs (NSAIDs and ACEI)
- remove or treat causative factors
  - ➤ Review present, recent and past drug use
  - ➤ Evaluate for infection – treat
  - ➤ Evaluate for systemic disease – treat
- Obtain ultrasound
  - ➤ check kidney size
  - ➤ echo density
  - ➤ rule out obstruction

SPECIFIC THERAPY

Depends on Cause:
- Drug induced-stop drug
- Infectious – treat infection
- Systemic disease – treat-underlying disease (Sarcoidosis, Sjogren's, SLE-treat with steroids)
- Idiopathic (TINU and true idiopathic cause -consider steroids)
  - ➤ if after stop drug BUN/Cr do not increase further, monitor conservatively.
  - ➤ keep patient euvolemic
  - ➤ adjust drug doses for decreased GFR
  - ➤ avoid nephrotoxins (NSAIDs and ACEI)

Acute TIN
- early treatment is essential
- acute TIN treated within the first 2 weeks, the post recovery serum Cr approx 1 mg/dl
- Cr for those treated after 3 weeks of acute TIN >3.0 mg/dl
- longer time between diagnosis and treatment, the worse the recovery creatinine
- late treatment after extensive fibrosis on biopsy less beneficial
- if renal function not improving after 2–3 days, proceed to biopsy
- with biopsy confirmation or strong history to suggest acute TIN (drug, some systemic diseases and idiopathic) – prednisone 1 mg/kg/day

- steroids shorten time to recovery-best if started early
- if no response to steroids after 2 weeks consider cyclophosphamide
- Discontinue steroids if no response after 3–4 weeks
- stop cyclophosphamide if no response after 4–6 weeks
- if anti TBM found on biopsy treat with steroids, cyclophosphamide and also consider 2-week trial of plasmapheresis
- initiate dialysis early if oliguric, uremic, volume overloaded.

Chronic TIN

- investigate cause and treat
- stop offending drugs (lithium NSAIDs),
- treat systemic disease
- relieve obstruction
- aggressive BP control
- biopsy not always indicated
- extent and severity of fibrosis on biopsy will predict GFR and prognosis

FOLLOW-UP

Acute TIN

- daily monitor of BUN/Cr, acid/base and electrolytes
- daily assess volume status, urine output, need for dialysis

Chronic TIN

- periodic charting of BUN/Cr
- periodic calculation of GFR refer to Nephrology when serum creatinine is sustained >1.5 mg/dl

COMPLICATIONS AND PROGNOSIS

Acute TIN

- post recovery serum creatinine if treatment started before 2 weeks, approx 1 mg/dl
- post recovery serum creatinine if treatment delayed after 3 weeks, approx 3 mg/dl

Chronic TIN

- may lead to chronic renal impairment and progression to ESRD without and even with aggressive management

TUMORS OF PARATESTICULAR AND SPERMATIC CORD STRUCTURES

ARTHUR I. SAGALOWSKY, MD

HISTORY & PHYSICAL
- round, smooth mass in epididymis or cord
- slow growth (likely benign) vs. rapid (concern for malignancy)

TESTS
- does not transilluminate
- ultrasound reveals solid mass

DIFFERENTIAL DIAGNOSIS
- benign adenomatoid tumor most common
- malignant – rhabdomyosarcoma, leiomyosarcoma, mesothelioma

MANAGEMENT
n/a

SPECIFIC THERAPY
- inguinal exploration
- simple excision of benign mass; inguinal orchiectomy for malignant lesions
- further staging and Rx of paratesticular malignancies beyond the scope of this chapter

FOLLOW-UP
n/a

COMPLICATIONS AND PROGNOSIS
n/a

TUMORS, INTRACRANIAL

MICHAEL J. AMINOFF, MD, DSc

HISTORY & PHYSICAL
- General: headache, poor concentration, memory disturbance, somnolence, nausea & vomiting, visual obscurations
- Focal: depend on tumor location
- May have family history of tumor
- General findings: Signs of increased ICP (papilledema, reduced attention, drowsiness, cognitive changes)

- False localizing signs – eg, 3rd or 6th nerve palsy or extensor plantar responses from herniation syndromes
- Focal deficits depending on tumor location
  - Frontal: focal & generalized seizures, intellectual changes, pyramidal weakness, aphasia
  - Temporal: complex partial seizures, personality change, memory disturbance, visual field defects, aphasia
  - Parietal: simple partial seizures (sensory or motor), sensory disturbances, sensory neglect, apraxia, visual field defects
  - Occipital: Field defects, visual hallucinations, seizures
  - Brain stem or cerebellar: diplopia, dysarthria, dysphagia, weakness or sensory disturbance (or both) in face or limbs, vertigo, ataxia

TESTS
- Cranial CT scan or MRI w/ contrast enhancement will detect, define & localize lesion
- If cerebral metastases are likely, screen for primary lesion
- Lab studies generally unhelpful; CSF studies of limited help; lumbar puncture may provoke herniation syndrome

DIFFERENTIAL DIAGNOSIS
- Other structural lesions are distinguished by imaging findings
- May be family history of neurofibroma, retinoblastoma, hemangioblastoma
- Medulloblastoma, brain stem glioma, craniopharyngioma, cerebellar astrocytoma occur most commonly in childhood
- Primary cerebral lymphoma is assoc w/ AIDS

MANAGEMENT
- Steroids reduce cerebral edema
- Herniation syndrome treated with dexamethasone; mannitol also effective short term
- Anticonvulsants if seizures occur

SPECIFIC THERAPY
- Treatment depends on tumor type, site & size
- Surgery permits histologic diagnosis; extra-axial tumors can often be removed; some other tumors can also be removed or debulked, w/ reduction in ICP; shunting procedures relieve obstructive hydrocephalus
- Irradiation or chemotherapy is indicated for certain tumor types

FOLLOW-UP
- Depends on type of tumor & whether complete surgical resection is possible

COMPLICATIONS AND PROGNOSIS

Complications
- Incidence depends on tumor type & location
- Cerebral edema: treat as above
- Herniation syndrome: treat as above
- Obstructive hydrocephalus: treat as above
- Seizures: anticonvulsants
- Tumor spread: irradiation or chemotherapy if feasible

Prognosis
- Depends on tumor type; extra-axial primary lesions often resectable completely (eg, acoustic neuroma, meningioma) w/ good prognosis; glioblastoma multiforme & brain stem gliomas have poor prognosis– usually inoperable or total removal not possible; oligodendroglioma & cerebellar hemangioblastoma have good prognosis if removed completely; metastases often multiple & not resectable–prognosis is of primary neoplasm

---

TUMORS, SPINAL

MICHAEL J. AMINOFF, MD, DSc

HISTORY & PHYSICAL
- Pain in back or limbs in radicular or diffuse distribution; worse on coughing or straining
- Weakness, numbness or paresthesias below level of lesion
- Bladder, bowel, sexual dysfunction
- Progression may be gradual, but acute deterioration may occur unpredictably
- Spinal tenderness sometimes present
- Lower motor neuron deficit may be evident at level of lesion: upper motor neuron deficit (spastic paraparesis) below lesion
- Sensory disturbance below level of lesion
- Brown-Sequard syndrome sometimes present (ipsilateral pyramidal deficit, hyperesthesia, impaired vibration and postural sense; contralateral analgesia)

TESTS

- Imaging studies (MRI or CT myelography) to localize lesion
- CSF may be xanthochromic w/ high protein concentration, especially if subarachnoid block is present

DIFFERENTIAL DIAGNOSIS

- Tumor may be primary or secondary, intramedullary or extramedullary (extra- or intradural); intramedullary tumors usually ependymoma or glioma; primary extramedullary tumors include meningiomas and neurofibromas; carcinomatous or lymphomatous deposits usually extradural
- Imaging studies help localize lesion & distinguish from other disorders (eg, disc protrusion, hematomas)

MANAGEMENT

- High-dose steroids (eg, dexamethasone) to reduce cord edema and relieve pain; analgesics may be needed; urgent decompression may be needed if sphincter function threatened

SPECIFIC THERAPY

- Extradural metastases: dexamethasone, w/ taper depending on response; irradiation; surgical decompression if poor response (or previously irradiated)
- Intramedullary tumors: surgical excision or irradiation
- Extramedullary primary tumors: surgical excision

FOLLOW-UP

- Depends on tumor site & type

COMPLICATIONS AND PROGNOSIS

- Prognosis is poor for extradural metastases; prognosis of intramedullary lesions depends on lesion type & severity of cord compression before treatment; prognosis good for primary extramedullary tumors, but degree of recovery depends on severity of deficit before surgery

---

TYPHUS FEVERS

RICHARD A. JACOBS, MD, PhD

HISTORY & PHYSICAL

- *Epidemic Typhus*: Body contact with body louse carrier 1 week before onset of symptoms. Living in unsanitary, crowded conditions, especially during cold weather.

- *Endemic (murine) Typhus*: History of flea bite or exposure to cats, oppossums, rabbits, skunks 1–2 weeks before the onset of symptoms, especially during late spring-summer in southern Texas or southern California.
- *Scrub Typhus*: Chigger bite 1–3 weeks before onset of illness. Travel to endemic areas in eastern Asia or western Pacific.

Symptoms:
- *Epidemic Typhus*: Abrupt onset of fever, severe headache, chills, myalgias +/− nonproductive cough.
- *Endemic typhus*: Abrupt onset of fever (100%), severe headache (45%), chills (44%), myalgias (33%), nausea (33%).
- *Scrub Typhus*: Abrupt onset of fever (100%), severe headache (100%), and myalgias.

Physical Signs:
- *Epidemic Typhus*: Fever (102–104°F), maculopapular rash begins in axillary folds and upper trunk 3–5 days after onset of illness and becomes progressively petechial and confluent, nonproductive cough with diffuse rales/rhonchi. Conjunctival injection, eye pain, skin necrosis, digit gangrene.
- *Endemic Typhus*: Macular/maculopapular rash beginning 3–5 days after disease onset on arms/axillae and spreading to trunk, extremities, occasionally including palms and soles, eventually 50% have rash, 35% nonproductive cough, 23% abnormal CXR, hepatosplenomegaly in 1–45%. Neurologic symptoms and signs may occur.
- *Scrub Typhus*: Eschar at site of tick bite, tender generalized or regional lymphadenopathy (85%), conjunctival injection, macular/maculopapular rash on trunk and extremities 5 days after onset of symptoms (34%), splenomegaly. Neurologic findings in <10% (ataxia, slurred speech, tremor, delirium, nuchal rigidity, deafness), fever to 40–40.5°C.

TESTS

Laboratory
- Basic Blood Tests:
- Early: Low Hematocrit and WBC
- Later: low platelets, elevated WBC (may be lymphocytic predominance), hyponatremia, low albumin and mild LFT abnormalities.
- Specific Diagnostic Tests: Clinical diagnosis. Treat while awaiting lab confirmation.

- *Epidemic Typhus*: Indirect immunofluorescent antibody (IFA) titer ≥1:128
- *Endemic Typhus*: IFA 4-fold rise to >1:64 or single titer of ≥1:128, usually 15 days after onset. Immunohistology of skin biopsy.
- *Scrub Typhus*: IFA titer >1:320 or 4-fold rise in titer. Early treatment may blunt antibody response.

Other Tests
- CXR in endemic typhus may be abnormal.
- CSF in scrub typhus may have 0–110 WBC/mm^3, and mildly increased protein.

DIFFERENTIAL DIAGNOSIS
- Rocky mountain spotted fever, brucellosis, meningococcemia, bacterial and viral meningitis, measles, rubella, toxoplasmosis, leptospirosis, typhoid fever, Dengue fever, flavivirus infection, relapsing fever, secondary syphilis, infectious mononucleosis, gastroenteritis, ehrlichiosis, Kawasaki's disease, toxic shock syndrome.

MANAGEMENT
What to Do First
- Consider rickettsial infections in patients with abrupt onset of fever, headache and myalgias with appropriate exposures. Examine carefully for rashes. Begin antirickettsial therapy.

General Measures
- General supportive measures as needed.
- 10% of patients with endemic typhus will require ICU hospitalization; these have a 4% mortality.
- Can give corticosteroids in patients with severe CNS disease.

SPECIFIC THERAPY
Indications
- Treat all suspected rickettsial infections.

Treatment Options
- Treat severely ill patients intravenously with the same drugs and dosages as oral regimens.
- *Epidemic Typhus*: Louse-borne typhus – Doxycycline. Indigenously acquired epidemic typhus or Brill-Zinsser disease – until patient afebrile 2–3 days.
- *Endemic Typhus*: Doxycycline or chloramphenicol 7–15 days.

- *Scrub Typhus*: Doxycycline or chloramphenicol 7–15 days. Chloramphenicol- and tetracycline-resistant strains of scrub typhus found in northern Thailand may respond to ciprofloxacin or azithromycin.
- Contraindications: Sulfa drugs should be avoided since they can increase the severity of endemic typhus.
- No tetracyclines in children < 9 years.
- In pregnancy, use chloramphenicol

FOLLOW-UP

During Treatment

- Fever usually abates rapidly with antibiotics: ≤48 hours in epidemic typhus, ≤72 hours in endemic typhus and ≤24 hours in scrub typhus.
- Inpatient care for only severely ill. Outpatients should be checked weekly until clinically improving. Patient education for prevention, especially for travelers to endemic areas. Effective vaccine available for those at high risk for epidemic typhus.
- Epidemic typhus may relapse if treated within 48 hours of the onset of symptoms. Recurrent disease responds to 2nd course of antibiotics.
- Scrub typhus may relapse if treatment given within the first 5 days of illness; treating for 2 weeks decreases the chance of relapse.
- Epidemic typhus can recrudesce years later from lymph nodes, causing milder, Brill-Zinsser disease.

COMPLICATIONS AND PROGNOSIS

Complications

- *Epidemic Typhus*: Renal failure/azotemia, CNS abnormalities/seizures, myocardial failure, deafness and tinnitus, respiratory failure, electrolyte abnormalities (low sodium, calcium and potassium), hypoalbuminemia, hypovolemia and shock.
- *Endemic Typhus*: Respiratory failure requiring mechanical ventilation, cerebral hemorrhage, hemolysis (with G6PD deficiency).
- *Scrub Typhus*: Heart failure, circulatory collapse and pneumonia cause mortality.

Prognosis

- *Epidemic Typhus*: Up to 40% mortality without treatment, highest in elderly. Without treatment, fever will lyse after 2 weeks.
- *Endemic Typhus*: Worse severity with old age, underlying disease, treatment with sulfa drug; case fatality 1–4%. Usually mild. May be fatal if misdiagnosed or inadequately treated.
- *Scrub Typhus*: Untreated, fever resolves in 2 weeks with mortality 0–30%. No mortality with appropriate treatment.

ULCERATIVE COLITIS

CHRISTINE A. CARTWRIGHT, MD

HISTORY & PHYSICAL

- History: bloody diarrhea, tenesmus, mucus, abdominal cramps, fever
- Trigger factors: NSAIDs, antibiotics, smoking cessation, stress, ?OCP
- Physical signs: fever, tachycardia, abdominal tenderness, bloody stools; extra-intestinal manifestations: peripheral arthritis, uveitis, episcleritis, scleritis, erythema nodosum, pyoderma gangrenosum

TESTS

Basic Studies: Blood

- CBC, ESR, albumin, LFTs

Other Studies

- stool studies: culture, O+P × 3, C. difficile × 3
- amebic ELISA serology
- colonoscopy and biopsies

DIFFERENTIAL DIAGNOSIS

- Crohn's disease or other causes:
- Infectious colitis (amebiasis, pseudomembranous, CMV, shigella, campylobacter, E. coli, salmonella)
- Ischemic colitis
- Radiation
- Drugs
- Cleansing agents

Differences between ulcerative colitis and Crohn's disease:

- ➤ ulcerative colitis: mucosal, diffuse, continuous, involves the rectum, limited to colon
- ➤ Crohn's: transmural, patchy, skip lesions, discrete ulcers, can occur anywhere in the GI tract but usually involves the distal ileum and right colon and spares the rectum; perianal disease, fistulae, abscesses, strictures, obstruction, granulomas

MANAGEMENT

What to Do First

- Assess severity and extent
- Severity:

> mild: <4 BMs/day, with or without blood, no systemic toxicity, CBC and ESR are normal
> moderate: >4 BMs/day with minimal systemic toxicity
> severe: >6 BMs/day, fever, tachycardia, anemia, thrombocytosis, elevated ESR, hypoalbuminemia

■ Extent:
> proctitis, proctosigmoiditis, left-sided colitis, pancolitis

General Management
■ Complete baseline evaluation: lab tests, colonoscopy, ?SBFT

SPECIFIC THERAPY
Maintenance therapy:
■ Mild-moderate colitis
> oral aminosalicylates:
  • sulfasalazine 2–4 g/day, mesalamine 4–4.8 g/day or balsalazide 6.75 g/day
  • effective maintenance drugs within 2–4 weeks in 40 to 80% of patients
  • intolerance to sulfapyridine moiety of sulfasalazine is common (headache, nausea), as are mild allergic reactions (skin rash); severe allergic reactions (e.g., fibrosing alveolitis, pericarditis, pancreatitis, agranulocytosis) are rare
  • abnormal sperm count, motility and morphology occur commonly with sulfasalazine (and not mesalamine) but are reversible with discontinuation of medication
  • low-grade hemolysis on sulfasalazine is not unusual but is rarely severe
  • sulfasalazine may interfere with folic acid absorption
  • interstitial nephritis from mesalamine is rare but may be irreversible
■ Moderate-severe colitis:
> Add azathioprine (Aza) or 6-mercaptopurine (6MP) – start at a low dose (50 mg/d) and slowly increase the dose by adding not more than 25 mg each month until 2.5 mg/kg/day for Aza or 1.5 mg/kg/day for 6MP or until leukopenia or elevated LFTs, whichever occurs first. Check CBC and LFTs every 2 weeks when starting or increasing the dose and every 3 months when on a stable dose. If TPMT enzyme activity is checked initially and is normal, then one can start at a higher dose and increase the dose at a faster rate to achieve earlier effect.

- side effects of Aza or 6MP: fatigue, nausea, bone marrow depression, opportunistic infections, pancreatitis, hepatitis, fever, rarely lymphoma
  - Methotrexate if intolerant to Aza or 6MP. Induction dose: 25 mg i.m. weekly for 16 weeks. Maintenance dose: 15 mg i.m. weekly.
- side effects of methotrexate: fatigue, nausea, diarrhea, leukopenia, opportunistic infections, liver disease
  - consider anti-TNF alpha if Aza, 6MP or methotrexate cannot be tolerated or is ineffective. Caution: we need more data on its effectiveness for maintaining long-term remission.

Active colitis:

Topical Therapy

- works faster and better than oral medication and less is absorbed
- mesalamine suppositories or enemas for mild proctitis or for maintenance therapy
- hydrocortisone enemas (100 mg) for more severe flares of proctitis or proctosigmoiditis (about one third of the enema is absorbed)

Oral Corticosteroids

- oral prednisone at 40 mg/day with gradual tapering – usually faster at higher doses and slower at lower doses (e.g., 5 mg/week initially and then 2.5 mg/week when <20 mg/day)
- short-term side effects include acne, night sweats, sleep and mood disturbances, appetite stimulation
- long-term side effects include hypertension, diabetes, acne, osteoporosis, osteonecrosis, glaucoma, cataracts, life-threatening infections, depression and obesity
- Budesonide (9 mg/d); Caution: may not be as effective as prednisone and has long-term steroid toxicities
- There is no place for frequent or long-term systemic steroids (including budesonide) in the management of IBD because the adverse effects outweigh the potential benefits.

Severe Colitis (Refractory to Oral Medications)

- admit to hospital; stool studies and colonic biopsies to rule out infectious diseases; abdominal CT scan
- iv corticosteroids (methylprednisolone 60 mg/day) and hydrocortisone enemas
- TPN is usually unnecessary in patients capable of eating.

- maximum 7–10 days observation on this regimen; watch for mega-colon or other signs of impending perforation; have a colorectal surgeon follow
- failure to improve mandates colectomy, or cyclosporine in highly selected individuals who decline surgery and agree to long-term maintenance therapy with Aza or 6MP (or methotrexate if unable to tolerate Aza or 6MP)
- start cyclosporine (CSA; only at a transplant center where daily accurate levels of CSA are available) at 4 mg/kg/day and follow whole-blood levels daily to maintain the level at 200–400
- if remission is achieved with iv CSA, start oral CSA, an oral aminosalicylate, Aza or 6MP (may take 3–6 months to work) and Bactrim (three times/week) for Pneumocystis prophylaxis
- taper off steroids and CSA over the next 3 months
- side effects of CSA include nephrotoxicity, seizures, hypertension, opportunistic infections, hirsutism, tremor and gingival hyperplasia

Colectomy
- Indications:
  - urgent or emergent:
    - failure to achieve remission with maximum medical management
    - perforation, or impending perforation
  - elective:
    - confirmed dysplasia and/or carcinoma
    - failure to maintain remission with immunomodulatory therapy and without long-term or frequent systemic steroids
    - pyoderma gangrenosum resistant to corticosteroids or cyclosporine
  - Procedures:
    - proctocolectomy with a one- or two-stage ileal pouch-anal anastomosis (IPAA)
    - for emergent surgery, subtotal colectomy with Brooke ileostomy and Hartmann procedure; later an elective IPAA
  - Complications:
    - multiple BMs (6–8/day), nocturnal incontinence (small amount), pouchitis (>50%; treat with metronidazole and cort enemas), pouch failure (5%), pouch dysplasia (requires surveillance)

FOLLOW-UP
- Frequent visits to assess symptoms and laboratory tests, particularly CBC, LFTs

COMPLICATIONS AND PROGNOSIS
- Extra-intestinal manifestations:
- Colitis-related: correlates with inflammatory activity of the bowel
  - arthritis:
    - peripheral
    - central – follows an independent course
      - associated with HLA haplotype B27
      - sacro-iliitis
      - ankylosing spondylitis
  - skin:
    - erythema nodosum
    - pyoderma gangrenosum
  - eye:
    - episcleritis
    - uveitis – may follow an independent course
      - often clusters with AS and SI
      - often associated with HLA-B27
- Not related to activity of colitis:
  - Hepatobiliary complications:
    - fatty infiltration
    - pericholangitis
    - chronic active hepatitis
    - cirrhosis
    - primary sclerosing cholangitis
    - cholangiocarcinoma

UNSTABLE HEMOGLOBINS

AKIKO SHIMAMURA, MD, PhD

HISTORY & PHYSICAL
- Family history of anemia, jaundice, splenomegaly, gallstones (usually autosomal dominant inheritance)
- Pallor, jaundice, dark urine, often precipitated by infection or oxidant drugs

Signs & Symptoms
- Pallor
- Jaundice
- Splenomegaly
- Cardiac flow murmur if anemic

TESTS

Blood

- Peripheral blood smear: hypochromia, poikilocytosis, anisocytosis, reticulocytosis, basophilic stippling
- Increased indirect bilirubin
- Increased LDH
- Decreased haptoglobin

Specific Tests:

- Supravital stain (methylene blue) may show Heinz bodies (may be minimal or absent if spleen is present)
- Isopropanol stability test may show excessive precipitation of abnormal hemoglobin at 37 degrees C in 17% isopropanol.
- Heat stability test may show hemoglobin precipitation at 50 degrees C.
- Some unstable hemoglobin variants may be detected by hemoglobin electrophoresis/isoelectric focusing.
- The above tests may be negative if the hemoglobin is too unstable to be released from the bone marrow into the periphery. Tests may be performed on bone marrow samples.

DIFFERENTIAL DIAGNOSIS

- Other hemolytic anemias
  - ➤ Glucose-6 phosphate dehydrogenase deficiency (low enzyme levels)
  - ➤ Immune hemolytic anemia (Coombs positive)
  - ➤ Hereditary spherocytosis (positive osmotic fragility test)
  - ➤ Red cell membrane defects (characteristic morphologies on peripheral smear)
  - ➤ Red cell enzyme defects (measure enzyme level)
- Thalassemias (hemoglobin electrophoresis)
- If nucleated red cells and teardrops on blood smear, consider congenital dyserythropoietic anemias, sideroblastic anemia (bone marrow aspirate and biopsy, including iron stain)

MANAGEMENT

- Red cell transfusions for symptomatic anemia (hemolysis may be exacerbated by illness, oxidant drugs)
- Splenectomy for: persistent severe anemia
  - ➤ risk of splenic rupture
  - ➤ hypersplenism

➤ Complications: increased risk of infection with encapsulated bacteria (immunize patient against pneumococcus, *Haemophilus influenzae*, and meningococcus prior to splenectomy, prophylactic penicillin)
■ General measures:
➤ Folic acid, 1 mg po qd
➤ Avoidance of oxidant drugs
• Antimalarials (primaquine, quinacrine, pentaquine, pamaquine)
• Sulfonamides
• Acetanilide
• Nalidixic acid
• Nitrofurantoin
• Toluidine blue

SPECIFIC THERAPY
n/a

FOLLOW-UP
■ Monitor CBC, MCV (increases in MCV may indicate folate deficiency), reticulocyte count, bilirubin (frequency determined by rate of hemolysis)
■ Children: monitor growth, development, and energy level
■ Monitor spleen size
■ Check CBC, reticulocyte count, bilirubin if patient develops increased pallor, jaundice, dark urine

COMPLICATIONS AND PROGNOSIS
■ Hypersplenism
■ Cholecystitis
■ Hemolytic crisis: increased rate of hemolysis may be precipitated by illness or oxidant drugs
➤ Treatment:
• Treat underlying infection
• Stop oxidant drugs
• Supportive care
• Transfusion if symptomatic anemia
➤ Prognosis: hematocrit improves with resolution of infections or discontinuation of inciting medication
■ Aplastic crisis: transient decrease in red cell synthesis may accompany certain infections (eg: parvovirus B19)
➤ Treatment: supportive care, monitor for symptomatic anemia
➤ Prognosis: hematocrit improves as infection resolves

UPPER URINARY TRACT OBSTRUCTION

MARGARET S. PEARLE, MD

HISTORY & PHYSICAL

History

- Acute obstruction
  - ➤ Severe flank pain with or without radiation to lower abdomen, nausea, vomiting
  - ➤ Oliguria/anuria if bilateral process
  - ➤ Fever if associated with infection
- Chronic obstruction
  - ➤ Unilateral or bilateral flank discomfort
  - ➤ Vague feeling of fullness
  - ➤ Anorexia
  - ➤ Flank pain with forced diuresis

Signs & Symptoms

- Elevated pulse and blood pressure secondary to pain in acute obstruction
- Low-grade fever not uncommon with acute obstruction; high fever suggests pyelonephritis
- Signs of volume overload such as pedal edema
- Tenderness over flank or anterior abdomen
- Palpable abdominal mass in some cases of extrinsic obstruction Elevated creatinine if bilateral, or unilateral with renal dysfunction

TESTS

Basic Blood Tests

- CBC: mild leukocytosis (10,000–15,000/mm2) common in acute obstruction
- Creatinine and blood urea nitrogen: to assess renal functional impairment
- Serum electrolytes
- Glucose

Basic Urine Tests

- Urinalysis: pH, microhematuria, pyuria, crystalluria, proteinuria, bacteria, hyphae
- Urine electrolytes: elevated urinary sodium and decreased urine osmolality in chronic obstruction
- Urine culture (bacterial and fungal)

Specific Diagnostic Tests
- Erythrocyte sedimentation rate (ESR): retroperitoneal fibrosis
- Prostate Specific Antigen (PSA): locally advanced prostate cancer
- Carcinoembryonic antigen (CEA): colon cancer
- Urine cytology (voided or wash): transitional cell carcinoma

Imaging
- Non-enhanced, thin-cut CT of kidneys and ureters
  - Study of choice for acute flank pain
  - Highly sensitive for ureteral stones
- Intravenous urogram (IVU)
  - Identifies presence and site of obstruction
- Renal sonogram
  - Rapid means of detecting hydronephrosis but nonspecific for site of obstruction
- Retrograde pyelogram
  - Identifies distal extent of obstruction
  - May differentiate intrinsic from extrinsic obstruction
- Diuretic renogram
  - Differential renal function
  - Quantifies degree of obstruction
- Whitaker test
  - Pressure-flow test of kidney
  - When renal scan equivocal

DIFFERENTIAL DIAGNOSIS

Intrinsic Obstruction
- Renal/ureteral calculi: non-enhanced helical CT highly sensitive
- Renal/ureteral tumor (most commonly transitional cell carcinoma): non-radiopaque filling defect on IVU, CT or retrograde pyelogram
- Sloughed papilla from papillary necrosis
  - Associated with urinary tract infection
  - Usually in diabetics
  - Associated with interstitial nephritis from analgesic abuse
  - IVU and history highly suggestive
- Fungus ball:
  - Commonly seen in immunocompromised patients
  - History and positive urine fungal culture suggestive
  - Filling defect on IVU, CT
- Ureteral stricture: IVU and retrograde pyelogram suggest intrinsic obstruction

➤ Congenital ureteropelvic or ureterovesical junction obstruction
➤ Secondary to ureteral injury or previous surgery

Extrinsic Obstruction
■ Retroperitoneal disease
  ➤ Idiopathic fibrosis
    • Insidious, dull, back/flank pain
    • Elevated ESR
    • IVU or CT urogram: medial deviation of ureters
    • CT: confluent fibrotic mass encasing great vessels and ureters from level of renal vessels to bifurcation of great vessels
  ➤ Tumor
    • IVU: ureter deviated laterally
    • CT: retroperitoneal mass
  ➤ Abscess
    • Positive "psoas sign" (pain with hip extension)
    • IVU: displacement of ureter
    • CT: psoas abscess in association with renal obstruction from stone
  ➤ Pelvic lipomatosis
    • IVU: elevation and elongation of bladder
    • KUB: radiolucent areas in pelvis
    • CT: pelvic fat
■ Gynecologic disease
  ➤ Pregnancy
    • Sonography: hydronephrosis, right side most common
  ➤ Benign or malignant tumor
    • CT: characterizes mass and demonstrates hydronephrosis
  ➤ Pelvic inflammatory disease or abscess
    • Sonography or CT: abscess and hydroureteronephrosis
  ➤ Endometriosis
    • IVU, sonography or retrograde pyelogram along with pelvic examination establish diagnosis
■ Gastrointestinal disease: CT establishes diagnosis of tumor or abscess
■ Vascular disease
  ➤ Abdominal aortic or iliac artery aneurysm
    • KUB: rim of calcification along aorta
    • IVU: deviation of ureter on IVU
    • CT: aneurysm
  ➤ Ovarian vein syndrome

- • IVU, CT urogram or retrograde pyelogram: obstruction at level of L3–4 where ovarian vein crosses ureter
- • CT: ovarian vein crosses at level of obstructed ureter
■ Iatrogenic injury
➤ IVU, CT or retrograde pyelogram: show point of obstruction

MANAGEMENT

What to Do First
■ Urgent decompression of collecting system in cases of obstruction associated with clinical signs of infection (ureteral stent or percutaneous nephrostomy tube)

General Measures
■ Acute renal colic
➤ Hydration
➤ Pain relief with narcotic analgesics
➤ Decompression of collecting system (ureteral stent or percutaneous nephrostomy tube) for pain control
■ Endoscopic inspection (ureteroscopy) if diagnosis not established with imaging

SPECIFIC THERAPY

Intrinsic Obstruction
■ Ureteral stone (see Urolithiasis)
■ Ureteral tumor
➤ Endoscopic resection or laser ablation
➤ Surgical resection (nephroureterectomy, segmental resection)
■ Sloughed papilla
➤ Antimicrobial agents if infection-related
➤ Cessation of analgesics if analgesic abuse
➤ Endoscopic retrieval of sloughed papilla for persistent obstruction
■ Fungus ball
➤ Systemic antifungal therapy (amphotericin B, fluconazole)
➤ Nephrostomy drainage
➤ Intra-renal irrigation with amphotericin B
■ Ureteral stricture
➤ Endoscopic incision or balloon dilation
➤ Laparoscopic or open surgical reconstruction

Extrinsic Obstruction
■ Segmental resection of ureter may be necessary

- Retroperitoneal fibrosis
  - ➤ Steroids with or without tamoxifen
  - ➤ Ureterolysis and intraperitonealization of the ureters
- Iatrogenic ureteral injury
  - ➤ Deligation of ureter with or without placement of a ureteral stent
  - ➤ Ureteral resection

FOLLOW-UP

- IVU, sonography or CT to assure resolution of obstruction and the underlying pathology

COMPLICATIONS AND PROGNOSIS

Complications

- Pyonephrosis and/or urosepsis
  - ➤ Prompt decompression of the collecting system
  - ➤ Initiation of broad-spectrum antibiotics
- Post-obstructive diuresis: loss of urinary concentrating ability
- Physiologic diuresis: self-limited, normal thirst mechanism maintains sufficient fluid replacement
- Pathologic diuresis (elevated BUN/Cr, signs of volume overload): supplement with intravenous 0.45% saline, matched $^1/_2$ cc per cc urine output
- Loss of renal function
- Hypertension
  - ➤ Unilateral ureteral obstruction: in rare cases, renovascular hypertension is associated with obstruction
  - ➤ Bilateral ureteral obstruction: usually resolves with resolution of obstruction and diuresis

Prognosis

- Depends on degree and duration of obstruction

URETHRITIS

JAMES W. SMITH, MD and DANIEL BRAILITA, MD

HISTORY & PHYSICAL

History

- History of urethral discharge may vary from significant to scanty.
- The discharge may be purulent, mucopurulent or clear.
- It may be noted continuously throughout the day or only with the first voiding in the morning.

- Patients could have painful urination throughout the stream or discomfort only with the initiation of stream.
- In women, it is often a prelude to a full-blown urinary tract infection.
- In elderly men with difficulty with urinary stream, symptoms could indicate urinary tract infection or prostatitis.

Signs & Symptoms
- The urethral meatus may have signs of dried crust, erythema, or moist discharge.
- Occasionally, discharge can be collected following gentle pressure along the dorsum of the penis.

TESTS
- A Gram stain smear of urethral exudate or an intraurethral swab specimen that reveals >5 PMN's/oil immersion field is presumptive for a diagnosis but insensitive.
- A first voided urine (first 5 ml) can be examined for leukocytes.
- A swab of urethral exudate or intraurethral swab specimen should be submitted for nucleic acid amplification test (NAAT, Gen-probe) for *Chlamydia* and *N. gonorrhoeae*.
- Either an LCR (ligase chain reaction) or PCR done on first voided urine specimen is a more sensitive and specific but more expensive test.

Other Tests
- Syphilis serology and HIV counseling and testing are indicated.
- Examine a wet mount of urethral material for Trichomonas.

DIFFERENTIAL DIAGNOSIS
- The principle causative agents of urethritis with polymorphonuclear leukocytes are *Chlamydia trachomatis* (25–40%) and *Neisseria gonorrhoeae* (approximately 20% of cases).
- Less frequent causative agents include Mycoplasma, Ureaplasma, Trichomonas, HSV, and genital candidiasis in diabetics.
- Urethritis can be a feature of systemic diseases, including Reiter's, Belicet's, Stevens-Johnson syndrome or Wegener's granulomatosis.

MANAGEMENT

What to Do First
- It is imperative to examine urethral specimen and provide care at the time of examination.
- If Gram stain evidence of gonococcal infection is not established, then treatment for both gonococcal and non-gonococcal causes of urethritis is to be administered.

General Measures

- Patients should be informed of importance of using barrier contraceptives to prevent sexually transmitted diseases.
- They should be counseled about HIV and informed of the increased likelihood of HIV transmission with urethritis.
- All sexual partners within 60 days of patients with urethritis should be referred for examination and treatment.
- Women <25 who are sexually active or women >25 who have new or multiple partners should have screening tests for both Chlamydia and gonorrhea.

SPECIFIC THERAPY

- All who have 5 or more leukocytes per oil immersion field in urethral fluid or sexual contact within the last 60 days with a person who has urethritis should be treated.
  - ➤ Give empiric treatment for high-risk patients who are unlikely to return for follow-up.

Treatment Options

- If the results of the nucleic acid amplification tests are not available, then patients should be treated with both ceftriaxone 125 mg IM in a single dose PLUS azithromycin 1 g orally in a single dose or doxycycline 100 mg orally twice a day for 7 days.
- Alternatively, ofloxacin bid or levofloxacin once daily for 7 days can be administered (but fluoroquinolone-resistant gonorrhea has been reported in Southeast Asia, Hawaii, California, New England and in men who have sex with men).
- If patients have recurrent or persistent urethritis, have a wet mount examination that shows trichomonas, or if an etiology is not determined, they should receive metronidazole p.o. in a single dose plus erythromycin qid for 7 days unless noncompliant with previous regimen.
- *Side Effects & Contraindications*
- Ceftriaxone
  - ➤ Side effects: rarely allergic reactions
  - ➤ Contraindications
    - Absolute: a patient who is allergic to penicillin
- Doxycycline
  - ➤ Side effects: nausea, vomiting, diarrhea, photosensitivity on exposure to sun
  - ➤ Contraindications

- Relative: if a patient is not likely to be compliant with the 7-day course of therapy. Then, treat with azithromycin single dose.

FOLLOW-UP

■ The patient should be instructed to return for evaluation if symptoms persist or if they recur after completion of therapy.

■ If symptoms recur, laboratory documentation of urethritis needs to be substantiated.

■ Patient should not have sexual intercourse until 7 days after therapy is initiated or until sexual contacts have been treated.

COMPLICATIONS AND PROGNOSIS

Complications

■ The major complication is a reaction to one of the antimicrobial agents. Rarely, urethral stricture occurs, if untreated. Post-Chlamydia, Reiter syndrome can develop.

Prognosis

■ Most patients respond promptly to appropriate therapy.

■ Re-infection usually relates to initiation of sexual intercourse with untreated sexual partner.

■ Prevention and treatment of urethritis is one of the mainstays of reducing sexually transmitted diseases.

■ Some authorities recommend re-examination within a year of all patients with urethritis because of high recurrence rates.

■ In some settings, such as adolescent women, re-examination within 3 months is indicated.

URINARY INCONTINENCE

ELIZABETH TAKACS, MD; GARY E. LEMACK, MD;
and PHILIPPE ZIMMERN, MD

HISTORY & PHYSICAL

History

■ Determine onset, duration, evolution and inciting event (cough, sneeze, laugh, change of position, sport, sex, urge to void, unaware)

■ Other symptoms: urge, frequency, nocturia, straining to urinate, hematuria, recurrent urinary tract infections

■ Detail patient's attempts to improve symptoms (medications, prevention by frequent voiding, Kegel exercises).

- Severity of incontinence (type and number of pads [day and night], Validated Quality of Life Questionnaire to assess the impact of incontinence on daily activities, such as Incontinence Impact Questionnaire [IIQ-7] or Urogenital Distress Inventory [UDI-6])
- Fluid intake (amount and type)
- Past urologic history (childhood and bedwetting problems)
- OB/GYN history (parity and types of delivery and complications – i.e., lacerations/episiotomies/forceps), symptoms of prolapse or prior procedures to correct incontinence or prolapse, hormonal deprivation, dyspareunia
- Bowel habits (constipation, fecal incontinence, vaginal splinting)
- Medical conditions interfering with urinary output (impaired renal function, diabetes, congestive heart failure)
- Neurological history (multiple sclerosis, Parkinson's disease, stroke, etc.)
- Prior surgical history (abdominal, back, brain)
- Medications with urinary side effects (diuretics, sedatives, cholinergics or anticholinergic drugs, hormones, and psychotropics)

Signs & Symptoms
A complete exam (abdominal, genital, pelvic, and neurologic) is essential in the evaluation of all incontinence in women.
- Genital examination: vaginal condition (scar from episiotomy; vaginal atrophy: loss of rugae, thin shiny vaginal wall)
- Urethral meatus: caruncle, condyloma, Skene's abscess
- Urethra: palpated for scarring or tenderness suggestive of urethral diverticulum
- Speculum examination looking for cystocele, uterine descent, vault prolapse, enterocele, or rectocele
- Ask patient to cough and strain, supine and/or standing. Leakage with effort indicates stress incontinence. Secondary leakage triggered by an effort suggests stress-induced instability.
- Careful neurologic exam
  ➢ Perineal examination (sensation)
  ➢ Bulbocavernosus reflex

TESTS

Basic Tests
- Lifestyle Questionnaires
- Voiding diary (3–7 days) – diary should include time of voiding, volume voided, number of pads used per day, leakage episodes and inciting events

- Urinalysis (with urine culture when UA positive for red and/or white cells)
- Uroflow to evaluate voiding dysfunction – outpatient and non-invasive (minimum volume voided 150 ml for proper interpretation)
- Post void residual (by catheterization or bladder scan)
- Blood tests: urea, creatinine, electrolytes when indicated

Specific Tests
- Urodynamic testing to assess severity of stress incontinence (Valsalva leak point pressure), identification of detrusor overactivity, and assessment of detrusor voiding function. Surface patch electromyogram for neurogenic bladder and in patients suspected of outlet obstruction.
- Cystoscopy to exclude etiology for urge incontinence (tumor, stone, etc.) or for assessment of urethral sphincter (indirect). The procedure can be followed by a stress test in supine and/or standing position to demonstrate stress incontinence.
- Imaging studies: voiding cystourethrogram in standing position to assess impact of gravity on urethral support and bladder base. Upper tract studies (i.e., CT or IVP) rarely needed unless hematuria or associated high-grade bladder prolapse.

DIFFERENTIAL DIAGNOSIS
- Pseudo-incontinence
  - ➢ Vaginal voiding (well documented on the post-void film of the cystourethrogram)
  - ➢ Post-void dribbling from a urethral diverticulum

Classification
- Stress urinary incontinence (urinary leakage secondary to an increase in abdominal pressure with cough, sneezing, laughing, etc.)
- Risk factors for stress incontinence
  - ➢ Aging
  - ➢ Hormonal changes
  - ➢ Traumatic delivery
  - ➢ Parity
  - ➢ Pelvic surgery
- Urge incontinence (urinary leakage associated with an abrupt desire to void – urgency that cannot be suppressed)
- Overflow incontinence – from overdistention of the bladder
- Total incontinence usually from extra-urethral sources (ectopic ureter or vesico-vaginal fistula)

■ Transient urinary incontinence (common in the elderly, especially when hospitalized)

MANAGEMENT

What to Do First

■ Exclude urinary tract infection.
■ Verify proper bladder emptying (uroflow and post-void residual).
■ Exclude neurologic disease.
■ General measures
  ➤ Adjust fluid intake if excessive.
  ➤ Teach pelvic floor exercises (Kegel).
  ➤ Consider biofeedback.
  ➤ Medical therapy
    • Alpha-agonist medication to increase outlet resistance
    • Anticholinergic drugs for urge incontinence
  ➤ Local and/or systemic hormonal replacement

SPECIFIC THERAPY

Pseudo-Incontinence

■ Transvaginal excision of urethral diverticulum
■ Vaginal voiding (spread labia or legs wide during voiding)

Stress Incontinence Not Responding to Nonsurgical Options

■ Surgical Treatment Options
  ➤ Periurethral injection therapy (collagen, fat, others)
  ➤ Vaginal surgery to restore proper urethral support
  ➤ Abdominal surgery (Burch-type procedure)
  ➤ Sling (source: autologous, synthetic, or cadaver tissue)

Urge Incontinence

■ Nonsurgical Treatment Options
  ➤ Anticholinergic medications: Ditropan and Detrol are the most common drugs prescribed because they have the longest track record, but many new medications have entered the market in recent years: Vesicare, Sanctura, Enablex.
  ➤ Timed voiding
■ Surgical Treatments
  ➤ New research drugs administered intravesically (capsaicin, resiniferatoxin, BoTox (B toxin)
  ➤ Open abdominal surgery (augmentation cystoplasty)

➤ Neuromodulation (Interstim implant)
➤ Supravesical diversion (continent or non-continent urinary conduit)

Overflow Incontinence

■ Bladder drainage with Foley catheter, suprapubic catheter or, if technically possible, intermittent catheterization
■ Search for etiology (idiopathic, neurogenic, psychogenic, drug-induced, viral).
■ Prognosis dependent on cause and urodynamic findings

Extra Urethral Cause of Incontinence

■ Vesico-vaginal fistula (closure transabdominally or transvaginally; consider tissue interposition [Martius, omentum] to reduce risk of recurrence)
■ Ectopic ureter (excision of upper pole moiety; distal ureteral excision)

FOLLOW-UP
n/a

COMPLICATIONS AND PROGNOSIS
n/a

URTICARIA AND ANGIOEDEMA (DERMATOLOGY)

CAROL L. KULP–SHORTEN, MD

HISTORY & PHYSICAL

Classification

■ **Immunologic**
  ➤ *Ig-E dependent (Type I hypersensitivity)*
    • Specific antigen sensitivities – e.g., latex, insect sting, medication, infection
    • Physical urticarias – e.g., dermatographism, pressure, solar, cold, cholinergic, aquagenic, vibratory
  ➤ *Complement mediated (Type III hypersensitivity)*
    • Hereditary angioedema (qualitative or quantitative C1 esterase inhibitor deficiency)
    • Acquired C1 esterase inhibitor deficiency (lymphomas, myelomas, systemic lupus erythematosus)
    • Serum sickness reaction
    • Urticarial vasculitis

- **Nonimmunologic**
  - ➤ *Direct mast cell degranulators* – e.g., opiates, polymyxin, tubocurarine, radiocontrast dye
  - ➤ *Indirect mast cell degranulators via arachidonic acid pathway or kallikrein–kinin system alteration,* e.g., aspirin, NSAIDs, tartrazine (yellow food dye), benzoate (food preservative)+
  - ➤ *Angiotensin–converting enzyme (ACE) inhibitors*
- **Autoimmune**
  - ➤ Due to histamine-releasing IgG autoantibodies to high-affinity IgE receptors
  - ➤ Associated with Hashimoto's thyroiditis, systemic lupus erythematosus, vasculitis, and/or hepatitis
- **Idiopathic** – etiology indeterminable in over 50–75% chronic urticarias

Signs & Symptoms
- Urticaria
  - ➤ Pruritic wheals appearing in crops that are transient and evanescent (individual lesions resolve in <24 h)
- Angioedema
  - ➤ Nonpruritic, painful swelling of eyelids, mouth, distal extremities
  - ➤ May involve larynx, tongue and GI tract
- Urticarial vasculitis
  - ➤ Wheals last >24 h
  - ➤ Wheals heal with purpura or postinflammatory hyperpigmentation
  - ➤ +/− constitutional symptoms

TESTS

Provocative Testing for Suspected Physical Urticarias
- Dermatographism: stroke skin with firm pressure
- Pressure: apply 15 lb. weight for 20 minutes, inspect at 48 hours
- Solar: phototesting with UVL and fluorescent light
- Familial cold: expose to cold air for 20–30 minutes
- Acquired cold: plastic wrapped ice cube to skin for 5 minutes
- Cholinergic: exercise patient
- Aquagenic: 35°C water compress to upper body skin for 30 minutes
- Vibratory: apply vortex vibration to forearm for 5 minutes

Laboratory
- Usually not necessary for acute urticaria (episodes <6 weeks)
- Basic: CBC with differential, ESR, urinalysis, LFTs
- Additional testing directed by history and physical exam

> stool for O and P, ANA, hepatitis profile, CH100, C4, C1 esterase inhibitor level and function, thyroid function tests, thyroid autoantibodies
> Sinus films, chest X-ray, other radiologic studies

*Evaluation for angioedema with urticaria is the same as urticaria alone; if angioedema alone, think hereditary or acquired C1 esterase inhibitor deficiency

■ Skin Biopsy
> Usually not necessary
> Helpful if urticarial vasculitis is suspected as vascular damage will be seen

DIFFERENTIAL DIAGNOSIS

■ Erythema multiforme – lesions are fixed, frequently targetoid, often palmar involvement
■ Bullous pemphigoid – urticarial plaques eventually become bullous
■ Dermatitis herpetiformis – grouped vesicles and excoriations are characteristic
■ Morbilliform drug eruption – confluent erythematous macules and papules rather than wheals

MANAGEMENT

■ Acute urticaria/angioedema
> Assess airway, breathing, circulation
> Identify and eliminate etiology if possible
> Sympathomimetics
> Antihistamines
> Systemic corticosteroids may be required but onset of action delayed
■ Chronic urticaria/angioedema
> Identify and eliminate etiology
> Avoid physical triggers
> Antihistamines
> Nontraditional therapies (IVIg, plasmapheresis, PUVA, immuno-suppressives such as cyclosporine, methotrexate, azathioprine, or mycophenolate mofetil)
> Avoid chronic systemic corticosteroids
> Avoid aspirin/NSAIDs, narcotics, benzoates, and ACE inhibitors

SPECIFIC THERAPY

■ Traditional H1 antihistamines
> Chlorpheniramine maleate
> Diphenhydramine HCl

- ➤ Hydroxyzine HCl
- ➤ Clemastine fumarate
- ➤ Cyproheptadein HCl
- Second-generation H1 antihistamines
  - ➤ Loratidine
  - ➤ Cetirizine
  - ➤ Fexofenadine
  - ➤ Desloratidine
- H2 antihistamines (must be used with H1 blocker)
  - ➤ Cimetidine HCl
  - ➤ Ranitidine HCl
- Combination H1 and H2 antihistamines
  - ➤ Doxepin HCl
- Leukotriene antagonists
  - ➤ Montelukast
  - ➤ Zafirlukast
- 5-Lipoxygenase inhibitors
  - ➤ Zileuton
- Corticosteroids
  - ➤ Short tapering course for autoimmune urticaria
- Immunosuppressives
  - ➤ Cyclosporine, methotrexate, azathioprine, and/or mycophenolate mofetil may be useful for chronic urticaria

FOLLOW-UP
- Laboratory reassessment as dictated by changes in history or physical exam

COMPLICATIONS AND PROGNOSIS
- Angioedema may be life-threatening
- 50% with urticaria alone free of lesions within 1 year; 20% have involvement >20 years
- 75% with combined urticaria and angioedema have episodes >5 years

---

URTICARIA AND ANGIOEDEMA (RHEUMATOLOGY)

ALLEN P. KAPLAN, MD

HISTORY & PHYSICAL
- Hives & swelling
- Acute: <6 weeks
- Probably chronic: 6–10 weeks

■ Chronic: >10 weeks
  ➤ 40% urticaria alone
  ➤ 40% urticaria & angioedema
  ➤ 20% angioedema alone

Chronic
■ Most are idiopathic, have no association
■ Duration of lesions
  ➤ Individual hives last <2 hrs: consider physical urticaria
  ➤ Individual hives last >2 hrs: any other cause
■ Physical Urticaria
  ➤ Linear hives lasting <2 hrs w/ generalized pruritus = dermato-graphism
  ➤ Hives w/ exercise, hot showers, acute anxiety = cholinergic urticaria
  ➤ Hives along belt line, tight garments, foot swelling or hives when walking & hives on buttocks with sitting = pressure urticaria
  ➤ Hives touching cold objects, wind blowing in face, lip swelling eating ice cream = cold urticaria
  ➤ Hives w/ exposure to sun = solar urticaria. If only outdoors, due to UV wavelengths. If indoors also, visible light wavelengths
  ➤ Hives touching warm/hot objects = local heat urticaria
  ➤ Swelling when rubbing with towel = vibratory angioedema
■ Angioedema typically lasts 1–3 days

TESTS

Acute Urticaria/Angioedema
■ CBC, ESR
■ Food skin tests
■ Penicillin skin testing and/or RAST assay, if suspect
■ Liver function tests or EB viral titer if either hepatitis or infectious mononucleosis suspected

Physical Urticaria
■ Hives w/ scratch: dermatographism
■ Hives w/ ice cube applied to forearm for 5 minutes; cold urticaria; obtain cold agglutinin titer & check for cryoglobulins
■ Hives after running in place or on treadmill for 15 minutes: cholinergic urticaria
■ Hives after application of test tube containing hot water to forearm for 5 minutes: local heat urticaria
■ Weighted carrying case with strap over shoulder for 15 minutes; hives on shoulder 4–8 hrs later: pressure urticaria

■ Laboratory vortex to vibrate forearm for 1 minute; prominent swelling of extremity: vibrating angioedema

Chronic Urticaria
■ Thyroid function tests (abnormal in 19%)
■ Antibody to thyroglobulin (8% positive), microsomal antigens (5% positive); antibodies to both in 14%
■ ANA, especially in young women
■ Autologous skin test w/ pnt serum is positive in about 35% & indicates the presence of antibody to the IgE receptor & in 5% anti-IgE. It is diagnostic of chronic autoimmune urticaria.
■ Research assay – histamine release upon incubation of pt serum w/ basophils indicates an autoimmune cause in 45%; the remainder have chronic idiopathic urticaria
■ Skin biopsy if vasculitis suspected (eg, hives >36 hrs, increased ESR, arthralgias & myalgias, petechiae or purpura w/ hives); angioedema alone – recurrent
■ Measure plasma C4 & C1 inhibitor (C1 INH) levels
  ➤ If normal: idiopathic, the most common form of angioedema
  ➤ If subnormal, consider hereditary angioedema or acquired C1 INH deficiency assoc w/ lymphoma, cryoglobulinemia, SLE, carcinoma or antibody to C1 INH

DIFFERENTIAL DIAGNOSIS
■ Acute urticaria: food allergy, drug reactions, prodrome of hepatitis B, infectious mononucleosis, transfusion reaction
■ Chronic urticaria and/or angioedema: cutaneous vasculitis (<1%)

MANAGEMENT
What to Do First
■ Note size, shape, distribution of any hives
■ Test for dermatographism
■ Check for angioedema: swelling of lips, tongue, pharynx, face, extremities, penis, scrotum
■ Emergency: epinephrine 1:1,000 subcutaneously, diphenhydramine IV; tracheotomy for laryngeal edema

SPECIFIC THERAPY
Acute Hives or Swelling
■ If mild: nonsedating antihistamines (cetirizine, fexofenadine, loratidine)
■ Moderate: diphenhydramine, hydroxyzine

■ Severe: prednisone for 3 days, taper by 10 mg/day plus diphenhydramine

Physical Urticaria
■ Dermatographism: any antihistamine; hydroxyzine in severe cases
■ Cold urticaria: ciproheptadine
■ Cholinergic urticaria: hydroxyzine
■ Local heat urticaria: any antihistamine in high dosage
■ Pressure urticaria: treat as for chronic urticaria (see below); often requires low-dose alternate-day steroid
■ Vibratory angioedema: diphenhydramine
■ Solar urticaria: antihistamines, sunscreen if due to UV light

Chronic Urticaria ± Angioedema
■ Nonsedating antihistamines if mild; hydroxyzine if severe
  ➤ H2 blockers (eg, ranitidine)
■ Leukotriene antagonists (eg, montelukast, Zafirlukast)
■ In refractory cases: low-dose alternate-day prednisone
■ If thyroid tests abnormal, treatment to achieve euthyroid state. Do not treat autoantibodies alone.

Chronic Recurrent Angioedema Without Hives
■ Diphenhydramine in full dose
■ Prednisone for acute episodes; discontinue w/o taper

Hereditary Angioedema
■ Attenuated androgens (eg, danazol) reverse the disease
■ Surgery prophylaxis: increased dose of androgen perioperatively; alternatively: IV infusion of fresh-frozen plasma or, if available, C1 INH concentrate

Acquired C1 INH Deficiency
■ Attenuated androgens
■ Treatment of underlying lymphoma or rheumatic disease
■ If due to antibody to C1 INH, stanazolol, E-aminocaproic acid; plasmapheresis, cyclophosphamide, C1 INH concentrate may be required

FOLLOW-UP
N/A

COMPLICATIONS & PROGNOSIS

Complications

- Hypotension: epinephrine, supportive therapy
- Laryngeal edema: tracheotomy may be required
- In hereditary angioedema: bowel wall edema mimicking intestinal obstruction is treated w/ IV fluids, nasogastric suction, not laparotomy

Prognosis

- Chronic urticaria & angioedema remits: 65% in 3 years, 65% in 3 years, 98% in 10 years
- Hereditary angioedema can be maintained symptom-free w/ impeded androgens

UVEITIS

HENRY J. KAPLAN, MD and SHLOMIT SCHAAL, MD

DEFINITIONS

The uvea (from the Latin uva, meaning grape) is a pigmented vascular structure consisting of the iris, ciliary body, and choroid.

Uveitis is an ocular inflammatory process that may have many different causes. Some uveitides are solely ocular, but many are associated with systemic diseases.

Uveitis that is primarily located in the front part of the eye is called anterior uveitis (or iritis). The inflammatory process may involve other parts of the eye as well, and then it is called either intermediate uveitis (inflammation in the vitreous body) or posterior uveitis (inflammation of the retina and/or choroid). Some patients have panuveitis, which is an inflammation of both the anterior and posterior segments of the eye.

Acute uveitis is defined as a disease <3 months in duration. After 3 months, the uveitis is defined as chronic.

HISTORY & PHYSICAL

History

- Previous episode of uveitis
- Exclude trauma or previous intraocular surgery
- Underlying systemic disease:
  - ➤ Immunocompromised: AIDS, cancer, immunosuppressive medications

➤ Nonimmunocompromised: spondyloarthropathies, TB, syphilis, sarcoidosis, autoimmune diseases, other infectious diseases

Signs & Symptoms

- Ocular pain, redness, photophobia
- Blurring of vision, floaters
- Red eye (conjunctival/ciliary injection) w/ excessive tearing & lid closure or quiet, white eye
- Cataract (posterior subcapsular cataract)
- Intraocular inflammation (anterior chamber &/or vitreous body)
- Macular edema
  ➤ Intraocular pressure (IOP) should be measured. IOP is most frequently decreased, although occasionally it may be increased.

The diagnosis requires slit-lamp examination to identify inflammatory cells floating in the aqueous humor or deposited on the corneal endothelium (keratic precipitates) in anterior uveitis. Intermediate, posterior, and panuveitis are diagnosed by observing inflammation in the vitreous, retina or choroid. They are more likely than anterior uveitis to be associated with an identifiable systemic disease.

TESTS

Basic Blood Tests

- CBC w/ differential
- VDRL, if sexually active; if positive, confirm w/ FTA

Other Basic Tests

- CXR (PA, lateral) to exclude sarcoidosis, TB

Specific Diagnostic Tests

- HLA B-27: w/ juvenile RA, spondyloarthropathy, unilateral acute anterior uveitis
- HLA A-29: w/ birdshot chorioretinopathy
  ➤ HLA B-51: w/Bechet disease
- Sacroiliac joint x-ray: w/ back pain, ankylosing spondylitis

Other Tests

- Serum antibody titers for suspected disease; eg, toxoplasmosis, Lyme, cat-scratch disease, AIDS
- ACE, gallium scan, biopsy of conjunctival or lid nodule, DTH (mumps, Candida, PPD intermediate): sarcoidosis

> Antinuclear antibodies (ANAs) in juvenile idiopathic arthritis
- Other lab tests as dictated by associated systemic disease

Imaging
- US (A-, B-) of eye to exclude retinal detachment if small pupil, cataract, or vitreous hemorrhage prevents visualization of retina
- CT of eye w/ penetrating trauma

Ocular Biopsy
- Not routine
- Anterior chamber paracentesis (to remove aqueous humor), vitreous paracentesis (to remove vitreous), or retinal biopsy for diagnostic culture, PCR & light/electron microscopy

DIFFERENTIAL DIAGNOSIS
- Viral conjunctivitis may mimic red, painful, photophobic eye; frequently associated w/ cold & swollen preauricular lymph nodes
- Intraocular infection after trauma (blunt, penetrating, surgical) immediately suspect; institute aggressive diagnosis & therapy
- Intraocular malignancy (retinoblastoma in childhood, lymphoma in elderly) may present as uveitis

MANAGEMENT
What to Do First
- Determine if uveitis localized to anterior segment, posterior segment, or both.
- Assess cause of decreased vision (cataract, macular edema).

General Measures
- Use history, physical, & lab tests to determine cause: most common causes of acute anterior uveitis are seronegative spondyloarthropathies (look for HLA-B27 and perform sacroiliac films). Most common cause of chronic anterior uveitis is juvenile rheumatoid arthritis (look for ANAs). Most common causes of posterior uveitis are infections such as toxoplasmosis, toxocariasis, syphilis, TB (perform antibody titer tests).
- If intraocular infection suspected, refer to ophthalmologist as emergency.
- Use eyeshield for blunt & penetrating trauma; refer immediately to ophthalmologist for diagnosis and treatment.

SPECIFIC THERAPY

Indications
- Control of inflammation w/in anterior segment to relieve symptoms

Treatment Options
- Topical corticosteroids:
  - Prednisolone acetate suspension 1%, while awake at onset of treatment; taper frequency to therapeutic response
- Topical mydriatic/cycloplegic: homatropine 5%
- Periocular steroids:
  - Used to supplement nonresponsive anterior segment inflammation (subconjunctival injection) or posterior segment inflammation (sub-Tenon injection)
  - Sub-Tenon or subconjunctival injection: triamcinolone
- Systemic anti-inflammatory & immunosuppressive drugs:
  - Systemic therapy w/ corticosteroids usually initiated for pts nonresponsive to topical corticosteroid therapy, severe visual loss, or inflammation of posterior segment
  - Immunosuppressive medications (methotrexate, cyclosporine, azathioprine) usually added to therapy to enhance effect of treatment & for steroid sparing
  - Systemic therapy directed at underlying systemic infection; eg, clindamycin for Lyme disease

Side Effects & Contraindications
- Topical corticosteroids:
  - Side effects: increased IOP (after 2 wks in corticosteroid responsive eyes); cataract w/ long-term therapy
  - Contraindications: herpes simplex keratitis requires concomitant antiviral topical therapy
- Topical mydriatic/cycloplegic drugs:
  - Side effects: dilated pupil, inability to accommodate, difficulty reading
  - Contraindications: angle-closure glaucoma
- Periocular steroids:
  - Side effects & contraindications: as for topical corticosteroids
  - Other contraindications: glaucoma filtering bleb, history of glaucoma or suspected glaucoma, scleral thinning

Newer treatments: Cytokine inhibitors such as etanercept and infliximab are being studied for treatment of various types of uveitis.

FOLLOW-UP

During Treatment

■ After 2–4 d after initiation of treatment; at 1- to 2-wk intervals after start of therapeutic response; less frequently thereafter

Routine

■ W/ return of symptoms or q 6–12 mo if asymptomatic & inactive

COMPLICATIONS AND PROGNOSIS

Complications

Uveitis is a potentially blinding condition that can result in serious complications in the eyes.

■ Posterior subcapsular cataract: may require surgery
■ Cystoid macular edema: if permanent, may decrease visual acuity
■ Ocular hypertension or glaucoma: may require medical/surgical treatment

Prognosis

■ Very good if not associated w/ underlying systemic disease & if each episode of intraocular inflammation promptly treated

VAGINITIS

SARAH STAEDKE, MD

HISTORY & PHYSICAL

History

■ Vaginitis is an infection or inflammation of the vagina
■ Three syndromes are described: bacterial vaginosis (BV) caused by overgrowth of normal vaginal flora by *Gardnerella vaginalis* and other anaerobes; vulvovaginal candidiasis (VVC) primarily caused by *C. albicans*, less commonly by *C. glabrata* and *C. tropicalis*; trichomoniasis, caused by the protozoan *Trichomonas vaginalis*
■ Risk factors include sexual activity (trichomoniasis is considered a sexually transmitted disease; BV is associated with sexual activity, but is not an STD); diabetes, antibiotics, and corticosteroids; VVC: physical agents such as synthetic undergarments and clothing, soaps and detergents; hormonal factors such as pregnancy and estrogen use

Signs & Symptoms

■ BV: frequently asymptomatic, symptoms include malodorous vaginal discharge, increased after coitus; signs: thin, gray/yellow discharge, vaginal pH > 4.5, amine "fishy" odor with KOH (+ whiff test)

■ VVC: symptoms: vaginal discharge, intense pruritus, dysuria; signs: thick, white discharge; vulvovaginal erythema, edema, erosions; vaginal pH 3.5–4.5; no odor with KOH

■ Trichomoniasis: symptoms: frothy malodorous vaginal discharge, vulvovaginal pruritus, dysuria; signs: profuse purulent discharge, vaginal inflammation, "strawberry cervix", vaginal pH > 4.5, +/− whiff test

TESTS

Basic Tests

■ Vaginal pH: normal 3.8–4.2, BV > 4.5, VVC ≤4.5, trichomoniasis > 4.5

■ "Whiff" test: apply KOH to vaginal secretions (can place a few drops onto speculum after removing from vagina) to inspect for amine "fishy" odor

Specific Diagnostic Tests

■ Vaginal wet mount: take sample from posterior vaginal sidewalls or pooled secretions and add to glass slide with 1 or 2 drops of sterile saline; clue cells (squamous epithelial cells coated in bacteria, particularly along cell edge creating a fuzzy appearance) = BV (sensitivity >90%); budding yeast and pseudohyphae = VVC; motile trichomonads and WBCs = trichomoniasis (sensitivity averages 45–60%)

■ Vaginal KOH preparation: add sample of vaginal secretions to glass slide with 1 or 2 drops of 10% KOH; improves visualization of yeast; budding yeast and pseudohyphae = VVC

■ Culture: yeast = Sabourand's medium; trichomoniasis = Diamonds TYM medium; no culture for BV

DIFFERENTIAL DIAGNOSIS

■ Atrophic vaginitis due to estrogen deficiency

■ Chemical vulvitis/vaginitis

■ Fixed drug eruption: multiple medications implicated

■ Foreign body: visible on exam

■ GC or CT cervicitis

MANAGEMENT

What to Do First

■ Examine patient; avoid empiric treatment

General Measures

■ Perform full pelvic examination to assess for vaginitis, cervicitis, PID
■ Obtain fresh samples for vaginal pH testing, microscopic evaluation of vaginal specimens by wet mount and KOH, cervical gram-stain
■ Consider pregnancy testing and evaluation for chlamydia, gonorrhea, syphilis, and HIV
■ Counsel regarding modifiable risk factors
■ Advise patient to abstain from sexual activity during treatment
■ Empirically treat all sexual partners of patients with trichomoniasis; BV and VVC do not typically require treatment of partner

SPECIFIC THERAPY

Indications

■ BV: diagnosis requires 3 of the following 4 criteria: homogenous gray-white vaginal discharge; pH > 4.5, amine odor, clue cells on wet mount; treat all symptomatic patients
■ VVC: fungal elements on KOH or wet mount; compatible clinical syndrome
■ Trichomoniasis: motile trichomonads on wet mount; sexual contact to patient with trichomoniasis

Treatment Options

■ BV
  ➤ Metronidazole for 7 days OR Metronidazole 0.75% gel intravaginally twice a day for 5 days OR Clindamycin 2% cream intravaginally each night for 7 days
  ➤ Alternatives: Clindamycin for 7 days OR Metronidazole orally once (less effective than 7 day course)
  ➤ In pregnancy: Clindamycin for 7 days OR Metronidazole for 7 days (after 1st trimester)
■ WC
  ➤ Fluconazole orally once OR intravaginal Butoconazole, Clotrimazole, Miconazole, Nystatin, Terconazole, Tioconazole (creams, tablets, suppositories) for 1–7 days
  ➤ Alternatives: Itraconazole orally once; OR Nystatin vaginal tablets for 14 days (less effective)
  ➤ Consider longer courses (14 days of topical treatment or Fluconazole for 4 days) for complicated infections
  ➤ In pregnancy: topical agents only, treat for 7 days
■ Trichomoniasis
  ➤ Metronidazole orally once OR for 7 days

Tinadazole orally once
- Alternatives: Metronidazole gel – much less effective; generally not recommended
- For recurrences: tinadazole, longer courses of Metronidazole
- In pregnancy: Metronidazole after 1st trimester OR Clotrimazole vaginal tablets

Side Effects & Contraindications
- Clindamycin: side effects: diarrhea, C. difficile colitis, rash, GI intolerance; caution in pregnancy but no risk with extensive experience; vaginal cream not recommended in pregnancy because of increased risk of premature delivery
- Fluconazole: side effects: GI intolerance, rash, diarrhea, elevated LFTs; drug interactions common (astemizole, calcium channel blockers, cisapride, coumadin, cyclosporine A, oral hypoglycemics, phenytoin, protease inhibitors, tacrolimus, terfenadine, theophylline, trimetrexate, rifampin); avoid in pregnancy (C)
- Metronidazole: side effects: disulfiram-like reaction with alcohol, GI distress, headache, metallic taste; pregnancy = B, avoid during 1st trimester

Tinadazole: metallic taste, GI distress, fatigue, avoid in first trimester of pregnancy (C)
- Topical imidazoles: side effects: local irritation, dyspareunia; avoid in first trimester

FOLLOW-UP
- Generally not necessary if symptoms resolve
- In pregnancy, repeat evaluation in 1 month to document successful treatment

COMPLICATIONS AND PROGNOSIS
- BV
  - Cure rate with 7 day Metronidazole therapy 75–90%
  - In early pregnancy, associated with preterm delivery and late miscarriage; some experts recommend BV screening at beginning of 2nd trimester and treatment of asymptomatic infection in high-risk women (those with prior preterm delivery)
  - BV associated with PID following invasive procedures (endometrial biopsy, IUD placement, dilatation and curettage, hysterosalpingography, hysterectomy, cesarean section)
- VVC
  - Treatment with azole regimen results in 80–90% cure

> For persistent/recurrent symptoms, re-examine and repeat therapy with longer course of topical therapy, different topical agent or oral therapy if topical originally used; consider infection with non-albicans candida
> Consider treatment of sexual partner; review hygiene
> For recurrent VVC (defined as ≥4 episodes of symptomatic disease per year), screen for diabetes and HIV; consider gynecological referral and long-term antifungal suppression therapy
- Trichomoniasis
  > Treatment with Metronidazole results in cure rates of 90–95%
  > Recurrent infections caused by organisms with decreased susceptibility to Metronidazole can usually be treated with higher doses
  > Associated with premature rupture of membranes and preterm delivery but routine screening in pregnancy not generally recommended

VALVULAR HEART DISEASE AORTIC STENOSIS (AS)

JUDITH A. WISNESKI, MD

HISTORY & PHYSICAL

Etiology
- Congenital bicuspid aortic valve (develops AS ages 40–60; more common in males)
- Senile calcified (normal 3 – leaflet valve; AS ages 70–80)
- Rheumatic heart disease (abnormality of mitral valve present)
- Congenital AS

History
- Symptoms of pulmonary congestion: PND, DOE or orthopnea (due to left ventricular (LV) diastolic impairment or systolic dysfunction)
- Angina (may be related to LV hypertrophy alone, or in combination with CAD)
- Syncope/near-syncope – usually associated with exertion (due to limited cardiac output secondary to aortic valve obstruction, vasodepressor response, or stress induced arrhythmia)

Signs & Symptoms
- Systolic murmur radiates to the right supraclavicular fossa
  > Mild to moderate AS: Murmur peaks early in systole

- Loud
- Post-PVC beat; loudness of murmur increases
- Systolic click (associated with opening of valve)
- A2 increased

➤ As AS progresses: Murmur peaks later; thrill may be present
  - Murmur becomes soft and may be absent later in course
  - Single S2 due to absence of A2.

■ Carotid Upstroke – delayed and decreased, but can be normal
■ PMI – forceful

TESTS
ECG
■ Left atrial abnormality
■ Left ventricular hypertrophy (LVH)

Chest X-Ray
■ Normal heart size or "Boot-shaped" heart (due to LVH)
■ Calcification of aortic valve (best seen in lateral view)
■ Post-stenotic dilation of the aorta
■ Pulmonary venous congestion may be present

Echo/Doppler
(If any symptoms, echo/Doppler should be obtained)
■ Decreased aortic valve leaflet mobility
■ Systolic gradient across aortic valve
■ Quantitate aortic valve area
■ Degree of LVH
■ LV systolic function
■ Mitral valve leaflets and mobility (can provide information concerning etiology of AS)

Cardiac Catheterization
■ Right heart catheterization – pulmonary capillary wedge pressure to assess LV function (*provided mitral valve function is normal*)
■ Quantitate LV/aortic systolic gradient
■ Gorlin formula: calculate aortic valve area using cardiac output and mean aortic valve gradient
■ Elevated LV end-diastolic pressure (LVEDP) – due to decreased compliance of hypertrophied LV wall
■ Coronary angiography – assess presence of stenoses in coronary arteries (Required by CT surgery prior to aortic valve replacement)

Exercise Testing
- Severe AS – Do not perform exercise test
- Mild AS with vague symptoms – perform cautiously under guidance of trained physician

DIFFERENTIAL DIAGNOSIS
- Idiopathic hypertrophic subaortic stenosis
- Discrete subaortic stenosis
- Supravalvular aortic stenosis
- Subclavian arterial bruit
- Pulmonic valvular stenosis
- Dilated aorta with systolic murmur
- Mirtal regurgitation

MANAGEMENT
Medical Treatment
- Antibiotic prophylaxis for all patients (asymptomatic included)
- Therapy for angina and congestive heart failure (**Use medical therapy cautiously – medication may mask symptoms**)

Surgical Treatment
- **Aortic valve replacement (AVR) only effective treatment to improve survival in adults**
- Indications for AVR:
  - Symptomatic (angina, syncope or congestive heart failure – aortic valve area (AVA) < or = 0.75 cm2; AVA may be 1.0 cm2 with CAD)
- Mechanical versus bioprosthetic AVR:
  - Mechanical AVR – requires warfarin, but more durable
  - Bioprosthetic AVR – older patients and patients not able to tolerate warfarin

Palliative Treatment
(*co-morbidity prohibits AVR*)
- Aortic balloon valvotomy may relieve symptoms (does not change overall mortality; survival without restenosis <50% at 1 year)
- Treatment for CHF may temporarily improve symptoms

SPECIFIC THERAPY
n/a

FOLLOW-UP
n/a

COMPLICATIONS AND PROGNOSIS

Complications

- Medical therapy – improves symptoms while LV dysfunction progresses (**medical therapy can mask severe symptomatic AS**)
- Aortic valve replacement
  - ➤ Acute
    - Complications of cardiopulmonary bypass surgery
    - Morbidity higher with poor LV function
  - ➤ Long-term
    - Warfarin therapy for mechanical AVR
    - Endocarditis
    - Thromboembolism
    - Deterioration of bioprosthetic AVR or mechanical valve malfunction (*bioprosthetic valve deterioration is more common than mechanical valve malfunction*)

Prognosis

- Asymptomatic – excellent prognosis (risk of sudden death < 1%/year)
- Symptomatic – survival rate decreases significantly unless aortic valve replaced
  - ➤ *Natural history related to symptoms of AS without AVR*
    - Angina – 50% survival at 5 years from symptom onset
    - Syncope – 50% survival at 3 years from symptom onset
    - Congestive heart failure – 50% survival at 2 years from symptom onset
- Post-AVR
  - ➤ Normal LV function – good prognosis

VALVULAR INJURY

JUDITH A. WISNESKI, MD

HISTORY & PHYSICAL

Trauma may cause:

- Rupture of papillary muscle with acute mitral regurgitation (MR) (see Valvular heart disease)
- Rupture of chordae tendineae with acute MR (see Valvular heart disease)
- Rupture of mitral valve with acute MR (see Valvular heart disease)
- Rupture of tricuspid valve with acute tricuspid regurgitation (see Valvular heart disease)

Symptoms & Signs
- New heart murmur following trauma
- Pulmonary congestion
- Hypotension
- Signs of right ventricular failure

TESTS
- Echo/Doppler – detect valvular abnormality and severity

DIFFERENTIAL DIAGNOSIS
n/a

MANAGEMENT
(see Valvular heart disease)

SPECIFIC THERAPY
n/a

FOLLOW-UP
n/a

COMPLICATIONS AND PROGNOSIS
- In general, prognosis for cardiac trauma depends on the severity of injury, early detection and initiation of effective treatment (which often includes emergency surgery)
- Myocardial contusion – prognosis worst with presence of CAD and arrhythmias

VARICELLA-ZOSTER

CAROL A. GLASER, MD

HISTORY & PHYSICAL

History
- Varicella – zoster virus (herpesvirus 3)
- Late winter, early spring
- Common childhood disease
- Human host only
- Person to person contact, or droplet or airborne spread of vesicle fluid
- Chickenpox
- Highly contagious, zoster – much less contagious

■ Incubation periods: usually 14–16 days (10–21 days) (may be prolonged after passive immunization)
■ Primary infection; chickenpox, reactivation; "shingles"

Signs & Symptoms
■ Chickenpox – primary infection varicella-zoster; acute, generalized viral disease
  ➤ Fever
  ➤ Mild constitutional symptoms
  ➤ Skin eruption; initially maculopapular, later vesicular ($\times$3–4 days)
  ➤ Lesions commonly occur in successive crops
  ➤ Lesions often high number covered versus non-covered area
  ➤ More severe in adults/adolescents
■ Shingles
  ➤ Local manifestation of latent varicella infection in dorsal root ganglia
  ➤ Vesicles restricted to skin areas of sensory nerves (1–3 sensory dermatomes)
  ➤ Severe pain/paresthesia common
  ➤ Systemic symptoms are few
  ➤ More common in elderly or immunosuppressed

TESTS
■ *Usually a clinical diagnosis*
  ➤ can culture vesicles but not practicable in most settings
  ➤ DFA/Tzanck smear of lesion
■ Serology (ELISA, IFA) limited utility in acute setting – can retrospectively confirm care
■ PCR is available in some settings

DIFFERENTIAL DIAGNOSIS
n/a

MANAGEMENT
■ Susceptible persons at high risk for developing severe varicella – give VZIG w/in 96 h, give as soon as possible with exposure.
■ May be treated with acyclovir, valacyclovir, famciclovir, and foscarnet
■ Therapy should be initiated early to maximize efficacy
■ Oral therapy can be used for otherwise healthy persons, persons on long-term salicylate therapy and persons on short course steroids.
■ Immunocompromised patients; intravenous therapy

- Some recommend oral acyclovir for secondary household cases - disease is more severe. Complications
- Pneumonia: viral/bacterial
- Secondary bacterial infections (esp. invasive group A strep)
- Bacterial superinfection of skin lesions
- Hemorrhagic complications
- Encephalitis
- Immunosuppressed individuals (esp. children with leukemia) High risk disseminated disease
- Maternal infection 1st trimester – congenital varicella syndrome
- Reyes syndrome (especially with use aspirin)

SPECIFIC THERAPY
n/a

FOLLOW-UP
Varicella vaccine – live attenuated virus. Recommended by ACIP for all children at 12 months. Efficacy 85–95%. Not currently recommended in immunosuppressed pts.

COMPLICATIONS AND PROGNOSIS
Bacterial skin infection, encephalitis and Reye syndrome, pneumonia (rare in children, but common cause of varicella morbidity in adults). Varicella is leading cause of vaccine-preventable pediatric death in US. Adults have higher rate of complications overall than children.

VARICOCELE

ARTHUR I. SAGALOWSKY, MD

HISTORY & PHYSICAL
- an anatomic dilation of the pampiniform plexus due to valvular incompetence
- prevalence – 10% of post-pubertal males
- left side most often affected
- may be associated with infertility
- sudden onset may be due to venous occlusion by retroperitoneal tumor (renal, lymphoma, other)
- characteristic "bag of worms" in scrotum when patient is upright

TESTS

Tests for Unclear Cases
- ultrasound
- Valsalva maneuver

DIFFERENTIAL DIAGNOSIS
n/a

MANAGEMENT
n/a

SPECIFIC THERAPY
- indicated if associated testis shrinkage, pain, infertility
- occlusion of spermatic veins by surgery or interventional radiology

FOLLOW-UP
n/a

COMPLICATIONS AND PROGNOSIS
n/a

VARICOSE VEINS

RAJABRATA SARKAR, MD

HISTORY & PHYSICAL

History
- Seen in 10–20% of adult population
- Familial component in 50% of patients
- May develop during pregnancy
- May be asymptomatic, or cause:
  - Aching pain
  - Early fatigue
  - Superficial thrombophlebitis
  - bleeding

Signs & Symptoms
- May range from telangiectasia ("venous spider") to protuberant vein
- Check for associated deep venous insufficiency
  - Pt may have history of prior DVT
  - Duplex scan if there are symptoms of leg swelling
- Trendelenberg test for superficial insufficiency:
  - Tourniquet at thigh with pt supine
  - Have pt stand – if varicosity still dilates then there is reflux from deep to superficial system

TESTS
- Duplex scan for deep venous insufficiency in selected pts

DIFFERENTIAL DIAGNOSIS
n/a

MANAGEMENT
- Cosmetic problem in most pts
- No risk of PE from varicose vein
- Some have a particular painful vein
- Compression stockings
  - Safe but not very effective
  - Provide some relief in a fraction of pts

Surgical Therapy
- >10 mm diameter – ligation and excision
- 4–10 mm – stab avulsion
- 1–4 mm – injection sclerotherapy
- <1 mm – laser treatment

Contraindications
- Severe deep venous occlusion
  - contraindication to excision of the superficial veins
  - superficial veins may be only drainage of leg
  - leg swelling and ulceration will worsen

Side Effects (of All Surgical Procedures)
- Ulceration of skin
- Superficial skin infection
- Recurrent varicosity (risk proportional to size)

SPECIFIC THERAPY
n/a

FOLLOW-UP
- None needed

COMPLICATIONS AND PROGNOSIS
- Rare patients have bleeding and ulceration
- Bleeding stops with gentle pressure
- Persistent ulceration is sign of chronic deep venous insufficiency
- Prognosis is excellent with most treatments (or no treatment)

VASCULAR DISEASE OF SPINAL CORD

MICHAEL J. AMINOFF, MD, DSc

HISTORY & PHYSICAL

- Sudden onset of back or limb pain & of neurologic deficit in limbs or sphincter disturbance
- Flaccid, areflexic paraparesis leading to spastic paraparesis w/ hyperreflexia & extensor plantar responses
- Sensory deficit in legs; typically is dissociated loss (impaired pinprick & temperature sensation, preserved postural & vibration sense) w/ cord infarction from occlusion of anterior spinal artery; may be more global sensory loss w/ hematomas compressing cord
- Brown-Sequard syndrome may occur w/ intrinsic or extrinsic hematomas or occluded branch of anterior spinal artery

TESTS

- Blood studies: CBC & differential count, ESR, PT & PTT, FBS, LFT, RPR, cardiac enzymes, cholesterol & lipids, antiphospholipid antibodies
- Imaging studies typically normal initially w/ cord infarction; show intramedullary, subdural or epidural hematomas

DIFFERENTIAL DIAGNOSIS

- Imaging studies distinguish btwn infarct & hematomas; pts may have history of bleeding disorder, anticoagulant use or recent trauma or lumbar puncture
- AVM of spinal cord causes myeloradiculopathy, cord infarction or spinal subarachnoid hemorrhage; myelogram is required if MRI is unrevealing

MANAGEMENT

- Urgent decompression for subdural or epidural hematomas
- Symptomatic measures, including catheterization for urinary retention

SPECIFIC THERAPY

- Subdural or epidural hematoma requires urgent evacuation.
- Treatment for cord infarction is purely symptomatic.
- AVM can usually be treated by embolization or surgery after angiographic delineation.

FOLLOW-UP
n/a

COMPLICATIONS AND PROGNOSIS
n/a

VENTILATOR MANAGEMENT IN THE ICU

MARK D. EISNER, MD, MPH

HISTORY & PHYSICAL

History
- Determine etiology of respiratory failure: history of asthma, chronic obstructive pulmonary disease, underlying malignancy, immuno-compromise (e.g., HIV infection), cardiac disease

Signs & Symptoms
- Signs indicating respiratory failure include:
  - nasal flaring
  - prominent activity of sternocleidomastoid muscles
  - paradoxical motion of abdomen
  - respiratory rate > 30
  - decreased level of consciousness
  - appearance of "tiring out"
- Wheezing suggests bronchospasm (e.g., asthma or chronic obstructive pulmonary disease exacerbation)
- Bronchial breath sounds, egophony suggest pneumonia

TESTS

Basic Blood Tests
- Arterial blood gas to assess hypoxemia, hypercapnea, and pH
- CBC to evaluate for anemia
- Serum potassium, phosphate, calcium, and bicarbonate

Specific Diagnostic Tests
- Chest x-ray to elucidate etiology of acute respiratory failure (e.g., pneumonia)
- After intubation, chest x-ray to confirm endotracheal tube placement, evaluate for complications (e.g., pneumothorax, pneumomediastinum)
- Continuous pulse oximetry to monitor oxygen saturation

- Peak and plateau airway pressures, to allow adjustment of respiratory rate, tidal volume, and ventilator mode
- Other thoracic imaging – ultrasound or CT scan to evaluate suspected pleural effusion
- With pulmonary infiltrates, consider fiberoptic bronchoscopy

DIFFERENTIAL DIAGNOSIS

n/a

MANAGEMENT

What to Do First

- Establish airway, usually by endotracheal intubation

General Measures

- Ventilate with $FIO_2 = 1.0$ (100% oxygen)
- Evaluate cause of acute respiratory failure by performing focused cardio-pulmonary examination
- Use etiology to guide choice of ventilator mode and settings

SPECIFIC THERAPY

Indications

- Acute hypercapneic respiratory failure, with rising PCO_2, respiratory distress, and / or somnolence (e.g., chronic obstructive pulmonary disease exacerbation)
- Acute hypoxemic respiratory failure, refractory to high levels of supplemental oxygen by face mask (e.g., pneumonia)
- Respiratory distress – physical signs suggesting distress or "tiring out"
- Depressed level of consciousness, inability to protect airway (e.g., stroke, subarachnoid hemorrhage, drug overdose)

Treatment Options

- Assist control (AC) ventilation, synchronized intermittent mandatory ventilation (SIMV), and pressure control ventilation (PCV)
- Ventilator mode should be guided by etiology of respiratory failure
- Tidal volume based on "predicted" body weight, not actual body weight
- For male patients, predicted body weight is 50+ 0.91 (centimeters of height-152.4); for female patients, 45.5+0.91 (centimeters of height-152.4).

Treatment for Specific Diseases

■ Acute respiratory distress syndrome (ARDS) or acute lung injury
  ➤ AC mode
  ➤ Low tidal volume (6 ml/kg predicted body weight) reduces mortality by 22% vs. traditional tidal volume (12 ml/kg)
  ➤ If plateau pressure > 30 cm of water reduce tidal volume stepwise by 1 ml per kg (minimum tidal volume 4 ml/kg)
  ➤ Low tidal volume ventilation requires careful attention to sedation and analgesia
  ➤ Refer to full ARDS-network protocol available at http://hedwig.mgh.harvard.edu/ardsnet

■ Acute respiratory failure with chronic obstructive pulmonary disease or asthma exacerbation
  ➤ Bronchospasm increases risk of high airway pressure, barotrauma, and auto-PEEP
  ➤ SIMV may be mode of choice; PCV is an alternative
  ➤ AC mode increases risk of "breath stacking" due to inadequate expiratory time, resulting in auto-PEEP (complications include barotrauma and hypotension)
  ➤ Set respiratory rate low (4–10), to allow adequate expiratory time with target I:E ratio
    • >1:3
  ➤ Set tidal volume 6–10 ml/kg
  ➤ Target the patient's "baseline" PaCO2, not a normal $PaCO_2$
  ➤ If ventilation is difficult due to high airway pressures, allow "permissive" hypercapnea; consider bicarbonate infusion if pH < 7.15
  ➤ Administer bronchodilators via endotracheal tube

■ Other forms of acute respiratory failure
  ➤ Most efficacious ventilator mode not established
  ➤ AC is easiest, because patient can achieve "desired" minute ventilation

Side Effects & Complications

■ General
  ➤ Barotrauma – pneumothorax, pneumomediastinum, subcutaneous emphysema
  ➤ Auto-PEEP (intrinsic PEEP or occult PEEP) – occurs when inadequate time for expiration; end-expiratory pressure rises; results in hypotension or pneumothorax; test by performing end-expiratory pause and measure airway pressure

➤ Patient-ventilator dyssynchrony – "bucking" the ventilator; adjust tidal volume, respiratory rate, inspiratory flow rate, ventilator mode, or increase sedation

➤ Hypoventilation – when minute ventilation is inadequate; from mucous plugging or atelectasis

➤ Hyperventilation – more common with AC; occurs with anxiety, dyspnea, fever, central causes; can result in respiratory alkalosis

➤ Oxygen toxicity – safe level not clearly established in humans; FIO2 <0.40 probably safe, $F_IO_2 > 0.8$ may be dangerous over prolonged period

➤ Ventilator-associated pneumonia – risk factors are prolonged mechanical ventilation, H_2-antagonists

■ *Endotracheal intubation*
➤ vocal cord trauma, tracheal stenosis

■ *Nasotracheal intubation*
➤ sinusitis

■ *Contraindications to treatment: relative*
➤ AC in patients with asthma or COPD exacerbation

➤ SIMV in Acute Lung Injury or ARDS (AC with low tidal volume reduces mortality)

➤ PCV in patients who have changing lung compliance or airway resistance

FOLLOW-UP

■ Key issue is when patient can be liberated from mechanical ventilation ("weaning"):
➤ Respiratory failure and/or underlying medical condition must be improving

➤ Reduce sedation and analgesia

➤ Assess ability to protect airway (underlying medical and neurologic status, level of consciousness, gag reflex)

■ Daily trial of spontaneous ventilation for 30 minutes to 2 hours – either CPAP with pressure support ≤5 cm water OR T-piece; terminate trial for overt distress, tachycardia, hemodynamic instability, respiratory rate > 30

■ Rapid shallow breathing index = respiratory rate (breaths/minute) / tidal volume (liters)
➤ index less than 105 associated with successful weaning from ventilator

- For difficult weaning, consider other strategies such as pressure support, neuromuscular problems (e.g., myopathy, neuropathy, diaphragm dysfunction), nutrition (e.g., malnutrition, over-feeding), electrolyte disturbance (e.g., hypokalemia, hypophosphatemia, hypocalcemia), acid-base disturbance (e.g., metabolic alkalosis), oversedation, retained secretions

COMPLICATIONS AND PROGNOSIS
- Pneumothorax – incidence depends on etiology of respiratory failure; about 10% of patients with ARDS; insert chest tube immediately
- Ventilator-associated pneumonia – 20–50% of patients; tracheal aspirate for gram stain and culture; consider bronchoalveolar lavage or protected specimen brush sampling; antibiotics based on culture results
- Prognosis – mortality depends on underlying condition and not mode of mechanical ventilation. ARDS mortality about 40%.

VENTRICULAR FIBRILLATION (VF) AND SUDDEN DEATH

EDMUND C. KEUNG, MD

HISTORY & PHYSICAL
History
- VF present in 75% of patients resuscitated from out-of-hospital cardiac arrest.
- Most commonly associated with coronary artery disease, acute myocardial infarction or ischemia, dilated cardiomyopathy with reduced LV function, CHF, severe metabolic derangement. Usually preceded by VT.
- Sudden cardiac death: unexpected, nontraumatic death in stable patients who die within 1 hour after onset of symptoms. 75% or more have significant coronary artery disease. First symptom in 20% of CAD patients.

Signs & Symptoms
- Immediate catastrophic cardiovascular collapse

TESTS
- Basic Tests
  - ➤ 12-lead ECG:
  - ➤ Fast, irregular, poorly organized QRS-T complexes with varying morphology and amplitude
- Specific Diagnostic Test
  - ➤ none

DIFFERENTIAL DIAGNOSIS
- Other causes of sudden collapse such as pulmonary embolism, seizure from neurological events and diabetic coma.

MANAGEMENT

What to Do First
- Immediate cardiopulmonary resuscitation: begin Advanced Cardiac Life Support protocol

General Measures
- Correction of electrolyte imbalance. Magnesium replacement. Evaluation and treatment for acute coronary syndrome or myocardial infarction.

SPECIFIC THERAPY
- Unsynchronous external DC shock with 360 J.
- Immediate infusion of IV amiodarone

Side Effects & Contraindications
- Drugs: proarrhythmia; heart block; CPR: rib fractures. Prolonged cardiac arrest: stroke, coma, death.

FOLLOW-UP
- Treatment of underlying diseases. Coronary angiography with revascularization. Implantation of an internal cardioverter defibrillator if no reversible causes are identified or VF occurs more than 24 hours after an acute infarction.

COMPLICATIONS AND PROGNOSIS
- Survival related to underlying diseases and improved with ICD therapy.

VENTRICULAR PREMATURE COMPLEXES

EDMUND C. KEUNG, MD

HISTORY & PHYSICAL

History

■ Common with structural heart diseases: coronary artery disease, hypertensive heart disease, rheumatic heart disease, myocarditis, and cardiomyopathy.

■ Also caused by electrolyte imbalance and digoxin toxicity.

■ In normals, often associated with stress, tobacco, excessive caffeine or alcohol intake.

■ Decreased intensity of heart sounds and peripheral pulse with the VPC. Abnormal splitting of the second heart sound.

■ Second heart sound is altered, depending on the VPC focus (see BBB above).

Signs & Symptoms

■ Often asymptomatic. Anxiety. Palpitation, irregular pulse. Fatigue and exacerbation of heart failure.

TESTS

■ Basic Tests
  ➤ 12-lead ECG:
  ➤ Premature and wide (>120 ms) QRS complex without preceding P wave, usually followed by a compensatory pause (R-R interval encompassing the VPC is twice the regular RR-interval).

■ Specific Diagnostic Test
  ➤ none

DIFFERENTIAL DIAGNOSIS

■ Atrial premature complex with aberrant conduction, junctional premature complex, pre-excited QRS complex.

MANAGEMENT

General Measures

■ No antiarrhythmic treatment because of increased mortality from such treatment.

■ Avoid caffeine, alcohol, tobacco, chocolate, caffeine-containing tea.

SPECIFIC THERAPY

■ none

FOLLOW-UP
- Treatment of underlying diseases

COMPLICATIONS AND PROGNOSIS
- Marker of sudden death in patients with infarction, especially in the presence of LV dysfunction.

VENTRICULAR SEPTAL DEFECT (VSD)

MARIA ANSARI, MD

HISTORY & PHYSICAL

History
- Rarely presents in adulthood unless small and hemodynamically insignificant or large and associated with Eisenmenger's physiology
- Associated with Down's syndrome and Holt-Oram syndrome
- 50% of cases associated with other cardiac anomalies such as tetralogy of Fallot, PDA, AI, TR or infindibular stenosis

Signs & Symptoms
- Symptoms usually do not develop until shunt ratio greater than 2:1
- Patients with Eisenmenger's will have dyspnea and cyanosis
- Holosystolic murmur at lower left sternal border
- Thrill at 4th ICS
- Enlarged LV and RV

TESTS

Screening
- Physical exam

Imaging
- CXR may show cardiomegaly and pulmonary venous congestion
- EKG may demonstrate biventricular hypertrophy
- Echocardiogram is diagnostic and defines location, size and physiology with 80% located in membranous septum
- Catheterization usually unnecessary unless there is a discrepancy between non-invasive and clinical data

DIFFERENTIAL DIAGNOSIS
- Physical exam murmur may be mimicked by mitral regurgitation or PDA

MANAGEMENT
■ Endocarditis prophylaxis indicated

SPECIFIC THERAPY
■ Surgical closure recommended when pulmonary to systemic shunt ratio >2:1, patient develops symptoms or significant aortic insufficiency is present

FOLLOW-UP
■ Leak of VSD patch may occur-detected by echocardiography
■ Endocarditis prophylaxis for first 6 months after surgery

COMPLICATIONS AND PROGNOSIS
Complications
■ Most common congenital heart defect to lead to Eisenmenger's syndrome (right-to-left shunting associated with pulmonary hypertension)

Prognosis
■ May close spontaneously up to age 20
■ Small VSDs ("maladie de Roger") have benign course
■ Uncorrected larger VSD's in adults have a 76% ten-year survival

VENTRICULAR TACHYCARDIA

EDMUND C. KEUNG, MD

HISTORY & PHYSICAL
History
■ Often associated with structural heart diseases, most commonly coronary artery disease, especially acute myocardial ischemia and infarction
■ Risk factors include prior myocardial infarction and reduced LV function.
■ Related to antiarrhythmic drug treatment (torsades de pointes)
■ Arrhythmogenic right ventricular cardiomyopathy
■ Can occur in the absence of structural heart disease: congenital long QT syndrome, Brugada syndrome, idiopathic left ventricular tachycardia and idiopathic right ventricular outflow tachycardia

Signs & Symptoms
■ Depending on co-existing cardiac conditions and rate of ventricular response: Dizziness, hypotension, shortness of breath, near syncope and syncope, exacerbation of CHF and angina

TESTS
■ Basic Tests
  ➤ 12-lead ECG:
  ➤ Regular wide QRS complexes tachycardia. No 1:1 P-QRS relationship
  ➤ Brugada criteria:
    • Rs complex in all precordial leads (100% specific for VT)
    • Beginning of R to nadir of S interval >100 ms in any precordial lead (98%)
  ➤ A-V dissociation (98%)
  ➤ RBBB QRS: V1: predominantly positive in (R, qR or Rs); V6: QS, qRs or R/S <1
  ➤ LBBB QRS: V1: R wave width >30 ms, notched downstroke of the S wave, onset of QRS to nadir of the S wave >60 ms; V6: QR, QS, QrS or Rr'
  ➤ Other diagnostic features: fusion or capture QRS during VT, presence of Q waves during tachycardia
  ➤ Special Cases:
    • Idiopathic left ventricular tachycardia: RBBB with R/S < 1 in V5 and V6; mostly superior QRS axis
    • Idiopathic right ventricular outflow tachycardia: LBBB with inferior QRS axis
    • Brugada Syndrome: elevated J wave in V1 to V2 (baseline ECG)
    • Right ventricular dysplasia: epsilon wave in V1 to V2, inverted T wave in V1 to V3, isolated increase in QRS (110 ms) in V1 to V2 (baseline ECG)
■ Specific Diagnostic Test
  ➤ Electrophysiology study for induction and mapping of VT, to diagnose bundle branch block and fascicular re-entrant VT
  ➤ Genotyping of congenital long QT-syndrome and arrhythmogenic right ventricular dysplasia (generally not required for clinical practice)

DIFFERENTIAL DIAGNOSIS
■ SVT with aberrantly conducted QRS complexes or SVT from WPW syndrome

MANAGEMENT

What to Do First

- 12-lead ECG to assess acute myocardial ischemia or infarction
- Vital signs to assess hemodynamic response
- Immediately begin cardiopulmonary resuscitation and Advanced Cardiac Life Support protocol if cardiopulmonary collapse occurs.

General Measures

- Correction of electrolyte imbalance
- Magnesium replacement
- Evaluation and treatment for acute coronary syndrome or myocardial infarction

SPECIFIC THERAPY

Immediate

- Emergency DC cardioversion (synchronized to R wave) to restore NSR in patients with a rapid ventricular response resulting in hemodynamic instability or angina
- Infusion of IV amiodarone
- Ventricular overdrive pacing

Chronic

- Implantation of an internal cardioverter defibrillator (ICD), Class I indications:
- Cardiac arrest due to VF or VT without a reversible cause
- Spontaneous sustained VT with structural heart disease
- History of syncope and hemodynamically significant VT or VF induced at EP study
- Nonsustained VT with prior MI and LV dysfunction and inducible VT at EPS
- Spontaneous sustained VT without structural heart disease and not amenable to other treatments
- RF ablation of VT focus, especially in idiopathic right or left ventricular tachycardia or refractory ischemic VT with recurrent shocks after ICD implantation

Side Effects & Contraindications

- Prorhythmic effects from drug therapy (not recommended)

FOLLOW-UP

- Treatment of underlying diseases. Coronary angiography with revascularization.

COMPLICATIONS AND PROGNOSIS
- Survival related to underlying diseases and improved with ICD therapy
- Best prognosis for idiopathic right or left ventricular tachycardia
- ICD: same as for pacemaker. Inappropriate shocks.

VIRAL ARTHRITIS

STEVEN R. YTTERBERG, MD

HISTORY & PHYSICAL

History
- Exposure to specific infectious agents
- Dependent on individual viruses
  - ➤ Parvovirus B19: children w/ fifth disease
  - ➤ Hepatitis B: IV drug use, sexual transmission
  - ➤ Hepatitis C: IV drug use
  - ➤ Rubella: infected individuals, postvaccination
  - ➤ Alphaviruses: mosquito-borne, in endemic areas
  - ➤ HIV infection often causes joint pain, occasionally an oligoarthritis involving lower extremities; self-limited

Risk Factors
- Exposure to specific viral infections, esp. being in an endemic area
- No known genetic factors
- Immunocompromised conditions

Signs & Symptoms
- Presentation depends on individual virus; symmetric polyarticular arthralgias or arthritis most common, some pts w/ oligoarticular or monoarticular
- Parvovirus B19: flu-like illness; typical "slapped cheeks" & fine reticular rashes in children, mild maculopapular rash in adults; arthralgia & arthritis in up to 80% of adult women, less common in men; symmetric polyaarticular joint involvement of small & large joints
- Hepatitis B: symmetric or migratory polyarticular arthritis often w/ rash during prodromal, preicteric phase of hepatitis; often improves w/ onset of jaundice
- Hepatitis C: often assoc w/ cryoglobulinemia–arthritis & palpable purpura; some pts w/ arthralgias or arthritis w/o cryoglobulins

- Rubella: flu-like illness; adenopathy; morbilliform rash; symmetric polyarticular arthralgia & arthritis more commonly in women than men; tenosynovitis, carpal tunnel syndrome, brachial neuritis or lumbar radiculoneuropathy (in children)
- Alphaviruses: arthropod-borne; commonly w/ constitutional symptoms, rash & arthralgia or arthritis – symmetric polyarticular or oligoarticular
- Other viruses assoc w/ joint involvement infrequently: mumps, adenovirus, CMV, EBV, HSV, varicella-zoster virus, coxsackieviruses, echoviruses, hepatitis A, smallpox

TESTS

Basic Tests

- General lab tests usually nonspecific: leukocytosis & elevated ESR & CRP possible
- Selected viruses may cause specific changes
  - ➤ Parvovirus B19: anemia, thrombocytopenia possible
  - ➤ Hepatitis B & C: elevated transaminases
  - ➤ Autoantibodies may be found w/ parvovirus B19 (ANA, RF, cardiolipin, ds-DNA, Ro, La) or hepatitis C (ANA, RF)
- Synovial fluid findings variable: inflammatory or noninflammatory

Specific Diagnostic Tests

- Serologic tests for specific agents
  - ➤ Parvovirus B19: B19 IgM antibodies indicate current infection
  - ➤ Hepatitis B: HbsAg usually detectable at time of arthritis
  - ➤ Hepatitis C: positive anti-HCV antibody confirmed by qualitative HCV RNA test
  - ➤ Rubella: IgM antibody or IgG seroconversion; culture from tissue
  - ➤ Alphaviruses: viral isolation or seroconversion

Imaging

- Imaging studies nonspecific: soft tissue swelling

DIFFERENTIAL DIAGNOSIS

- Inflammatory arthritis: early-onset connective tissue disease (eg, RA or SLE, early seronegative spondyloarthropathy)

MANAGEMENT

What to Do First

- Exclude other possibilities, esp. bacterial infection; must consider new-onset connective tissue disease, RA or spondyloarthropathy

■ Symptomatic treatment: NSAIDs for the inflammatory symptoms, acetaminophen or other analgesics may be needed

General Measures
■ Long-term therapy usually not needed as these conditions are generally self-limited, lasting for days to a few weeks
■ Chronic arthropathy may require corticosteroids

SPECIFIC THERAPY

Indications
■ Joint pain & swelling; systemic symptoms

Treatment Options
■ Symptomatic therapy: NSAIDs, occasionally low-dose prednisone or hydroxychloroquine for more persistent joint inflammation
■ Interferon & ribaviron used for hepatitis C; no specific antiviral therapy available for other infections
■ IVIg reported for persistent parvovirus B19 infection in immunocompromised hosts

Side Effects & Complications
■ NSAID complications: GI bleeding & pain, renal insufficiency, platelet inhibition
■ Prednisone: osteoporosis, immunosuppression
■ Contraindications
  ➤ Usual contraindications to use of NSAIDs or prednisone

FOLLOW-UP

During Treatment
■ Follow-up should document resolution of symptoms & permit discontinuation of therapy

Routine
■ Recurrent episodes of arthritis reported, esp. w/ parvovirus B19

COMPLICATIONS & PROGNOSIS
■ Viral arthritis is generally self-limited w/ a good long-term prognosis
■ Chronic arthropathy occurs occasionally following parvovirus B19 infection, at times w/ positive RF, raising question of the relationship of infection to RA

VISCERAL LARVA MIGRANS

J. GORDON FRIERSON, MD

HISTORY & PHYSICAL

History
- Exposure; Ingestion of eggs of *Toxocara canis* or *cati*, through contaminated fingers, objects, or eating dirt. The eggs hatch in the intestine, producing larvae which migrate through intestinal wall and to all organs of body.

Signs & Symptoms
- Usually seen in small children or mentally ill. Mild infections asymptomatic. Symptoms include fever, hepatomegaly, abdominal pain, myalgias, sometimes wheeze or cough, urticaria.

TESTS
- Basic tests: blood: eosinophilia, may be very pronounced.
- Basic tests: urine: normal
- Specific tests: Diagnosis usually clinical. Biopsy of liver or other tissue may show larva.
- Other tests: Serology by ELISA (done at CDC and other labs) helpful, but can be elevated in 1–10% of "normal" children. Rising titer more specific.

DIFFERENTIAL DIAGNOSIS
- Migratory phase of several nematodes, such as hookworm, ascaris, strongyloides. Hypereosinophilic syndromes.

MANAGEMENT

What to Do First
- Assess severity. IV fluids if needed.

General Measures
- Determine source of infection, and remove it.

SPECIFIC THERAPY

Indications
- Patient with significant symptoms.

Treatment Options

■ No treatment is established as highly effective. Recommended are:
> ➤ Albendazole for 5 days
> ➤ or: Diethlycarbamazine for 10–20 days.
> ➤ Corticosteroids helpful in sick patients to reduce inflammatory response.

Side Effects & Complications

■ Allergic reactions to medications. Some GI side effects from medications.

■ Contraindications to treatment: absolute: allergy to medications

■ Contraindications to treatment: relative: mild infections.

FOLLOW-UP

■ During treatment: Monitor vital signs, general status

■ Routine: follow eosinophilia, hepatomegaly. Serology stays elevated long time and not useful in follow.

COMPLICATIONS AND PROGNOSIS

■ Ocular larva migrans is main complication. Usually occurs in lightly infected children. Vision reduced, and tumor and/or edema of retina seen. Needs to be distinguished from retinoblastoma and other tumors, trauma, other inflammatory conditions. Treatment is with steroids.

VITAMIN A DEFICIENCY

ELISABETH RYZEN, MD

HISTORY & PHYSICAL

History

■ prolonged dietary deprivation of carotene-rich foods, malabsorption syndrome, celiac disease, cystic fibrosis, pancreatic disease, cirrhosis, kwashiorkor

Signs & Symptoms
- night blindness, xerophthalmia, keratomalacia, hyperkeratosis, urinary calculi

TESTS
Laboratory
- Basic blood studies:
  - ➤ plasma retinol <10 mcg/dL

DIFFERENTIAL DIAGNOSIS
n/a

MANAGEMENT
n/a

SPECIFIC THERAPY
- Vitamin A 10,000–25,000 U/day

Side Effects & Contraindications
- birth defects, dermatitis, dry skin, coarse hair, weakness, pseudotumor cerebri, hepatosplenomegaly, headaches, hypercalcemia

FOLLOW-UP
n/a

COMPLICATIONS AND PROGNOSIS
- Completely reversible

VITAMIN C DEFICIENCY

ELISABETH RYZEN, MD

HISTORY & PHYSICAL

History
- poor diet, GI disease; pregnancy, lactation, inflammatory diseases, burns, diarrhea increase requirements

Signs & Symptoms
- Severe = scurvy: poor wound healing, bruising, splinter hemorrhages, fractures, abnormal dentin, weakness, myalgias, arthralgias, swollen gums, lower extremity edema

TESTS

Laboratory
- Basic blood studies:
  - ➤ plasma ascorbic acid <0.2 mg/dL

DIFFERENTIAL DIAGNOSIS

n/a

MANAGEMENT

n/a

SPECIFIC THERAPY
- Vitamin C protective; treatment plus dietary measures. No evidence huge doses decrease incidence or severity of common cold

Side Effects & Contraindications
- nephrolithiasis (oxalosis) at doses > 4 gm/day

FOLLOW-UP

n/a

COMPLICATIONS AND PROGNOSIS
- Completely reversible

VITAMIN E DEFICIENCY

ELISABETH RYZEN, MD

HISTORY & PHYSICAL

History
- rare; premature infants, fat malabsorption, chronic cholestatic hepato-biliary disease, celiac disease, genetic abnormality of vitamin E metabolism

Signs & Symptoms
- infants, mild hemolytic anemia, spinocerebellar disease with DTR loss, ataxia

TESTS

Laboratory
- Basic blood studies:
  - tocopherol level <5 mcg/mL

DIFFERENTIAL DIAGNOSIS
n/a

MANAGEMENT
n/a

SPECIFIC THERAPY
- Vitamin E. No evidence Vitamin E prevents heart disease or cancers.

Side Effects & Contraindications
- None, perhaps increased tendency for bleeding

FOLLOW-UP
n/a

COMPLICATIONS AND PROGNOSIS
- Completely reversible except in genetic defects

VITAMIN K DEFICIENCY

ELISABETH RYZEN, MD

HISTORY & PHYSICAL

History
- newborns; marginal dietary intake, extensive surgery, trauma, prolonged TPN, biliary obstruction, malabsorption, liver disease; anticonvulsant, anticoagulant use, cephalosporins, salicylates, megadoses vitamins A or E

Signs & Symptoms
- bleeding, easy bruising, epistaxis, hematuria, GI bleeding, signs of anemia or menorrhagia, puncture site blood oozing

TESTS

Laboratory
- Basic blood studies:
  - ➤ PT, INR, PTT prolonged

DIFFERENTIAL DIAGNOSIS
- Warfarin use
- Liver disease
- Dysfibrinogenemia
- Lupus anticoagulant
- Factors V, X, II deficiency
- Disseminated intravascular coagulation

MANAGEMENT
n/a

SPECIFIC THERAPY
- phytonadione IM (can use IV in emergencies, do not exceed 1 mg/min); response detectable within 1–2 hours

Side Effects & Contraindications
- None

FOLLOW-UP
n/a

COMPLICATIONS AND PROGNOSIS
- Reversible with replacement

VITILIGO

KAREN GOULD, MD and
JEFFREY P. CALLEN, MD

HISTORY & PHYSICAL

History
- autoimmune mechanism with genetic predisposition likely cause
  - ➤ possible environmental triggers are trauma sun exposure, systemic illness
  - ➤ 1–2% population

> all races affected, but darker skin tones more common
> peak onset 10–30 years
> 21% have affected first-generation family members
- associated disorders
  > thyroid disease, diabetes mellitus, Addison's disease, pernicious anemia

Signs & Symptoms
- depigmented, white round to oval macules and patches without surface change
- Predilection for periorificial, acral and genital involvement
- other associated cutaneous findings
  > halo nevi, leukotrichia
  > alopecia areata may be more common in patients with vitiligo
- segmental – unilateral macules in dermatomal pattern
  > more common in children
  > usually nonprogressing
  > nonfamilial, earlier onset
  > not associated with other autoimmune disorders
  > 50% associated with poliosis
  > trigeminal area most common site
- generalized – few to many macules and patches
  > most common type
  > extensor surfaces usually symmetric
  > common sites include IP joints, MCP, MTP, elbows, knees, periorificial
- universal – widespread vitiligo with few remaining normal pigmented areas
  > associated with multiple endocrinopathy syndrome

TESTS

Specific Diagnostic Tests
- Diagnosis clinical
- wood's lamp showing accentuation of sharply bordered macules

Other Tests as Appropriate
- Thyroid panel in patients with generalized or universal vitiligo
- consider work-up for associated diseases if symptomatic
- consider ophthalmologic examination

➤ associated ocular abnormalities are uveitis, chorioretinitis, choroidal abnormalities, iritis

DIFFERENTIAL DIAGNOSIS

■ chemical leukoderma, leprosy, mycosis fungoides, piebaldism, pityriasis alba, tinea versicolor, tuberous sclerosis, nevus depigmentosus, idiopathic guttate hypomelanosis, post-inflammatory hypopigmentation

MANAGEMENT

General Measures

■ workup for associated disorders if indicated
■ sunscreen use especially of non-pigmented macules
■ cosmetic products to cover up discoloration

SPECIFIC THERAPY

■ topical glucocorticoids
  ➤ potent glucocorticoids
    • use for 3 weeks, then stop for 1 week
    • for nonfacial, nonaxillary, non-groin
  ➤ mild glucocorticoids
    • face, groin, and axilla, especially in kids
■ topical calcineurin inhibitors – tacrolimus or pimecrolimus
■ Phototherapy
  ➤ PUVA
  ➤ Topical – isolated small macules 1–2% BSA
    • 1:10–1:100 mixture of 8-MOP in petrolatum or ethanol
    • apply 30 minutes prior to UVA irradiation
    • twice a week
  ➤ Systemic – widespread vitiligo in people > 10 years old
    • 8-MOP 1–2 hours prior to UVA 2–3 times per week for 50–100 treatments (not on consecutive days)
    • 50% substantial repigmentation
  ➤ Narrowband UVB phototherapy – either localized (excimer laser) or generalized therapy may result in repigmentation equal to that of PUVA therapy.
■ Surgical
  ➤ mini-grafting-1–2 mm punch grafts for isolated small macules
■ Depigmentation of normally pigmented skin
  ➤ used in extensive vitiligo

- ➤ MBEH (monobenzylether of hydroquinone) 20% cream
  - permanent and irreversible depigmentation
  - BID application for 9–12 months
  - must avoid subsequent sun exposure
- ➤ Q-switched ruby laser
- ■ alternative therapies
  - ➤ multivitamin therapy (folic acid/vitamin B12/vitamin C)
    - L-phenylalanine with UVA or UVB
    - Pseudocatalase with UVA or UVB
    - Khellin with UVA
- ■ *Side Effects & Complications*
- ■ topical PUVA
  - ➤ severe sunburns, phototoxic response, hyperpigmentation,
- ■ depigmentation with monobenzyl ether of hydroquinone
  - ➤ erythema, dryness, burning, pruritus
  - ➤ contact dermatitis in 15%

FOLLOW-UP
- ■ During Treatment – every 6–8 weeks

COMPLICATIONS AND PROGNOSIS
- ■ cosmetic appearance is main complication
  - ➤ Squamous cell carcinoma may occur in depigmented skin
- ■ prognosis excellent for segmental and focal vitiligo
- ■ spontaneous regression is rare in generalized and universal vitiligo

---

VOLUME DEPLETION AND EDEMA

BIFF F. PALMER, MD

HISTORY & PHYSICAL

Volume Depletion
- ■ clinical setting and history usually can localize site of volume loss
  - ➤ gastrointestinal loss: vomiting, diarrhea, external gastrointestinal drainage
  - ➤ renal losses: diuretic use, uncontrolled diabetes
  - ➤ skin or respiratory losses: insensible losses, sweating, burns
- ■ Signs & Symptoms

➤ decreased body weight, orthostatic change in blood pressure and pulse, decreased skin turgor, flat neck veins, dry mucous membranes

Edema

■ clinical setting, history and physical usually can identify abnormality

➤ congestive heart failure: dyspnea, orthopnea, paroxysmal nocturnal dyspnea

➤ cirrhosis: history of chronic liver disease, ethanol abuse, hepatitis B or C

➤ nephrotic syndrome: diabetes

➤ end-stage renal disease

■ Signs & Symptoms

➤ pitting edema, increased body weight, hypertension, distended neck veins, S3 gallop, ascites, jaundice

TESTS

■ hemodynamic monitoring

➤ central venous pressure

➤ pulmonary capillary wedge pressure

■ blood tests

➤ BUN/creatinine ratio >20 (normal ratio 10:1): low effective arterial blood volume (EABV)

➤ hemoconcentration of hematocrit and albumin: low EABV

➤ increased serum uric acid concentration: low EABV

➤ assess acid base status

• normal gap metabolic acidosis: diarrhea

• metabolic alkalosis: vomiting, diuretics (loop or thiazide)

■ urinary tests

➤ renal response to contracted EABV is to conserve sodium and water

➤ urine [Na] or [Cl] < 10–15 mEq/L is appropriate response to extrarenal volume loss

➤ fractional excretion of Na or Cl <.005-.01 is appropriate response to extrarenal volume loss

• $FENa = (UNa \times PCr)/(UCr \times PNa)$ $FECl = (UCl \times PCr)/(UCr \times PCl)$

➤ special situations where either urine [Na] or [Cl] or FENa or FECl are not reflective of existing volume depletion

• increased [Na] and increased [Cl] or increased FENa and increased FECl

- diuretics, salt wasting nephropathy, decreasedmineralocorticoid activity
- increased [Na] and decreased [Cl] or increased FENa and decreased FECl (effect of nonreabsorbable anion)
  - vomiting (bicarbonaturia), ketonuria, urinary excretion of penicillin salts
- decreased [Na] and increased [Cl] or decreased FENa and increased FECl (effect of increased UNH4V)
  - chronic diarrhea
- ➤ Other tests indicative of increased renal reabsorption of Na and water
  - urine:plasma creatinine >40:1
  - increased U_{osm} and increased urine specific gravity

DIFFERENTIAL DIAGNOSIS
- ■ decreased total body Na, decreased EABV
  - ➤ extrarenal loss
    - diarrhea, fistula, vomiting/nasogastric suction, excessive sweating
  - ➤ renal loss
    - diuretics
    - adrenal insufficiency
    - cerebral salt wasting
- ■ increased total body Na, decreased EABV (edematous disorders)
  - ➤ congestive heart failure
  - ➤ cirrhosis
  - ➤ nephrotic syndrome
  - ➤ third-spacing
    - pancreatitis
    - peritonitis
    - extensive burns
- ■ increased total body Na, increased EABV
  - ➤ acute glomerulonephritis
  - ➤ acute oligo-anuric renal failure
  - ➤ advanced end stage renal disease

MANAGEMENT
- ■ first ensure hemodynamics are stable

- determine whether there is increased or decreased total body Na
- if decreased total body Na, determine whether there is renal or extrarenal Na wasting
- if increased total body Na, determine reason for renal Na retention
- treat underlying cause of the disorder

SPECIFIC THERAPY
- disorders with decreased total body Na that are hemodynamically stable
  - ➤ encourage increased PO intake with salt containing foods (bouillon)
  - ➤ if unable to take PO, administer intravenous fluids
    - if hyponatremic or normonatremic: use isotonic saline
    - if hypernatremic: use 0.45% normal saline
  - ➤ if metabolic acidosis is present: can use D5W with 1–2 ampules NaHCO3 added
- disorders with increased total body Na and decreased EABV
  - ➤ dietary Na restriction, diuretics
  - ➤ transfuse to keep hematocrit >30
  - ➤ colloid solutions such as albumin more effective that crystalloids to expand EABV
- disorders with increased total body Na and increased EABV
  - ➤ dietary Na restriction, diuretics, renal failure patients may require dialysis if refractory to maximal medical therapy

FOLLOW-UP
- ensure hemodynamics remain stable
- attempt to treat underlying disorder
- monitor serum [Na] in those patients with either hyponatremia or hypernatremia

COMPLICATIONS AND PROGNOSIS
- administration of salt containing solutions can lead to volume overload if not closely monitored
- loop diuretics complicated by hypokalemia, metabolic alkalosis, and pre-renal azotemia
- prognosis of conditions with decreased total body Na is good
- prognosis of conditions with increased total body Na dependent upon underlying disorder

VON WILLEBRAND DISEASE

MORTIMER PONCZ, MD and MICHELE LAMBERT, MD

HISTORY & PHYSICAL

- Easy bruising
- Recurrent epistaxis or other mucosal bleeding
- Menorrhagia
- Hemorrhage after injury or surgery; especially tonsillectomy, adenoidectomy, dental extraction
- Hemarthrosis (only with certain subtypes)
- Associated with congenital hemorrhagic telangiectasia (Osler-Weber-Rendu syndrome) and can see acquired vWD with Wilms tumor
- Family history of excessive bleeding (particularly menometrorrhagia) or vWd (most common type [type 1] is autosomal dominant)

TESTS

- CBC, PT, PTT: PTT usually normal but can be prolonged; platelets can be decreased in type 2B vWD
- Bleeding time: usually prolonged but can be normal (rarely done)*
- von Willebrand factor (vWf) level: normal values depend on blood type. Can be artificially increased by high-dose estrogens (OCP or pregnancy) or high stress levels
- Factor VIII level: lower in type 2N vWd
- vWf activity (ristocetin cofactor): low in vWd – levels do not depend on blood type; may also be elevated with high-dose estrogen; ristocetin induces vWf binding to platelet GPIb; lower ratio of ristocetin cofactor to vWf level with normal multimers in type 2M vWd
- Willebrand factor multimers: all multimers decreased in type 1 (most common variant – 5% of the general population); all multimers absent in type 3 (autosomal recessive or compound heterozygous inheritance); high-molecular-weight multimers decreased in type 2B and platelet-type pseudo vWd, absent in type 2A vWd
- Low-dose ristocetin-induced platelet aggregation: increased in type 2B vWd. vWf and ristocetin cofactor can intermittently be normal: if significant bleeding history, repeat labs at least 3 times over 3–6 months.

DIFFERENTIAL DIAGNOSIS

- Significant bleeding history: hemophilia, other factor deficiency, qualitative platelet defect, thrombocytopenia, collagen-vascular defect, aspirin use
- Prolonged PTT: acquired inhibitor, antiphospholipid antibody, intrinsic coagulation pathway factor deficiency, hemophilia
- Decreased high-molecular-weight vWf multimers: DIC, TTP, HUS

MANAGEMENT

- Avoid aspirin.
- Head injury precautions; avoid contact sports
- Assess efficacy of DDAVP intranasal (must use Stimate brand) or intravenous in increasing vWf activity (ristocetin cofactor) only if multimers are normal.
- Avoid use DDAVP in type 2B vWd: risk of increased thrombosis.
- Patient education on use of Stimate at home for epistaxis, oral bleeding, menorrhagia; Stimate + / − epsilon-aminocaproic acid for minor dental work
- For major surgery, IV DDAVP 30 min prior to procedure, repeat 12 and 36 h later. For tonsillectomy and adenoidectomy, extra dose given 5–7 days later when eschar falls off. May also require epsilon-aminocaproic acid.
- Severe bleeding in type 3, 2N, 2M, or in type 1 vWD that does not have a good therapeutic DDAVP trial: treat with plasma-derived vWf/factor VIII concentrate to maintain ristocetin/vWf activity at least 50%
- Platelet-type pseudo vWd: treat severe bleeding with platelet transfusion.
- Acquired inhibitor to vWf in Wilms tumor: treat with DDAVP, cryoprecipitate, plasma-derived vWf/factor VIII concentrate, IVIG, or platelets; inhibitor resolves with treatment of Wilms tumor.

SPECIFIC THERAPY
n/a

FOLLOW-UP
n/a

COMPLICATIONS AND PROGNOSIS
Pts usually do well; associated with a normal life expectancy.

WALDENSTROM'S MACROGLOBULINEMIA

KENNETH C. ANDERSON, MD

HISTORY & PHYSICAL
- Symptomatic anemia and hyperviscosity
- Adenopathy and organomegaly

TESTS

Basic Blood Studies
- Anemia, leukopenia, thrombocytopenia, renal insufficiency, quantitative monoclonal protein, hepatitis, elevated serum viscosity

Specific Diagnostic Tests
- Excess monoclonal lymphoplasmacytoid cells in bone marrow
- Computerized tomographic scan of chest/abdomen/pelvis to demonstrate organomegaly/adenopathy
- Cold agglutinins, cryocrit
- Hepatitis serology

DIFFERENTIAL DIAGNOSIS
- Monoclonal gammopathy of unknown significance: low level IgM without any other manifestations of Waldenstrom's macroglobulinemia
- Non-Hodgkin's lymphoma: distinct histopathology
- Chronic lymphocytic leukemia: circulating mature lymphocytes
- Primary amyloidosis: plasma cells in marrow, distinct viscera involved
- Other lymphoproliferative disorders: distinct histopathology

MANAGEMENT

What to Do First
- Plasmapheresis for sympomatic hyperviscosity

SPECIFIC THERAPY

Indications
- Symptomatic hyperviscosity
- Anemia, pancytopenia
- Bulky adenopathy or symptomatic organomegaly
- Symptomatic cryoglobulinemia or neuropathy

Treatment Options
- Alkylating agents: high response rates, but compromise stem cell reserve; dysmyelopoiesis with prolonged use

- Nucleoside analogs: high response rates, but prolonged immuno-suppression
- Rituxan alone or with chemotherapy.
- Bortezomib.

FOLLOW-UP
- Quantitative immunoglobulins and quantitation of monoclonal protein and serum viscosity every 2 cycles
- Complete blood count, differential, platelets
- CT scans (if abnormal at presentation) every 3–6 mo

COMPLICATIONS AND PROGNOSIS

Progressive Disease
- Nucleoside analogs
- in patients who progress despite treatment with alkylating agents
- in patients who respond to but relapse within 6 months after alkylating agent therapy
- in patients who relapse more than 6 months after treatment with nucleoside analogs
- Alkylating agent therapy
- in patients who relapse more than 6 months after treatment with alkylating agents
- in patients who progress despite treatment with nucleoside analogs
- in patients who respond to but relapse within 6 months after nucleoside analog therapy

Prognosis
- Median survival of 50 months, similar to best reported myeloma series
- Prolonged indolent course not requiring therapy in some patients
- Higher risk with older age, male sex, general symptoms, and cytopenias

WARTS

ROBERT T. BRODELL, MD and SANDRA MARCHESE JOHNSON, MD

HISTORY & PHYSICAL

History
- Exposure to the Human Papillomavirus, direct contact
- 2/3 of sexual contacts with genital warts develop genital warts
- Peak incidence: 12–16 years
- Incubation: few weeks to more than 1 year, average: 2.8 months

Signs & Symptoms
- Firm rough papules with tiny surface papillations, 1 mm to >1 cm on any mucocutaneous surface
- Paring of the thick surface may show pinpoint bleeding ("seeds," thrombosed capillaries)

TESTS
- Skin biopsy: Rarely needed
- Research tools: PCR to determine HPV type

DIFFERENTIAL DIAGNOSIS
- Common warts: squamous cell carcinoma, molluscum contagiosum, deep fungal infection (blastomycosis), epidermal nevi, seborrheic keratoses, fibroepithelial polyps
- Flat warts: acne comedones
- Plantar warts: callus, clavus/corn
- Genital warts: condyloma lata (secondary syphilis), squamous cell carcinoma including giant condyloma of Buschke-Lowenstein, bowenoid papulosis

MANAGEMENT
- Avoid potentially scarring therapies when possible.
- Virtually all warts should be treated considering inhibition of function, cosmetic factors, potential for decreasing spread, and the fact that small warts are more easily cleared.
- The natural history of warts is not favorable (only 40% of patients are free of wart in 2 years without treatment).

SPECIFIC THERAPY
- First-line therapies:
- Over the counters: 17% salicylic acid qd to moist skin; file with emery board or pumice stone prior to application
- Cryotherapy: liquid nitrogen applied to wart for 2 freeze/thaw cycles each about 15–30 seconds with a thaw time of 20–30 seconds. Repeat every 2–3 weeks.
- Cantharidin: apply to warts, cover with occlusive tape for 24 hours, then wash with soap and water. Repeat every 2–3 weeks.
- Cantharidin plus salicylic acid plus podophylin: Apply to warts, cover with occlusive tape ×2 hours, then wash off with soap and water.
- Imiqimod (Aldara): applied three times a week to genital warts, left on overnight and washed off in the morning (inducer of interferon alpha).
- Contact sensitizers: squaric acid, diphecypropenone (DCP). For DCP: Apply test patch of 0.1% solution to flexor arm and cover for 24

hours to sensitize. One week later, apply 0.1% to warts and cover for 6 hours.
- Podophyllin: 25–50% applied weekly to warts by physician, washed after 6 hours. Repeat every 1–2 weeks.
- Podophyllotoxin (Condylox) can be applied at home twice daily for 3 days, then not treated for 4 days, then repeated each week until clear. Avoid in pregnant women.
- Vascular Lesion Laser (585 nm) - 20 W, two or three pulses to each wart. Repeat every 2–3 weeks until clear.
- Tretinoin: may be applied once a day to flat warts
- For recalcitrant warts:
- Intralesional alpha interferon: reserve for recalcitrant warts, inject each wart 2x/week for up to 8 weeks or until clear
- Surgical excision: reserve for large warts to remove tumor burden. HPV in clinically normal skin results in frequent recurrence.
- CO_2 laser ablation: Scarring possible; recurrences likely
- Electrosurgery: best for small warts, use a smoke evacuator to avoid inhalation of aerosolized viral particles
- Bleomycin: injected intralesionally or applied topically and instilled with an allergy needle excoriating surface. Avoid injecting the distal digits because of a risk of necrosis.
  - Candida antigen: into warts: Inject 0.3 ml into one of the larger warts every 2–4 weeks until wart resolves. Discontinue if no response after 5 treatments. Warts distant to the treatment site often resolve as the target lesion disappears.

FOLLOW-UP
- Self-exam weekly after clearing; follow up with physician with any sign of recurrence for physician-applied therapies
- Periodically every 2 weeks to 2 months for patient-applied therapies

COMPLICATIONS AND PROGNOSIS
- "Doughnut wart": treated wart clears but a new wart may occur encircling the prior wart as viral particles within blister fluid infect the skin at the periphery of the blister initiated by previous treatment
- Scarring: occurs more commonly with destructive therapies: electrosurgery, CO_2 laser, cold-steel surgery
- Side effects of treatment may include pruritus, local skin necrosis
- Prognosis is excellent when treatment is tailored to each patient and adjusted according to response. Immune surveillance will clear warts in some cases even without treatment.

WHIPPLE'S DISEASE

GARY M. GRAY, MD

HISTORY & PHYSICAL

History
- Fatigue, abdominal bloating/distention, large volume loose stools, arthralgias and arthritis, weight loss, mental changes

Physical
- Smooth, red tongue; cracking at mouth corners; evidence of weight loss; cardiac murmur; mental slowing

TESTS

Basic Blood:
- anemia (iron deficiency; folate/vitamin B_{12} deficiency); hypoalbuminemia

Basic Urine:
- none usually helpful; see xylose test under specific diagnostic tests

Special Diagnostic Tests
- Functional tests of malabsorption: elevated quantitative fecal fat (72-hour); reduced xylose absorption (25 g ingested; 5-hour urine excretion)
- Small intestinal biopsy (via upper GI endoscopy to distal duodenum): prominent and irregularly shaped folds; microscopic: broadened and shortened villi, often with normal surface enterocytes; prominent infiltration of lamina propria with large round cells (macrophages; PAS-positive)
- Positive PCR test for responsible genetic material of the bacterial agent (Tropheryma whippelii) in intestinal biopsy
- Identification of PCR-positive material in other tissues involved (cerebral-spinal fluid, joint aspirates, liver, heart valves)
- Altered heart valves on cardiac ECHO (if heart valve involvement)

DIFFERENTIAL DIAGNOSIS

Differential Diagnosis
- Other intestinal enteropathies, especially celiac sprue, a more common disease
- Other causes of arthritis, especially immunologic (rheumatoid arthritis)

- Maldigestion due to pancreatic insufficiency (chronic pancreatitis) or pancreatic duct obstruction (pancreatic carcinoma): fecal fat elevated but xylose absorption normal
- Irritable bowel syndrome (multiple stools but scanty quantity and no malabsorption)

MANAGEMENT
What to Do First
- If intestinal biopsy reveals PAS-positive macrophages and positive PCR for T. Whippelii, then CSF fluid should be obtained for PCR also

General Measures
- Add vitamin supplements for 2–3 months (multivitamins, folic acid, fat-soluble vitamins [A,D,E])
- Initiation of appropriate long-term antibiotic therapy (see below)

SPECIFIC THERAPY
- Long-term treatment with oral antibiotics (trimethoprim 160 mg/ sulfamethoxazole 800 mg p.o. b.i.d. for 1 to 2 years)
- If cerebral involvement, parenteral Penicillin G 1.2 million units and streptomycin 1 Gm daily should be given initially for 14 days, followed by the oral drugs

FOLLOW-UP
- Response to antibiotic therapy usually prompt, within a week or so
- Monitoring of improvement in functional absorptive parameters (xylose, fecal fat); serum albumen, correction of anemia
- Repeat intestinal biopsy for histology and PCR analysis for T. whippelii at 6–12 months
- Long-term monitoring: yearly assessment of nutrition, cardiac and neurologic status
- Prompt thorough evaluation at any suggestion of enteric, cardiac or neurologic recurrence over the years

COMPLICATIONS AND PROGNOSIS
- At least 90% of patients have a complete and sustained response to antibiotic therapy
- Relapse rate 15–20% in earlier years when oral penicillin was most widely used; now relapse much lower after trimethoprim/ sulfamethoxazole therapy
- CNS recurrence may be severe and extensive, mimicking more common diseases such as ischemia, stroke or dementia

- Cardiac involvement may be devastating, especially valvulitis or myocarditis
- Yearly monitoring of nutritional, cardiac, and neurological status prevents most complications

WILSON'S DISEASE

ERIC LEONG, MD, FRCPC

HISTORY & PHYSICAL

Risk Factors
- Family history of liver, neurologic, and/or psychiatric disease

Symptoms and Signs
- Symptoms rare before 5 years of age
- Hepatic disease
  - Asymptomatic with biochemical abnormalities
  - Chronic hepatitis, with or without fatigue
  - Cirrhosis with symptoms & signs of liver failure
  - Fulminant hepatitis with or without intravascular hemolysis
- Neurologic disease
  - Kayser-Fleischer rings in 90–100% with neurologic disease
  - Dystonia with rigidity, contractures, bradykinesia, & cognitive impairment
  - Tremors & ataxia
  - Dysarthria, dyskinesia, & organic personality syndrome
- Psychiatric disease
  - Symptoms present in almost all patients with neurologic disease
  - Early symptoms: subtle behavioral changes, with deterioration of academic or work performance
  - Late symptoms: emotional lability, depression, impulsive behavior, personality changes
  - Rare: schizophreniform psychosis, anxiety, cognitive impairment
- Symptomatic arthropathy
- Azure lunulae (blue discoloration of fingernail base)
- Abdominal pain related to cholelithiasis

TESTS

Basic Tests: Blood
- Low serum ceruloplasmin in 90% of all patients & 65–85% of patients with hepatic manifestations

- Serum alkaline phosphatase often low in fulminant hepatitis
- Serum free copper concentration typically >0.25 mg/L in symptomatic patients

Basic Tests: Urine
- 24-hour urine copper excretion may be normal in asymptomatic patients; usually >100 μg per day in symptomatic patients & frequently >1,000 in fulminant hepatitis

Specific Diagnostic Tests
- Incorporation of radiolabelled copper into ceruloplasmin: rarely used; may be useful when liver biopsy contraindicated
- DNA linkage analysis: expensive; can be performed only within families with established diagnosis of Wilson's in one member

Imaging
- Abdominal sonogram or CT scan: nondiagnostic

Liver Biopsy
- Hepatic copper concentration >250 μg per gram of dry liver tissue AND low ceruloplasmin usually seen in homozygous Wilson's

DIFFERENTIAL DIAGNOSIS
- Elevated hepatic copper concentration <250 μg/g in cholestatic disorders, Indian childhood cirrhosis, and idiopathic copper toxicosis
- Other causes of chronic liver disease

MANAGEMENT
What to Do First
- Evaluate severity of liver disease, extrahepatic complications, and patient's candidacy for therapy

General Measures
- Adjust or avoid potentially hepatotoxic agents
- Evaluate liver disease with history, physical, CBC, LFTs, INR
- Check serum ceruloplasmin & 24-hour urine copper excretion; if possible, liver biopsy for hepatic copper quantitation

SPECIFIC THERAPY
Indications for Treatment
- Medical therapy to improve symptoms & prevent disease progression.
- Liver transplantation for fulminant hepatitis or decompensated cirrhosis

Treatment Options

- D-penicillamine: give vitamin B6 also
  - ➤ Initial therapy: 250–500 mg PO daily; gradually increase to 1,000–1,500 mg daily, in 3–4 divided doses
  - ➤ Maintenance: 750–1,250 mg daily, in 3–4 divided doses
- Trientine
  - ➤ Initial therapy: 1–2 grams PO daily, in 3–4 divided doses
  - ➤ Maintenance: 750–1,000 mg daily, in 3–4 divided doses
- Zinc salts
  - ➤ Maintenance: 150 mg PO daily, in 3 divided doses
- Ammonium tetrathiomolybdate
  - ➤ Initial therapy: 120–420 mg per day for 8 weeks
  - ➤ Maintenance: use zinc salts

Side Effects & Contraindications

- D-penicillamine
  - ➤ Side effects: hypersensitivity reaction, bone marrow suppression, proteinuria, lupus-like reaction, myasthenia, may worsen neurologic symptoms, pemphigoid-type skin reaction
  - ➤ Contraindications
    - Absolute: history of penicillamine-related aplastic anemia or agranulocytosis
    - Relative: concomitant therapy with gold salts, antimalarial or cytotoxic drugs, oxyphenbutazone, phenylbutazone
- Trientine
  - ➤ Side effects: sideroblastic anemia, rhabdomyolysis
  - ➤ Contraindications
    - Absolute: known hypersensitivity
- Zinc salts
  - ➤ Side effects: gastric intolerance, headache
  - ➤ Contraindications: none
- Ammonium tetrathiomolybdate
  - ➤ Side effects: bone marrow suppression, elevation of aminotransferases

FOLLOW-UP

During Treatment & Routine

- With penicillamine and trientine, aim for 24-hour urine copper >250 mcg per day or serum free copper <0.1 mg/L, checking every 3–6 months; with zinc therapy, urine copper usually <150 mcg per day & urine zinc >1,000 mcg per day.

- CBC & urinalysis every 2 weeks during first 2 months of penicillamine therapy
- CBC, AST, and ALT every 2 weeks during therapy with ammonium tetrathiomolybdate
- Annual slit-lamp examination

COMPLICATIONS AND PROGNOSIS

- Hepatic: occurs at mean age of 8–12 years; 5–30% of patients with Wilson's present with chronic hepatitis; consider liver transplantation for fulminant hepatitis or decompensated cirrhosis.
- Neurologic: often occurs in 2nd to 3rd decades of life; initial presentation in one-third of patients
- Psychiatric: occurs in one-third of patients; requires chelation therapy
- Acute intravascular hemolysis: presenting feature in up to 15%; often seen with fulminant hepatitis; usually transient
- Renal: includes renal tubular acidosis, nephrocalcinosis, hematuria, aminoaciduria; chelation improves renal function.
- Symptomatic arthropathy: occurs in 25–50% of all patients, resembling premature osteoarthritis; 50% have osteomalacia, osteoporosis, or both
- Cardiac: arrhythmias & cardiomyopathy may develop; rarely clinically evident
- Cholelithiasis: pigment & cholesterol gallstones
- Malignancy: cholangiocarcinoma, HCC, and adenocarcinoma of indeterminate origin may develop in 4–15% of patients, regardless of treatment

Prognosis

- Generally excellent in patients compliant with therapy

X-LINKED HYPOPHOSPHATEMIA

MICHEL BAUM, MD

HISTORY & PHYSICAL

- Rickets resistant to vitamin D therapy, failure to thrive, short stature, dental abscesses, males more severely affected

TESTS

- Hypophosphatemia, inappropriately normal serum 1,25 dihydroxy vitamin D

- High fractional excretion of phosphate (>20% of filtered phosphate)
- Rickets on X-ray
- Increased levels of FGF-23 and likely other phosphatonins

DIFFERENTIAL DIAGNOSIS
- X-linked dominant disorder due to defect in PHEX gene (phosphate regulating neutral endopeptidase of the X chromosome)
- Distinguish from other causes of rickets.

MANAGEMENT
n/a

SPECIFIC THERAPY
- Phosphate and pharmacologic doses of Vitamin D improve growth and rickets.
- Growth hormone improves growth.

FOLLOW-UP
To ensure optimal growth and healing of rickets

COMPLICATIONS AND PROGNOSIS
Hypercalcemia, hyperparathyroidism and nephrocalcinosis can be complications of therapy.

ZINC DEFICIENCY

ELISABETH RYZEN, MD

HISTORY & PHYSICAL

History
- pica, vegetarianism, alcoholism, malabsorption syndromes, prolonged TPN, sickle cell anemia, autosomal recessive genetic abnormalities

Signs & Symptoms
- non-specific in mild cases; growth retardation & delayed sexual maturation in children; hypogeusia; impaired wound healing; immune dysfunction, anorexia, night blindness, acrodermatitis enteropathica

TESTS

Laboratory
- Basic blood studies:
  - ➤ plasma zinc <70 mcg/dL

DIFFERENTIAL DIAGNOSIS
n/a

MANAGEMENT

General Measures
- Treat underlying cause

SPECIFIC THERAPY
- Oral zinc

FOLLOW-UP
n/a

COMPLICATIONS AND PROGNOSIS
- None
- Completely reversible

ZOLLINGER-ELLISON SYNDROME

SHAI FRIEDLAND, MD and ROY SOETIKNO, MD

HISTORY & PHYSICAL
- less than 1% of patients with gastroduodenal ulcers have ZE syndrome
- consider ZE with multiple ulcers, ulcers distal to duodenal bulb, or ulcers that do not respond to treatment
- more than 30% have diarrhea (due to excessive acid secretion)
- 90% of gastrinomas are malignant; liver metastases common
- 85% are found in gastrinoma triangle (most in pancreas or duodenal wall)
- consider multiple endocrine neoplasia (MEN) type I with hyperparathyroidism, pituitary adenomas, or family history of ZE

TESTS
- Serum gastrin (fasting)
  - greater than 1000 pg/ml with gastric pH <3 is diagnostic
  - 150–1000 pg/ml is nonspecific; can be caused by gastric atrophy, antisecretory drugs, H pylori
  - secretin stimulation test: increase by 200 pg/ml is diagnostic
- Localization
  - contrast CT with pancreatic protocol: sensitive for pancreatic-gastrinomas larger than 1.5 cm and for metastases
  - endoscopic ultrasound sensitive for smaller pancreatic lesions

➤ octreotide scans are 80%–90% sensitive
➤ selective arteriography, venous sampling also used

DIFFERENTIAL DIAGNOSIS
- peptic ulcer disease
- *H. pylori* infection with ulcer
- NSAID-induced ulcer disease
- other hypersecretory states
  ➤ systemic mastocytosis can cause high gastric acid output due to histamine release by infiltrating mast cells
  ➤ islet cell tumors can secrete substances that increase acid output
  ➤ antral gastrin cell hyperplasia can cause high gastrin level and high acid secretion

MANAGEMENT

What to Do First
- Consider diagnosis as alternative to standard peptic ulcer disease
- Arrange diagnostic tests for ZE syndrome

General Management
- Initiate antisecretory therapy

SPECIFIC THERAPY
- Omeprazole to heal ulcer
- Octreotide is sometimes used
- Surgery indicated for localized disease; controversial in MEN type Igastrinomas
- Chemotherapy can decrease symptoms in metastatic disease and mayprolong survival

FOLLOW-UP
n/a

COMPLICATIONS AND PROGNOSIS
- Omeprazole treatment is highly successful for healing ulcers, decreasing diarrhea, and preventing ulcer recurrence
- Complete surgical removal is possible in 40% of patients
- When tumor is resected completely, >90% 5 year survival
- With liver metastases, 20% 5-year survival and 10% 10-year survival